Practical Manual of Hysteroscopy

Enlan Xia
Editor

Practical Manual of Hysteroscopy

河南科学技术出版社
HENAN SCIENCE AND TECHNOLOGY PRESS

Springer

Editor
Enlan Xia
Hysteroscopy Center
Fuxing Hospital, Capital Medical University
Beijing, China

ISBN 978-981-19-1331-0 ISBN 978-981-19-1332-7 (eBook)
https://doi.org/10.1007/978-981-19-1332-7

B&R Book Program
Jointly published with Henan Science and Technology Press

This Springer imprint is published by the registered company Springer Nature Singapore Pte Ltd.
The registered company address is: 152 Beach Road, #21-01/04 Gateway East, Singapore 189721, Singapore

Foreword to the Third Edition

It has been 6 years since the publication of the second edition of *Practical Manual of Hysteroscopy*. During this period, hysteroscopy has been widely practiced in clinics and has developed rapidly. Hysteroscopic diagnosis with localized biopsy is the golden standard for modern diagnosis of intrauterine pathologies. Hysteroscopic surgery has been widely accepted because of its low traumatic ratio, high potency ratio, excellent efficacy, and irreplaceability. It has been described as a model of successful modern minimal traumatic surgery and has been one of four main gynecological surgeries which are commonly used (hysteroscopy, laparoscopy, laparotomy, and transvaginal surgery). By retrieving hysteroscopic-related literatures published in these 6 years, 7925 papers were found from China National Knowledge Infrastructure (CNKI), and 1520 papers from MEDLINE, which showed active academic activities and wide applications in the field of hysteroscopy. By writing the third edition of *An Atlas of Hysteroscopy*, we undergo some supplement and revision according to the advancements of basic research and clinical application at home and abroad in recent years, combining with our own practical experience in our center. We hope that this book will be of great benefit to gynecologists in studying, grasping, advocating, and even teaching hysteroscopic technique.

In total, there are 16 chapters, more than 380,000 words, and 760 pictures included in this book. The revised item is Sect. 2.4, Chap. 2—Cleaning, Sterilization, and Maintenance of Hysteroscopic Instruments. It introduced the disinfection of hysteroscopic instruments in the second edition, including bacteriostasis and sterilization. In the third edition, the sterilization of hysteroscopic instruments is described, as bacteriostasis was obsoleted. The contents added include: (1) A new classification of uterine malformation: there is a new classification system of female genital malformations and jointly published by European Society of Human Reproduction and Embryology (ESHRE) and European Society for Gynecological Endoscopy (ESGE). This system is simple and memorable with high practicability and achieves the approval of most clinical gynecologists. (2) Metroplasty for a rare form of uterine malformation: it includes Robert uterus, complete bicornuate uterus, unicornuate uterus, and "T"-shaped uterus. Transcervical uterine incision (TCUI) excises the excessive myometrial tissues on uterine lateral walls or cuts the thickened myometrium on one or two lateral walls so as to improve the shape of the uterus, enlarge the uterine cavity, relieve intrauterine pressure, improve endometrial blood supply to facilitate the implantation of fertilized eggs, prevent miscarriage, and improve the reproductive outcomes. Combined hysteroscopic and laparoscopic metroplasty for complete bicornuate uterus is performed under laparoscopic monitoring, the hysteroscopic electrode is used to incise the intrauterine plate and the fundus to serosal layer, causing artificial perforation. Then transversely incise the full layer of the fundus and suture the incised wall longitudinally by laparoscopy to achieve a normal shape cavity and increase the possibility of fertility. Some infertile women who were treated in our center for these malformations have delivered healthy infants after metroplasty. (3) The advancement of diagnosing and treating adenomyosis: it includes the findings under hysteroscopy, which can make the diagnosis in early stage; hysteroscopic surgery for cystic adenomyosis can replace the removal of uterine corpus or partial uterus, and obtain the possibility of fertility; the joint application of phloroglucinol dehydrate, narrow band imaging (NBI) hysteroscopy, levonorgestrel-releasing intrauterine system (LNG-IUS), GnRH analog, and hysteroscopic endometrial resection for treatment of adenomyosis, which can enhance the effect of GnRH-a and TCRE and meet the patients' desire to preserve the uterus. (4) Transcervical resection of diffuse uterine leiomyomatosis (DUL): after operation, the endometrium can recover within 2 to 3 months, the improvement of menstruation achieved 93.5%, the recurrence rate was 32.3%, and some patients obtained conception and birth. (5) The prevention of adhesion recurrence after transcervical resection of intrauterine adhesions (TCRA): adjunctive therapies such as postoperative hormone treatment, intrauterine placement of balloon catheter, insertion of human amnion graft, instillation of auto-cross-linked HA (ACP) gel, application of prophylactic antibiotics, and second-look hysteroscopy have been discussed. (6) NBI hysteroscopy: NBI utilizes the light absorption properties of hemoglobin at a certain wavelength to improve the contrast of blood vessels in superficial endometrial layer and well display the mini-structure of the endometrium; therefore it could facilitate the identification of endometrial atypical lesions. It can be used in hysteroscopy so that it can discover the endometrial lesions in early stage, make localized biopsy, and increase the discovery rate of precancerous lesion and endometrial cancer. (7) Pretreatment of cervix with phloroglucinol: it is a pro-muscle non-atropine non-papaverine class pure smooth muscle antispasmodic agent, which is applied in hysteroscopic examination and operation, and has analgesic and cervical looseness effects. (8) Paradoxical emboli caused by venous air embolism with gas emboli entering the left heart: in 2008, Rademaker et al. first reported on one case of fatal paradoxical gas embolism with gas emboli entering the left heart from the right heart through atrial septal defect, open foramen ovale, pulmonary arterio-venous malformations, or arterio-venous fistula.

I would like to express my acknowledgment to all people who provided us with generous help during my compilation of this book, such as Li Jing and Zhong Qin from Scientific Research Office of Fuxing Hospital; Mr. Liu Xuegang and Mr. He Baijiang, who are former managers of Endoscope Marketing Department, Olympus (Beijing) Ltd.; and Mrs. Zhang Zhen from Endoscope Marketing Department, Olympus (Beijing) Ltd. I would also like to thank all colleagues, advanced training physicians, and graduate students in our department for their cooperation!

Any mistake and deficiency due to our limited experience will hopefully be pointed out and forgiven!

Beijing, China Enlan Xia
August 31, 2014

Foreword to the Second Edition

With the development of a holistic concept of surgical treatment in the 1970s, an aggregative indicator, including patients' physiological condition, social activities, and mental outlook, has become an important indicator for the assessment of surgical outcomes and a research object. The introduction of advanced technology prompts the minimally invasive concept and minimally invasive surgery to develop gradually and boom. As an important part of the minimally invasive surgery, the development of hysteroscopy has changed the diagnosis and treatment pattern of the traditional gynecological diseases, which can not only bring about the benefits of minimally invasive surgery, including less trauma, less intraoperative bleeding, few complications, low cost, short hospitalization, and quick recovery, but also preserve the uterus, improve the reproductive prognosis, and cope skillfully with such intractable conditions as vaginal foreign body, cervical/intrauterine lesions, asymmetric septate uterus, and oblique vaginal septum, which is hard to deal with even in an open surgery. Hysteroscopy can be used to diagnose almost all the intrauterine benign diseases like intrauterine lesions, dysfunctional uterine bleeding, submucous myoma, septal deformities, endometrial polyps, intrauterine adhesions, removal of foreign bodies, et al. and can replace, even be superior to traditional open surgery. So hysteroscopy has become a revolutionary event and a milestone in the developmental history of gynecology. Hysteroscopic technology is characterized by its minimal invasiveness, which offers doctors a golden platform to open up new fields of application, and thus making their professional career prolonged and more colorful.

Over the past 10 years, there has been a rapid development of hysteroscopic technology in our country, the gap with the international advanced level has been narrowed ceaselessly, and both the hysteroscopic philosophy and technique have been greatly improved. Encouraged by Henan Science and Technology Press, 5 years ago, we edited a book *An Atlas of Hysteroscopy* together with experts in hysteroscopy at home and abroad, and this book has been widely appreciated by readers.

Time slipped away little by little, and 5 more years passed away unnoticed. There have been a lot of new advances in hysteroscopic technology over time. Firstly, the improved instruments and devices—the integrated hysteroscope has integrated the double advantages of flexible and rigid hysteroscope, which can not only further relieve patients' pains and improve the therapeutic effects but also make doctors feel more intuitively the motive force of the progress in instruments on the development of therapeutic techniques and clinical treatment. Secondly, the application of transvaginal endoscope has turned hysteroscopic examination into a noninvasive procedure. Hysteroscopy has been widely used in the diagnosis and treatment of infertility, and a consensus has been reached that hysteroscopic surgical treatment for intrauterine abnormalities is superior in reproductive prognosis to traditional surgery. In 2006, plasma bipolar resectoscope came into being in China. The use of bipolar resectoscope with saline as irrigation fluid is unlikely to cause hyponatremia and safer than monopolar resectoscope. A second look following resection of severe intrauterine adhesions may prevent reformation of adhesion and multiple surgeries and can restore the normal morphology of uterine cavity, which has been widely accepted. And the postoperative pregnancy rate may reach 28.7%–53.6%. With the wide application of operative hysteroscopy and accumulation of experiences, it has become a safe and minimally invasive surgery with excellent prognosis and few complications and is easy to learn. There has been a change in the sequence of complication occurrence, the risk of false passage and uterine perforation rises to be the first. Gas embolism is the most dangerous complication and can be prevented if strict precautions are taken. Second-generation endometrial ablation procedure is simpler and quicker than first-generation monopolar electroresection, but similar in satisfaction rate and the effect of reducing blood loss. And complications occur after both first-generation and second-generation endometrial ablation. On the occasion of the reprinting of this book, the above advances in hysteroscopy will be expatiated in the related chapters for readers.

I dedicate this book to my first teacher in hysteroscopy Prof. Lin Yuanying and also to Prof. Song Hongzhao, Prof. Zhou Suwen, Prof. Li Zixin, and Prof. Liu Zongtang, who gave me a lot of support and encouragement. And my most sincere gratitude goes to Mr. Liu Xuegang, Mr. He Baijiang, Mrs. Li Jihong, Mrs. Liu Ya'an, and Mrs. Zhang Meng from Japan's Olympus Corp., who helped me in collecting images and providing equipment and technical support.

December 20, 2008 Enlan Xia

Foreword to the First Edition

The application of diagnostic hysteroscopy and operative hysteroscopy and other new techniques provides an economic, feasible, simple, and effective way in the clinical treatment of intrauterine benign lesions. At present, diagnostic hysteroscopy is the gold standard for diagnosing intrauterine lesions and is gradually replacing the blind diagnostic curettage. And operative hysteroscopy has become the optimal surgical procedure in treating dysfunctional uterine bleeding and also the standard surgical procedure for the treatment of uterine septum and the gold standard for treating endometrial polyps. A great deal of follow-up study has confirmed the efficacy of hysteroscopic electroresection in the treatment of benign intrauterine lesions. Operative hysteroscopy has the minimal ratio of internal trauma and the maximal ratio of cost and effect, so it is called a model of successful minimally invasive surgery. In our country, as the clinical application of hysteroscopic diagnosis and therapeutics has been popularized day by day, the hysteroscopic technique has been applied more extensively in recent years.

Tracing back to the developmental history of hysteroscopic techniques in China, we could not forget the late specialist in obstetrics and gynecology, Prof. Lin Yuanying, PhD. He was the first person to advocate the development of hysteroscopy in China, who had ever worked in the Department of Gynecology and Obstetrics of former Shanghai Municipal First People's Hospital. I had the honor to be admitted to this hospital for further education between 1964 and 1965 and was instructed by respectful Professor Lin. At that time, he was there to guide the joint development of hysteroscope with the medical instrument factory and to observe an isolated uterus. Professor Lin's careful thinking, rigorous style of work, and relentless pursuit impressed me deeply. Inspired by his spirit, I inherited my teacher's unfulfilled wish. Since 1990, I have committed myself to the introduction, clinical application, and basic research of hysteroscopy, and I have accumulated a large number of image data. Today, hysteroscopic technique has already been mature. To popularize this procedure in our country and benefit the broad masses of women, the Ministry of Health has listed hysteroscopic techniques as one of 10-year 100 projects of 2001. In view of fewer related works at present and lack of systematic atlas monographs, well-known experts and scholars domestic and abroad were invited to edit this book under the energetic support of Henan Science and Technology Press.

I dedicate this book to my first teacher in hysteroscopy Prof. Lin Yuanying and also to Prof. Song Hongzhao, Prof. Zhou Suwen, Prof. Li Zixin, and Prof. Liu Zongtang, who supported and encouraged me a lot. And my most sincere gratitude goes to Mr. Liu Xuegang, Mr. He Baijiang, Mrs. Li Jihong, Mrs. Liu Ya'an, and Mrs. Zhang Meng from Japan's Olympus Corp. Beijing Office, who helped me in collecting images and providing equipment and technical support.

I sincerely welcome colleagues domestic and abroad to give me more valuable advice so as to make it better in time if there are some careless omissions.

In April 2001, the tenth meeting of the International Society for Gynecologic Endoscopy held in Chicago, USA, put forward a target to the gynecological workers of the whole world: "To 2025, most of gynecological surgeries will be replaced by endoscopic operations." This will inspire and guide us to develop our hysteroscopic techniques and render unremitting efforts to the implementation of international standards.

June 2002 Enlan Xia

Preface

This is a delicate book with precious atlas and a fruit of hard work. As a monograph on medicine, we'd rather attach much importance to great amounts of data obtained through long time of practice, accumulation and summarization combined with scientific analyses and elaboration in relation to academic viewpoints. In view of clinical medicine involving highly practical technology, especially the laboratory techniques and operating techniques, their popularization is of great significance. And clear elaboration, lucid expression, and justified statement on the latter are extremely difficult to make.

However, after I read through the book *An Atlas of Hysteroscopy*, edited by Prof. Xia Enlan, I felt shocked and greatly excited! The reason is that this is just the kind of professional works on technology that we have expected. And its contributors are all experienced experts in hysteroscopy especially those from the hysteroscopic center under the leadership of Prof. Xia, who are richly experienced and have achieved brilliant achievements. And more valuably, this center has constantly recruited visiting physicians and postgraduates and has trained a large number of professional and technical personnel throughout the year, so this is a well-deserved training center and a cradle of specialists.

Hysteroscopy and laparoscopy, being a major tool and technical source of gynecological endoscopy, have been widely extended in their diagnosis and treatment and have promising prospects. If you'd like to make good use of them, first, you should know well about their indications and contraindications, then, have a good command of their techniques and skills, and you also should be always on guard against the occurrence of complications. Standardization of techniques and training for operators are indispensable "double-track railway" in the progress of technology. Endoscope-related accessories, energy source, and limited space and vision have posed new problems for surgery, so it seemingly becomes a "double-edged sword," that is, a minimally invasive surgery may be turned into a maximally invasive surgery. And through reading this book you may grasp its gist and understand its meanings. So when such kind of book is often called "cookbook," I beg to differ. And what's more, even though it is a cookbook, the ingredients and procedures described, if managed by different hands, may have quite different flavors! How important the cooking skill and cooking temperature control is! Let alone the much more complex hysteroscopic technique. Illness differs from person to person, so we can't "look for a steed with the aid of its picture"; it depends on individual's power of understanding, intelligence, experience, and personal skill. Learning from others through reading improves one's own ability, in a sense, as the saying implies, "Laymen are overwhelmed by the fun while professionals try to find out the trick" and "A master may teach, but progress is up to the hard work of an individual." We are running after a lot of new dreams (they are not necessarily all splendid), but more importantly, we need calmness and reflection, including summarization, analysis, and deduction from our daily work, just as the book contributed by Prof. Xia together with other authors.

Professor Xia is our respectable senior. Upon her order, I wrote these out of my own heart, which aren't be but a preface.

Beijing, China Jinghe Lang

Chinese Gynecological Endoscopy Group
Beijing, China

Chinese Academy of Medical Sciences
and Peking Union Medical College
Beijing, China

Obstetrics and Gynaecology in Peking Union
Medical College Hospital
Beijing, China

At Mid-Autumn of 2002

Abstract

The book is made up of 16 chapters, in which a systemic introduction is made to the history of hysteroscopy, hysteroscopic equipment and instruments, applied anatomy and histology in relation to hysteroscopy, distention media and perfusion system, anesthesia for hysteroscopy, and so on. This book elaborates on the application of diagnostic hysteroscopy and operative hysteroscopy in the treatment of gynecological diseases, combined hysteroscopy and laparoscopy, and hysteroscopic surgery under ultrasound monitoring. This book also expounds incisively on the technical training and the trend in the future development of hysteroscopy. At the end of this book, a report sheet of hysteroscopic examination, routine orders in hysteroscopic ward, patient consent form prior to hysteroscopic surgery, and operating manual for hysteroscopic electroresection are attached so as to help readers to standardize the hysteroscopic examination, diagnosis, and surgeries.

This book is based on rigorous and scientific research with emphasis on a combination of theory and practice, in which various typical cases are redisplayed clearly by more than 700 color photos to facilitate readers' understanding and grasp of hysteroscopy. Meanwhile, it is also a professional and reference book for medical students, gynecologists, and nurses at all levels to use.

Cataloguing in publication (CIP) data

An Atlas of Hysteroscopy/Edited by Xia EnLan—the third edition

An Atlas of Hysteroscopy/Editor-in-chief: Xia EnLan.—third edition.—Zheng Zhou: Henan Science and Technology Press, 2015.4

ISBN 978-7-5349-3958-7

I. Hysteroscopy II. Xia EnLan III. Hysteroscopy—Atlas IV.R711.740.4–64

Chinese Version Library CIP Data Reg. No. 118839 (2008)

Published and issued by: Henan Science and Technology Press

Address: Jingwu Road No. 66, Zhengzhou City, China

Postcode: 450002

Tel: 0086-(0)371-65737028 65788627

URL: www.hnstp.cn

Editor in charge: Ma Yanru

Proofreader in charge: Ke Jiao

Cover designer: Zhang Wei

Layout designer: Sun Song

Printed by: Zhengzhou New Coast Computer Color Printing CO., Ltd

Distributed by: National Xinhua Book Stores

Page size: 185 mm × 260 mm

Printed sheet: 29.5 Number of words: 580,000

Edition: Third published in May 2015. First Printed in May 2015

Contents

Editor and Contributors

About the Editor

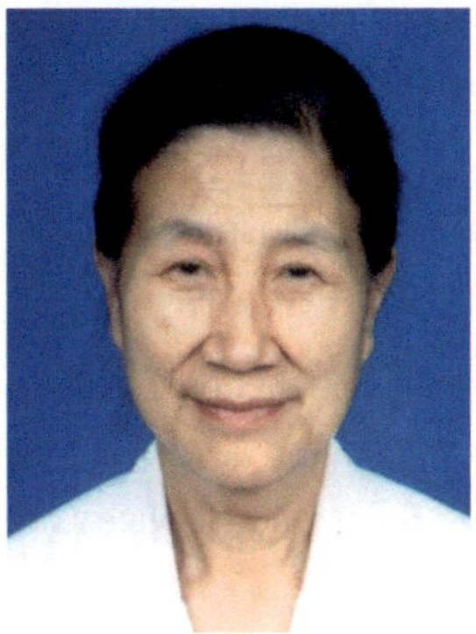

Enlan Xia, graduated from Northwestern Medical College in 1955, has been engaged in teaching and research on clinical obstetrics and gynecology for more than 50 years. Nowadays she is a professor of Obstetrics and Gynecology in Capital Medical University, supervisor of graduate students, head of the Hysteroscopic Center of Fuxing Hospital, Capital Medical University, director of Beijing International Hysteroscopic Training Center, member of American Association of Gynecological Laparoscopists (AAGL), a lifetime member of the International Society for Gynecologic Endoscopy (ISGE), an editorial board member of *Chinese Journal of Obstetrics and Gynecology*, *Chinese Journal of Practical Gynecology and Obstetrics*, *Journal of Practical Obstetrics and Gynecology*, and *Foreign Medical Science: Section of Obstetrics and Gynecology*. She has won 22 governmental awards for scientific and technological progress at all levels from the Ministry of Health, Beijing Municipal Science and Technology Commission, Beijing Municipal Health Bureau, and Xicheng District Government. In 1992, she started to enjoy special government allowances of the State Council. Under her drive, "hysteroscopic technology" was listed as 10-year 100 projects for popularization by State Ministry of Health in 2000 and the key project in 2001 and 2003. The research project "Clinical application and basic research of hysteroscopy" won the second prize of 2004 State Scientific and Technological Progress Award.

Professor Xia Enlan is the founder and pioneer of gynecologic endoscopy—hysteroscopic diagnosis and therapeutics in China. In 1990, she took the lead in the introduction and implementation of hysteroscopic electroresection in China. In 1993, the first domestic hysteroscopic center was established to further clinical practice and scientific research. Since then, 20,000 diagnostic hysteroscopies, more than 8000 procedures of hysteroscopic electroresection, more than 3000 cases of laparoscopic surgeries, and 1000 cases of hysteroscopy combined with laparoscopy have been performed over more than 10 years. Professor Xia has extremely proficient skills in hysteroscopic surgeries and has formed her unique style, which is praised as "Xia's style" by counterparts domestic and abroad, and the success rate of hysteroscopic surgeries has been at the international advanced stage. And many a time she has paid visits to the United States, France, Germany, Japan, Holland, Switzerland, and other countries and Hong Kong, Taiwan, and other regions for communication and lecturing. She has held 12 Beijing International Academic Symposiums and 90 workshops in different places of China and has trained more than 400 physicians from our country and other countries like Australia, Philippines, and others for advanced learning.

Professor Xia is notable for her noble medical ethics and medical skills. She has long been diligently committed to the popularization of hysteroscopy and enhancing China's international status in the scientific community of obstetrics and gynecology so as to relieve pains for many more patients.

Contributors

Handong Cai Department of Anesthesiology, Fuxing Hospital, Capital Medical University, Beijing, China

Hua Duan Minimally Invasive Center, Beijing Obstetrics and Gynecology Hospital, Capital Medical University, Beijing, China

Limin Feng Department of Obstetrics and Gynecology, Beijing Tiantan Hospital, Capital Medical University, Beijing, China

Baijiang He Endoscope Marketing Department, Olympus (Beijing) Sales and Service Co., Ltd, Beijing, China

Xiaowu Huang Hysteroscopy Center, Fuxing Hospital, Capital Medical University, Beijing, China

Baoliang Lin Department of Obstetrics and Gynecology, Kawasaki Municipal Hospital, Kawasaki, Japan

Xuegang Liu Endoscope Marketing Department, Olympus (Beijing) Sales and Service Co., Ltd, Beijing, China

Yuhuan Liu Hysteroscopy Center, Fuxing Hospital, Capital Medical University, Beijing, China

Ning Ma Hysteroscopy Center, Fuxing Hospital, Capital Medical University, Beijing, China

Xuebing Peng Hysteroscopy Center, Fuxing Hospital, Capital Medical University, Beijing, China

Yan Quan Operating Room, Fuxing Hospital, Capital Medical University, Beijing, China

Rafael F. Valle Department of Obstetrics and Gynecology, Northwestern University Medical School, Chicago, IL, USA

Enlan Xia Hysteroscopy Center, Fuxing Hospital, Capital Medical University, Beijing, China

Dan Yu Hysteroscopy Center, Fuxing Hospital, Capital Medical University, Beijing, China

Dan Zhang Department of Ultrasound, Fuxing Hospital, Capital Medical University, Beijing, China

Jie Zheng Hysteroscopy Center, Fuxing Hospital, Capital Medical University, Beijing, China

Translators

Tin Chiu Li Department of Obstetrics and Gynaecology, The Chinese University of Hong Kong, Hong Kong, China

Dan Yu Hysteroscopy Center, Fuxing Hospital, Capital Medical University, Beijing, China

History and Development of Hysteroscopy

1

Enlan Xia

The history of hysteroscopy could be traced back to 150 years ago. Under the influence of low productivity, the hysteroscopic technique was developed very slowly. Until the twentieth century, it improved gradually, especially in recent 20 years, the evolution of operational hysteroscopy brought epoch-making revolution in the treatment of some gynecological diseases. The advances of hysteroscopic technique are owing to the contributions made by many innovators, whose years of continuous efforts innovated the means of diagnosis and treatment for today's gynecologists and obstetricians. This chapter will describe several different historical periods, especially the important stages in which the uterine cavity could be revealed in front of us (Table 1.1).

Table 1.1 Milestones in the development of hysteroscopy

Year	Inventor	Contributions
1807	Bozzini	First endoscope (sunlight source)
1869	Pantaleoni	First hysteroscopy on human body
1879	Nitze	Cystoscope with distal source of light
1889	Clado	First designer of hysteroscopic instruments
1907	David	First contact hysteroscope
1914	Heineberg	Uterine distention system
1925	Rubin	Uterine distention with carbon dioxide (CO_2)
1926	Seymour	Hysteroscope with separate inflow and outflow channels
1927	Mikulicz-Radecki	Functions of biopsy and intrauterine cornual electrocauterization
1928	Gauss	Uterine distention with the help of the height of fluid
1934	Schroeder	Measurement of intrauterine pressure
1934–1943	Segond	Distention system and biopsy
1936	Shack	Verification of its clinical application
1942–1970	Norment	Rubber balloon, practical irrigating system, cutting loop, fiberoptics
1952	Forestier	First cold quartz light source
1953–1978	Mohti and Mohri	Fiber hysteroscope, falloposcope
1957	Englund etc.	Evaluation of abnormal uterine bleeding with hysterography, curettage, and hysteroscopy
1962	Silander	Research focused on endometrial cancer
1965	Hopskin	Development of optical fiber system
1968	Menken	Hysteroscopic tubal occlusion with polyvinyl pyrrolidone (PVP)
1970	Edstrom and Fernstrom	32% dextran as distending medium
1970	Quinones et al.	Hysteroscopic tubal catheterization
1972	Lindemann	Set a safe flow rate of CO_2 in distending uterine cavity and applied cervical vacuum cup
1974	Edstrom	Therapeutic hysteroscopy
1974	Parent et al.	Contact hysteroscopy
1978	Sugimoto et al.	Normal saline as distending medium
1978	Neuwirth	Use of resectoscope
1980	Quinones-Guerrero	5% glucose solution as distending medium
1980	Hamou	Microcolpo-hysteroscope
1981	Goldrath et al.	Laser endometrial ablation
1981	Feng Zanchong et al.	First diagnostic and therapeutic hysteroscopy in China
1988	Lin Baoliang	Roller-ball endometrial ablation
1989	Magos et al.	Transcervical resection of endometrium
1990	Xia Enlan et al.	First hysteroscopic resection in China
1997	Glasser	Hysteroscopic vaporizing electrode
1997	Bettocchi	Vaginoscopy
1999	Vilos	Use of coaxial bipolar electrode
2005	Olympus Ltd	Saline plasma bipolar resectoscope
2005	Emanuel and Wamsteker	Intrauterine morcellator
2009	Papalampros et al.	Mini-resectoscope

E. Xia (✉)
Hysteroscopy Center, Fuxing Hospital, Capital Medical University, Beijing, China

E. Xia (ed.), *Practical Manual of Hysteroscopy*, https://doi.org/10.1007/978-981-19-1332-7_1

1.1 The First Hysteroscope

The key to invent hysteroscope is how to introduce the instrument into the uterine cavity and use the external light source to view the interior of the uterus.

Philip Bozzini (1773–1809) first invented an instrument, which could be used to see hollow organs inside the body. The light conductor he designed was to refract the external light through a channel and this channel was separated into two parts by a vertical concave mirror, by which the light was refracted into the uterine cavity. He developed different types of such devices so as to adapt to the different hollow organs of the human body, such as oral cavity, nasal cavity, external auditory meatus, vagina, cervix and uterus, ureter and bladder, and rectum. Although Bozzini published a brief description of this instrument in Frankfurt's newspaper in 1804, it was not until 1805 that he declared the accomplishment of his design in German newspaper, which enabled people to visualize the interior cavities of human body. Only in 1807, a formal and elaborate report about such devices was published.

Bozzini had been in dispute with the bureaucrat and intellectuals over his inventions, but today he was recognized as the father of endoscope. On the wall of Frankfurt Cathedral, Bozzini's epitaph was written in Latin: *"To the devote soul of Philip Bozzini, doctor of medicine, who was the first to explore the inside of organs through his ingenious light projector. He was able to tenaciously fight fever in other people, with a great sense of duty, and succumbed on the night from the 4th to the 5th day of April 1809, in his 36th year of life. His faithful friend F.F."*

In 1853, a French urologist, Antonin J. Desormeau, first introduced a truly workable cystoscope to the French Academy of Medicine. With this, he could observe through a central channel. The light source was a turpentine oil lamp which was refracted into this channel through a mirror. When the light got to the halfway of it, it could be refracted through a concave mirror to any cavity observed. This device permitted the observation of a full bladder through a lens at the distal end of the endoscope, and other operative instruments could be introduced through the side channel. 12 years later, Cruise, from Dublin, improved Desormeaux's endoscope. He applied a petroleum lamp with a mixture of a bit of dissolved camphor instead of turpentine oil lamp, and added a glass chimney to hold the vapor. In 1869, Pantaleoni, who had learned how to manipulate the endoscope from Cruise, underwent hysteroscopy for a patient with postmenopausal abnormal uterine bleeding. Polypoid tissues were detected at the fundus of the uterine cavity, and were cauterized with silver nitrate under the hysteroscopic guidance.

After Pantaleoni performed the first hysteroscopic examination and treatment, many doctors began to utilize this new technique. However, poor light conduction, impaired vision owing to intrauterine bleeding, and inadequate distention of the uterine cavity impeded the application of hysteroscopy and its popularization.

In 1879, Nitze invented the cystoscope, which used an incandescent lamp with platinum wire for illumination, and flowing water for cooling of the lamp. Because of the thin bladder wall and the avascular cavity, such kind of endoscope was very suitable for the bladder examination.

1.2 Contact Hysteroscope and Modern Contact Hysteroscope

In 1907, David first invented a contact hysteroscope that permitted a direct visualization of endometrial surface without distention of the cavity. Because infection might be spread through the distending medium, the contact hysteroscope had a great advantage in preventing infections. It was commonly used in postmenopausal or post-abortion patients.

After that, many scholars improved the magnification of David's contact hysteroscope, including Palmer (1942), Norment (1947), Marleschki (1966), Parent (1974), Hamou (1980), and so on. Although the contact hysteroscope has been getting simple, it still could not assess the whole uterine cavity accurately and comprehensively. Therefore, it is only suitable for inspections of cervical mucosa or the areas suspected of pathological lesions under panoramic hysteroscopy, and observation of endometrial blood vessels.

In the middle of the twentieth century, when doctors were at a loss which was the best, Parent and his colleagues (1974) reported an improved technique. It was a modified instrument of David and Marleschki's contact hysteroscope by enclosing a glass rod in a metal sheath, which could reflect the external light for the illumination of the uterine cavity. In order to meet the requirements of examinations, the instrument was made of different sizes, of which the outer sheath was 4 mm, 6 mm, or 8 mm, respectively. This technique seemed to be simple and immediate, but could not make a comprehensive and accurate assessment of the uterine cavity. Furthermore, direct biopsy was impossible with it and could only be used in diagnosis.

The emerge of panoramic hysteroscope dwarfed the contact hysteroscope. In 1983, Hamou made some improvements on the contact hysteroscope, called vaginal-hysteroscope. Such hysteroscope could be a contact type or a panoramic one, and its magnification ranged from 1 to 150 times. When doing panoramic hysteroscopy, if endometrium was found suspicious, it could be switched to a contact type to magnify the tissue by 80–150 times to be inspected. At present, such kind of method is used to observe the endometrial blood vessels, especially of the cancerized area, but not as a routine examination.

1.3 Hysteroscope with a Balloon at the End

Based on Norment's design, the redesigned hysteroscope had a transparent balloon attached to the distal end, which was of plastic or silicone rubber instead of a rubber balloon, and it was thinner, more transparent, and more difficult to rupture. Wulfsohn (1958) and Bank (1960) conducted the first evaluation of this hysteroscope. Although it had a clear vision and avoided the distention medium infiltrating into the peritoneal cavity, the compression of balloon on the endometrium distorted and twisted the endometrial tissues. In addition, biopsy and resection remained inaccessible. Thus people soon realized its limitations and then forbidden its use. Soon modern hysteroscope turned to the use of distention medium to distend the uterine cavity.

1.4 Fluid Irrigation Mode (Original Continuous Irrigation System) and Uterine Distending Medium

Like cystoscope, to observe uterine cavity required distention medium to distend the cavity. Heineberg in 1914 and Seymour in 1926 developed the hysteroscope with integrated fluid inflow and outflow channels, which founded the basis for later continuous flow hysteroscope. Inspired by bronchoscope, in 1926, Seymour modified the hysteroscope to diagnostic type and operative type, and the latter can be used for the resection of submucous myomas and other intrauterine lesions. He had conducted a 6-mm-diameter bronchoscope with its distal end connected to a suction device, and continuous suction helped to observe the uterine cavity. A 9-mm endoscope had been applied, through which a biopsy forceps could be used to remove the intrauterine tissues. Later Seymour adjusted the diameter of endoscopic sheath to 6 mm, which appeared to be very practical, but there are no more clinical reports to confirm it.

In 1928, Gauss reported that a diagnostic hysteroscopy was performed using low-viscosity fluid and gained a clear image of uterine cavity. On this basis, Schroede tested out the most suitable pressure so as to get the best view and avoid the leakage of distention fluid from fallopian tube. He found that the container with distention fluid could be placed at the different heights along with the change of the intrauterine pressure. The most suitable pressure was 25–30 mmHg, and when the pressure exceeded 55 mmHg, the fluid would flow into the abdominal cavity via fallopian tubes. In addition, he applied hysteroscopic coagulation for tubal sterilization.

In 1936, Shack sought to clarify the hysteroscopic indications, and he attributed the failure of hysteroscopy to poor view. Almost at the same time, Segond used fluid as distention medium in France in 1934. They readjusted fluid inflow channel and outflow channel so as to obtain optimal uterine distending effects and reduce the fluid into the peritoneal cavity. The object lens of telescope obliqued forward, which made it easy to view the uterine cornua and tubal ostia, but intrauterine bleeding remained a major obstacle to observe the uterine cavity.

American scholar Norment developed an air bag being introduced into the uterine cavity when conducting intrauterine observations, which avoided the infiltration of fluid into the peritoneal cavity, and obtained the expansion of uterine cavity without distention medium. The low-viscosity continuous fluid infusion system that Norment designed was the model of modern continuous flow hysteroscope and resectoscope. In 1957, Norment designed an electric resectoscope which used a cutting loop to remove the submucous myomas and polyps. Eighteen years later, he finalized the design.

Friedrich-Carl Menken (1968) firstly used high-viscosity uterine distention medium—polyvinyl pyrrolidone (PVP). Compared with the low-viscosity distention medium, it rarely infiltrated into the abdominal cavity. However, because PVP could not be degraded, and the liquid was light yellow after dissolution, it was not widely applied.

In 1970, Edstrom and Fernstrom used dextran with 70,000 molecular weight (MW) to distend the uterine cavity. The reduced volume of its usage could greatly reduce infiltration of the liquid into the peritoneal cavity and high-viscosity dextran could not mix with blood, so it might not interfere with the view because of bleeding, and could keep the uterine cavity with a certain pressure as well.

When the researchers engaged in the research on tubal ostia sterilization by diathermy (1972), Quinones-Guerrero and his colleagues began to perform operative hysteroscopy using low-viscosity distending medium. They adopted Norment's design to pumping liquid into the uterine cavity with the tourniquet or pressurized pump. Sugimoto (1978) used low-viscosity liquid like saline, connected the syringe to the joints, and increased the pressure according to the requirements of the uterine cavity. However, the problem of excessive fluid absorption through blood vessels still remained to be solved.

1.5 Distention of Uterus with CO_2

In 1925, Rubin attempted CO_2 to distend the uterine cavity, which made him the father of tubal insufflations with CO_2. Nevertheless, most doctors would still like to apply low-viscosity distention fluid. In 1927, Mikulicz-Radecki reported the hysteroscopic diagnosis and treatment with fluid distention. These procedures included biopsy, resection of lesions in the cavity, and diathermy of tubal interstitial for contraception, etc.

In 1971, Lindemann reported the use of CO_2 in expanding the cavity. A normal flow rate of CO_2 in distending uterine cavity was 40–100 mL/min, with the pressure <200 mmHg. CO_2 is clean and capable of gaining a clear view, and it may help to provide high definition pictures of the uterine cavity. Hence Lindemann thought it was the best distension medium. With the improvement of the equipment, and the automatic control of gas flow rate and pressure, the fatal complications due to excessive gas injection and higher pressure were avoided.

1.6 Invention of Fiber Hysteroscope

In 1954, Basil I. Hirschowitz first invented optical fiber. Later, he applied it to flexible hysteroscope. Fiberoptic endoscope was also applied to the hysteroscope with a plastic airbag at the end, which permitted the examination of embryo and fetus outside the amniotic membrane without distention medium (1968). In 1975, Mohri first used flexible hysteroscope with the optical fiber to observe early pregnancy embryos. When using the miniaturized fiber endoscope to observe fallopian tube, falloposcope was born. In 1973, M. Hayashi also evolved a similar mini fiber endoscope for the observation of fallopian tube and successfully visualized the fallopian tube lumen.

1.7 Continuous Flow Hysteroscope

A lot of medical apparatus and instruments companies attempted to design continuous flow systems with many different plans to make the low-viscosity fluid distention simpler. Continuous flow system could also be applied to hysteroscope with 4–6 mm outer sheath. In addition, with the developments of instruments and maintenance, hysteroscopic diagnosis and operation were moved from the operation room and hospital to outpatient department. With the improvement of telescope, 2–3 mm mini hysteroscopy can also be used without continuous flow system.

Hysteroscope with continuous flow started to replace the one-way irrigating hysteroscope, by which the flow rate and intrauterine pressure could be controlled. These improvements led to the development of accessorial instruments, such as monopolar electrode and bipolar electrode. Vaporization electrode can make the tissue fragments vaporized. In addition, bipolar electrode allows for ionic liquid to distend uterine cavity, thus avoiding hyponatremia caused by the liquid absorption.

1.8 A Clinical Review

In addition to Norment, Mohri, and Palmer, many other researchers had been indulged in the development of equipment and techniques, but few of them focused on how to use these techniques. Englund et al. published a valuable article about patients who had abnormal uterine bleeding and underwent hysteroscopy followed by curettage. In total, 165 women had diagnostic curettages during hysteroscopy, of which 21 cases had hysterography beforehand. Among 109 women who had hysteroscopy and curettage, the accuracy of hysteroscopic diagnosis was 93%. They found hysteroscopy was superior to hysterography in diagnosis. Among 124 women who had diagnostic curettage, only 44 cases (35%) were confirmed by operation, and most pathologies including abnormal tissue, polyps, and submucous myomas were missed by hysterography. Over 5 of 46 cases who had second hysteroscopy were found to have disagreement with the operational results.

1.9 Other Innovations

In 1976, Neuwirth applied prostatic resectoscope to remove submucous myomas, whereas continuous irrigation was not used in the original resectoscope, so myoma fragments could not be cleared promptly. Later, Iglesias and his colleagues changed the sheath of resectoscope to be round, and utilized the continuous flow system, therefore the operation view was clean and clear. These evolutions created a new field for electric surgeries in uterine cavities.

In 1981, Goldrath performed Nd-YAG laser endometrial ablation on patients who had abnormal uterine bleeding and did not respond to drug therapy. This therapy, which was approved by FDA in 1986, seemed to be very effective, especially for those who had hysterectomy contraindications. But soon, laser was replaced by electric surgery. In 1989, FDA formally approved the use of electric resectoscope.

The emergence of new techniques at the end of the 1980s also made successive improvements on equipment. The most important breakthroughs were:

1. Both operative and diagnostic hysteroscopy adopted continuous flow system, which could effectively control the flow rate and intrauterine pressure;
2. Imaging technique was also developed rapidly. Most problems baffled doctors were solved in the early 1980s. The invention of couple charge device (CCD) solved the problem of miniaturizing the video camera, which could be connected with the eyepiece and transmit the image on the TV screen. It could greatly improve the definition of images, relieve the fatigue of operator's neck and back when observing and operating through the eyepiece, and

reduce the doctors' labor intensity. Television monitoring system could also record and playback the procedure of operation, which might be used in analysis and review after operation. The fluid infusion pump which was specially designed for hysteroscopic resection could set the pressure and flow rate, so that the operation could be done under satisfactory distension of uterus and clear vision. Its fluid outflow collection device could provide the fluid deficit by accurately calculating the amount in inflow and outflow containers, thus preventing TURP syndromes effectively.

3. A vaginoscopic approach was adopted for hysteroscopy. In 1997, Bettocchi first reported the use of vaginoscopic hysteroscopy. It was introduced into vagina without speculum. Under the help of vaginal expansion with normal saline irrigation, it could clearly visualize both the vaginal wall and cervix. Then it progressed into uterine cavity through cervical canal. All the abnormalities from vagina, cervical canal, and intrauterine cavity could be detected and managed. This technique avoided the introduction of speculum, dilation of cervical canal, and measurement of endometrial cavity length, and therefore preserved the integrity of hymen in young girls and virgins. In recent years, it has become a commonly used diagnostic and operational technique for young girls, virgins, and older women due to its reduction of injury and discomfort caused by speculum.
4. The utilization of bipolar resectoscope. In 2005, Olympus Corporation in Japan produced a plasma bipolar resectoscope. It used saline as distention medium so that it greatly reduced the occurrence of TURP syndrome, it avoided the use of a negative plate so that it had no risk of burning the human body. SURGMASTER high frequency current generator was utilized. The high frequency current could convert saline to electric plasma with a high density of free electron particles, used for precise cutting, accurate, and clean coagulating, and thus made the operation more convenient. The decrease of thermal conductivity can bring down the depth of coagulation, thereby reducing the tissue charring. There is only minimal current passing through the human body when using bipolar technique without bearing the risk of conventional monopolar resection. Compared with conventional monopolar operation, bipolar technique improves the safety of operation, and is a great innovation of hysteroscopic surgery.
5. Evolution of intrauterine morcellator. In 2005, Emanuel and Wamsteker invented an intrauterine morcellator which was introduced through a working channel of a 9 mm bipolar resectoscope. Polyps and myomas were cut and suctioned by morcellator during the procedure, therefore both the operation time and study curve were shorter than conventional resection. It had a clear view of operation, prevented air embolism which resulted from many times of insertion and withdrawal of hysteroscope for taking out intrauterine myoma fragments, and significantly decreased the risk of some severe complications including excessive fluid deficit, hyponatremia, and uterine perforation. In 2009, an improved instrument named "MyoSure" was developed for removal of intrauterine tissues. It was more convenient for outpatient operation because of its small diameter and fast cutting speed.
6. The development of Mini-resectoscope. In 2009, Papalampros et al. reported the application of a 5.3 mm diameter monopolar resectoscope, which was used to remove endometrial polyps and small type 0 or 1 submucous myomas, and achieved a satisfying treatment result.

When looking back on 180 years of hysteroscopy, many of the early problems, such as poor view of operation, inappropriate distending medium, inadequate expansion of uterine cavity, the larger diameter of endoscope, have been gradually settled. This technique has evolved for a long time, so today we can smoothly perform operations inside the uterine cavity. When recalling the history of hysteroscopy, we paid great and deep respects to all the pioneers. It was their innovations together that brought us such a safe, simple, and effective hysteroscopic technique.

Suggested Reading

1. Aguero O, Aure M, Lopez R. Hysteroscopy in pregnant patients. A new diagnostic tool. Am J Obstet Gynecol. 1966;94:925–8.
2. Bettocchi S, Selvaggi L. A vaginoscopic approach to reduce the pain of office hysteroscopy. J Am Assoc Gynecol Laparosc. 1997;4:255–8.
3. Burnett JE. Hysteroscopy controlled curettage for endometrial polyps. Obstet Gynecol. 1964;24:621–5.
4. Cohen MR, Dmowski WP. Modern hysteroscopy: diagnostic and therapeutic applications. Fertil Steril. 1973;24:905–11.
5. David C. Endoscopie de l'uterus apres l'avortement et dans les suites de couches normales et pathologiques. Soc Obst de Paris. 1907;10:288–97.
6. Desormeaux AJ. Del'Endoscope et de ses application au diagnostic et au traitement des affections de l'urethre et de la vessie. Paris: Balliere; 1865.
7. Emanuel MH, Wamsteker K. The Intra Uterine Morcellator: a new hysteroscopic operating technique to remove intrauterine polyps and myomas. J Minim Invasive Gynecol. 2005;12:62–6.
8. Englund S, Ingelman-Sundberg A, Westin B. Hysteroscopy in diagnosis and treatment of uterine bleeding. Gynaecologia. 1957;143:217–22.
9. Glasser MH. Endometrial ablation and hysteroscopic myomectomy by electrosurgical vaporization. J Am Assoc Gynecol Laparosc. 1997;4:369–74.
10. Goldrath MH, Fuller TA, Segal S. Laser photovaporization of endometrium for the treatment of menorrhagia. Am J Obstet Gynecol. 1981;140:14–9.
11. Gribb JJ. Hysteroscopy. An aid in gynecologic diagnosis. Obstet Gynecol. 1960;15:593–601.

12. Hamou J. Microhysteroscopy. A new procedure and its original applications in gynecology. J Reprod Med. 1981;26:375–82.
13. Harrison RM. The development of modern endoscopy. J Med Primatol. 1976;5:73–81.
14. Heineberg A. Uterine endoscopy: an aid to precision in the diagnosis of intra-uterine disease. A preliminary report with the presentation of a new uteroscope. Surg Gynecol Obstet. 1914;18:513–5.
15. Iglesias JJ, Sporer A, Gellman AC, Seebode JJ. New Iglesias resectoscope with continuous irrigation, simultaneous suction and low intravesical pressure. J Urol. 1975;114:929–33.
16. Leidenheimer H. Office gynecologic hysteroscopy. S Louisiana State M Soc. 1969;121:319–21.
17. Levine RU, Neuwirth RS. Evaluation of a method of hysteroscopy with the use of thirty per cent dextran. Am J Obstet Gynecol. 1972;113:696–703.
18. Lindemann HJ, Mohr J. CO_2 hysteroscopy: diagnosis and treatment. Am J Obstet Gynecol. 1976;124:129–33.
19. Lindemann HJ. Historical aspects of hysteroscopy. Fertil Steril. 1973;24:230–42.
20. Lindemann HJ. Pneumometra für die hysteroskopie. Geburtsbilfe Frauenbeilkd. 1973;33:18–23.
21. Lindemann HJ. The use of CO_2 in the uterine cavity for hysteroscopy. Int J Fertil. 1972;17:221–4.
22. Lyon FA. Intrauterine visualization by means of a hysteroscope. Am J Obstet Gynecol. 1964;90:443–9.
23. Marleschki V. Die moderne zervikoskopie und hysteroskopie. Zentralbl Gynaekol. 1966;20:637.
24. Menken FC. Endoscopy procedures and their combined application in gynecology. J Reprod Med. 1974;12:250.
25. Mohri T, Mohri C, Yamadori F. Tubaloscope flexible glass fiber endoscope for intratubal observation. Endoscopy. 1970;4:226–30.
26. Neuwirth RS. A new technique for and additional experience with hysteroscopic resection of submucous fibroids. Am J Obstet Gynecol. 1978;131:91–4.
27. Nitze M. Über eine neue behandlungs—methode der hohlen des menslichen korpers, vol. 26. Wien: Med Press; 1879. p. 851.
28. Norment WB, Apple ED. The diagnosis of submucosal myomas and polyps of the uterus. South Med Surg. 1941;103:373–5.
29. Norment WB, Sikes CH. Photographing tumors of the uterine canal in patients. JAMA. 1956;160:1014–7.
30. Norment WB. A method of study of the uterine canal. South Surg. 1947;13:885–9.
31. Norment WB. A study of the uterine canal by direct observation and uterogram. Am J Surg. 1943;60:56–62.
32. Norment WB. Diagnosis of tumors of the uterine canal. N C Med J. 1951;12:607–10.
33. Norment WB. Hysteroscope in diagnosis of pathological conditions of uterine canal. JAMA. 1952;148:917–21.
34. Norment WB. Improved instruments for the diagnosis of pelvic lesions by the hysterogram and water hysteroscope. N C Med J. 1949;10:646–9.
35. Norment WB. The hysteroscope. Am J Obstet Gynecol. 1956;71:426–32.
36. Norment WB. Visualization and photography of the uterine canal. N C Med J. 1948;9:619–23.
37. Palmer R. L'hysteroscopie cervicale. Rev Franc Gyn Obst. 1942;403:88–92.
38. Pantaleoni D. On endoscopic examination of the cavity of the womb. Med Press Cir. 1869;8:26–7.
39. Papalampros P, Gambadauro P, Papadopoulos N, Polyzos D, Chapman L, Magos A. The mini-resectoscope: a new instrument for office hysteroscopic surgery. Acta Obstet Gynecol Scand. 2009;88(2):227–30.
40. Parent B, Toubas C, Doerler B. L'hysteroskopie de contact. J Gynecol Obstet Biol Reprod. 1974;3:511–20.
41. Quinones-Guerrero R, Alvarado-Duran A, Esperanza-Aguilar R. Histeroscopia: (Reporte preliminar). Ginecol Obstet Mex. 1970;27:683–91.
42. Rathert P, Lutzeyer W, Goddwin WE. Philipp Bozzini (1773~1809) and the Lichtleiter. Urology. 1974;3:113–8.
43. Rubin IC. Uterine endoscopy. Endometroscopy with the aid of uterine insufflation. Am J Obstet Gynecol. 1925;10:313–27.
44. Schack L. Unsere Erfahrungen mit der Hysteroskopie. Zentralbl Gynakol. 1936;31:1810–5.
45. Schroeder C. Über den Ausbau und die Leistungen der Hysteroskopie. Arch für Gynäk (Berlin). 1934;156:407–19.
46. Segond R. L'hysteroscopie. Bull Soc Obst Gyn. 1934;23:709–11.
47. Seymour HF. Endoscopy of the uterus: with a description of a hysteroscope. J Obstet Gynecol Br Emp. 1926;33:52–5.
48. Siegler AM, Kemmann E. Hysteroscopy. Obstet Gynecol Surv. 1975;30:567–88.
49. Silander T. Hysteroscopy through a transparent rubber balloon. Surg Gynecol Obstet. 1962;114:125–7.
50. Sugimoto O. Hysteroscopic diagnosis of endometrial carcinoma. Am J Obstet Gynaecol. 1975;121:105–13.
51. Valle RF, Sciarra JJ. Diagnostic and operative hysteroscopy. Minn Med. 1974;57:892–6.
52. Valle RF. A manual of clinical hysteroscopy. London: Parthenon Publishing Group; 1998. p. 11–4.
53. Valle RF. Hysteroscopy. Obstet Gynecol Annu. 1978;7:245–83.
54. Wulfsohn NL. A hysteroscope. J Obstet Gynecol Br Emp. 1958;65:657–8.

2 Equipment and Instruments for Hysteroscopy

Xuegang Liu, Baoliang Lin, and Yan Quan

Since Pantaleoni applied the first hysteroscopy in 1869, with the help of candlelight and concave mirror on human living body and found cervical polyps in a woman with postmenopausal vaginal bleeding, quite a few scholars have committed to exploring the mystery of uterine cavity in the next 100 years. But due to the physiological and anatomical characteristics of uterus and the limitation of instruments and optical-electrical system, optimal results were hardly achieved. Until 1970s, with the emergence of fiber-optic devices, cold light sources, and modified uterine-distending method, the research and application of hysteroscopy regained attention and underwent rapid development.

In the early 1990s, a new hysteroscopy video system was applied in clinical practice. Modern hysteroscopic system basically consists of several parts: hysteroscope and its instruments (including diagnostic and therapeutic hysteroscope, and hystero-resectoscope), lighting system, distention/irrigation system, camera imaging system, and power system (high frequency electrosurgery, laser, etc.). Just as "A craftsman must sharpen his tools if he is to do his work well," a handy telescope and instruments, a bright and clear imaging system, good uterine distension, and a safe and convenient power system are premises and foundations to smoothly carry out hysteroscopic diagnosis and treatment.

X. Liu (✉)
Endoscope Marketing Department, Olympus (Beijing) Sales and Service Co., Ltd, Beijing, China

B. Lin
Department of Obstetrics and Gynecology, Kawasaki Municipal Hospital, Kawasaki, Japan

Y. Quan
Operating Room, Fuxing Hospital, Capital Medical University, Beijing, China

2.1 Equipment for Hysteroscopy

Xuegang Liu

2.1.1 Power System

Power system is also called the energy system. The most commonly used energy sources for hysteroscopy are high frequency electricity and laser. Compared with mechanical operative hysteroscopy, their applications have broadened the type and extent of surgery inside the uterine cavity.

2.1.1.1 High-Frequency Current Generator

A high-frequency current generator can generate current for cutting tissues and (or) electro-coagulating vessels. Generally, low frequency current may cause muscle and nerve stimulation, while high frequency current does not, and cannot induce ventricular fibrillation, but may cause tissue to heat up, carbonize, and be vaporized, resulting in coagulation and incision. The current frequency usually reaches hundreds of kilohertz. When the current passes intensively through the tissue, it produces Joule heating, which may make water evaporate from cells. As the water evaporates, the tissue impedance increases further, and more heat is produced. Thus it causes tissue protein to be denaturized and dried, and then coagulated. As the temperature elevates further, the tissue begins charring, and then arc discharge is generated and vaporizes the tissue, which achieves the effect of incision. Hysteroscopic operation is conducted in liquid with relatively high impedance, thus it is necessary to be equipped with a large power electric generator which has a power display and return power monitoring system. Modern power generators are all equipped with an alarm system, hence it is safe and reliable when in use. However, the connecting parts of high-frequency current generator should be carefully checked before operation to make sure not to burn the patients, for example, whether the electrode plate is placed appropriately or not, and whether

E. Xia (ed.), *Practical Manual of Hysteroscopy*, https://doi.org/10.1007/978-981-19-1332-7_2

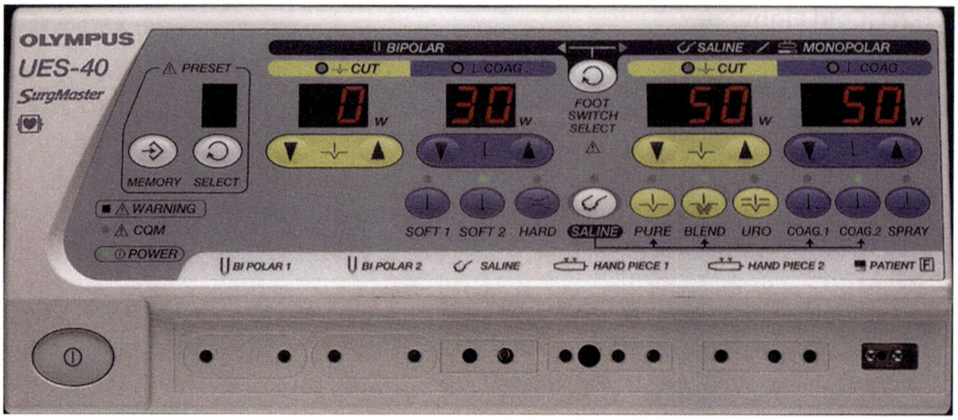

Fig. 2.1 SurgMaster Electrosurgical Unit (UES-40)

there is loose contact or wire falling off. Multifunctional high-frequency electrosurgical device may depend on changes in tissue impedance and be controlled by computer to adjust output automatically instead of manually. This technique ensures that electric knife can maintain the same cutting and coagulating effects no matter what tissues are. This device also has the digitalized power output display, the power-on self-test system, the automatic standby system, the poor circuit alarm, the overload output alarm, and the overtime output alarm. The power output stops automatically when it alarms, which ensures the safety of surgery. Because its energy attenuation in liquid is faster than that in air, so high-frequency electrosurgical device is specially provided with the tissue cutting mode in liquid (panel display URO), which ensures that it can do as fast and effective cutting in liquid as in air. UES-40 multi-functional high-frequency electrosurgical device (Fig. 2.1) covers almost every need of electrosurgery. It is applicable in conventional monopolar resectoscope as well as bipolar and monopolar instruments, and also allows the procedure of cutting in saline.

2.1.1.2 Nd-YAG Laser

The laser used for intrauterine surgery has been the neodymium:yttrium aluminum garnet (Nd:YAG) laser, which has the property of being attracted by the purplish-colored tissue. The coagulating effect produced when in contact with the tissue will lead to protein denaturalization and deactivation of its front and lateral tissues, which is ideal to destroying the endometrium. Therefore it was most suitable for endometrial ablation. However, this laser is an invisible light and located in the infra-red portion of the spectrum, with the wavelength 1064 nm, so it requires a guide of He-Ne light to reach the treatment area. When compared with CO_2 laser, it has more power, stronger penetrating, and more destructive effects on tissues. Fiberoptic lasers may deliver the laser energy through the operation channel of the hysteroscope. After being processed into the uterine cavity, it is conducted in fluid medium and act on lesions without attenuation of energy.

When the fiberoptic laser is used for other intrauterine surgery except for endometrial ablation, "bare" fibers must be avoided to reduce the depth of coagulation. New sculptured or extruded fibers, which can concentrate and focus the laser to prevent scattering, have been introduced that permit dissection or cutting with little coagulation. Such laser fibers can be used to divide intrauterine adhesions or a intrauterine septum, or for removal of a pedunculated submucous myoma. There is another kind of optical fiber, of which the sapphire tip is attached to the quartz fiber of the Nd:YAG. This special sapphire tip need to be cooled in liquid or gas medium during the procedure. In contrast, it is safer to use liquid distending medium than a gas medium when doing laser operative hysteroscopy, but the liquid medium used must have very strong cooling capacity. Safety is relative, and improper use will lead to excess absorption of distention medium. Improper use of the gaseous coolants, including CO_2, may also lead to air embolism. In short, the fiberoptic laser with sapphire tips must do with the high velocity of liquid or gas exchange so as to cool its tips. The velocity of thermal exchange medium requires about 1 L/min. A non-refrigerant gas or cooling through air is never allowed to use inside the uterine cavity.

2.1.2 Lighting System

Because the outer diameter of the telescope used in intrauterine operation is very small, only an extremely strong light can make the vision clear. So far, the light guided through the light cable has high brightness and low heat dissipation, with a piece of insulating glass located between light bulb and optical fibers, therefore, it is traditionally called "cold" light source. The commonly used cold light-source bulbs are halogen lamps, metal halide lamps and xenon lamps. These light sources with high color temperatures may produce high brightness, natural colors, and clear images. Xenon light with a higher color temperature is close to natural daylight and its bulb can be used for a long time, therefore it is more suitable for endoscopic lighting, and an ideal light source for hysteroscope.

2.1.2.1 Cold Light Source

1. Xenon cold light source (Fig. 2.2): The high power 300 W Xenon light source is equipped with both manual and automatic brightness adjusting modes to maintain best lighting, and higher brightness mode to increase the amount of light by nearly 2 times. At the same time, a 150 W emergency Halogen lamp is equipped so as to be switched on automatically to complete the necessary procedures when the main light is going off. The brightness can be automatically adjusted when the light source is connected to video systems via a light control cable. A standby illumination can be set through the use of a switch on the front panel or a remote control switch on the camera heads. With intensity-mode memory, when the light source is turned off no matter in what intensity mode, it will still be in that mode when turned back on. It can be also used in a variety of other flexible or rigid endoscopes in addition to hysteroscope. There is a record form for the use of light bulbs, and a waterproof panel with concise and cozy design, which is easy to clean. The brightness of light sources is quantized display.
2. Metal halide light source (Fig. 2.3): This high power metal halide lamp has high brightness with color temperature close to natural light, and a long lamp life with smooth consumption curve. The Olympus CLD-S is a multifunctional light source with its brightness adjusted automati-

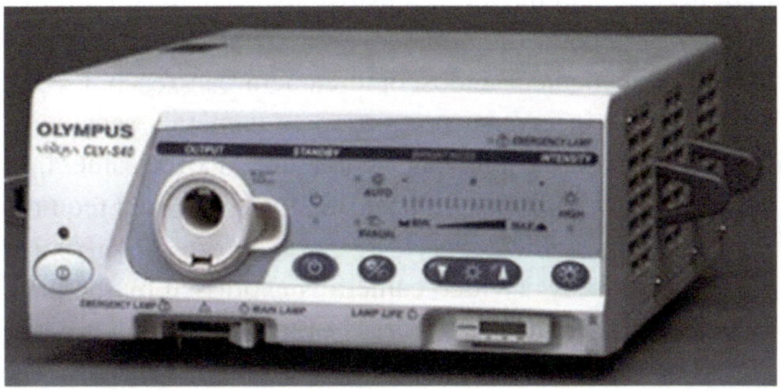

Fig. 2.2 CLV-S40 light source

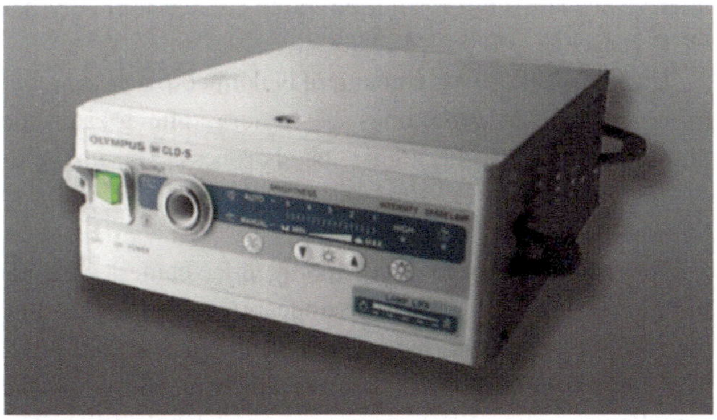

Fig. 2.3 CLD-S light source

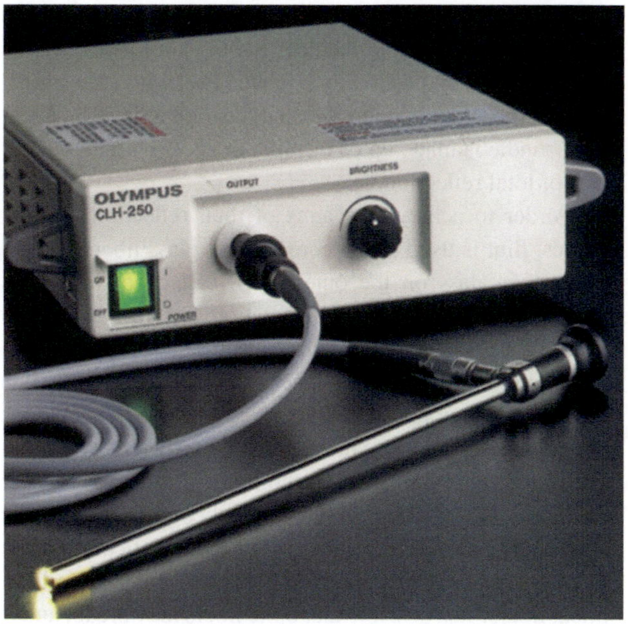

Fig. 2.4 CLH-250 light source

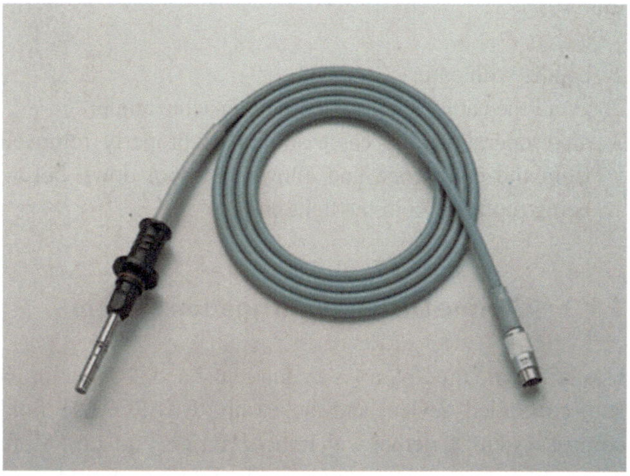

Fig. 2.5 Light guide bundle

cally or manually. It also has an emergency lamp (150 W halogen lamp) which ensures the safety of surgeries.

3. Halogen light source (Fig. 2.4): This high power 250 W halogen lamp has high brightness and good color temperature. It is convenient and intuitive in brightness adjustment, and also has an emergency bulb (250 W).

2.1.2.2 Light Guide Bundle

Light guide bundle (Fig. 2.5) is also known as light cable, consisting of a bundle of optical fibers with both ends to be curved. It is a part of camera imaging system, which has high quality to transmit light and connects the endoscope with light source. When the light passes from one medium into another, the reflection and refraction can be seen at the boundary surface. If the incident light cannot pass into the second medium, but is totally reflected back into the original medium, this phenomenon is called the total reflection. Light guide bundle is made up of the optical fibers with characteristics of total reflection.

In order to achieve the aims of total reflection of fiber bundles, flint is used as the core fiber of glass fibers, coated with crown glass on the outer layer, called coating layer, which solves the problem of insulation. Because refraction rate of flint glass is higher than that of the crown glass, the irradiation of light on the inner surface of flint glass is reflected to the opposite side of inner surface. Crown glass acts as a coating layer, which solves the problem of the so-called insulation and prevents the light from leaking. After repeated total reflection, the light shoots out from the other end of the fiber. The diameter of each optical fiber is 10–25 μm, and each of the cables contains over one million optical fibers. It is possible that optic fibers may break, and if damaged, it can be found when optical cable is checked in the daytime. The damaged fiber appears to be a black point. In order to extend the life of optical fibers, suggestions are as follows:

1. handle with care;
2. avoid the cable being folded into an acute angle;
3. after operation, the cable should be properly removed from the endoscope and allowed to cool down before being replaced from the light unit.

2.1.3 Uterine Distention/Irrigation System

Hysteroscopic fluid pump is an automatic and accurate pressure controlled device, and makes up "UTEROMAT fluid control system" together with its accessories (Fig. 2.6). More values like intrauterine pressure, flow rate, and liquid level

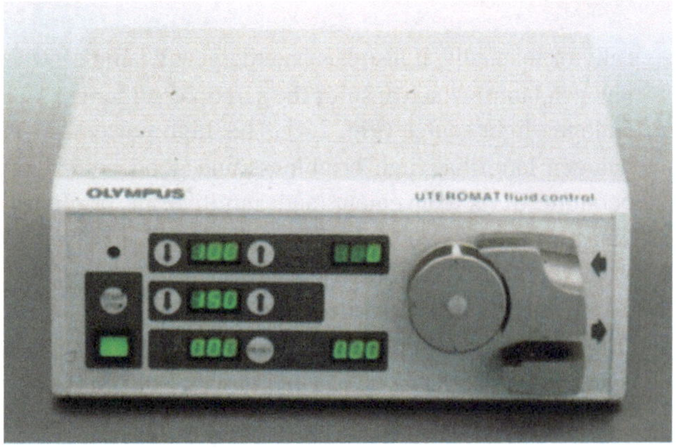

Fig. 2.6 UTEROMAT fluid control system

can be preset and stored; automatic monitoring of fluid deficit and alarming when exceeding the preset values ensure its safety. All these are very important in endometrial resection. Generally, fluid distending pressure is set at 80–100 mmHg and the flow rate at 200–400 mL/min.

2.1.4 Camera Imaging System

2.1.4.1 Imaging System

Imaging system is to take the endoscopic images by camera, analyze and process images by image processor, and then display them on the monitor, which includes CCD (charge coupled device) camera, video recorder, and monitor, etc. The camera image sensor can turn a real image into an digital image, and display it on the screen. Nowadays, CCD image sensor is used in all cameras. However, it cannot recognize color signals. Therefore, in order to obtain the color images, the presence of color must be realized through the prism or color filter. In China, hysteroscopic camera is of PAL signal system.

Most of video cameras in use now have VIDEO, Y/C, and RGB output, and the high quality cameras have SDI or HDMI output.

Camera sensitivity, also known as the minimum illumination, is the sensitivity degree of CCD to ambient light, or the darkest light that CCD normal imaging requires. The unit of illuminance is lux (Lx). The smaller the values are, the less light needed, and the more sensitive the camera is. Lx 2 to 3 belongs to general illuminance, and now the minimum illumination of medical endoscopic camera can reach 1.4 Lx. Lux value is in inverse proportion to camera's sensitivity. Therefore, 10 Lx camera is clearer than 15 Lx camera, of which the lower the Lux value is, the lower the light required for a satisfactory image.

The sharpness of video camera is expressed by the pixel value, which decides the accuracy of the sensor, and is determined by the number of the points forming the images. The larger the pixel value is, the better the clarity of the image. Therefore, low resolution video cameras of the earliest 150,000 pixel were replaced by high resolution cameras in later years. This high-resolution video camera normally has CCD sensor of 400,000–470,000 pixels.

The sharpness of video camera is defined by the number of horizontal scanning lines of camera. The greater the numerical value is, the higher the sharpness. The image of video camera with existing CCD sensor can achieve 1080 lines and above.

The television image generated by video camera contains the so-called noise. The noise appears in the form of fine particles in the image, particularly in the dark or red zone. The noise volume of video camera can be measured by the signal/noise ratio (S/N), expressed in decibels (dB). The higher the ratio is, the smaller the noise of the image.

Some video cameras are equipped with imaging system under dim light. This system works through adding auto gains, thereby improving the brightness of image. However, it is much better if there is a strong light source than the video cameras with auto gains function.

Finally, the video camera is generally equipped with automatic shutter so that the video camera can adjust the shutter speed to adapt to the light conditions. The shutter speed is usually regulated between 1/30 and 1/10,000 s, thus allowing video cameras to be used in all light conditions. If such a video camera is used, it is not necessary to apply an adjustable light source.

The focal length of most video camera lenses is between 20 and 40 mm. Usually the lens has 110° optical angle, 35 mm focal length, and allows for full screen images. Some cameras have a focusing function, which can magnify the image. Therefore, even a minor diameter lens or a narrow angle lens may also obtain full screen images. If it is a 35 mm lens, full screen images usually can be achieved. The use of light focusing means high consumption of light. Therefore, if the camera has focusing function, stronger light source will be required. Operative hysteroscopy is implemented through video monitor, and high resolution video camera can display the images of uterine cavity on the monitor, through which assistants and other staff at the operating room can understand the progress of operations and cooperate with surgeons. It is also convenient for doctors to explore and summarize the operational skills. The new hysteroscopic imaging system makes the vision more extensive, the image clearer, and observation and identification of lesions more detailed. Meanwhile, operators do not need to look through tiny telescope to observe uterine cavity, thus relieving the fatigue of operator's neck and back when operating, and obviously reducing the doctors' labor intensity.

The advanced modern 3CCD system makes its resolution greater than 1080 lines, thus ensures a perfect image quality. Each CCD will only take in one color of RGB according to its features. These three signals are processed in the camera individually to ensure the balance and reality of color reproduction, just as the eyes see. The first focusing free video camera in the world has a permanent and clear vision, and is freed of trouble in adjusting the focus. 10 Lx digital processor makes the signal-to-noise ratio greater than 62 dB and the clear images greatly relieve our visual fatigue. The first CF electric protection video camera can reduce electric leakage.

2.1.4.2 Monitor

The monitor is an important part of the monitoring system, and should be selected according to the resolution of video camera system, but the key is to indicate the quality of video camera. The number of horizontal scanning line of the monitor must be at least equal to the number of the lines of the video camera, and it will be better if the monitor resolution is greater than that of video camera system. The size and resolution of the monitor are two different concepts, so the requirement on the size of monitor is very subjective and 34 to 49 cm (14–20 in.) monitor could be chosen to one's personal preference. Generally, a monitor with 44 cm (18 in.) screen diagonal is suitable for performing high quality operations.

The video camera is like the surgeon's eyes, therefore, the best video camera should be provided.

2.1.4.3 High Definition Digital Camera System

High definition digital camera system (Fig. 2.7) is a new-type digital camera system, which has high signal-to-noise ratio, high image resolution (1080 p), and true color reproduction. There are vertical and curved types of standard video camera (Fig. 2.8a, b), respectively, for hysteroscopy and laparoscopy. Different adapters (Fig. 2.9a, b) may be chosen and applied in different endoscopes. In order to meet the sterilization requirements of modern minimally invasive surgery, the cameras (Fig. 2.10) which can be sterilized under high temperature and high pressure are developed. The high resolution video camera with 470,000 pixels ensures a clear and natural image, and has the doubled sensitivity function and a new additional automatic metering function, which may ensure the brightness of the images in various conditions. It also has a display function of wide depth of field, making both distance and near vision clear and bright. Two kinds of light adjusting modes - electronic shutter dimmer and dimming cable dimmer - ensure the best brightness of the images. Three-degree contour enhancement and white balance functions help to adjust the color match according to the user's preference. It has extremely strong adaptability to different light sources, and the corresponding parameters can be set according to the chosen light source. The waterproof panel simply and clearly designed is easy to operate and con-

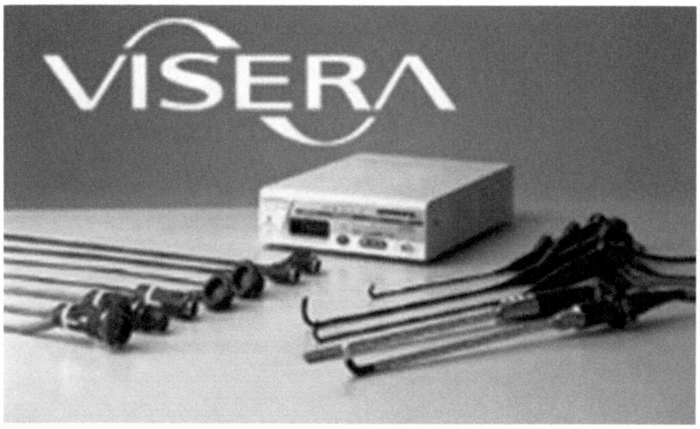

Fig. 2.7 OTV—S7 digital camera system

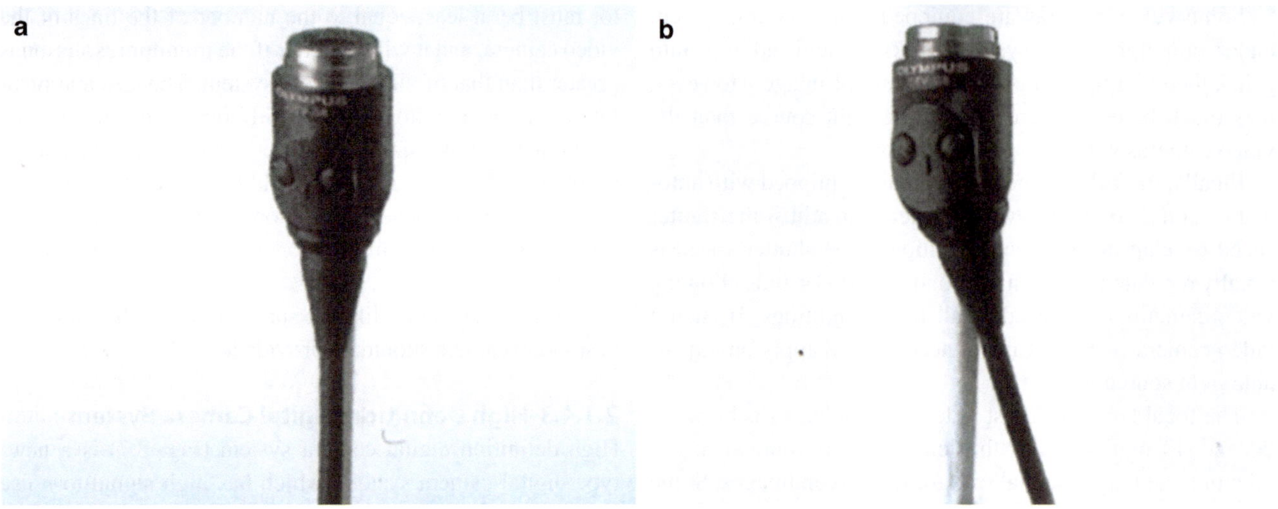

Fig. 2.8 Standard camera head. (**a**) Vertical. (**b**) Curved

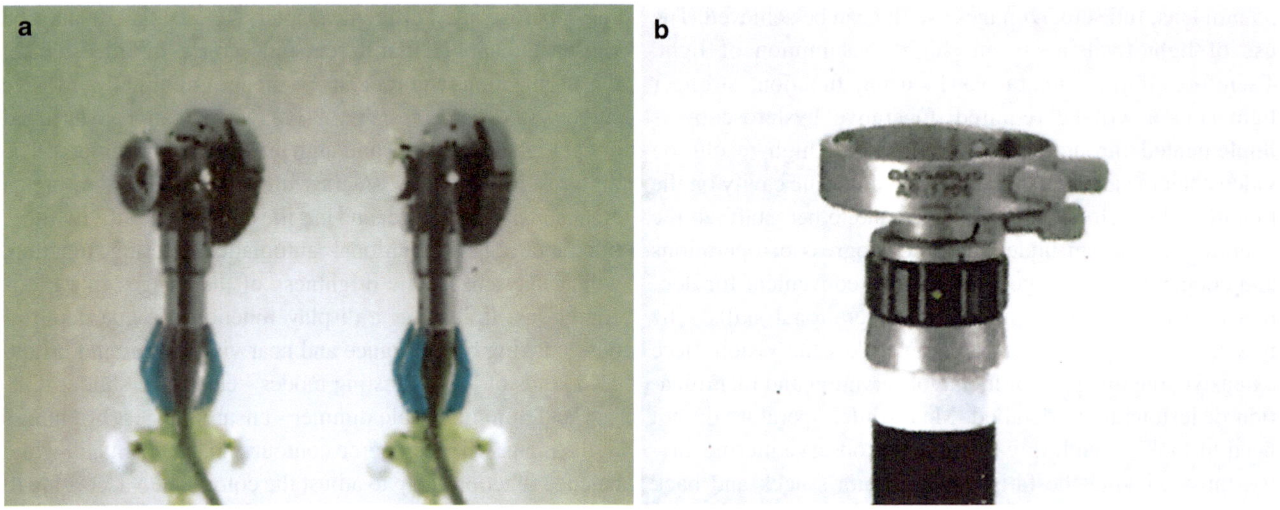

Fig. 2.9 Adapter. (**a**) 0.8 magnification. (**b**) 1.2 magnification

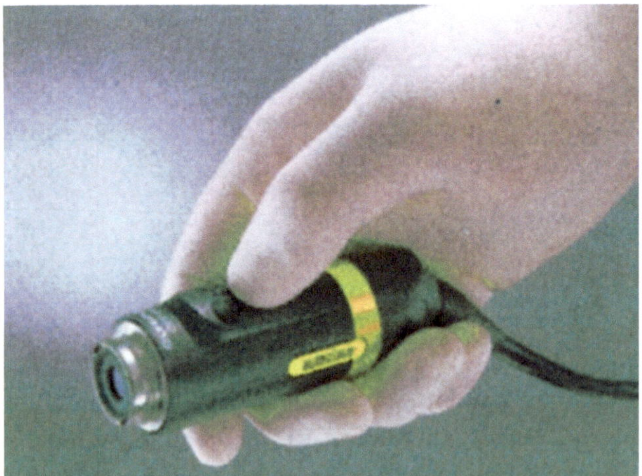

Fig. 2.10 Autoclavable camera head

venient for cleaning. The video camera head is waterproof so it can be immersed and fumigated for sterilization. It has professional red, green, and blue (RGB) output, and also the Y/C (S- video) and component video output. Its integrated digital image capturing system (Fig. 2.11) can do digital recording. In addition to the standard camera, a lightweight camera head with only 45 g is developed for being connected to the telescope.

2.1.4.4 Other Application Systems

With the development of technology, various application systems have emerged, such as voice-activated video camera system (Fig. 2.12) and an integrated modern minimally invasive operating room (Fig. 2.13) with a variety of instruments.

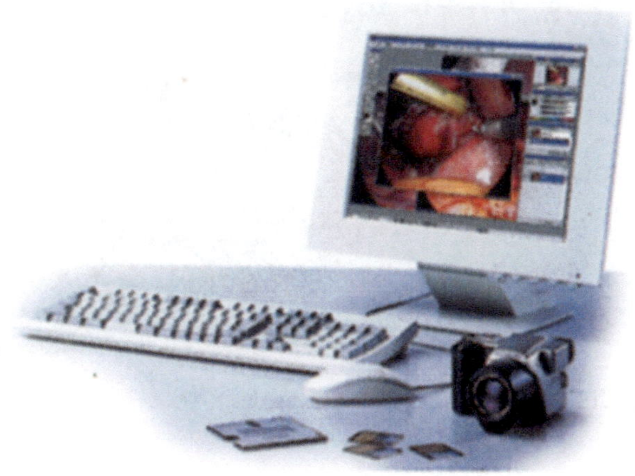

Fig. 2.11 Digital image capturing system

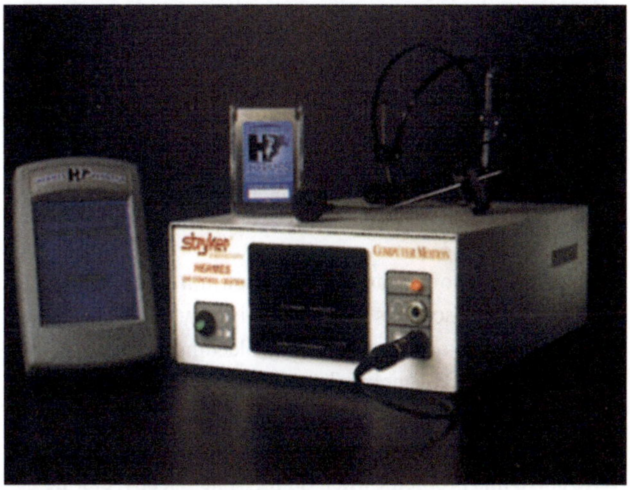

Fig. 2.12 Host machine of voice-activated camera system

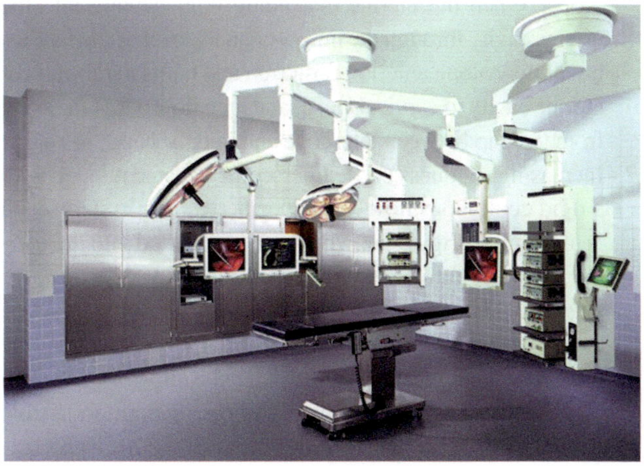

Fig. 2.13 Modern minimally invasive operating room

2.2 Instruments for Hysteroscopic Diagnosis and Treatment

Baoliang Lin

There are two types of hysteroscope according to different features—fiber hysteroscope (flexible hysteroscope) and rigid hysteroscope.

2.2.1 Fiber Hysteroscope

The fiber hysteroscope is flexible, and both the image and light are conducted by glass fiber bundles, so when the image is enlarged, it appears to be meshy. This is its weakness when compared with rigid hysteroscope. However, when using glass fiber, the hysteroscope can be finely-made with both sides of its tip fixed with steel wire and the direction of its tips adjusted and controlled by the manipulators at its handle. Anatomically, uterus appears to be in positions of anteflexion or retroflexion. Thus fiber hysteroscope is easier to be inserted into uterine cavity than rigid hysteroscope, and easier to view both tubal ostia. This is the advantage of fiber hysteroscope over rigid hysteroscope. The comparison between them is given in Table 2.1.

According to the functions, fiber hysteroscope can be divided into the following two types:

2.2.1.1 Diagnostic Fiber Hysteroscope (Fig. 2.14)

1. Total flexible fiber hysteroscope: The diameter of insertion tube is 3.1 mm. In early stage, the examination of uterine cavity was done by tracheal fiberscope or urethral fiberscope instead of fiber hysteroscope. Because the fiberscope was soft, it was often a problem to be inserted into the uterine cavity. Therefore, a modified fiberscope was developed by increasing its rigidity to facilitate the insertion. Another characteristic is maintaining a clear

Table 2.1 Comparison between rigid hysteroscope and fiber hysteroscope

Index	Rigid hysteroscope	Fiber hysteroscope
Image	Bright	Poorer
Magnification of the image	Yes (through camera head)	Yes (through camera head)
Procedure	Simple	Slightly difficult
Insertion into the uterine cavity	Sometimes difficult	Easy
Reaching the target directly	Possible	Slightly difficult
Observation of tubal ostia	Sometimes difficult	Easy
Duration of procedure	Long	Short
Price	Less expensive	More expensive
Uterine perforation	Possible	Rare
Operator's posture	Uncomfortable	Comfortable

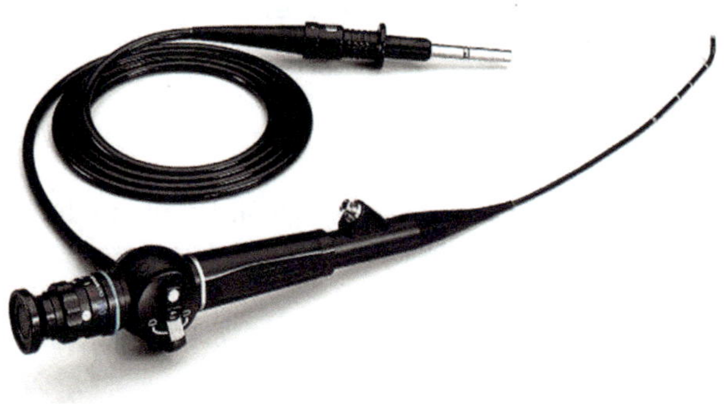

Fig. 2.14 Diagnostic fiber hysteroscope

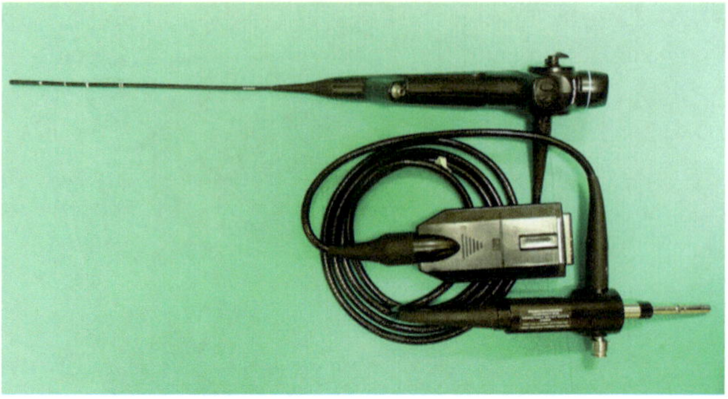

Fig. 2.15 New diagnostic fiber hysteroscope

vision when fixed with Lin's outer sheath for continuous-flow system.

2. Soft and rigid diagnostic fiber hysteroscope: The front section of telescope is soft and flexible, the middle rigid, and the rear flexible. Because the middle section is rigid, it is easier to perform procedures in uterine cavity or insert the telescope directly into the uterine cavity than the total flexible fiber hysteroscope.
3. Diagnostic fiber hysteroscope without light guide bundle: It is one of the total flexible fiber hysteroscopes, whose characteristic is the light source integrated with the hysteroscope. It is installed in itself with small bulb light source and a dry cell battery for 1H continuous use. The set of hysteroscope becomes very light and easy to carry because it need neither a long light guide bundle nor a heavy cold light source.
4. Flexible video hysteroscope: This is a total flexible fiber hysteroscope with the light conducted by fiber bundles and the images transformed into RGB digital signals by mini-CCD which is fixed to the rear of fiberscope. Then the digital signals are transmitted into processor for processing through wire lines. Therefore there are two main advantages: the first is that it does not apply fiber bundles for transmitting images, thus could provide superior quality images as that achieved from rigid telescope, as well as avoids the defect that a black point will appear on the image when a fiber is broken. The second is that the front tip of this hysteroscope can bend up and down as other fiberscope. The outer diameter of insertion tube is 3.8 mm (Fig. 2.15).

In 1997, Japanese scholar Lin Baoliang developed a continuous flow outer sheath (Fig. 2.16) and changed the history of fiber hysteroscope, thus making the fiber hysteroscope into an era of continuous flow system. This continuous flow outer sheath has two kinds, flexible and rigid. Their functions are as follows.

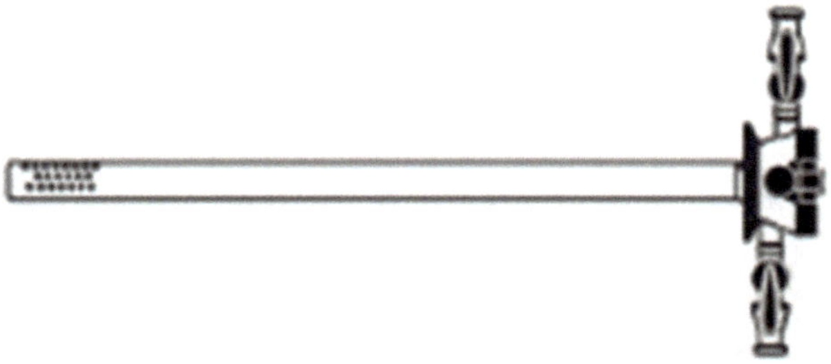

Fig. 2.16 Continuous flow outer sheath

1. Continuous flow features: Endometrium is easy to bleed. When hysteroscope is inserted, its tip may touch the cervical canal or endometrium and cause bleeding, which may lead distending fluid sanguinolent and obscure the observation. Therefore, in general, hysteroscopy would not be done if there is abnormal uterine bleeding or menstruation. In order to solve this problem, when doing hysteroscopy, uterine distending fluid will be frequently renewed if tainted with intrauterine blood. The continuous flow outer sheath can be assembled surrounding the insertion tube of fiber hysteroscope. When the uterine distending fluid flowing into the uterine cavity through the inflow channel reaches the fundus, it will flow along anterior, posterior, and both lateral walls of uterine cavity to cervical canal, and then flow out of the body from the gap between telescope and outer sheath.
2. Increasing rigidness of the fiberscope: When equipped with a rigid continuous flow outer sheath, the fiber hysteroscope is made into a rigid one, which can be inserted into the uterine cavity by force and reaches the target location. If there is trouble in inserting the telescope, only fiber hysteroscope can be sent into the uterine cavity for observation under the protection and guidance of the outer sheath.
3. Easy to handle the fiber hysteroscope: Continuous flow outer sheath is installed with a control handle, which is convenient for holding.

4. Diagnostic flexible hysteroscope using Lin polyp snare system: For endometrial polyps which are detected by diagnostic flexible hysteroscope in the office, a traditional management is curettage with requirements of cervical dilation and anesthesia. Another treatment is to perform management by changing the diagnostic hysteroscope to an operative one. However, the operative hysteroscope is larger and also needs cervical dilation and anesthesia. It has been an ambition to hysteroscopic surgeons for a long time that endometrial polyps could be removed at the time of being discovered with diagnostic flexible hysteroscope. In 2011, Lin polyp snare system was developed to resolve this problem. When an endometrial polyp is detected by a diagnostic flexible hysteroscope in the office, it can be simultaneously removed using a Lin polyp snare system under direct vision of hysteroscope without requirements of cervical dilation and anesthesia (Fig. 2.17a, b).

2.2.1.2 Therapeutic Fiber Hysteroscope

The telescope is equipped with a working channel, through which a biopsy forceps or a grasping forceps can be inserted. Therefore, a biopsy can be done by a pair of biopsy forceps under direct vision or an intrauterine foreign body or IUD can be removed by a pair of grasping forceps. Therapeutic fiber hysteroscope has two types as follows.

1. Flexible therapeutic fiber hysteroscope (Fig. 2.18): It has 4.9 mm outer diameter of the front tip, 120° field of view, 100° up/down angulation, and 2.2 mm diameter of working channel.
2. Soft and rigid therapeutic fiber hysteroscope (Fig. 2.19): The front section of telescope is soft and flexible, the middle rigid, and the rear semi-rigid. In addition to the above advantages of total flexible fiber hysteroscope, the middle rigid part can be used to hold the scope, and can do 180° left/right shaft rotation. The semi-rigid part of the rear segment can do 45° bending in all directions and free fixation. The operator can take advantage of these functions to insert mini-instruments into the working channel for treatment in a relaxed posture.

Usually, the diameter of flexible forceps used for therapeutic hysteroscope is 1.8 mm, two are commonly used.

1. Biopsy forceps: Intrauterine tissues are taken under the direct vision of hysteroscope for pathological examination. Because of small blades and very small samples, pathological examination is often far from satisfactory.
2. Grasping forceps: It is used to take out the intrauterine foreign bodies or remove the IUD. The forceps can only clamp the tail string of the IUD because it is too small to hold an IUD.

These traditional flexible forceps are very small and can do very little work. Japanese Lin's flexible forceps include

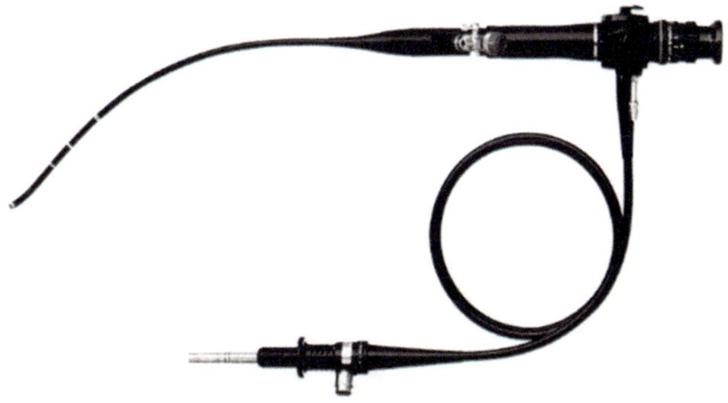

Fig. 2.18 Flexible therapeutic fiber hysteroscope

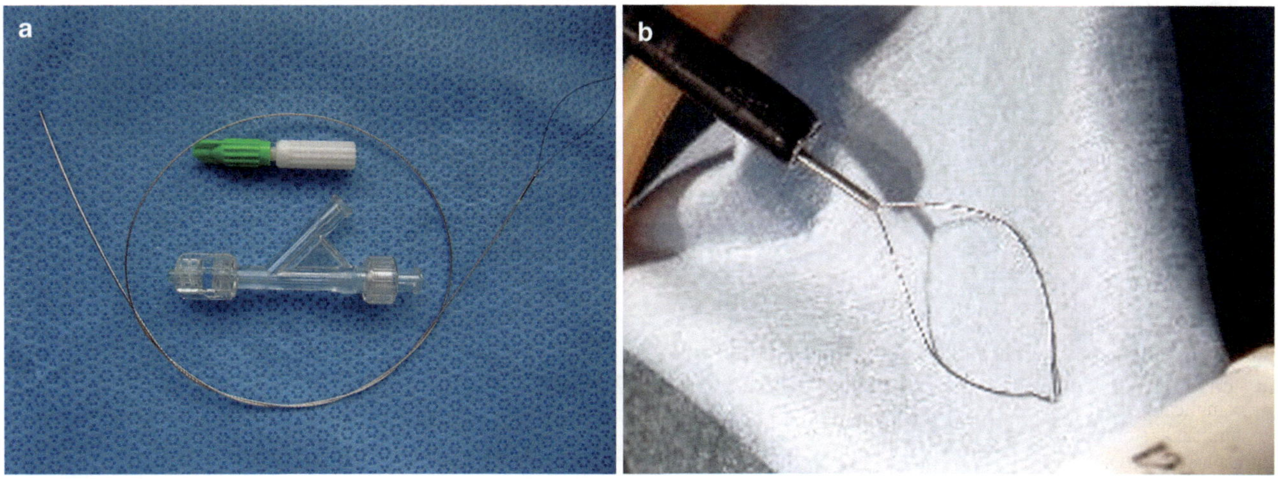

Fig. 2.17 (**a**) Lin polyp snare system. (**b**) The snare is extended from the hysteroscope

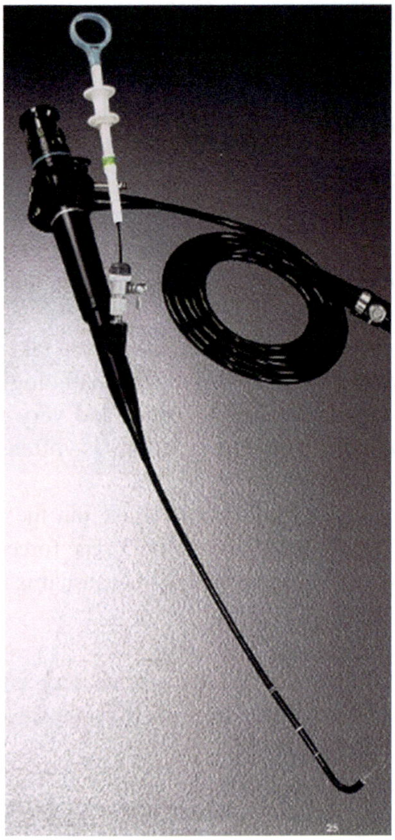

Fig. 2.19 Soft and rigid therapeutic fiber hysteroscope

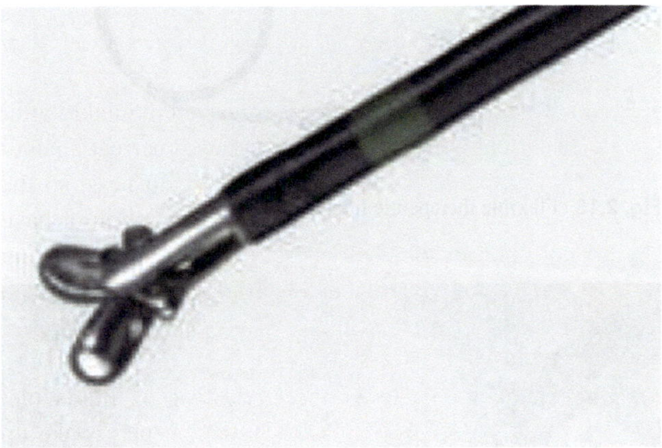

Fig. 2.20 Biopsy forceps

biopsy forceps (Fig. 2.20), grasping forceps, and scissors. They are larger instruments and do not go through the working channel but are fixed at the front of scope. The use of Lin's flexible forceps improves the capacity of therapeutic hysteroscopy.

2.2.2 Rigid Hysteroscope

Such hysteroscope has a rigid appearance, consists of an outer sheath, inner sheath, and telescope itself. The rigid telescope is composed of lens transmitting images and optic fibers delivering light. It is easy to manipulate, suitable for beginners, but one should be very careful of uterine perforation any time. According to its function, rigid hysteroscope can be divided into two types as the following.

2.2.2.1 Diagnostic Rigid Hysteroscope

The diameter of the telescope is 2–4 mm, and the diameter of the outer sheath supporting its use is 3–5 mm, which is exclusively used to examine the uterine cavity. It can be done in office and does not need anesthesia, dilatation of the cervical canal, and grasping cervix with clamps. A 30° oblique viewing telescope is preferred to observe the uterine cavity, and dilation of cervical canal is needed when a continuous flow hysteroscope with 5.5 mm diameter outer sheath is used.

2.2.2.2 Therapeutic Rigid Hysteroscope

A 4.5 mm therapeutic rigid hysteroscope with continuous irrigation is made up of 30° and 3 mm optical tube, and the tubal sheath. Its 4.5 mm outer diameter makes examination of uterine cavity possible without dilation of cervix. Its 30° wide-angle scope allows to observe two tubal ostia and the whole uterine cavity simultaneously by rotating the telescope. The design of double valves and double sheaths ensures smooth and continuous irrigation, and always a clear vision. On this basis, if equipped with a 6.5 mm outer sheath, it is a standard 6.5 mm therapeutic hysteroscope. There is a 2.2 mm operating channel on the outer sheath, and treatment can be done if inserting hysteroscopic forceps. 8 mm continuous flow operative rigid hysteroscope consists of 30°, 4 mm telescope, the tubal sheath, working channel, and operative instruments. It has a clearer vision, elevating working platform, greater distention flow, and 2.2 mm operating channel (Fig. 2.21). The forceps can be classified into rigid, semi-rigid, and flexible ones according to its feature, and semi-rigid forceps is the most suitable for intrauterine treatment. According to the purposes, operative instruments can be sorted into biopsy forceps, grasping forceps, and scissors, etc. A biopsy forceps can also be fixed on the outer sheath of the hysteroscope or a special bending device (Albarran bridge) is installed onto the hysteroscope to adjust the direction of inserting a flexible forceps. This procedure requires to be done under anesthesia.

2.2.2.3 Mini-Hysteroscope

Flexible hysteroscope can well meet the patients' needs of comfort during a minimally invasive surgery. The new

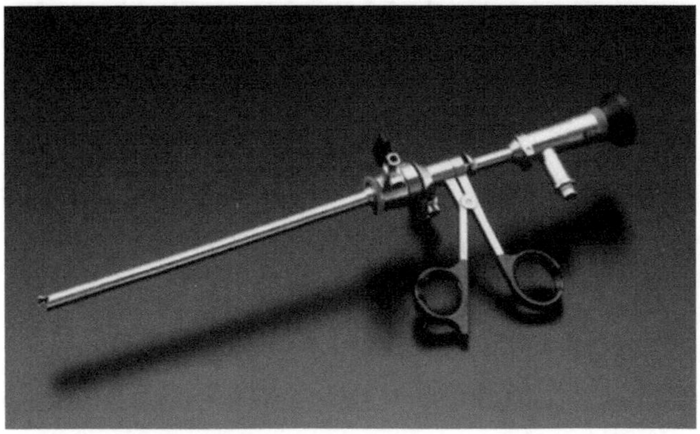

Fig. 2.21 Therapeutic rigid hysteroscope

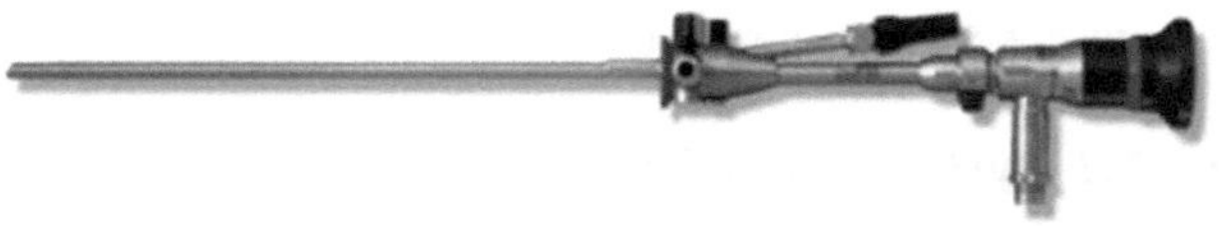

Fig. 2.22 Mini-hysteroscope

1.9 mm mini-telescope system integrates advantages of both flexible and rigid hysteroscopes: patients' comfort improved (thin outer diameter), easiness in cleaning (can have autoclave sterilization), and effective treatment (5Fr or 7Fr working channel) (Fig. 2.22).

2.2.2.4 Hamou Hysteroscope

Hamou micro-contact hysteroscope is equipped with magnifying lens, which cannot only see normal object images, but also can magnify the object by 20 times, 60 times, and even 150 times. The disadvantages are that the hysteroscope is too heavy, and one needs specialized knowledge about intrauterine pathology when doing contact hysteroscopy.

2.2.3 Integrated Hysteroscope

With the development of hysteroscopic technique, the instruments used for hysteroscopy are also in constant progress and are being perfected. In the minimally invasive surgery, flexible hysteroscope can well meet the patients' needs for comfort, but there is a slight defect in treatment. Now, integrated hysteroscope (Fig. 2.23) integrates the double advantages of both flexible and rigid hysteroscopes, and its thin diameter elevates greatly the patient's comfort, simple ways of sterilization make it easier to clean, and operative channel meets the need of effective treatments.

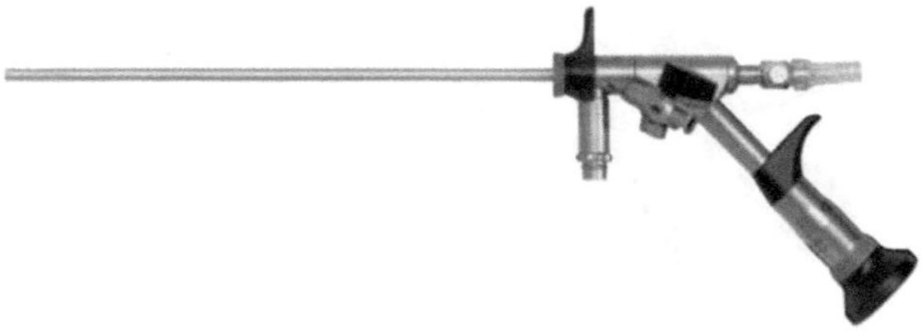

Fig. 2.23 Integrated hysteroscope

2.3 Instruments for Hysteroscopic Surgery

Xuegang Liu

At the beginning of hysteroscopic surgery, the pioneers, such as Magos from Britain, Lin Baoliang from Japan, Xia Enlan from China, used prostatic resectoscope or bladder resectoscope from department of urology to perform hysteroscopic surgery. It was until 1992 that the hystero-resectoscope exclusive for gynecological surgery was developed.

2.3.1 Hystero-Resectoscope (Fig. 2.24)

Hystero-resectoscope for gynecological surgery originated from urological resectoscope, and on this basis the shape and size of its outer sheath was modified and continuous flow system was added in order to adapt to the operational characteristics inside uterine cavity (Fig. 2.24). Its whole length is 30–35 cm and working length 18–19.5 cm, and the working length of super-long hystero-resectoscope is 22 cm or 26.5 cm, which can be used in enlarged uterus. The outer diameters of different hystero-resectoscopes are 21Fr (7 mm), 24Fr (8 mm), 25Fr (8.3 mm), 26Fr (8.7 mm), 27Fr (9 mm), and 28Fr (9.3 mm), respectively.

2.3.1.1 Telescope (Fig. 2.25)

It provides a panoramic view with diameter 3 mm or 4 mm and depth of focus 30–35 mm. Angle options of different objective lens are 0°, 12°, and 30°, with visual field 70°–120°. The modes of 12° and 30° are commonly used so as to observe the uterine cornua and lateral walls easily. The 21/24Fr (7/8 mm) hystero-resectoscope is equipped with a 3 mm telescope, with the others 4 mm telescope. The eyepiece has an insulated shaft which can be connected to a teaching scope, a camera, a video camera or an adapter.

2.3.1.2 Working Element (Fig. 2.26)

It is an elastic hand control mechanical device, which can control the operation of electrode. There are channels for the insertion of telescope and working electrode on it, and also

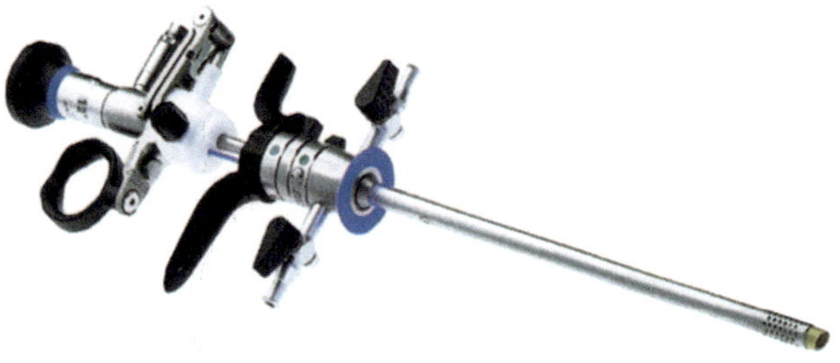

Fig. 2.24 Hystero-resectoscope

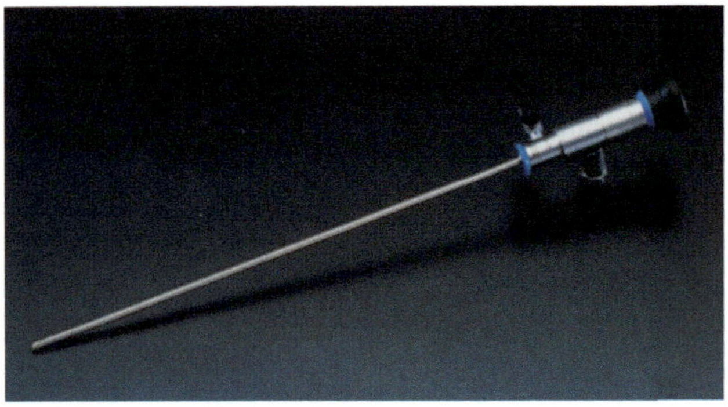

Fig. 2.25 Telescope

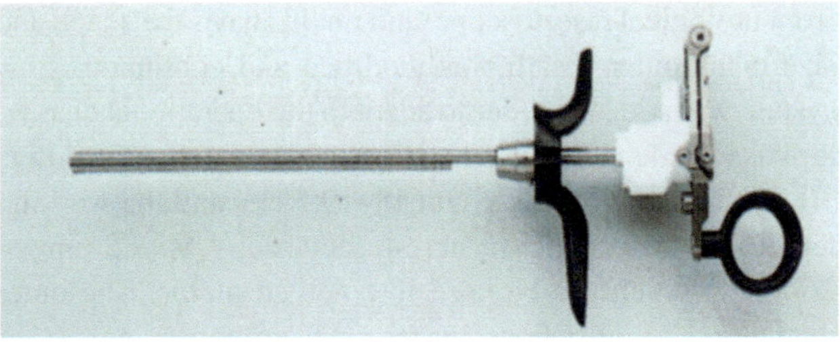

Fig. 2.26 Working element

the connector connected with a high frequency current generator. Since the telescope has fore oblique angle, thus when installed, the port of light source should be upward and electrode downward. And the direction of the electrode port may also be upward or sideward. When fingers are pulling on the trigger, the working electrode may move forward or backward. The hystero-resectoscope adopts a passive rebound device with the resting position of electrode inside the sheath. When pulling the trigger by hand, the electrode tip moves out of the sheath and then moves back into the sheath by the force of the spring. The cutting is to be done when the electrode tip is returning to the sheath. The electrode may move 30–40 mm within the visual field of hysteroscope. It should be paid attention that only when operation field is totally in sight and the electrode tip is on the way back to the sheath, electricity current may be powered on. At present, only

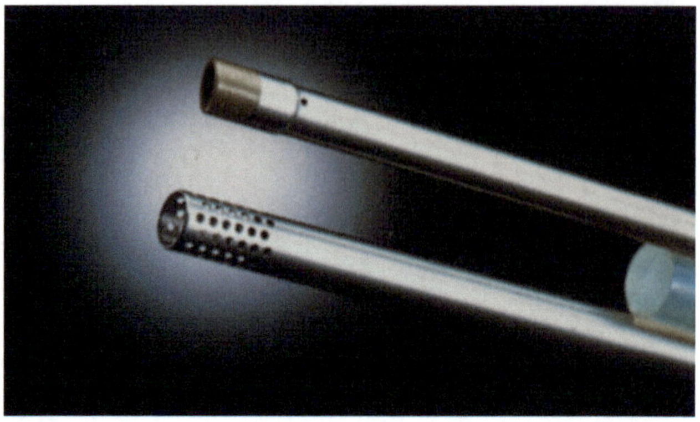

Fig. 2.27 Hysteroscopic sheath

Olympus and the like have special video camera for electric resectoscope with panoramic view.

2.3.1.3 Hysteroscopic Sheaths (Fig. 2.27)

The resectoscope has two concentric circular sheaths to introduce working element. The outer sheath and the inner sheath can rotate between each other and prevent damage to the cervix.

1. Outer sheath: Its diameter is 8–9 mm and there are sieve holes at its front end and a stopcock at the rear end for fluid outflow.
2. Inner sheath: Its front beak is embedded with oblique ceramic insulation, and its rear end is fitted with a stopcock for fluid inflow. The design of the oblique ceramic insulation greatly increases the effective irrigation of the telescope and its durability, and can prevent leakage of electricity. Olympus ABS (anti-blocking system), which was a patent, integrates a micro-hole in the inner sheath of hystero-resectoscope (Fig. 2.28), and ensures a certain amount of distention flow even if the irrigation holes are blocked by tissues, thus a smooth operation is possible.

After the inner sheath is inserted into the outer sheath, the irrigation fluid flows from the tip of the inner sheath into the uterine cavity and makes it distending, and then retunes via the sieve holes of the distal end of the outer sheath into the gap between the outer and inner sheaths. The gap between the inner and outer sheaths is very small, and this design is to reduce the resistance of water inflow and slightly elevate resistance of water outflow. The continuous flow resectoscope allows a great deal of low viscosity distending medium to flow continuously and rapidly, thus maintaining a proper pressure and a moderate distention of uterine cavity. The vision becomes clear and the visibility is increased. There was a hysteroscope applying intermittent irrigation, which had only one sheath and might be used with high viscosity distending medium.

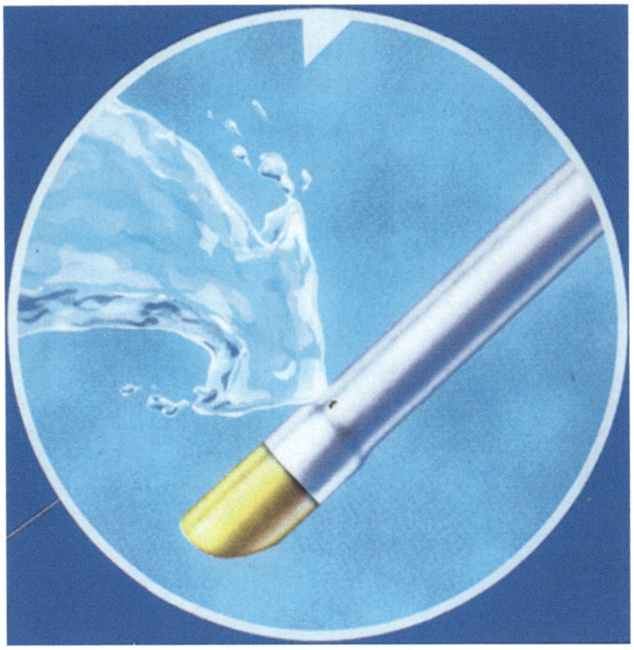

Fig. 2.28 ABS (anti blocking system)

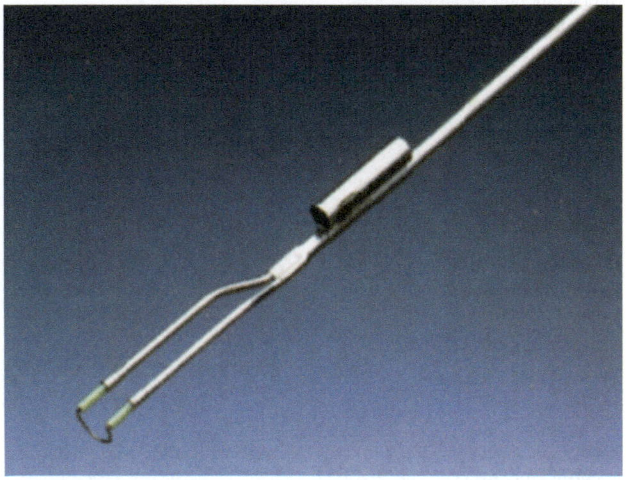

Fig. 2.29 Wire loop electrode

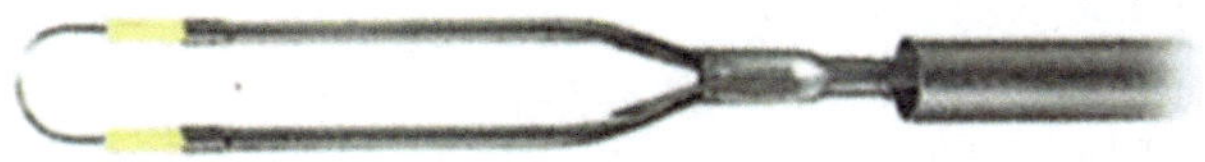

Fig. 2.30 Forward angled loop electrode

2.3.1.4 Obturator

It is the core of the sheath with its head oval-shaped. It can close the window of the beak of resectoscope, and suits the shape of cervical channel for an easy insertion.

2.3.2 Active Electrodes

The resectoscope is often used with a monopolar electrode and the power is 70–100 W.

2.3.2.1 Wire Loop Electrode

It is also known as wire loop electrode (Figs. 2.29 and 2.30), and has two types, open (U-shape) and closed (O-shape), with different angles like 0°, 12°, and 30°. 12° open wire loop appears to be vertical, usually 6.2 mm wide and 4.1 mm deep, which is mainly used for resection of endometrium, cutting and removal of myomas and polyps. 0° open wire loop electrode is used for incision of uterine septum and splitting large myomas so that they may be clamped out easily. 21Fr (7 mm) resectoscope adopts closed wire loop (Fig. 2.31), and this small wire loop is very suitable for the resection of small polyps, division of intrauterine adhesions, resection of uterine septum, and removal of intrauterine foreign bodies.

2.3.2.2 Needle Electrode (Fig. 2.32)

It is suitable for cutting uterine endometrium and myometrium, removing intramural myoma by fenestration.

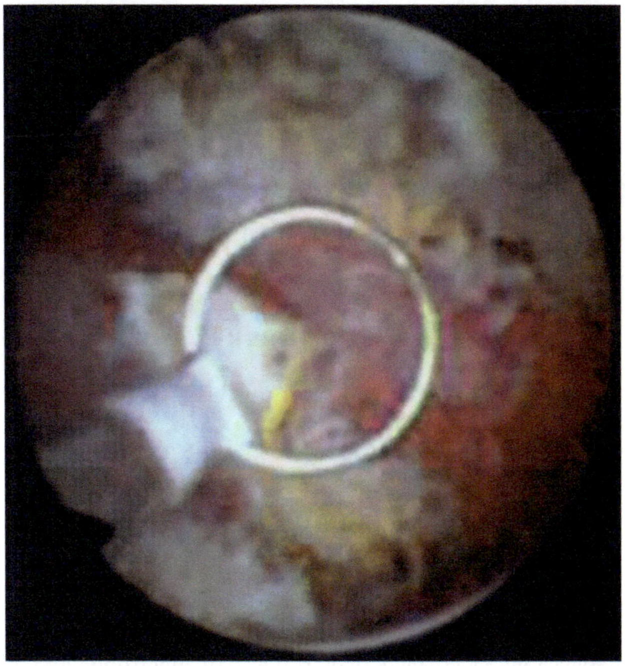

Fig. 2.31 Closed wire loop electrode

2.3.2.3 Roller Ball Electrode

Its diameter may be 2 mm or 3 mm (Fig. 2.33). It can rotate around the axis with focused current and is mainly used for coagulation of bleeding or ablation of uterine endometrium.

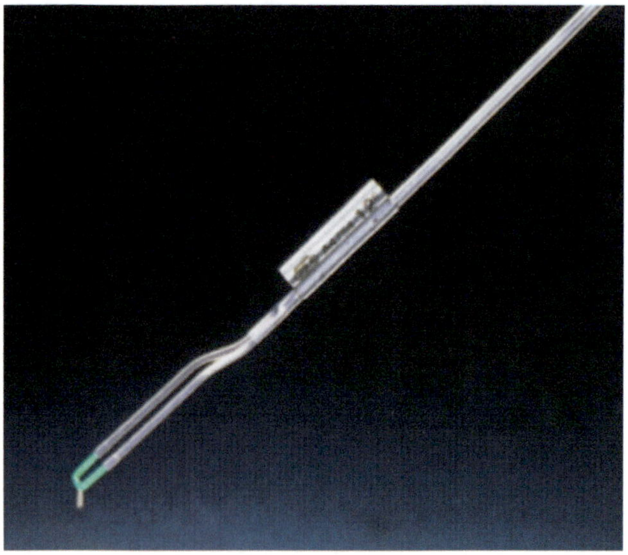

Fig. 2.32 Needle electrode

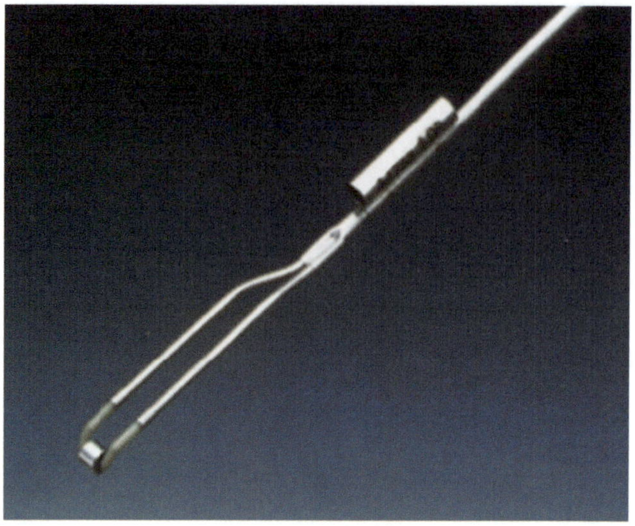

Fig. 2.34 Roller barrel electrode

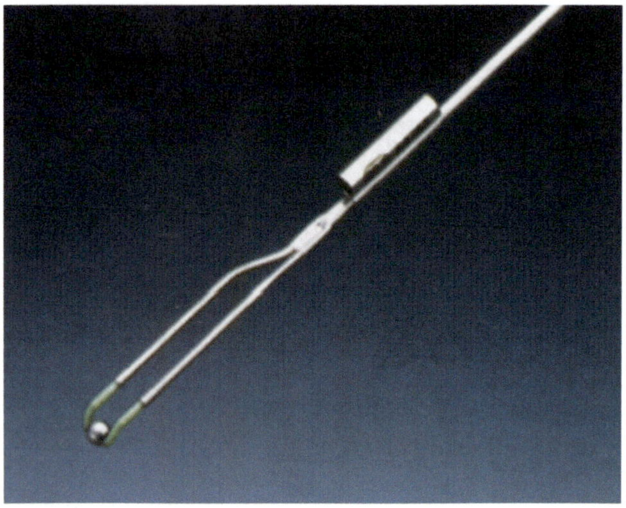

Fig. 2.33 Roller ball electrode

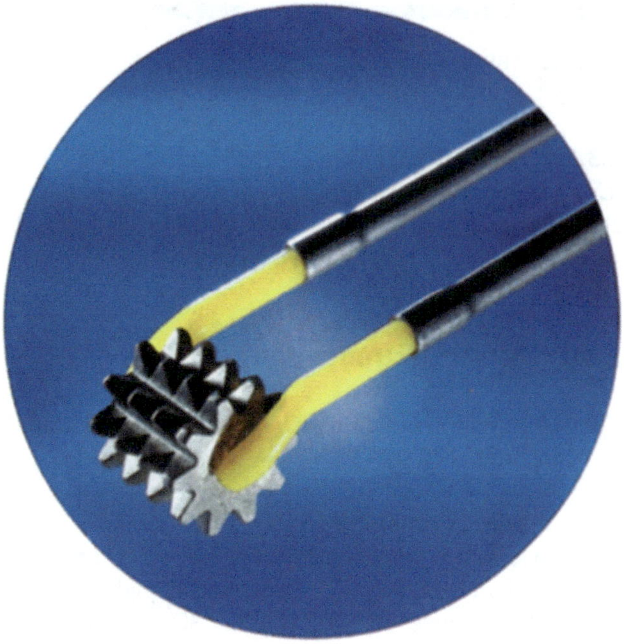

Fig. 2.35 Vaporizing electrode

2.3.2.4 Roller Bar/Roller Barrel Electrode (Fig. 2.34)

There are different sizes of roller bars, like 2 mm, 3 mm, and 5 mm, which may rotate around the axis. It has a wider contact surface than roller ball electrode, and is more suitable for endometrial ablation and coagulation of bleeding.

2.3.2.5 Vaporizing Electrode/Vaportrode (Fig. 2.35)

Vaporizing electrode appears to be groove-shaped with the working power 200 W, which is different from the electrodes above and may be used to vaporize endometrium and small intrauterine myoma.

2.3.2.6 Band Electrode (Fig. 2.36)

It is similar to open wire loop, but wider, using pure cutting current and 200 W power. It shares the advantages of the wire loop and the vaporizing electrode, and there is no bleeding when resects endometrium and other tissues. In addition, the tissue resected can be sent for histopathological examination.

2.3.3 Accessory Instruments and Equipment

The accessory instruments and equipment include a catheter, vaginal speculum or hammer, vaginal retractor, cervical clamps, cervical dilator, myomas grasping forceps, polypus forceps, oval forceps, a curette, uterine suction head, suction tube, and uterine suction cart, etc. Complex operations should be monitored by ultrasonography and (or) laparoscopy.

2.3.4 Plasma Bipolar Resectoscope (Fig. 2.37)

The plasma bipolar resectoscope allows the surgeon to perform transcervical resection in saline (TCRis), with a special multifunctional high-frequency current generator (Olympus SurgMaster Electrosurgery Generator) (Fig. 2.38). SurgMaster high-frequency electrosurgery generator is equipped with the resection mode in saline, and when combined with transcervical resectoscope in saline, plasma electric resection may be done. Compared with conventional monopolar operation, SurgMaster generator can use high frequency energy to convert the saline into electron plasma with a high density of free electric particle for precise cutting of tissue. In addition, the decrease of heat conduction can reduce coagulation depth, thereby reducing the tissue charring. And there is no need to take the risk of conventional high-frequency monopolar resection.

Clinically, TCRis has the following characteristics:

- Cutting in saline can be done without TURP syndrome, and super large tissues can be removed;
- Bipolar current, which goes only through the local part of patient's body without hazard of burning;
- Safe for pacemaker;

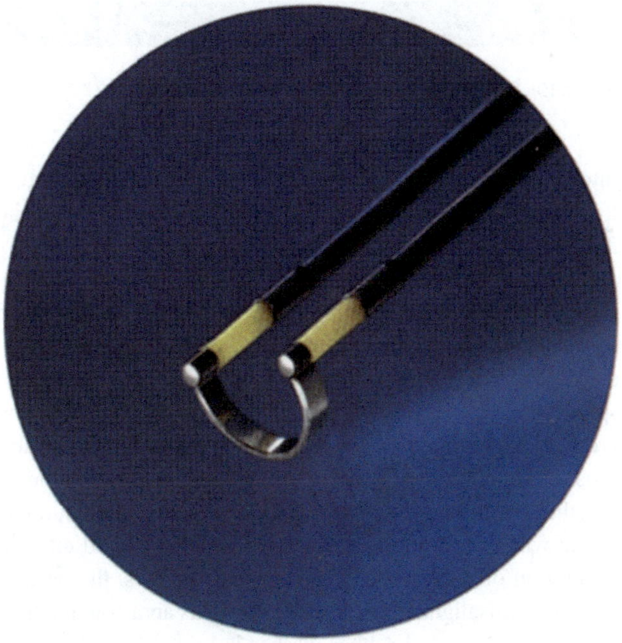

Fig. 2.36 Band electrode

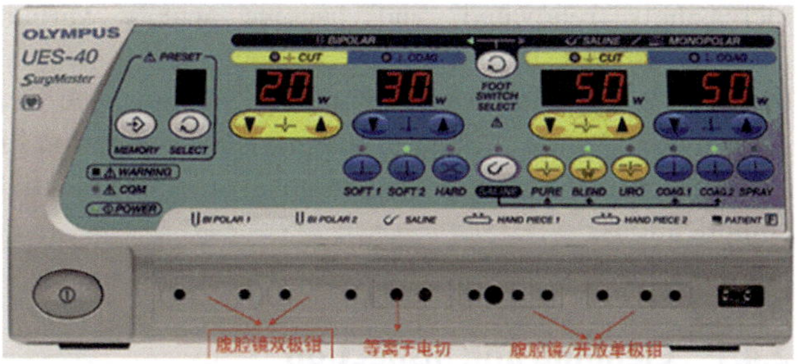

Fig. 2.38 SurgMaster multifunctional high-frequency electrosurgery generator

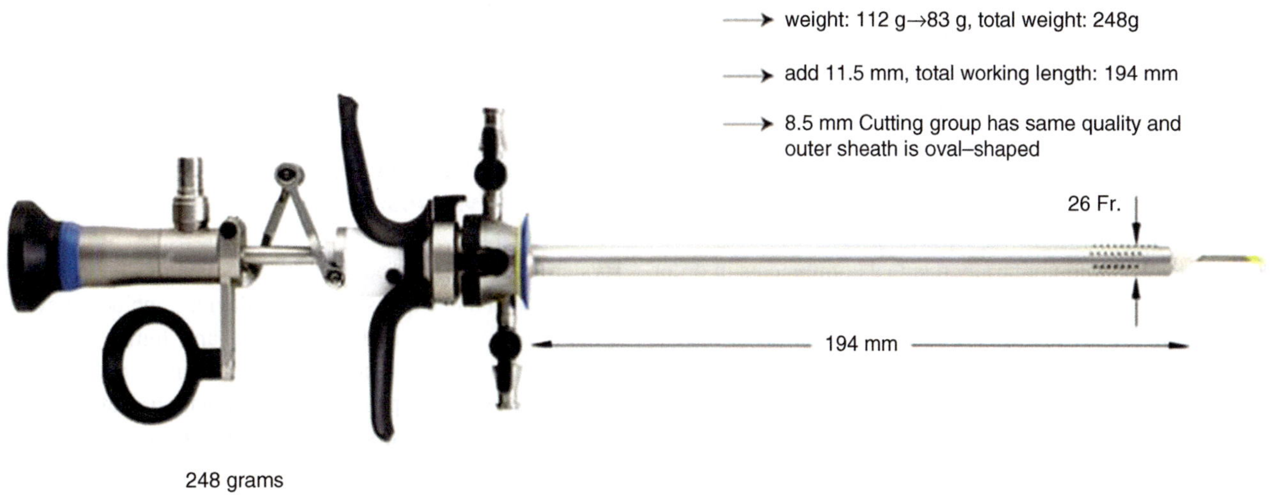

Fig. 2.37 Plasma bipolar resectoscope, also known as transcervical resection in saline (TCRis)

- Avoidance of obturator nerve reflex;
- Accurate resection of the tumor (using a small wire loop), especially mosslike floating tumor;
- No tissue adhesion, no need to clean up, and cutting more smoothly;
- Decreased depth of thermal tissue damage with no charring, and convenience for pathological examination;
- Clean operating surface, and more accurate tissue identification;
- Bipolar current, accurate coagulation, and more reliability;
- First choice for Diabetic patients.

2.4 Cleaning, Sterilization, and Maintenance of Hysteroscopic Instruments

Yan Quan and Xuegang Liu

With the continuous development and improvement of micro-mechanical, electronical, and optical instruments, the instruments and equipment for hysteroscopy are also increasingly renovated, and become widely varied. Because of their high accuracy and complex functions, their proper cleaning, sterilization, and maintenance can not only ensure the successful diagnosis and operation of hysteroscopy, but also is critical to avoid the potential complications.

2.4.1 Cleaning and Inspection of Hysteroscopic Instruments

One should keep in mind being gentle is very important when cleaning the hysteroscope and its accessories.

After the operation, place the instruments in cleaning solution, and be sure not to hit, fold, and press. Then disassemble all the instruments completely and clean all the blood clots and mucus deposits inside the channels with a special brush or a cleaning gun. As for the cleaning of the exterior surface of endoscope, one can use soft scrubs to brush clean the telescope and its head, especially the lens of hysteroscope. There should not be any residual components in order that the lens is kept clear. If the lens is blurred, cleanliness can be done by scrubbing it with mixed solution including ethanol and diethyl ether (95% ethanol 7 mL + ether 3 mL). When wiping the lens, it is proper to use lens paper or soft gauze.

After cleaning, place the hysteroscope and its accessories in a rinse sink, and rinse the channels with flowing water for at least 10 s. Then wash the surfaces of hysteroscope and all instruments and accessories with flowing water, insufflate air into the channels with a compressed air gun or a syringe to flush out water. Finally, wipe the surface of hysteroscope and its accessories to keep the channels dry.

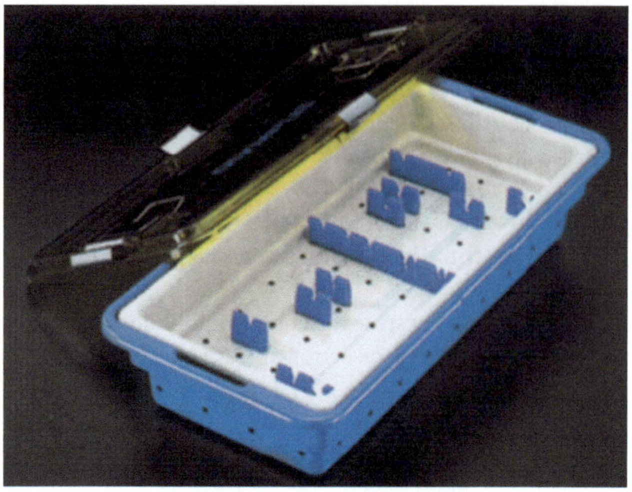

Fig. 2.39 Specialized storage box for instruments

Different kinds of hysteroscopic operative instruments, such as biopsy forceps, scissors, foreign body forceps, and grasping forceps, must be cleaned after being used. Open each stop-cock, clean the interior of the channels using cotton swabs or special cleaning agents for hysteroscope; scrub the holes and grooves of instruments using a long thin brush or cotton swabs, brush the joints of forceps using special soft brush. After cleaning, the instruments should be inspected carefully and routinely to see whether or not the lens is cracked, the sealed end has infiltration of water droplets which blur the lens, the jaws of forceps is misaligned, the insulated part has abrasion, the telescope is broken; and rubber washer is broken and damaged, etc. After inspection, the instruments are wiped dry, and placed in a special box for spare use (Fig. 2.39).

The cleaning and inspection of instruments is a critical factor affecting the operation, therefore, a person should be specially assigned to be in charge.

2.4.2 Sterilization Methods for Instruments of Hysteroscope

Hysteroscopic telescope and its accessories are a set of sophisticated and expensive optical devices, including cylindrical lens system, light-guide fiber, and lighting system. Sterilization methods recommended currently are as follows and can be chosen depending on the situation. Before sterilization, first open each stop-cock of the sheaths, coil up the light guide bundles, and inflow/outflow tubes. Cables and tubes cannot be folded and all channels should be kept open. All instruments should be put in a specialized sterilization box (Fig. 2.40).

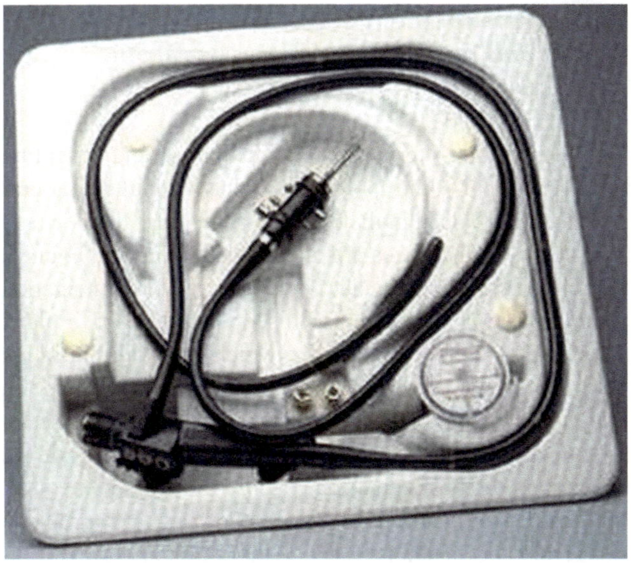

Fig. 2.40 Sterilization box for flexible hysteroscope

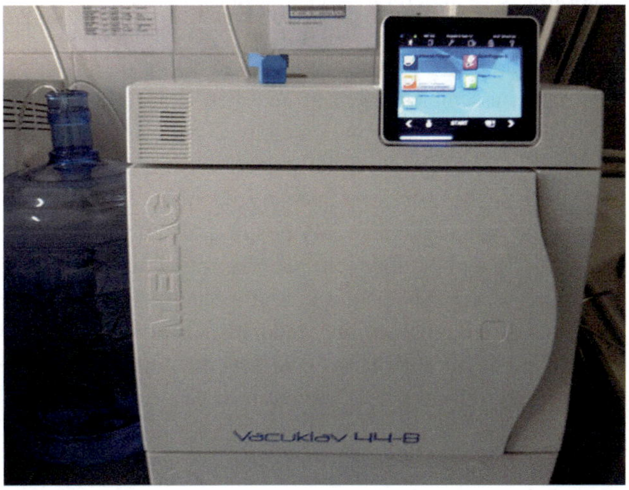

Fig. 2.41 Autoclave

2.4.2.1 Autoclave Sterilization

It is a preferred and the most reliable method for sterilization, and is recommended to use 2.3 bar (1 bar = 10^5 Pa = 101.325 kPa, 1 kPa = 7.5 mmHg), 134 °C, and 5 min for sterilization (Fig. 2.41).

2.4.2.2 Low Temperature Sterilization

1. Low temperature plasma sterilizers: Plasma is the forth fundamental states of matter in nature except for solid, liquid, and gas. It is generated by ionizing gas state of matter under a strong electric field. Hydrogen peroxide (H_2O_2) plasma, which is used as a media of sterilization, includes a variety of active species such as hydroxyl radical (HO), hydroperoxyl radical (HO_2), excited hydrogen peroxide (H_2O_2), active oxygen atoms (O), active hydrogen atom (H), etc. These active ions and abundant ultraviolet (UV) radiation have a high thermal kinetic energy, so that it can greatly increase the effectiveness on microprotein and nucleic acids, and kills the microorganisms in a very short time so as to achieve the aim of sterilization for instruments.

   Low temperature hydrogen peroxide plasma sterilization system is based on the above intrinsic properties of plasma. At low temperature (lower than 60 °C) and vacuum state, a regular plasma field is created in the sterilization chamber under the influence of high-frequent electrical field. During this procedure, abundant UV radiation is generated, which can directly damage the genetic materials of microorganisms. Photolysis of UV radiation breakdowns the chemical bonds of microbe-molecules, and finally generates volatile compound. Through the effect of plasma etching, free radicals within the plasma field are capable of interacting with nitrogen/hydrogen and nucleic acid of microorganisms, which may inactivate the microorganisms and disrupt the metabolism of microorganisms.

   No toxic product remains after the use of hydrogen peroxide, eliminating the need for ventilation and drainage. Nowadays, it is a widely used low temperature sterilization method (Fig. 2.42).
2. Ethylene Oxide (EtO) sterilizer: The mechanism of EtO killing varies microorganisms is alkylation reaction, which can alkylate free radicals of protein including carboxyl (-COOH), amino ($-NH_Z$), sulfhydryl, and hydroxyl, leading to disruption of normal biochemical reaction and metabolism of protein, resulting in the death of microorganisms. Ethylene glycol (EG), a secondary product of EtO after hydrolyzing, can also be used as a sterilizing agent. However, the shortcomings of EO are that it needs

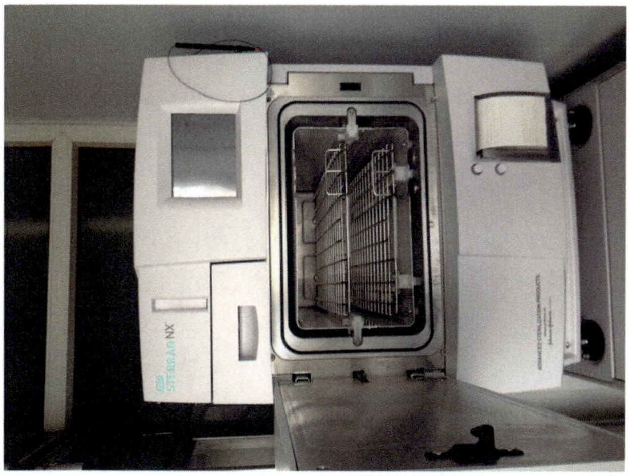

Fig. 2.42 Plasma sterilizer

a long sterilizing time and is harmful to environment and human bodies (Fig. 2.43).

3. STERIS low temperature rapid sterilizer: It uses peracetic acid as sterilizing agent to damage the microorganisms by changing the pH value or killing them by high oxidation. There are no toxic residuals on instruments after sterilization, and the second-product is not harmful to humans, but has corrosive and bleaching effect.

   To use STERIS, the instruments should be rinsed by sterilant repeatedly for 30 min with the sterilization temperature at 45 °C (Fig. 2.44a, b).

Light guide bundles, adaptors, and accessories can be disinfected by scrubbing their surfaces with a piece of 75% alcohol-dampened gauze, or dressed in a sterile disposable plastic suit to isolate for sterilization purposes, but the contact area should still be scrubbed with alcohol.

The video camera head can be sterilized through scrubbing with alcohol or dressing in a sterile disposable plastic set.

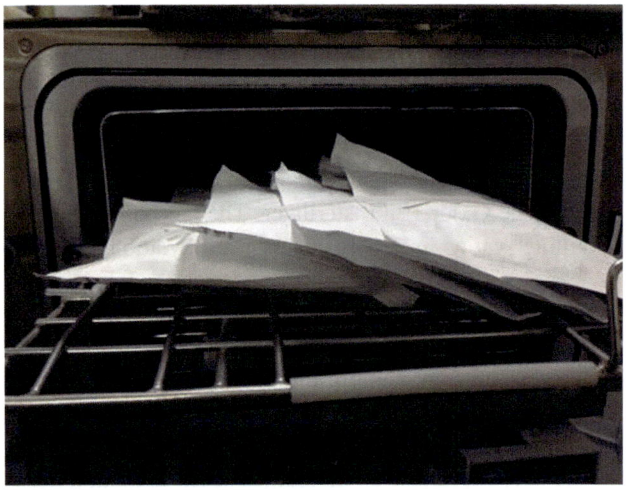

Fig. 2.43 Ethylene Oxide (EtO) sterilizer

2.4.3 Arrangement of Device and Instruments for Hysteroscopic Surgery

Video monitors, uterine distending pump, and irrigating medium are put in the appropriate place, with ultrasonography machine placed in the opposite side. After the power is switched on, all devices are at "ready" state. Then connect them with the camera head, power cable, uterine irrigation tubing, electric cable for resectoscope, and negative plate. Put in the distention medium, of which 0.9% normal saline and mannitol are often used. At the first time of using the telescope, white balance should be adjusted after the scope is connected with camera to ensure that the clarity of the scope is in the best condition. Record patients' name, age, medical history, and operation name with a specialized image-text workstation. When using a monopolar resectoscope, switch on the electric generator after a negative plate being well placed and then set the power at 80 W for resection and 60 W for coagulation. When using a bipolar, the generator is switched on and set at plasma mode.

Sterilized instruments, such as telescope, cutting loop, roller ball, working elements and obturator, are placed on the instrument table, assembled together, and then connected with the video camera and optical cable carefully. Use the sterilized gauze to wipe the telescope from the object lens to eyepiece. Then place them on the instrument table in order of use (Fig. 2.45).

Lay the patient in lithotomy position, disinfect her vulva with 0.5% iodophor, and then spread aseptic towels over legs and hips. When the operation begins, pay attention to the supply of distending medium, and make sure there is no stop of flow and no air embolism occurs. At the same time record the amounts of fluid inflow and outflow. When the amount of inflow exceeds far too much the amount of outflow, the surgeon should be alerted that TURP syndrome might occur (Figs. 2.46, 2.47 and 2.48).

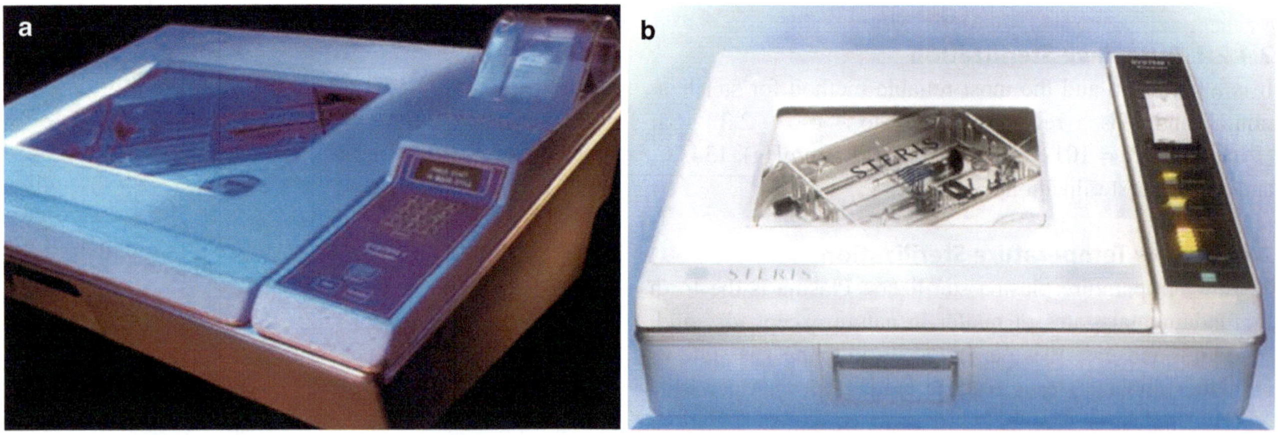

Fig. 2.44 (**a**, **b**) Low temperature rapid sterilizer for Endoscope

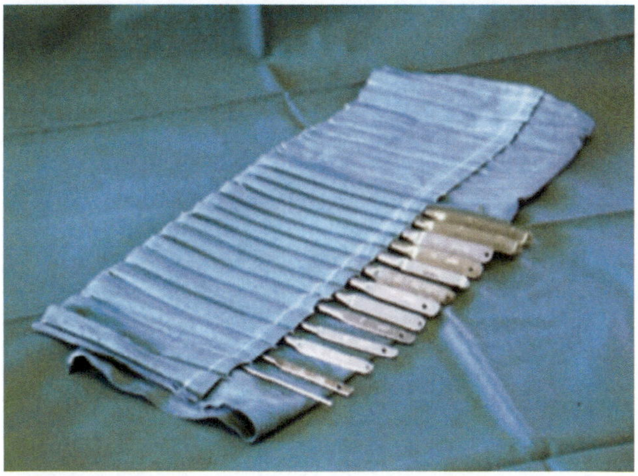

Fig. 2.45 Whole set of cervix-dilator (No. 4–12)

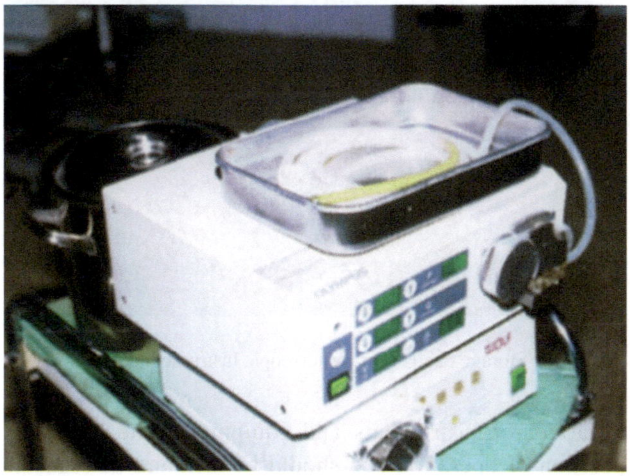

Fig. 2.46 Sterilized irrigation tubing

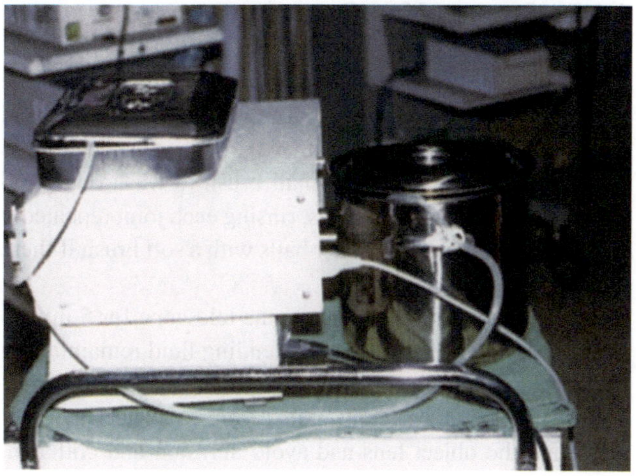

Fig. 2.47 Connection of distention medium with irrigation tubing

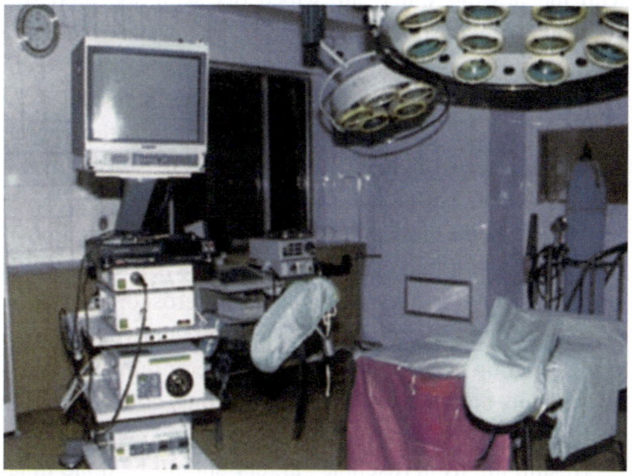

Fig. 2.48 Layout of hysteroscopic devices

2.4.4 Maintenance of Hysteroscopic Equipment

As there are various kinds of hysteroscopes, the common features will be generalized in this section so as to enable the user to master principles of maintenance.

2.4.4.1 Optical Lens

There are lots of optical products in the hysteroscopic operative system, such as endoscopic lens, camera system, and condenser and filter built in cold light source, etc. It is absolutely forbidden to touch or wipe the surface of these products with fingers, but one should use absorbent cotton dipped in alcohol and ether mixture to scrub gently, and avoid using rigid cloth to wipe so as to prevent scratching and injuring lens.

2.4.4.2 Electronic Equipment

The electronic equipment in endoscopic operational system includes cold light source, video camera system, uterine distending pump, and high-frequency electric generator, etc. Because the performance and purposes of different equipment varies, so its maintenance must be done in accordance with the requirements listed in the instructions, and only the common features of these equipment are singled out for description.

1. The power supply used must be consistent with power 220 V and 50 Hz specified in the instructions, and grounding power socket must be reliable.
2. Hysteroresectoscope belongs to high frequency electrical appliances, should be checked regularly each year, and its performance, electrode plates, and foot switch must be monitored and checked by professionals to see whether they are normal or not.
3. It is forbidden to move an equipment when it is on operation or run an instrument when its sheath is broken.
4. The total power supply must be turned off when equipment are not in use.

2.4.5 Storage After Operation

After use, all instruments are immediately immersed in the enzymatic solution for 30 min to dissolve blood clots and residual tissues adhering to them. All blood and stains should be cleaned, such as using a small brush to wash out blood clots from the interior channels, rinsing each joint repeatedly with syringes, scrubbing roller balls with a soft brush if there are charring tissues.

Use the flowing water to rinse the telescope for 5 min so as to wash out completely the distending fluid remaining on the telescope and flush out any residues and blood stains. Then wipe dry it with gauze. Take care to protect the eyepiece and the object lens and avoid abrasion and collision. The lens on eyepiece should be scrubbed with 70% alcohol swab, thus preventing the damage to its surface.

The hysteroscope and instruments, after being cleaned with the flowing water, are wiped dry with specified soft cloth, with their surface blown dry. The water remaining inside the channels and stop-cocks is blown dry as well. Then place them in boxes separately. The telescope needs to be placed into the scope case and kept in the box, then stored and kept in the equipment cabinet by the person in charge (Figs. 2.49 and 2.50).

Any patient with hepatitis B virus surface antigen positive should be arranged to be the last one in whole day's operations. After the operation, hysteroscope and its instruments are immersed in 2% glutaraldehyde for 1 h, then stored up according to the above requirements. Other instruments and dressings are sterilized as anti-O-positive routine.

To sum up, hysteroscopic surgery should be done in an operation room specialized for endoscopic surgery. Operation room should be relatively large to accommodate a variety of instruments and equipment. The lithotomy position of operation bed should be firm and be ready to adjust various angles. The nurses who assist in performing hysteroscopic operation must have specialized training and strong responsibility. Not only should they have cooperation experiences in a routine operation, but also they should command a comprehensive grasp of the use, sterilization and maintenance of hysteroscopic instruments. Only when they have a loving heart for patients and a highly responsible spirit, could they complete the cooperative work very well in hysteroscopic operation.

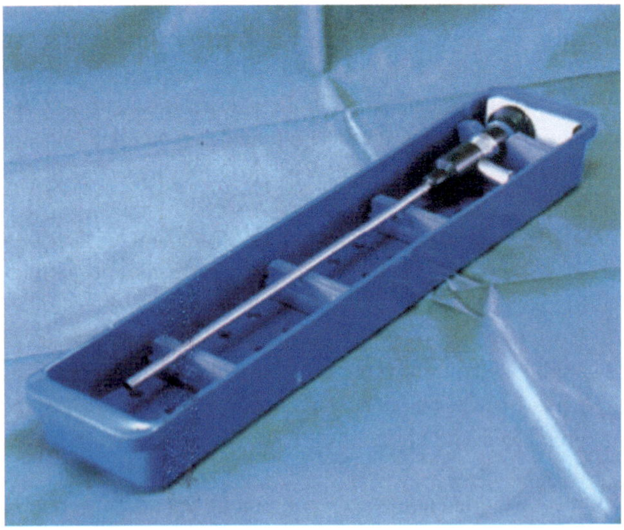

Fig. 2.49 Storage box for hysterscope

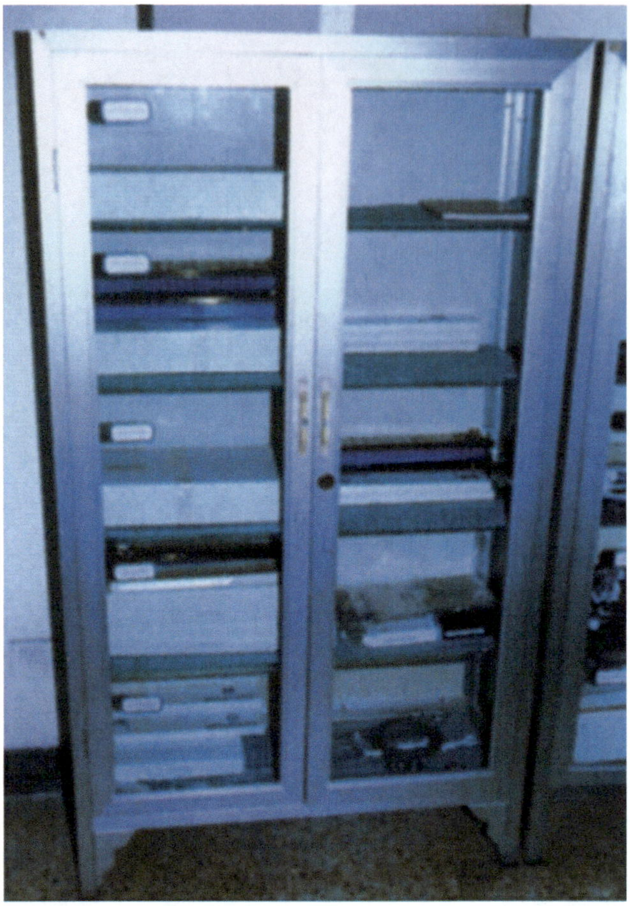

Fig. 2.50 Storage cabinet for hysterscopic instruments

Suggested Reading

Equipment for Hysteroscopy

1. Baggish MS. Establishment of a hysteroscopy program. In: Baggish MS, Barbot J, Valle RF, editors. Diagnostic and operative hysteroscopy. 2nd ed. St Louis: Mosby; 1999. p. 367–90.
2. Peng Y. Medical endoscope image transverse striation elimination algorithm simulation. Comput Simul. 2013;30:417–20. Chinese.
3. Xia EL. Latest development of hysteroscopy. Chin J Pract Gynecol Obstetr. 2000;16:180–2. Chinese.

Instruments for Hysteroscopic Diagnosis and Treatment

4. Lin BL, Miyamoto N, Tomomatsu M. Development and clinical application of flexible hysteroscope. Jpn J Gynecol Obstet. 1987;39:649–54. Japanese.
5. Lin BL, Miyamoto N, Tomomatsu M. Development of the scope of new resectoscope for women—application of transcervical resection and endometrial ablation (EA). J Jpn Assoc Endosc Maternity. 1988;4:56–61. Japanese.
6. Lin BL, Tomomatsu M, Su L. Development and clinical application of new hystero-fiberscope. Jpn J Gynecol Obstet. 1988;40:1733–9. Japanese.
7. Lin BL, Ishikawa H, Komiyama M. Development of flexible outer sleeve for hystero-fiberscope. Japan J Gynecol Obstet Endosc. 1997;13:169–72. Japanese.
8. Lin BL, Iida M, Yabuno A, Higuchi TY, Murakoshi Y, Iwata SK, Zhao Y. Removal of Endometrial polyps through a small caliber diagnostic flexible hysterosocpe using a Lin polyp snare system. Gynecol Minim Invasive Ther. 2013;2:18–21.
9. Lin BL, Iwata Y, Valle RF. Clinical applications of Lin's forceps in flexible hysteroscopy. J Am Assoc Gynecol Laparosc. 1994;1(4 Pt 1):383–7.
10. Murman RJ, Norris HJ. Endometrial carcinoma. In: Blaustein's pathology of the female genital tract. 3rd ed. New York: Springer-Verlag; 1987. p. 338–9.
11. Tanizawa O, Miyake A, Sugiki O. Revaluations on diagnostic hysteroscopy prior to operation of endometrial carcinoma. Jpn J Gynecol Obstet. 1991;43:622–6.

Instruments for Hysteroscopic Surgery

12. Glasser MH. Endometrial ablation and hysteroscopic myomectomy by electrosurgical vaporization. J Am Assoc Gynecol Laparosc. 1997;4:369–74.
13. Magos AL, Baumann R, Turnbull AC. Transcervical resection of the endometrium in women with menorrhagia. Br Med J. 1989;298:1209–12.
14. Pantaleoni D. On endoscopic examination of the cavity of the womb. Med Press Cir. 1869;8:26–7.
15. Xia EL. Latest development of hysterscopy. Chin J Pract Gynecol Obstetr. 2000;16:180–2. Chinese.

Cleaning, Sterilization, and Maintenance of Hysteroscopic Instruments

16. Laurey D, Luke J, Mayette B. Care and maintenance of hysteroscopes and nursing procedures. In: Baggish MS, Barbot J, Valle RF, editors. Diagnostic and operative hysteroscopy. 2nd ed. St. Louis: Mosby; 1999. p. 147–54.
17. Ma W, He JF, Shen W, Wang X. Experimental observation on sterilization effect of a desktop ethylene oxide sterilizer on medical instruments. Chin J Disinfect. 2013;30(1):25–6. Chinese.
18. Winer W. Role of the operating room nurse. In: Sutton C, Diamond MP, editors. Endoscopic surgery for gynecologists. 2nd ed. London: WB Saunders; 1998. p. 38–40.

3 Anatomy and Histology in Hysteroscopy

Enlan Xia

3.1 Anatomy of a Normal Uterus

The uterus is a hollow organ, inverted pear-shaped, and located in the center of the pelvis. It is made up of three parts, the fundus, the corpus, and the cervix. The narrow portion between the corpus and the cervix is called isthmus, and its upper portion is internal orifice of the uterus, that is, anatomical internal os; the lower portion is histological internal os, which marks the transition from the endometrium to the endocervix. The size and shape of the uterus may vary with age and fertility. The uterus of normal non-childbearing women measures 7–8 cm in length, 4–5 cm in width, and 2–3 cm in thickness. The volume of uterus increases in women after parturition. The proportion of the uterus to the cervix changes with age. At adolescence, the corpus is as long as the cervix; in women of child-bearing age, the length of the corpus is about twice that of the cervix; in postmenopausal women, the corpus and the cervix are equal in length.

3.1.1 Uterine Corpus

The upper portion of uterus is broader, which is known as the uterine body or corpus. The dome-shaped upper portion is called fundus, the middle space is called the uterine cavity, which is shaped in an inverted triangle with upper part broad and lower part narrow. The structure of uterine wall is composed of three layers.

3.1.1.1 Endometrium

Endometrium lines the uterine cavity and is influenced by ovarian hormones from adolescence to menopause. It presents slightly differently with the changes of menstruation cycle in its color, thickness, and crease, and is related to the degree of uterine expansion. Its color may be pale white, brown yellow, light pink, peach-pink, or dark red. Sometimes it is accompanied by small petechiae. Its thickness may grow to 5–6 mm at late secretory phase. The upper 2/3 of endometrium is the functional layer, which is shed and passed out of the body during menstruation. Inferior 1/3 adjacent to the myometrium is the basal layer, in which there is no periodic shedding and a new endometrial lining from it grows after the menstruation.

3.1.1.2 Myometrium

It is the thickest layer of the uterine wall, approximately 10–15 mm in thickness. It consists of bundles of smooth muscle fibers and a few intermixed connective tissues, which contain undifferentiated interstitial cells, macrophages, fibroblasts, and mast cells. The muscular layers are four in number.

1. Submucosal layer: It is a thinner layer, located under the mucous membrane, mostly composed of the longitudinal muscle fibers and intermixed with a small amount of circular and oblique muscle fibers. Conspicuous circular muscle fibers develop at the uterine cornua of fallopian tube.
2. Vascular layer: It is located 5–6 mm beneath the mucous membrane and mostly composed of circular muscular fibers with fewer oblique muscle fibers, through which there are plenty of blood vessels, called vascular layer.
3. Subvascular layer: It is located underneath the vascular layer with the muscle fibers disposed longitudinally and transversely.
4. Subserosal layer: It is located beneath the serosa and composed of longitudinal muscle fibers.

3.1.1.3 Serosa

It is also known as perimetrium, which covers the corpus and fundus of the uterus. The outer layer of the rest of the uterus is fiber membranes.

E. Xia (✉)
Hysteroscopy Center, Fuxing Hospital, Capital Medical University, Beijing, China

E. Xia (ed.), *Practical Manual of Hysteroscopy*, https://doi.org/10.1007/978-981-19-1332-7_3

3.1.1.4 Uterine Horn and Ostium of Fallopian Tube

At either side of the uterine fundus there is a uterine horn, connected to each of the fallopian tubes, where the muscular wall is thinner, only 5–6 mm. The cornu is deep and funnel-shaped when not expanded. When fully expanded, tubal ostium is visible at its top end, but it is not necessarily at the medial top end, sometimes slightly lateral. Most ostia appear to be round, oval, crescent-shaped, even astral. When uterus does not expand fully, it appears to be a brown hole, and contraction of fallopian tube can be observed occasionally.

3.1.2 Uterine Cervix

The lower portion of the uterus is narrow and cylindrical in shape, called cervix. Its upper portion is the internal os of cervix, which is round or oval in contour, and the edge of which is neat or mildly irregular. The cervix varies in length and width from person to person, and the proportion of the uterine body to the cervix of an adult is 2:1.

3.2 Cyclical Changes in Endometrium

3.2.1 The Menstruation Phase

It refers to the first to the fifth day of the menstruation cycle, during which the endometrium is fragmented, and endometrial gland shrinks and is hydrolyzed. Disintegrated endometrium can be seen under hysteroscope, as well as the glandular regeneration.

3.2.2 Early Proliferative Phase

It refers to the sixth to the seventh day of the menstruation cycle. During this period, the endometrium is thinner, only about 1 to 2 mm; its glands are sparse and dispersed and the lumina are also small. The epithelial cells present low columnar shape with cell nuclei oval-shaped. The stroma is loose with less cytoplasm. This period is the optimal time for hysteroscopy and surgery.

3.2.3 Late Proliferative Phase

It refers to the eighth to the 14th day of the menstruation cycle. The thickness of endometrium becomes 3–4 mm; the glands increases and are curved; the shape of the epithelial cell is tall columnar; and the cell nuclei are long oval and lie in the cell center. The endometrium presents pseudostratified structure without secretion, with stromal proliferation. Sometimes small spiral arteries may be seen.

3.2.4 Early Secretory Phase

It refers to the 16th to the 19th day of the menstruation cycle. At this phase, the endometrium gets thickened to 5–6 mm, and the glands proliferate and dilate further with indented appearance. The glandular epithelia change to simple short columnar cells, and the presence of vacuoles below the nuclei is characterized.

3.2.5 Late Secretory Phase

It refers to the 20th to the 28th day of the menstruation cycle. During this period, the endometrium becomes reddish or pink, and edematous. Exuberant glandular secretion can be observed by microscopic examination, and there is secretion within the glandular lumina, with the upper epithelium incomplete, stroma edematous, and interstitial cells change to decidual-like cells.

4 Effects of Preoperative Medication for Hysteroscopy and Commonly Used Drugs in Gynecology on Endometrium

Xiaowu Huang

4.1 Preoperative Medication for Hysteroscopy

During hysteroscopic surgery, particularly when the uterus is distended with distention medium, the endometrial shedding fragments are prone to block the sieve holes of hysteroscopic outer sheath, which may cause the blockage of return flow. Together with intraoperative bleeding, the operation view is hindered, which is not helpful for the operation to run smoothly. The preoperative administration of drugs can make endometrium thinner, and endometrial blood vessels decreased, thus achieve a good vision that facilitates the operation and shortens the operation time. Pretreatment with drugs was originally used for hysteroscopic endometrial ablation. In 2014, the French clinical guidelines indicated that, pretreatment with drugs may achieve a good vision, but cannot decrease the occurrence of complications, therefore it should not be considered as a routine use.

At present, pretreatment with drugs is mainly used for women who have submucous fibroids and menorrhagia. Pretreatment with drugs may induce amenorrhea, which is beneficial for the correction of anemia. In addition, some drugs may decrease the volumes of the uterus and fibroids, as well as shorten the operation time.

Commonly used drugs for pretreatment and their mechanisms are elaborated below.

4.1.1 Mechanism of Pretreatment with Drugs Prior to Surgery

Clinically, the basis for pretreatment of endometrium with drugs is nearly the same as the treatment of endometriosis, including pseudo-pregnancy therapy, pseudo-menopause therapy, and medical oophorectomy.

X. Huang (✉)
Hysteroscopy Center, Fuxing Hospital, Capital Medical University, Beijing, China

4.1.1.1 Pseudo-Pregnancy Therapy

In 1953, Meigs first found that, during pregnancy, decidualization might appear in the endometrial tissues outside the uterus, followed by liquefaction, necrosis, and absorption. In 1956, Kistner began to apply synthetic progesterone in combination with estrogen to elevate the hormone levels of serum to a state similar to pregnancy, called the pseudo-pregnant therapy, and first reported its clinical effects in 1958.

The administration of low dose progesterone does not inhibit ovulation and the endometrium retains thickening; and that of high-dose progesterone could cause most women's endometrium to atrophy, but occasionally irregular bleeding. Progesterone is tolerable for most women. Clinically, the commonly used synthetic progesterone is divided into two categories according to its basic structure.

1. Testosterone derivatives: Norethisterone is commonly taken orally with 5 mg, twice a day. It is clinically used for the treatment of dysfunctional uterine bleeding. The endometrium always manifests endometrial thickening, yellow color, flocculent, and sometimes wave-like under hysteroscope. The manifestations of endometrial histology are highly secretory, and even stromal decidualization. This medication is rarely used in pretreatment.
2. Progesterone derivatives: Medroxyprogesterone acetate is often used orally with 30–50 mg, once a day. Its possible mechanism is to inhibit ovulation, which suppresses the growth of endometrium and has a continuous but immature secretory response. If used for a long term, the secretory phenomenon can be less obvious, the endometrium is atrophied, the gland is reduced and sometimes disappears, and the stromal cells are fusiform. In addition, progesterone has some anti-estrogen effects by stimulating the activity of 17β-hydroxysteroid dehydrogenase and sulfotransferase resulting in turning estradiol into estrone sulfate, which may be discharged quickly out of

E. Xia (ed.), *Practical Manual of Hysteroscopy*, https://doi.org/10.1007/978-981-19-1332-7_4

the cell. Through the inhibition of estrogen receptor, progesterone can also reduce the biological effect of estrogen on target cells, thereby inhibiting the growth of endometrium. Its adverse effects are menstrual abnormalities, headache, abdominal discomfort, mental stress, and loss of libido, etc.

3. Oral contraceptives: It is clinically used for adjusting and reducing menstrual blood loss, which was reduced to 40% of that before medication from clinical report. Take the estrogen-progesterone components, short-acting oral contraceptives as example, its progesterone may resist estrogen continuously. By hysteroscopy the endometrium appears to be thinner, smooth, red-pink, or red-yellow. Although their endometrial thickness is thinner than that in ovulatory women, most patients' estrogen stimulation could not be completely suppressed, the endometrium still affects the hysteroscopic view, and the basal layer is difficult to be destroyed during operation. Its continuous use can cause decidualization and amenorrhea, resulting in pseudo-pregnancy. Because the individuals respond to this medication is different, its application as a preoperative medication is restricted. However, the administration of estrogen-dominant long-acting contraceptives may cause endometrium to appear to be proliferation or hyperplasia. By hysteroscopy, the endometrium appears to be thickened or with uneven thickness, and polypoid hyperplasia, wave-like, red-pink or red-yellow in color are visible. This medication is not usually used as pretreatment.

There were also some clinical reports on successful endometrial pretreatment with oral contraceptives prior to hysteroscopic surgeries. Grow et al. reported that from the early follicular phase, the patient took oral contraceptives with 150 μg of desogestrel combined with 30 μg of ethinyl estradiol for 18–20 days. The thickness of endometrium achieved 4.1 ± 1.6 mm after pretreatment by ultrasonography monitoring, so they could be used for endometrial pretreatment before hysteroscopic surgery. In recent years, Cicinelli et al. carried out some studies to evaluate the effect of pretreatment. From the first day of menstruation cycle, desogestrel was given orally combined with raloxifene vaginally 60 mg for 10 days. In another group, oral danazol was taken 200 mg, 3/day for 10 days. On the 11th day of the cycle, endometrial thickness was measured by ultrasonography. The results showed that the application of desogestrel combined with raloxifene was better than that of danazol group, and it is a fast, cheap, and satisfactory pretreatment prior to hysteroscopic surgeries.

Raloxifene is a selective estrogen receptor modulator, and its known therapeutic role is to exert estrogen-like effects on the bone and cardiovascular system, increase bone density and inhibit bone loss, but it may have an anti-estrogenic effect in breast and uterine tissues. Desogestrel is the third generation of new contraceptive drugs and is likely to replace norgestrel currently used.

4.1.1.2 Pseudo-Menopause Therapy

Danazol is a synthesized derivative of 17alpha ethynyl testosterone, and its chemical name is (17α)-Pregna-2,4-dien-20-yno[2,3-d]isoxazol-17-ol. It can block the synthesis and release of GnRH, FSH, and LH, and directly inhibits the synthesis of ovarian steroid hormone. And it may also be combined with the sex hormone receptors of target organs, thus causing the endometrium to atrophy, and resulting in temporary amenorrhea. That's why people call the treatment with danazol the pseudo-menopause therapy.

Danazol cannot only inhibit the synthesis and release of GnRH, FSH, and LH, suppress the activity of cholesterol cleavage enzyme and 3β-hydroxysteroid dehydrogenase, but also depress the conversion of estrone sulfate (E1S) to estradiol (E2), which forms a low estrogen environment, and thus prevents the growth of endometrium. Studies have shown that it can also inhibit the endometrial growth directly. Application of danazol 200 mg, twice a day for 3 months can transform the endometrial hyperplasia into atrophic or proliferative endometrium. Read and Sharp reported that after the application of danazol 200 mg, 3 times a day for 6 weeks, the average endometrial thickness reduced to 1.2 mm; while in the untreated group, the average endometrial thickness is 3 mm at the proliferative phase, 7 mm at the secretory phase. Under hysteroscope, the endometrium appears to be atrophic or mildly hyperplasia, similar to menopausal atrophic endometrium, being white or pink, and bilateral tubal ostia are often visible.

Taking danazol for a long time may affect the liver function, and taking danazol for 2 to 4 weeks will increase serum glutamic pyruvic transaminase (SGPT) level. Generally, SGPT level may decrease rapidly after stopping taking danazol, and return to normal 2–4 weeks later. Commonly, there are no abnormal changes in bilirubin and acid phosphatase. In addition, during the medication, one may have adverse reactions like increased sebum, voice coarsening, hairiness, breast enlargement or reduction, hot flashes, and excessive sweating. In a comparison study, danazol was given vaginally 400 mg/day. In another group, danazol was given orally 600 mg/day. The medication was taken for 30 days in both groups. The results showed that the thickness of endometrium in vaginal group was thinner than that in oral group, with adverse effects less in vaginal group.

4.1.1.3 Medical Oophorectomy

GnRH-analogs (GnRH-a) are similar to GnRH in structure, can compete for the pituitary GnRH receptors. When the pituitary GnRH receptors are all occupied and drained by GnRH-a, it may have a descending regulatory effect on the pituitary, namely, the pituitary secretion of gonadotropins decreases, thus the sex hormone levels secreted by the ovaries decline significantly, the effect of which is similar to surgical resection of the ovaries, called medical oophorectomy. Commonly used drugs are leuprorelin acetate (trade name: Enantone), buserelin, nafarelin, goserelin, and triprelin.

Only at the early period of the first administration, the GnRH-a can transiently promote the secretions of FSH, LH, and estrogen. Thereafter, due to the decline of the reactivity of pituitary and ovary, the secretions of FSH, LH, and estrogen are inhibited. Take goserelin as an example. After administration of sustained-release goserelin with the dose of 3.6 mg for once, the levels of FSH and LH can decline below the basal values within 14 days and continue to be suppressed in the following 5 or more weeks. In healthy women and patients with benign gynecologic diseases, the estrogen levels can be reduced approximately to the level in menopausal women or women after gonadectomy. The first injection of goserelin 3.6 mg is commonly given at the late luteal phase and the second injection 4 weeks later. The operation is to be done at the fifth to the sixth week. At the fourth to the fifth week, the estrogen levels are low enough to make the endometrial thinning similar to that in menopause women, with the uterine volume reduced and the total endometrial area decreased. Under hysteroscope, the endometrium appears as that of menopausal women.

After comparing danazol with goserelin for preoperative medication prior to hysteroscopic surgeries, some scholars found that the pretreatment with goserelin had better endometrial thinning, less bleeding, less absorption of distention medium, and was better than that with danazol. There was no difference in uterine dilation time between two groups prior to operations. Another study showed that through fixing and slicing endometrial biopsy specimens, and marking endometrial vascular epithelial cells with anti-CD34 antibody, there was no significant difference in microvascular density between the natural menopause endometrial atrophy and endometrial atrophy induced by danazol and goserelin.

As for the cases with intrauterine fibroids over 5 cm, intramural fibroids or secondary anemia, GnRH-a may be applied to reduce the size of fibroids, decrease the blood supply, control bleeding, and improve the anemia (see Fig. 9.52, Sect. 9.3, Chap. 9), so as to help the anemic patients with prolonged bleeding to increase their hemoglobin level. It was reported that after medication, the volume of the uterus could be reduced by 30% to 50% and that of the fibroid could be reduced by 10% to 60%. It cannot only lessen the difficulty in surgery, but also reduce the intraoperative bleeding, both of which are beneficial to the operation running smoothly and operation time shortening. Therefore, the occurrences of the TURP syndromes are reduced and more patients may have the opportunity of treating uterine fibroids by the hysteroscopic operation. The duration of drug administration is usually 3–6 months.

Campo et al. found that, for submucous myoma patients, the pretreatment with GnRH-a did not improve postoperative short-term or long-term effects except those with severe anemia. After pretreatment, the uterus was contracted and the cervix was narrowed, which caused difficulties in dilating the cervix. The operation time was significantly longer than that of the untreated group. Clinical practices proved that this shortcoming could be overcome by placing laminaria tent into cervix to soften it prior to operation. Most scholars believed that GnRH-a could facilitate the removal of larger fibroids by hysteroscopic surgery. Even so, at present the high prices of GnRH-a have limited its widespread clinical applications.

The adverse effects of GnRH-a are due to its low estrogenic properties, including hot flashes, vaginal dryness, headache, loss of libido, and so on. These symptoms can be relieved or disappear after stopping taking medicines. The bone losses of lumbar spine and proximal femur are also the side effects of GnRH-a, which are apparent when the drug is used for 3 months or more. A study showed that the related low estrogen symptoms could be lessened when the treatment was combined with the application of tibolone.

4.1.1.4 Other Anti-Estrogen, Anti-Progesterone, and Endometrial Growth-Inhibiting Drugs

Gestrinone, a 19-nor-testosterone derivative, has some properties, such as agonistic interaction with progesterone receptors, anti-progesterone, anti-estrogen, inhibition of FSH and LH secretion, suppression of ovulation, and atrophy of endometrium. It was first synthesized in 1965 by Roussel-UCLAF and was the earliest oral contraceptives. It is now mainly used for treatment of endometriosis.

Laboratory studies showed that gestrinone in a weekly dose of 10 mg could result in the suppression of ovulation and subsequent disturbance of the luteal phase formation. The histological characteristics of endometrium under the influence of gestrinone presented the features of secretory phase after ovulation. Its therapeutic effect was dependent on high affinity to estrogen and progesterone receptors. Mettler thought that gestrinone could not cause the ectopic endometrial lesions to disappear completely, but might lead to a pause of proliferative or secretory phase. Its ultrastructural characteristics showed intraepithelial lysosomal deformation with increases in its activities, numbers and sizes, which contained amorphous cell debris or lipid moieties. These presentations were similar to premenstrual liposomal degradation in the endometrium. Its usage was twice weekly in a dose of 2.5 mg for 4 to 6 weeks.

Gestrinone-induced side effects are less than that of danazol, with better tolerability. The main side effects are amenorrhea, breast reduction, and acne, which are all moderate. Its price is higher than that of danazol.

In recent years, ulipristal acetate, a selective progesterone receptor modulator, was reported to be used as pretreatment for hysteroscopic surgery. When comparing oral ulipristal acetate (5 mg or 10 mg) taken everyday for 3 months, with injection leuprorelin acetate (3.75 mg) taken monthly for three times, ulipristal acetate is not inferior to leuprorelin acetate in controlling uterine bleeding in women with fibroids and menorrhagia. For women receiving ulipristal acetate at a dose of 5 mg or 10 mg, the median times to amenorrhea are 5–7 days, the volumes of fibroids are reduced by 36%–42%, and the possibility of hot flashes is significantly decreased. For those receiving leuprorelin acetate, the median time to amenorrhea is 21 days and the volumes of fibroids are reduced by 53%.

Most scholars believed that the ideal depth of hysteroscopic endometrial resection involved the endometrium and 2.5–3 mm superficial muscular layer of the uterus. If the lesions were resected or ablated superficially, which cannot effectively destroy the functional layer of endometrium and blood supply underneath, recurrence would occur easily after operation. The most optimistic outcome after transcervical resection of endometrium is amenorrhea, but currently it can only be achieved in 50%–62% of the women after operations. When goserelin is applied prior to operation, the average endometrial thicknesses before and after treatment are 3.7 mm/1.9 mm, with the mean thickness ratio 2.7. For endometrial resection, Kriplani believed that the pretreatment with danazol was not necessary in improving the prognosis. Although the endometrial thickness after medication is not relevant to the success or failure of surgery, and thickened endometrium indicates its activity, currently the pretreatment prior to operation could not be abandoned. It is most apparent that the endometrial pretreatment is advantageous in choosing the size of cutting loop. The 26 Fr (8.67 mm) hystero-resectoscope is suitably fitted with 24 Fr (8 mm) cutting loop, and the cutting depth is nearly 4 mm. When the endometrial thickness is less than 1–2 mm, the basal layer can be completely resected once for all, therefore, each site of uterine cavity can be cut only once. So it is quick and easy to operate with a desired expectation. Others held that hysteroscopic surgeries should be performed at early proliferative phase when endometrium was the thinnest. However, this scheme is hard to put into practice for women with disordered menstruation, because there is no way to predict the state of the endometrium. After medication, the endometrium gets atrophied and thinner, and the absorption of distension fluid during hysteroscopic surgery are less than that without pretreatment, thus reducing the occurrence of the operative complication—TURP syndrome, which is a series of severe life-threatening systemic symptoms resulting from hypervolemia and hyponatremia caused by absorption of a great amount of uterine distension fluid into the blood circulation system. Another scholar stated that after pretreatment with GnRH-a, low estrogen state might enhance the activities of endometrium and cerebral Na^+ and K^+ –ATP enzyme, decrease the patients' susceptibility to hyponatremia, prevent the brain damage, reduce the levels of antidiuretic hormone, and prevent the excessive absorption of distention fluid, all of which formed the protective mechanism against hyponatremia.

Endometrial pretreatment with drugs have some potential problems, that is to say, if the diagnosis is determined, the operation should be done at a particular time after the medication; the patients also need to pay more for these expensive drugs; and all of them have side effects. While the endometrial pretreatment with the suction aspiration by negative pressure will neither be affected by menstruation cycle nor influenced by the time of operations, and can be done on those who are reluctant to accept drug therapy or with acute massive hemorrhage. Since there is no need for medication, the patients' economic burden is lightened, and the impact and the interference of the drugs on the endocrine system are avoided, so it is a fast, simple, effective, and safe method of endometrial pretreatment, which is applicable to a variety of hysteroscopic operation.

In 1997, Hugo et al. published a report about a proposal that the pretreatment with drugs should be unnecessary, but the mechanical pretreatment could get thin endometrium. In addition, it did not interfere with the operation view due to the increase in bleeding during operation, and also would not cause the increase in the absorption of distention medium. Moreover, the completion of uterine suction needed only 2 min or less, which could reduce the endometrial thickness and expose the basal layer quickly and effectively. Suction aspiration can cause the endometrium thinning, which could be confirmed by histological studies. Regardless of any period in the menstruation cycle, the suction aspiration can remove almost all the functional layer and reduce the function named "protection barrier" of thickened endometrium on the basal layer. However, some scholars insisted that preoperative uterine suction might lead to bleeding and incomplete uterine suction could affect surgery. For beginners, it is better to apply endometrial pretreatment with drugs.

4.2 Nolvadex

Nolvadex is styrene derivative, also known as tamoxifen (TMX). It competitively inhibits the endogenous estrogen by binding to the estrogen receptor of target cytoplasma, and the receptor complex entering into the nucleus, so the number of free estrogen receptors decreases. At the same time, the receptor complexes are binding to DNA to inhibit the synthesis of the estrogen receptor, thus decreasing the number of the receptors and having anti-estrogen effects. It is clinically applied to postmenopausal women who have metastatic estrogen receptor positive breast cancer as adjunctive therapy and palliative treatment.

Clinical and laboratorial study found that TMX had weak estrogenic effects on bone and endometrium. Its mechanism has not been fully elucidated and may be associated with continued low estrogen activity induced by the TMX/estrogen receptor complexes. TMX may stimulate endometrial proliferation in patients, and its role may differ with the change of the peripheral estradiol concentration. When the estradiol concentration is low, it shows a weak estrogen effect. As the estradiol concentration increases, the anti-estrogenic effect becomes more outstanding. And when the estradiol concentration reaches a certain level, its inhibitory effect is reversed, and it shows a stimulating effect on endometrial growth, causing endometrial hyperplasia, and even cancerization. In addition, the change of endometrial proliferation induced by TMX in postmenopausal patients with breast cancer may vary with time, long-term exposure to TMX can increase estrogenic effects and sensitivity of estrogen on TMX in the body itself.

It was reported that the occurrence rate of endometrial hyperplasia (thickness > 8 mm) after the postoperative application of TMX in postmenopausal women with breast cancer was 35.9% to 84%. Its histological characteristics were nearly the same as those in normal women with endometrial hyperplasia. While the occurrence rate in postmenopausal women who have breast cancer without medication and ordinary female population is only 0% to 10%. The occurrence rate of TXM induced endometrial polyp is 25% to 51%, and its incidence is higher than that of untreated patients [(8%–36%)/(0–10%)].

Another study was reported on applications of TXM in postmenopausal women who have breast cancer. Prior to medication, the endometrium was examined to exclude endometrial lesions. During 60 months of follow-up after taking TXM, the endometrium had pathological changes in 30.4% of patients, most of which were simple hyperplasia, and none of them was atypical hyperplasia. Therefore, it is suggested that for postmenopausal patients with breast cancer, endometrial assessment should be done by vaginal ultrasonography before the application of TMX. If the thickness of double layer endometrium is measured >4 mm, curettage or hysteroscopic biopsy under direct vision should be performed. If the lesion is found, corresponding treatment should be conducted, and close follow-up of drug usage should be implemented. The patients should be paid careful attention to any vaginal bleeding during medication; and also vaginal bleeding after the drug withdrawal.

Anastrozole and other aromatase inhibitors (AI) can also prevent the recurrence of breast cancer. Such drugs can play a role in affecting the synthesis of estrogen through the inhibition of key enzyme required in estrogen synthesis—aromatase. Garuti G applied aromatase inhibitors for treatment of breast cancer, and found that the occurrence rate of endometrial lesions was low, and it could reverse the endometrial thickening induced by TMX.

Under hysteroscopy, the endometrium of TXM induced endometrial hyperplasia appears as thickening and edema with unevenness, and polypoid hyperplasia visible, of which the surface is smooth, soft, and elastic with the gland ostia visible. Sometimes hemorrhagic and necrosis spots with different sizes can be seen. Endometrial polyps (Fig. 4.1a–c) is oval or ligulate, with its surface smooth, usually white, pink, or purple. Sometimes tiny dendritic blood vessels can be seen with the regular appearances. In patients having endometrial carcinoma, the endometrium manifests as fragile, being pale or yellow-dirtiness, with large and irregular blood vessels seen on its surface. Target biopsy should be done in these cases.

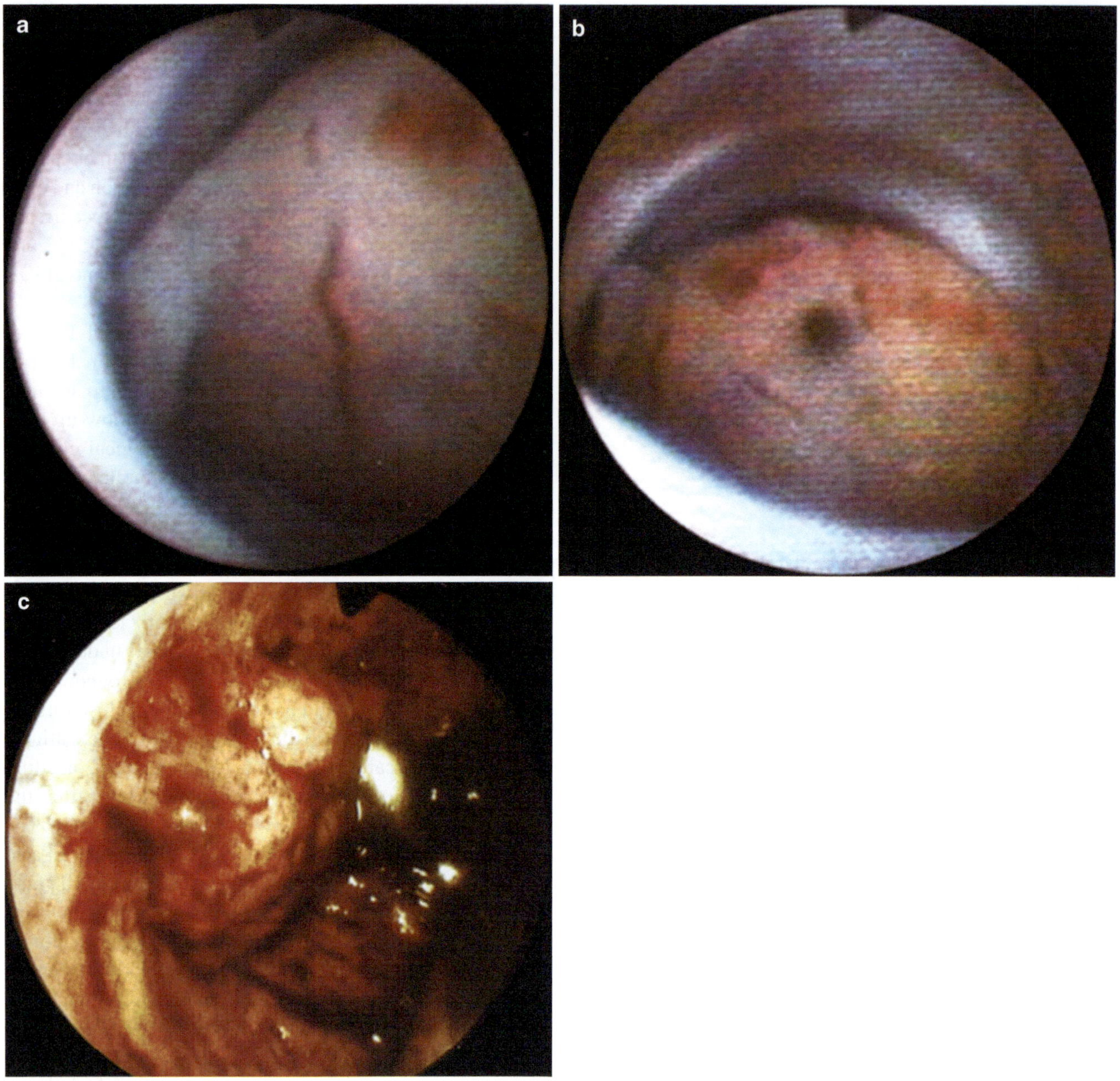

Fig. 4.1 (**a**–**c**) Endometrial polyps induced by TMX

4.3 Clomiphene

Clomiphene, also known as clomifene or Clomid, is chlorotrianisene derivatives and similar to tamoxifen in structure. It competes with estrogen for receptor, blocks the negative feedback effect of endogenous estrogen in the hypothalamus, which leads to increase of GnRH secretion, prompts the pituitary to secrete gonadotropins, thus starting or inducing the follicle growth. When follicle becomes mature, a sufficient amount of estrogen prompts a peak secretion of FSH and LH to stimulate ovulation through the positive feedback effect to hypothalamus. It is clinically used in women who have ovulatory dysfunction infertility. However, clinical observations found that ovulation rate was high after application of Clomiphene, but the pregnancy rate was lower, which might be associated with its other effects.

Regarding endometrium, Clomiphene may not only competitively bind to estrogen receptor within endometrial target cells to inhibit physiological effect of estrogen on the endometrium and cause the endometrial glandular dysplasia, it may also inhibit the induced synthesis of estrogen or progesterone receptors, affect normal reaction of endometrial glands to progesterone concentrations in circulating blood, thus decrease the gland secretory function and endometrial decidual reaction ability, and further influence the endometrial thickness.

Hysteroscopy should be done in ovulation and secretory phase, combining with ultrasonography, histological and immunohistochemical methods to comprehensively determine the influences of drugs on the endometrium, so as to guide proper clinical usage of drugs. Under hysteroscopy, the endometrium appears to have some nonspecific changes including unevenness, local edema, and inconspicuousness of gland ostia in secretory phase.

4.4 Levonorgestrel-Releasing Intrauterine System (LNG-IUS)

Levonorgestrel-releasing intrauterine system (LNG-IUS, trade name Mirena) is a new intrauterine contraceptive system which has been available since 1990s, and has been approved of application for contraception by more than 120 countries. LNG-IUS consists of a T-shaped intrauterine contraceptive, with the main body a T-shaped plastic frame (32 mm in length) and the vertical stem a steroid reservoir (50% in weight). The reservoir is 19 mm in length, contains a total of 52 mg Levonorgestrel (LNG) with polydimethylsiloxane covering the outer surface, and is a vital part to control the release of LNG. After the insertion of LNG-IUS into the uterine cavity, it provides an constant release rate of 20 μg/24 h of LNG, which results in very high concentrations in endometrium (470–1500 ng/mL). In contrast, the concentrations are 1.8–2.4 ng/mL in myometrium and 0.1–0.2 ng/mL in serum. The local concentration is over a thousand times higher than that in circulatory system. The high local LNG concentration suppresses the growth of endometrium, leading to atrophy of endometrial glands, and edema and decidualization of the stroma. LNG can inhibit the expression of an endometrial proliferation antigen Ki-67, causing cell apoptosis of endometrial glands and the stroma, the result is the thinning of endometrium under its long-term effects. After the placement of it for 1 year, under the light microscope, the number of endometrial glands is decreased, with its shape cubical or flat, the stroma decidualized and the blood vessels expanded.

LNG-IUS has little effect on the ovary, therefore the significant reduction of menses and amenorrhea are mainly due to direct inhibition of local LNG on the endometrium, rather than suppression of ovulation. Only when LNG intrauterine release is more than 50 μg/24 h, a complete suppression of ovulation can be achieved, which influences the ovary function. When 20 μg/24 h LNG is released, ovulation is maintained in 85% of women using the LNG-IUS. Because the LNG-IUS can release the LNG into uterine cavity during a long period, its clinical application has been developed from simple contraception into a variety of gynecological pathologies, such as menorrhagia, endometriosis and adenomyosis, endometrial hyperplasia and atypical hyperplasia, and endometrial protection, etc., with good effects.

To evaluate the efficacy of LNG-IUS compared with oral norethisterone acetate for treatment of simple and complex endometrial hyperplasia in perimenopausal women, a randomized controlled trial (RCT) was carried out and found that, after treatment for 12 months, the endometrial regression rate was 88.1% in the LNG-IUS group, and 55.7% in oral drugs group, with a significant difference achieved.

A prospective observational study was carried out on administration of GnRH-a and Mirena for 6 months in 14 young women who had early-stage endometrial cancer and wished to preserve their fertility, and discovered that endometrial regression was found in eight women, progression of the disease in four, and recurrence in two. Therefore, patients should be adequately counseled prior to conservational treatment, and have close follow-up during and after treatment. In hysteroscopic center of Fuxing hospital, Capital Medical University, for young women who have atypical endometrial hyperplasia and eager to have children, a partial endometrial ablation is performed just removing the functional layer of the endometrium and maintaining the basal layer. High-dose progesterone is given and a Mirena is placed in uterine cavity for adjuvant therapy post-operation. After endometrial regression, active fertility treatment is conducted (Fig. 4.2a–c).

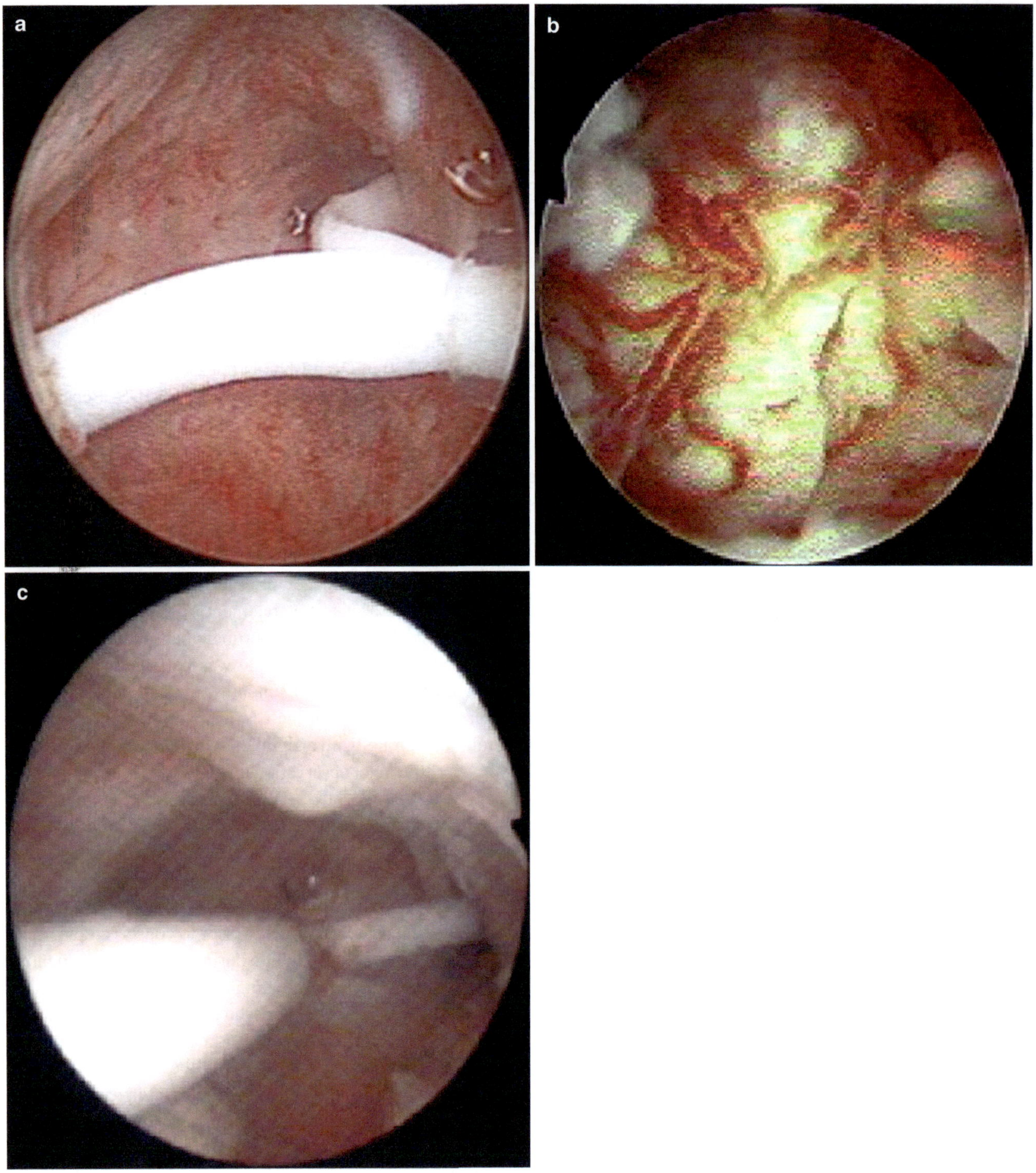

Fig. 4.2 (**a**) Hysteroscopic view after the placement of Mirena for 3 months in women with complex endometrial hyperplasia. Endometrial histology: endometrial glandular epithelium is flat and the stroma is decidualized. (**b**) Hysteroscopic view of complex atypical hyperplasia. (**c**) Hysteroscopic view of applying GnRH-a and Mirena for 3 months after partial endometrial ablation in women with complex endometrial hyperplasia. Endometrial histology: decidualization of the endometrial stroma

Suggested Reading

1. Abu Hashim H, Zayed A, Ghayaty E, El Rakhawy M. LNG-IUS treatment of non-atypical endometrial hyperplasia in perimenopausal women: a randomized controlled trial. Gynecol Oncol. 2013;24(2):128–34.
2. Bongers MY. Endometrial electrosurgical resection by hysteroscopy in 32 menorrhagic patients: endometrial preparation with a GnRH agonist may have some effect on results. J Gynecol Surg. 1995;11(2):65–70.
3. Brooks PG, Serden SP, Davos I. Hormonal inhibition of the endometrium for resectoscopic endometrial ablation. Am J Obstet Gynecol. 1991;164(6 Pt 1):1601–6.
4. Brun JL, de Chaballer F, Marmie S. Results and factors influencing the outcome of 203 transcervical endometrial resection. J Gynecol Surg. 1997;13:57–64.
5. Campo S, Campo V, Gambadauro P. Short-term and long-term results of resectoscopic myomectomy with and without pretreatment with GnRH analogs in premenopausal women. Acta Obstet Gynecol Scand. 2005;84(8):756–60.
6. Cicinelli E, Pinto V, Tinelli R, Saliani N, De Leo V, Cianci A. Rapid endometrial preparation for hysteroscopic surgery with oral desogestrel plus vaginal raloxifene: a prospective, randomized pilot study. Fertil Steril. 2007;88(3):698–701.
7. Colacurci N, de Franciscis P, Mollo A, Mele D, Fortunato N, Zarcone R. Preoperative GnRH analogue in hysteroscopic metroplasty. Panminerva Med. 1998;40(1):41–4.
8. Crosignani PG, Vercellini P, Meschìa M, Oldani S, Bramante T. GnRH agonists before surgery for uterine leiomyomas. A review. J Reprod Med. 1996;41(6):415–21.
9. De Falco M, Staibano S, D'Armiento FP, Mascolo M, Salvatore G, Busiello A, Carbone IF, Pollio F, Di Lieto A. Preoperative treatment of uterine leiomyomas: clinical findings and expression of transforming growth factor-beta3 and connective tissue growth factor. J Soc Gynecol Investig. 2006;13(4):297–303.
10. Deffieux X, Gauthier T, Menager N, Legendre G, Agostini A, Pierre F, French College of Gynaecologists and Obstetricians. Hysteroscopy: guidelines for clinical practice from the French College of Gynaecologists and Obstetricians. Eur J Obstet Gynecol Reprod Biol. 2014;178:114–22.
11. Dequesna JG. Use of GnRH agonist in hysteroscopic surgery. J Am Assoc Gynecol Laparosc. 1994;1:S10.
12. Dmowski WP. Endocrine properties and clinical application of danazol. Fertil Steril. 1979;31:237–51.
13. Donnez J, Gillerot S, Bourgonjon D, Clerckx F, Nisolle M. Neodymium: YAG laser hysteroscopy in large submucous fibroids. Fertil Steril. 1990;54(6):999–1003.
14. Donnez J, Nisolle M, Clerckx F, Casanas-Roux F, Saussoy P, Gillerot S. Advanced endoscopic techniques used in dysfunctional bleeding, fibroids and endometriosis, and the role of gonadotrophin-releasing hormone agonist treatment. Br J Obstet Gynaecol. 1994;101(Suppl 10):2–9.
15. Donnez J, Tomaszewski J, Vázquez F, Bouchard P, Lemieszczuk B, Baró F, Nouri K, Selvaggi L, Sodowski K, Bestel E, Terrill P, Osterloh I, Loumaye E, PEARL II Study Group. Ulipristal acetate versus leuprolide acetate for uterine fibroids. N Engl J Med. 2012;366(5):421–32.
16. Ducarme G, Davitian C, Zarrouk S, Uzan M, Poncelet C. Intérêt du gel d'acide hyaluronique dans la prévention des synéchies intra-utérines après hystéroscopie opératoire: étude cas-témoin [Interest of auto-cross-linked hyaluronic acid gel in the prevention of intrauterine adhesions after hysteroscopic surgery: a case-control study]. J Gynecol Obstet Biol Reprod (Paris). 2006;35(7): 691–5. French.
17. Erian J. Endometrial ablation in the treatment of menorrhagia. Br J Obstet Gynecol. 1994;101(supl 11):19–22.
18. Fedele L, Bianchi S, Gruft L, Bigatti G, Busacca M. Danazol versus a gonadotropin-releasing hormone agonist as preoperative preparation for hysteroscopic metroplasty. Fertil Steril. 1996;65(1):186–8.
19. Feng LM, Gao W, Zhang H, Xia EL. Hysteroscopic diagnosis and treatment of tamoxifen-induced endometrial lesions. J Pract Obstetr Gynecol. 2005;21(7):399–401. Chinese.
20. Filicor M, Flanigni C. GnRH agonists and antagonists. Current clinical status. Drugs. 1988;35:63–82.
21. Filicori M. Gonadotropin-releasing hormone agonists, a guide to use and selection. Drugs. 1994;48:241–58.
22. Florio P, Filippeschi M, Imperatore A, Mereu L, Franchini M, Calzolari S, Mencaglia L, Litta P. The practicability and surgeons' subjective experiences with vaginal danazol before an operative hysteroscopy. Steroids. 2012;77(5):528–33.
23. Fraser IS, Healy DL, Torode H, Song JY, Mamers P, Wilde F. Depot goserelin and danazol pre-treatment before rollerball endometrial ablation for menorrhagia. Obstet Gynecol. 1996;87(4): 544–50.
24. Garry R, Khair A, Mooney P, Stuart M. A comparison of goserelin and danazol as endometrial thinning agents prior to endometrial laser ablation. Br J Obstet Gynaecol. 1996;103(4):339–44.
25. Gimpelson RJ, Kaigh J. Mechanical preparation of the endometrium prior to endometrial ablation. J Reprod Med. 1992;37: 691–4.
26. Grow DR, Iromloo K. Oral contraceptives maintain a very thin endometrium before operative hysteroscopy. Fertil Steril. 2006;85(1):204–7.
27. Guan Z. Modern hysteroscopic diagnosis and therapeutics. Beijing: People's Military Medical Press; 2001. p. 130–7. Chinese.
28. Hickey M, Lau TM, Russell P, Fraser IS, Rogers PA. Microvascular density in conditions of endometrial atrophy. Hum Reprod. 1996;11(9):2009–13.
29. Nathanson HG, Phillips DR, Milim SJ, Haselkorn JS, Kapra A. Relationship of endometrial thickness with the menstrual timing of leuprolide acetate administration for preoperative preparation for hysteroscopic surgery. J Am Assoc Gynecol Laparosc. 1997;4(2):191–4.
30. Fraser IS. Added health benefits of the levonorgestrel contraceptive intrauterine system and other hormonal contraceptive delivery systems. Contraception. 2013;87(3):273–9.
31. Kesim MD, Aydin Y, Atis A, Mandiraci G. Long-term effects of the levonorgestrel-releasing intrauterine system on serum lipids and the endometrium in breast cancer patients taking tamoxifen. Climacteric. 2008;11(3):252–7.
32. Kodama M, Onoue M, Otsuka H, Yada-Hashimoto N, Saeki N, Kodama T, Wakasa T, Funato T. Efficacy of dienogest in thinning the endometrium before hysteroscopic surgery. J Minim Invasive Gynecol. 2013;20(6):790–5.
33. Kriplani A, Manchanda R, Nath J. A randomized trial of danazol pretreatment prior to endometrial resection. Eur J Obstet Gynecol Reprod Biol. 2002;103(1):68–71.
34. Lefler HT Jr, Sullivan GH, Hulka JF. Modified endometrial ablation: electrocoagulation with vasopressin and suction curettage preparation. Obstet Gynecol. 1991;77(6):949–53.
35. Lumsden MA, West CP, Thomas E, Coutts J, Hillier H, Thomas N, Baird DT. Treatment with the gonadotrophin releasing hormone-agonist goserelin before hysterectomy for uterine fibroids. Br J Obstet Gynaecol. 1994;101(5):438–42.
36. Maia H, Calmon LC, Margues D, Oliveira M, Coutinho E. Endometrial resection after vacumm curettages. Gynaecol Endosc. 1997;6:353–7.
37. Mettler L. Medicosurgical treatment of genital endometriosis focusing on gestagens and antigestagens together with surgical pelviscopy. Ann N Y Acad Sci. 1990;27:341–66.
38. Milton H, Goldrath. Use of danazol in hysteroscopic surgery for menorrhagia. J Reprod Med. 1990;35:91–6.

39. Minig L, Franchi D, Boveri S, Casadio C, Bocciolone L, Sideri M. Progestin intrauterine device and GnRH analogue for uterus-sparing treatment of endometrial precancers and well-differentiated early endometrial carcinoma in young women. Ann Oncol. 2011;22(3):643–9.
40. Muneyyirci-Delale O, Richard-Davis G, Morris T, Armstrong J. Goserelin acetate 10.8 mg plus iron versus iron monotherapy prior to surgery in premenopausal women with iron-deficiency anemia due to uterine leiomyomas: results from a phase III, randomized, multicenter, double-blind, controlled trial. Clin Ther. 2007;29(8):1682–91.
41. Muzii L, Boni T, Bellati F, Marana R, Ruggiero A, Zullo MA, Angioli R, Panici PB. GnRH analogue treatment before hysteroscopic resection of submucous myomas: a prospective, randomized, multicenter study. Fertil Steril. 2010;94(4):1496–9.
42. Rock JA, Truglia JA, Caplan RJ. Zoladex (goserelin acetate implant) in the treatment of endometriosis: a randomized comparison with danazol. The Zoladex endometriosis study group. Obstet Gynecol. 1993;82(2):198–205.
43. Römer T, Schmidt T, Foth D. Pre- and postoperative hormonal treatment in patients with hysteroscopic surgery. Contrib Gynecol Obstet. 2000;20:1–12.
44. Shaw RW. An open randomized comparative study of the effect of goserelin depot and danazol in the treatment of endometriosis. Fertil Steril. 1992;58:265–72.
45. Sutton CJG, Ewen SP. Thinning the endometrium prior to ablation: is it worthwhile? Br J Obstet Gynecol. 1994;10:10–2.
46. Tantini C, Tiso E, Ayub AV, Vizioli CB. Preoperatory treatment with Triptorelin LA in hysteroscopic metroplastic. Acta Eur Fertil. 1994;25(5):299–301.
47. Tapanaien JS, Hovatta O. Pituitary down-regulation with goserelin for in vitro fertilisation. Br J Obstet Gynecol. 1994;101:27–8.
48. Taskin O, Buhur A, Birincioglu M, Burak F, Atmaca R, Yilmaz I, Wheeler JM. Endometrial Na+, K+-ATPase pump function and vasopressin levels during hysteroscopic surgery in patients pretreated with GnRH agonist. J Am Assoc Gynecol Laparosc. 1998;5(2):119–24.
49. Triolo O, De Vivo A, Benedetto V, Falcone S, Antico F. Gestrinone versus danazol as preoperative treatment for hysteroscopic surgery: a prospective, randomized evaluation. Fertil Steril. 2006;85(4):1027–31.
50. Vercellini P, Antonio P. Treatment with a gonadotrophin releasing hormone agonist before endometrial resection: a multicentre, randomised controlled trail. Br J Obstet Gynecol. 1996;103:562–8.
51. Vercellini P, Trespidi L, Bramante T, Panazza S, Mauro F, Crosignani PG. Gonadotropin releasing hormone agonist treatment before hysteroscopic endometrial resection. Int J Gynaecol Obstet. 1994;45(3):235–9.
52. Vercellini P, Bocciolone L, Colombo A, Vendola N, Meschia M, Bolis G. Gonadotropin releasing hormone agonist treatment before hysterectomy for menorrhagia and uterine leiomyomas. Acta Obstet Gynecol Scand. 1993;72(5):369–73.
53. West CP, Lumsden MA, Baird DT. Goserelin (Zoladex) in the treatment of firbroids. Br J Obstet Gynecol. 1992;99:27–30.
54. Xia EL. Gynecological endoscopy. Beijing: People's Medical Publishing House; 2001. p. 29–34. Chinese.
55. Ye H, Weng X, Li Y. Obstetrician-gynecologists' series of books for further education. Beijing: People's Military Medical Press; 1996. p. 173–4. Chinese.

Application of High Frequency Electricity in Hysteroscopic Surgery and Its Thermal Effects on Tissues

5

Hua Duan

In 1924, Wyeth first found that high power and high frequency (HF) damped waves were able to incise tissues, and then high frequency damped wave electrotome was developed and applied in surgery by Anderson et al. In 1928, Bovieh and Cushing developed a high frequency undamped wave electrotome, which laid the basic foundation of high frequency electricity in the surgical treatment. In recent years, high frequency electricity has been proved to be safe, efficient, easily handled, and manipulated, and has been widely used in hysteroscopic surgery and improved quickly.

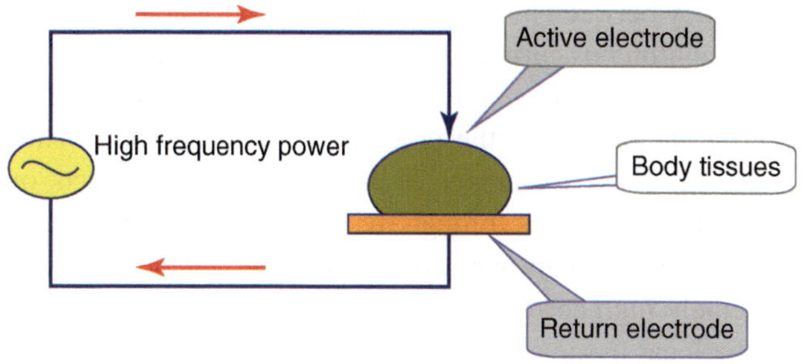

Fig. 5.1 Electrical circuit and its role

5.1 The Electronic Circuit Compositions and Current Types in Hysteroscopic Electrosurgery

5.1.1 The Electronic Circuit Compositions in Hysteroscopic Electrosurgery

High frequency electrosurgery refers to that the electric current of a certain intensity runs under the set voltage through the active electrode into the biological tissue to produce the electrothermal effects and cause expected damage to the target tissues, thus achieving the purpose of treatment. As shown in Fig. 5.1, in high frequency circuit system of hysteroscopic surgery, a part of the body tissue exposes to the median of two electrodes: one is an active electrode and the other is a return electrode (negative plate). In operation, high frequency current runs in the direction of the arrow along the tissues. Since there is only a narrow surface area between the active electrode and the body tissues, the current density is relatively high; but the return electrode has a larger contact area with the body tissues, so the current density is relatively low.

The changes of the temperature in human tissues are proportional to the square of current density. Therefore, when the high frequency current passes, the temperature of human tissues under the active electrode rises very quickly, while less heat is produced at the negative plate, which can be neglected. Thus, in a closed high frequency electrical circuit, the electric cutting, electrocoagulation, electrocautery, or other high frequency electrosurgery on body tissues are limited to the areas in contact with active electrode, so that high frequency electrosurgery could be done smoothly.

Electrocautery is different from electrosurgery. Electrocautery is to heat the metal conductor by electricity, and then acts on the tissues. Through the physical transfer of heat, the thermal destructive effect is achieved. Usually, the thermal effect temperature between the heated metal conductor and the biological tissues can reach 60 °C to 90 °C, therefore, it can only be used for coagulating tissues. However, electrosurgery is to have high frequency current of a certain intensity run under the set voltage through the active electrode into the biological tissue, achieving the electrothermal effect. The electrothermal temperature can be up to 100 °C–500 °C, thus the expected destruction and treatment can be implemented to the pathological tissues.

H. Duan (✉)
Minimally Invasive Center, Beijing Obstetrics and Gynecology Hospital, Capital Medical University, Beijing, China

E. Xia (ed.), *Practical Manual of Hysteroscopy*, https://doi.org/10.1007/978-981-19-1332-7_5

5.1.2 Current Types in Hysteroscopic Electrosurgery

The commonly used types of high frequency electrical current in hysteroscopic operation are mainly cutting current and coagulating current.

5.1.2.1 Cutting Current

The high frequency current that maintains a continuous output and produces cutting effects on biological tissues in electrosurgery is known as cutting current. The characteristics of its wave pattern are continuous undamped sine waves. As shown in the graph (Fig. 5.2), one may see that at a certain voltage, the current is oscillating at an extremely high frequency between the positive and negative electrodes. Due to the continuous current output, the cutting current has relatively higher average energy, and it also has no electric energy attenuation in the process of current output. When this continuous, undamped high frequency current acts on the biological tissues through the tiny active electrode (cutting electrode in hysteroscopic operation), it produces an extremely high current density on local tissues so as to heat up the local tissue rapidly, and causes vaporization and cell rupture, thus producing the cutting effect. During the cutting process, on the one hand, the intracellular heat is dispersed by the cell rupture resulting from high temperature, which prevents the heat transfer and infiltration from the site with high temperature to the adjacent tissues, producing "autonomous cooling effect." On the other hand, the high temperature carbonization of the tissue cells beneath the cutting surface increases tissue resistance and limits the conduction of electrothermal effects to the deeper tissues.

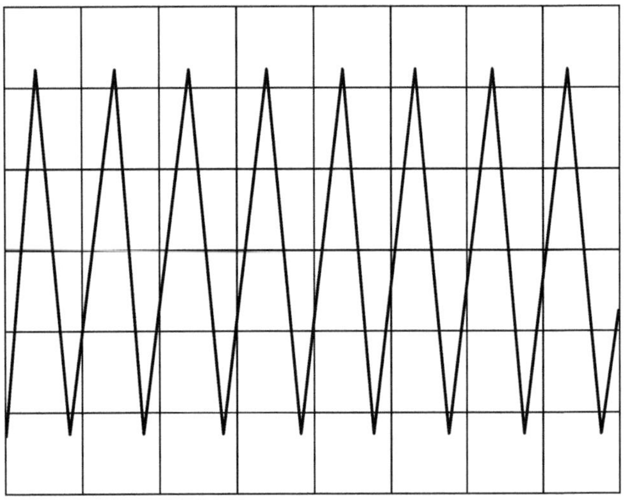

Fig. 5.2 Wave pattern of cutting current (continuous undamped waves)

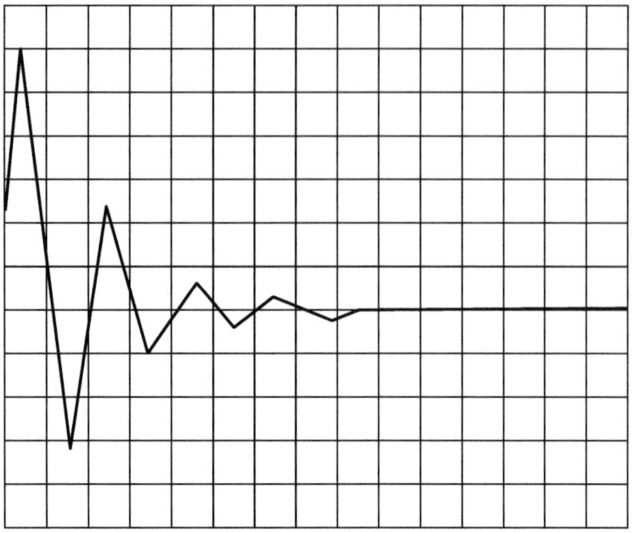

Fig. 5.3 Wave pattern of coagulating current (pulse damped wave)

5.1.2.2 Coagulating Current

Contrast to the cutting current, the high frequency current that changes the continuous output forms and produces coagulating effects on biological tissues is known as coagulating current. Its wave pattern characteristics are intermittent pulse damped waves (Fig. 5.3) and electric energy attenuation occurs in the process of current output. It is due to the electric energy attenuation of the coagulating current, the quantity of heat produced by tissues is reduced more significantly than the undamped current at the same voltage. In electrosurgery, the roles of coagulating current include desiccation and fulguration. When the coagulating current produces coagulating effect through the contact of rollerball electrode with tissues, because the contact area is larger than that of the cutting current, the current density passing through the contact surface is less than that of the cutting current. Therefore, at a higher voltage output, a wide range of tissue thermal damages may be resulted. Along with the increased distance away from the active electrode, the temperature conduction of its tissue thermal effect drops gradually. And when the temperature is over 45 °C, the thermal damage to tissue cells is closely related to the action time of the electrode.

5.1.2.3 Blended Current

Since the cutting current is different from the coagulating current in wave pattern characteristics, the electrothermal effect on tissues is also different. Therefore, cutting tissues combined with some coagulating current can often achieve a better clinical effect. This blended current usually manifests as blended damped and undamped waves (Fig. 5.4).

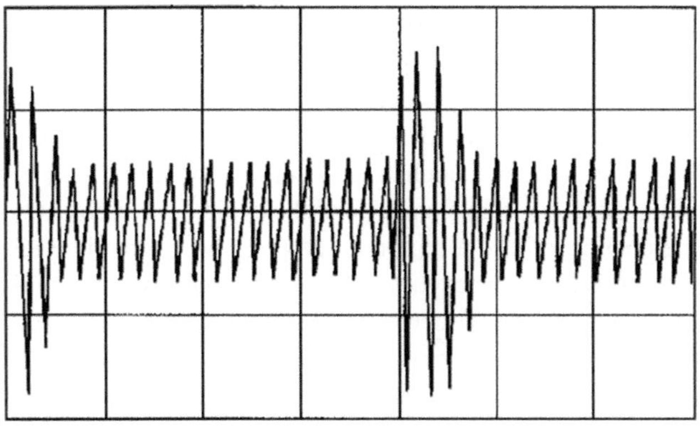

Fig. 5.4 Blended wave pattern of cutting and coagulating current

5.2 Electrothermal Effects in Hysteroscopic Surgery and Its Impact on the Tissues

5.2.1 The Changes in Tissue Cells Caused by Electrothermal Effects

5.2.1.1 Influence of Electrothermal Effect on Protein

Protein has high molecular weight and a complex composition and structure. The bond energy of secondary bonding (non-covalent) which maintains the molecular conformation is relatively low, thus its molecular structure is unstable and easily influenced by physical and chemical factors, leading to the destruction of its spatial conformation, change of its physicochemical properties, decrease of its stability and loss of the biological functions. All of them result in the denaturation of protein. High temperature can make the protein molecules denatured by rupturing the secondary bond. Generally, protein denaturation may occur at 60 °C. However, the usual active cells may die by producing protein denaturation when they are at the temperature of 600 °C for only 1 s.

5.2.1.2 Influence of Electrothermal Effect on Enzymes

Enzyme is one kind of protein with catalytic properties produced by active cells. In the metabolic process of the living organisms, almost every chemical reaction is induced by some enzymes. Enzyme is biological catalyst, so enzyme-induced reaction is similar to the general chemical reaction, that is, the temperature increases, the reaction speed is quickened. However, the enzyme is also a type of protein, and will denature at high temperatures. When the temperature reaches 60 °C, the enzymatic activity is obviously lower, and at 80 °C, the enzymatic activity is completely lost.

5.2.2 Influence of the Electrothermal Effect on Uterine Tissues

The thermal damage to the tissues during hysteroscopic surgery has been a focus of attention of gynecologic endoscopic surgeons. Due to the complexity of the factors related to the study, especially living tissue specimens are not easy to get, the further knowledge of this issue is restricted. The scholars who studied the isolated uterine specimens and some living uteruses drew the following conclusions: the depth of the endometrial damage is not related to the power of the electrode; there are variations in the depth of tissue thermal damage caused by different current waveforms; the tissue damages are related to the action time of the electrode. Indman et al. carried out studies of the electrothermal effects on the uterus in vivo and found that when the cutting current was 19 W and 59 W, and the coagulating current was 57 W and 28 W, the depths of the thermal damage into the uterine myometrium were 1.5 mm, 2.7 mm and 6.1 mm, 1.8 mm, respectively. Thus the depths of the tissue thermal damage caused by cutting and coagulating current were different even at the same power.

A clinical and laboratory study of electrothermal effects on tissues during hysteroscopic surgeries was carried out in the Hysteroscopy Center of Fuxing Hospital, Capital Medical University. Based on the study of isolated uterus, different current wave patterns were selected and different electric power and the action time were preset, then electric resection or coagulation was performed on the endometrium and the myometrium hysteroscopically. The tissue specimens obtained after operation were examined by histological and histochemical methods to observe and analyze the correlations among varieties of factors including the electric power, the action time, the thickness of the tissues by cutting or coagulating, and the depth of tissue thermal damages, and to study the histopathologic changes and the depth of electrothermal damages in uterine tissues by electrical thermal effect, as well as to discuss the changes in ultrastructure of cells influenced by the electrothermal effect at the subcellular level under the electron microscope. The aims are to find the appropriate operation power setting and the depth and scope of tissue thermal damage under this set power, and to discuss the action rules and related mechanisms of electrothermal effects on tissues during hysteroscopic surgeries, which can provide references and bases for clinical treatment and the improvement of the safety and effectiveness of hysteroscopic surgery.

5.2.2.1 Influence of Current Wave Patterns on the Thermal Damage to Tissues

In this study, a variety of powers and action times with different currents were set to work on endometrial tissues, it was found that at the same power and the action time, the depth of the tissue thermal damage beneath the cutting electrode was less than that of a coagulating electrode ($P < 0.05$).

5.2.2.2 Influence of Electrode Powers and Action Times on the Thermal Damage to Tissues

It was found from studies of the isolated uterus or hysteroscopic surgery that, (1) at the preset power and the action time, the depth of thermal damage to the tissues beneath the cutting electrode has no correlations to the electric power and the action time ($P > 0.05$); (2) in the isolated uterus, the depth of thermal damage to the tissues beneath the coagulation electrode does not correlate with the electric power and is positively related to the action time; (3) in hysteroscopic surgery, the depth of thermal damage to the tissues caused by coagulating current has significant correlations with electric power and the action time ($P < 0.001$), which is negative with the power and positive with the action time.

The effects of active electrode of different power output on thermal damage depth of uterine tissues can be seen in Tables 5.1 and 5.2.

5.2.2.3 Setting of Electrode Power

There is no uniform standard about the electric power settings in hysteroscopic surgery. The settings of electric powers range from 30 W to 160 W with the power of resection larger than that of coagulation. According to the mechanisms of the electrothermal damage and the clinical requirement on therapeutic effects, a minimum output power should be utilized to achieve the expected therapeutic purpose. The clinical studies in the Hysteroscopy Center of Fuxing Hospital, Capital Medical University indicated that the depth of the uterine tissue thermal damage caused by cutting current was unrelated to the electric power and the action time ($P > 0.05$); when the minimum output power of cutting current was set at 60 W, it could achieve the aim of damaging the whole endometrial layer, but sometimes there might be a phenomenon that the electric wire loop sticks to the endometrium when performing the operation and the speed and the depth of resection might be affected when cutting lasts longer; such phenomenon would be unlikely if the power was increased to 80–100 W, whether the electrode action time is long or short, therefore it was considered a suitable cutting power. The depth of the tissue thermal damage caused by coagulation current is closely correlated to the electric power and the action time. Its correlation could be expressed by regression equation: $Y = 2.666–0.021$ (W) +0.723 (T) ($P < 0.001$), namely, the depth of thermal damage is negatively correlated to power, but positively correlated to electrode action time. In our clinical studies, on the effects of the

Table 5.1 Thermal damage to the isolated uterus and its actual damage depth (mm, $\bar{x} \pm s$)

			Endometrium	Thermal damage depth		Actual destruction depth	
Type	Power (W)	Cases in total	Removal depth	Action 3–5 s	Action 6–8 s	Mean	Maximum
Cutting	60	8	2.422 ± 0.106	0.328 ± 0.130	0.516 ± 0.102	3.109 ± 0.126	3.790
	80	10	2.986 ± 0.341	0.375 ± 0.144	0.310 ± 0.082	3.824 ± 0.233	4.262
	100	10	3.325 ± 0.084	0.402 ± 0.121	0.325 ± 0.221	3.819 ± 0.611	4.412
Coagulating	30	8	0.084 ± 0.013	2.643 ± 0.416	3.290 ± 0.422	3.325 ± 0.240	3.948
	60	10	0.132 ± 0.066	2.763 ± 0.162	3.512 ± 0.625	3.610 ± 0.401	4.195
	80	10	0.863 ± 0.147	1.963 ± 0.312	3.020 ± 0.160	3.284 ± 0.138	4.212
	100	8	0.746 ± 0.211	2.041 ± 0.511	2.294 ± 0.242	3.016 ± 0.326	3.884

Note: In the table, the value of the average and maximum damage depth is taken from that of 6 to 8 s groups

Table 5.2 Thermal damage to the uterus in vivo and its actual damage depth (mm, $\bar{x} \pm s$)

			Endometrium	Thermal damage depth		Actual destruction depth	
Type	Power (W)	Cases in total	Removal depth	Action 3–5 s	Action 6–8 s	Mean	Maximum
Cutting	60	10	2.047 ± 0.045	0.324 ± 0.125	1.075 ± 0.233	3.081 ± 0.302	3.632
	80	14	2.683 ± 0.216	0.351 ± 0.142	0.536 ± 0.146	3.605 ± 0.423	3.993
	100	12	2.465 ± 0.243	0.447 ± 0.156	0.532 ± 0.186	3.249 ± 0.526	3.920
Coagulating	30	11	0.035 ± 0.007	2.609 ± 0.516	3.474 ± 0.444	3.546 ± 0.520	4.160
	60	13	0.101 ± 0.014	2.533 ± 0.310	3.118 ± 0.537	3.277 ± 0.534	3.788
	80	10	0.362 ± 0.087	1.354 ± 0.318	2.144 ± 0.606	2.514 ± 0.665	3.537
	100	8	0.519 ± 0.239	1.454 ± 0.551	2.106 ± 0.384	2.696 ± 0.485	3.338

Note: In this table, the value of the average and maximum damage depth is taken from that of 6 to 8 s groups

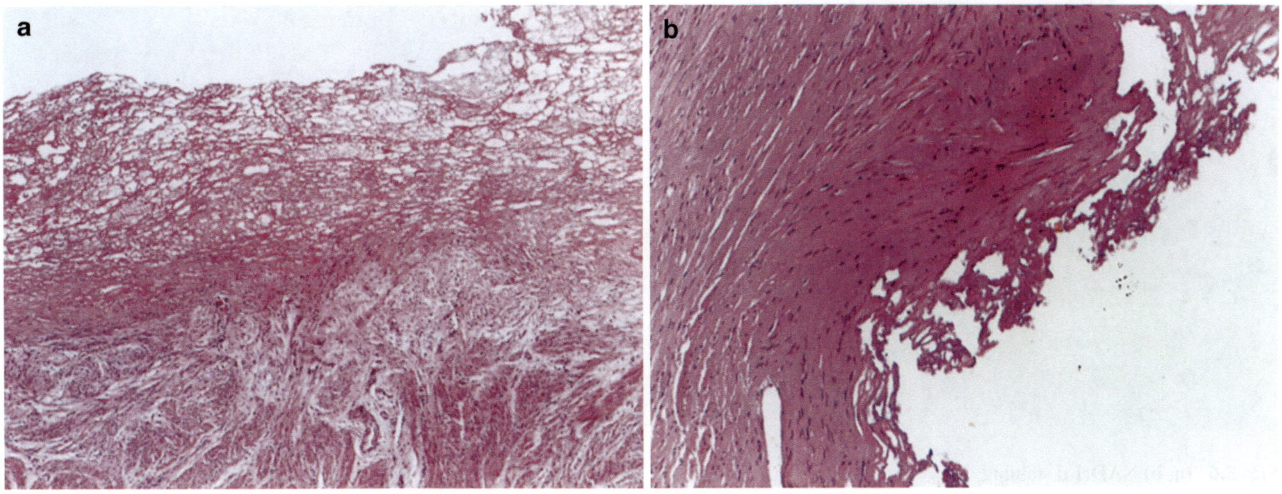

Fig. 5.5 (**a**, **b**) HE staining

four preset coagulation electrode powers on uterine endometrium, respectively, we found that at the same action time, the depth of tissue thermal damage decreased as the power increased; at the same power, it increased as the action time was prolonged. Thus 30–60 W should be a suitable coagulating power. In the clinical operations, when the endometrium is thicker or at a thicker position of the uterine wall, low power active electrode can be used and action time prolongs, thus producing its effect of deep tissue thermal damage. However, if the location is prone to perforation, such as uterine cornua, fundus or a thin uterine wall, the electrode action time should be shortened in order to avoid perforation or even damage to adjacent organs.

5.2.3 Histopathological Changes of Electrothermal Injury

5.2.3.1 Light Microscope

Through light microscopic observation, the pathological changes in thermal tissue damage caused by cutting and coagulation current manifest as a thermal damage zone which is made up of the coagulative and partial muscle necrosis layer from the surface to the inside. The thermal damage zone beneath the coagulating electrode is deeper than that under the cutting electrode.

1. HE (Hematoxylin and Eosin) staining: With HE staining, the coagulative necrosis layer shows that the tissue structure is damaged and cell structure disappears, forming an amorphous eosinophilic pink substance. This layer is thicker in the coagulating group, while thinner in the cutting group, intermixed with blue necrosis nuclear fragments. The characteristics of partial necrosis layer are that the amorphous necrotic cells coexisted with normal cells. Though some cells maintain the normal structure, the eosinophilic cytoplasm is increased, vacuole is formed, cell membrane disappears, and also nuclear pyknosis, karyorrhexis and karyolysis are present (Fig. 5.5a, b).

   The above pathological changes are more apparent in the coagulating group than those in the cutting group. The cutting current does not make any differences in tissue injury at different power and the action time, but in the coagulating group, the less the electric power is and the longer the action time is, the more serious is thermal damage to the tissues.
2. NADH-d (nicotinamide adenine dinucleotide diaphorase) staining: With NADH-d staining, under the action of electrode, the edge of the surface layer with tissue thermal damage appears to be yellowish-brown. A thick colorless tissue strip is visible to the underlying layer. At the bottom layer, the normal uterine smooth muscle cells and the vascular smooth muscle cells are dark blue; between the colorless tissue strip and normal deep blue tissue strip, there is a thin pale blue staining region, which is the transition zone for tissue injuries; the colorless layer of damaged tissue by coagulation is significantly thicker than that by resection, and its thickness is different along with the different power and the action time. The tissue thickness of thermal damage by coagulation is the most at 30 W and the least at 100 W, but the thickness is the most at 80 W and the least at 60 W by resection (Fig. 5.6a, b).
3. Masson's staining: By Masson's staining, the coagulative necrosis layer appears to be orange-red (necrotic smooth muscle), and blue non-cell structure (extracellular collagen fiber) substance. The underlying partial smooth muscle necrosis layer is orange-red denaturized necrotic muscle fibers intermixed with the light blue collagen fibers. At the bottom layer, it is the pink muscle fiber bundles and deep blue intra-bundle collagen fibers (Fig. 5.7a, b).

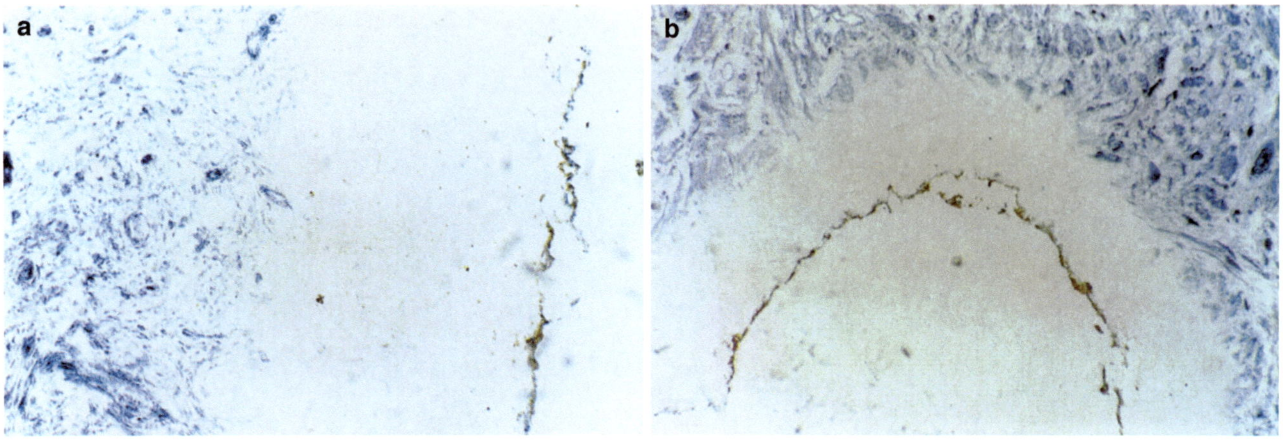

Fig. 5.6 (**a**, **b**) NADH-d staining

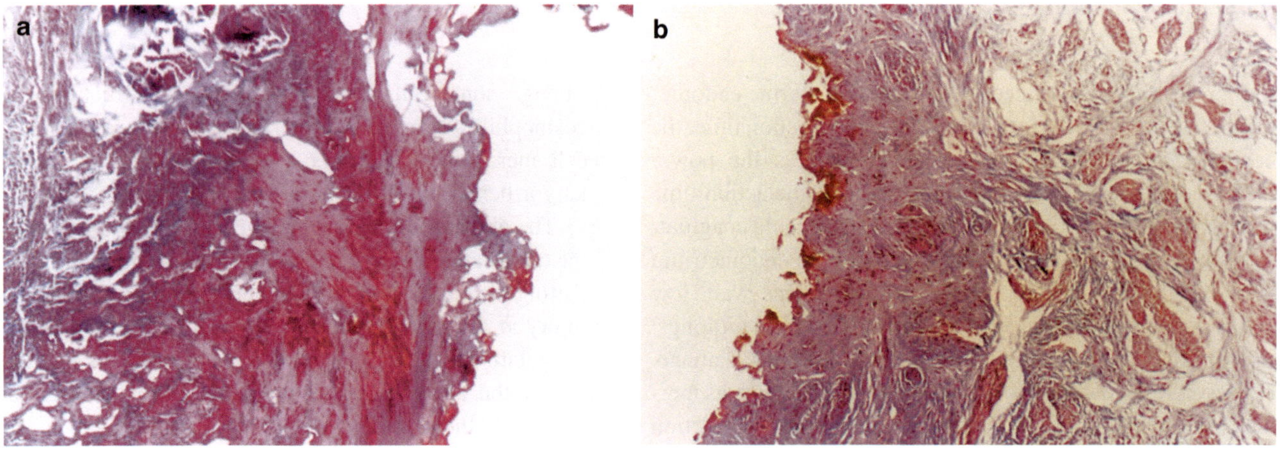

Fig. 5.7 (**a**, **b**) Masson's staining

5.2.3.2 Findings Under Electron Microscope

1. Tissue structure is destroyed by thermal energy, normal cell morphology disappears, only fragments without shapes and structures can be seen.
2. A variety of ultrastructure abnormalities can be seen in transition zone between necrotic zone and normal cells. The changes in nucleus mainly manifest as nuclear pyknosis, karyorrhexis, karyolysis, peripheral clumping of heterochromatin, etc., while in the cytoplasm, vacuoles, mitochondrial swelling, and endoplasmic reticulum expansion and degranulation develop (Fig. 5.8a, b).

5.3 Clinical Application of Hysteroscopic Electrosurgery

After comparing the outcomes of high frequency electrosurgery with laser operations, Gaillard et al. concluded that both techniques were similar, and that the electric energy had its advantages, including being economical and cheap, simple equipment, easy operation, and abundant histopathologic specimens obtained during the operation. Therefore, high frequency electricity has become the superior therapeutic energy source and has been widely used in clinical practice.

5.3.1 Application of Cutting Current in Hysteroscopic Electrosurgery

Cutting current is widely used in gynecological endoscopic surgery. In recent years, hysteroscopic resection of endometrium in treatment of abnormal uterine bleeding has substantially replaced laser endometrial ablation. Cutting current can resect endometrial layer and its underlying superficial myometrial tissues, which can effectively prevent endometrial regeneration. At the time of cutting, if appending some coagulating current, it can effectively coagulate the blood vessels in tissues underneath the cutting surface to achieve a hemostatic effect. Some scholars believed that the clinical effect using cutting current was

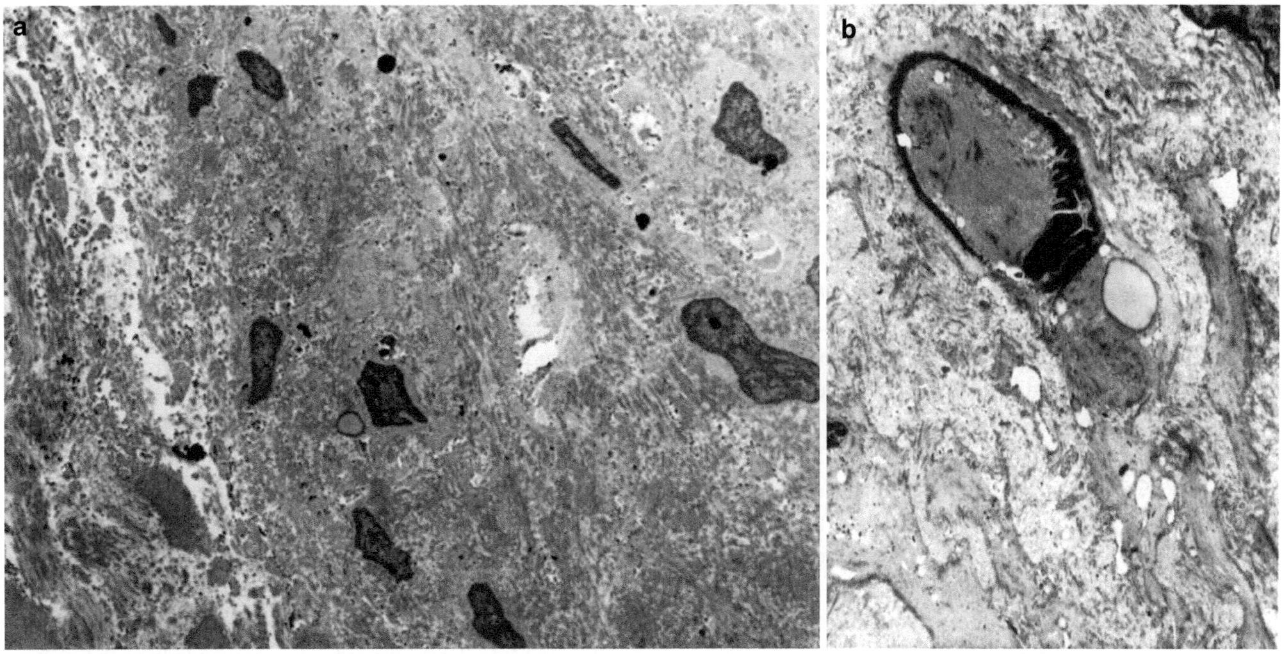

Fig. 5.8 (**a**, **b**) Transition zone between necrotic zone and normal cells

better than that using coagulating current. A cutting electrode could reach directly into the myometrium, which might not only ensure the removal and destruction of the endometrial glands, but also prevent its proliferation effectively. Meanwhile, prior to operation, the endometrium did not need to be pretreated with hormone, which could not only reduce the cost of treatment, but also avoid the side effects of drugs. Almost all the resected endometrial tissues should be taken for histological examination. Some authors reported that some endometrial lesions which were not suspected before the operation were detected from the resected specimens, which included endometrial focal atypical hyperplasia and focal endometrial cancer. This indicated that it helped to reduce the rate of missed diagnosis of endometrial precancerous lesions and endometrial cancer. In addition, the submucosal myoma of uterus and endometrial polyps can be resected continuously, without changing instrument halfway.

Since the uterus is an organ with very rich blood supply, uterine cavity is relatively narrow, and the uterine fundus and bilateral cornual portions have special anatomical and histological features, difficulties are brought about in the intrauterine operations with cutting electrode. In addition, pure cutting current cannot be used directly to coagulate the vessels. Therefore, clinically cutting current is commonly blended with certain coagulating current, which can not only ensure the effective cutting of the benign pathological changes in uterine cavity and endometrium, but also coagulate the blood vessels under the cutting site to achieve hemostasis.

5.3.2 Application of Coagulating Current in Hysteroscopic Electrosurgery

Coagulating current is also an indispensable form of power function in hysteroscopic surgery. Due to its strong thermal penetration, it gets a wide range of tissue damage and good hemostatic effects. Moreover, it is also a relatively simple operation and has small technical difficulty. It is a new approach of treatment for menorrhagia by endometrial ablation resulting from its electric coagulation effects under hysteroscope. Its therapeutic effects are essentially the same as that of laser endometrial ablation, but its postoperative amenorrhea rate is not as high as that by laser. On the one hand the tissue penetrating capability of coagulating current is less than that of laser; on the other hand there are more factors that influencing endometrial destruction by coagulating current, such as the setting of electric power, the shape and the force of the electrode, the action time and the endometrial pretreatment, etc. Thus, the depth of the tissue thermal damage by coagulating electrode is neither as intuitive as the cutting electrode nor easy to evaluate.

Electrocautery, a special form of coagulating current, is mainly used clinically to stop bleeding of a larger area. This electrode uses the higher output voltage of coagulating current to produce spark discharge, at the same time, some of the electrical energy is lost in the form of light. Therefore, it does not have the same depth of the tissue thermal effect as that of coagulating current. Electric spark coagulation is seldom used in hysteroscopic operation.

5.3.3 Application of High Frequency Vaporization in Hysteroscopic Electrosurgery

It is not rare to destroy the endometrium and intrauterine benign lesions in operative hysteroscopy by vaporization principle. However, it is just beginning that vaporization with high frequent electricity is applied in operative hysteroscopy. Since 1980s, laser vaporization has mostly been applied in gynecological endoscopic operation to destroy the lesions. In a comparative study of the removal of endometrium by laser vaporization and high frequency electricity, some scholars found that there was no difference in clinical effects between the laser group and the electrical cutting group. However, due to the complexity of laser equipment, being expensive energy, and failure to obtain specimens for histopathologic examination, it is gradually replaced by cutting and coagulating techniques with high frequency electricity. Compared to cutting and coagulating electrodes, operation by vaporization is relatively simple, easy, and can not only be used to remove larger neoplasm in uterine cavity, but also avoid repeatedly interruption of surgery to take out intrauterine tissue fragments. Furthermore, the electrical energy is cheap and the equipment is easy to use. Hence electric vaporization can yet be regarded as a better method for treatment.

The working principle of high frequency electrical vaporization is similar to that of laser, but the energy source is different. Vaporization current is an undamped current with high power output. Its power setting is well over that of cutting and coagulating current. Vaporization electrode used in hysteroscopic operation is a cylindrical electrode, which has equal spacing grooves. This structure can enlarge the contact areas between the electrode and the tissues, thus increasing the extent of the tissue damaged by the electrode. When the electrode is in operation, the strong output current may generate higher current density inside the contacted tissue with the electrode. Its electrothermal effect can elevate the temperature inside the tissues to vaporization temperature (≥100 °C). Glasser et al. recently reported that by using high frequency current to vaporize the endometrium, the depth of the tissue vaporization might reach 3–4 mm, and by clinical observation, the coagulating range of both the tissues underlying vaporization surface and the surrounding tissues is 1–3 mm. Therefore, a conclusion was drawn that the depth of the tissue damage by vaporization was similar to that by electric cutting. However, in the regions of the uterine cornua or with larger vessels, coagulation with a rollerball electrode is still used so as to avoid uterine perforation and intraoperative hemorrhage. In addition, due to failure to obtain tissue specimens during operation, only when combined with cutting and coagulation electrodes, the vaporization can gain a satisfactory outcome.

5.3.4 Application of High Frequent Bipolar System in Hysteroscopic Electrosurgery

The major difference in monopolar and bipolar circuit system in clinical treatment lies in that they pass through the whole body or local tissues in the current circuit loop. The biggest advantage of bipolar circuit is that it does not need the return electrode plate, and the active electrode is mutually adjacent to the return electrode, the current can only pass through the tissues between them, therefore, the electrothermal effect is relatively limited. Bipolar circuit system is applied quite a lot in laparoscopic surgery, with satisfactory outcomes and low occurrence of intraoperative and postoperative complications. The use of bipolar coagulation system in the treatment of uterine myoma and pelvic endometriosis does not only produce less damage to the adjacent tissues, but also gets better coagulating hemostatic effects, thus rarely causing accidental electric damage to adjacent organs.

Conventional bipolar circuit cannot produce the cutting effect, but the birth of bipolar needle electrode enables endoscopic surgeons to perform effective cutting and coagulation on pathological tissues in the bipolar circuit. The structure of a bipolar needle is shown in Fig. 5.9. The needle electrode is located at the top of return electrode, and the active electrode is 3 mm in length. The current acts on tissues through the active electrode and completes the circle via return electrode.

The animal experimental study by Isaacson et al. indicated that, at the same power output, the effects of both monopolar and bipolar systems on tissues were similar, and there was no difference in thermal damage degrees through their histological evaluations. Since the bipolar system must work in an electrolyte solution, the complications like hyponatremia may be avoided, which is caused by the use of nonionic distending medium. At present, the hysteroscopic bipolar vaporization system has been applied clinically. When the active electrode is activated, a circuit is closed by the electrolyte's ions in distending medium, and the return electrode does not touch the tissues of human body, thus increasing the safety of operation, and harvesting a good prospect of clinical application.

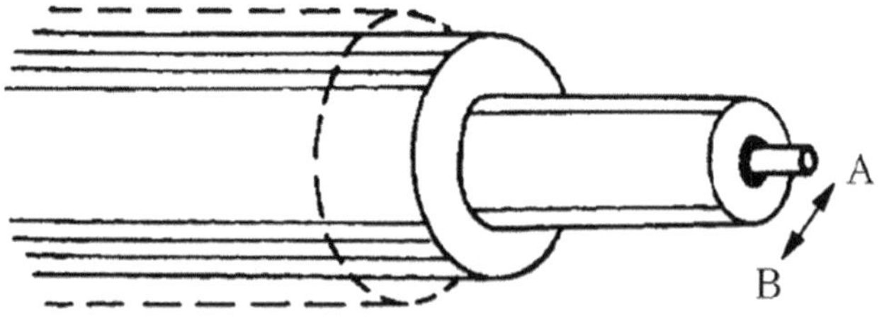

Fig. 5.9 The structure of bipolar needle electrode. (**a**) Active electrode. (**b**) Return electrode

Suggested Reading

1. Duan H, Xia EL, Liang Y. Influence of the thermal effects of hysteroscopic endometrial ablation on tissues. Chin J Pract Gynecol Obstetr. 1999;34:479–81.
2. Daniell JF, Kurtz BR, Ke RW. Hysteroscopic endometrial ablation using the rollerball electrode. Obstet Gynecol. 1992;80:329–32.
3. Glasser MH. Endometrial ablation and hysteroscopic myomectomy by electrosurgical vaporization. J Am Assoc Gynecol Laparosc. 1997;4:369–74.
4. Goldfarb HA. Bipolar laparoscopic needles for myomacoagulation. J Am Assoc Gynecol Laparosc. 1995;2:175–9.
5. Holm-Nielsen P, Nyland MH, Istre O, Maigaard S, Forman A. Acute tissue effects during transcervical endometrial resection. Gynecol Obstet Invest. 1993;36(2):119–23.
6. Indman P, Brown W. Uterine surface changes caused by electrosurgical endometrial coagulation. J Reprod Med. 1992;37:667–70.
7. Indman PD, Soderstrom RM. Depth of endometrial coagulation with the urologic Resectoscope. J Reprod Med. 1990;35:633–5.
8. Kaplan SA, Te AE. Transurethral electrovaporization of the prostate. A novel method for treating men with benign prostatic hyperplasia. Urology. 1995;45:566–72.
9. Loffer FD. Removal of large symptomatic intrauterine growths by the hysteroscopic resectoscope. Obstet Gynecol. 1990;76:836–40.
10. Isaacson K, Nardella P. Development and use of a bipolar resectoscope in endometrial electrosurgery. J Am Assoc Gynecol Laparosc. 1997;4:385–91.
11. Duan H, Xia EL. Application of HF electricity in hysteroscopic surgery and its development. China J Endoscopy. 2000;6:18–20.
12. Luciano AA, Soderstrom RM, Martin DC. Essential principles of electrosurgery in operative laparoscopy. J Am Assoc Gynecol Laparosc. 1994;1:189–95.
13. Luciano AA. Power sources. Obstet Gynecol Clin North Am. 1995;22:423–43.
14. Neuwirth RS, Amin HK. Excision of submucous fibroids with hysteroscopic control. Am J Obstet Gynecol. 1976;126:95–9.
15. Neuwirth RS. Hysteroscopic submucous myomectomy. Obstet Gynecol Clin North Am. 1995;22:541–58.
16. Onbargi LC, Hayden R, Valle RF, Del Priore G. Effects of power and electrical current density variations in an in vitro endometrial ablation model. Obstet Gynecol. 1993;82(6):912–8.
17. Pittrof R, Darwish DH, Shabib G. Nearfatal uterine perforation during transcervical endometrial resection. Lancet. 1991;338:197–8.
18. Serden SP, Brooks PG. Treatment of abnormal uterine bleeding with the gynecologic resectoscope. J Reprod Med. 1991;36:697–9.
19. Soderstrom RM. Electricity inside the uterus. Clin Obstet Gynecol. 1992;35:262–9.
20. Townsend DE, Richart RM, Paskowitz RA, Woolfork RE. "Rollerball" coagulation of the endometrium. Obstet Gynecol. 1990;76(2):310–3.
21. Tucker RD, Kramolowsky EV, Platz CE. In vivo effect of five french bipolar and monopolar electrosurgical probes on the porcine bladder. J Urol Res. 1990;18:291–4.
22. Valle RF. Hysteroscopic treatment of partial and complete uterine septum. Int J Fertil Menopausal Stud. 1996;41:310–5.
23. Wortman M, Daggett A. Hysteroscopic endomyometrial resection: a new technique for the treatment of menorrhagia. Obstet Gynecol. 1994;83:295–8.
24. Gaillard MC, De Grandi P. Endometrectomy: comparison of Nd-Yag laser and resectoscope. Gynakol Geburtshilfliche Rundsch. 1994;34(1):7–16. Germanica.
25. Gong Z, Zhan R. Pathological tissue specimen making and staining technique. Shang Hai: Shanghai Science & Technology Press; 1994. p. 343–53.
26. Qibo L. Practical pathological special staining and histochemical technique. Guang Zhou: Guangdong Higher Education Publish House; 1989. p. 1–32.
27. Liu F. Principle, structure and maintenance of medical electronic instruments, vol. 14–25. Beijing: China Medical Science and Technology Press; 1997. p. 339–49.
28. Nan D. Principles and maintenance of medical instruments. Shang Hai: Shanghai Science & Technology Press; 1985. p. 2–15.
29. Brill AI. What is the role of hysteroscopy in the management of abnormal uterine bleeding? Clin Obstet Gynecol. 1995;38:319–45.
30. Brooks PG. Resectoscopic myoma vaporizer. J Reprod Med. 1995;40:791–5.

Distention Medium in Hysteroscopy

6

Limin Feng

Hysteroscopic examination and operation are effective methods for the diagnosis and treatment of the dysfunctional uterine bleeding and other benign lesions in the uterine cavity. The sufficient distention and clear visualization of the uterine cavity is one of the most important factors for examination and treatment, so an appropriate distention medium is necessary for either diagnostic or operative hysteroscopy. The most commonly used distension media include gaseous medium (CO_2), low viscosity liquids (such as glycine, glucose, mannitol or sorbitol, and normal saline), and high viscosity liquids (such as dextran-70). However, due to the serious allergic reactions, the use of high viscosity liquids has already been prohibited. The procedures of hysteroscopic resection are performed under the continuous irrigating of distention media. It is done after the resectoscope being inserted into the uterine cavity through the cervical canal, with both the whole endometrial layer and 2–3 mm myometrial layer underlying the endometrium being resected so as to achieve the aim that the endometrium cannot regenerate. This operation is quite similar to transurethral resection of the prostate (TURP) in that a large amount of liquid distension medium (irrigating fluid) can be absorbed via the intraoperative open veins into the circulation. Furthermore, the uterus is different from the bladder in that the uterus is an organ with certain thickness and a hidden cavity which needs a very high distending pressure. What's more, there is much richer blood supply in the uterine wall than in the bladder wall, so there will be more absorption of distention medium during hysteroscopic surgery than that during TURP, resulting in the syndrome of transurethral resection of the prostate (TURP syndrome). This syndrome leads to the occurrence of hyponatremia, and if not corrected immediately, it could further cause the damage to cardiovascular system, serious neurologic and mental abnormalities, and even death, which are serious complications of endoscopic electro-resection.

During the hysteroscopic surgery, on the one hand, the uterine vessels are cut off when the endometrium and myometrium are resected, so the distention medium with a certain pressure flows into the body through the open vessel. On the other hand, the distention medium can flow into the abdominal cavity via the fallopian tubes and then is absorbed by the peritoneum, but its absorptive ability seems to be quite little. In many countries, a hysteroscopic surgery is always monitored by laparoscopy. Either laparoscopic suction of the distending fluid flowing into the abdominal cavity via the fallopian tubes at the end of hysteroscopic surgery or intraoperative ligation of both fallopian tubes laparoscopically cannot prevent the complications caused by the absorption of the distention medium, unless the hysteroscopy is complicated by the perforation of the uterus and then a large amount of distention medium flow into the abdominal cavity, which are then absorbed by the peritoneum and lead to a change in electrolytes. However, Istre held that an apparent absorption by the peritoneum might occur within 4 h after operation. The hysteroscopic surgery can also be monitored with ultrasonography, so it can be used to examine the distention medium during the operation, which flows into the abdominal cavity through the opening tubes and gathers in the posterior fornix and then disappears. With years of clinical observation, gynecologists of the Hysteroscopy Center in Fu Xing Hospital, Capital Medical University believed that the amount absorbed via the abdominal cavity is quite little.

The damage caused by the absorption of distention medium firstly raised concern in the 1950s when Creevy reported the first hemolytic reaction resulting from the absorption of the sterile distilled water which was used as irrigating fluid in a patient who had TURP. To prevent this complication, Creevy proposed the idea of using a "non-toxic and non-hemolytic distention medium." The other features of an ideal distention medium are isotonicity and high visualization, and that the increase in plasma and extracellular fluid caused by the absorption of distention medium is temporary and minimum. In addition, a distention medium should not crystallize on the surface of surgical instruments.

L. Feng (✉)
Department of Obstetrics and Gynecology, Beijing Tiantan Hospital, Capital Medical University, Beijing, China

E. Xia (ed.), *Practical Manual of Hysteroscopy*, https://doi.org/10.1007/978-981-19-1332-7_6

6.1 CO_2 Gas Insufflation

CO_2 is a colorless gas. It is handy, and its safety can be guaranteed if there is an appropriate gas insufflating machine. Linderman and Mohr reported that there was no complication happened in more than 1200 cases using CO_2 gas insufflation for hysteroscopy. The gas insufflation machine can perfuse gas continuously. After pre-setting the pressure, the flow rate can be automatically adjusted to an optimal state. If the pressure increases, the flow rate could be automatically reduced so as to prevent the complications induced by excessive pressure. The maximum flow rate and pressure in the uterine cavity of CO_2 gas insufflation are 100 mL/min and 200 mmHg respectively, while the most suitable flow rates range between 40 and 60 mL/min, and the most suitable pressures range between 40 and 80 mmHg.

The laparoscopic insufflators must never be connected to a hysteroscope, as they supply the abdominal pressure by L/min, which is far higher than the flow rate of uterine distention (mL/min) for hysteroscopy. The complications of CO_2 uterine distention—tubal rupture, hydrosalpinx and mediastinal rupture—are mainly caused by improper use of gas insufflation machine. Cardiac arrhythmia and cardiac arrest are also reported, which may be caused by too much absorption of CO_2. However, animal experiment models confirmed a wide range of its safety. A large volume of CO_2 entering the abdominal aorta almost did not cause cardiovascular complications, but the endoscopic surgeons should remember to use the minimum flow rate so as to achieve the optimal effect of insufflation.

According to a survey conducted by the American Association of Gynecologic Laparoscopists (AAGL) in 1991, the incidence rate of CO_2 embolism during hysteroscopic surgery was 0.1/1000. Although these cases were not described in detail, it was clear that both the embolism and death occurred in Nd: YAG laser operations cooled by CO_2. The flow rate of CO_2 when it is used for cooling the tip of laser is comparable to that of gas insufflators, which is 500–1000 mL/min. The fact that the CO_2 embolism may cause serious cardiovascular damage and death prompted the FDA to prohibit strictly the use of CO_2-cooled laser in hysteroscopy.

CO_2 is an ideal distention medium for diagnostic hysteroscopy, which can be done with CO_2 distention of the uterine cavity under local anesthesia of the patient. Jong et al. reported that hysteroscopies were performed in 152 outpatients under cervical block anesthesia with 1% lidocaine. Although some patients were extremely nervous, such as nulliparous women and women who had undergone cervical conization, most of them believed that this procedure was durable, and 90% thought that the degree of discomfort was lower than that of dysmenorrhea.

A number of cases proved that CO_2 insufflation could make a clear visualization, with the hysteroscope being directly placed into the uterine cavity through the cervical canal without the requirement of dilating the cervical canal, and CO_2 was insufflated continuously by irrigating through the inflow channel of the hysteroscope from the insufflator. The gas leakage could be prevented by using an appropriate cervical suction cup or holding forceps.

Performing the diagnostic hysteroscopy carefully during the luteal phase can improve the sharpness of the vision, decrease the bleeding and reduce the obstruction of mucus to the vision. Due to the lower refractive index of CO_2, it can make a clear vision, but its magnification is lower than that in the liquid distending media. Moreover, the CO_2 bubbles can be mixed with the blood, which may develop into the foam and affect the vision. In addition, it can make the endometrial debris float in the uterine cavity which leads to the difficulty of sampling. For multipara and patients who have had cervical conization, gas leakage can affect the surgeon's observation so other distending media are strongly suggested.

6.2 High Viscosity Distention Medium: Hyskon

Hyskon is a mixed solution of 32% dextran-70 in 10% glucose, and is produced by the fermentation of bacterial polysaccharides. The average molecular weight of dextran in Hyskon is 70,000, which belongs to a middle-molecular-weight dextran and is a colloidal solution. The dextran developed in 1940s was firstly used in blood volume expansion, which is to expand the blood volume by the absorption of the extravascular water under its colloid osmotic pressure. As a distending medium, Hyskon has the advantage of not mixing with blood. The metabolism of dextran is determined by its molecular weight. The low-molecular-weight dextran (<50,000u) can be filtered by the kidney so only minute quantity may be absorbed; the middle-molecular dextran should be gradually degraded into low-molecular-weight dextran and then be discharged through the kidney; and the high-molecular-weight dextran can be metabolized by the reticuloendothelial system.

It was reported in recent years that the absorption of Hyskon into blood vessels might cause anaphylactic shock and non-cardiogenic edema, and even there was a reported case of instant anaphylactic shock when Hyskon was used. According to the immunology, allergic reactions may be caused by the second encounter with the allergen after the antibody has already been produced by the first contact with antigen. The allergen of Hyskon may be sugar, and cross-reaction may occur with the bacterial antigens, such as streptococcus, pneumococcus, and salmonella. Although the incidence of such kind of anaphylactic shock is quite low, being only 1/10,000, Ahmed et al. reported that three such cases occurred in their hospital during only half a year. The amount of Hyskon administered in these three cases was all <100 mL, and skin test was negative in the postoperative dextran allergic reactions. Moreover, the risk of anaphylactic reaction in allergic patients did not increase compared with that in nonallergic people. As a result, the occurrence of allergic reactions cannot be predicted when dextran is in use.

Most reports of pulmonary edema caused by absorption of Hyskon suggested that it was related to the effect of dextran in pulmonary vessels, and such direct toxicity reaction also occurred when other molecular weight dextrans were in use.

The most possible cause of pulmonary edema secondary to absorption of Hyskon is the increased blood volume. Clinically, dextran has been used as a plasma substitute for the plasma volume expansion, but high-molecular-weight dextran is prohibited in expanding the blood volume. Because dextran has the property of slow metabolism, it can significantly increase plasma colloid osmotic pressure, which can promote a further increase in blood volume, leading to the movement of fluid and electrolytes. Each gram of dextran −70 can carry 20–27 mL of water into the blood circulation, so the absorption of only 100 mL of Hyskon can lead to the expansion of blood volume by 860 mL. Therefore, the blood expanding volume can be ten times more than the amount of Hyskon absorption (e.g. When 100 mL of Hyskon is absorbed into the blood, the blood volume will be expanded by 100 mL of Hyskon and 860 mL of fluid moving from the interstitial space into vessels). However, in the published literatures, it was not described in details about the amount of Hyskon absorption. Therefore there will be fold increases in the blood volume when Hyskon is absorbed, with 350 mL of Hyskon absorption leading to 3.5 L of volume expansion.

Unlike the low viscosity distending fluid, Hyskon does not cause water intoxication, and more specifically, fluid imbalance is secondary to the absorption of colloid osmolytes (dextran) whose half-life may last for several days. Excessive absorption of dextran −70 may lead to the movement of body fluids and electrolytes into vessels, so dextran causes fluid overload by changing the colloid osmotic pressure.

6.3 Low Viscosity Distention Medium

Bradycardia and hypertension may occur in patients with TURP syndrome, followed by hypotension, nausea, vomiting, headache, impaired vision, excitement, mental disorders, and lethargy, all of which resulting from the dilutional hyponatremia and a reduction in plasma osmotic pressure. If not diagnosed and treated in time, they can induce seizures, coma, collapse, and even death. The use of low viscosity distending fluid in hysteroscopic surgery, including glycine, sugar alcohol such as mannitol and sorbitol, is also prone to the occurrence of TURP syndrome, and its incidence is reported at a maximum of 50% and a minimum of 5%.

6.3.1 Research on Complications Induced by Glycine Absorption

Glycine ($CH_2{\cdot}NH_2{\cdot}COOH$) is a water-soluble small amino acid with the commonly used concentration of 1.5%. And it is hypotonic non-electrolyte solution with the osmotic pressure of 200 mOsm/L. The water intoxication caused by its absorption via the blood vessels appears as hypervolemia and hyponatremia. The incidence of these complications is up to 2% in TURP procedures.

During hysteroscopic surgery, when larger vessels in uterine cavity are cut off, glycine, a distention medium with certain distending pressure, can be absorbed quickly via the open veins. When glycine enters the circulatory system, the serum sodium levels are declined. Under normal circumstances, sodium and other positive ions play a decisive role in plasma osmotic pressure. Rapid reduction in the serum sodium often leads to the prompt reduction in plasma osmotic pressure, but the initial absorption of the glycine molecules contributes to the maintenance of plasma osmotic pressure. However, glycine cannot remain in the blood vessels for long, and the half-life of its molecules after being absorbed into vessels is 85 min. The longer the operative time is and the wider the excised tissues are, the more the glycine absorption will be, which eventually leads to an increase in free water. If this free water cannot be metabolized quickly, hypotonic hyponatremia will occur. Because of the adverse effect of the antidiuretic hormone in hysteroscopic surgery, diuretics are rarely used in surgical procedures. In addition, because of the effect of the female hormone on sodium-potassium adenosine triphosphate anhydride, female patients are more susceptible to hyponatremia, for example, progesterone can inhibit this kind of Na^+–K^+ ATPase in several different tissues.

The dangers of hyponatremia lie in inevitable brain damage, because the water molecules can pass freely through the cell membrane, and quickly establish intravascular, intracellular and extracellular equilibriums of osmotic pressure. Inside and outside the cells, it is easy for water to move from that being hypotonic (high water content) to that being hypertonic (low water content), so that the equilibrium of osmotic pressure is maintained both inside and outside the cells. Water molecules can also pass across the brain barrier freely, and the animal experiments and human observations both confirmed that hyponatremia most easily hurt the brain barrier. Therefore, a rapid increase of free water in vessels will lead to a drop in osmotic pressure and the transfer of water into the brain cells. When suffering from the cerebral edema, brain tissues can be damaged due to the narrow space of the cranial cavity. Increased intracranial pressure can reduce the blood flow velocity, resulting in hypoxia. An increase in the intracranial pressure by 5% can lead to brain herniation, while an increase by 10% can be life-threatening.

Hyponatremia may be an independent factor for TURP syndrome. Na^+ can affect the metabolism of cardiac smooth muscles and skeletal muscles, the release of nerve impulses, cell membrane potential and the permeability of cell membrane. Animal model experiments have confirmed the damage of hyponatremia to the central nervous system. In this study, when the experimental animals got severe hyponatremia under the normal osmotic pressure, they would always been in states of lethargy, twitching, or coma. Thus the authors believed that hyponatremia rather than low osmotic pressure was the main factor for its onset.

In addition to the low osmotic pressure and hyponatremia, another complications induced by glycine are caused by the products of glycine metabolism. The oxidative deamination of glycine is catalyzed by methyltransferase in the liver, forming glyoxylate and ammonia in the kidney. Then the glyoxylate is further metabolized into oxalic acid, forming oxalic acid crystals in the urine. There were many reports on the use of glycine causing hyperammonemic encephalopathy in urologic surgery. If hyponatremia and low osmotic pressure cannot account for patients' symptoms of central nervous system disorders, possibility ammonia poisoning should be considered. The incidence of hyperammonemia in patients with combined preoperative liver disease does not increase. In patients with severe ammonia poisoning, L-arginine can be used to stimulate the ammonia metabolites moving into the urea cycle.

The absorption of glycine may also affect the visual acuity. In a prospective study of 18 patients who underwent TURP, a transient decrease in visual acuity occurred in four patients. It might be caused by the secondary impact of glycine on neurotransmitters, with the formation of the inhibitors of the neurotransmitters in the retinal ganglion and horizontal cells. On the contrary, the blood ammonia levels in the asymptomatic group are significantly higher, which might be due to the fast metabolism of glycine in asymptomatic group. Some scholars have confirmed the significant individual differences in the speed that amino acid is produced through the metabolism of glycine in human body.

Some other scholars reported that glycine, as uterine distention medium, could cause obvious alterations in the function of blood coagulation, which mainly included the reductions of the platelets, fibrinogen, and the erythrocyte binding rate; the extension in partial thromboplastin time and prothrombin time; the presence of fibrin degradation products; a temporary reduction in oxyhemoglobin saturation; and hypercapnia. However, the reasons were not clear. Glycine had been considered as a safe and atoxic distention medium for many years, but the recent literature studies held a negative attitude.

6.3.2 Research on the Complications Induced by Absorption of Sorbitol and Mannitol

Sorbitol and mannitol can also be used as irrigating fluid in hysteroscopic surgery. Cytal, the most commonly used solution, includes 2.7% sorbitol and 0.54% mannitol, and the use of higher concentrations has also been reported. However, high concentrations of sorbitol and mannitol can be melted into caramel under high temperature when doing electric cutting, so it is rarely used clinically. Sorbitol and mannitol are six carbon isomers. Sorbitol is metabolized into fructose and glucose in the liver. Mannitol itself is inactive, only 6–10% can be absorbed and metabolized, and the rests are filtered through the kidney and excreted into the urine as prototype. Therefore, mannitol can produce the effect of osmotic diuresis, which theoretically helps to improve the symptoms of fluid overload and secondary hyponatremia. However, the half-life of mannitol in plasma is 1.5 h in patients with normal renal function, which is unhelpful to fluid equilibrium and recovery of cardiac function. The half-life can be further extended due to the blockage of excretion if patients have kidney disease. The isotonic mannitol 5% has ever been used as irrigating fluid for hysteroscopic surgery in the hysteroscopic center of Fuxing Hospital, Capital Medical University. It was found that the mannitol had the advantage of having the effect of diuresis when it enters the circulation, which might reduce the side effects caused by fluid overload, and it has the drawbacks of both forming a layer of crystal on all contacted surfaces after it is dried and possibly leading to postoperative hypotension after it produces diuresis and dehydration.

6.3.3 Research on the Safety of 5% Glucose as Irrigating Fluid

After years of research, many scholars have believed that an ideal distention medium is supposed to be sterile, non-toxic, and able to maintain the osmotic pressure of an organism; it should have good transparency and not mix with blood, and could ensure a clear operational view; it is non-conductive, low viscosity, easy to prepare, and relatively inexpensive; and its metabolites are very few and harmless. In recent years, the latest progress in hysteroscopic electro-resection with continuous irrigation is to use low viscosity distention media. However, according to the criteria above, those commonly used distention media abroad are not very satisfactory. Since 1990, 5% glucose has been used as distention medium in the Hysteroscopy Center of Fuxing Hospital, Capital Medical University and found:

1. Serum sodium level decreased gradually to the lowest point 1 h after operation and began to recover 4 h later. All changes were within normal range, without any clinical symptoms of hyponatremia.
2. Serum potassium level decreased gradually to the lowest point 1 h after operation, began to recover 4 h later and resumed normal 24 h later. All changes were within normal range, without any change in hypokalemia.
3. The level of blood chloride decreased gradually to the lowest point 1 h after operation and began to recover to normal from 4 h after operation.
4. Blood glucose levels significantly increased to the highest point 1 h after operation and returned to preoperative levels 4 h after operation.
5. The plasma osmotic pressure decreased gradually to the lowest point 1 h after operation and began to recover 4 h later.

The focus of whether 5% glucose can be applied in the irrigation for hysteroscopy lies in the influence of the changes in blood glucose level on the human body. We believe that there is significant increase in blood glucose level after surgery, which is highly correlated with the absorption of the irrigating fluid. If the patients did not have diabetes, the transient hyperglycemia would not produce significant physiological changes. We found that the level of blood glucose began to increase at the end of the operation, and peaked 1 h after operation, and returned to preoperative levels 4 h after operation, which recovered faster than the levels of potassium, sodium, and chlorine. Some scholars doubted that hyperglycemia would cause hypertonic and dehydration, and even aggravate hyponatremia, leading to the symptoms of central nervous system disorders. However, because of the great molecular weight of glucose, its osmotic pressure is limited. If the blood glucose increases by 10 mmol/L (180 mg%), the osmotic pressure will increase by 10 mOsm/L. If the blood glucose increases by 20 mmol/L (360 mg%), the osmotic pressure will increase by 20 mOsm/L. In our study, the maximum level of blood glucose is 469 mEq/L, and in theory, the osmotic pressure should increase by 26 mOsm/L. Animal experiments have confirmed that if the plasma osmolality is >350 mOsm/L, the animals will develop anxiety and irritability; if it is within 375–400 mOsm/L, they will have nystagmus, ataxia, and limb shaking; if it is >400 mOsm/L, they will have startle and develop tonic limb spasms; and if >435 mOsm/L, no animals will survive. Thus even if the plasma osmolality increases by 26 mOsm/L due to hyperglycemia, it does not produce significant pathophysiological changes and the patients do not have any complaints of discomfort according to clinical observations. Animal experiments have also confirmed that there is significant increase in blood glucose level in 5% glucose group, while there is no increase in blood glucose level in 5% mannitol group, but a high mortality. Therefore, high blood glucose is not the cause of death in experimental animals. If a transient increase in blood glucose could lead to a transient increase in plasma osmolality and water movement from the intracellular to the extracellular space, it would be the theoretical basis for some scholars' belief that the glucose as irrigating fluid may aggravate hyponatremia. However, we think this just partially offsets the extracellular hypotonicity and blocks some tendency of water movement from the extracellular space to the intracellular, so a transient increase in blood glucose will not aggravate the reaction of hyponatremia, but reduce the cell swelling and decrease the onset of hyponatremia. Of course, the use of 5% glucose as irrigating fluid for hysteroscopic surgery is not recommended in patients with diabetes and the elderly ones due to their hypoinsulinism.

Some studies suggested that 5% glucose was non-electrolyte solution with the osmotic pressure of 278 mOsm/L which was close to the tension of the blood plasma (280–320 mOsm/L), so it was known as isotonic solution. After being absorbed into the blood, it does not affect the tension in the red blood cells, so the red blood cells will neither swell nor shrink, but maintain its original integrity. However, glucose in the body is soon oxidized to CO_2 and H_2O, and supplies the energy at the same time, or it is stored in liver cells in the forms of glycogen, both of which leading to the loss of the original tension. Therefore, 5% glucose solution is isotonic solution apparently, but it can be used as tension-free solution due to its shortly-lasting tension in the body. Glucose returns to preoperative levels 4 h after operation, so the high metabolic rate would not cause the pathophysiological changes in the body.

Two phase contrast ultrasonography is applied in the monitoring of the whole surgical process of hysteroscopy. That is, the bladder is filled and the distention medium is injected into the uterine cavity, and strong echogenic band of light is formed under the high-frequency electric effect on the inner wall of the uterus. This unique change in the sonogram is an effective indication for ultrasonography monitoring of intrauterine electro-resection. Meanwhile, it is found in some patients that the irrigating fluids infiltrating into the muscle wall present cloudy strong echo, forming a special ultrasonic image (Fig. 6.1). A statistical analysis has been made for this phenomenon. According to other scholars' research, adverse effects may occur when absorption of distention medium is >900 mL, so we also took this as the standard. The result showed that in patients with infiltration of distention medium revealed by ultrasonography, there was a significant increase in the absorption of the distention

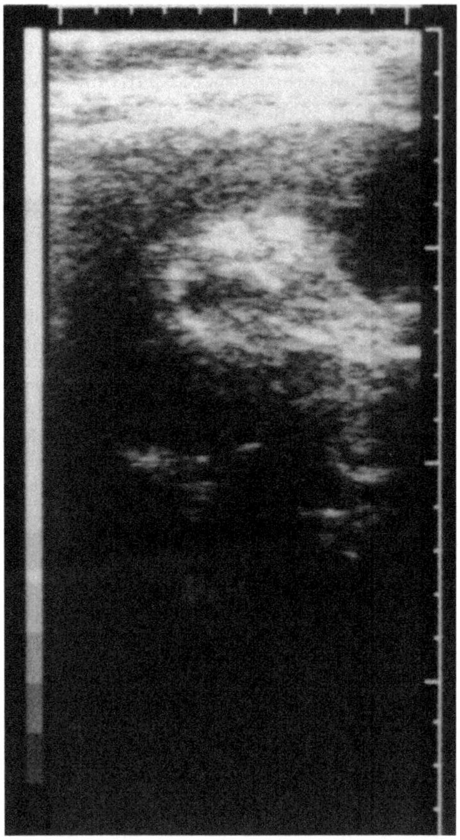

Fig. 6.1 The irrigating fluid infiltrates into the muscle wall, presenting cloudy strong echo under ultrasonography

medium. It was thought that such patients may have adenomyosis. The formation of strong echo when irrigating fluid infiltrates into the muscle wall may result from the direct extension of the basal endometrium into the myometrium and the reactive hyperplasia of uterine muscle fibers. If the glandular tubes in the muscle wall communicate with the uterine cavity, under ultrasonography, the irrigating fluid can be seen infiltrating into the focal areas of the uterine wall, and the bubbles can be detected accumulating in the cavity below the anterior wall, thus forming a special ultrasonic image. This is also another way of distention medium absorption, which cannot be neglected and needs to be further studied and confirmed.

6.4 Etiology and Clinical Presentation of TURP Syndrome

6.4.1 Etiology of TURP Syndrome

TURP syndrome has been the most serious complication of transurethral electro-resections. It refers to a series of symptoms in the whole body caused by hypervolemia and hyponatremia, which results from excessive absorption of irrigating fluid into the blood circulation. Though very rare, it may lead to a death rate of 15–40% once occurring. Early in 1946, Greevy et al. reported that, during a transurethral electro-resection, the distilled water was used as irrigating fluid, which entered blood circulation through the open veins caused by resection and increased the blood volume rapidly in a short time, leading to the destruction of large numbers of erythrocytes and then production of great quantities of hemoglobin, which finally resulted in impaired renal function. Afterwards, many scholars conducted the experimental studies by injection of the hemoglobin into the blood of animals, and the results showed that a large amount of hemoglobin in blood circulation did not cause impaired renal function. And when hemoglobin 50 g was injected into blood of human body at one time, it would be completely discharged out of the body after 30 h, causing no damage to the renal function. In 1955, Hagstrom firstly named transurethral resection of the prostate syndrome (TURP syndrome), described the typical clinical symptoms, and pointed out clearly that the true cause of the syndrome was the sudden decrease in plasma sodium. After more than 20 years of clinical practice and research, the mechanism of TURP syndrome has been clearly understood theoretically. Among them, Guy et al. conducted quite a lot of animal experiments and clinical observations and confirmed that the cause of TURP syndrome when glycine was used as distention medium was neither hyperammonemia nor low osmotic pressure hyperlipidemia, but hyponatremia. The clinical manifestations of TURP syndrome are bradycardia and hypertension secondary to hyponatremia, followed by hypotension, nausea, vomiting, headache, impaired vision, excitement, mental disorders, and lethargy. If not cured immediately, it can result in cerebral edema, herniation, leading to seizures, coma, collapse, and even death. All these symptoms are caused by dilutional hyponatremia and hypervolemia. And it is also suggested that the low osmotic pressure is also one of the causes of this syndrome.

To verify that a transient hyperglycemia does not aggravate hyponatremia, the researchers in the Hysteroscopy Center of Fuxing Hospital, Capital Medical University designed an animal experiment, the results were as follows:

1. There was a drop in plasma sodium in Wista rats of 5% glucose group, 5% mannitol group and the balanced solution group, and the most significant drop was in mannitol group.
2. There was an increase in plasma potassium levels in all three groups, and the most significant increase was in mannitol group.
3. There was an increase in plasma chloride levels in three groups, and the most significant increase was in mannitol group.

4. There was an increase of varying degrees in the blood glucose level in three groups, and the most significant increase was in glucose group.
5. There was a drop in plasma osmotic pressure in three groups, and the most significant drop was in mannitol group.
6. Status of animal survival: 2 died within 1 h and 4 died within 2 h in the group of 5% mannitol, 1 died in the group of 5% glucose, and 14 died in the group of mannitol within 24 h.

In recent years, the use of low viscosity uterine distending medium during hysteroscopy with continuous irrigating has been more and more advocated. The most frequently used media abroad are 1.5% glycine, Cytal solution and 5% mannitol. There is no 1.5% glycine and Cytal solution available in our country presently, so 5% mannitol and 5% glucose are used in our study.

As to the research on low viscosity fluid, it is found that 1.5% glycine cannot only easily lead to TURP syndrome, but also cause an increase in blood ammonia levels by its metabolites, resulting in a series of neurological and psychiatric symptoms and a transient decrease in visual acuity, which has been increasingly concerned by the hysteroscopists. The deep studies on the application of 5% mannitol as the irrigating fluid in the hysteroscopic resection are obviously inferior to that of 1.5% glycine. Although complications of water intoxication and hyponatremia induced by mannitol are similar to those of 1.5% glycine, only 6–10% of mannitol are absorbed and metabolized due to its inactive ingredient, and the rest is filtered by kidney and excreted into the urine as prototype. Therefore, mannitol can produce an effect of osmotic diuresis, and theoretically helps to reduce the dangers of the fluid overload and secondary hyponatremia. Thus Arieff believed that the isotonic mannitol was the most suitable for irrigating during electro-resection because it is non-conductive with only a little amount being metabolized in the body and will not cause a change in low osmotic pressure. However, the animal experiment confirmed the fact that the severity of hyponatremia, hypokalemia, low chlorine, and low osmotic pressure caused by the absorption of 5% mannitol was significantly higher than that of 5% glucose group. With respect to the recovery of animal behavior and survival rate, there was also significant difference between two groups. In addition, these experimental results showed that there was an obvious increase in blood glucose only in the group of 5% glucose, which confirmed that the increase in blood glucose would not increase the reaction of hyponatremia and mortality of animals. Therefore, the researchers believed that application of 5% glucose in hysteroscopic electro-resection was superior to 5% mannitol with regard to biochemical changes, the economic burden, the convenience of preparation, or the confirmation of clinical observations.

Surgical treatment of intrauterine disorders has become a trend in gynecological surgery, which has greatly decreased the administration of hysterectomy in many developed countries. In the past, 20% of the patients with dysfunctional uterine bleeding (DUB) needed to undergo hysterectomy, but hysteroscopic surgery can cure or effectively reduce the irregular vaginal bleeding in 80–90% of patients with DUB. In addition, treatment of uterine septum, submucous myoma, and intramural myoma can achieve therapeutic purposes without laparotomy so as to avoid the short-term and long-term complications caused by open surgery. The hysteroscopic surgery has fewer complications, shorter operative time, and shorter length of hospital stay and rapid recovery after operation. Since a high viscosity uterine distending medium may cause serious complications such as allergic-like reaction, non-cardiogenic edema, and coagulation disorders, nowadays people tend to use low viscosity uterine distending media which have fewer complications. The most frequently used distending medium abroad is 1.5% glycine, but the occurrence of hyponatremia has increasingly caught people's attention. Recently, there have also been continuous reports on hyperammonemia or death caused by great amounts of absorption of 1.5% glycine.

As to the application of 5% glucose as irrigating fluid in hysteroscopic electro-resection, there have been 13 cases reported by Lin about hysteroscopic resection of submucous myoma, but without any discussion on its safety. Sandra et al. performed hysteroscopic surgery using 5% glucose as the distention medium on four patients experimentally in the year of 1989, and the results discovered that all four patients developed hyperglycemia, with 2 of whom associated with serious hyponatremia. Therefore, it was believed that high blood glucose could aggravate hyponatremia. However, after analyzing Sandra's study, we believe that the distention pressure up to 150–250 mmHg they used was the inevitable reason for the aggravation of hyponatremia in patients. According to many years' research on hysteroscopic electro-resection, some scholars thought that the best distention pressure was 60 mmHg. However, Quinones declared that the bilateral tubal ostia could not be seen until the intrauterine pressure was raised to 100–110 mmHg. However, it is generally acknowledged by most scholars that the intrauterine pressure should not be higher than 100 mmHg, and even some scholars thought that there would be rare complications if the distention pressure was <100 mmHg.

We used 5% glucose as irrigating fluid in various hysteroscopic intrauterine operations, and found no TURP syndrome occurred, even in women complicated with renal failure, kidney transplantation, heart failure, cardiac valve replacement surgery, blood diseases, and so on. Amratage held that the procedure of hysteroscopic electro-resection should be stopped if the absorption of irrigating fluid was more than 1000 mL. However, in our study, the largest volume of irrigating fluid absorption was 1520 mL, and no hyponatremia was found to occur by either clinical observation or biochemical tests. With the measurements of the plasma electrolytes, blood glucose and plasma osmotic pressure and a contrast study conducted with 5% mannitol, it was further confirmed that 5% glucose used as irrigating fluid in intrauterine surgery was safe and economical, and was worthy of popularization. Of course, in order to avoid excessive fluid absorption, the operative time should be shortened as much as possible and the irrigating pressure should be controlled. If the infiltration of fluid into the uterine muscle wall was detected during operation, the absorption of irrigating fluid and the electrolyte balance should be closely monitored. In addition, close observation after operation should be done so as to avoid the occurrence of electrolyte disturbances post-operation.

6.4.2 Clinical Presentation of TURP Syndrome

The pathophysiological changes of TURP syndrome are dilutional hyponatremia and acute hypervolemia, with the clinical presentations mainly appearing as increased heart rate and increased blood pressure; lowered blood pressure, nausea, vomiting, headache, blurred vision, restlessness; dyspnea, pulmonary edema; arrhythmia, decreased heart rate, elevated CVP, heart failure, and hemolysis. Then, there may be more serious dyspnea, metabolic acidosis induced by excessive lactic acids produced by tissues; and shock due to worsened heart failures. Ventricular arrhythmias, mental confusion, lethargy, and death may follow in severe cases.

6.5 Treatment of TURP Syndrome

The treatment of TURP syndrome includes monitoring of the vital signs, management of disorders such as hyponatremia, heart failure, pulmonary edema, and cerebral edema, and correction of electrolyte disturbance and acid-base imbalance.

6.5.1 Treatment of Hyponatremia

Treatment of hyponatremia is aimed at potent diuresis and sodium replacement.

The precautions in the use of potent diuretics are: pay attention to its dosage, which can be decided through measurement of the hemoglobin content and relative density of urine, and through measurement of the central venous pressure as well. And attention should also be paid to serum electrolytes for prevention of hypokalemia.

6.5.1.1 Calculation of the Serum Sodium Deficit

$$\text{Sodium replacement required} = (\text{normal sodium} - \text{Patient's sodium}) \times 52\% \times \text{kg body weight}$$

52% refers to the ratio of person's body fluids to the total weight.

6.5.1.2 Key Points in the Replacement of Sodium

1. Rapid and high concentrations of intravenous sodium replacement should be avoided.
2. During the acute phase of hyponatremia, the replacement rate with serum sodium ions increased by 1–2 mEq/L per hour can relieve the symptom.
3. Increase in plasma osmotic pressure cannot exceed 12 mOsm/L in 24 h.
4. Dynamic monitoring of blood electrolytes and urinary output is needed.
5. Usually hypertonic saline solutions should not be used to correct hyponatremia, but correction with normal saline could be extremely effective. Generally, 1/3 or 1/2 of the sodium deficient is given at first so as to increase the osmotic pressure of extracellular fluid, transfer the water from the intracellular to extracellular space, and restore the cellular function. Observation of the patient is made for half an hour, which includes consciousness, mental status, blood pressure, heart and lung function, and serum sodium concentration. Those are basis to determine the replacement amount of the rest deficient, when hypertonic saline is always used.
6. Sodium replacement can just maintain serum sodium concentration at 130 mEq/L (mild hyponatremia).

Some authors believed that the best treatment for the body fluid overload was to restrict water intake and promote spontaneous diuresis, especially when patients had no obvious symptoms. This treatment may be inappropriate for patients with severe hyponatremia, which may lead to rapid deterioration of the symptoms. Arieff and Ayus reported that symptomatic hyponatremia occurred in 15 women who underwent surgery. Eight of the patients developed epileptic seizures and respiratory inhibition without any warning. Because there is usually no warning before the attack of these serious symptoms, immediate intervention should be taken. However, there is still much dispute over what is the proper therapy. The consensus of the researchers is that the serum sodium level should be corrected, but the correction rate has always been the focus of dispute. Rapid correction of sodium may lead to an intractable brain damage—central pontine myelinolysis (CPM). CPM refers to a phenomenon that after correction of hyponatremia, the symptoms of which would be firstly improved, but several days later, the patients' neurological conditions may worsen, and the new clinical symptoms are completely different from the original symptoms caused by hyponatremia, which can even lead to death. CPM was firstly defined and described by Adamas et al.

As CPM progresses, patients may develop spastic quadriplegia, aphasia, pseudobulbar palsy, behavioral impairment and movement disorders. Although the onset of symptoms may occur 4 h after surgery, CT and MRI can help to make diagnoses in the early stage of pathological process. Autopsy ascribes the destruction of myelin sheath at pons and outside the pons. In order to describe this pathological process more accurately, Arieff recommended the name of "demyelination disorders." Animal experiments have confirmed that too rapid correction of chronic hyponatremia can lead to brain demyelination, but gradual correction may prevent this disorder.

Brain demyelination disorders induced by rapid correction of hyponatremia are the corresponding pathological changes in brain tissues secondary to changes in osmotic pressure. The brain can relatively resist osmotic swelling, because when the intracranial pressure rises, the brain tissue can discharge water into the cerebrospinal fluid. The capacity to drain water and avoid osmotic swelling is time dependent. In patients with hyponatremia, as the pressure in the inter-tissue space increases, water is released into the cerebrospinal fluid by the effects of osmosis. Almost at the same time, the sodium and water is forced into the cerebrospinal fluid through the extracellular channel, so the liquid then enters the central nervous system. Secondary disorders of the brain occur at the cellular level. Unlike other tissues, brain cells discharge intracellular solute in a hypotonic state. Intracellular K^+ moves with the water from inside the cell to outside the cell within 3–4 h, and this movement may reach a peak within 24 h. A few days later, there may be a loss of the cytoplasmic organic solutes (formerly called as "spontaneous infiltration"), including taurine, creatine phosphate, and glutamate, and so on.

This adaptation to hyponatremia and low osmotic pressure can account for the changes of the brain in the rapid correction of hyponatremia. In order to reduce the swelling, the brain tissue achieves balance with plasma osmotic pressure by reducing the intracellular solute content. If the plasma osmotic pressure increases quickly, the brain tissue will dehydrate, because the rapid increase in osmotic pressure can lead to transfer of water from brain cells into plasma, causing brain dehydration.

Plasma osmotic pressure cannot be corrected rapidly because the intracellular spontaneous infiltration and K^+ release will last for a few days. Moreover, these ions re-enter the cells more slowly than being discharged. CPM is considered to be caused by brain cells "shrinkage" due to the rapid correction of hyponatremia. Thus, CPM is also known as "osmotic demyelination syndrome."

In addition, it is worthwhile to note that the mortality of acute hyponatremia is much higher than that of chronic one. When the serum sodium level is 120 mmol/L, acute hyponatremia can lead to death, while the chronic one would not. If the low sodium state lasts for 48 h, it can be recognized as chronic. Within 48 h, the brain cells can balance the hypotonic state through the release of solute. In an acute state, a rapid correction of serum sodium rarely causes damage, because no "shrinkage" is developed in brain cells. Animal experiments showed that a rapid correction of serum sodium within 24 h was feasible and would not cause either the "shrinkage" of brain cells or demyelination disorders. However, the same treatment for hyponatremia 3 days later can lead to the "shrinkage" of brain cells, demyelination disorders, and death.

Hyponatremia induced by hysteroscopic surgery is an acute process. Close intraoperative and postoperative monitoring, timely diagnosis, and advance treatment should be administered, and it is not appropriate to limit the fluid intake solely and wait for spontaneous diuresis. Rapid correction in serum sodium levels often leads to overcorrection, and the use of diuretics can usually cause hypernatremia. Minor increase in plasma osmotic pressure can offset the hazards of cerebral edema. Assuming that the serum sodium concentration drops to 120 mmol/L, and if it is raised to 126 or 132 mmol/L (increase rate 5–10%), cerebral edema could be effectively relieved. The serum sodium concentration can be raised from 1 to 2 mmol/L per hour in the first several hours and an increase in serum sodium concentration within the first 24 h should be <12 mmol/L. If hyponatremia is not diagnosed in the postoperative 24–48 h, subsequent treatment must be implemented cautiously so as to avoid CPM. If a large amount of irrigating fluid was absorbed via peritoneum, a series of symptoms of hyponatremia would be delayed, including cerebral edema.

To prevent the development of CPM in the treatment of chronic hyponatremia, some scholars believed that the serum sodium level could be raised by <25 mmol/L within first 48 h of treatment. Similarly, some scholars held that the correction rate of serum sodium should not exceed 12 mmol/L per hour. It is unnecessary to pursue the normal serum sodium level at the risk of overcorrection, and it is appropriate just to reach the level of mild hyponatremia. The correction rate per hour is still controversial currently. Earlier reports suggested that serum sodium levels should be slowly corrected, and the correction rate per hour be <0.6 mmol/L. Other reports indicated that the hourly rate of correction was not important, but excessively slow correction of the brain status could also lead to death.

In the treatment of acute hyponatremia, there are many different ways, including intravenous infusion of normal saline, 3–5% sodium chloride and potent diuresis. Hypertonic saline with concentration more than 5% is strictly prohibited, which may worsen the body fluid overload further. Some scholars advocated substituting furosemide or mannitol for diuretics, of which mannitol was preferred due to osmotic diuresis, and very small quantities of Na^+ in the urine might be lost. However just as hypertonic saline, mannitol is an effective intravascular osmotic agent, which can also cause unnecessary increase in blood volume. For this reason, some people advocated the use of furosemide. The diuretic effect can work a few minutes after intravenous infusion of furosemide. 20 mg is sufficient to achieve the diuretic effect in patients with normal renal function, but large doses of furosemide are required for patients with renal insufficiency. The amount of urine and urine sodium content should be accurately calculated, and a proper blood volume should be maintained in the treatment.

6.5.2 Treatment of Acute Heart Failure

The patient is placed in a semi-sitting position, and digitalis preparation is needed in addition to diuretics. Its principles are to strengthen the cardiac contractility so as to increase the cardiac output and slow down the heart rate, and to promote peripheral vasoconstriction and hepatic venous contraction so as to reduce venous return. Dosage: lanatoside C: 0.4 mg, slow intravenous injection; digitalis preparation: 1.0–1.2 mg, slow intravenous injection.

6.5.3 Treatment of Pulmonary Edema

1. Treatment of hypoxemia: Oxygen uptake through nasal catheter is given at a flow rate of 6 L/min; mask oxygen inhalation is administered to patients with obnubilation. If the above-mentioned treatment is ineffective and PO_2 is under 50 mmHg, trachea cannula is suggested. If the intermittent positive pressure breath at the beginning is still ineffective, positive end expiratory pressure is recommended so as to increase the functional residual capacity and effectively prevent the expiratory alveolar collapse. Application of defoaming agent: during the oxygen uptake through nasal catheter, 75–95% ethanol is put into the filter bottle and taken in together with the oxygen, while 20–30% alcohol used in mask oxygen inhalation.
2. About morphine: Morphine is suggested for patients with heart failure and lung edema due to other causes. However, it is not appropriate if lung edema is caused by TURP, because morphine may lead to the release of ADH (antidiuretic hormone), which reduces urine output, aggravating water intoxication.

6.5.4 Treatment of Cerebral Edema

1. High concentration urea—osmotic diuretic: Intravascular fluid osmotic pressure is higher than that in tissues, thus water enters from brain tissue into the blood vessels.
2. Corticosteroid hormone—dexamethasone: It may stabilize cell membrane, reduce capillary permeability, and relieve cerebral edema.

6.5.5 Correction of Electrolyte Imbalance

1. Hypokalemia: Excessive use of diuretics may cause low potassium and arrhythmia, serum potassium should be measured, and ECG monitoring should be taken.
2. Metabolic acidosis: pH value is measured and intravenous drip of 4% sodium bicarbonate injection is administered.

6.6 TURP Syndrome: Prophylactic Measures

Clinically, there are many effective ways to prevent excessive absorption of the distention medium. First of all, no matter what kind of distention medium is in use, the absorption should be closely monitored intraoperatively, and the volume of fluid input and output must be accurately measured. An resectoscope with double channels (i.e. the fluid inlet channel and the outlet channel are separated) should be used in surgery, which can effectively allow outflow of the fluid accumulating in the uterine cavity and also help drainage the fluid with vacuum aspiration. If not combined with laparoscopic monitoring, the surgery under non-general anesthesia is helpful in the observation of the complications, such as nausea, vomiting, and altered mental status which may be suggestive of hyponatremia and foamy sputum which may be suggestive of pulmonary edema. Moreover, the low temperature irrigating fluid can stimulate vascular contraction and reduce the absorption of distention fluid. If hysteroscopic resection of uterine fibroids is to be undertaken, preoperative administration of GnRH agonists can reduce the size of myoma and decrease the blood flow, which can be helpful to shorten the operative time and lower the volume of irrigating fluid. Finally, although the operative time is closely related to the absorption of irrigating fluid and hyponatremia, many scholars believed that the operation should be terminated when excessive absorption of fluid was threatening the safety of the operation, and another time should be selected for a second operation.

6.6.1 Prevention of Complications Caused by High Viscosity Distention Medium

The irrigating pressure of Hyskon, which is a high viscosity distention medium, should not be higher than 150 mmHg. Pulmonary edema occurs when the input volume is >500 mL, so the absorption volume should be limited within 300 mL. The absorption volume of 300 mL can increase the blood volume of 2900 mL, so the operative time should be less than 45 min when Hyskon is used as distention medium.

6.6.2 Prevention of Complications Caused by Low Viscosity Distention Medium

When low viscosity distention medium is used, such as glycine and mannitol solution, the absorption volume of fluid is easy to be underestimated, because the irrigating fluid usually leaks from the cervix and the leaked fluid is often underestimated or over calculated. Therefore, an accurate method of surveillance is needed. In order to monitor closely the balance of body fluid, many scholars suggested adding ethanol into the irrigating fluid to measure the ethanol content in breathing so as to calculate the absorption of irrigating fluid.

In TURP syndrome, the amount of irrigating fluid absorption is related to the weight of resected tissues and the duration of operation and the pressure of distention. In hysteroscopic surgery, the absorption of irrigating fluid is related to the intrauterine pressure, so the pressure should be confined to that achieving a clear vision. Mclucas held that the distention pressure should be limited to 60 cm H_2O (44 mmHg). Istre et al. believed that it could be considered as safe if the pressure was lower than 100 mmHg. Moreover, some scholars believed the highest pressure in the uterine cavity should be matched with the patients' blood pressure. The same irrigating pressure can produce different intrauterine pressure, which is also very important. Vulgaropulos et al. discovered that the intrauterine pressure could continue to be at a low level if the fluid outlet pipe remained to be open intraoperatively. On the contrary, if the fluid outlet pipe was closed and the height difference of the fluid was 2.44 m (8 ft) and 4.27 m (14 ft), the intrauterine pressure would be 230 and 280 mmHg, respectively. However, the author did not think this pressure would lead to absorption of fluid since it only lasted for 30—60s, and the author did not describe clearly what operative procedures were done under these pressures. Some authors suggested keeping the fluid output pipe unobstructed and the intrauterine pressure at 60–75 mmHg, which would be helpful for prevention of the fluid absorption. More attention should be paid especially when the extent of surgery became greater.

When low viscosity distention medium is used, if the absorption volume is greater than 500 mL, the surgeons should closely observe the conditions of the lungs and check the levels of serum electrolyte. The amount of fluid absorption should be accurately measured by the intake and outflow volume. Some scholars reported that there was an average decline in serum sodium concentration by 2.5 mEq/L (0–10 mEq/L)when the absorption volume of glycine was <500 mL, and there was an average decline by 8 mEq/L (0–25 mEq/L) when the absorption volume was >500 mL. In this research, the absorption volume in two patients was 2300 and 2700 mL, respectively, while the decrease in serum sodium was 16 and 25 mEq/L, respectively.

6.7 Equipment for Uterine Distention with Fluids

In order to continuously monitor the inflow and the absorption volumes of the fluid, the Olympus Cooperation designed and produced a continuous flow irrigation pump. Its operational principle is that the low viscosity irrigation fluid enters the uterine cavity through a rotating pump via resectoscope, the pressure and flow rate of the pump can both be previously set. The fluid flowing out of the uterine cavity is collected in a container with scales. The difference between the inflow and the outflow is the amount of absorption. These figures are all displayed on the screen of the monitor. If the amount of absorption is more than a certain standard volume (usu. 1 L), the pump should sound the alarm in order to remind the surgeon to terminate the operation immediately.

The distending pressures of the pump range from 0 to 150 mmHg, and the flow rate range from 0 to 450 mL/min. According to our experience, the pressure should be set at 100 mmHg and the flow rate at 200–250 mL/min, the average intrauterine pressure could be at 70–75 mmHg. If the effect of distension is not satisfied, leading to a blurry operation field, the pressure can be set lower than the patient's systolic arterial pressure according to the blood pressure. Low pressure and high flow rate are the guarantee of safe hysteroscopic electro-resections.

Suggested Reading

1. Adams RD, Victor M, Mancall EL. Central pontine myelinolysis: a hitherto undescribed disease occurring in alcoholic and malnourished patients. AMA Arch Neurol Psychiatry. 1959;81(2):154–72.

2. Ahmed N, Falcone T, Tulandi T, Houle G. Anaphylactic reaction because of intrauterine 32% dextran-70 instillation. Fertil Steril. 1991;55(5):1014–6.
3. Amratage RJ, Farquharson RG. Endometrial resection. Br J Hosp Med. 1995;53:90–3.
4. Arieff AI, Ayus JC. Treatment of symptomatic hyponatremia: neither haste nor waste. Crit Care Med. 1991;19:748–51.
5. Baba T, Shibata Y, Ogata K, Kukita I, Goto T, Hamada Y, Maehara A, Matsukado Y. Isotonic hyponatremia and cerebrospinal fluid sodium during and after transurethral resection of the prostate. J Anesth. 1995;9(2):135–41.
6. Bøe Engelsen I, Woie K, Hordnes K. Transcervical endometrial resection: long-term results of 390 procedures. Acta Obstet Gynecol Scand. 2006;85(1):82–7.
7. Brooks PG. Complications of operative hysteroscopy: how safe is it ? Clin Obstet Gynecol. 1992;35:256–61.
8. Goldenberg M, Zolti M, Seidman DS, Bider D, Mashiach S, Etchin A. Transient blood oxygen desaturation, hypercapnia, and coagulopathy after operative hysteroscopy with glycine used as the distending medium. Am J Obstet Gynecol. 1994;170(1 Pt 1):25–9.
9. Creevy CD. Hemolytic reactions during transurethral prostatic resection. J Urol. 1947;58:125–31.
10. De Jong P, Doel F, Falconer A. Outpationt diagnostic hysteroscopy. Br J Obstet Gynaecol. 1990;97:299–303.
11. Duleba AJ. Review of major complications related to devices used to treat abnormal uterine bleeding. J Am Assoc Gynecol Laparosc. 2004;11:S72.
12. Feng LM, Chen RF, Xia EL. Application of hysteroscopic resection in diagnosis of adenomyosis. Chin J Obstet Gynecol. 1998;33(7):435–6. Chinese.
13. Feng LM, Xia EL. Safety study of applying 5% glucose infusion fluid in hysteroscopic electroresection. Chin J Obstet Gynecol. 1996;31(5):302–4. Chinese.
14. Feng LM, Xia EL. Several focus issues of diagnosing intracavitary lesions with hysteroscope. Chin J Clin Obstet Gynecol. 2004;5(3):163–5. Chinese.
15. Foul CG. Absorption of irrigation fluid during transcervical resection of endometrium. Br Med J. 1990;300:748–52.
16. Garry R. Hysteroscopic alternatives to hysterectomy. Br J Obstet Gynecol. 1990;97:199–207.
17. Garry R. Safety of hysteroscopic surgery. Lancet. 1990;336:1013–4.
18. Guy TB, Kevin RL, Ruben FG. The physiologic basis of the TUR syndrome. J Surg Res. 1989;46:135–41.
19. Hagstrom RS. Studies on the fluid absorption from the bladder during transurethral prostatic resection. J Urol. 1955;73:852–3.
20. Hahn RG, Anderson T, Sikk M. Eye symptoms, visual evoked protentials and EEG during intravenous infusion of glycine. Acta Anaesthesiol Scand. 1995;39:214–9.
21. Hahn RG, Shemais H, Essén P. Glycine 1.0% versus glycine 1.5% as irrigating fluid during transurethral resection of the prostate. Br J Urol. 1997;79(3):394–400.
22. Hahn RG. Irrigating fluid in endoscopic surgery. Br J Urol. 1997;79:669–80.
23. Hahn RG. Prevention of TUR syndrome by deception of trace ethanol in the expired breath. Anesthesiology. 1990;45:581–3.
24. Huang Y, Huang W, Ou X, Huang Z, Xiao Q, Bai J. Analysis hysteroscopic transcervical resection of submucous myoma and transurethral resection of prostate (TURP) syndrome. Matern Child Health Care China. 2006;21(7):998–1000. Chinese.
25. Istre O, Skajaa K, Schjoensby AP, Forman A. Changes in serum electrolytes after transcervical resection of endometrium and submucous fibroids with use of glycine 1.5% for uterine irrigation. Obstet Gynecol. 1992;80(2):218–22.
26. Jedeikin R, Olsfanger D. Disseminated intravascular coagulopathy and adult respiratory distress syndrome: life-threatening complications of hysteroscopy. Am J Obstet Gynecol. 1990;162:44–5.
27. Jiang Z. Clinical water, electrolyte and acid-base balance. Chong Qing: Chong Qing Press; 1992. p. 56. Chinese.
28. Joel O, Robert GH. Simulated intraperitoneal absorption of irrigating fluid. Acta Obstet Gynecol Scand. 1995;74:707–13.
29. Joseph M, Dermot K, Sorin JB. Dilutional hyponatremia during endoscopic curettage: the "Femal TURP Syndrome"? Anesth Analg. 1994;78:1180–1.
30. Jeroen K, Henny R, Liesbeth B, Sjarlot K. Excessive fluid overload with severe hyponatremia, cardiac failure, and cerebral edema complicating hysteroscopic myomectomy: a case report and review of the literature. J Pelvic Med Surg. 2007;13(6):367–73.
31. Kirwan PH, Nakepace P, Layward E. Hyperammonaemia after transcervical resection of the endometrium. Br J Obstet Gynecol. 1993;100:600–4.
32. Lin BL. Transcervical resection of submucous myoma. Nippon-Sanka-Fujinka-Gakkai-Zasshi. 1986;38:1647–52. Japanese.
33. Lindemann HJ, Mohr J. CO2 hysteroscopy:diagnosis and treatment. Am J Obstet Gynecol. 1976;12:129–33.
34. Loffer FD. Complications of hysteroscopy-their cause, prevention, and correction. J Am Assoc Gynecol Laparosc. 1995;3:11–26.
35. Magos AL, Baumann R, Lockwood GM, Turnbull AC. Experience with the first 250 endometrial resections for menorrhagia. Lancet. 1991;337(8749):1074–8.
36. Maner P, Holl D. Transcervical endometrial resection for abnormal uterine bleeding. Aust N Z J Obstet Gynecol. 1990;30:357–60.
37. McLucas B. Intrauterine applications of the resectoscope. Surg Gynecol Obstet. 1991;172:425–31.
38. McSwiney M, Hargreaves M. Transcervical endometrial resection syndrome. Anaesthesia. 1995;50:254–8.
39. Mizutani AR, Parker J, Katz J, Schmidt J. Visual disturbances, serum glycine levels and transurethral resection of the prostate. J Urol. 1990;144(3):697–9.
40. Molnar BG, Broadbent JAM, Magos AL. Fluid overload risk score for endometrial resection. Gynaecol Endosc. 1992;1:133–8.
41. Morrison DM. Management of hysteroscopic surgery complication. ARON J. 1999;69(1):193–4.
42. Olsson J, Nisson A, Hahn RG. Symptoms of the irrigant. J Urol. 1995;154:123–8.
43. Qin X, Lu Y. Transurethral resection of prostate syndrome. Hua Xi Med. 2000;15(1):118–9. Chinese.
44. Quinones RG. Hysteroscopy with a new fluid technique. In: Siegler AM, Lindemann HJ, editors. Hysteroscopy. Principals and practice. Philadelphia: Lippincott; 1984. p. 41–2.
45. Carson SA, Hubert GD, Schriock ED, Buster JE. Hyperglycemia and hyponatremia during operative hysteroscopy with 5% dextrose in water distention. Fertil Steril. 1989;51(2):341–3.
46. Schäfer M, Von Ungern-Sternberg BS, Wight E, Schneider MC. Isotonic fluid absorption during hysteroscopy resulting in severe hyperchloremic acidosis. Anesthesiology. 2005;103(1):203–4.
47. Schlumbrecht M, Balgobin S, Word L. Pyometra after thermal endometrial ablation. Obstet Gynecol. 2007;110(2, Part 2 Suppl):538–40.
48. Shveiky D, Rojansky N, Revel A, Benshushan A, Laufer N, Shushan A. Complications of hysteroscopic surgery: "beyond the learning curve". J Minim Invasive Gynecol. 2007;14(2):218–22.
49. Singer M, Patel M, Webb AR, Bullen C. Management of the transurethral prostate resection syndrome: time for reappraisal? Crit Care Med. 1990;18(12):1479–80.
50. Stern RH. The management of symptomatic hyponatremia. Semin Nephrol. 1990;10:503–14.
51. Stern RH. The treatment of hyponatremia: first, do no harm. Am J Med. 1990;88:557–60.
52. Tao Z. Hypotonic hyponatremia. J Postgrad Med. 2000;23(7):54–7.
53. Vulgaropoulos SP, Haley LC, Hulga JF. Intrauterine pressure and fluid absorption during continuous flow hysteroscopy. Am J Obstet Gynecol. 1992;167:386–91.

54. Witz CA, Silverberg KM, Burns WN, Schenken RS, Olive DL. Complications associated with the absorption of hysteroscopic fluid media. Fertil Steril. 1993;60(5):745–56.
55. Xia EL, Felix W, Li Z. Gynecologic endoscopics. Beijing: People's Medical Publishing House; 2001. p. 220–2. Chinese.
56. Xia EL, Zhang M, Duan H. Analysis of 140 hysteroscopic electroresection. Chin J Pract Gynecol Obstet. 1994;(Suppl):135–6. Chinese.
57. Xia EL. Advances in hysteroscopic clinical applications. Chin J Pract Gynecol Obstet. 2006;22(1):18–23. Chinese.
58. Xia EL. Modern views on prevention of complications of hysteroscopy. J Int Obstet Gynecol. 2008;35(5):387–90. Chinese.
59. Xu G. Relations between hyposmolality and prognosis of congestive heart failure. Clin Focus. 2000;15(2):77–8. Chinese.
60. Ye Y, Wang Y. National guide to clinical laboratory procedures. Nan Jing: Southeast University Press; 1991. p. 168–9. Chinese.
61. Zhang Q, Zhao S, Chen X. Chronic pulmonary heart disease acute phase accompanied by moderate and severe hyonatremia in 35 cases. J Shanxi Med Univ. 2000;31(3):224–5. Chinese.
62. Zhang W, Ekengren J, Hahn RG. Large-sized bladders reduce intravesical pressure and fluid absorption during TURP using the suprapubic trocar. Urol Int. 1996;56(1):28–32.

7 Anesthesia for Hysteroscopy

Handong Cai

Hysteroscopy is a new technique for treatment of gynecological diseases which was developed in 1990s. It integrates optical fiber, photoelectricity, mini camera, image analysis, and imaging as a whole. When these high-tech instruments are in clinical use, due to its characteristic technique, adverse effects and severe complications may occur. Therefore, anesthetists must have sufficient knowledge related to this field and possess emergency treatment skills to deal with intraoperative accidents and complications.

7.1 Pre-anesthetic Assessment

Although the pre-anesthetic assessment of hysteroscopy is very similar to that of other surgery, large quantities of epidemiological studies showed that inadequate preparation before surgery was one of the main causes of postoperative complications and death. The saying "There is only a minor operation but no minor anesthesia" admonishes people to administer anesthesia cautiously and more importance should be attached to the pre-anesthetic assessment. The pre-anesthetic assessment should be conducted as follows.

7.1.1 Preoperative Visits on Patients and Participation in Preoperative Discussions

One to three days before the surgery, the anesthetist should go into the ward to visit the patient or participate in preoperative discussion. An anesthesia outpatient clinic should be established in hospitals with better conditions so as to conduct a pre-anesthetic assessment. This helps to establish the patient's senses of security and trust, relieve the possible physical and psychological damage to the patient caused by fear and tension, and also figure out the operation site, method, scope and position so that the anesthetic method, equipment, and pharmaceutical preparations can be determined. The patient should be told not to eat and drink 8–12 h before surgery, and both the patient and her family should be informed of the dangers of anesthesia, especially the occurrence of an anesthetic accident, which might endanger the patient's life. Their understandings and written signatures should be obtained before the surgery. As the legal system in our country has been gradually perfected, some hospitals have already implemented a notarized signature on the consent for anesthesia, which is helpful in the implementation of anesthesia.

7.1.2 Getting Familiar with the Patient's Medical History and Conducting a Systematic Physical Examination

The anesthetist must be especially clear about the patient's history of present illness and whether there is concomitant medical diseases, such as heart disease, hypertension, diabetes, liver and kidney disease, asthma, anemia, blood diseases, blood coagulation disorders, and anticoagulant therapy, whether they are already cured or still being treated, what medications are used, the therapeutic reactions, any history of drug allergy, which are directly related to the safety of anesthesia. Much importance should be attached to the past history and family history, like whether the patient has received anesthesia or not, its frequency, mode, and effect, and whether her family has had hereditary diseases, myasthenia gravis or malignant hyperthermia, which is directly related to the effects of anesthesia and prognosis. Therefore, the patient's general conditions must be systematically examined before surgery, including vital signs, heart and lung auscultation, extremities and spine, and nervous system so that an anesthetic plan can be determined.

H. Cai (✉)
Department of Anesthesiology, Fuxing Hospital, Capital Medical University, Beijing, China

E. Xia (ed.), *Practical Manual of Hysteroscopy*, https://doi.org/10.1007/978-981-19-1332-7_7

7.1.3 Examining and Checking the Essential Laboratory Parameters

1. Routine blood and urine test: It is mainly to find out whether the patient is anemic or not, and the degree of anemia and functions of the kidney.
2. Biochemical examination: It is to focus on the liver function, plasma protein, and albumin/globulin ratio, and serum concentration of potassium, sodium, and glucose. Some medical treatments like cardiotonic, diuretic, and hypoglycemic can lead to electrolyte imbalance.
3. Electrocardiogram (ECG) and chest X-ray: ECG and chest X-ray are to understand the cardiac electrophysiological activity, myocardial blood supply, and lung condition.
4. Other special examinations: Patients with heart and lung diseases should undergo examination of lung function, cardiac echocardiography, and blood gas analysis when necessary. Patients with a history of blood disease and anticoagulant therapy must have blood coagulation function.

7.1.4 Assessment of Anesthesia Risks

Anesthetists should consider whether the patient receives anesthesia in her best physical conditions before surgery, and whether the benefits brought to the patient by this surgery are more than the risks of anesthesia for surgery induced by the coexistent illnesses. Each of the following items may lead to complications during and after surgery and increase the danger of death.

1. Clinical assessment of American society of Anesthesiologists (ASA) is above grade III.
2. Heart failure, digitalis therapy, electrolyte imbalance.
3. Goldman's cardiac risk index is >25.
4. Lung disease and pulmonary abnormalities confirmed by chest X-ray.
5. Renal failure or metabolic acidosis.
6. Abnormal ECG.
7. Acute respiratory tract infection.
8. Severe anemia and hypoproteinemia.
9. Blood diseases related to blood coagulation dysfunction and inevitable anticoagulation therapy.

7.2 Anesthetic Methods and Choices for Hysteroscopy

Although hysteroscopy restricts its stimulation in cervical dilatation and intrauterine operation, since the splanchnic nerves governing the uterus are mainly from the sympathetic nerves of T_{10-12} and $L_{1\,\&\,2}$ and from the pelvic plexus composed of parasympathetic nerves of S_{2-4}, it easily leads to general reactions like reaction of artificial abortion syndrome (RAAS) (that is, bradycardia, arrhythmia, lowered blood pressure, nausea, vomiting, chest tightness, pale, sweating, and so on). Therefore, the anesthetic methods and choices are determined by the following points:

1. Whether diagnostic or therapeutic hysteroscope, flexible or rigid.
2. Non-hospitalized or hospitalized patients.
3. Whether the patients are cooperative mentally and psychologically.
4. The patients' requirements for anesthesia.
5. The surgeons` requirements for anesthesia and proficiency in operation techniques.
6. Duration of operation.

7.2.1 Topical Anesthesia

Topical anesthesia is a kind of anesthetic method by local spray of the anesthetics which has strong penetration and immediate effect into the cervical canal or into the uterine cavity. The commonly used medications are 0.5–1% tetracaine or 2% lidocaine by tamponade with cotton sticks into the cervical canal or by injection into the uterine cavity. Although the topical anesthesia can relieve the pain caused by uterine dilation and systemic adverse reactions, it cannot well relieve the nerve reflex symptoms during intrauterine operation, because it cannot completely block up the nerve reflex of submucosal layer and muscle layer to compression, stretching, and thermal effects of resection or coagulation. However, combined with neuroleptanesthesia, this method can be used for hysteroscopic biopsy and examination, TCRP, and other minitraumatic procedures.

7.2.2 Paracervical Nerve Block

Paracervical nerve block is administered with the cervical injection of 0.5 ml to 1 ml of 2% lidocaine at 4, 8, and 10 o'clock position and 0.5 cm to outer edge of cervix with 3 cm deep of the needle insertion, which can loosen cervical canal in 92% of patients and reduce the incidence of RAAS significantly. Theoretically the paracervical nerve block with high concentration and high volume can be more effective, but there exists injection pain and systemic toxic reactions, and the nerve reflexes of the fundus and the corpus cannot be completely released.

7.2.3 Epidural Anesthesia and Subarachnoid Block

Epidural anesthesia consists of continuous epidural anesthesia and single epidural anesthesia, and is a widely used and skillful anesthetic method. It can modify the duration and the level of anesthesia freely according to the length of operative time and the doctor's proficiency. The advantages are: (1) the block is perfect and can be easily controlled after successful puncture; (2) it can release the stress reaction and reduce the occurrence of increased blood pressure and tachycardia; (3) the gastrointestinal peristalsis can be improved, the abdominal distention can be reduced, and the tension of parasympathetic nerves is increased due to a sympathetic nerve block; (4) the patients remain conscious during operation so they can tell about the possible adverse effects immediately, such as TURP syndrome; (5) nausea, vomiting, and lethargy are decreased after operation; (6) it can also be used to provide analgesia after operation. However, there are also some disadvantages. The failure rate is higher because of the higher requirement for skills in anesthetic procedures. The onset time for anesthesia is relatively longer and there's possibility of total spinal anesthesia. Some patients may have coagulation disorders, hemodynamic instability or spinal deformity, which should be contraindications for epidural or spinal anesthesia. Although the subarachnoid block can be easily administered and perfect block can be achieved, it is not suitable for the non-hospitalized patients, and it can produce great effects on hemodynamics, especially in the young and adults. Due to a higher incidence of postoperative headache, it is rarely used clinically.

7.2.4 General Anesthesia

Hysteroscopic surgery is limited inside the uterine cavity and the operation time is shorter, so general anesthesia is not necessary. However, with the improvement of people's life quality, knowledge, and awareness, more and more patients demand to spend the perioperative period quietly, smoothly, and painlessly, so general intravenous anesthesia is usually adopted. The anesthetic agent should be selected with a short acting time, rapid recovery, good analgesic effect, and few side effects. Ketamine in sub-anesthetic dose was adopted more often in the past, which had the analgesic effect of 80–90%. However, it could not totally inhibit RAAS, and an increase in muscular tension might cause difficulty in uterine dilatation. Vomiting and more secretions in oral cavity and respiratory tract are more likely to cause upper airway obstruction and aspiration. And the patients may become excited, dysphoria, develop nightmare, and disturbance in psychology, so ketamine is rarely used now.

7.2.4.1 Intravenous Anesthesia

With the development and application of new intravenous anesthetics in recent years, clinical anesthesiologists can choose general anesthetic drugs more flexibly in according to the patient's condition. The more commonly used anesthetic drugs in China are etomidate and propofol, while a single dose of alfentanil or sufentanil is more frequently used abroad. These anesthetics have relatively fewer side effects, safe and reliable, and the patients can wake up quickly after operation. Alfentanil is especially good with perfect analgesia, and can separate analgesia from consciousness, so the patients seldom feel painful at the end of operation or have any memory of the process of operation. It has a short acting time, but may cause transient respiratory depression at a large dose, most of which can be relieved spontaneously.

1. Etomidate: Etomidate is the derivative of imidazole. Given a dose of 0.1–0.3 mg/kg, a patient may wake up naturally in 7–14 min, without any mental disorders but high incidence of vomiting. The patient may feel pain at the injection position and may have body movement as well. This drug can also inhibit the adrenal cortex function. If used together with low dose of fentanyl, etomidate can produce perfect analgesia, immediate wake up, and fewer side effects.
2. Propofol: Propofol works quickly and has a short duration. The patients may recover quickly and smoothly, meanwhile, this drug is antiemetic to a certain extent. The commonly used dosage is 2.5–3 mg/kg, which can last 8–10 min. After first administration, an intravenous drip of 3–4 mg/(kg·h) is given continuously, which can optionally prolong the duration of anesthesia without changing the time of waking up. However, there has also been transient respiratory and circulatory depressions. Therefore, the anesthetists are required to be armed with the assisted ventilation equipment and techniques.
3. Alfentanil: The potency ratio of alfentanil to fentanyl is 8:1, and its onset of effects and the duration of action is 1/3 of that of fentanyl. Alfentanil does not accumulate, has little influence on cardiovascular system, and separates the analgesic effect from the patient's consciousness. The usual dosage is 30–50 μg/kg and the analgesic effect maintains for 15–20 min.
4. Ketamine: It has strong analgesic effect with the usual dosage at hysteroscopy 0.3–1.3 mg/kg, and it is administered via intravenous injection after dilution. Ketamine with such a sub-anesthetics dose has little influence on breathing with rapid wake up time, but its disadvantages include muscle tension, vomiting, more respiratory secretions, excitement, nightmares, and so on.
5. Remifentanil: It is an ultrashort acting opioid μ-receptor agonist, with features of prompt onset of effect, short duration of action, and no accumulation, so it is widely used clinically. Its advantages are that it is metabolized and eliminated rapidly with $t_{1/2}$Keo[1] 3–4 min; it is metabolized through non-specific plasma and tissue esterases so it can be safely used in patients with liver and kidney dysfunction. Its analgesic potency is 50–100 times that of

[1]Keo, the rate constant of medicine transferring from effect compartment to central compartment; $t_{1/2}$keo, half-time of equilibration between drug concentration in the blood and effect compartment.

fentanyl and 20–50 times that of alfentanil. The usual dosage of Remifentanil is 0.25–1 μg/kg via intravenous drip, and its analgesic effect may last 3–10 min. Larger dosage or too fast intravenous drip may also result in bradycardia, nausea, vomiting, and respiratory depression.

6. Target-controlled infusion (TCI) of propofol-opioid: With the development of computer technology, in 1992, Kenny et al. produced computer-assisted titration intravenous anesthetics and microcomputer-controlled infusion pump, which target the plasma or effect compartment as the regulation index and simultaneously display the target plasma concentration, the effect compartment concentration, the administration time, and the cumulative dose, and the maximum dosage can be restricted as well. At present, target-controlled infusion of propofol-opioid has been widely used in clinical anesthesia and analgesia. There are two kinds of commonly used TCI systems, that is: Diprifusor and Fresenius base primea, which can administer dual or multichannel target-controlled infusion of analgesia-sedatives. Nowadays, the target-controlled infusion of propofol-remifentanil is usually used with propofol 0.8 μg/L and remifentanil 0.2–2 μg/L. They have better analgesic and sedative effects, and is also suitable for examination and surgical treatment for old and weak women or women with more complications.

7.2.4.2 General Anesthesia Using Laryngeal Mask Airway

Laryngeal Mask Airway (LMA), which was developed by British anesthesiologist Dr. Brain in 1981, was an artificial airway device basing on the study of the anatomy of the adult's upper airway. LMA is divided into three categories according to its sequence of development and its applications: the first generation is a simple airway tube; the second generation is intubating LMA (LMA-Fastrach); the third generation is LMA double tube (ProSeal-LMA). The advantages of LMA are: (1) it is convenient and speedy to use, and easy to maintain the airway; (2) it does not need a laryngoscope, and there are less difficulty and higher success rate for beginners when compared with tracheal intubation; (3) for long time operations without the requirement of relaxing the muscles, LMA takes over the function of a mask; (4) it can establish an airway so as to permit a spontaneous or a controlled ventilation; (5) the patency of the airway can be maintained even if the position of LMA is not optimal; (6) the damage to mucous membrane of the trachea is avoided; (7) the patient can tolerate the LMA at a lighter level of anesthesia, which need less dosage of anesthetic than an endotracheal catheter; (8) the stability of hemodynamics is increased during the anesthetic induction and recovery period, the degree of increased intraocular pressure is reduced when inserting the tube, the occurrence of cough is lessened and the oxygen saturation is increased at recovery period, and the occurrence rate of throat pain after operations in adult is reduced.

For various hysteroscopic operations such as removal of submucous fibroid, severe intrauterine adhesions, endometrial polyps and hyperplasia, and congenital uterine abnormalities, due to their long duration of procedures, LMA should be inserted under intravenous anesthesia to ensure the effective ventilation. In addition to ensuring the ventilation, it can also reduce the possibility of both reflux and aspiration, and perform mechanical ventilation and inhalation anesthesia. However, it is necessary to obtain the indications of LMA. Patients who have the probability of reflux and aspiration, including maxillofacial or oropharyngeal deformation, adenoidal hypertrophy, and satiety intestinal obstruction, should be considered to be absolute contraindications.

7.2.4.3 Inhalation Anesthesia

Some of hysteroscopic surgery may be completed under simple inhalation anesthesia. The anesthetic gas is taken with a certain concentration via respiratory tract to keep a proper depth of anesthesia. At present, the inhaled anesthetic gas is nitrous oxide, and the volatile agents are fluorine-containing anesthetics including enflurane, isoflurane, sevoflurane, desflurane, etc. Because nitrous oxide has a weak anesthetic effect and a risk of oxygen lack when being taken at a high concentration, it is hardly used by itself to maintain the anesthesia. The volatile anesthetics (e.g. sevoflurane, desflurane) has a strong anesthetic effect and cause the patient to lose her consciousness and sense of pain when being taken at a high concentration, so it can maintain the anesthesia on its own. However, its muscle-relaxing effect is not satisfying. If the muscle-relaxing effect was blindly pursued, an anesthetist certainly would increase the concentration of inhalation drugs. The higher the concentration of inhalation drugs are, the more serious the influence of it on physiology is. Therefore, nitrous oxide (N_2O) is often administrated in combination with oxygen (O_2) clinically, with the concentration of nitrous oxide 50–70%. The concentration of the volatile anesthetics can be regulated as required and adding some muscle relaxants when muscle relaxation is needed. Muscle relaxants cannot only relax the muscles, but also enhance the anesthetic effect so that it can reduce the influence of deep anesthesia to physiology. When nitrous oxide is applied, the flow meter of anesthesia machine must be precise. The fraction of inspired oxygen and oxygen saturation (SPO_2) should be monitored with the fraction of inspired oxygen no more than 30% being considered as safety. Volatile anesthetics should adopt special evaporator to control the concentration of inhalation. The concentration of the anesthetics should be monitored continuously if it is possible, which permit a better control of the depth of anesthesia.

General anesthesia with endotracheal intubation can be performed if it is necessary so as to ensure the patient's safety.

7.3 Intraoperative Surveillance During Hysteroscopic Surgery

The specificity of anesthesia for hysteroscopy lies in that the anesthesiologists should know about some potential adverse reactions (such as TURP syndrome) and complications related to surgical operation. Therefore, through surveillance and analysis of the physiological parameters and its changes, the anesthesiologists may detect the problem as early as possible, judge its seriousness, and provide early diagnosis so as to provide better anesthetic support and physiological protection for treatment of surgical complications.

7.3.1 Routine Monitoring

7.3.1.1 Electrocardiogram (ECG)

ECG need to be routinely monitored in the elderly or the patients with congenital or acquired heart disease. Due to the influence of electric cutting or electrocoagulation on cardiac electrophysiology in the process of anesthesia and operation, ECG can detect the changes in myocardial ischemia and cardiac arrhythmia as early as possible.

7.3.1.2 Blood Pressure

Blood pressure is determined by the cardiac output, blood volume, and systemic vascular resistance. Hypotension may occur due to relatively insufficient blood volume after the spinal anesthesia, and hypertension would result from high blood volume if the operative time is long and the perfusion pressure is high when fluid is used for uterine distention. Once hypertension or hypotension occurs, the anesthesiologists should determine the underlying cause as early as possible so as to administer the correct treatment.

7.3.1.3 Monitoring of Pulse Oxygen Saturation (SpO_2)

It may detect hypoxic hypoxia and pulsatile blood flow, and displays continuously gas exchange in the lungs, such as oxyhemoglobin saturation and central oxygenation status. Quite a few gynecologic patients are anemia when they have hysteroscopy. If the patient's hemoglobin is 5–6 g, the oxygen content will be insufficient but the oxygen saturation will be satisfactory; if the patient suffers from hypotension or low cardiac pump function, the pulsatile blood flow will decrease but the oxygen saturation will be normal. Therefore, there is less value and fewer importance for oxygen saturation in the diagnosis of anemic anoxia and early hypotension.

7.3.1.4 Auscultation in the Precordium and Inside the Esophagus

Heart sounds, respiratory rate, and ventilation can be monitored but the respiratory mode cannot be recognized. When gas is used for uterine distention, gas embolism can be easily induced, which can be detected early by this kind of auscultation. If abnormal breath sound and heart sound are detected with auscultation, the operation should be terminated immediately and timely treatment should be given without any delay.

7.3.2 Special Monitoring

7.3.2.1 Monitoring of Electrolyte

It is mainly the monitoring of the sodium concentration. 98% of osmotic pressure is provided by electrolyte, in which sodium takes up almost half. Nausea and discomfort will occur if sodium concentration is <125 mmol/L; headache, fatigue, and unresponsiveness will occur if it is between 110 mmol/L and 120 mmol/L; convulsions and coma will occur if it is <110 mmol/L. During hysteroscopic resection of uterine fibroids, if the uterine distension pressure is >100 cmH_2O at a large perfusion flow rate or the patient is in a state of low blood pressure, dilutional hyponatremia is apt to occur, which may provide a sound basis for prevention and treatment of acute water intoxication.

7.3.2.2 Blood Glucose Monitoring

There are three kinds of uterine distending media for hysteroscopy. The commonly used fluid presently is 5% glucose, so it is quite necessary to determine the blood glucose concentration quickly at regular time interval. Once there is significant increase in the blood glucose, it is suggestive of excessive absorption of irrigating or distending fluid.

7.3.2.3 Monitoring of Central Venous Pressure (CVP)

An increase in CVP indicates the increase in effective blood volume, and there is an earlier change in CVP than in blood pressure, which can be accordingly taken as the pre-symptom of dilutional hyponatremia. However, its sensitivity is not the same as in monitoring of pulmonary capillary wedge pressure (PCWP), so it would be safer to instruct the treatment if it is in line with the monitoring of PCWP.

7.3.2.4 Noninvasive Estimation of Extravascular Lung Water (EVLW)

Any changes in capillary wall filtration and differences between capillary internal and external hydrostatic pressure and colloid osmotic pressure caused by any reasons may all lead to pulmonary edema monitoring of the thoracic fluid index (TFI) by use of impedance cardiogram (ICG) can distinguish cardiogenic edema from noncardiogenic edema.

7.4 Prevention and Treatment of Complications During Hysteroscopy

The following complications are usually found out by anesthetists first.

7.4.1 Mechanical Injury

The statistical data showed that the incidence of uterine perforation was about 2% in hysteroscopic examination and surgery, which resulted from physiological and pathological causes, including those being related to abnormal positions of the uterus, such as anteverted or retroverted uterus, anatomical abnormalities, uterine atrophy or hypoplasia, intrauterine adhesions and cervical stenosis, and also those being related to unsatisfactory uterine distension during surgical operation. Uterine rupture can occur due to cervical perforation and tearing, and creation of false passages, during the process of cervical dilation or intrauterine operation. For instance, if perforation occurs due to electrocautery, electroresection, laser knife or some sharp instruments, the damaged sites might not heal spontaneously; if the perforated sites were near the uterine cornua and adnexa, heavy bleeding may occur because of the rich blood supply; if a large amount of distention medium (gas or fluid) was absorbed into the circulation, metabolic, and circulatory disorders such as anemia could happen. As a result, the surgeons must cautiously select suitable patients undergoing hysteroscopy, master the hysteroscopic instruments skillfully, use uterine distention pump with adjustable flow rate to expand the uterine cavity, so that they can achieve an optimal surgical view and improve the safety of surgery.

7.4.2 Bleeding

Heavy bleeding induced by hysteroscopy is relatively rare unless there is simultaneous uterine perforation. However, some patients are suffering from coagulation disorders or have been taking non-steroidal anti-inflammatory drugs and anticoagulant therapy due to cardiovascular diseases for a long term, especially aspirin, which may lead to heavy bleeding. Coagulation disorders should be treated preoperatively, and surgical treatment can be administered in patients only after 7–14d discontinuation of aspirin. Some literatures reported that the duration of discontinued use of aspirin should be more than 20 days.

7.4.3 Gas Embolism

It mostly occurs in cases using gas (CO_2) as uterine distending medium. Some literatures showed that a gas flow of 90 mL/s could be produced when the pressure gradient between vein cut and distending pressure was >4 mmHg. Obvious symptoms would appear if it was absorbed by air bubbles [0.5 mL/(kg·min)]. And it may cause death in patients with poor cardiac function. Its main manifestations are abnormal ECG and blood gas values, hypotension, characteristic heart murmurs—metal murmur or water-wheel murmur. Once suspected gas embolism occurs, uterine cavity distension should be stopped immediately, and the surgical position should be changed to left lateral decubitus position or head-down tilt position in order to elevate the venous pressure, and the bubbles should be suctioned via right heart catheter when necessary.

7.4.4 TURP Syndrome

Excessive absorption of uterine distending fluid during hysteroscopy under the elevated pressure may also lead to acute water intoxication which is similar to TURP syndrome. The occurrence of TURP syndrome is subject to the type of distention fluid, as well as the amount and the rate of absorption. Acute water intoxication is mostly caused by intravascular absorption, that is, the distending medium directly enters the blood vessels via injured small vein or sinusoids. However, the absorption of distention fluid via defective endometrium or extravascular absorption of distention fluid which enters the abdominal cavity via fallopian tubes can promote the hypotonic solution into the extravascular space, resulting in delayed hyponatremia.

The amount and the rate of fluid absorption are determined by the following situations. (1) pressure of distention fluids: It is a key factor for the amount of absorption. Large amounts of distention medium can also be absorbed even if the pressure is less than 60 cmH_2O. And an equally important factor is the duration of pressure. (2) Operative time: The duration of operation is mainly related to the amount of intravascular absorption. It is generally believed that severe TURP syndrome would not occur if the operative time is within 60 min, but there is also a report on the occurrence of acute water toxication only 15 min after the start of surgery. (3) The volume of the fibroids and the area of the endometrium to be resected. (4) Blood loss: The amount of distention medium absorption is positively correlated with blood loss, as the flow rate of perfusion fluid needed is also larger when there's more blood loss. (5) the looseness of cervical canal and the opening degree of the outflow stopcock of hysteroscope: Poor drainage and elevated intrauterine pressure can also lead to great volume and fast rate of fluid absorption.

Generally speaking, elevated blood pressure, slow pulse, and mentally abnormal excitement are the three early signs of acute water intoxication. Significant decrease in plasma colloid osmotic pressure can lead to noncardiogenic pulmonary edema, and the patient will manifest as hypoxemia, such as shortness of breath, pink frothy sputum, lips cyanosis, and so on. Serious reduction in serum sodium concentration can lead to low electrolyte cardiovascular collapse, and the patient will manifest as hypotension, headache, nausea, vomiting, blurred vision, disturbance of consciousness, and even tonic convulsions and coma if not treated in time.

Once TURP syndrome occurs, operation should be stopped immediately, the normal blood volume should be actively recovered, and the venous return should be reduced. The serum sodium concentration and plasma osmotic pressure should be monitored frequently, and excessive water should be excreted so as to correct hyponatremia.

1. Application of furosemide: The volume of distention fluid absorption dilutes the Na^+ in the blood, which inhibits the diuretic action of the osmotic diuretic substances in distention fluid. Therefore, furosemide should be given routinely and cardiac therapy is necessary if the patient is with severe pulmonary edema.
2. Application of hypertonic saline solution: 3–5% sodium chloride solution can be used to correct the abnormal blood volume and hyponatremia, and can also have a function of osmotic diuresis so as to relieve the intracellular edema.
3. In case of non-cardiogenic pulmonary edema, the patient may have great amounts of pink frothy sputum and cyanosis. The transfusion of crystalloid solution should be limited, and colloidal solution should be given appropriately together with 40% ethanol atomization oxygen inhalation.
4. Maintaining a lower intraoperative distention pressure at about 60 cmH_2O whenever possible, using non-hemolytic isotonic or hypotonic uterine distention medium and shortening the operation time as far as possible are the main measures for prevention of TURP syndrome.

Suggested Reading

1. Gustorff B, Hoechtl K, Sycha T, Felouzis E, Lehr S, Kress HG. The effects of remifentanil and gabapentin on hyperalgesia in a new extended inflammatory skin pain model in healthy volunteers. Anesth Analg. 2004;98(2):401–7.
2. Jeffery LP. Complications of endoscopic and laparoscopic surgery. New York: Lipincott Raven; 1997. p. 233–41.
3. Liu X, Cao J, Zheng L. Clinical anesthesia implementation program. Bei Jing: The People's Medical Publishing House; 2000. p. 94–9. Chinese.
4. Viviand X, Fabre G, Ortéga D, Dayan A, Boubli L, Martin C. Target-controlled sedation-analgesia using propofol and remifentanil in women undergoing late termination of pregnancy. Int J Obstet Anesth. 2003;12(2):83–8.
5. Wiebe ER. Comparison of the efficacy of different local anaesthetics and techniques of local anaesthesia in therapeutic abortions. Am J Obstet Gyneol. 1992;167(1):131–4.
6. Wiebe ER, Rauling M. Pain control in abortion. In J Gynecol Obstet. 1995;50(1):41–6.

8 Diagnostic Hysteroscopy

Enlan Xia and Dan Yu

Diagnostic hysteroscopy can be used to directly investigate intrauterine lesions and localize them for biopsy, so it is more intuitive, accurate, and reliable than traditional diagnostic dilatation and curettage (D&C), hysterosalpingography (HSG), and ultrasonography. Hysteroscopy can reduce the rate of missed diagnosis, significantly improve the accuracy of diagnosis, and has been reputed to be the golden standard of modern diagnosis of intrauterine lesions. Dotto et al. classified the endometrial images under hysteroscope into five categories: normal endometrium, benign lesions, low-risk endometrial hyperplasia, high-risk endometrial hyperplasia, and endometrial cancer, which were highly consistent with the findings of endometrial biopsy. Clark et al. reviewed 65 articles and studied the accuracy of hysteroscopy in diagnosis of endometrial cancer and hyperplasia in women with abnormal uterine bleeding. They found that in all patients included, the pretest probability of endometrial cancer was 3.9%, which was increased to 71.8% by a positive result of hysteroscopy and was reduced to 0.6% by a negative result. Thus, it was considered that the accuracy of hysteroscopy for endometrial cancer was high, but was only applicable to endometrial disease. Agostini et al. made a review and analysis of 17 cases who were diagnosed pathologically to have endometrial atypical hyperplasia after hysteroscopic resection. One case was discovered to have endometrial adenocarcinoma, with the risk of 5.9% (1/17). Nowadays, diagnostic hysteroscopy has become a new and valuable gynecological diagnostic technique. Applications of micro-devices and non-invasive techniques have expanded the use of hysteroscopy from out-patient clinic to movable stations. Nagele et al. suggested that outpatient hysteroscopy had a high detection rate for intrauterine lesions and simple hysteroscopic surgeries could be performed at the same time. Therefore, just as D&C in the twentieth century, hysteroscopy has been considered as a routine method for diagnosis of intrauterine lesions in the twenty-first century.

E. Xia (✉) · D. Yu
Hysteroscopy Center, Fuxing Hospital, Capital Medical University, Beijing, China

8.1 Hysteroscopy

Enlan Xia and Dan Yu

8.1.1 Indications for Hysteroscopy

Any intrauterine pathologies which are suspected in any form or need to be diagnosed and treated are indications of hysteroscopy.

8.1.1.1 Abnormal Uterine Bleeding (AUB)

It is abnormal bleeding occurring in women of child-bearing age, or in perimenopausal women and postmenopausal women, which includes menorrhagia, epimenorrhea, prolonged menstruation, irregular bleeding, and pre-menopausal and post-menopausal uterine bleeding, all of which are the main indications for hysteroscopy. Nagele et al. reported that AUB was the most common indication for hysteroscopy (87%). For women of child-bearing age with abnormal bleeding, abnormal pregnancies, such as threatened abortion, ectopic pregnancy, etc. should first be excluded. As for pre-menopausal and post-menopausal abnormal bleeding, the patient should be alerted to the possibility of endometrial carcinoma and the uterine-distending pressure cannot be too high during hysteroscopy so as not to cause the cancer cells to spread into the abdominal cavity.

8.1.1.2 Abnormal Sonographic Findings in Uterine Cavity

A number of imaging techniques such as ultrasound, HSG, CT, MRI, sonohysterography (SHSG), saline infusion sonohysteroscopy (SIS), and television color doppler (TVCD) may be used to indirectly visualize the endometrial activity. With diagnostic hysteroscopy, intrauterine lesions can be

E. Xia (ed.), *Practical Manual of Hysteroscopy*, https://doi.org/10.1007/978-981-19-1332-7_8

directly identified, evaluated, and located, while the suspected lesions can be biopsied for histological and cytological examination. As for patients with infertility and recurrent pregnancy loss, under hysteroscopy, anatomical morphology of the uterine cavity and the tubal ostia should be observed to see whether there are uterine malformations, intrauterine adhesions, submucous myomas, etc. In addition, the mucosa of endometrium should be observed to see whether there is endometrial hyperplasia or endometrial polyp, and target biopsy should be done on suspected areas.

8.1.1.3 Infertility

Intrauterine factors for infertility can be found under hysteroscopy. Li analyzed the results of diagnostic hysteroscopy in 259 patients with infertility. The results showed that 120 cases (46.33%) had intrauterine lesions, with endometrial polyps in 42 cases (35%), uterine malformation in 37 cases (30.83%), intrauterine adhesions in 23 cases (19.17%), endometrial diseases in 10 cases (8.33%), intrauterine foreign body in one case (0.83%), and submucous myoma in 6 cases (5%).

8.1.1.4 Physiological or Characteristic Changes Caused by Tamoxifen or Hormone Replacement Therapy (HRT)

Due to the estrogen effect of the drugs, long-term use of tamoxifen or estrogenic hormones can lead to endometrial hyperplasia, formation of polyps, and even endometrial carcinogenesis, which need assessment under hysteroscope.

Abnormal findings of endometrial aspiration cytology or endometrial histopathology. Sometimes hysteroscopy is needed for localization of the lesions and sampling.

8.1.1.5 Secondary Dysmenorrhea

It is often caused by intrauterine abnormalities including submucous myomas, endometrial polyps or intrauterine adhesions, and hysteroscopy should be the preferred diagnostic method.

8.1.1.6 After Complex Intrauterine Operations

Secondary hysteroscopy is done 6–8 weeks after the original operation so as to diagnose and divide early filmy adhesions.

8.1.1.7 Staging of the Endometrial Carcinoma

Diagnostic hysteroscopy can be used to observe whether there is any invasion on the mucosa of the cervical canal. Garuti et al. reported that the predictive values of hysteroscopy on cervical spreading of endometrial carcinoma had a sensitivity of 100% and specificity of 87.3%. Hysteroscopy was highly accurate in excluding the spread to cervix.

8.1.1.8 Uterine Myomas

When an operation is to be determined in a patient with multiple myomas, hysteroscopy should be used to detect the existence of submucous myomas.

8.1.1.9 Examination of Intrauterine Device

Hysteroscopy can be used to observe the location of IUD, and detect whether there is embedment.

8.1.1.10 Abnormal Vaginal Discharge

Patients with endometrial cancer sometimes visit the hospital due to abnormal vaginal discharge. In Fuxing hospital, ultrasonography showed no abnormality in a patient who has had vaginal discharge of colorless and transparent liquid for 2 years. High-differentiated adenocarcinoma was confirmed by diagnostic hysteroscopy.

8.1.2 Contraindications for Hysteroscopy

8.1.2.1 Absolute Contraindications

It has been said that there were no absolute contraindications for diagnostic hysteroscopy. As the procedure of hysteroscopy would spread the inflammation, some surgeons considered the following points as absolute contraindications. In these cases, anti-infective treatment should be given firstly, and the hysteroscopy deferred until the infection is controlled.

1. Acute endometritis.
2. Acute salpingitis.
3. Acute pelvic inflammatory disease.

8.1.2.2 Relative Contraindications

Some scholars did not consider the following conditions as contraindications but only as precautions during hysteroscopy.

1. Massive uterine bleeding: The vision of hysteroscopy may be all covered by blood when there are heavy bleeding, which not only makes lesions difficult to be detected, but also increases bleeding.
2. Pregnancy: The hysteroscopy may cause abortion.
3. Chronic pelvic inflammatory disease: The hysteroscopy may cause the spread of inflammation.

8.1.3 Preoperative Evaluation

Comprehensive evaluations and preparations should be done on patients who are going to undergo hysteroscopy, which includes the confirmation of examination indications:

whether the patient has hypertension or diabetes, whether the patient can tolerate the discomfort caused by a relatively longer period of lithotomy position and uterine distension, the degree of cervical relaxation, whether there are risk factors such as damage and infection of viscera, whether it is possible to be treated in one procedure, etc. Therefore, decision should be made on whether an anesthesia is needed and which is the best anesthesia; selecting and preparing the equipment, and whether it is necessary to use prophylactic antibiotics; etc.

8.1.3.1 Patient's History

The patient's general condition and past history should be inquired in detail, and attention should be paid to whether the patient has suffered from some important viscera diseases, such as heart, lung, liver and kidney, etc.; and whether there is a bleeding tendency or a history of diabetes. In addition, the possibility of pregnancy must be excluded before operation in patients with irregular menstruation.

8.1.3.2 Physical Examination

Blood pressure, pulse, and temperature should be routinely measured and the cardiorespiratory function should be checked. Attention should be paid to whether there is pelvic inflammation and acute vaginitis. For patients with inflammation, treatment must be administered first, and hysteroscopy cannot be performed until the inflammation is controlled.

8.1.3.3 Laboratory Examination

Routine urine and blood tests should be done. If the patient's urine glucose is positive, the fasting blood glucose should be measured so as to choose a proper distending fluid. The tests of the vaginal secretions include cleanliness, candida, trichomonas, etc. If necessary, cervical secretions should be taken to detect chlamydia pneumoniae, mycoplasma pneumoniae, and neisseria gonorrhoeae. Routine examination of the cervical cytology and some indicators such as liver and kidney function, and hepatitis B surface antigen should be carried out.

8.1.3.4 Psychological Counseling

Doctors should carefully explain the process of hysteroscopy and the necessity of hysteroscopy so as to get the patient's understanding and cooperation, which may be helpful in getting a satisfactory diagnosis result and successful completion of operation, and even reduce the demand for anesthesia. It has ever been said that the doctors' explanation is the best medicine and the noninvasive technique is the best anesthesia, which supports the importance of psychological counselling.

8.1.4 Uterine Distention System in Hysteroscopy

Under normal conditions, the anterior and posterior walls of uterine cavity are close to each other. So the observation of the uterine cavity can only be achieved when the uterine cavity is distended artificially by injection of the distending medium.

8.1.4.1 Fluid Medium for Uterine Distention

Uterine Distending Equipment

An infusion bottle may be used to connect with the inflow pipes and distend the uterine cavity with the pressure produced by gravity, that is, the height difference between the cavity and the fluid surface. Or an automatic fluid uterine-distending pump can be used to distend the cavity, with which the pressure and the flow rate can be set to keep the uterine cavity expanded continuously. The distending pressure should be set less than 100 mmHg. If there is no automatic distension pump and the uterine cavity had to be distended by the pressure caused by liquid level differences, the compression belt or the three-tee tubes could be used to elevate the pressure when it is not high enough.

Distention Medium

Sufficient distension of the uterine cavity and clear bloodless vision are the important factors for hysteroscopic examination and surgery. The fluid distention medium cannot only expand the uterine cavity, but also flush the objective lens so as to avoid being stained by blood, mucus, and intrauterine floaters, thus the field of view is kept clear.

1. Normal saline: It is isotonic solution, with the refractive index of 1.37, and can wash away the intrauterine debris and blood clot easily, but it has a worse viscosity and can be blended with the blood easily, which affects the field of view.
2. 5% glucose solution: It has a relatively high viscosity and clear field of view, but it makes the surfaces of equipment and gloves sticky when used, which is uncomfortable.
3. Hyskon solution: It is a high-viscosity uterine distending medium, and is a mixture of 32% dextran-70 and 10% glucose. Its advantages include high viscosity, fewer amount used, not easy to mix with blood and mucus, and it is especially applicable to patients with metrorrhagia. The disadvantages are its expensiveness, difficulty in cleansing, and that all equipment must be soaked in hot water after being used so as not to form deposit on the surface of the pipes or the lens because the deposit could lead to damage of the equipment easily. Moreover, there had also been reports of cases with allergy.

8.1.4.2 Gas as Uterine Distention Medium

1. Uterine distending equipment: When an automatic CO_2 insufflation machine is used (Fig. 8.1), the distention pressure and flow rate can be controlled and regulated according to the requirement of the procedures. When CO_2 was originally used to expand the uterus, gas embolisms had occurred which resulted in death in some cases. The invention of CO_2 insufflator has greatly increased the safety of CO_2 distention, which is now very popular and mostly used in Europe and America. The flow rate of CO_2 insufflation is set at 30–80 mL/min and the pressure is set below 100 mmHg. During the hysteroscopic procedures with CO_2 insufflation, if there is intrauterine bleeding, the objective lens would be contaminated by blood, which could not be removed and would make the observation impossible, and this is its shortcoming.
2. Uterine-distending gas: The ideal gas used as distending medium should be highly soluble, non-flammable, non-explosive, easy to be absorbed and have no adverse reaction. CO_2 is a natural gas inside human body and can be quickly absorbed after being insufflated. Due to its high viscosity, CO_2 is not likely to cause gas embolism after entering the blood. Furthermore, it does not cause any damage to the equipment, is effective in distending the cavity and does not produce any allergic reaction. The refractive index of CO_2 is 1.00. Compared with other media, it has a relatively large field of view and high definition. All of these make it the most ideal uterine distending gas.

The shortcomings of CO_2 as a distention medium include: (1) A special insufflating machine is needed, which is not as simple and convenient as that required for fluid distention medium; (2) it may cause intrauterine bubbles or an increase in mucus secretion; (3) it can be dangerous if improperly used. If the distending pressure is too high, the chances of CO_2 entering the blood vessels would increase, which lead to potential dangers including acidosis, arrhythmia, heart failure, and gas embolism, and is even life-threatening in severe cases.

CO_2 is a kind of excellent uterine distending medium, especially for diagnostic hysteroscopy or hysteroscopy without intrauterine operation. The field of view is especially clear with the use of gas insufflation. However, in the implementation of hysteroscopic operation, gas medium is not very satisfactory. Intraoperative bleeding and smoke or bubble produced by cauterized tissue make the field of view blurred, which hinders the accomplishment of the operation. Therefore, gas distending medium is rarely used in operative hysteroscopy.

A comparison of distention media between CO_2 and fluid is made in Table 8.1.

Table 8.1 Comparison of distention media between CO_2 and fluid

Items	CO_2	Fluid
Definition of image	Relatively good	Good
Angle of view	Wide	Relatively narrow
Hysteroscopic embryo transplantation or artificial tubal insemination	Applicable	Not applicable
Examination when bleeding	Difficult	Easy
Insertion of the scope under direct vision	Difficult	Easy
Observation of blood vessels in the diseased area	Difficult	Easy
Difficulty in observation induced by bubbles	Often occur	No
Contamination of objective lens	Often occur	Few
Observation of myomas or polyps in the posterior wall of uterine cavity	Difficult	Easy
Pain after examination	Relatively strong	Few
Distention equipment	Necessary	Not necessary
Gas embolism	Possible	Impossible
Floor contamination	No	Often

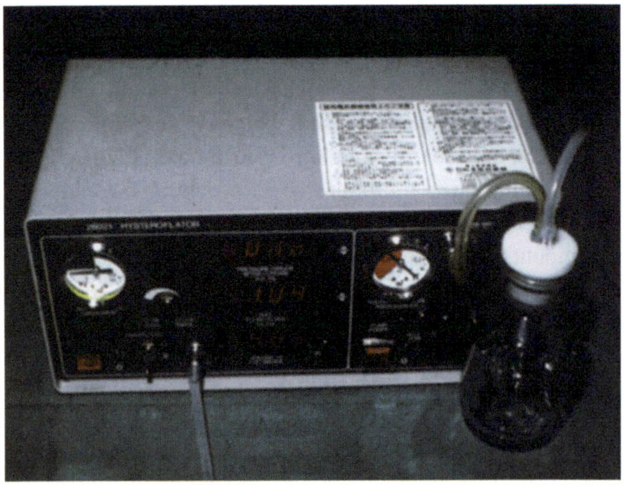

Fig. 8.1 CO_2 insufflator

8.1.5 Timing of Hysteroscopy

Generally, the ideal time for doing hysteroscopy is within 5 days after menstruation except for special conditions. During this early proliferative phase, the endometrium is thin with less mucus and not easy to bleed, so the intrauterine lesions are more easily seen, which makes a satisfactory observation. For the patients with irregular bleeding, hysteroscopy can be done at any time after the bleeding has stopped. If hysteroscopy is necessary to be done during uterine bleeding period, it can be performed after administration of antibiotics as appropriate.

8.1.6 Anesthesia and Analgesia in Hysteroscopy

In order to reduce the intraoperative reaction, analgesics and tranquilizers or intramuscular injection of atropine can be given preoperatively. It is also possible not to use anesthesia in patients with relaxed cervical canal or when a flexible hysteroscope is applied. The commonly used analgesia and anesthesia methods are as follows.

8.1.6.1 Indomethacin Suppository

Normally, indomethacin suppository of 50–100 mg can be inserted deep into the rectum 20 min before examination. Indomethacin could inhibit the synthesis and the release of prostaglandin, and eliminate the sensitizing effect of pain fibers, so it has a good analgesic effect. Its plasma half-life is 20 min, thus the duration of analgesia is not long. Therefore it is appropriate for minor operations in the uterine cavity and the patients can leave the hospital quickly after operation.

8.1.6.2 Kaflan

Kaflan of 25–50 mg may be taken orally 30 min before examination.

8.1.6.3 Paracervical Nerve Block

1% procaine of 5–10 mL or 0.5% lidocaine of 5–10 mL can be injected into both sides of cervix, and the injection can only be administered if blood cannot be aspirated from the injection needle.

8.1.6.4 Surface Anesthesia of Cervical Mucosa

It is done by inserting a cotton swab which had been dipped in the 2% lidocaine solution into the cervical canal up to the level of the internal os for 1 min.

8.1.6.5 Endometrial Spraying Anesthesia

1% lidocaine of 5 mL or 0.25% bupivacaine of 8 mL can be sprayed on the surface of endometrium through a special lumen injector, and the procedure could be done 5 min later.

8.1.6.6 Intravenous Anesthesia

Propofol or ketamine can be given via intravenous injection.

8.1.7 Procedures of Hysteroscopy

8.1.7.1 Preparation Before Hysteroscopy

1. Before hysteroscopy, the bladder is emptied, the patient is examined to determine the position and size of the uterus. If the procedure of hysteroscopy needs to be combined with ultrasonography, the bladder should be kept moderately full.
2. A lithotomy position is taken, and vulvo-vagina is sterilized with 0.25% or 0.5% iodophor. If intrauterine mucus is too much and difficult to be removed, a 2 mL syringe can be used to suck it out so as not to disturb the hysteroscopic vision.
3. The air inside the inflow pipe and between the sheath and the scope must be emptied before insertion of the hysteroscope. The fluid distention pressure is set at 80–100 mmHg (10–13 kPa) and the flow rate is at 200–300 mL/min, while the pressure of CO_2 uterine distension is 60–80 mmHg (about 10 kPa) and the flow rate is 20–30 mL/min.
4. During the operation, noninvasive technique should be used as much as possible, including not using a speculum, neither clamping or dilating the cervix, not sounding the uterus, and performing low pressure distension of uterine cavity, etc.

8.1.7.2 Procedures

Fiber (Flexible) Hysteroscopy

1. Control of the operating lever results in the up and down movement of the objective lens. The tip of the hysteroscope is inserted through the cervical os under the direct vision and is guided by the flushing of distention fluid, which permits a comprehensive observation of cervical canal (Fig. 8.2a, b). Then the hysteroscope is introduced into the cavity and the direction of its tip is regulated by rotating the scope or moving the lever, so observations of the cavity can be achieved sequentially, which include anterior wall, left cornua, left tubal orifice, posterior wall, right cornua, right tubal orifice, and then fundus. When retracting the scope after inspecting the cavity, the cervical canal should be carefully observed again as this part is difficult to expand and easy to be misdiagnosed.
2. If insertion of telescope into the uterine cavity meets resistance, the pressure of the distending fluid can be increased so that the tip of the hysteroscope is pushed along with the water flow. If still unsuccessful, the insertion direction could be explored with a uterine probe with the cervix held with cervical forceps. When the probe could be introduced through the cervical canal but the

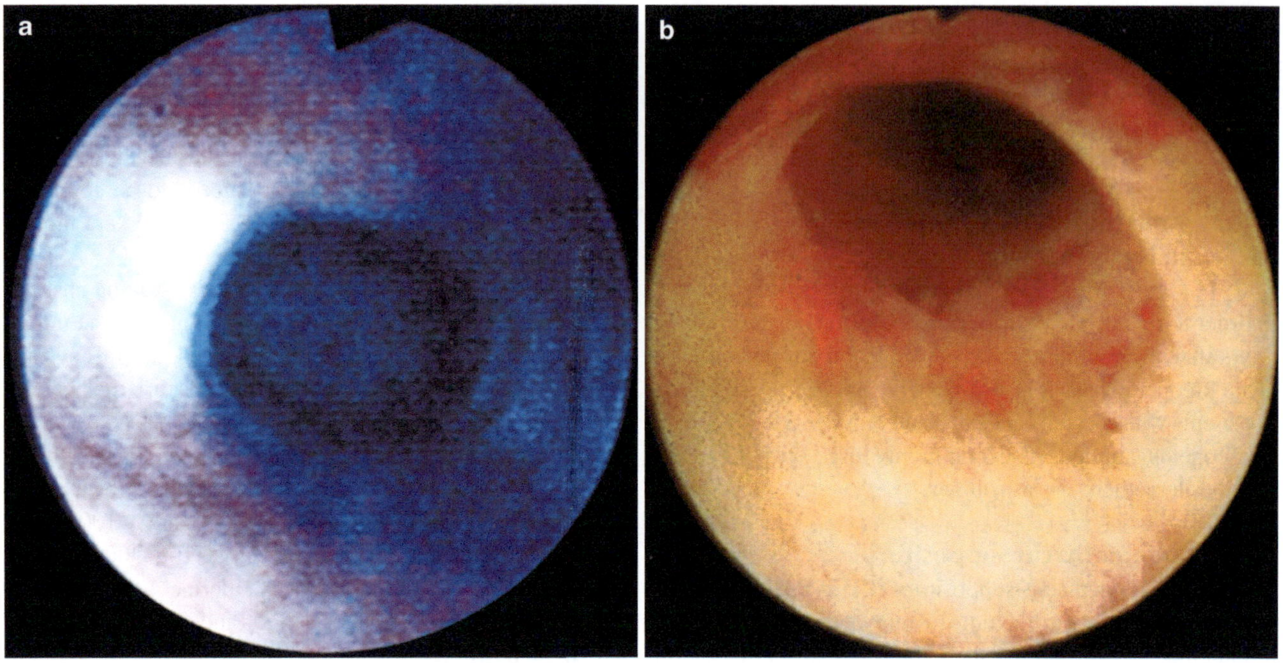

Fig. 8.2 (**a**, **b**) Observation of the cervical canal with fiber hysteroscope

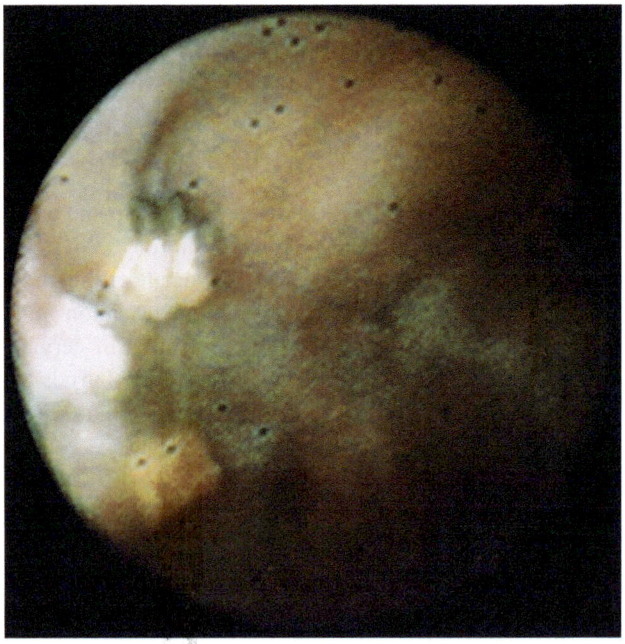

Fig. 8.3 The optical fibers of the hysteroscope are broken, and little black dots appear on the screen. (This is of a menopausal woman whose removal of IUD was not successful. Under hysteroscope, the residual IUD is seen embedded in the right uterine wall)

internal os was seen to be narrow under hysteroscope, a cervix dilator could be used to dilate it slightly. Be sure not to push forward the hysteroscope by force, otherwise the glass optical fibers inside the telescope might break, resulting in blurred images and little dots appearing on the screen. (Fig. 8.3).

Rigid Hysteroscopy

1. It is mainly used when a more detailed observation of intrauterine lesions, a bigger uterine cavity, and larger or more complicated intrauterine lesions are needed.
2. The scopes of modern rigid hysteroscope are 12° or 30° for oblique lens, so when the telescope is pushed forward via the cervix, it should be rotated and the observation should be done as well. After inserting the telescope into the uterine cavity, the scope should be turned over, aiming the oblique lens at the target to conduct the observation. For example, when the objective lens has reached the uterine fundus, aiming oblique lens at the left side, the left uterine cornua and tubal orifice can be observed, then continue to rotate the scope mandrel 90° clockwise, the uterine posterior wall maybe observed, and by analogy, the observation sequence is the same with the fiberscope.
3. The outer diameter of a rigid hysteroscope is larger, therefore it is often necessary to do the cervical dilatation and anesthesia to apply this noninvasive technique, excluding the conditions of chronic uterine bleeding or some major intrauterine space-occupying lesions, in which the cervical canal is relatively relaxed.

Comparison Between Fiber Hysteroscopy and Rigid Hysteroscopy

Unfried et al. made a comparison of imaging properties and the patient's acceptance between fiber hysteroscopy and rigid hysteroscopy using a grading system. The results showed that during the introduction and the examination using rigid hysteroscope, the discomforts were significantly greater than those of fiber hysteroscope (P = 0.003 and $P < 0.001$ respectively), but the imaging properties were far better ($P < 0.001$) and the duration of operations was significantly shorter (P = 0.003). Therefore it was concluded that fiber hysteroscope seemed to cause less pain and was preferred to be applied in outpatient setting. Nevertheless, rigid hysteroscope could provide good imaging quality, short procedure, a higher success rate and a lower cost.

"No Touch" Technique

"No touch" hysteroscopy techniques, means the procedure does not use speculum, not clamp the cervix, not dilate the cervical canal, not sound the uterine cavity, not need anesthesia, use the miniature instruments, and use low pressure to distend the cavity, thus it could be performed in an outpatient office. If the surgeon is quite experienced in discerning the lesions under the hysteroscope, treatment and surgery could be continued. This "no touch" technique is called vaginoscope, which needs a disinfected saline soaked gauze pad to cover the vulva so as to prevent the leakage of distending medium from the vulva. It uses mini hysteroscope and is applicable to young girls, unmarried women, women with intact hymen, postmenopausal women, and those with vaginal and cervical stenosis. Bettocchi reported his experience of vaginoscopy in 9093 cases during 10 years, all of them were successful with a satisfactory rate of almost 100%.

8.1.8 Hysteroscopy Combined with Ultrasonography

The joint use of hysteroscopy and ultrasonography has made these two advanced diagnostic techniques complementary to each other. It has altered the limitations of hysteroscopy for simple diagnosis of intrauterine lesions and the limitations of ultrasonography for simple diagnosis of lesions within or outside the uterine wall. It also has solved the problems of no access to the relationship between the submucous myoma and myometrial wall by hysteroscopy, and no way to detect the intrauterine space-occupying lesions smaller than 1–2 mm and to locate the submucous leiomyoma by only ultrasonography. The patient's conditions of the uterine cavity, uterine wall and pelvic cavity can be determined immediately, comprehensively and accurately at one combined examination. The joint inspection provides reliable information for diagnosis, expands the indications for hysteroscopy and ultrasonography, and establishes new ways of rapid and accurate diagnosis of gynecologic disorders.

8.1.8.1 Indications for Hysteroscopy Combined with Ultrasonography

1. Anybody with indications for hysteroscopy.
2. Patients who have pelvic masses with which the relationship of the uterus need to be determined.
3. The operation methods of uterine myomas are to be decided.

8.1.8.2 Procedures for Hysteroscopy Combined with Ultrasonography

1. The bladder should be moderately filled so that the uterine fundus could be seen by ultrasonography.
2. Before the start of hysteroscopy, a transabdominal ultrasonography should be first performed in order to detect size and position of the uterus, thickness of the uterine wall, location and thickness of the endometrium, any dents at the fundus, any malformation of the uterus, any myomas, size, number and location of myoma, and the state of the adnexa.
3. The hysteroscope is inserted along with the orientation of the uterine cavity under the guidance of ultrasonography. While the uterine cavity is examined by hysteroscopy, abdominal ultrasound probe should be used to do horizontal and vertical scanning up over the symphysis pubica and make the full range of observation, taking the intrauterine distention fluid and hysteroscope as the reference object. If the fallopian tubes are patent, sometimes ultrasound scan images with water flowing through the tubes or over the fimbria could be seen. While the telescope is retracted, attention should be paid to the sonographic changes before and after the uterine distention and whether there is any uterine distention medium going into the uterine wall.

8.1.8.3 Abnormal Findings in Hysteroscopy Combined with Ultrasonography

Intrauterine Lesions

1. Uterine malformation: After the uterine cavity is distended adequately by the distention medium, ultrasonographic imaging can display whether there is a dent in the contour of the uterine fundus, whether there is a septum at the fundus of the cavity, and its length, width, and thickness, etc. Ultrasonography with high resolution can also show the myometrium within the septum, accurately establishing the diagnosis of uterine septum.
2. Intrauterine hematocele: Hysteroscopy can only detect the intrauterine adhesion but cannot view the conditions

above the adhesive band, while the joint inspection can view simultaneously the location, extent, single cavity or multi-cavities of intrauterine hematocele induced by adhesions.
3. Intrauterine foreign body: The joint inspection can accurately locate the foreign bodies, such as an IUD which is totally embedded in the uterine wall or covered by endometrium.

Lesions on the Uterine Wall or Outside the Uterus
1. Intramural myoma: The joint inspection would combine the intrauterine morphological changes detected by hysteroscopy with the location, size, and protruding degree of the intramural myoma shown by ultrasonography, through which the inward-protruding intramural myoma is accurately located.
2. Adenomyosis: During the joint inspections, if the opening of ectopic glands of adenomyosis originates from the uterine cavity, the uterine distention medium can flow into the uterine wall thus the area of lesion is shown as inhomogeneous cloudy strong echoes on the ultrasonogram.
3. Subserous myoma and adnexal masses: The joint inspection can observe clearly the relationship between them and the uterus or uterine cavity.

8.1.9 A Normal Uterus Under Hysteroscopy

8.1.9.1 Various Images Seen by Hysteroscopy
Except for the especially obvious conditions, judgment and histopathologic examination are still needed in deciding whether the observed target is normal or not.

1. Endometrium: It can be normal endometrium in menstrual cycles such as menstruation, proliferative phase and secretory phase, and atrophic or hyperplastic endometrium.
2. Protrusion of the endometrium: It includes endometrial polyps, thickened endometrium, and polypoid, papillary, nodular, hemispherical and spherical protrusions of the endometrium (Fig. 8.4).
3. Endometrial glandular opening: It can be presented as punctiform, rotiform, and tubular (Fig. 8.5).

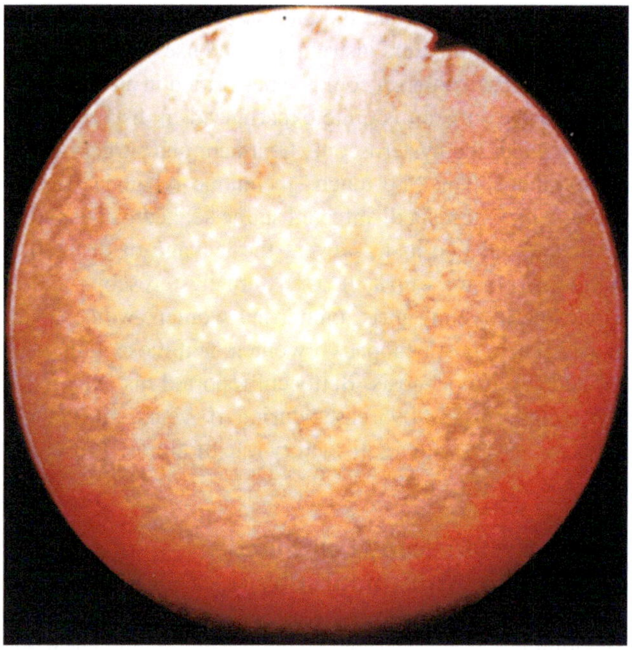

Fig. 8.5 Endometrial glandular opening

Fig. 8.4 Protrusions of endometrium (the figure was kindly provided by Dr. Takashima Hideyo)

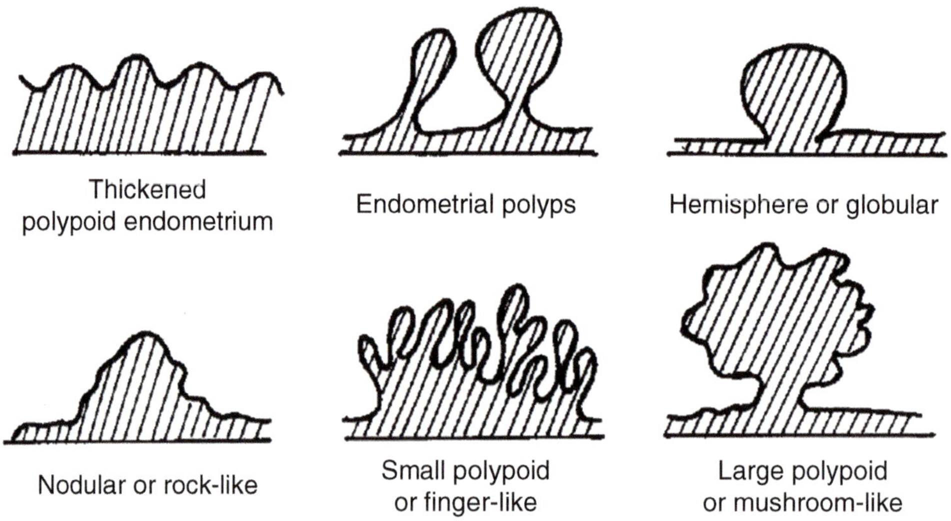

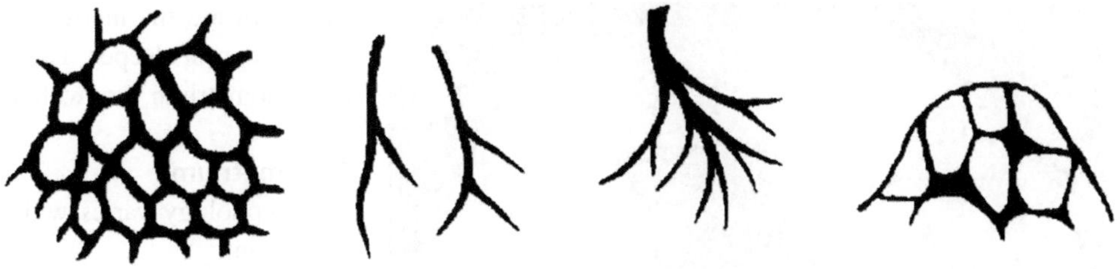

Fig. 8.6 Normal or benign blood vessels. (The figure was kindly provided by Dr. Takashima Hideyo)

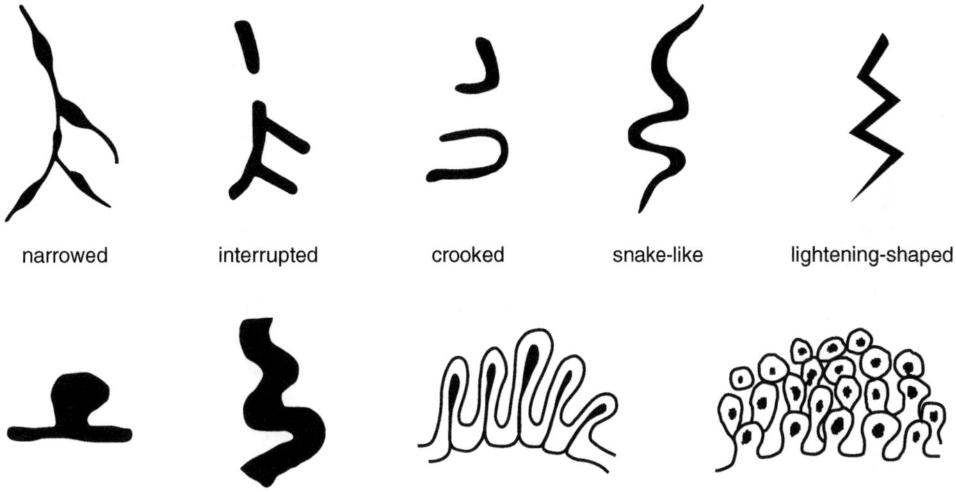

Fig. 8.7 Atypical blood vessels. (This figure was kindly provided by Dr. Takashima Hideyo)

4. Endometrial surface: It can be smooth, rough or uneven.
5. Transparency: It includes transparent, translucent or opaque.
6. Color: The endometrium can be white, gray-white, yellow-white, brown, light red, and red.
7. Texture: The endometrium can be hard, soft, and fragile.
8. Necrosis: The endometrium may develop necrosis with punctiform, patchy, and lamellar features.
9. Normal blood vessels or benign blood vessels: It can be divided into the capillary network, small blood vessels, and dendritic vascular and flattened shape of vessels (Fig. 8.6). The capillary network can often be seen on the normal endometrium and sometimes the small blood vessels and other vessels shaped like willow branch are also benign blood vessels. Flattened shape of wide vessels can be seen over the submucosal myoma.
10. Atypical vessels: Atypical vessels are mainly vessels which are expanded and run irregularly (Fig. 8.7). The latter refers to the vessels which appear to be partly narrow, run intermittently or with interruption, bending abruptly, or be snake-like or lightning-shaped winding. All the above-mentioned vessels and vascular engorgement are often seen in malignant tumor. In addition, the main feature of the papillary adenocarcinoma is that the central blood vessel can be seen in its long and short papillae.

8.1.9.2 Normal Morphology of the Uterine Cavity Viewed by Hysteroscopy

Cervical Canal

It is a circular or oval-shaped tube, and its shape may change with the degree of uterine distention. The mucosa is pale red, whitened or red, with more vertical and horizontal folds, which are significantly different from the uterine endometrium, and typical palm-like folds are occasionally seen (Fig. 8.8). The internal orifice is mostly round or oval, with its edge being tidy, smooth, and slightly irregular occasionally. The internal orifice tilts forward or backward in those uteri with obvious anteflexion or retroflexion. Compared with the endometrium, cervical mucosa is a little pale, so many intrauterine interventions such as abortion, curettage, placement or removal of IUD, and D&C can easily cause injuries and lead to adhesions of cervical canal.

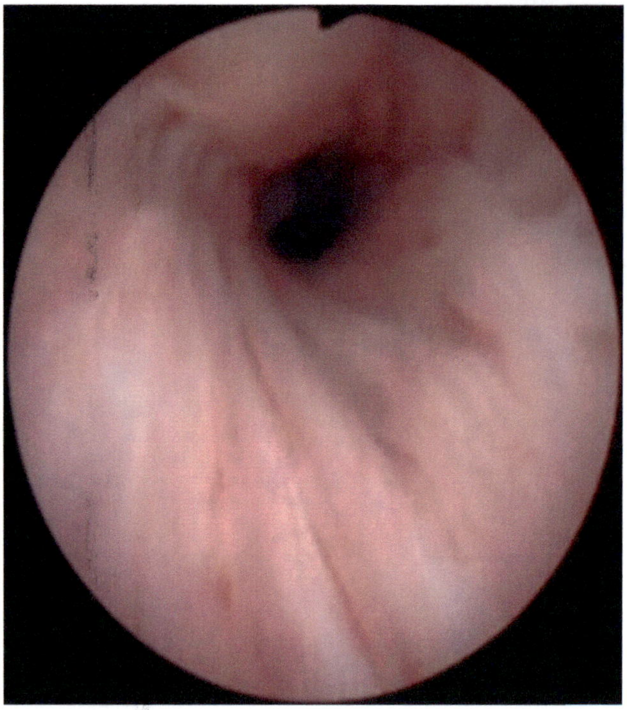

Fig. 8.8 Normal cervical canal

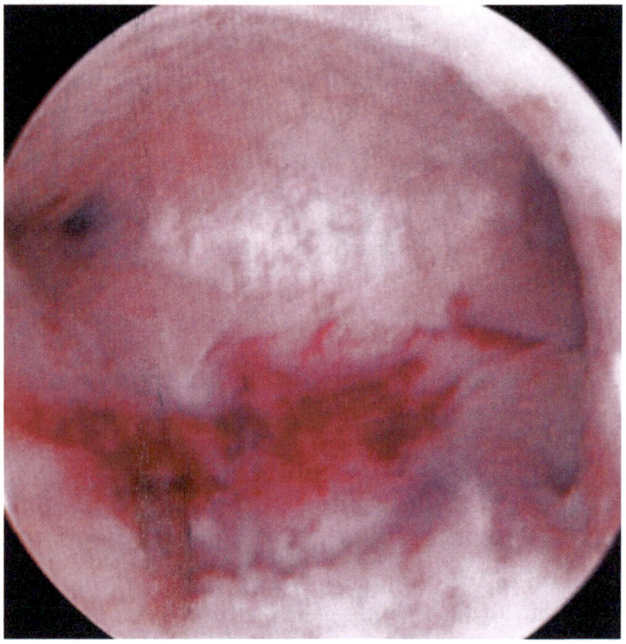

Fig. 8.9 The uterine fundus is flattened when it is well distended

Uterine Cavity

With an ideal uterine distention, the uterine fundus is flattened (Fig. 8.9), but sometimes it is slightly arc-shaped and protrudes toward the uterine cavity so as to make both uterine cornua appear deeper. The color, thickness, and wrinkles of the endometrium vary with the menstrual cycle (Fig. 8.10a–d).

Endometrium

Its morphology varies with the age and menstrual cycle of the patient.

Endometrium of Women in Reproductive Age

1. Endometrium in repair phase: It generally refers to the fifth to sixth days of menstruation, during which the entire uterine cavity is covered by the new epithelium with the thickness of 0.5–0.9 mm. The endometrium appears to be smooth, yellow-red, with rare vascular veins, scattered bleeding spots and unclear glandular openings (Fig. 8.11).
2. Endometrium in the early and middle proliferative phase: Its thickness is 2–5 mm, and the endometrium gradually turns into a red color, more wrinkled, and uneven. The glandular openings become clearer and are distributed equally with the endometrium being like a strawberry (Fig. 8.12a, b).
3. Endometrium in late proliferative and early secretory phase: It is 2–3 days before and after ovulation. The endometrium is thickening and swelling, being light yellow-red with translucent polypoid protrusions. The subepithelial vessels might be visible. The glandular openings can be unclear, wavy, and particularly evidently concave (Fig. 8.13a–c).
4. Endometrium in secretory phase: The endometrium is thickening to 7–8 mm and is undulating. Due to the interstitial edema, the endometrium is yellowish-white or yellowish-red translucent with hemispherical or polypoid protrusions, with clear capillary network, and the white punctiform glandular openings are not obvious or even almost undistinguishable (Fig. 8.14a, b).
5. Premenstrual endometrium: Interstitial edema subsides, the endometrium becomes thinner again, and there are more small wrinkles on its surface, with scattered red plaque hematoma underlying the endometrium, which is fragile and easy to bleed (Fig. 8.15).
6. Menstrual endometrium: The endometrium is shed, accompanied by punctiform bleeding spots and moss-like pale stripped surface, and coarse vessels and glands stump are visible (Fig. 8.16a, b).

Endometrium of Women in Postmenopause

The endometrium appears atrophic and becomes thinner, smooth, yellow-white and opaque, and ecchymosis are often visible (Fig. 8.17).

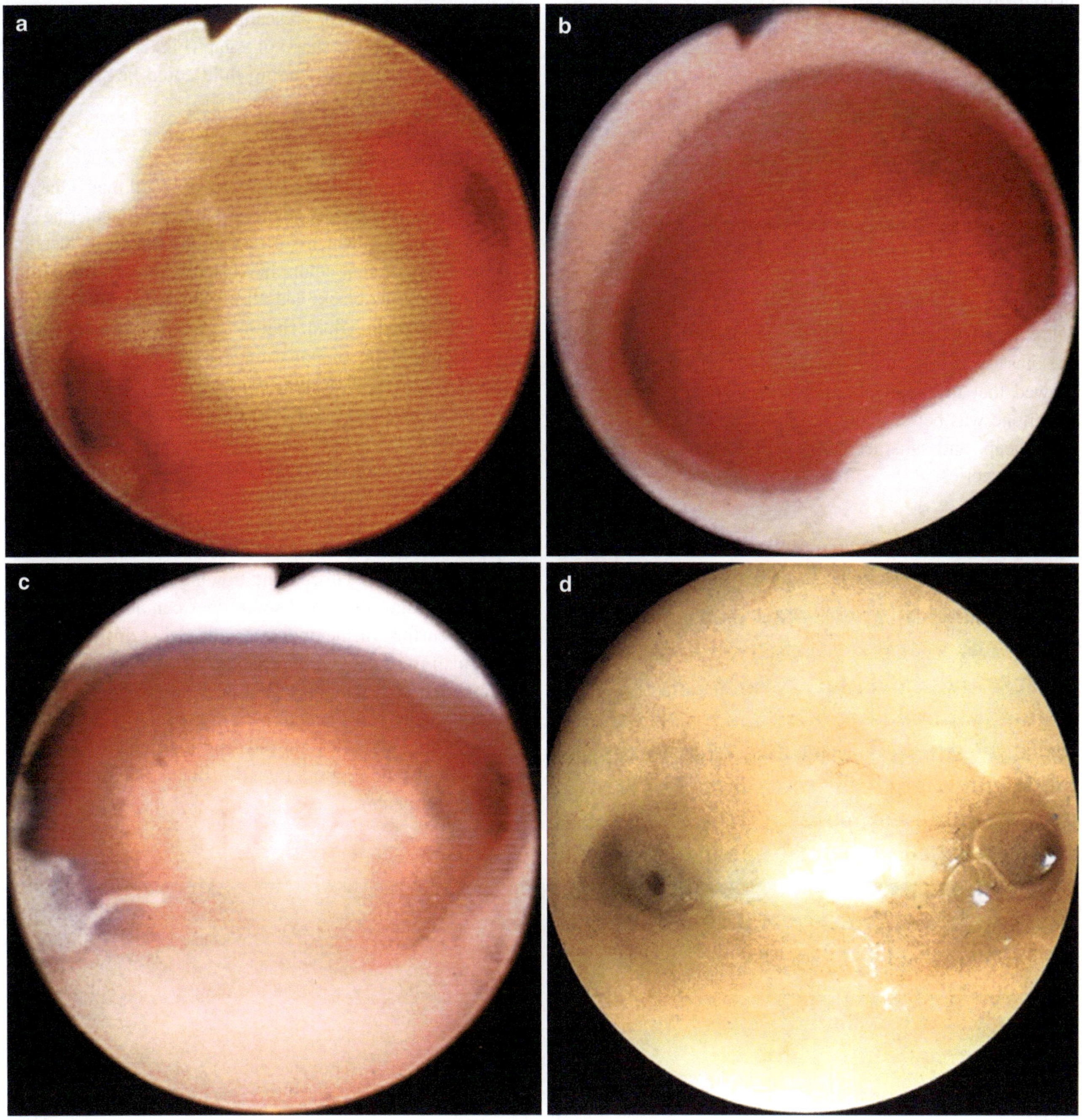

Fig. 8.10 (**a**–**c**) Normal uterine cavity. (**d**) Normal uterine cavity (CO_2 uterine-distension)

Uterine Cornua and Fallopian Tubal Orifice

The uterine cornua present as deep and dark funnels before the uterine cavity unfolds (Fig. 8.18a, b), while the fallopian tubal orifice can be seen on top of or at the inner side of the top of the cornua after the cavity totally unfolds (Fig. 8.19a–d). The tubal orifices are mostly round or oval (Fig. 8.20), occasionally like star or crescent. Sometimes it can also be seen to shrink into the shape of a gap (Fig. 8.21). If the tube is patent, the uterine distending fluid could be seen to flow into the fallopian tubal ostia.

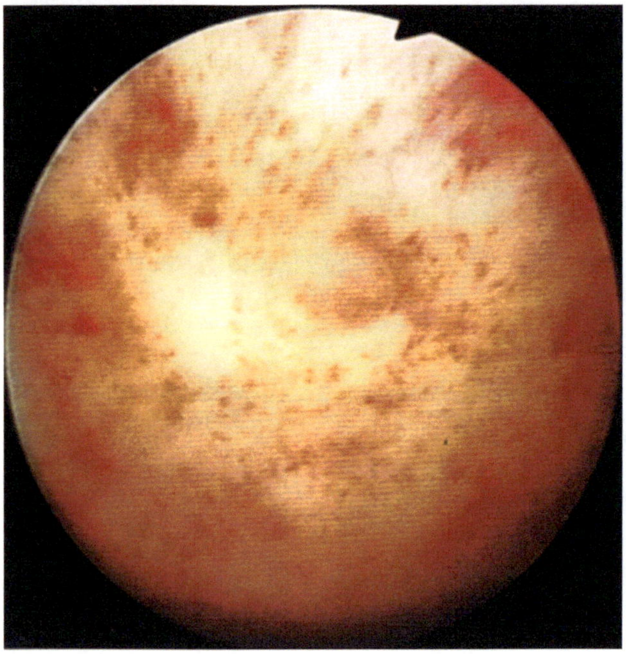

Fig. 8.11 Endometrium in repair phase

Other Intrauterine Findings

1. Bleeding: Slices, streaks, and clots of blood may adhere to the endometrial surface or be suspending in the uterine cavity, the color of which varies with the length of bleeding time with different colors like bright red, dark red, violet-red, and purple-black, and all of which can shift with the flow of distending fluid. Hemorrhagic spots or hemorrhagic marks under the endometrium may be scattered or fused together into patches, being red or dull red hemorrhagic foci with their surfaces covered by the endometrium, so they do not shift with the flow of the distending fluid. If small veins or blood capillary actively bleed, the blood can be seen oozing out slowly. Arteriolar bleeding is associated with pulsation. If there is heavy bleeding, the blood will mix with the distending fluid, resulting in a blurred red vision.
2. Mucus: It is white flocculent, flowing and deforming with the distending fluid, and sometimes can also be attached to the surface of the endometrium and is difficult to distinguish from the endometrial debris.
3. Endometrial fragments: They are partly attached to the uterine wall, partly hang down in the uterine cavity, with the color of pale or light red, and their shapes are more rigid in distending fluid than the mucus. It can be shaken but does not shift.

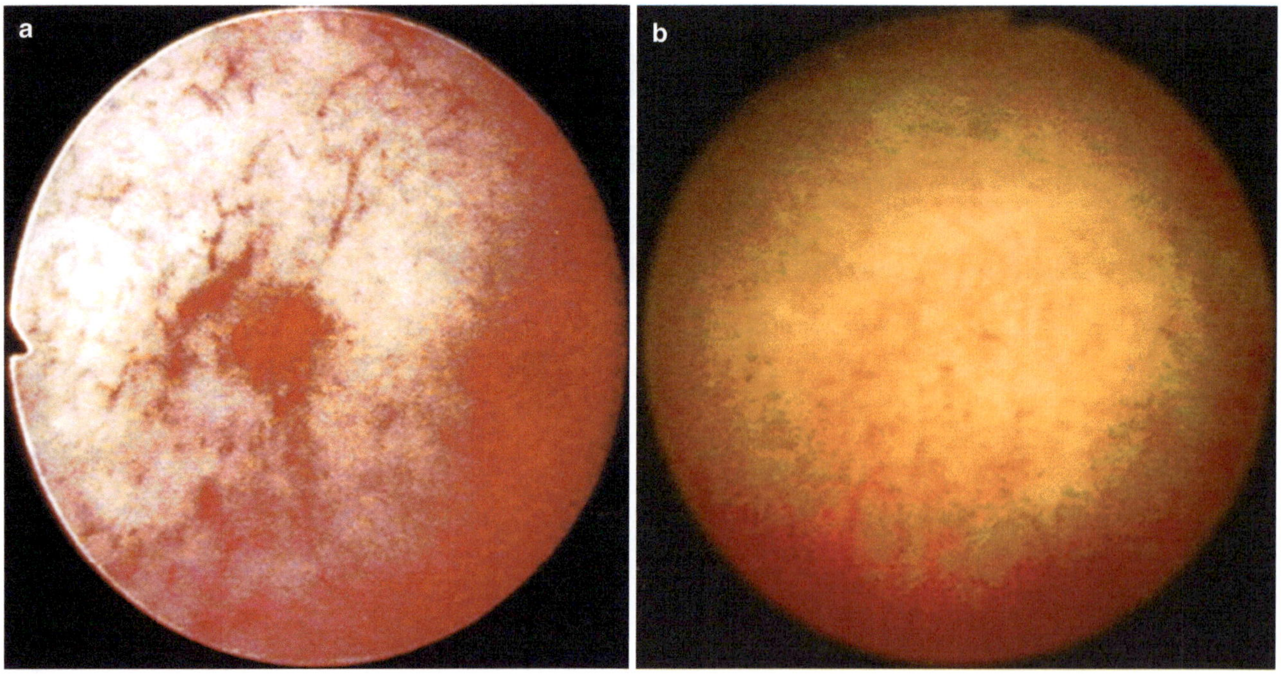

Fig. 8.12 (**a**) Endometrium in early proliferative phase. (**b**) Endometrium in middle proliferative phase

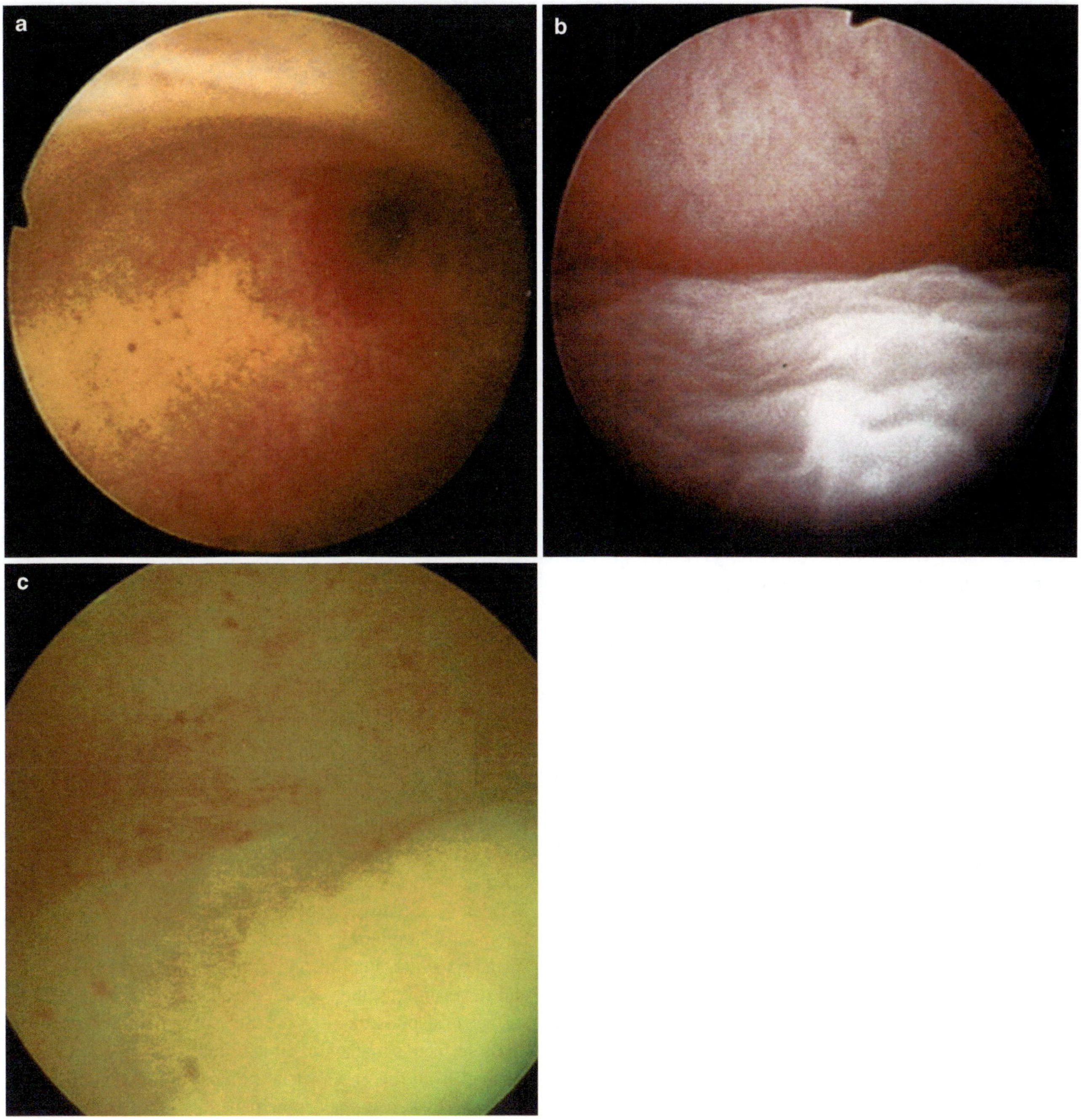

Fig. 8.13 (**a**) Endometrium on the 12th day in a menstrual cycle. (**b**) Endometrium in early secretory phase. (**c**) Endometrium in early secretory phase

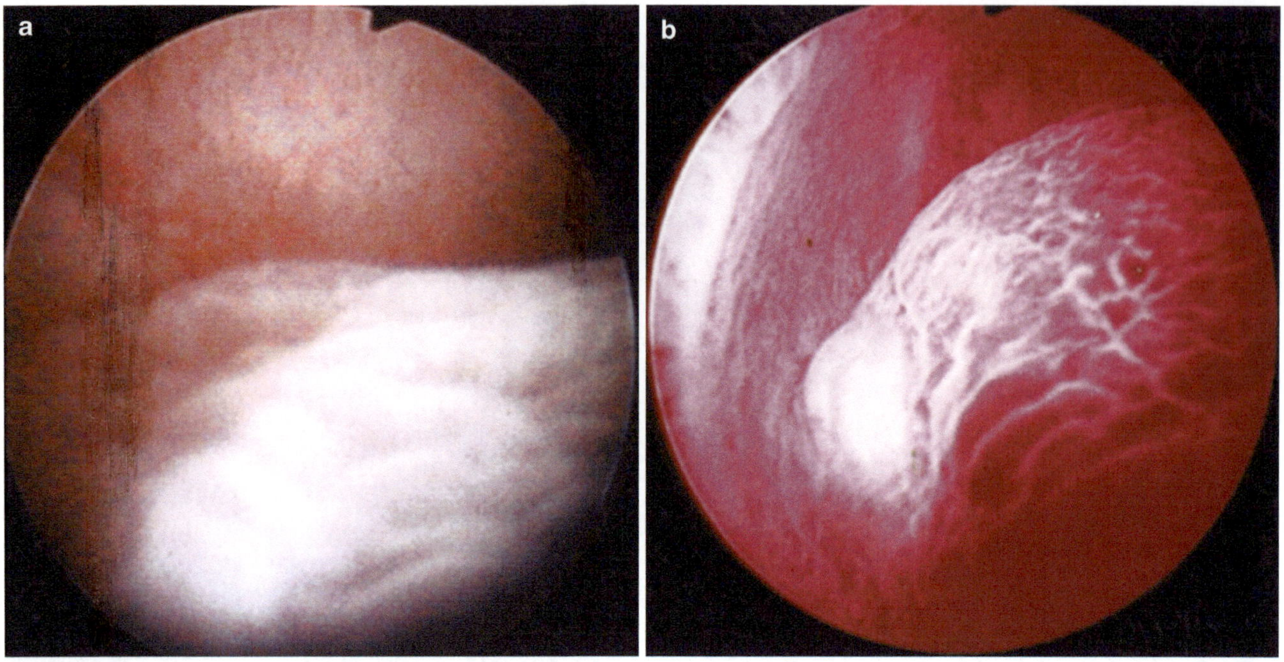

Fig. 8.14 (**a**, **b**) Endometrium in secretory phase

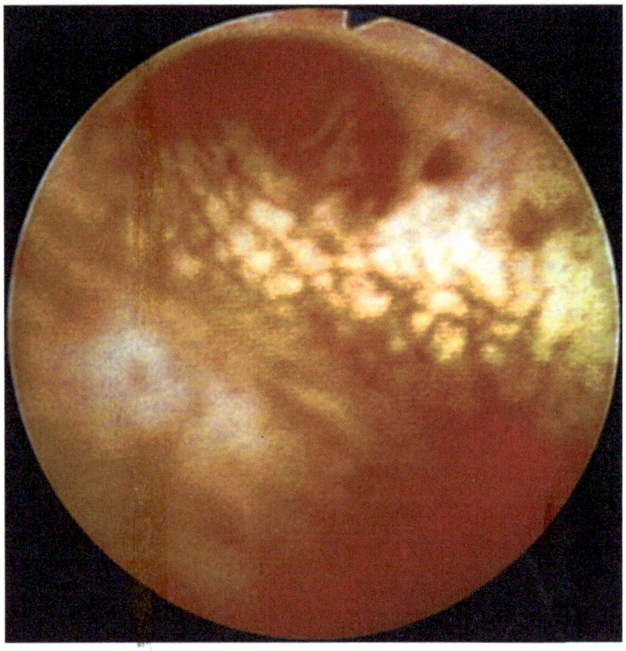

Fig. 8.15 Endometrium on the 27th day in a menstrual cycle

4. Bubbles: When the air in inlet pipes is not totally emptied, it would flow into the uterine cavity and gather at the anterior wall or the fundus of the uterus in the forms of microvesicles.

8.1.10 Abnormal Findings Under Hysteroscope

8.1.10.1 Submucosal Myoma

Submucosal myoma is round or oval in appearance and its surface is white, smooth, and shiny, on which relatively thick and dendritic vascular or vascular network running over its surface is also visible (Fig. 8.22a, b). When the endometrium on its surface is thickening, it is usually difficult to be distinguished from the endometrial polyps. In this condition, the tip of the hysteroscope can be penetrated into this thickened endometrium so that the white myoma nodules behind it could be visible. The thickness of the pedicle and the degree of protrusion toward the cavity of the myoma should be observed carefully.

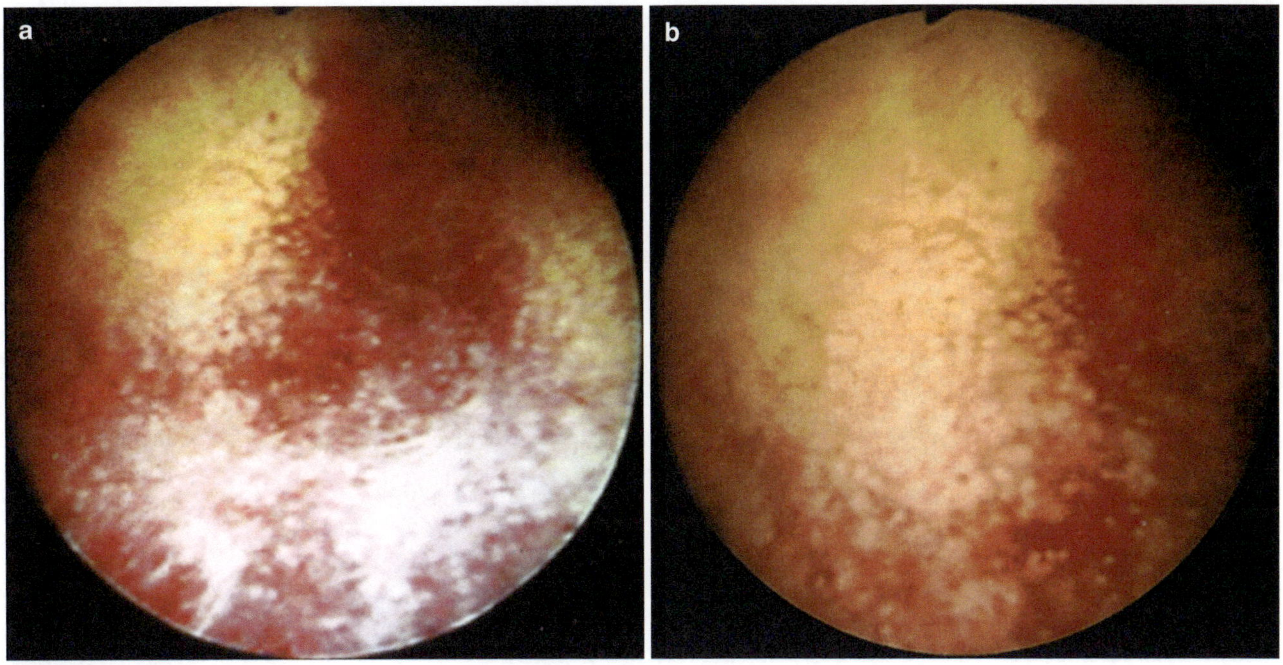

Fig. 8.16 (**a**, **b**) Endometrium on the first day of menstruation

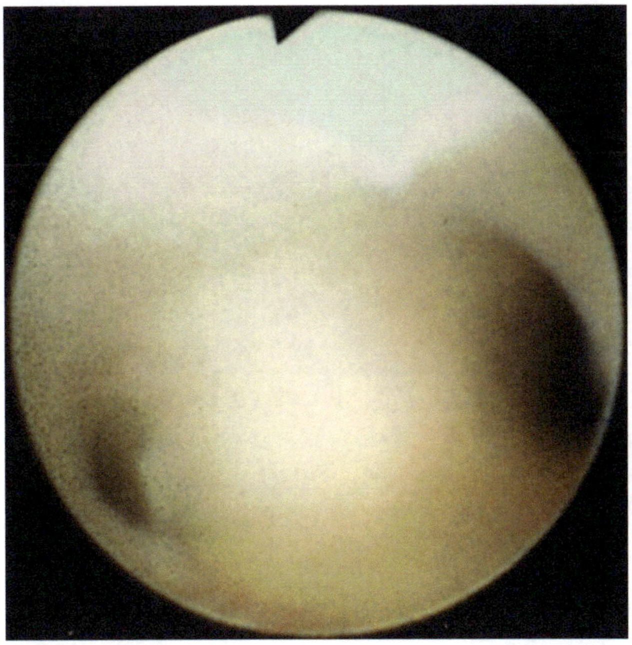

Fig. 8.17 Endometrium in postmenopause

According to the relationship between myomas and the myometrium, Haarlem international hysteroscopy training center in Netherlands classified the submucous myomas into three types, which has been commonly applied clinically and was described in detail in Chap. 9, Sect. 9.3.

1. Type 0 submucosal myoma: It is pedunculated and does not extend into the myometrium. A typical image under hysteroscope is a round or similar round mass, which protrudes into the cavity (Fig. 8.22c).
2. Type I submucosal myoma: It is sessile and extends less than 50% into the myometrium. A typical image under hysteroscope is a hemispheric protrusion, which produces an acute angle between the myoma and the uterine wall (Fig. 8.22d).
3. Type II submucosal myoma: It is sessile and extends more than 50% into the myometrium. A typical image under hysteroscope is a hemispheric or an arc-shaped protrusion, which produces an obtuse angle between the myoma and the uterine wall (Fig. 8.22e).

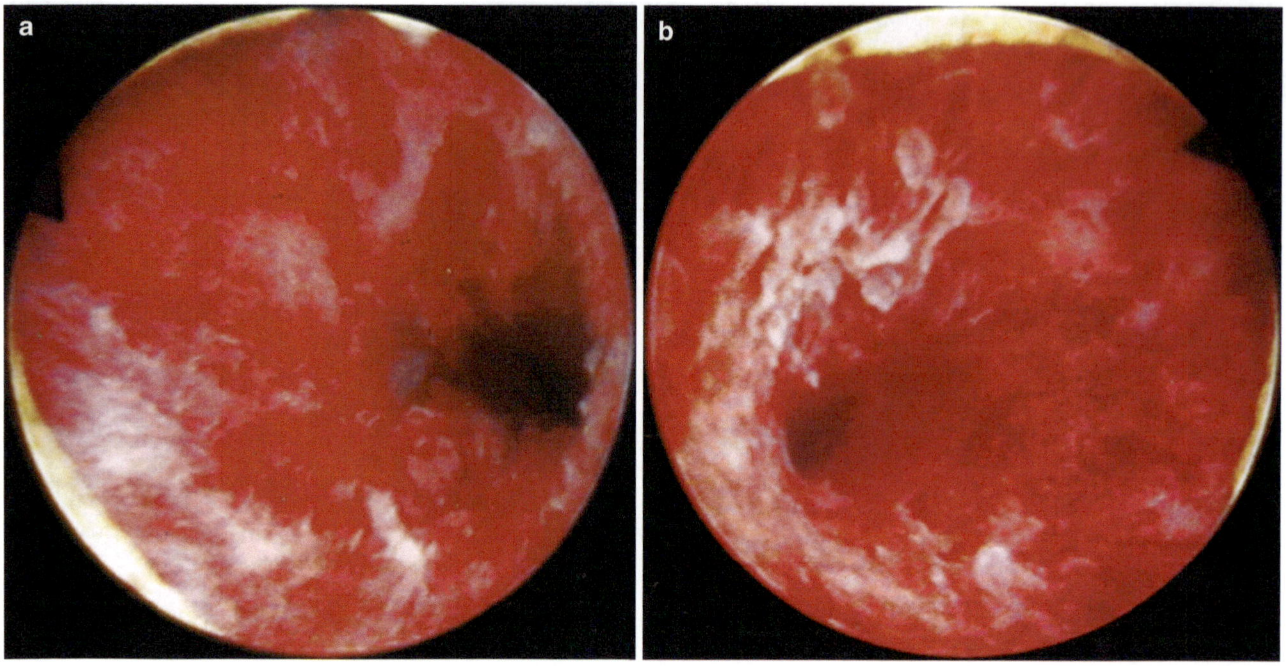

Fig. 8.18 (**a**) Left uterine cornu under hysteroscope. (**b**) Right uterine cornu under hysteroscope

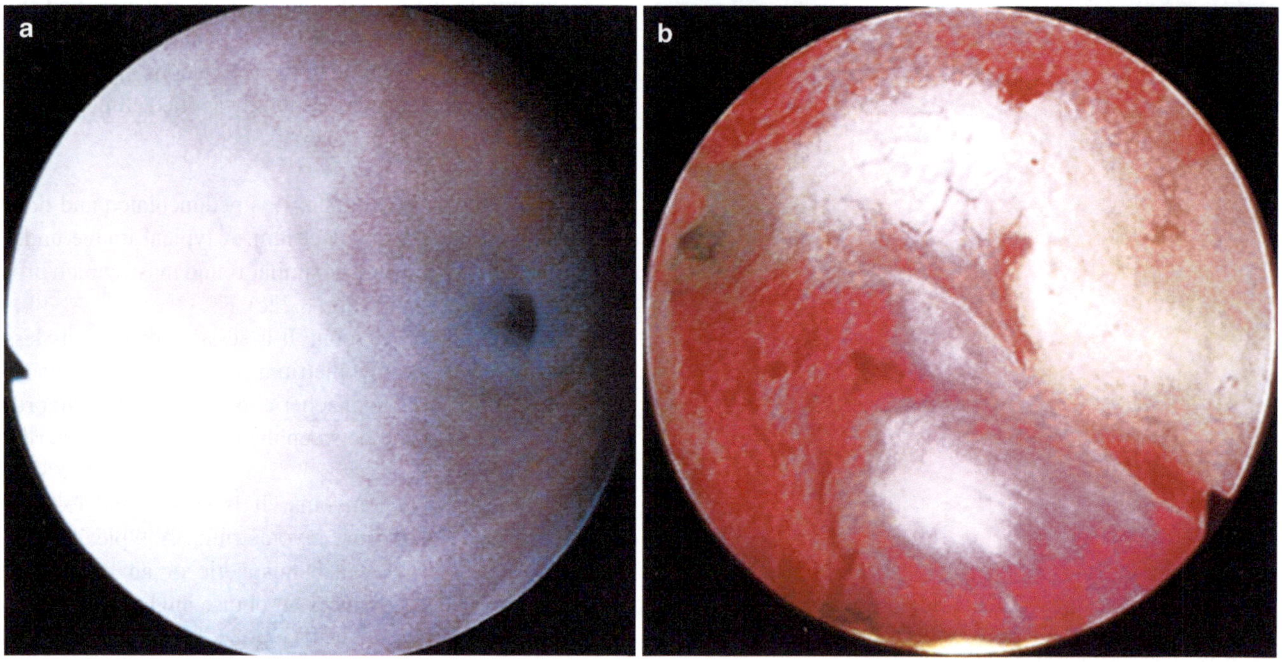

Fig. 8.19 (**a–c**) Fallopian tubal ostium under hysteroscope. (**d**) Fallopian tubal ostium under hysteroscope (Interstitial segment of fallopian tube is visible)

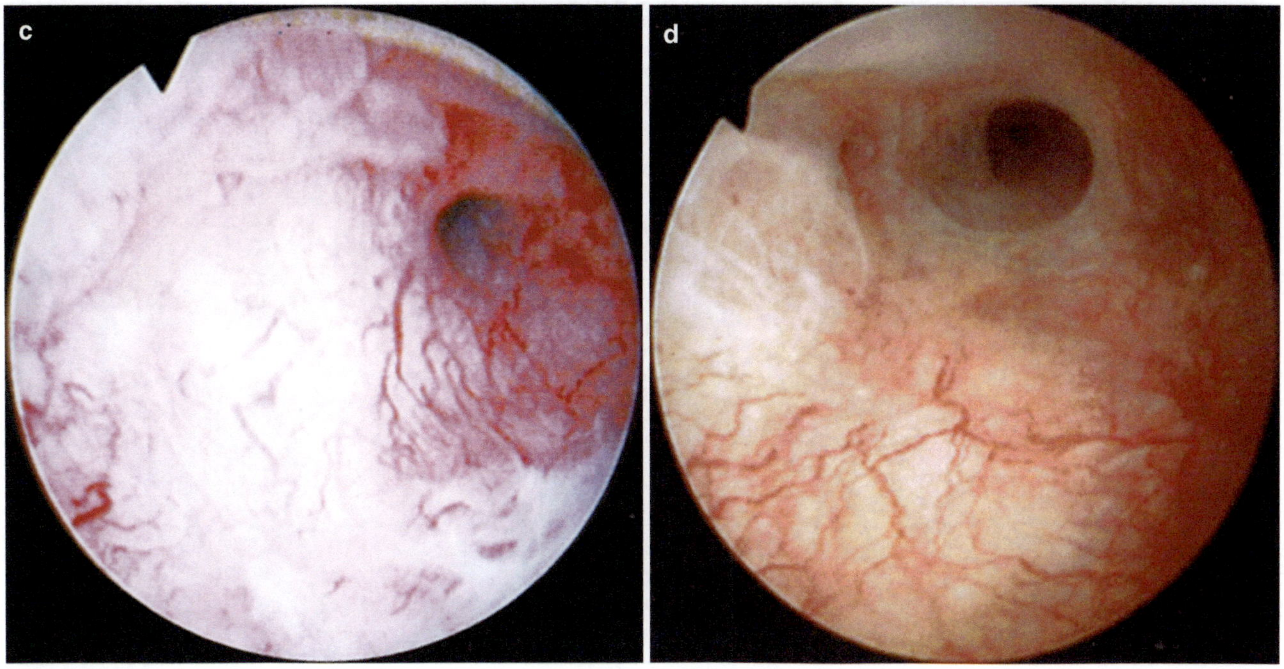

Fig. 8.19 (continued)

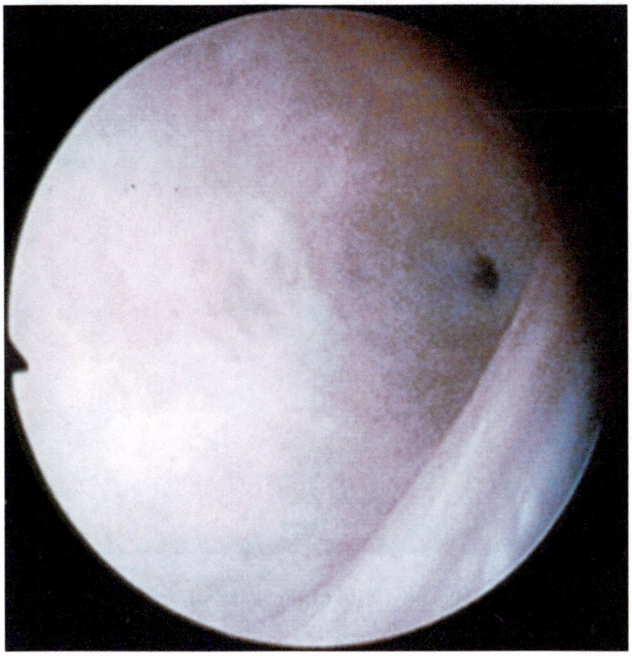

Fig. 8.20 Fallopian tubal ostium is oval-shaped under hysteroscope

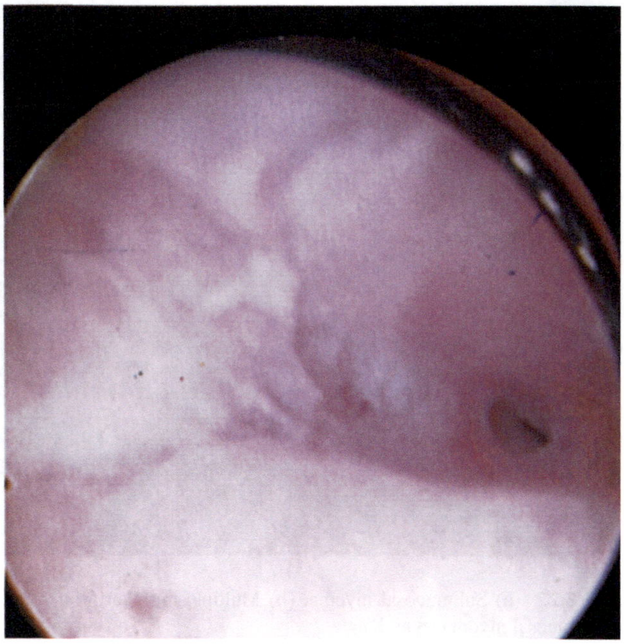

Fig. 8.21 Fallopian tubal ostium presents as a gap under hysteroscope

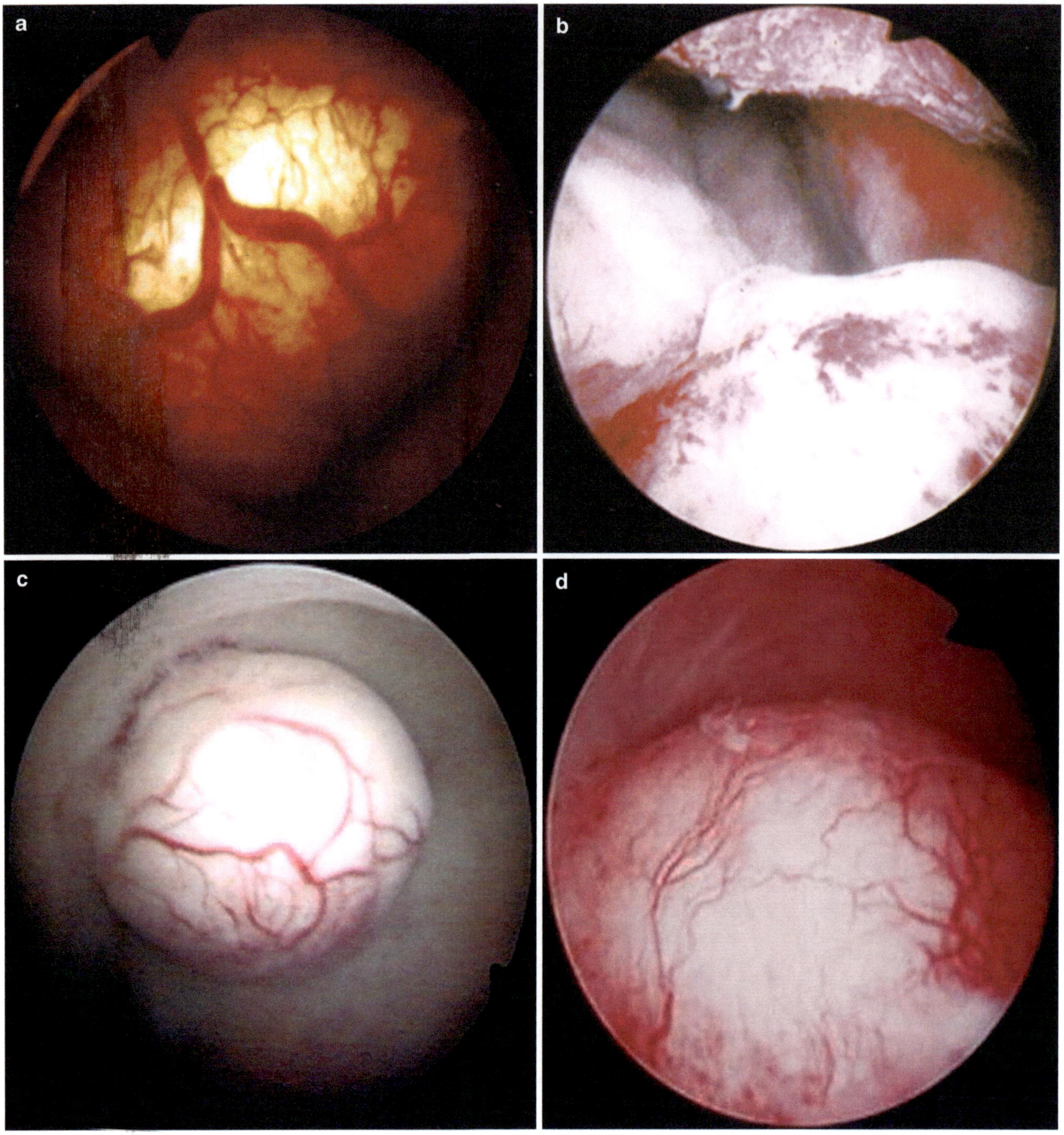

Fig. 8.22 (**a**) Submucosal myoma. (**b**) Multiple intrauterine myomas. (**c**) Submucosal myoma (type 0). (**d**) Submucosal myoma (type I). (**e**) Submucosal myoma (type II)

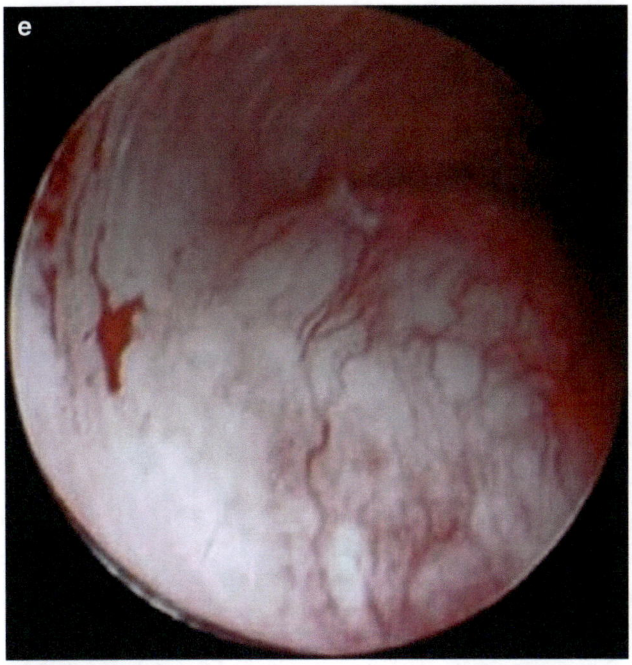

Fig. 8.22 (continued)

8.1.10.2 Intrauterine Adhesions

Intrauterine adhesions are adhered tissues between anterior and posterior walls, and mostly locate either in the center or at the margins of the cavity (Fig. 8.23a, b). The intrauterine adhesions can be classified into endometrial adhesions, fibromuscular adhesions, and connective tissue adhesions. The surface of endometrial adhesions looks similar to the surrounding endometrium, which is easy to be divided by hysteroscope (Fig. 8.23c). Fibromuscular adhesions, being light red or yellowish-white, grid-shaped or ledge-shaped, is covered by the endometrium, so it has smooth surface, is hard and tough, and is not easy to be divided but prone to uterine perforation (Fig. 8.23d). The connective tissue adhesion is a kind of relatively coarse and scarred tissue with pale white surface, which is not covered with endometrium (Fig. 8.23e). It should usually be distinguished from the uterine septum if it is in the center of the uterine cavity. The extensive adhesions inside the uterine cavity cannot be comprehensively investigated by hysteroscopy, so other adjunctive investigations such as HSG are usually needed.

8.1.10.3 Congenital Uterine Abnormalities

Congenital uterine abnormalities include malformations like didelphic uterus, unicornuate uterus, bicornuate uterus, arcuate uterus, saddle form uterus, septate uterus, Robert uterus, infantile uterus, and T-shaped uterus, etc.

1. Septate Uterus: A uterine septum is formed by the disturbance of the absorption process of the midline septum during the fusing process of the two Müllerian ducts. Septate uteri can be classified into complete and incomplete septate uteri. The intrauterine septum extending from the fundus to midline of the cavity can be detected under hysteroscopy. A complete septate uterus is defined as a septum extending to the internal os or cervical canal, which fully divides the uterine cavity from the fundus to the level of the internal os (Fig. 8.24a). A partial or incomplete septate uterus is defined as a septum not reaching the internal os, which partly divides the uterine cavity from the fundus to the cavity (Fig. 8.24b, c).
2. Bicornuate Uterus: A bicornuate uterus is developed by incomplete fusion of the middle segment of the Müllerian ducts, which forms the bifurcate abnormity in the upper part and the fundus of the cavity. The bicornuate uterus can be classified into complete and incomplete bicornuate uteri, of which the concrete criteria are still disputed. Observations under hysteroscope can discover that there are various degrees of convexities of the fundus, the midline septum is similar to that of septate uterus, and the septum can extend to the upper, middle or lower part of the cavity, internal cervical os, or even cervical canal (Fig. 8.24d).
3. Unicornuate Uterus: Unicornuate uterus is caused by asymmetric development of two Müllerian ducts, with unilateral duct developing normally and the contralateral duct absent or failing to form a cavity. Under hysteroscopy, the cavity of a unicornuate uterus is long and narrow, and only unilateral tubal ostium can be seen. Sometimes it does not communicate with the rudimentary uterus (Fig. 8.24e).
4. Robert Uterus: It was first reported by Robert in 1970 and was named after him. In the stage of embryonic development, the absorption of the septum is disturbed during the fusing process of the two Müllerian ducts. The septum remained is not in the midline but on one side of the cavity, which totally blocks it, leading to a blind cavity non-communicating with the vaginal or contralateral cavity. Under hysteroscope, a long and narrow cavity and an ipsilateral tubal ostium can be seen (Fig. 8.24f).
5. T-shaped Uterus: A T-shaped uterus is a developmental anomaly of myometrial constriction bands formation which are caused by the influence of intrauterine exposure of diethylstilbestrol (DES) or other hazardous factors for patients in fetal period. Under hysteroscope, the whole cavity is T-shaped with the upper part narrow and the fundus arced, the smallest distance between the middle of the fundus and the lateral walls is less than 2 cm, and the myometrium of both lateral walls of middle and lower cavity is thickened which leads to a tubular cavity (Fig. 8.24g).
6. Arcuate Uterus: The arcuate uterus is a form of uterine anomaly that the intrauterine septum cannot be totally absorbed after the fuse of the two Müllerian ducts, which

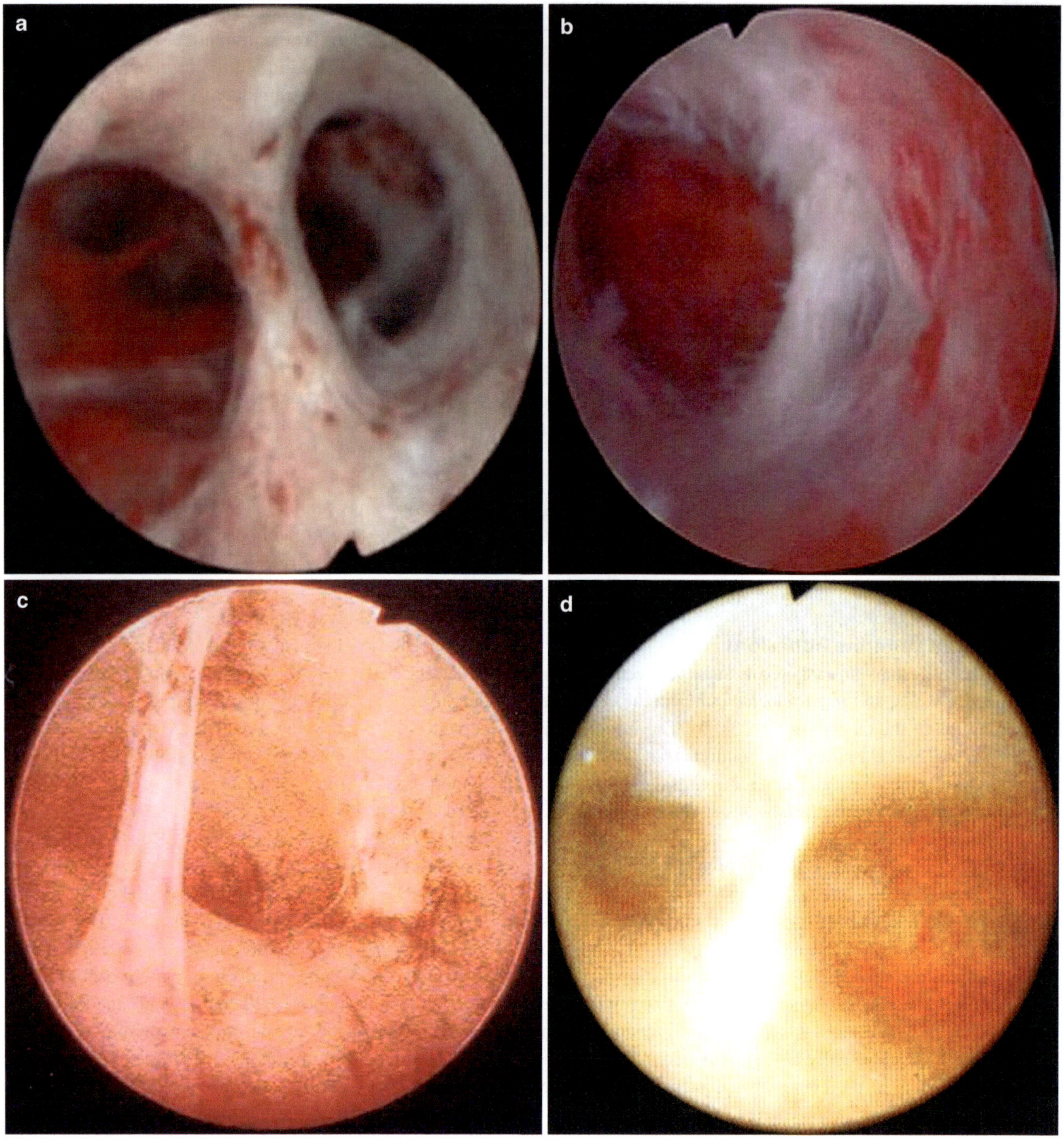

Fig. 8.23 (**a**) Intrauterine adhesions (central). (**b**) Intrauterine adhesions (marginal). (**c**) Intrauterine endometrial adhesions. (**d**) Intrauterine fibro-muscular adhesions. (**e**) Intrauterine connective tissue adhesions

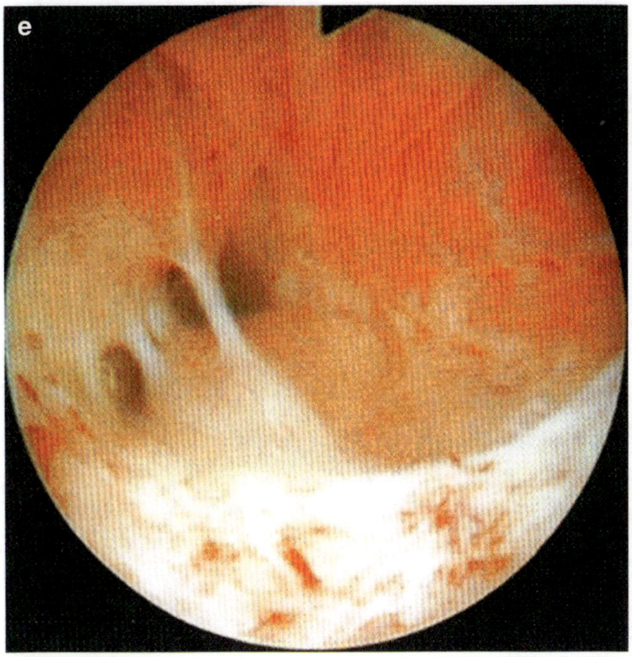

Fig. 8.23 (continued)

leads to myometrial thickening and protruding of the fundus but does not form a specific septum. Under hysteroscopy, the fundus is wide and thick, and protrudes to the cavity without any definite septum (Fig. 8.24h).

7. Saddle form Uterus: The saddle form uterus is a kind of uterine anomaly that occurs when incomplete middle segment fusion of the two Müllerian ducts forms slightly external fundal indentation and internal fundal protrusion. Similar to arcuate uterus, measurements under 3-D ultrasonography indicate that, taking the connecting line between bilateral tubal ostia as base line, the vertical distance between the midpoint of the fundal protrusion and the base line is ranged from 0.5 to1.5 cm.

8.1.10.4 Intrauterine Foreign Bodies

The intrauterine foreign bodies include intrauterine device (IUD), fractured cervical dilators, residual fetal bone, and embryonic remnants after induced labor in second trimester, or residual silk thread after cesarean section. It is usually not difficult to diagnose according to the external appearance of

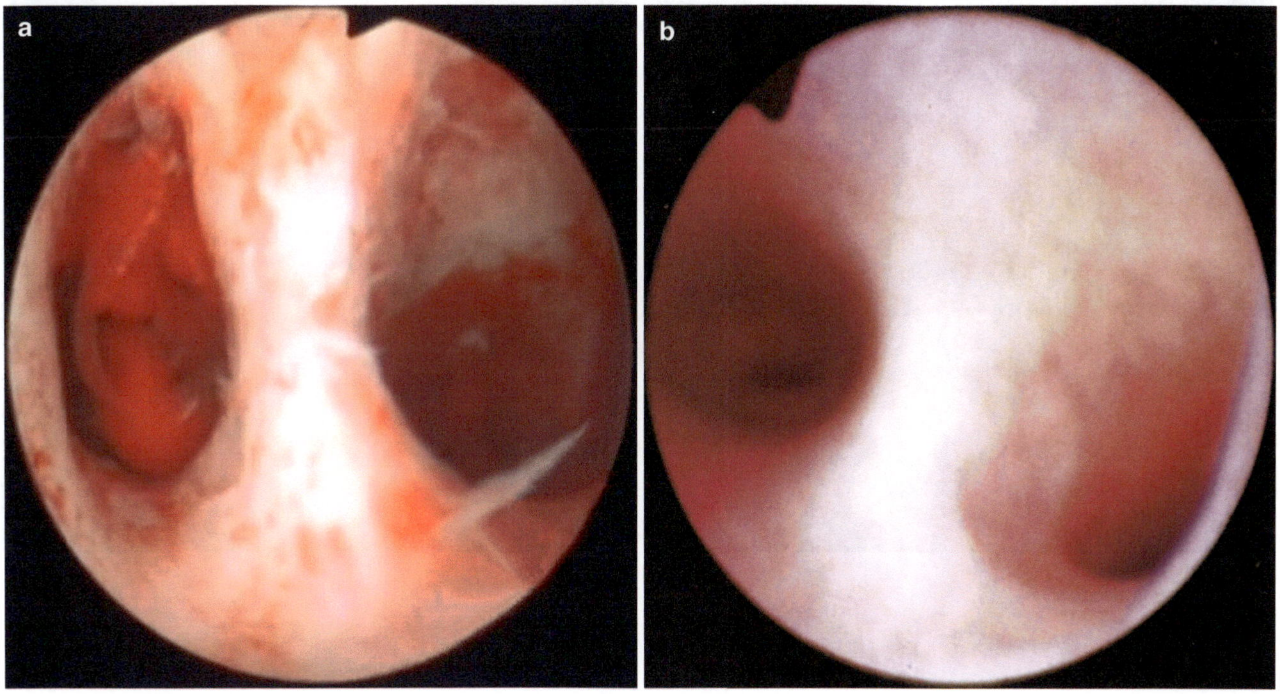

Fig. 8.24 (**a**) Complete uterine septum. The long and narrow septum extends to the internal cervical os. (**b**) Incomplete uterine septum. (**c**) Incomplete uterine septum. (**d**) Bicornuate uterus. A wide and short plate in uterine cavity is seen under hysteroscope. (**e**) Left unicornuate uterus. A long and narrow cavity with a tubal ostium at its top is seen under hysteroscope. (**f**) Left Robert uterus. The telescope goes into the left cavity with its shape unicornual, and the left tubal ostium can be seen. (**g**) T-shaped uterus. A narrow, cylindrically shaped uterus is seen with the upper part stenosis and middle and lower parts constriction. (**h**) Arcuate uterus. The fundus is wide and thickened, and protrudes to the cavity without any definite septum under hysteroscope

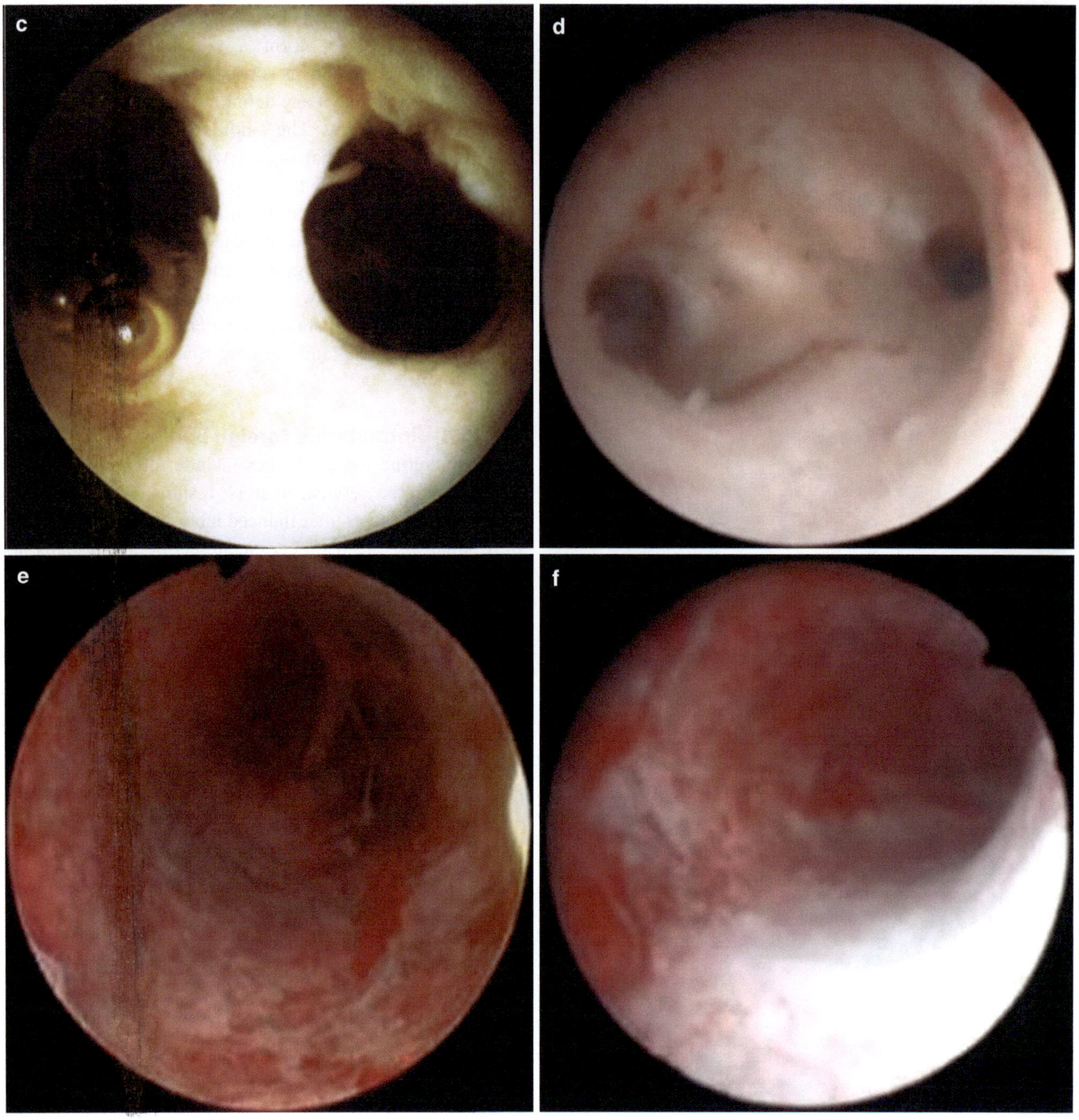

Fig. 8.24 (continued)

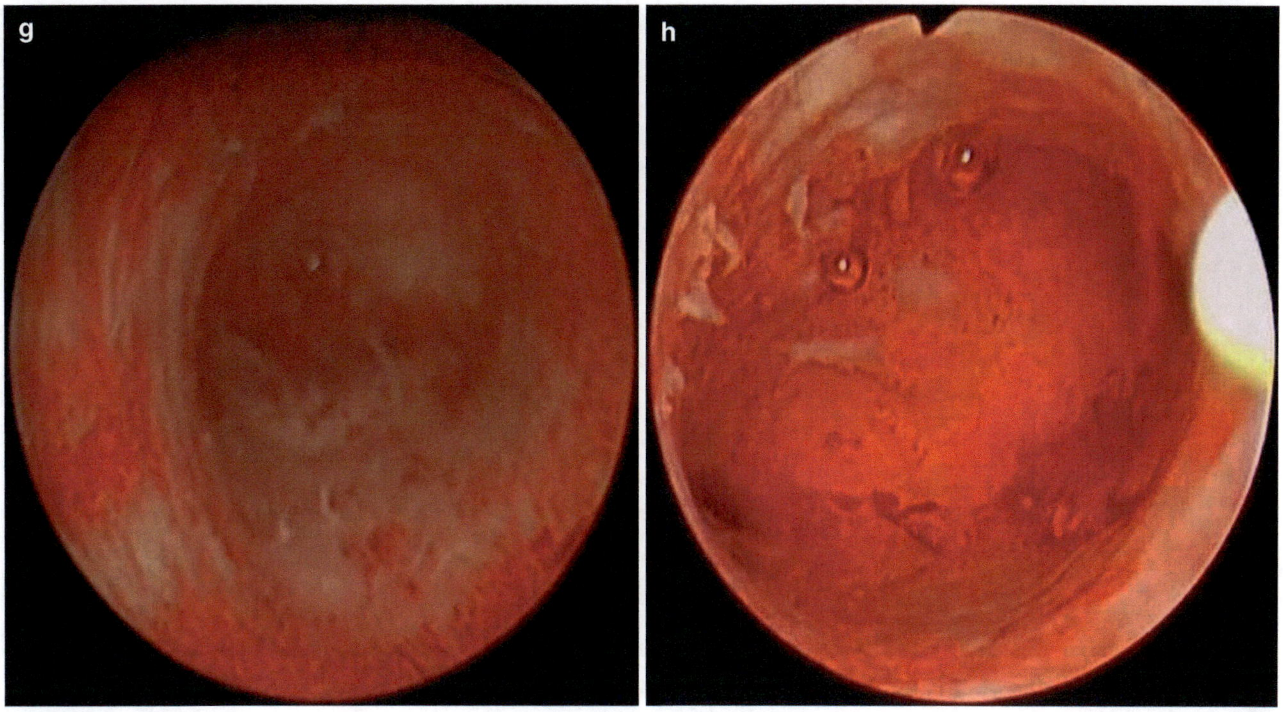

Fig. 8.24 (continued)

various foreign bodies. Occasionally, misdiagnosis or missed diagnosis may occur when the foreign bodies are too small, or when they are hidden by intrauterine hemorrhage, mucus, endometrial debris or some lesions.

1. Intrauterine contraceptive device (IUD): Diagnostic hysteroscope can observe the location and integrity of IUD in uterine cavity. Normally, an IUD is located in the center of the cavity. If there are two arms, they should sit at two cornua. Hysteroscopic examination can discover IUDs which are displaced, partly remained after a failed removal, embedded in myometrium or on the surface of an occupying lesion, etc. (Fig. 8.25a–h).
2. Intrauterine embryonic materials: Hysteroscopic examination may observe the gestational sac, or discover residual embryonic materials in uterine cavity such as delayed miscarriage, incomplete miscarriage, adherent placenta, and placenta accrete. Diagnosis can be achieved hysteroscopically in cooperation with the histopathological examination. Under hysteroscope, intrauterine gestational sac is an irregular mass with its surface full of vessels and its color dark-red (Fig. 8.26a). Sometimes fetal pole and even fetus can be detected. When the pregnancy is in one cornu, the cornu on this side is bulky and filled with irregular embryonic materials (Fig. 8.26b). Usually, the residual embryonic materials are irregular dark-red tissues with a nodular or floccular shape, and the surface white, yellow, or yellow-brown in color (Fig. 8.26c, d). In addition, hysteroscopy can also discover the pregnancy in a cesarean scar. Under hysteroscopy, the embryonic materials are attached to the anterior scar at lower part of the cavity, and protrude to the cavity. Its surface could be white, light yellow or dark-red (Fig. 8.26e). When performing a hysteroscopic examination, if the uterine cavity is normal, but the embryonic materials lie in the cervical canal with its color white, light yellow or dark-red, cervical pregnancy could be diagnosed (Fig. 8.26f).
3. Residual fetal bone and endometrial ossification: In patients with remained fetal bone, yellow-white firm bony tissues in uterine cavity can be observed under hysteroscopy, with a rod-like, flat, or irregular shape (Fig. 8.26g). In patients with endometrial ossification, sand-like rigid tissues can be detected scattering locally in the cavity under hysteroscopy, with varying sizes, colors, and shapes, and the largest diameter 1–2 cm (Fig. 8.26h).
4. Other foreign body remnants: By hysteroscopic examination, fractured cervical dilators or Laminaria tent may be detected in cervical canal or uterine cavity, or residual silk suture or suture knot can be observed in the anterior wall at the level of internal cervical os in patients with previous cesarean section, over which inflammatory tissues are adhered and wrapped (Fig. 8.26i).

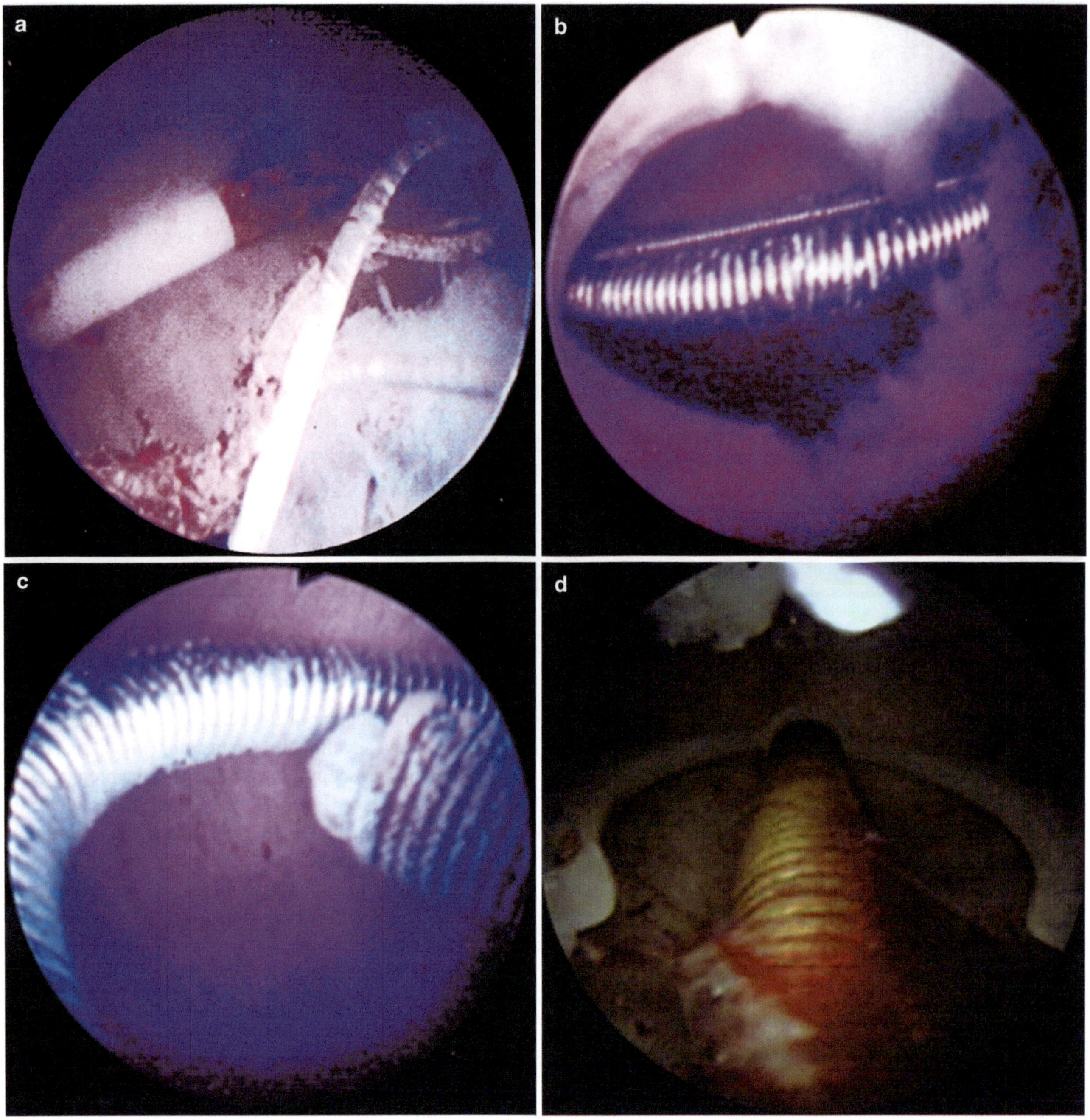

Fig. 8.25 (**a**) T shaped copper intrauterine device and tail string. (**b**) Intrauterine device (metal single-ring). (**c**) Cooper-bearing 250 intrauterine device. (**d**) Intrauterine device (multiload). (**e**) Intrauterine device (Ota's). (**f**) Intrauterine device ("Y" shape). (**g**) A metal single-ring IUD is embedded in longitudinal adhesive band of uterine cavity. (**h**) A metal single-ring IUD is embedded on the surface of myoma from anterior wall

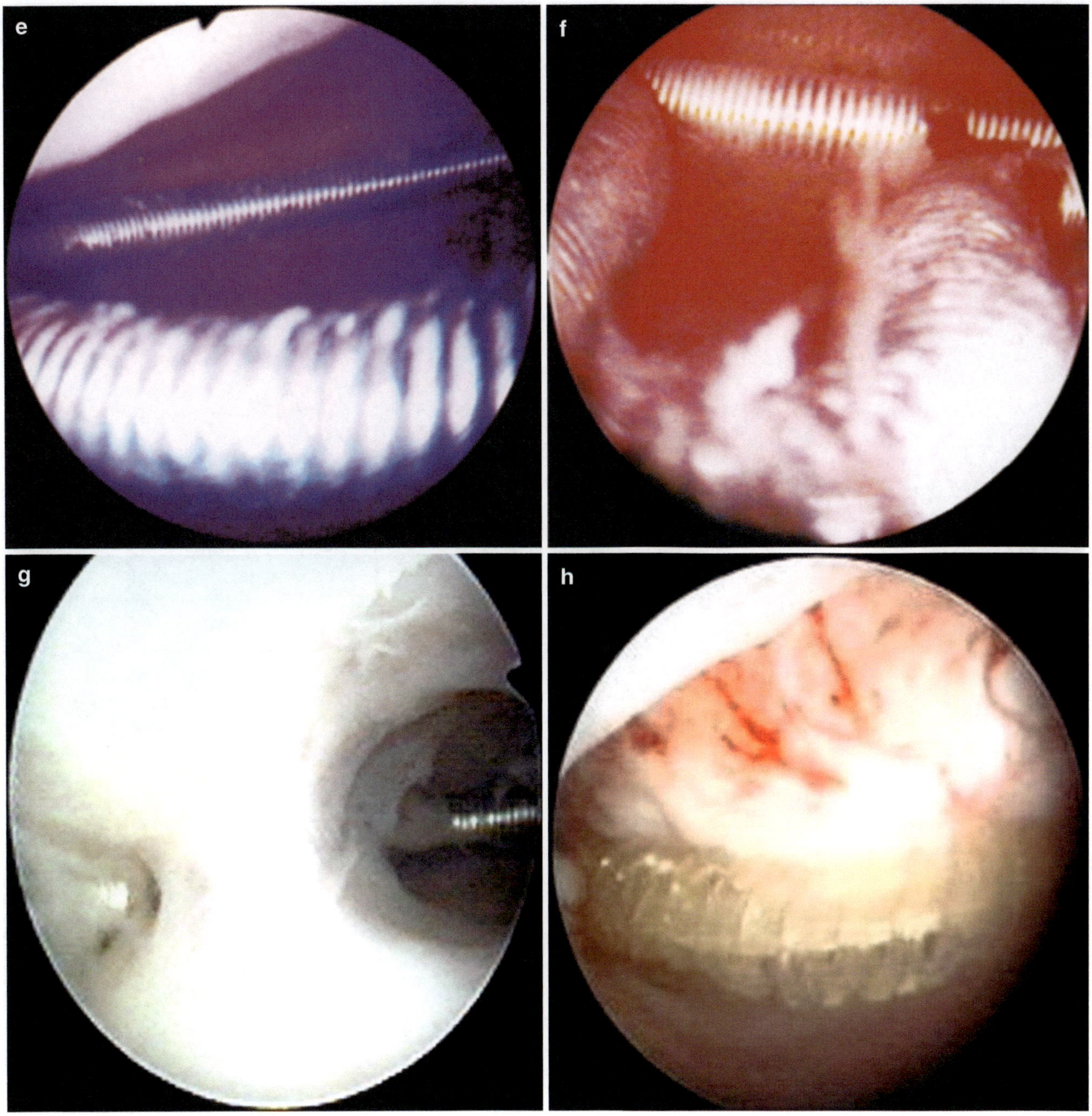

Fig. 8.25 (continued)

8.1.10.5 Endometrial Polyps

Endometrial polyps are benign nodules projecting from the surface of endometrium, which is made up of endometrium, glands, and stroma, and generally contains some fibrous tissues. It has a slender cone or oval-shaped appearance and a smooth surface, on which there are often blood vessels. It may be single or multiple, large, or small. The large one may prolapse out of the external orifice of cervix and the small one can only be seen with a microscope. It may appear to be ball-shaped occasionally and must be differentiated from submucous myomas (Fig. 8.27a, b). The gland of endometrial polyps may be inactive, sometimes proliferative or secretory. In addition, varied metaplasia or other kinds of hyperplasia may also occur. Sometimes cancer or other malignancies may develop from the polyps. According to Kurman's report, endometrial polyps can be classified into hyperlastic, atrophic, functional, mixed endometrial-endocervical, adenomyoma, and atypical polypoid adenomyoma. Takashima Hideyo divided them into four types, which is more practical clinically.

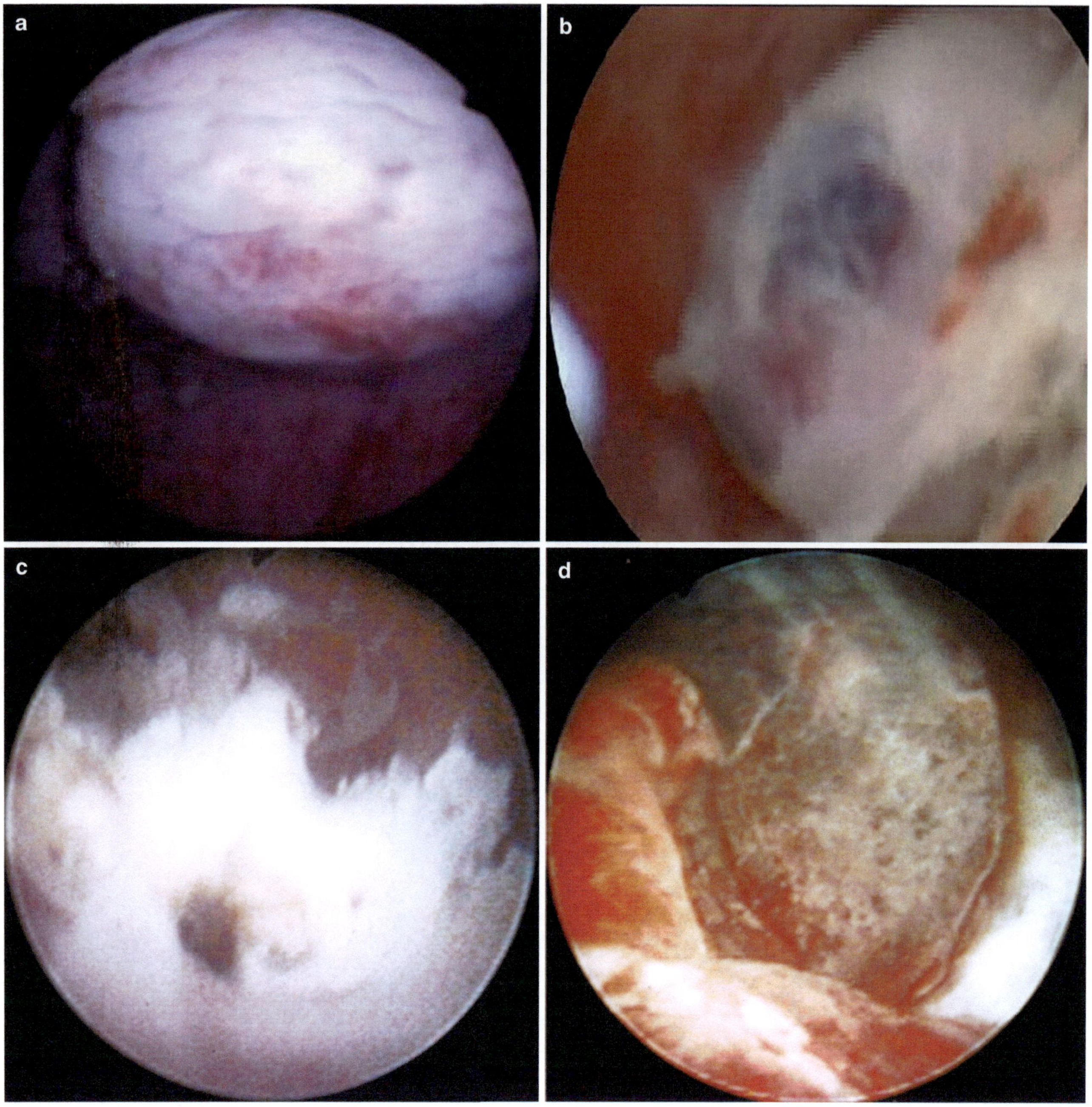

Fig. 8.26 (**a**) Intrauterine embryonic materials (on the 44th day of pregnancy). By hysteroscopy, a mass is shown on anterior wall, with plenty of vessels on its surface. (**b**) Left cornual pregnancy. Irregular embryonic materials are identified in the left cornu of the cavity, with a diameter of 1.5 cm. (**c**) Residual embryonic materials are detected in uterine cavity under hysteroscope half a year after artificial abortion. (**d**) Bleeding, gestational sac, and decidual tissues are visible under hysteroscope after two failed suction aspirations in a patient who had amenorrhea for 2 months and failure in medicine abortion for early pregnancy. (**e**) Pregnancy in cesarean scar. The irregular embryonic materials lying in the lower anterior wall protrude to the cavity with a dark-red surface. (**f**) A cervical pregnancy. The irregular embryonic materials are detected in cervical canal with dark-red color. (**g**) Intrauterine fetal bone remnant. A bony tissue in uterine cavity is seen under hysteroscopy, which is flat, yellow-white and rigid. (**h**) Endometrial ossification. Sand-like small nodules are scattered in the cavity under hysteroscope, which are firm and white. (**i**) Fractured silicone dilator. A translucent light brown tent is detected in the cavity

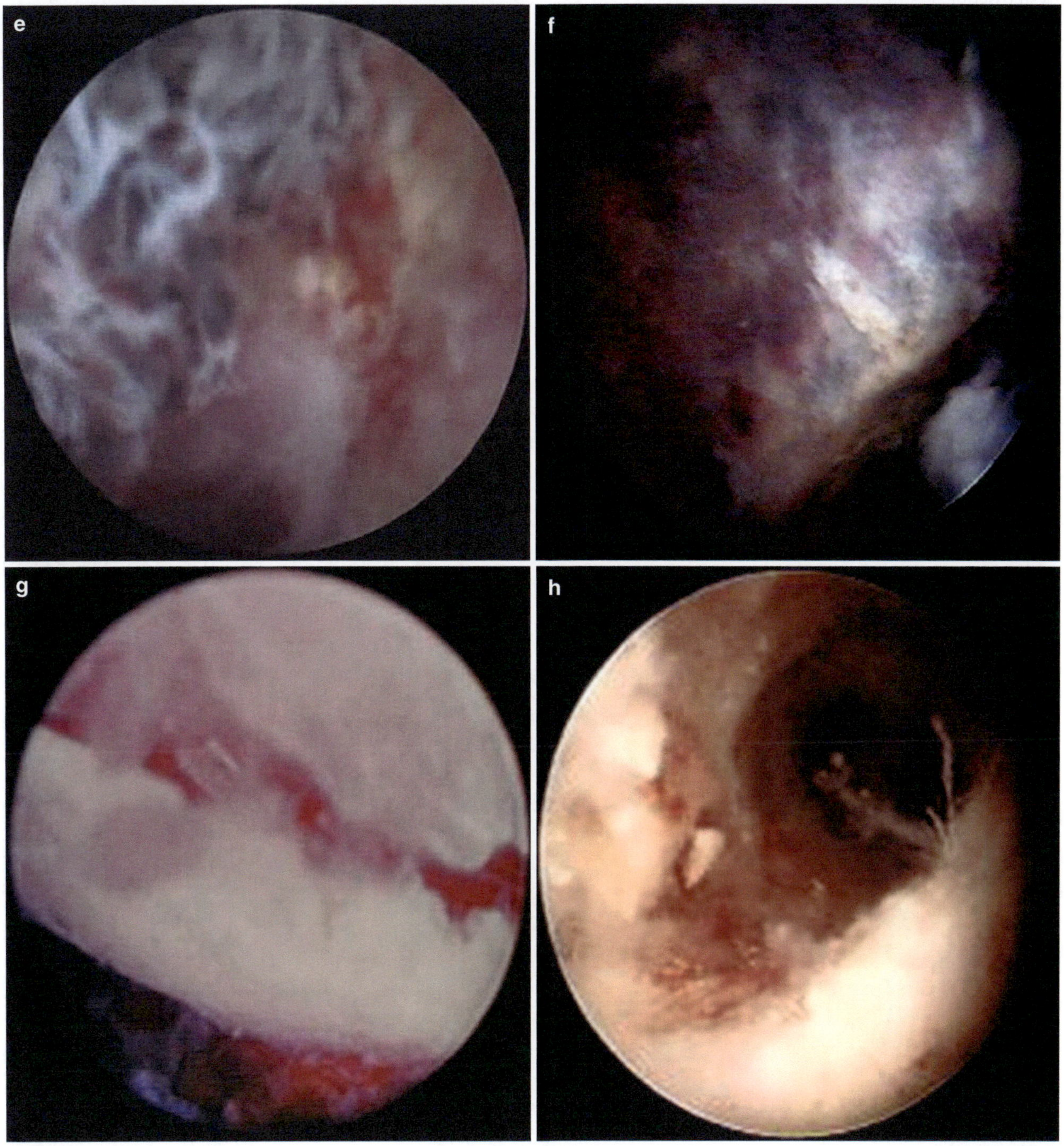

Fig. 8.26 (continued)

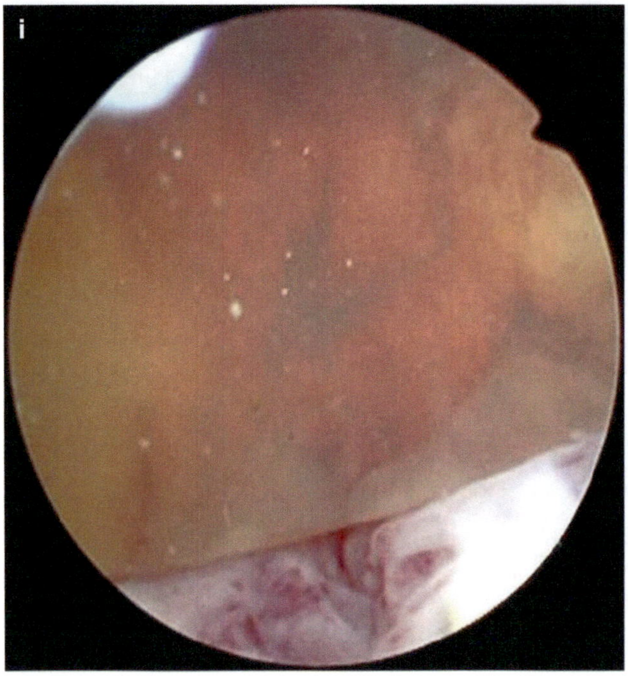

Fig. 8.26 (continued)

1. Hyperplastic polyps: They are common in patients of age 40–50. The polyps have much more hyperplasia of glands, with smooth surface, no atypical vessels, and scattered glandular openings (Fig. 8.28a). They are inactive to progestogen with their tips usually flushing and bleeding.
2. Functional polyps: The glands present the same changes as those in menstrual cycle, so the color and the state are the same as that of surrounding endometrium. During the proliferative phase, the endometrium is light red or ash gray with most glandular openings visible. During secretory phase, the polyps are edematous, pale yellow or grey white, glandular openings are not clear with the subepithelial vessels visible (Fig. 8.28b).
3. Atrophic polyp: After the menopause, hyperplastic or functional polyps degenerate, and show similar changes to the surrounding endometrium. Histologic features are atrophic glandular epithelium, dilatated gland duct, and fibrosed interstitial substance. The light reddish white polyps with smooth surface can be seen under hysteroscope, vascular dilatation is not obvious, but sometimes scattered translucent vesicles and dendritic dilated blood vessels are also visible (Fig. 8.28c).

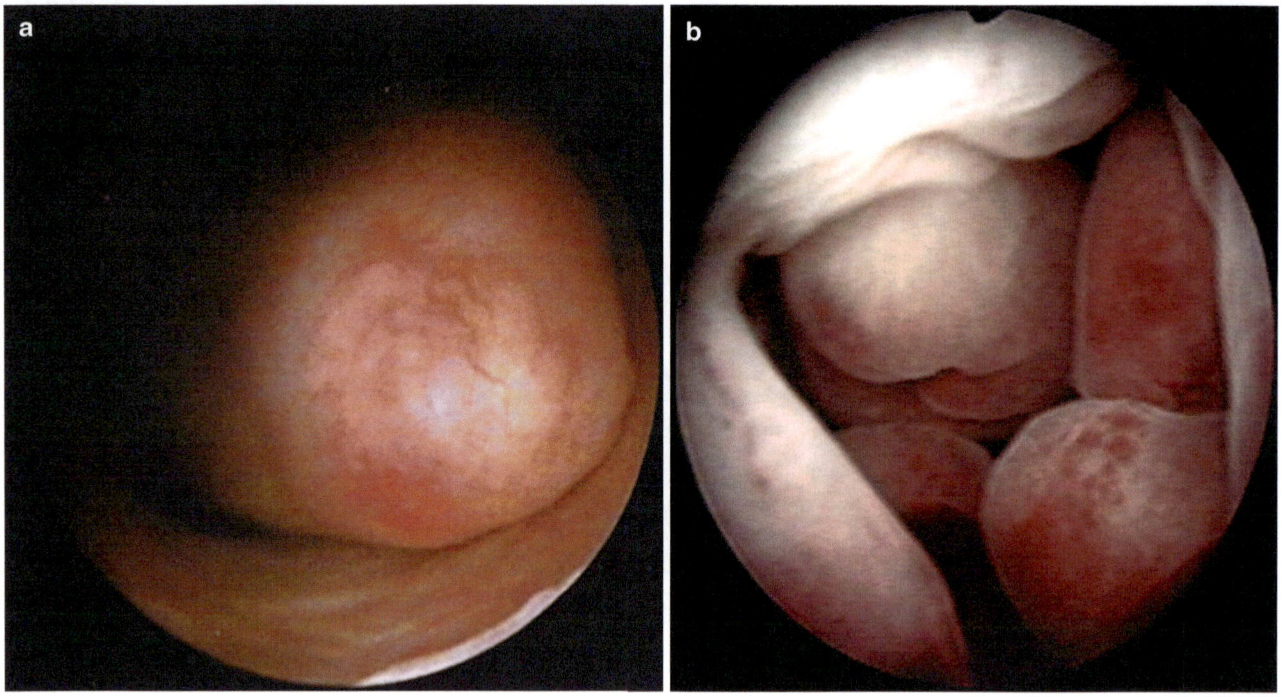

Fig. 8.27 (**a**) Endometrial polyp. (**b**) Multiple endometrial polyps

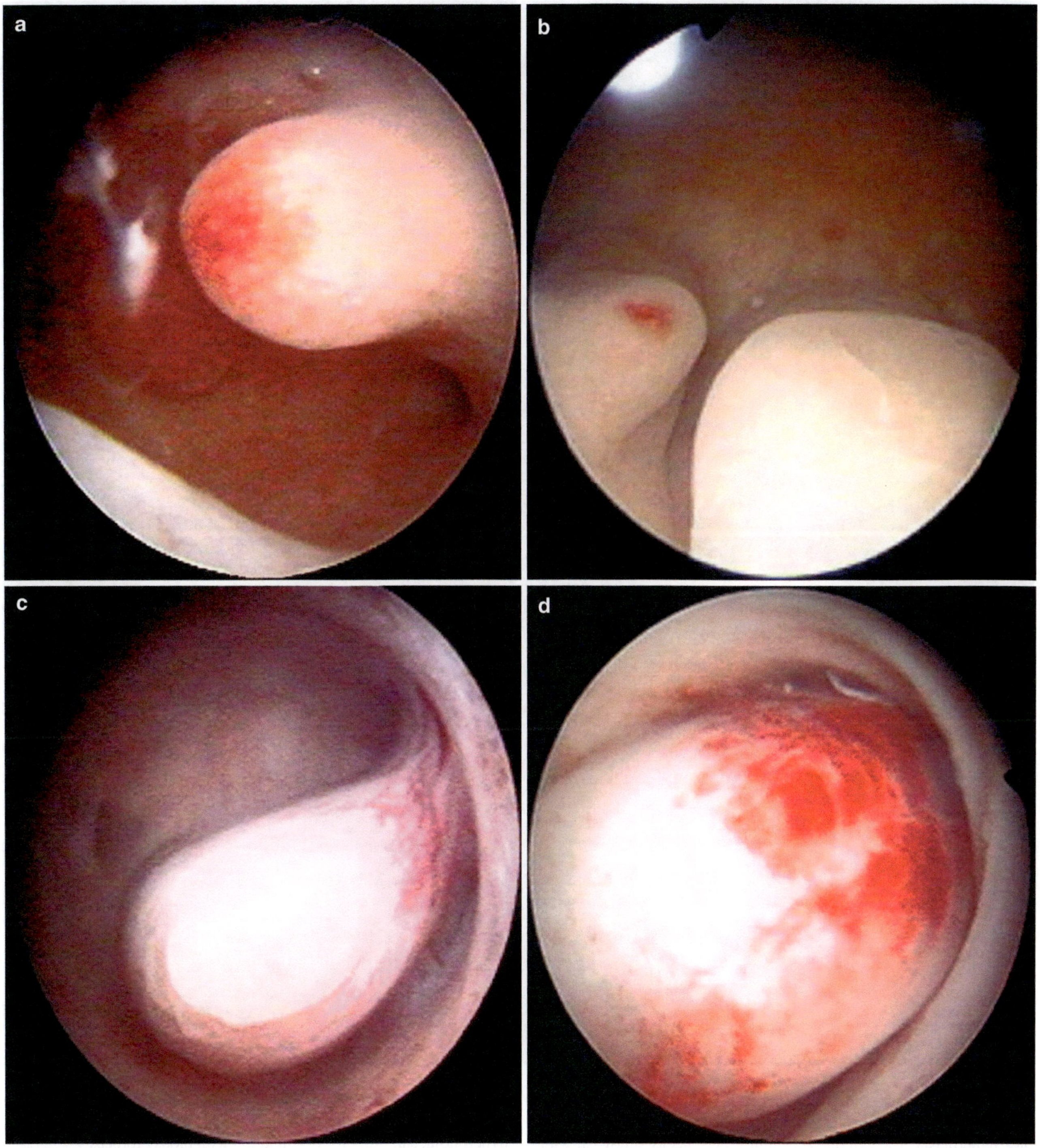

Fig. 8.28 Endometrial polyps. (**a**) An endometrial hyperplastic polyp. (**b**) Endometrial functional polyps. (**c**) An endometrial atrophic polyp. (**d**) An adenomatous polyp

4. Adenomatous polyps: Adenomatous polyp is one kind of endometriosis, with endometrium on its surface, and a muscular fiber mass mixing with endometrium inside. It has the same appearance as submucous myoma, so the histopathological examination is often needed for the differentiating diagnosis (Fig. 8.28d).

8.1.10.6 Endometrial Hyperplasia

Endometrial hyperplasia (Fig. 8.29a–d) refers to the excessive proliferation of the endometrial glands without atypical cells. The hyperplasia of glands is sometimes focal (Fig. 8.30a–c), sometimes diffuse (Fig. 8.31a–c). Endometrial hyperplasia can be classified into the following two types.

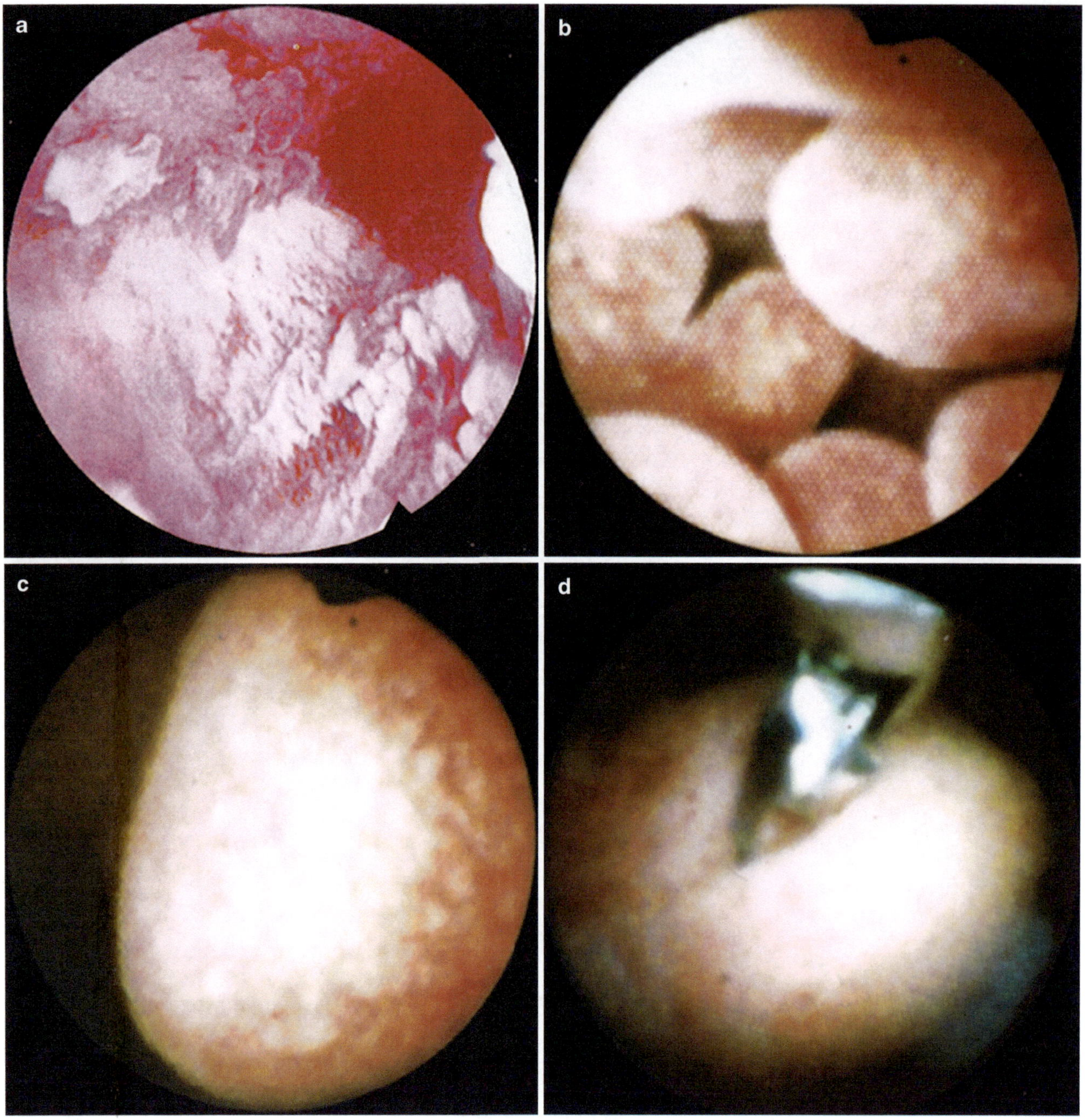

Fig. 8.29 (**a**) Endometrial hyperplasia. The endometrium is grey, and presents as tiny, coarse and irregular protrusions. (**b**) Endometrial complex hyperplasia. The external appearance presents as yellowish-white or red opaque polypoid or lichenoid protrusions. (**c**) Endometrial complex hyperplasia. Glandular openings with different sizes and uneven distributions can be seen on its surface. (**d**) Endometrial complex hyperplasia, sampling for examination with biopsy forceps

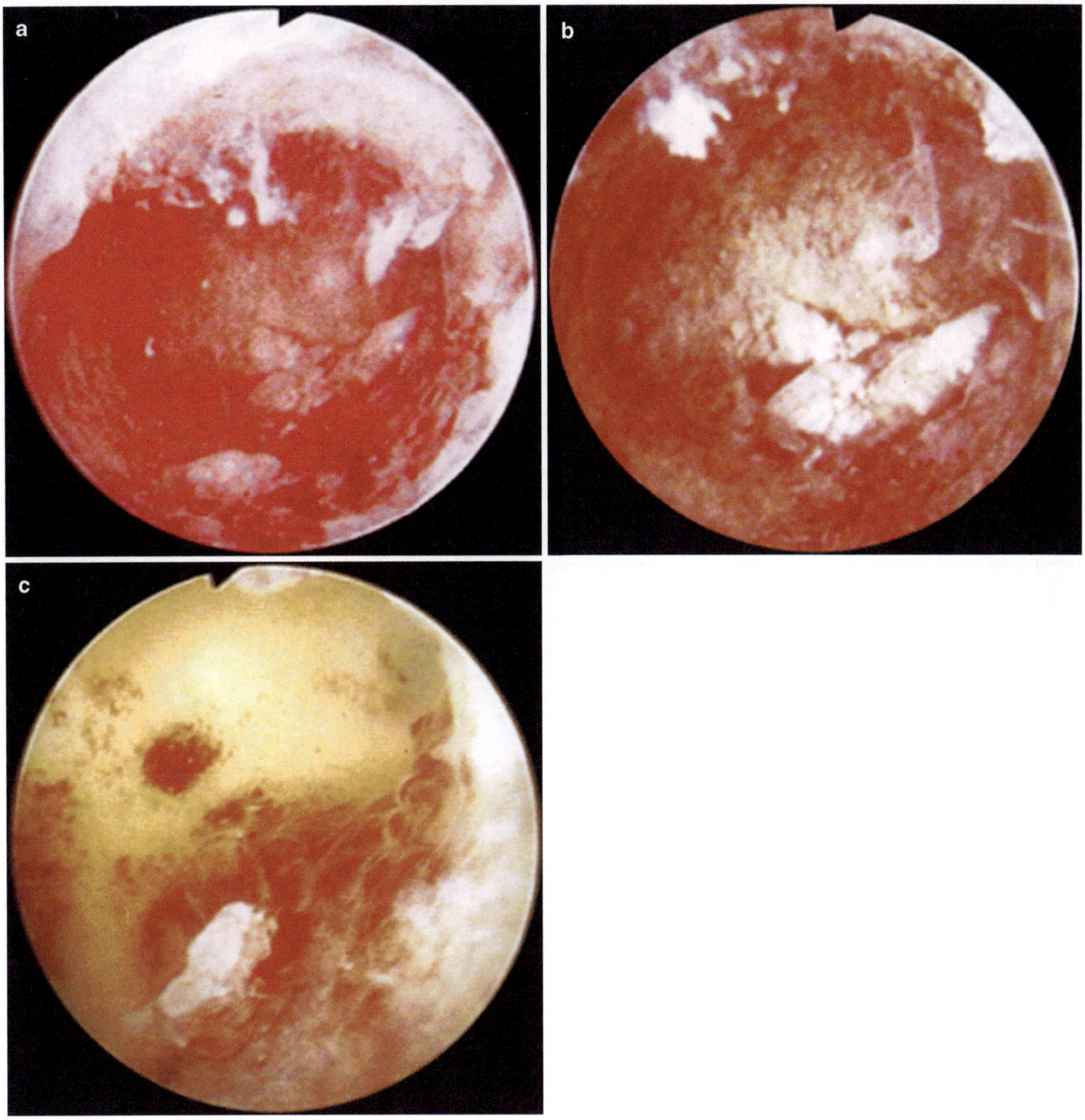

Fig. 8.30 (**a**) Focal hyperplasia of endometrial glands (far view). (**b**) Focal hyperplasia of endometrial glands (close view). (**c**) Secretory endometrium and focal hyperplasia of endometrial glands in posterior wall

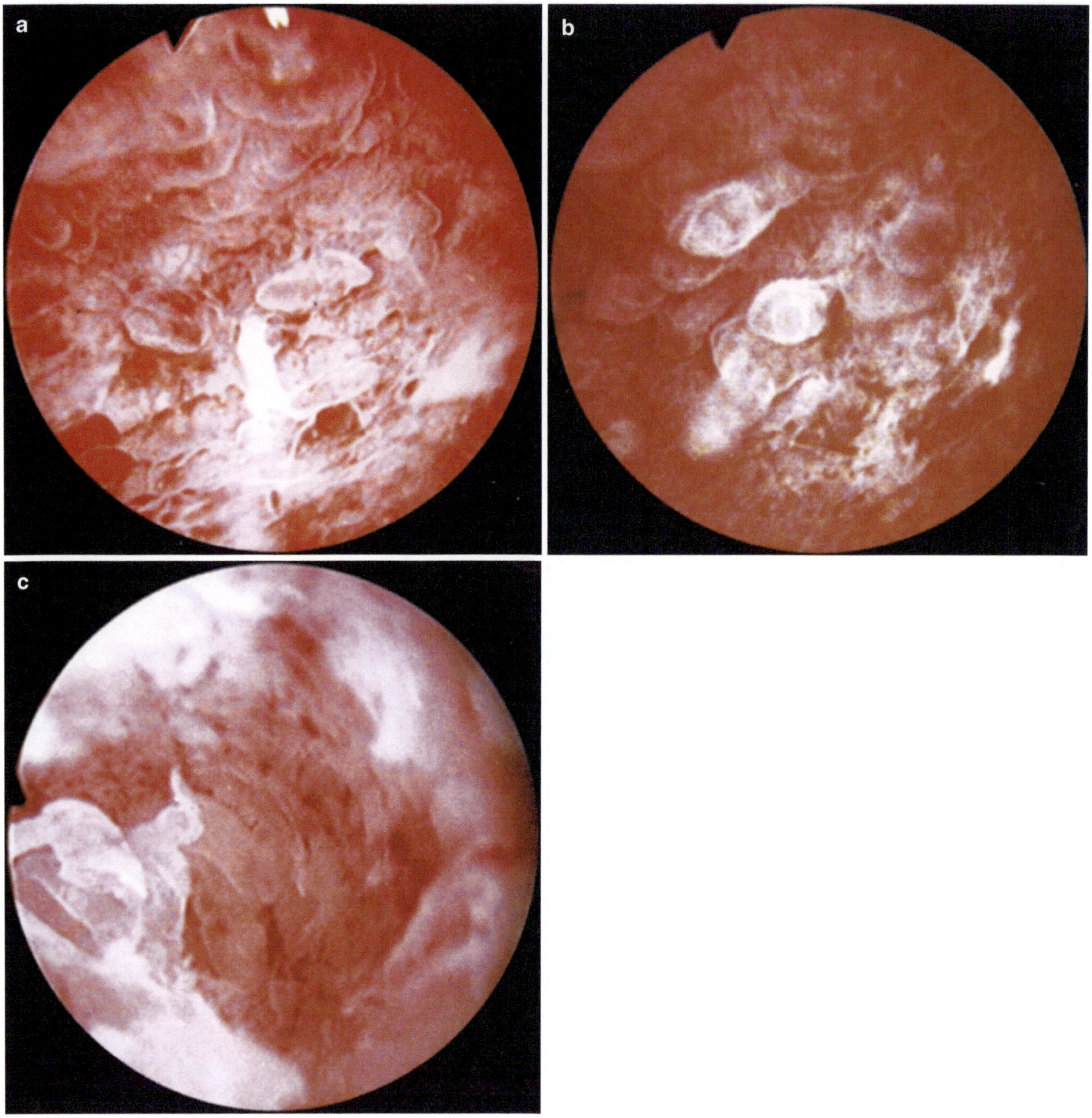

Fig. 8.31 (**a**–**c**) Diffuse hyperplasia of endometrial glands

1. Simple hyperplasia: It is equivalent to cystic endometrial hyperplasia according to the old classification, and it usually has glands expansion and stromal hyperplasia, so it shows mild irregular morphology. Multiple small polyps or solitary large polyp and mossy uplift are visible under hysteroscope. The surface of the endometrium is smooth and opaque, with small round translucent vesicles visible, presenting various colors from red to pale grey. The blood vessels on its surface are smaller and appear regular (Fig. 8.32a–d).
2. Complex hyperplasia: It is equal to the adenomatous endometrial hyperplasia according to the old classification, with obvious glands hyperplasia, loss of gland polar-

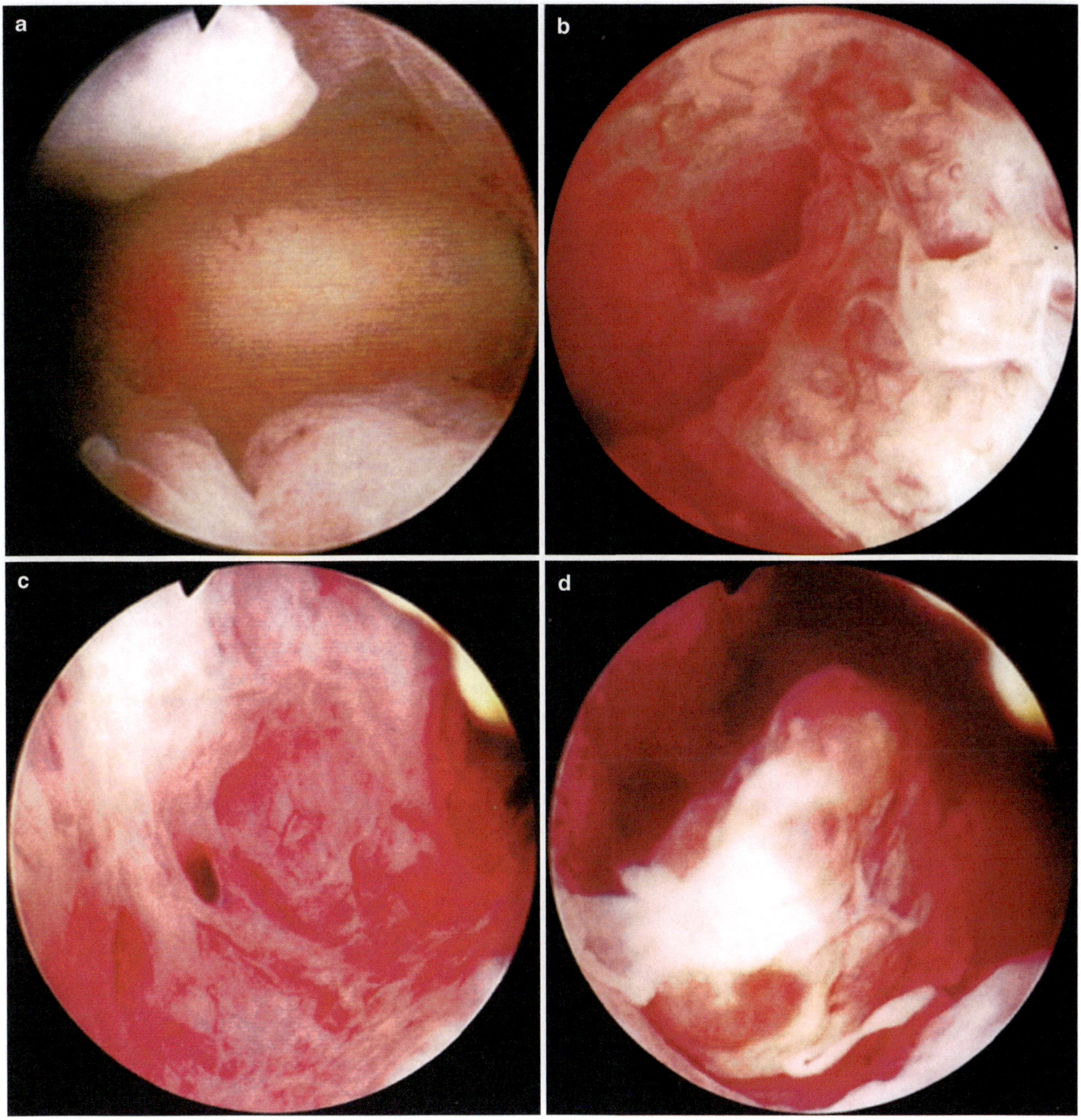

Fig. 8.32 (**a**) Polypoid endometrium, with polypoid and moss-like protrusions of endometrium visible on both anterior and posterior walls in uterine cavity. Simple hyperplasia of endometrium. (**b**) with tiny blood vessels running regularly on its surface. (**c**) with the surface smooth and opaque, and tiny blood vessels running regularly. (**d**) with irregular polypoid protrusions

ity, and irregular alignment. The appearance consists of yellowish white or red opaque polypoid or moss-like protrusions, with atypical vessels and various sizes of unevenly distributed glandular openings visible on the surface (Fig. 8.33a–i).

8.1.10.7 Atypical Endometrial Hyperplasia

Atypical endometrial hyperplasia refers to excessive hyperplasia of endometrial glands containing heterocyst. Polypoid or moss-like protrusions, with yellowish white or ash grey opaque surface and atypical vessels, are visible under the

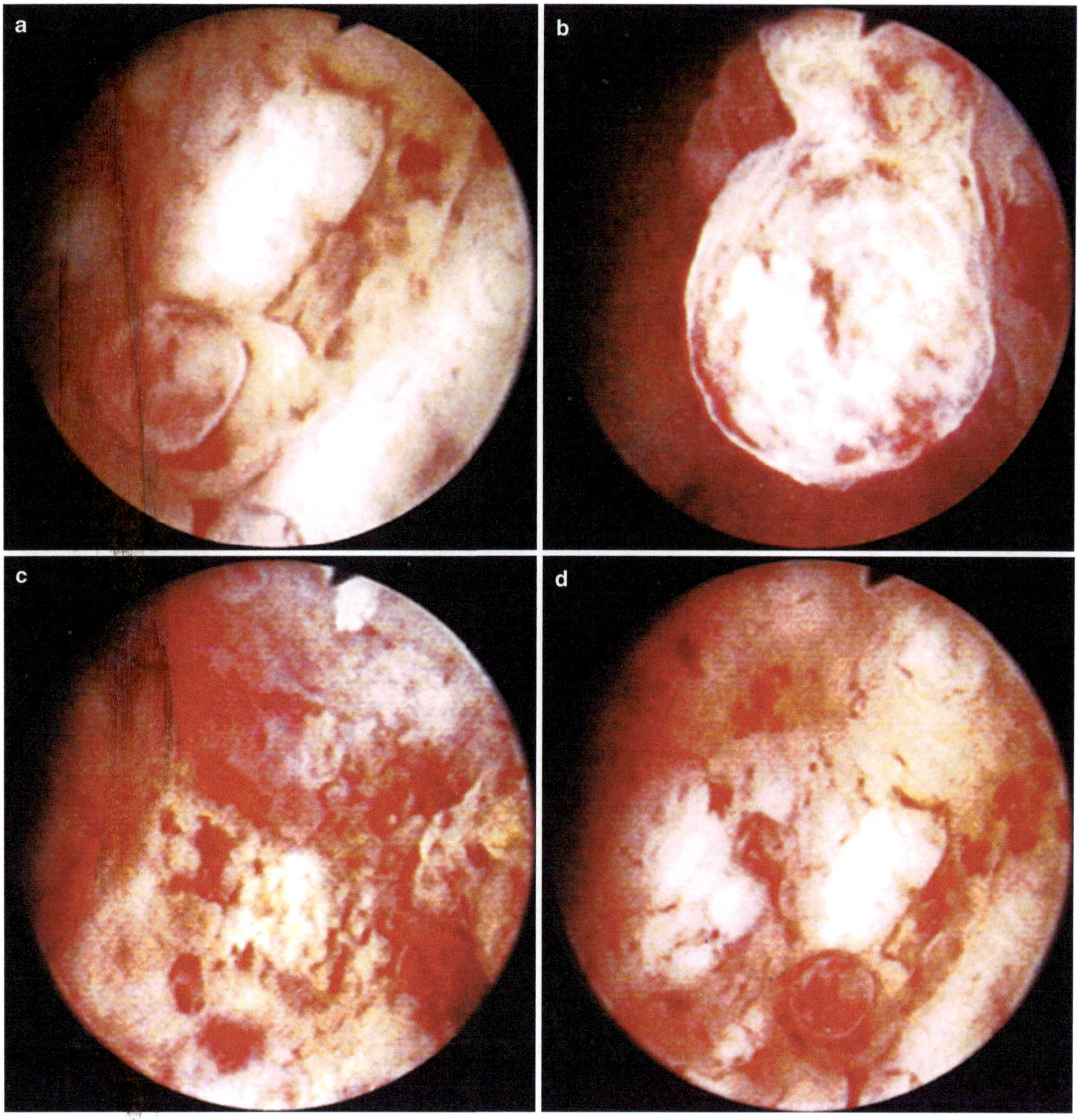

Fig. 8.33 Complex hyperplasia of endometrium. (**a**) Irregular polyps and moss-like protrusions are visible, with blood vessels enlarged and running in a disorderly fashion. (**b**) Presenting with white opaque polypoid protrusions. Focal complex hyperplasia of endometrium. (**c**) With atypical blood vessels and bleeding points visible. (**d**) With enlarged and irregular blood vessels visible. (**e**) With atypical blood vessels visible. (**f**) With atypical blood vessels and bleeding points visible. (**g**) With focal and irregular protrusions on the posterior wall and its surface appears yellowish-white. (**h**) With coarse surface, irregular morphology and a little enlarged blood vessels. (**i**) With several polypoid or moss-like protrusions on the posterior wall and atypical blood vessels on its surface

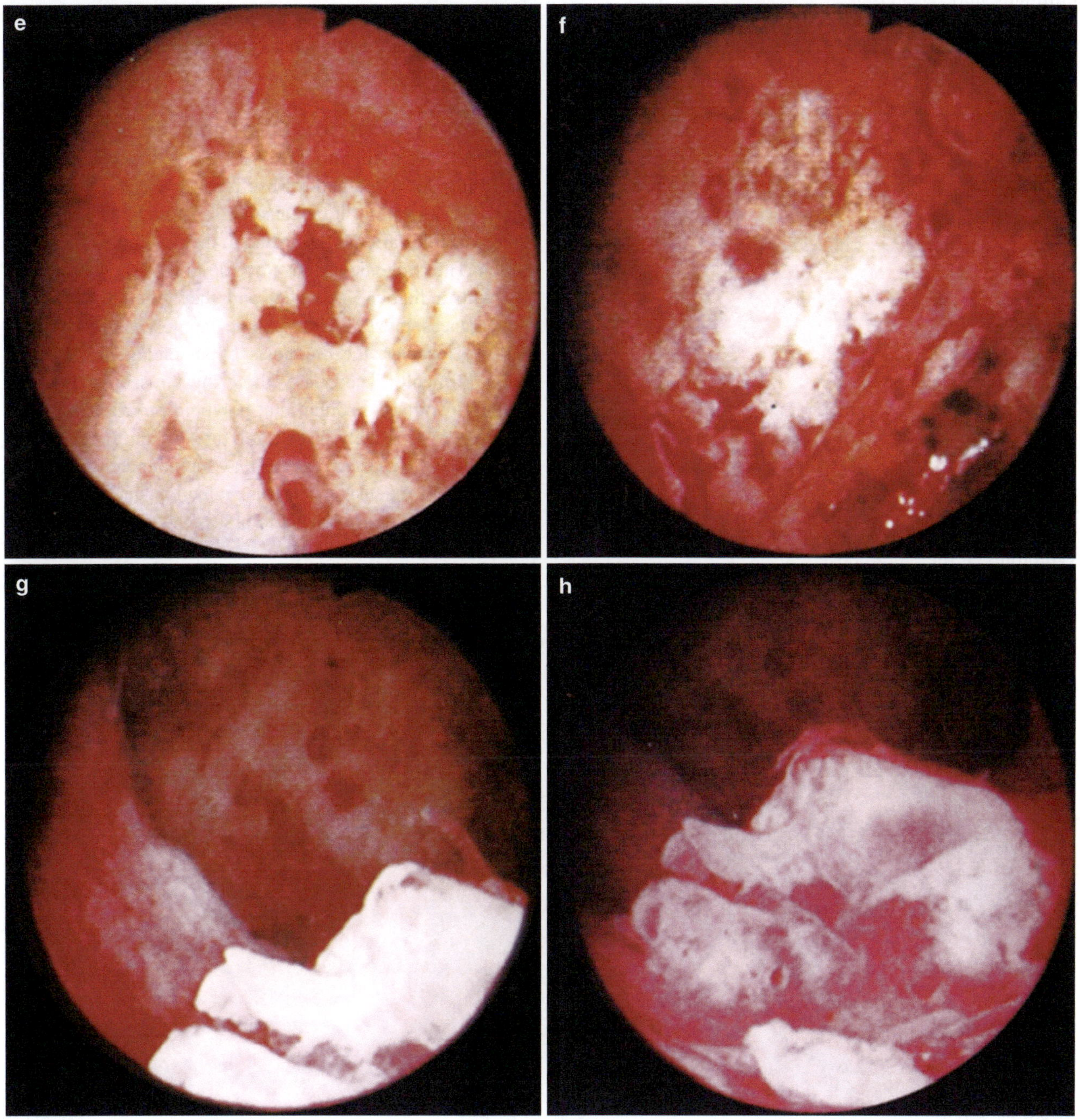

Fig. 8.33 (continued)

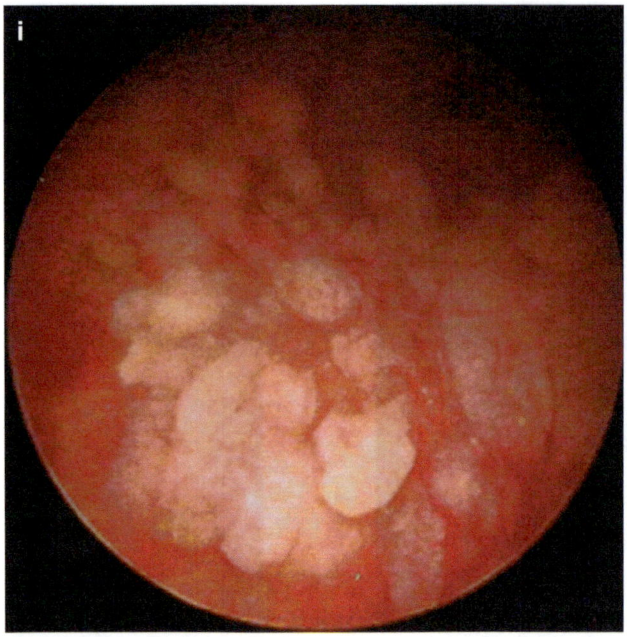

Fig. 8.33 (continued)

hysteroscope (Fig. 8.34a–d). It is usually difficult to be differentiated from endometrial carcinoma by hysteroscopy only.

8.1.10.8 Endometrial Carcinoma

Endometrial carcinoma (Figs. 8.35 and 8.36a–d) can be classified into localized and diffuse types according to its morphology and extent. It can also be separated into endogenic and exogenic varieties according to the developmental orientation. The exogenic lesions develop toward the uterine cavity with a higher incidence, and they often have special appearances, most of which can be diagnosed under hysteroscope. However, the diagnosis of an endogenic lesion is more difficult. There are three hysteroscopic findings, namely papillary, nodular, and polypoid protrusions, which can appear separately or as a mixture. When the pathology progresses, a focal carcinoma may be extended to diffused lesions, and extensive necrosis, infection and ulcers may develop, which can be used to assess the depth of myometrial infiltration.

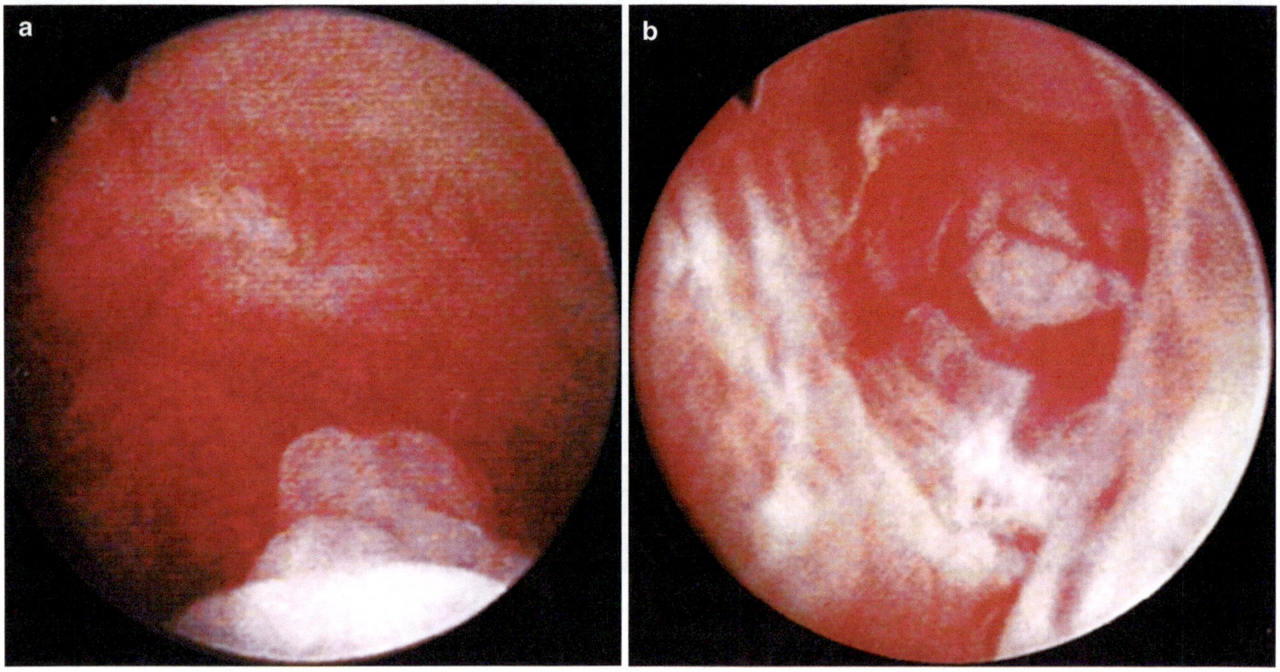

Fig. 8.34 Atypical endometrial hyperplasia. (**a**) With grey-colored moss-like protrusions on the posterior wall. (**b**) With atypical vessels visible. (**c**) With atypical vessels and bleeding visible under hysteroscope. (**d**) A localized area over the posterior wall is congested, with blood vessels enlarged and running irregularly

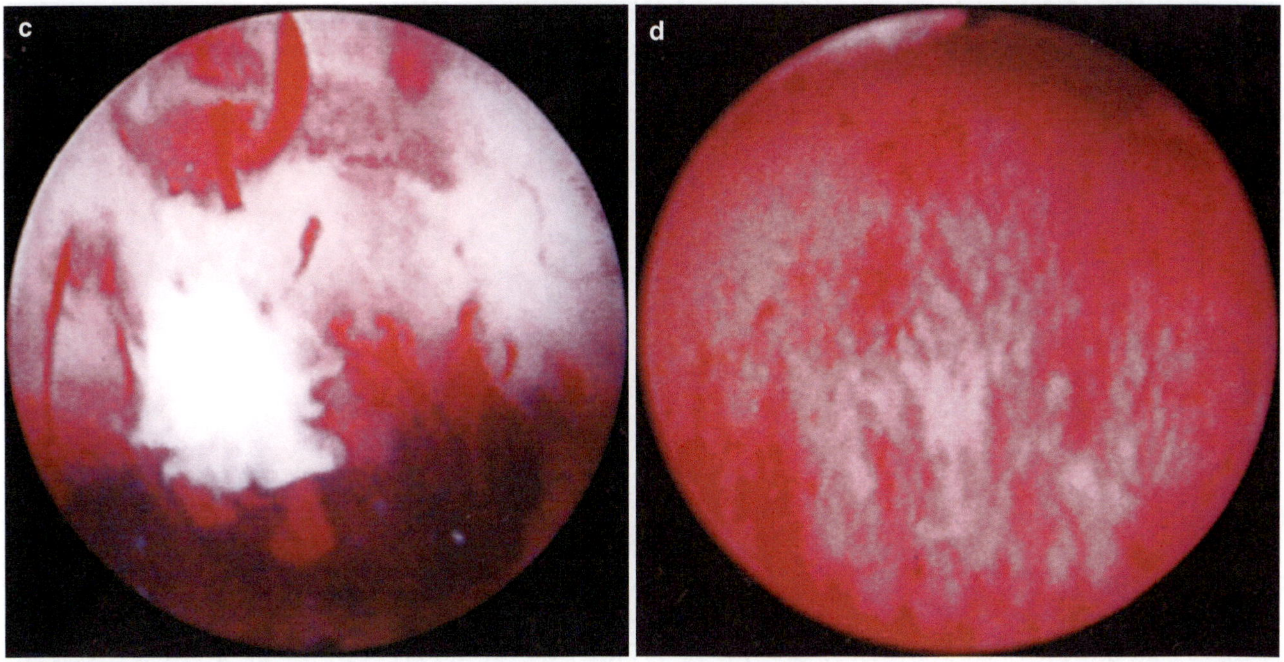

Fig. 8.34 (continued)

Fig. 8.35 Endometrial carcinoma

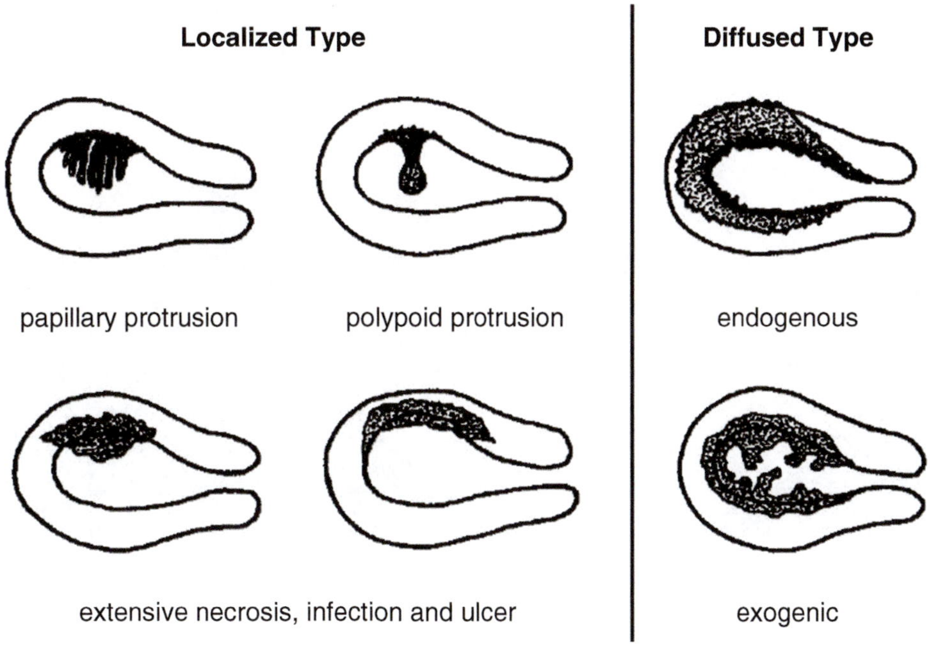

Hysteroscopic Findings

1. Nodular protrusions (Figs. 8.37 and 8.38): They are the most common findings of endometrial carcinoma, with uneven nodular protrusions in appearance, and opaque yellowish-white or ash grey in color. On its surface the engorging blood vessels present irregular snake-like winding, and white punctiform or maculosus necrosis is often visible.
2. Papillary protrusions (Fig. 8.39): They are made up of translucent villiform protrusions with central vessels. As specific findings in well differentiated adenocarcinoma, the villiform protrusions are varied in length and often accompanied by white punctiform necrosis.
3. Polypoid protrusion (Fig. 8.40a–c): It may be large or small, and appear to be an oval or sphere-shaped eminence. The base may be thin or thick. There are no vessels

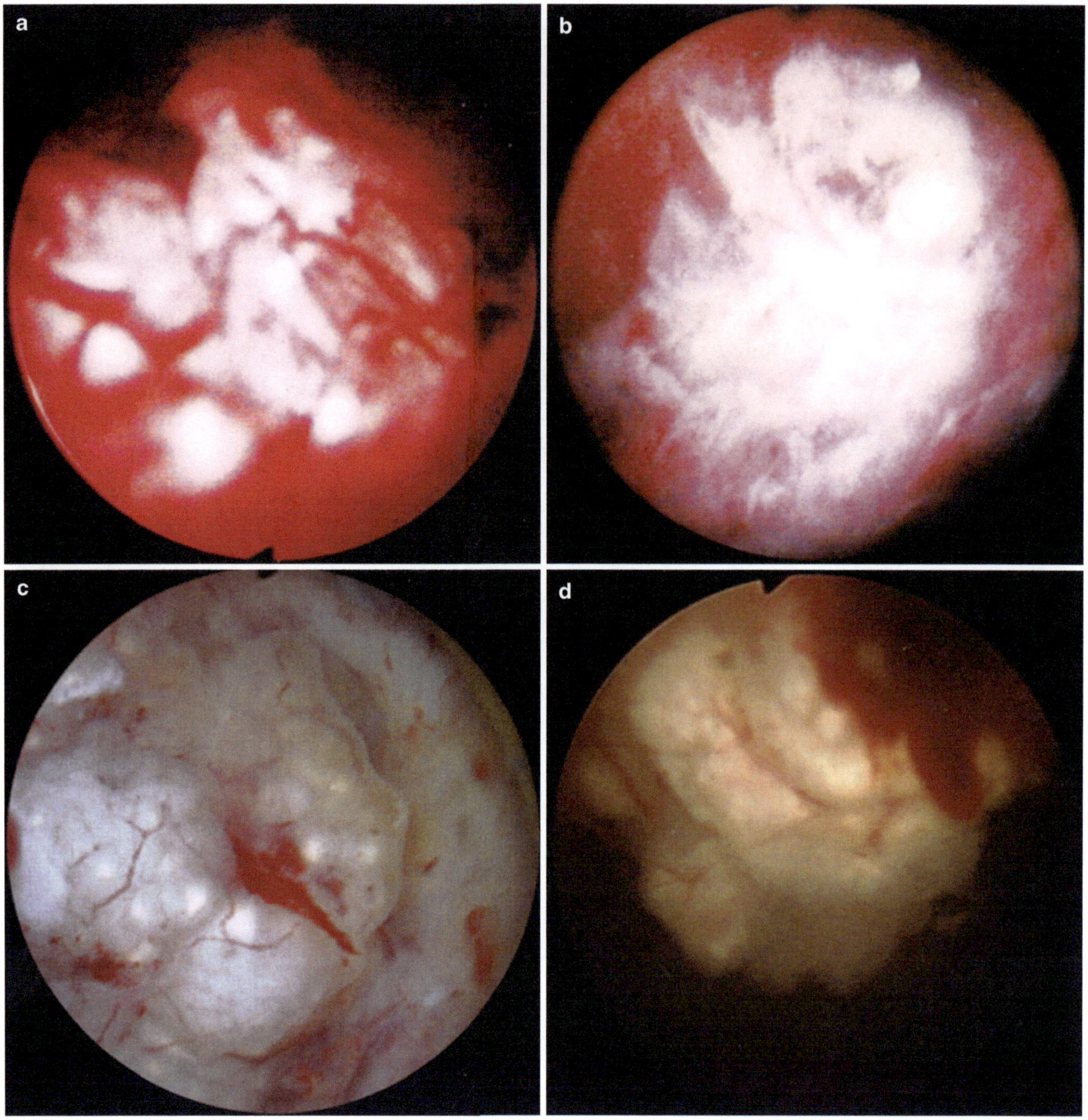

Fig. 8.36 (**a**–**d**) Endometrial carcinoma

visible on its surface or irregular expanded vessels visible occasionally.

4. Necrosis and ulcer: There are white punctiform or maculosus necrosis tissues. Repeated inflammations, suppuration, and necrosis may lead to irregular and rough ulcer-like appearance.
5. Cervical canal infiltration: If the cancer tissues invading the cervix are closely related to the intrauterine foci, it can be classified as infiltrating carcinoma, which is stage II endometrial carcinoma. However, it is more difficult to make the diagnosis of cervical infiltration if there is only a single lesion in the cervical canal. In addition, endometrial cancer tissues may be hanging from the cavity into the cervical canal, which is non-infiltrative and must be differentiated from invasion.

Keypoints of Diagnosis Under Hysteroscope

The following findings may be indications for endometrial carcinoma and so a biopsy specimen must be sent for histopathological examination.

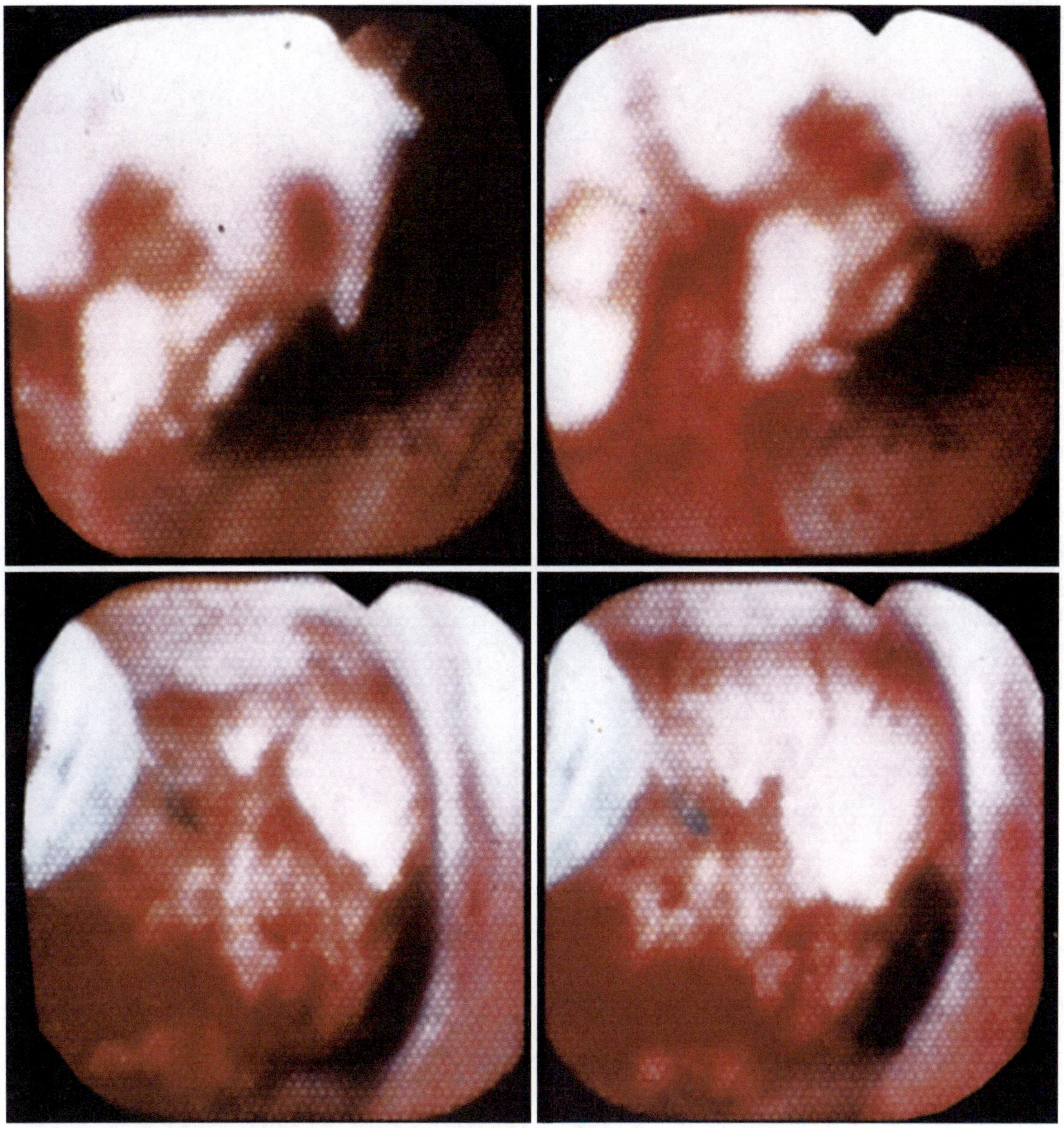

Fig. 8.37 Nodular protrusions of endometrial carcinoma

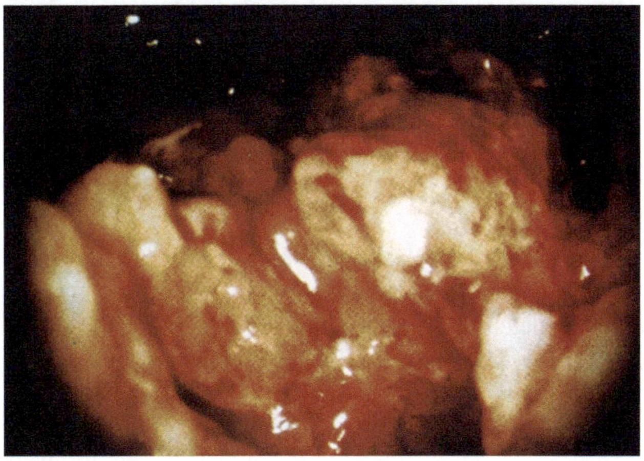

Fig. 8.38 Nodular protrusions of endometrial carcinoma

1. Translucent villiform protrusions with central vessels are highly likely to be well-differentiated endometrial adenocarcinoma.
2. There are atypical vessels and especially irregularly expanded vessels (Fig. 8.41).
3. Nodular or polypoid eminences with a fragile texture.
4. There are white punctiform or maculosus necrosis tissues.

Precautions During Hysteroscopy

Whether diagnostic hysteroscopy may cause metastasis of cancer into the peritoneal cavity is always a problem worried by hysteroscopic surgeons. In a large-scale investigation conducted in Japan, the conclusion reached was that diagnostic hysteroscopy did not affect the five-year survival rate.

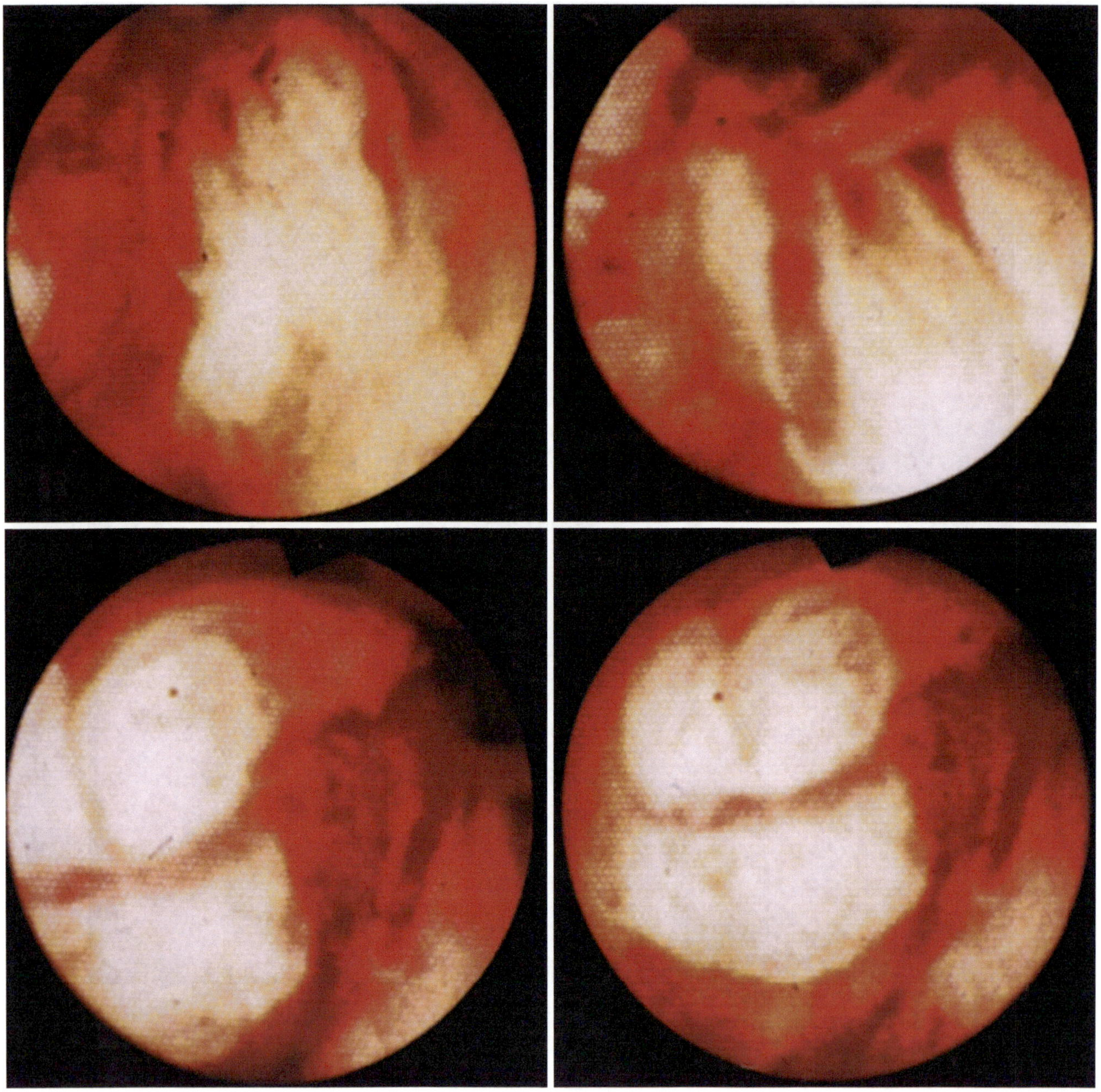

Fig. 8.39 Papillary protrusions of endometrial carcinoma

But even so, the uterine distention pressure must be lowered to a minimum and the increase of pressure should be avoided as much as possible. Moreover, resectoscope is sometimes used to obtain a large volume of specimens for histopathological examination, but there is also a possibility of pulmonary metastasis of cancer cells through blood vessels under high-pressure irrigation, so some people believe that it should be regarded as an absolute contraindication.

Practicability of Hysteroscopy

1. Sometimes endometrial carcinoma can be judged from the specific appearance of the eminence under hysteroscope.
2. The histopathological types or the degrees of histological differentiation can be inferred in some lesions.
3. After determining the location of the foci, a biopsy should be done under direct vision, thus even small lesions can

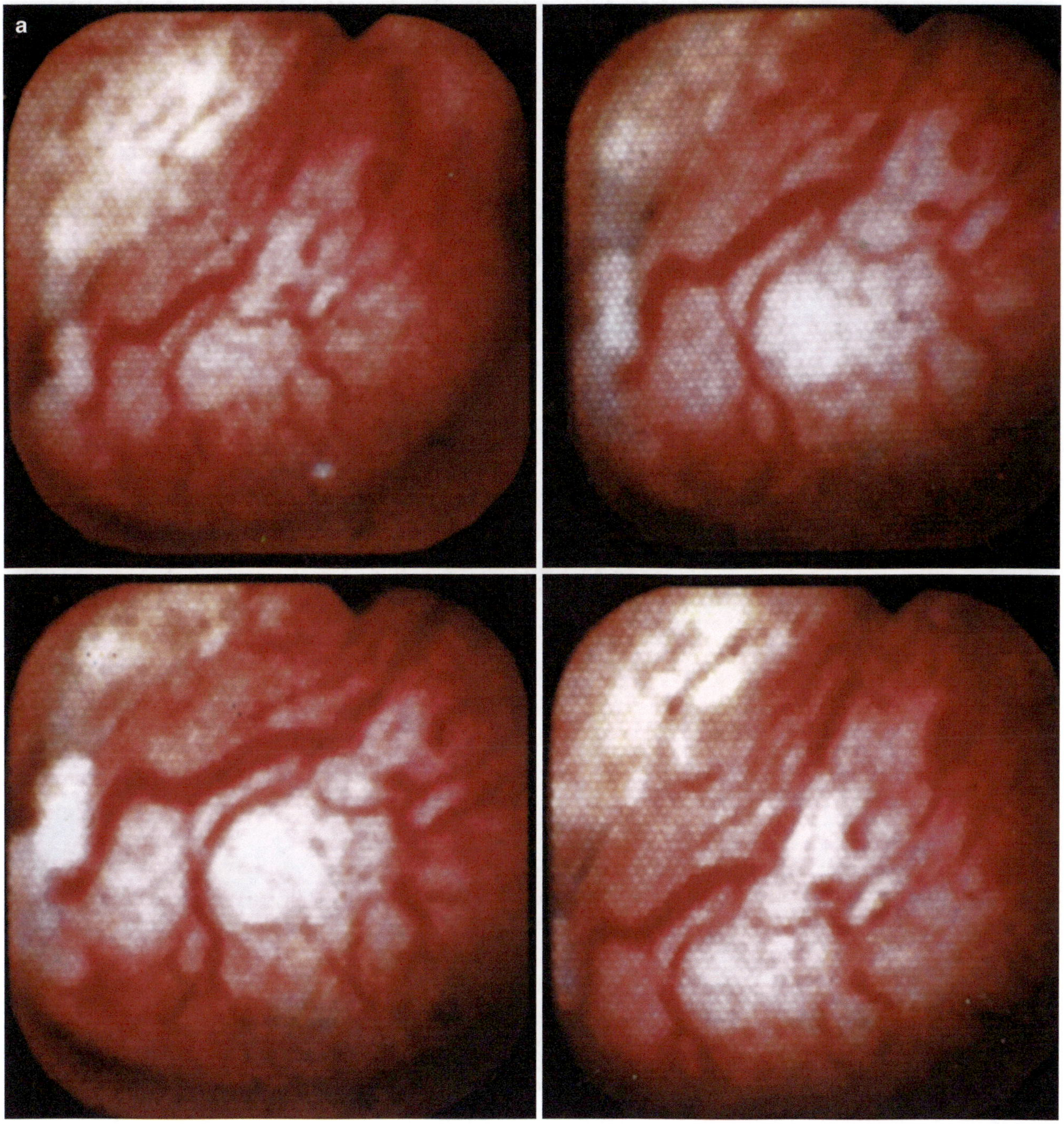

Fig. 8.40 (**a**) Large polypoid protrusions of endometrial carcinoma. (**b**) Small polypoid protrusions of endometrial carcinoma. (**c**) Diffused polypoid endometrial carcinoma

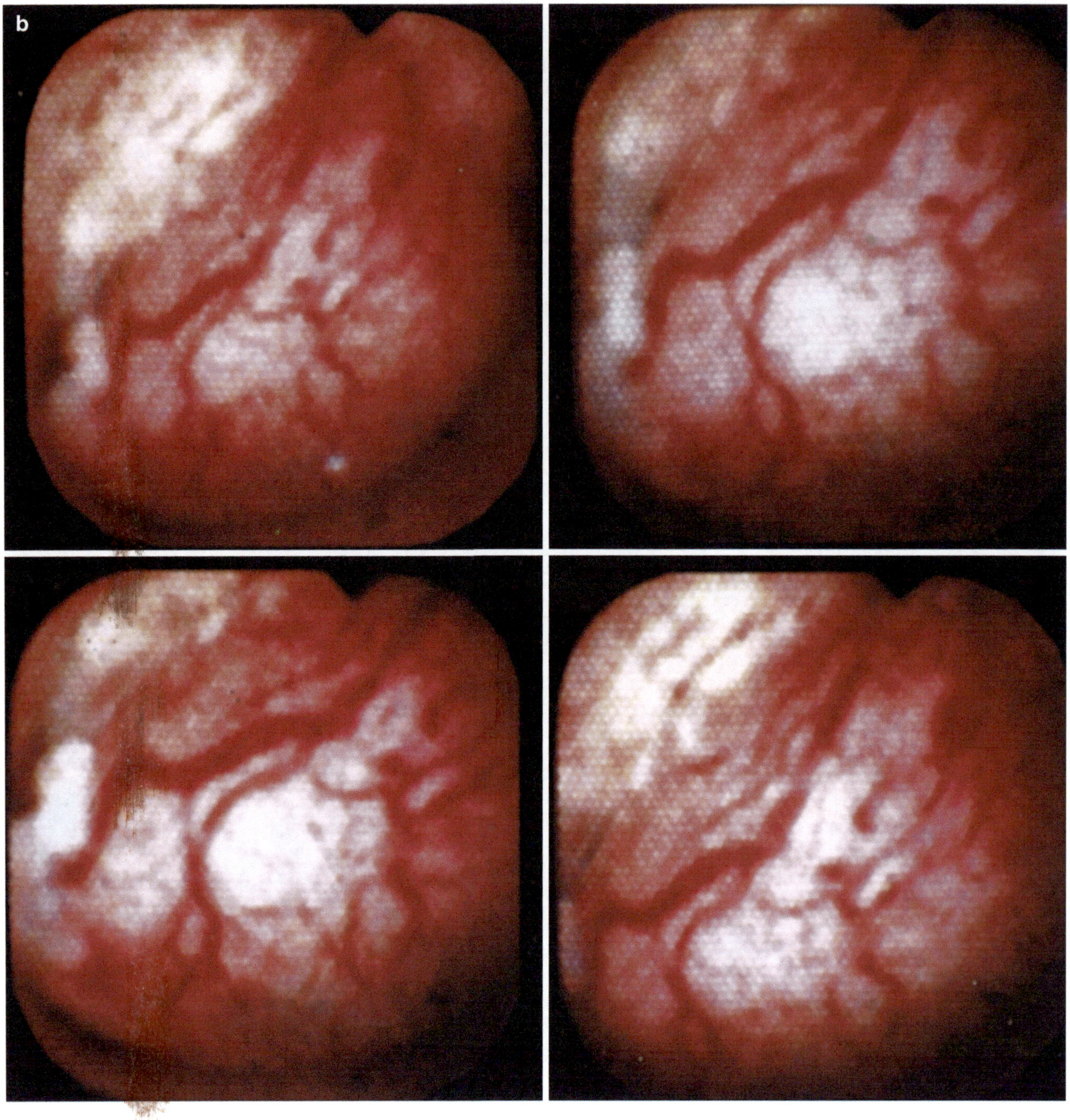

Fig. 8.40 (continued)

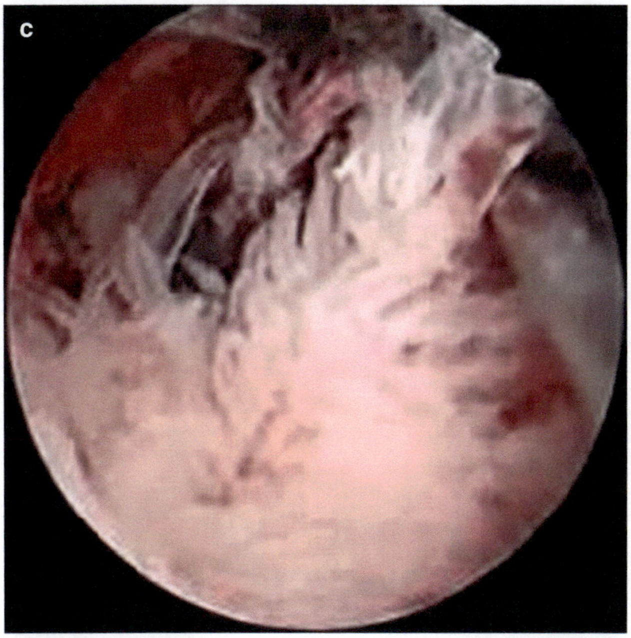

Fig. 8.40 (continued)

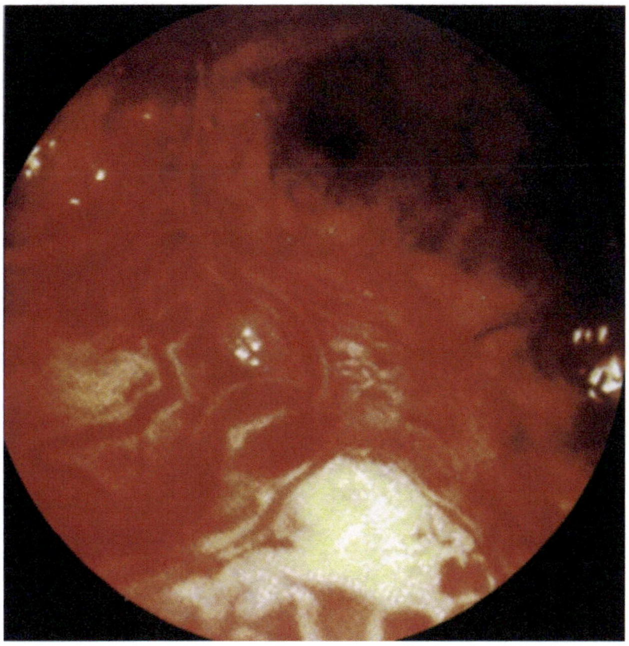

Fig. 8.41 Thick and irregular blood vessels on the surface of carcinoma

be diagnosed correctly and a blind curettage can be avoided.

4. Judging whether there is cancer infiltration within the cervical canal and staging for endometrial carcinoma.

8.1.10.9 Intrauterine Inflammatory Disease

1. Acute endometritis: It is a contraindication for hysteroscopy. Cravello reported endometrial edema and bleeding covered by abnormal mucus under hysteroscope in a patient with acute endometritis.
2. Chronic nonspecific endometritis: It is mostly common in post-menopausal women with the endometrium congestion being crimson or ignitus. Cravello reported that the endometrium was "strawberry-like" with white points in its center. The subepithelial vascular network becomes intensified and increased, with slightly wrinkled surface (Fig. 8.42a–c). The endometrium around the intrauterine lesions such as foreign body or cancer etc. is mostly accompanied with chronic inflammation, presenting as hyperemia (Fig. 8.43a–c), edema, exudation or even necrosis.
3. Uterine empyema: The surface of uterine cavity is covered by a thick, brown, or yellow-green crust when pus builds up, and dark red or brown-red inflamed granulo endometrium with coarse surface exposed after flushing, which is usually associated with other intrauterine organic lesions, such as endometrial carcinoma.
4. Endometrial tuberculosis: It manifests as uterine cavity stenosis and irregularity, and the cavity is filled with yellowish white or isabelline tissue unorderly and fragile polypoid neoplasm, associated with bilateral uterine cornua blockage (Fig. 8.44). For patients in more advanced stages, the uterine cavity is seriously deformed and adhered with quite firm scar tissues which are difficult to be expanded and separated.
5. Granulomatous endometritis: Colgan et al. studied the endometrial healing process after endometrial ablation (EA). Among 19 cases who underwent EA, 15 cases were treated for dysfunctional uterine bleeding (DUB), while the other four had EA due to atypical hyperplasia revealed during TCRE. The specimens of the uterus were obtained from 1 to 48 months after EA and were sent for histopathological examinations. Among six cases examined within 3 months after ablation, myometrial necrosis, red foreign body, granulomatous reaction, myometrial necrosis, thermal damage, and acute inflammation with varying degrees were found in five cases. Myometrial necrosis was never exhibited in the specimens at 3–16 months after ablation of the remaining 13 cases. Persistent granulomatous and/or foreign-body reaction were detected in five cases. Obvious endometrial scarring were found in nine cases. It was thought that the postoperative reactions of EA should be recognized as granulomatous endometritis. It was reported that a patient with postoperative granulomatous endometritis had been cured by uterine

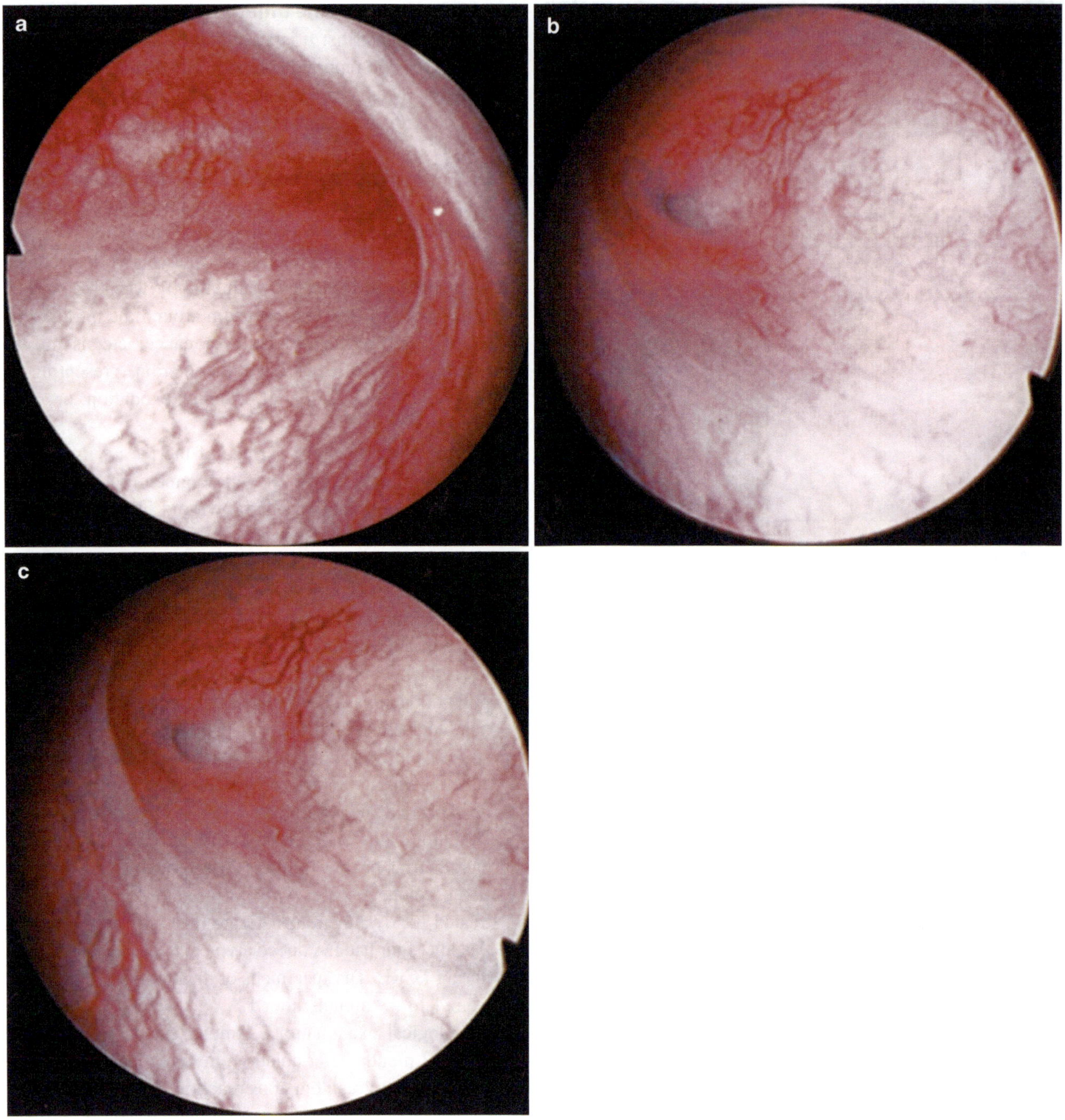

Fig. 8.42 (**a**–**c**) Endometritis

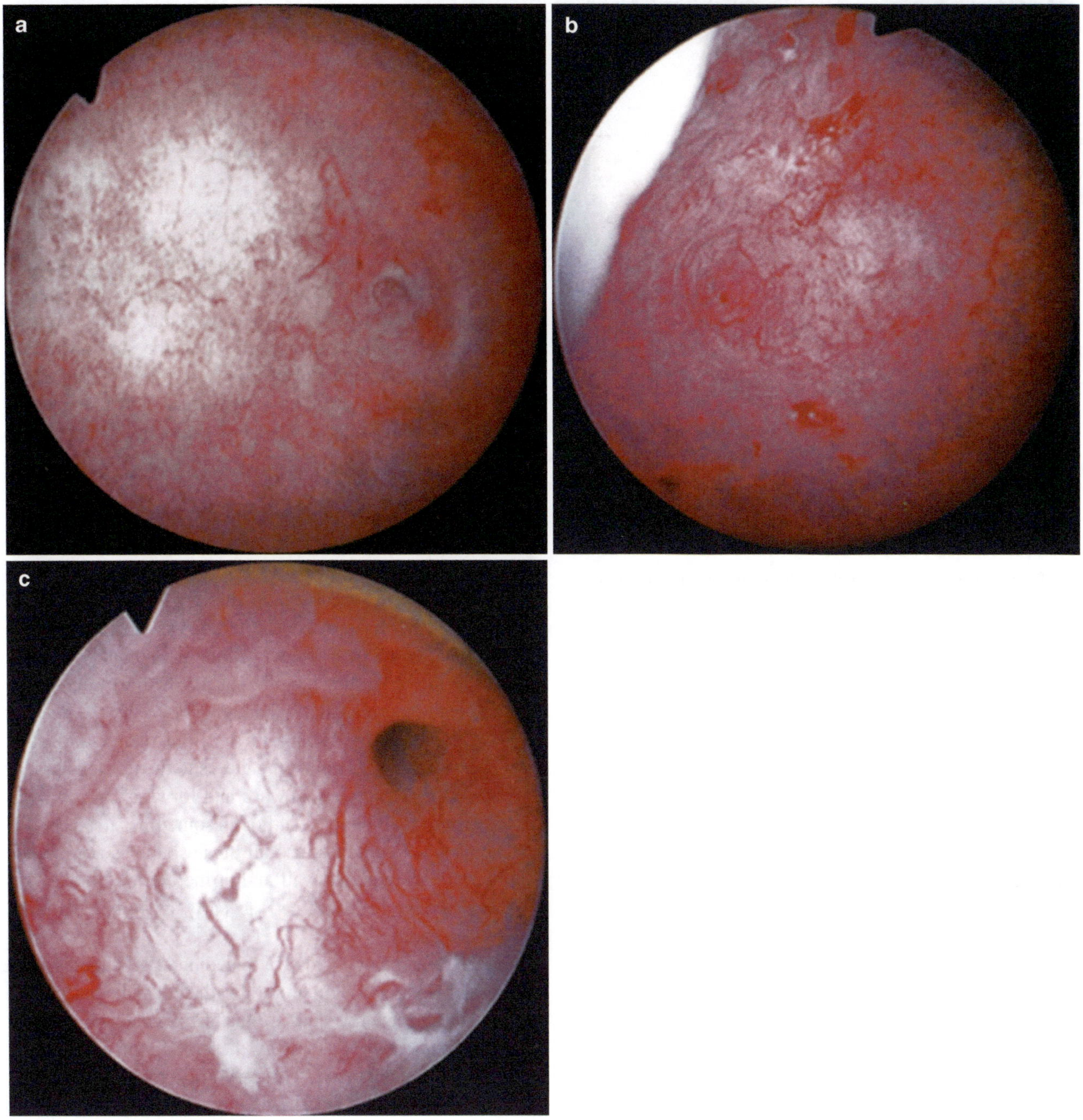

Fig. 8.43 (**a**–**c**) Endometrial congestion

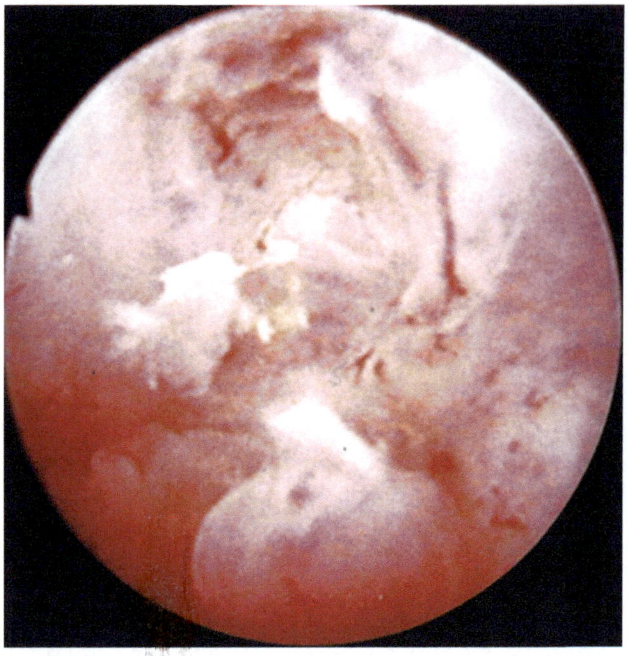

Fig. 8.44 A narrow uterine cavity with endometrial tuberculosis

curettage in the Hysteroscopy Center of Fuxing hospital, Capital Medical University.

8.1.10.10 Denomyosis

On the endometrial surface in cases with adenomyosis, ectopic glandular openings are visualized as punctiform diverticula, small hematoceles are shown as purple-blue glandular openings or purple-blue points hidden underlying the mucosa. Sometimes thickened vessels with thin walls and adhesive or scarring changes are visible in the uterine cavity (Fig. 8.45a–c).

8.1.11 Principles of Endometrial Biopsy for Histopathologic Examination During Hysteroscopy

There are four principles:

1. As for a normal uterine cavity, especially in menopausal women, sampling may not be needed.
2. As for common benign lesions, uterine aspiration or random curettage of endometrium is suggested.
3. As for obviously focal lesions, hysteroscopic biopsy or target sampling for examination is suggested (Fig. 8.46).
4. As for obviously diffuse lesions, the whole functional layer of the endometrium should be resected with wire loop electrode for examination. Garuti et al. recommended that endometrial sampling be obtained in cases of thickened and uneven endometrium, distorted uterine cavity, and obscure visualization.

8.1.12 Causes of and Solutions to Hysteroscopic Failures

Sometimes hysteroscopy is not successful. Van Trotsenburg et al. reported on 317 premenopausal patients who had outpatient hysteroscopies due to abnormal uterine bleeding. The procedures succeeded in 305 cases (96.2%), but the success rate increased up to 98.9% when lidocaine spray was routinely used. Nagele et al. reported that the success rate of outpatient hysteroscopy was 96.4%, while Unfried et al. reported a success rate 87.5% with fiber hysteroscope and 100% with rigid hysteroscope. The causes for failure are as follows:

1. Difficulty in insertion of the hysteroscope: If the cervix is narrow, the Hegar dilator can be used to expand it under the guidance of ultrasonography. If the flexion degree of the uterus is too great and the dilating of the cervix is difficult, a fiber hysteroscope could be used instead.
2. Bubbles in the uterine cavity: The incompletely emptied air in the irrigating tube or sheath of the hysteroscope enters the uterine cavity and gathers beneath the anterior wall or at uterine fundus in the form of microvesicles. The operators can adjust the uterus to the retroposition or move the telescope backward and forward quickly so as to drive out air bubbles, although sometimes it is very difficult to take effect. Since all the air bubbles accumulate beneath the anterior wall and at the uterine fundus, this area should be examined as early as possible during hysteroscopy.
3. Intrauterine blood clots or bleeding: For patients with more bleeding, a rigid urethral catheter can be placed into the uterine cavity, and normal saline may be injected quickly so as to wash away the blood clots, and then a hysteroscope is inserted quickly to perform the examinations. For patients with much more bleeding, the pressure and/or flow rate of uterine distending fluid can also be increased so as to wash out the blood clots and the blood. If the internal os is relaxed, a rigid urethral catheter can be placed beside the hysteroscope in order to accelerate the circulation of uterine distending fluid so as to keep a clear vision. Spraying adrenaline into the uterine cavity has been reported to reduce bleeding.
4. Unclear visualization: It is mostly due to the inadequacy of uterine distension which may be caused by a relaxed internal os and leakage of uterine distending fluid. In this condition, a bigger hysteroscope can be used instead, and clamping the cervical os with a cervical clamp or elevat-

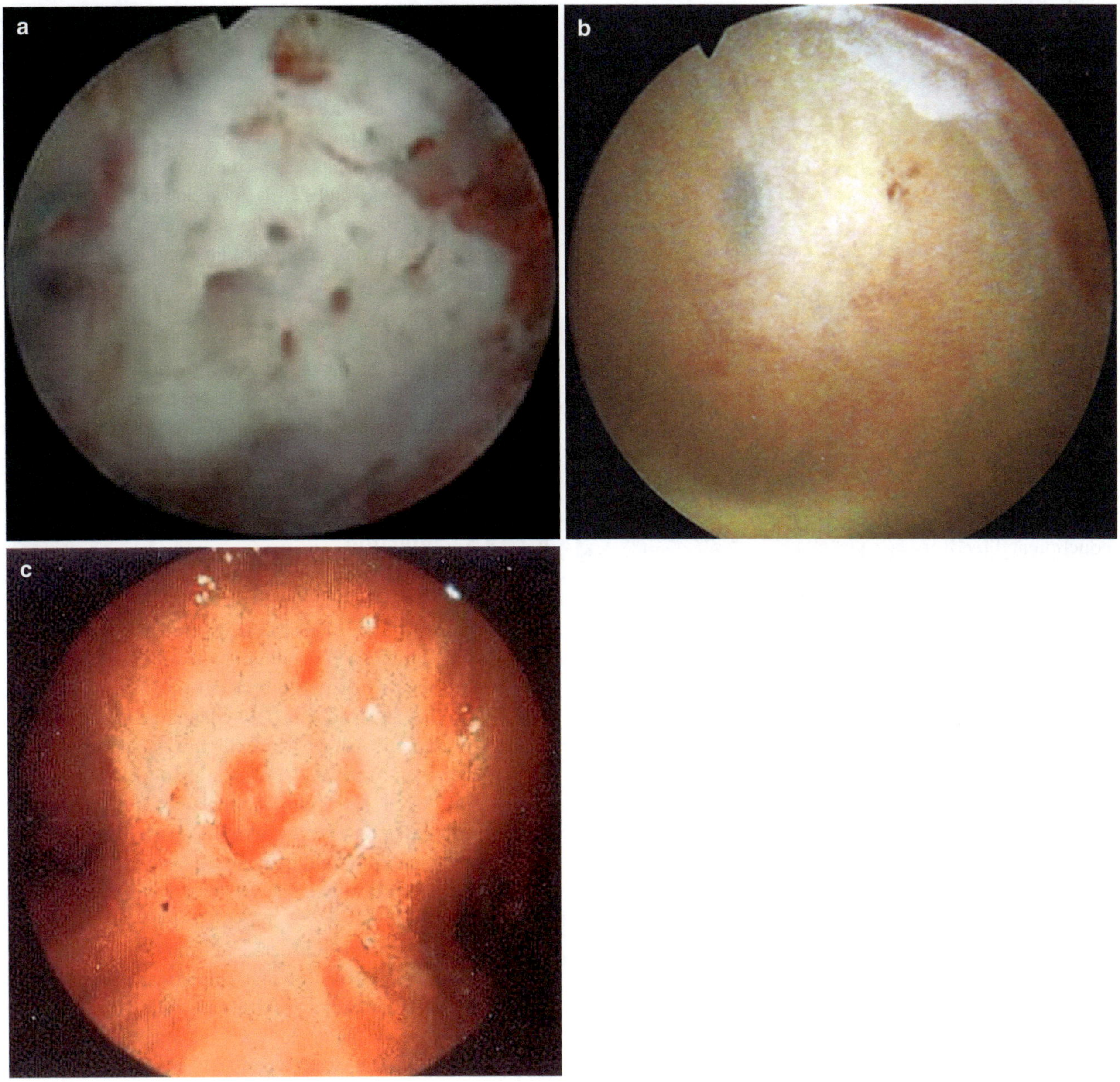

Fig. 8.45 (**a**) Ectopic glandular openings on the endometrium in a patient with adenomyosis. (**b**) Ectopic focus underlying the endometrium in a patient with adenomyosis. (**c**) Intrauterine adhesions and scars in a patient with adenomyosis

ing the pressure and flow rate of distending fluid can be applied. In some individual cases when the lens are stained, 0.5% iodine or 95% ethyl alcohol can be used to swab it.

5. Intrauterine lesions such as endometrial hyperplasia, uterine malformation or intrauterine adhesions, which affect a full inspection of fallopian tubal ostia. A joint examination with ultrasonography may be helpful.
6. If quite a large amount of fluid is injected, endometrium edema may result, which may affect the observation.
7. If a patient is too nervous, anesthesia may be needed.

8.1.13 Management After Hysteroscopy

During hysteroscopy, the patients may complain of lower abdominal pain. Uterine distention with CO_2 may cause slight shoulder pain, which can be mostly relieved 1 h later. There may be low-grade fever for several days post-operation or small amount of bleeding within 1 week after the operation. Therefore, sexual activity should be avoided for 2 weeks after the operation, and antibiotics should be used for prevention of infection when necessary, the underlying diseases should also be treated.

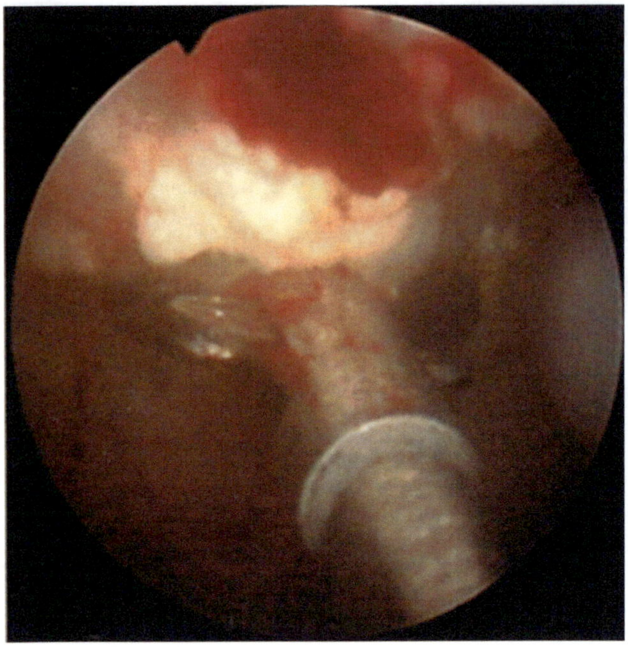

Fig. 8.46 Localizing and sampling for examination with biopsy forceps

8.1.14 Prevention and Treatment of Complications in Hysteroscopy

Hysteroscopy is safe and reliable with relatively few complications, most of which can be prevented.

8.1.14.1 Damage

1. Causes and symptoms: During the dilation of cervix and insertion of the sheath of hysteroscope, cervical laceration and uterine perforation may occur, most of which are related to rough operation. The patients may have increase vaginal bleeding and other symptoms like abdominal pain, but some patients may be asymptomatic. Once the sheath of hysteroscope is inserted through the internal os of cervix, the occurrence of perforation will decrease. Excessive uterine-distending pressure may lead to rupture of fallopian tubes.
2. Prevention measures: (1) Ultrasonography guidance: Insertion of the hysteroscope under Ultrasonography guidance may reduce or prevent the damages caused by incorrect direction of inserting. (2) Be alert to high-risk factors for uterine perforation, such as excessive uterine flexion, suspected carcinoma and tuberculosis, breastfeeding or post-menopausal women. Cervical dilator may be inserted into the cervix or 200 μg misoprostol may be placed in vagina 4 h before the examination to soften the cervix and prevent damage. (3) The use of automatic uterine-distention control device: The continuous distention pressure should always be set below 100 mmHg to prevent rupture of fallopian tubes caused by excessive pressure. (4) When there is heavier bleeding and/or abdominal pain, Ultrasonography should be used to scan the pelvic cavity comprehensively, and the operator should note whether there is free fluid around the uterus, and observe carefully whether the images under hysteroscope are what it is in the uterine cavity to determine or exclude uterine perforation and formation of false passage. Figure 8.47a–g are images when the hysteroscope is inserted into the right broad ligament during hysteroscopy.

8.1.14.2 Bleeding

Generally, slight hemorrhage occurs after hysteroscopy, which can be cleared within 1 week. No heavy bleeding has ever been observed in patients who underwent diagnostic hysteroscopy. Symptomatic treatment is needed for the patients with more bleeding.

8.1.14.3 Infection

The occurrence of infection is quite rare. Franklin reported that its incidence was 0.2%, most of which was related with improper sterilization of instruments. Some sporadic cases had previous chronic pelvic inflammatory disease. Therefore, case history should be queried in detail, and attention should be paid to whether there was pelvic tenderness and adnexal thickening or not. If so, proper antibiotics should be administered intraoperatively and postoperatively. Bracco et al. studied the infectious complications after hysteroscopy. Among 253 cases that were followed up for 20 days after procedures, bacteria from the cervical canal were detected in 35 cases and the positive rate decreased with age. Pelvic inflammatory disease was identified in two cases (0.79%) with Chlamydia trachomatis detected from the cervical canal in both. The conclusion was that patients at higher risk of developing pelvic inflammatory disease following hysteroscopy were patients under 35 years of age, infertility and those with pelvic pain. Meae's data indicated that application of hysteroscopy on patients suffering from salpingitis before the examination may lead to severe pelvic infection. Severe postoperative infections had occurred in four cases following hysteroscopic examinations in the Hysteroscopic Center of Fuxing Hospital, Capital Medical University, with the processes given in Table 8.2. Of them, the first case with previous pelvic inflammatory disease had acute episode caused by hysteroscopy, and antibiotics were administered preoperatively and postoperatively. The second to forth cases were all examined with fiber hysteroscope, which was disinfected with 75% ethanol at that time and now it is disinfected with Swashes immersion instead.

8.1.14.4 Vaso-Vagal Syndrome

Dilation of cervix and distention of uterine cavity may lead to increased tension of vagus nerve, and the same symptoms

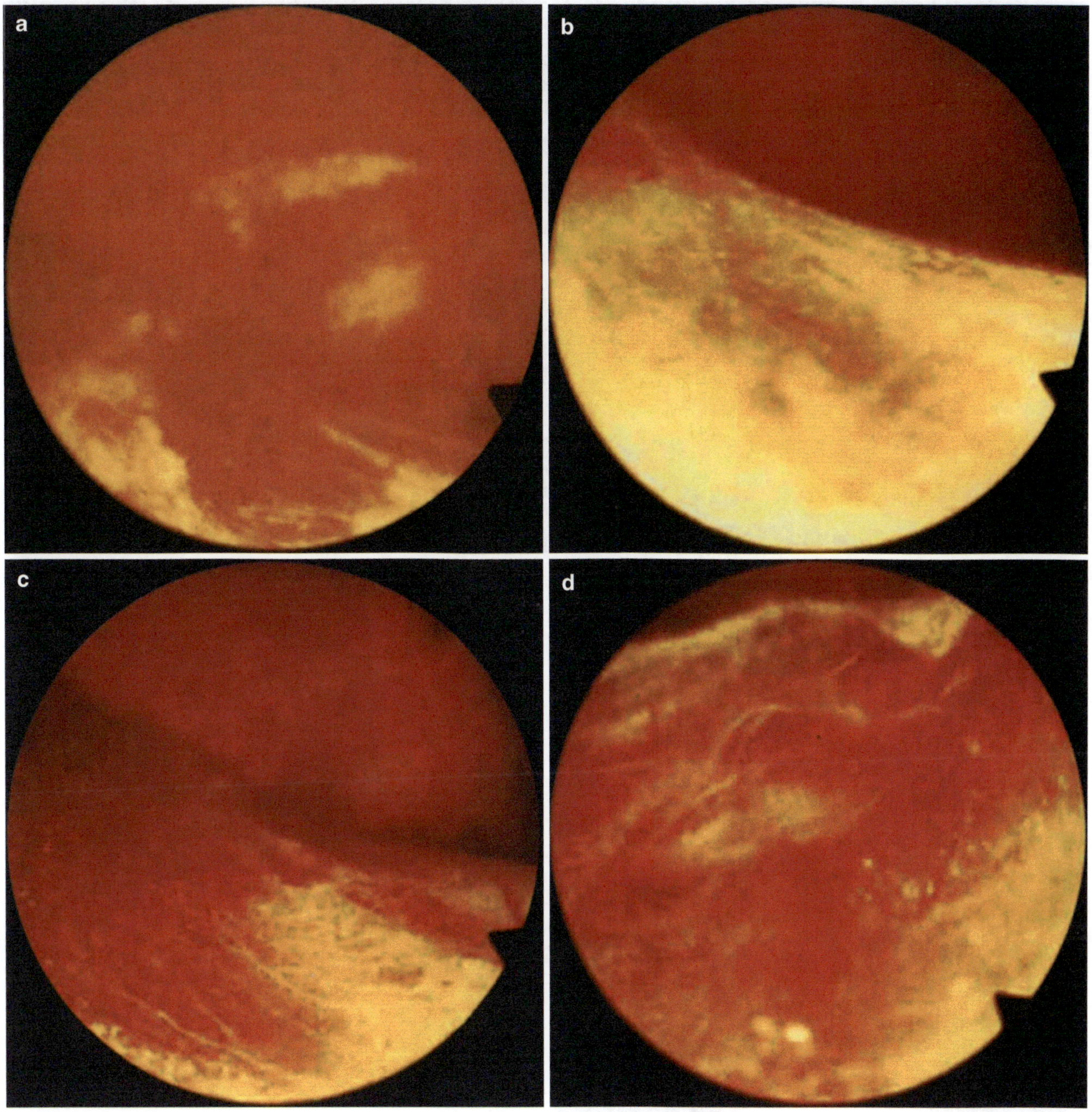

Fig. 8.47 Perforation at left uterine isthmus with rigid hysteroscope. (**a**) Diffuse effusion of blood is seen after inserting a 4.5 mm rigid hysteroscope. The uterine cavity mistakenly entered is actually the place between left parauterus and broad ligament. (**b**) After the flow rate of uterine-distending fluid is accelerated and the blood is washed out, pale yellow adipose tissues can be seen in the posterior wall of the cavity. (**c**) Bleeding is visible from upper area of view with separation of tissues. (**d**) After washing with the uterine-distending fluid, the amount of bleeding decreases and the base surface is clearly seen. (**e**) After the right-side cavity is washed thoroughly, yellow adipose tissues are visible. (**f**) After the hysteroscope is moved backward, the surface of cavity is seen to be blood-staining. (**g**) After the telescope is moved backward, the surface of cavity is blood-staining. Compressed by the telescope, there is no obvious bleeding in the left lower area, with pale yellow appearance

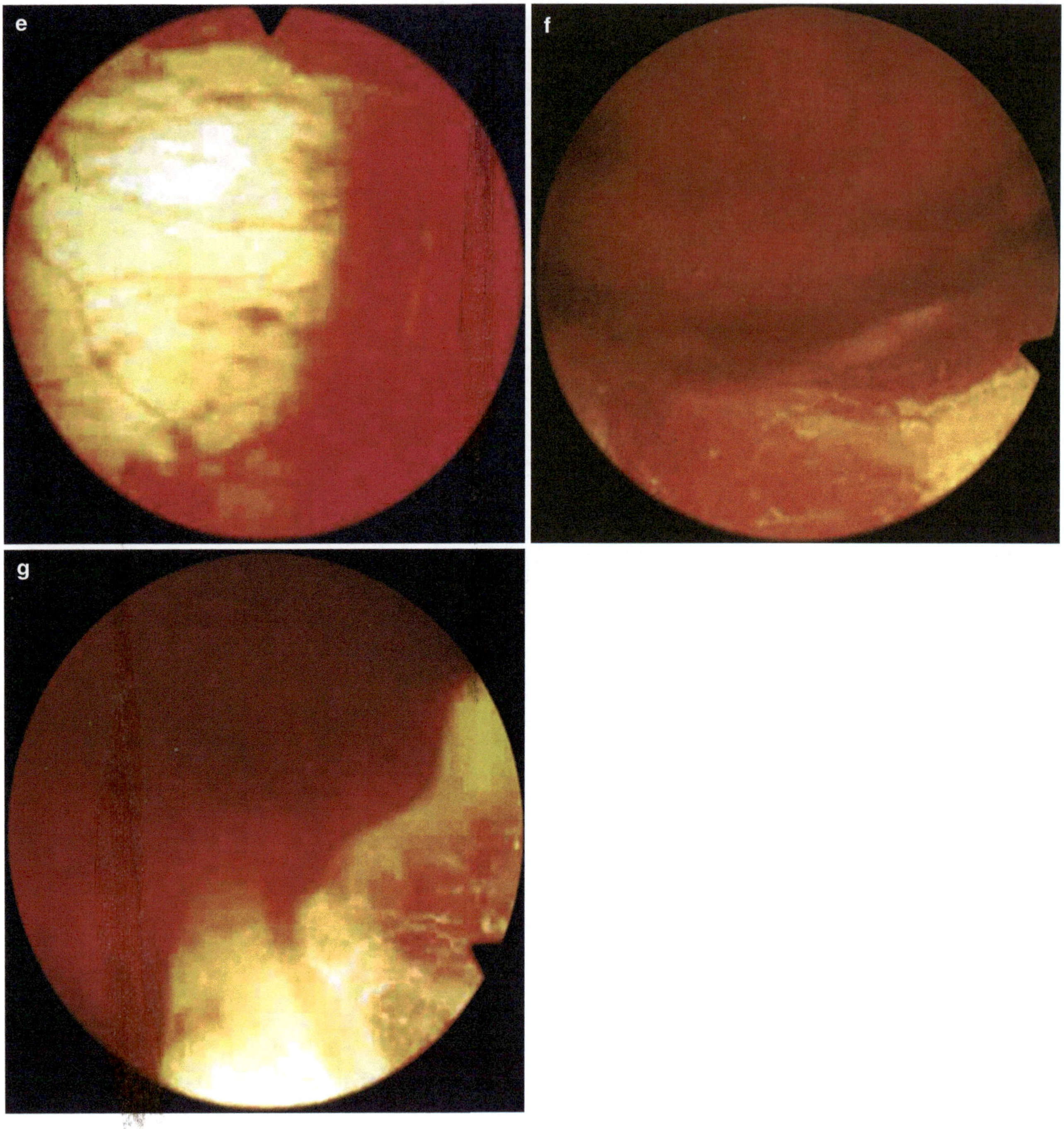

Fig. 8.47 (continued)

of Vaso-Vagal Syndrome are as those in induced abortion. It is quite rare and can be treated symptomatically.

8.1.14.5 Allergic Reaction

Very few people are allergic to dextran, causing symptoms like rashes and asthma, etc., to whom Hyskon solution or sodium carboxymethyl cellulose cannot be applied.

8.1.14.6 Gas Embolism and Pneumoperitoneum

Air embolism may be caused when air in the inflow pipe is not emptied completely during the use of fluid distention medium, or CO_2 embolism can occur when CO_2 is applied as distention medium. The manifestations include shortness of breath, chest distress and coughing, etc. The operation should

Table 8.2 The morbidity and treatment of infections in four cases following hysteroscopy

No.	Clinical diagnosis	Types of hysteroscope	Clinical manifestations	Treatment processes
1	DUB, PID history	Rigid hysteroscope(immersion disinfection with swashes)	Fever, mass on right adnexa on the third day	No improvement in response to conservative treatment. Right adnexa removed by laparotomy. Chronic inflammation of right fallopian tube with tiny purulent foci, and right ovarian chocolate cyst confirmed by histopathological examination.
2	DUB	Fiber hysteroscope (disinfection with 75% ethanol)	High fever, lower abdominal tenderness, rebound tenderness and increased vaginal discharges on the second day	Conservative treatment, cured by antibiotics.
3	DUB, adenomyoma	Fiber hysteroscope (disinfection with 75% ethanol)	High fever, lower abdominal pain, enlarged uterus and obvious tenderness on the second day	No improvement in response to conservative treatment. The uterine corpus was removed by laparotomy. Adenomyoma with local purulent foci in the uterine wall was confirmed by histopathological examination.
4	DUB, adenomyoma	Fiber hysteroscope (disinfection with 75% ethanol)	High fever, lower abdominal pain, enlarged uterus and obvious tenderness on the second day	No improvement in response to conservative treatment. The uterine corpus was removed by laparotomy. Adenomyoma with local purulent foci in the uterine wall was confirmed by histopathological examination.

be stopped immediately to avoid life-threatening risk. Pneumoperitoneum is resulted from too much absorption of CO_2, may cause abdominal distention and shoulder pain, and will disappear after CO_2 is absorbed.

8.1.15 Experiences and Evaluation of Hysteroscopy

Owing to the direct inspection of the uterine cavity with hysteroscope, most intrauterine diseases can now be diagnosed accurately and quickly. It is estimated that use of hysteroscopy in patients with indications may increase the diagnostic rate of intrauterine abnormalities from 28.9% by other traditional ways to 70%, among whom quite a few abnormalities detected by hysteroscopy cannot be diagnosed by other traditional ways.

8.1.15.1 Comparisons of Hysteroscopy and HSG

During X-ray radiographic study (HSG), false positive diagnosis may result from intrauterine small blood clots, mucus, endometrial debris and insufficient contrast medium, etc. In addition, misdiagnosis may also be caused by technical factors, the choice of the contrast medium and differences in the interpretation of the images. According to statistics, only 43–68% of the patients who were found to be abnormal by HSG could be confirmed by hysteroscopy. There were several reports comparing the diagnosis of intrauterine abnormalities by HSG and the confirmation by hysteroscopy (Table 8.3). As hysteroscopy can only inspect the uterine cavity, but is not able to find out the conditions of the uterine walls and the fallopian tubes, hysteroscopy cannot replace HSG absolutely.

8.1.15.2 Comparisons of Hysteroscopy and D&C

D&C is a blind operation, which solely relies on the surgeon's feeling and experience, so missed diagnosis is easy to happen. The intrauterine lesions, especially soft polyps, often cannot be scraped, and focal lesions cannot be located, which may lead to missed diagnosis. There had been reports that even when D&C was performed by experienced gynecologist, the residual rate of endometrium after curettage reached up to 20–25%, while hysteroscopy was able to make up for the inadequacies of curettage. Gebauer et al. reported the results of hysteroscopy and simple uterine curettage in 83 patients. The indications for hysteroscopy were postmenopausal bleeding and/or abnormal endometrium detected by ultrasonography. Endometrial polyps were revealed in 51 patients by hysteroscopy and in 22 patients by simple curettage (43%). Epstein et al. studied postmenopausal women with the thickness of endometrium ≥ 5 mm by TVS. By hys-

Table 8.3 Diagnosis of intrauterine abnormalities by HSG and hysteroscopy in published literatures

Year	Authors	No of cases with abnormal HSG	Percentage of cases confirmed by hysteroscopy (%)
1956	Norment	50	60
1957	Englund et al.	21	52
1970	Guerrero et al.	41	65
1973	Neuwirth and Levine	10	60
1973	Porto	76	5
1974	Porto	134	70

teroscopy or hysterectomy, intrauterine lesions were found in 80% of the patients, among them, 98% of the lesions were detected by hysteroscopy. In 87% of the women with focal lesions in the uterine cavity, the lesions were not completely removed by D&C. 58% of polyps, 50% of hyperplasia, 60% of complex atypical hyperplasia, and 11% of endometrial carcinoma were missed by D&C. Brooks reported that the false-negative rate of D&C in women with AUB was 10–15% with the missed diagnosis of submucous myoma remarkably high. Luo from China reported that about 35% area of uterine cavity could not be scraped during the D&C procedure. Therefore, it is believed that D&C should no longer play a significant role in the endoscopy era. Seamark even declared its death. In some developed countries, there has already been trend of the hysteroscopy replacing blind dilatation and curettage. However, it still should be realized that hysteroscopy also has limitations, as simple hysteroscopy alone may also miss diagnosis such as hormone affected endometrium or atypical hyperplastic endometrium, the reason is that these changes may not have reached the identifiable degree with naked eyes. Therefore, hysteroscopy must be combined with histopathological examination so as to improve the diagnosis.

8.1.15.3 Comparisons of Hysteroscopy and Ultrasonography

In cases with uterine myomas suggested by ultrasonography, if the endometrial lining is obscure, it would be difficult to identify whether the myomas is submucous or intramural, and be difficult to locate which sides or walls they were in; if the endometrial lining is thickened obviously, the endometrial polyps could not be excluded, while hysteroscopic examination can solve the above problems clearly. Granberg et al. believed that transvaginal ultrasonography is an effective way to diagnose endometrial and intrauterine abnormalities, so it can be taken as the first routine examination for patients with abnormal uterine bleeding. For patients with abnormal or unidentifiable ultrasonic images, or with normal ultrasonographic images but continuous symptoms, hysteroscopy must be performed together with further biopsy so as to exclude or identify pathologic conditions. Paschopoulos et al. compared the accuracy of diagnosis of intrauterine lesions between vaginoscopic hysteroscopy and TVS in women with abnormal uterine bleeding. Findings of 397 patients were compared with histopathologic results. The sensitivity and the specificity for hysteroscopy were 92% and 95%, with the positive and the negative likelihood ratios 18.4 and 0.08, respectively. Those for TVS were 67% and 87%, with the positive and the negative ratios 5.15 and 0.38, respectively. Therefore, it was concluded that hysteroscopy had the advantages of rapid diagnosis and well tolerated, which was more accurate than TVS in detecting lesions in uterine cavity. Deckardt compared the examination results with TVS, hysteroscopy, and D&C in 1286 perimenopausal and postmenopausal women with bleeding. Among 29 cases (2.26%) who were histopathologically diagnosed of endometrial carcinoma, the thickness of endometrium was ≤5 mm in 2 cases (7.14%), and the diagnosis of endometrial carcinoma by hysteroscopy was missed in 10 cases (34.5%). Therefore, in perimenopausal and postmenopausal women who were suspected of endometrial carcinoma, it could not be reliably excluded by TVS or hysteroscopic examination alone.

8.1.15.4 Comparisons of Hysteroscopy and Transvaginal Color Doppler (TVCD)

Bidzinski et al. investigated the application of color flow Doppler (CDF) and hysteroscopy to evaluate the endometrium status in 33 patients who had endometrial cancer and were treated by radiotherapy alone. Hysteroscopy was confirmed to be highly accurate, with sensitivity of 89% and specificity of 91%. The sensitivity and specificity of CDF were 69% and 75%, respectively. The lack of the endometrial flow signal was related to the absence of uterine malignant pathology. The CDF indexes of pulsatility and resistance were not correlated with the endometrial histopathology.

8.1.15.5 Comparisons of Hysteroscopy and Sonohysterosalpingography (SHSG) or Saline Infusion Sonogram (SIS)

Rogerson et al. conducted a prospective and comparative study of the accuracy in diagnosis of the intrauterine pathologies with hysteroscopy and SHSG, and believed that both examinations were well tolerated. SHSG had a higher failure rate, but less pain scores than hysteroscopy. De Kroon et al. conducted a prospective observational study of SHSG in 180 cases, with failed examination of SHSG in 12 (5.6%), and inconclusive diagnosis in 22 (10.3%). They concluded that SHSG was able to replace 84% of the hysteroscopy, which could be applied only when SHSG was failed or could not make a diagnosis. Descargues et al. compared the results for examination of abnormal uterine bleeding with SHSG and hysteroscopy. The SHSG had a positive predictive value of 89% and a negative predictive value of 100%. The difficulties of cervix cannulation occurred in 13% of the cases, which limited the application of SHSG. Krampl et al. compared the diagnostic accuracy for 88 patients with abnormal uterine bleeding by means of TVS, SHSG, and hysteroscopy with biopsy. The diagnostic rate of intrauterine lesions was 100% with hysteroscopy and biopsy, 94.1% with SHSG, and 23.5% with TVS. None of the above methods were able to accurately diagnose the endometrial hyperplasia in about 75% of all cases. However, endometrial pathologies detected by TVS and SHSG still needs direct biopsy under hysteroscope.

8.1.15.6 Comparisons of Hysteroscope and Magnetic Resonance Imaging (MRI)

The research outcomes reported by Dueholm et al. indicated that MRI had the same accuracy as hysteroscopy for exclusion of intrauterine abnormalities, and were slightly superior to TVS. Both MRI and TVS tend to miss endometrial abnormalities, which were inferior to hysteroscopy. Dykes et al. reported that the diagnosis of severe intrauterine adhesions with MRI were correlated with hysteroscopy.

8.1.16 Minimally Invasive Diagnostic Hysteroscope

Following the advent of micro-hysteroscope, the Olympus Corporation of Japan released minimally invasive diagnostic hysteroscope in 2001 with the telescope of 1.9 mm and the outer sheath of 3 mm. Non-invasive techniques were driven by the equipment miniaturization, so that the hysteroscopy can be safely carried out in outpatient setting. Fiber hysteroscope has its unique characteristics among many available hysteroscopes, whose objective scopes have different sizes of 3.1 mm, 3.6 mm, and 4.9 mm in outer diameter. Generally, dilation of cervix and anesthesia are not needed during examination, except for a few menopausal women and some patients with extremely narrow cervical canals caused by adhesions. The front tip of fiber hysteroscope can be bent for 90°–120° towards both sides, so that it is convenient to show the uterine cornua and the fallopian tubal ostia, and has fewer blind spots of examination compared with rigid hysteroscope. Due to its small diameter and flexible front tip, it is easy to pass through the hymen in young girls or unmarried adult women and into the vagina to inspect the cervix, and sometimes may enter the uterine cavity via the cervical canal for visualizing the cavity (Figs. 8.48 and 8.49). In the Hysteroscopic Center of

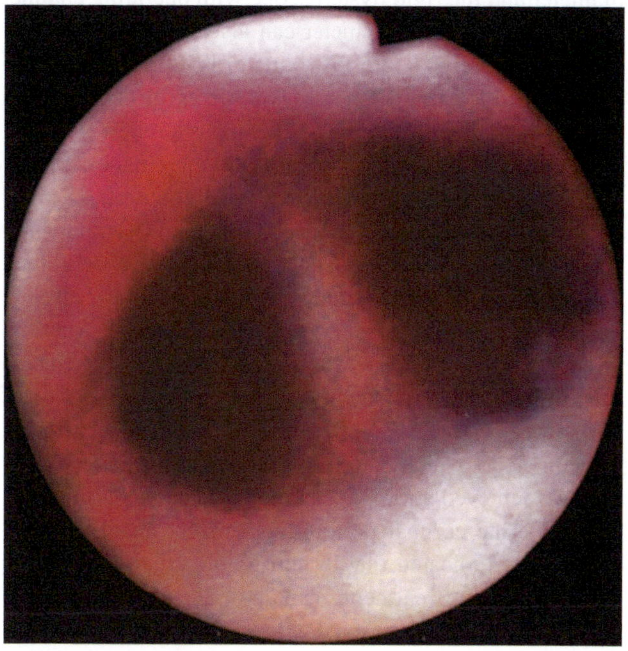

Fig. 8.48 Uterine septum under fiber hysteroscope

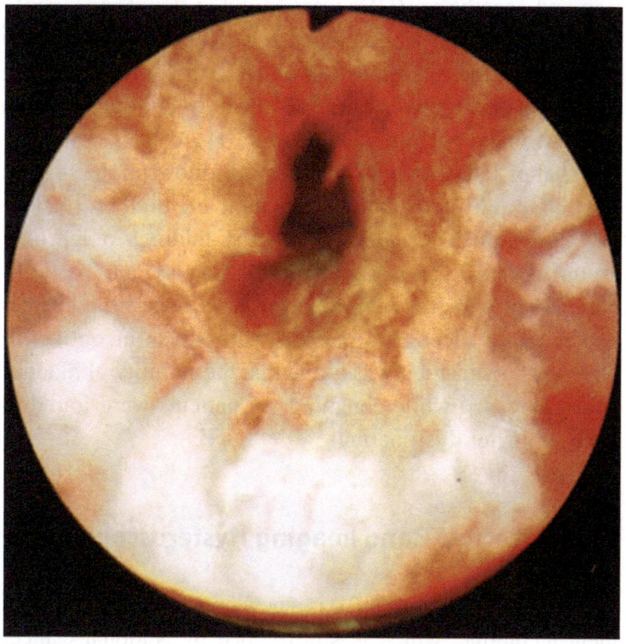

Fig. 8.49 Intrauterine adhesions under fiber hysteroscope

Fuxing Hospital, Capital Medical University, the flexible fiber hysteroscope has also been used for inspection of the vaginal wall cyst. In an unmarried woman with a ruptured cyst in the vaginal wall, the telescope was inserted from the defect of the cyst to look into the intracapsular structure and take samples of the cystic wall tissues, which was diagnosed pathologically to be Mullerian duct cyst. HYF-1T fiber hysteroscope with an insertion tube of 4.9 mm in outer diameter and the rigid hysteroscope with operating channel and 4.5 mm in outer diameter can also be used to remove the vaginal foreign bodies of young girls. If the uterine cavity is too wide, it will not be easy to control the direction when using a fiber hysteroscope, as it has a relatively small visual field. Therefore, it is not suitable to be used in patients with large uterine cavity, large intrauterine lesions or complicated conditions. Burke applied an Olympus flexible hysteroscope with a Cook catheter and a combined laparoscopy to perform a tubal cannulation in the treatment of 120 women with bilateral interstitial tubal obstruction. After treatment, post-operative tubal patency was achieved in 96 cases, and pregnancy occurred in 48 cases, two of which were ectopic. Reocclusions of the tubes occurred in 12 women, of which 8 were retreated with catheterization and two achieved normal pregnancy. The only complication was a uterine cornual perforation with the tubal catheter. The results indicated that hysteroscopic tubal cannulation was effective in treatment of interstitial tubal obstruction. Lin et al. reported their experiences of removing intrauterine devices (IUDs) in 33 cases of early pregnancy. When the IUDs were not visible from cervical canal, it could be removed with flexible hysteroscope without cervical dilatation and anesthesia. IUDs were found in the uterine cavity in 30 women, and were removed in 28. There was no IUD observed in the remaining 3 women. All women were followed-up until delivery, with 24 healthy children born. 6 other women performed curettage 1–2 weeks after the removal of IUDs. Others were lost to follow-up. Ross used flexible minihysteroscopes to examine the urethra, bladder and colon in 225 patients, with the findings of chronic urethritis in 13 cases, significant urinary symptoms in 18 patients, of which 3 were found to have interstitial cystitis and mucosal ulcer. 194 patients with stress incontinence were examined and it was found that the stability of bladder neck decreased while coughing. 17 patients were found to have sphincter dysfunction.

8.1.17 Narrow Band Imaging Hysteroscopy

Narrow band imaging (NBI) is a new optical image enhancement technique, which was developed by National Cancer Center Hospital East, Japan and Olympus Medical Systems (Tokyo, Japan). It utilizes the light absorption properties of hemoglobin at certain wavelengths to improve the contrast of blood vessels in superficial endometrial layer and well display the mini-structure of the endometrium, therefore it could facilitate the identification of endometrial atypical lesions and achieve the aim of early diagnosis.

8.1.17.1 Principles of NBI

Xenon, which is known as "White light," is applied as light source in traditional endoscopic surgery, with its spectrum being composed of three-primary colors - red, green, and blue, and its wavelengths range from 400 nm to 700 nm. In NBI system, white light is filtered through an optical filter to produce blue light (the central wavelength of 415 nm) and green light (the central wavelength of 540 nm), both of which are prone to be absorbed by hemoglobin. The hemoglobin obtains the first absorption peak at 415 nm wavelength (blue) and the second peak at 540 nm (green), so the blood vessels containing much more hemoglobin will be darken after the absorption of blue and green lights, while the surrounding endometrium appears to be relatively bright, which highlight the contrast of vessels. In addition, light has the characteristic that its penetration ability is directly proportional to wavelength. The capillary vessels in the surface of endometrium mainly absorbs blue light and appears blue, while blood vessels in deep layer of endometrium or in submucous layer absorb green light and appear green, both of which make the visualization of blood vessel distributions in endometrium clearer.

8.1.17.2 Clinical Applications of NBI

Folkman firstly carried out several pieces of research and found that both the occurrence and the development of tumors relied on the generation of blood vessels, and the intensity of the vessels suggested the presence of malignant tumors. In 2001, Sano et al. first reported the administration of NBI in gastrointestinal endoscopy to infer the extent and the degree of the lesions from displaying the abnormal vessels in pathological areas, thus helping gastrointestinal endoscope to diagnose digestive system tumor and precancerous lesions, and increase the accuracy ~~rate~~ of biopsy. Nowadays NBI is mostly applied in diagnosis of digestive system disorders, and is more and more utilized in diseases of otolaryngology, respiratory system and urinary system. However, there are relatively few research of its application in gynecology and obstetrics. In 2007, Farrugia et al. first applied NBI in gynecologic endoscopic surgery, and in recent years they mainly studied the use of NBI in laparoscopic removal of pelvic endometriosis and removal of peritoneum metastasis of ovarian carcinoma. In 2009, Surico et al. first used NBI in hysteroscopy to diagnose endometrial pathologies, and concluded that NBI could clearly identify the structures of capillary vessels and diagnose endometrial lesions via the observation of irregular and thickened vessels. In 2010, Fujii et al. reported the use of NBI in colposcopy, which could increase the diagnostic rate of cervical cancer in situ and cervical adenocarcinoma.

8.1.17.3 Characteristics of Intrauterine Pathology Under NBI Hysteroscopy

1. Normal proliferative endometrium: The endometrium appears to be smooth and flat with an even color and without abnormal vascular networks (Fig. 8.50a, b).
2. Endometrial polyps: The neoplasm is characterized by a vascular axis and longitudinal dendritic branch vasculars which derive from the pedicle (Fig. 8.51a, b).
3. Postmenopausal atrophic polyps: The neoplasm is characterized by a vascular axis and irregular vascular network (Fig. 8.52a, b).
4. Uterine leiomyomas: Large main vessels and branching vasculars deriving from them can be visualized on the surface of the white neoplasm (Fig. 8.53a, b).
5. Chronic endometritis: In these cases, the endometrium is interspersed with uneven blue petechiae, with the superficial or subepithelial vascular network expanding, or tiny papillary foci with vascular axis existing (Fig. 8.54a, b).
6. Low risk endometrial hyperplasia (simple and complex hyperplasia): The endometrium is thickened and uneven with subepithelial vascular network visible (Fig. 8.55).
7. High risk endometrial hyperplasia (atypical hyperplasia): The endometrium is thickened with its surface uneven or polypoid. The number of vessels is increased with irregular and messy vascular branches visible (Fig. 8.56).
8. Endometrial cancer: The neoplasm appears to be polypoid, gyriform or cauliflower-like. The blood vessels are increased in numbers and distributed irregularly with the calibers uneven in thickness and the shapes curly and spirally (Fig. 8.57a–c).

8.1.17.4 Clinical Applications of NBI Hysteroscopy

Both endometrial hyperplasia and endometrial cancer are common in gynecological disorders, and the early diagnosis and treatment have significant influence on prognosis of endometrial cancer and precancerous lesions. Trimble et al. reported that in women who had been previously diagnosed as atypical endometrial hyperplasia by biopsy and histopathologic examination, the morbidity of endometrial cancer was up to 42.6%. Thus, a precise target biopsy is the key to increase the diagnostic rate, and the hysteroscopy has been an optimal technique in diagnosing intrauterine pathology, which can be detected under direct vision and facilitate target biopsy. However, it was reported that the sensitivity of diagnosing endometrial hyperplasia and endometrial carcinoma by traditional hysteroscopy under white light was 56.3% and 80%, respectively. The properties of NBI technique provide us a possibility of early detection of endometrial diseases. In 2009, Surico et al. firstly utilized NBI technique in hysteroscopy to perform NBI diagnostic hysteroscopy in patients with postmenopausal abnormal uterine bleeding, and discovered that micro-vascular structures could be clearly visualized under NBI, which could help sur-

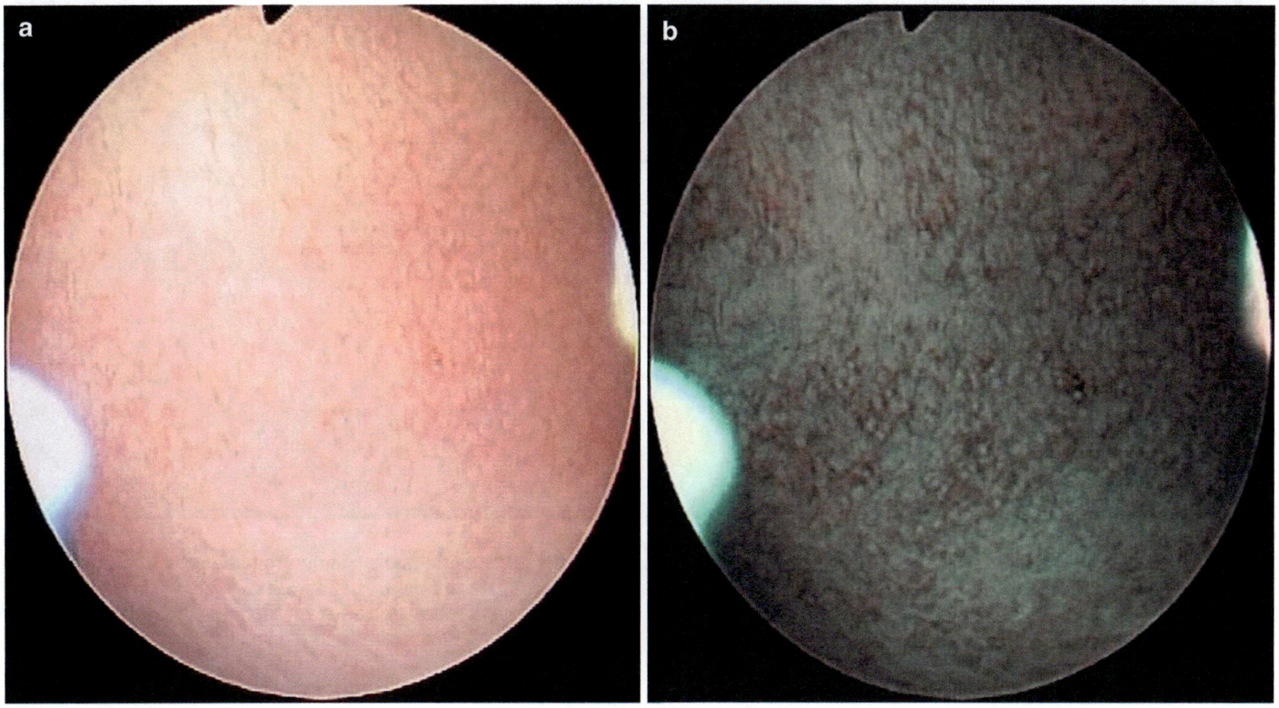

Fig. 8.50 (**a**) Normal proliferative endometrium under white light. (**b**) Normal proliferative endometrium with NBI

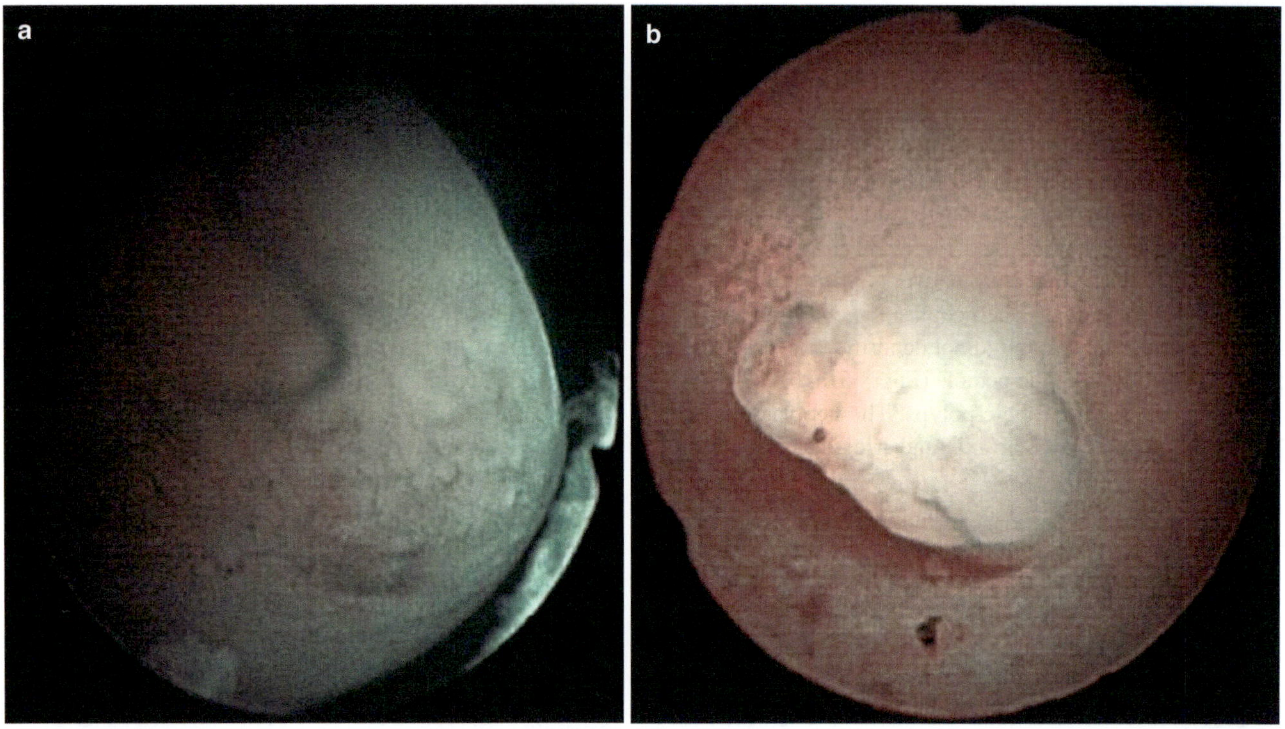

Fig. 8.51 (**a**) An axial blood vessel in an endometrial polyp with NBI. (**b**) Branch vessels in an endometrial polyp with NBI

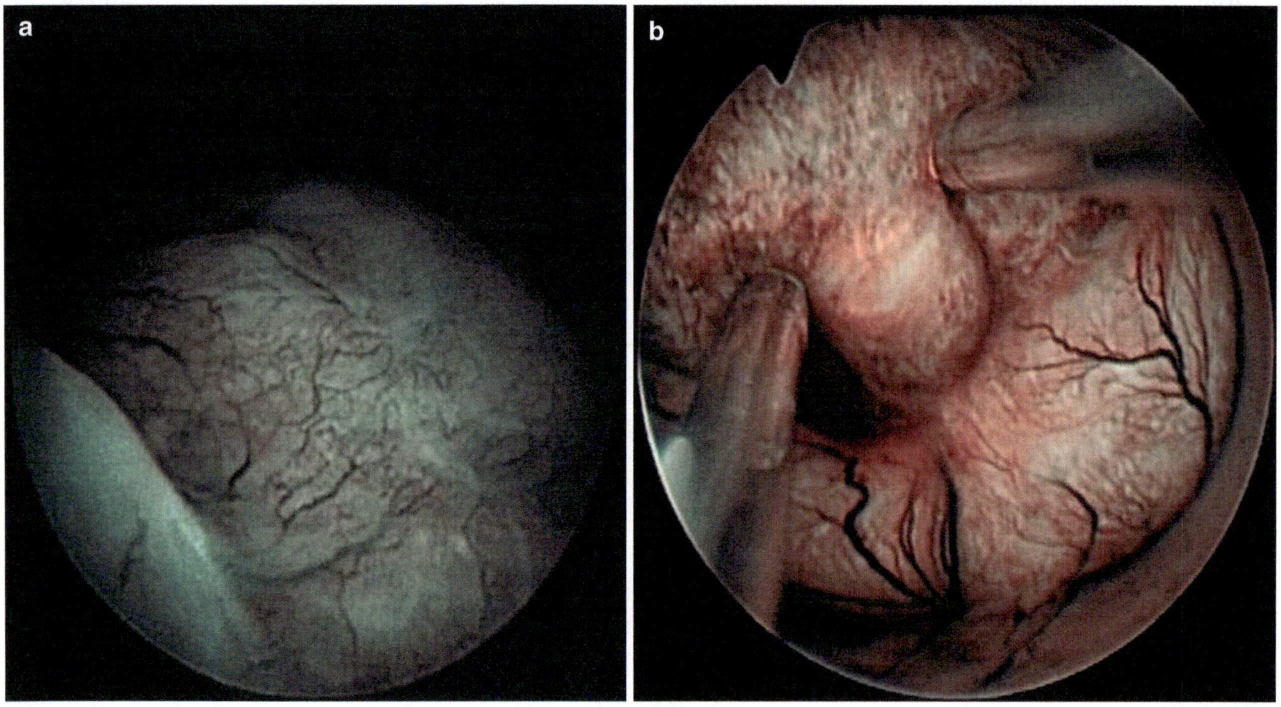

Fig. 8.52 (**a**) Vascular networks in a postmenopausal endometrial polyp with NBI. (**b**) Blood vessels coming from the pedicle in a postmenopausal endometrial polyp with NBI

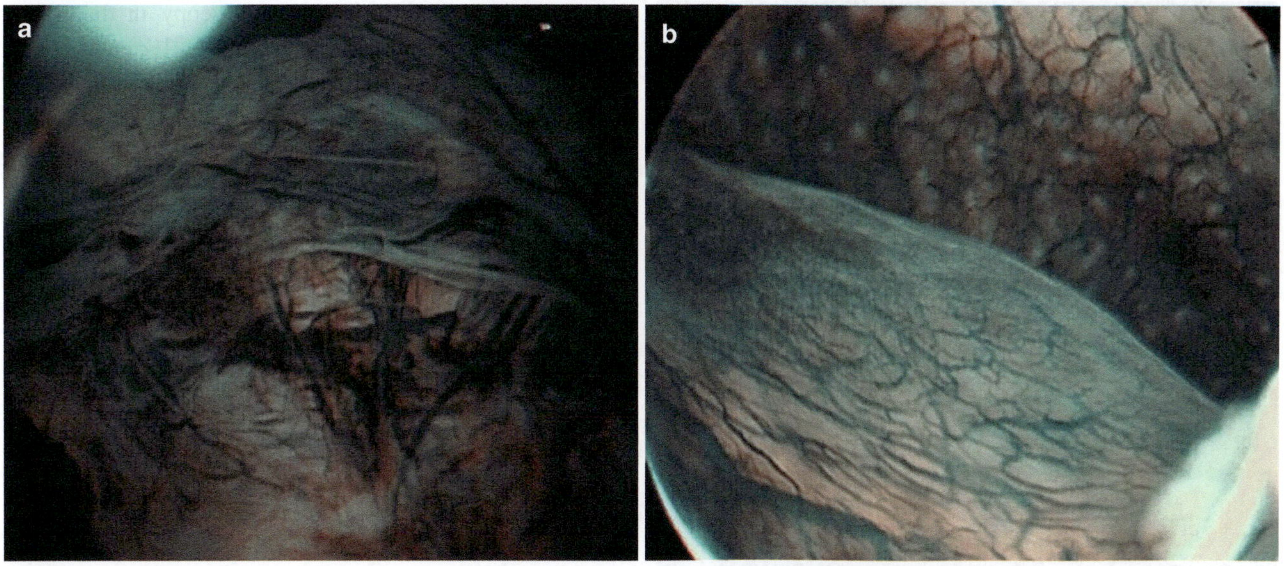

Fig. 8.53 (**a**) Thick and large blood vessels in an uterine myoma with NBI. (**b**) Regular branch blood vessels in an uterine myoma with NBI

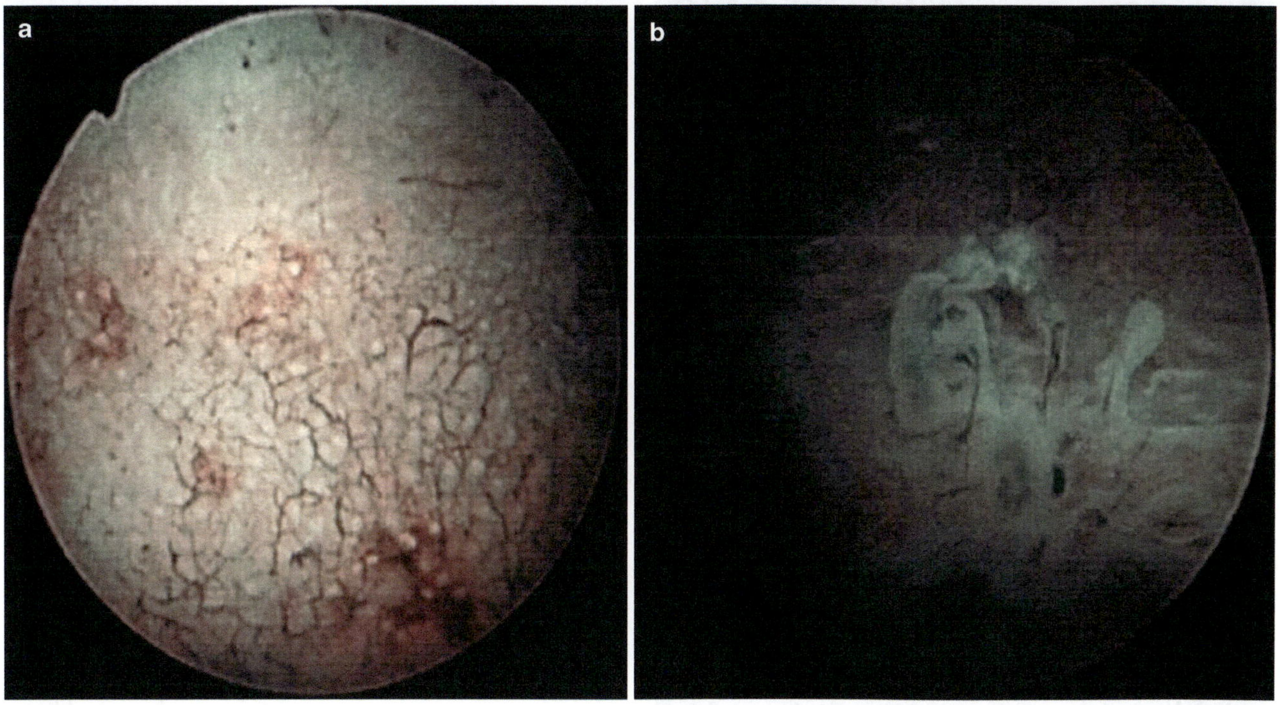

Fig. 8.54 (**a**) Expanded vascular network and scattered bleeding spots in chronic endometritis with NBI. (**b**) Tiny polyps in chronic endometritis with NBI

geons to identify the suspicious foci with very tiny, intensive and irregularly arranged micro-vasculars. These indicated that NBI could improve the accuracy of the identification of endometrial cancer and endometrial hyperplasia, and could be considered as an effective auxiliary method for early diagnosis of endometrial lesions. In 2010, Surico et al. carried out a prospective study on 209 women with abnormal uterine bleeding. Diagnostic hysteroscopy with white light and NBI was taken in each woman, and endometrial direct biopsy followed. The results indicated that the sensitivity and specific-

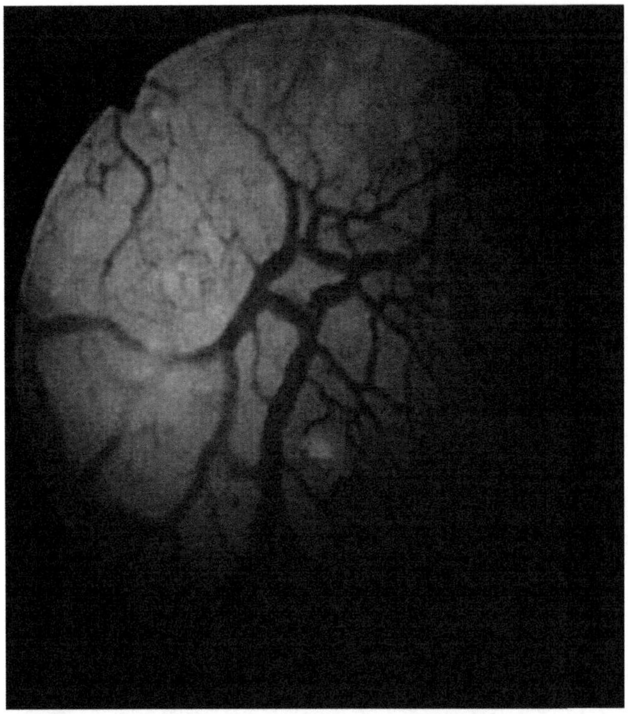

Fig. 8.55 Vascular networks in endometrial simple hyperplasia with NBI

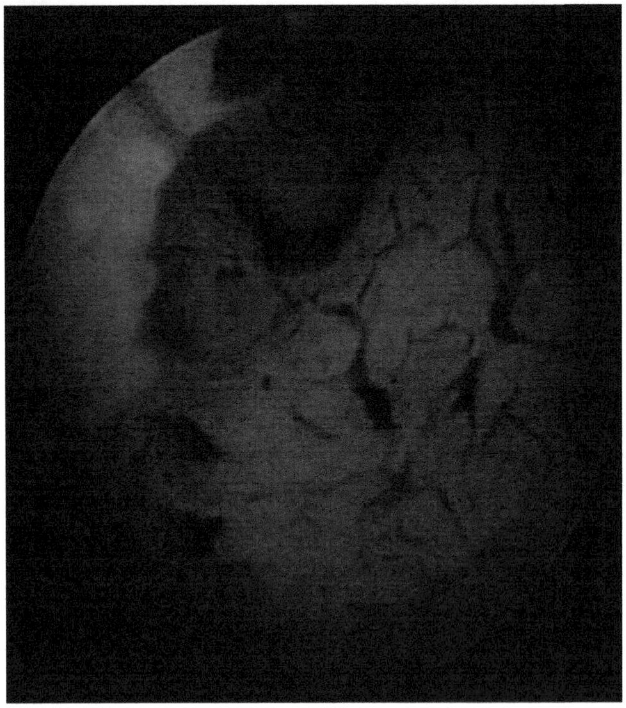

Fig. 8.56 Uneven in thickness and messy in distribution of blood vessels in endometrial complex atypical hyperplasia with NBI

ity of traditional white light hysteroscopy in diagnosing endometrial cancer were, respectively, 84.21% and 99.47%, and those in diagnosing endometrial hyperplasia were 64.86% and 98.77%. However those of NBI hysteroscopy were 94.74% and 98.36%; 78.38%, and 98.88%, respectively, therefore NBI could significantly increase the diagnostic sensitivity. Cicinelli et al. reported that diagnostic hysteroscopy was taken in 395 women and NBI hysteroscopy was discovered to have a higher specificity (0.93:0.78) and negative predictive value (0.92:0.81) than white light hysteroscopy to make diagnosis of disorders. Thus it can be concluded that the diagnostic accuracy of normal endometrium with NBI hysteroscopy was higher than that with white light hysteroscopy, both of which could achieve a higher diagnostic accuracy for diagnosing endometrial polyps and myomas (95.3–100%). NBI hysteroscopy could obtain higher sensitivity than white light hysteroscopy for the diagnosis of chronic endometritis (0.88:0.70), low risk endometrial hyperplasia (0.88:0.70), and high risk endometrial hyperplasia (0.60:0.40). Furthermore, NBI could improve the positive predictive values of endometritis (0.95:0.69) and high risk endometrial hyperplasia (0.75:0.40), and decrease the false negative values as well. Tinelli et al. reported a multicenter study about NBI hysteroscopy being applied in 801 outpatient women. It was found that, with NBI hysteroscopy and white light hysteroscopy, the sensitivity in diagnosing low risk hyperplasia was 82% and 56%, respectively; in detecting high risk atypical hyperplasia was 60% and 20%; and in diagnosis of endometrial cancer was 93% and 81% which indicated that NBI hysteroscopy could decrease the missed diagnosis of endometrial severe lesions thus improving the diagnosis of precancerous lesions and malignant tumors. In addition, NBI may also be applied in flexible hysteroscope and can achieve a higher diagnostic rate of endometrial atypical hyperplasia and endometrial cancer than white light hysteroscopy. In 2011, Ercan et al. studied the application of NBI for evaluating the intrauterine abnormalities of infertility. Diagnostic hysteroscopy was performed in women who failed in IVF treatment. Among 8 women with no endometritis identified under white light hysteroscopy, 3 were diagnosed as endometritis when NBI hysteroscopy was applied. Therefore NBI hysteroscopy is also useful in examination of women with unexplained infertility.

Although the NBI technique has not been applied for a long time in diagnostic hysteroscopy, the above studies suggest that it could improve the sensitivity of early detection for endometrial carcinoma and precancerous lesions. Therefore NBI holds promise to be a commonly used technique in hysteroscopy.

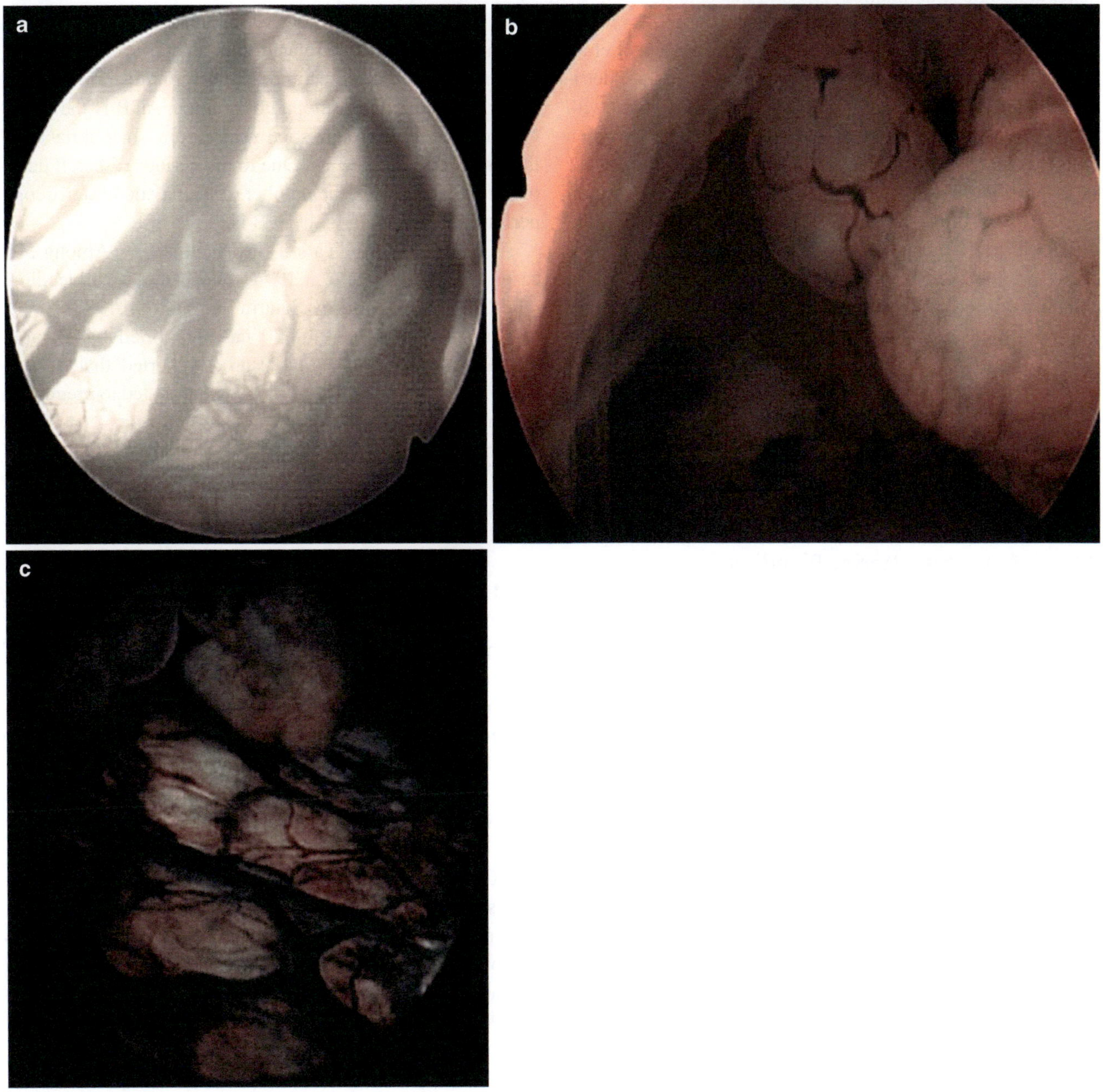

Fig. 8.57 (**a**) Uneven in thickness and messy in distribution of blood vessels in endometrial adenocarcinoma with NBI. (**b**) Polypoid endometrial cancer with NBI. (**c**) Endometrial adenosarcoma with NBI

8.1.18 Does Diagnostic Hysteroscopy Facilitate the Dissemination of Tumor Cells?

Whether diagnostic hysteroscopy facilitates the dissemination of tumor cells has always been the most concerned and controversial question among scholars. There have been several reports on endometrial tumor cells disseminating into the abdominal cavity, which was suspected to be caused by hysteroscopy with fluids distention and irrigation. Obermair et al. evaluated the incidence of positive peritoneal cytology in patients who underwent hysteroscopy and D&C, or D&C without hysteroscopy. They conducted a multicentric, retrospective cohort analysis of 113 patients with endometrial carcinoma staging Ia or Ib in the year of 1996–1997. Positive peritoneal cytology was obtained during laparotomy and was defined as detection of malignant or suspicious cells. The results showed that peritoneal cytology was suspicious or positive in 10 of 113 patients (9%), which was associated with an intrauterine procedure of hysteroscopy ($P = 0.04$) but had no relationships with myometrial invasion ($P = 0.57$), histological types ($P = 1.00$), staging ($r = 0.16$, $P = 0.10$), or the intervals between D&C and laparotomy (r = 0.04, P = 0.66). The research outcomes published by Kuzel et al. were concordant with those by Kobilkova, that is, no detrimental result was found by cytological examination with hysteroscopy being followed with target biopsy in women with endometrial cancer, while the tumor cells would appear at posterior fornix after the curettage. These limited literatures strongly support the point that hysteroscopy with fluid distention and irrigation do facilitate tumor cell dissemination, but it has not been verified whether it will cause tumor cell invasion and metastasis, thus further studies are required.

8.2 Applications of Hysteroscopy in Gynecological Diseases

Enlan Xia

8.2.1 Abnormal Uterine Bleeding

Abnormal uterine bleeding (AUB) is the earliest and the most common indication for hysteroscopy. Nagele et al. performed 2500 hysteroscopies in an outpatient setting, 87% of which were indicated because of abnormal uterine bleeding. The indication for the first successful hysteroscopy performed by Pantaleoni in 1869 was menopausal uterine bleeding. Endometrial polyps on the fundus of uterus was discovered and cured by hysteroscopy as well. Because the problem with suboptimal visualization caused by intrauterine bleeding during diagnostic hysteroscopy was not resolved for more than one century, the development of hysteroscopic technology has been postponed. As a result, D&C and the HSG had remained the two major methods of examination for women with hypermenorrhea until recently. However, now a great number of research have confirmed hysteroscopy to be the most accurate and reliable way of intrauterine examination.

By direct observation of the bleeding lesions, not only can hysteroscopy improve the gynecologists' understanding of AUB, but also a variety of intrauterine lesions can be managed by the advanced hysteroscopic surgery, which totally changes the previous therapeutic procedures. The conventional interventions, such as repeated curettage and hysterectomy, have not been applied any longer. For most cases, high-frequency electric or laser surgery, which have a long-term effectiveness on intrauterine benign lesions, have become conservative treatment modalities for intrauterine benign lesions.

8.2.1.1 AUB Among Indications for Hysteroscopy

AUB is the most common complaint of the women who come to the gynecologic outpatient clinic, and it may appear sooner or later as a warning symptom of most intrauterine lesions. Since it is often related to pregnancy, AUB in young women has tended to become less as an indication for hysteroscope, while for menopausal women, AUB is the strongest indication for diagnostic hysteroscopy since it has very little relation with fertility. Due to the various research fields of each gynecologist, the number of diagnostic hysteroscopy performed on women with AUB is different.

AUB is a main indication for hysteroscopy. Among 500 cases reported by Porto in 1974, 48% had uterine bleeding. Of 320 cases reported by Sciarra and Valle in 1977, 49.6% had uterine bleeding. Of 680 cases reported by Hamou, 37.5% had uterine bleeding. Barbot reported that, in one study group of 810 patients who were unrelated to pregnancy and had examinations by contact hysteroscope, 64.8% of whom mainly complained of AUB. Among his later report of 1500 cases of hysteroscopy, AUB took up 52.1% of the cases, so roughly one in two hysteroscopies was performed for AUB.

8.2.1.2 Hysteroscopic Techniques Related to Uterine Bleeding

Diagnostic hysteroscopy can be performed very easily if there is no uterine bleeding. However, if there is, high-level techniques are required for both emergency and bleeding following ineffective medication. The degrees of difficulty are varied, which depend on: (1) the amount of bleeding; (2) the properties of the equipment used; (3) the technique applied; and (4) the experiences of the surgeon.

1. CO_2 uterine distension: When CO_2 is used as the uterine-distending medium, intrauterine blood may lead to the formation of bubbles, blurring of the vision and even obstacle to the whole vision field. The solution is to insufflate gas through the outer sheath of hysteroscope with an inflow channel opened at the front tip so that the airflow may clean the surface of the objective lens and remove bubbles and blood. If this method cannot provide a clear vision either, the end of objective lens can be attached to the mucosa of the uterine fundus, by which a satisfactory vision can usually be restored. If it fails again, the telescope should be taken out and soaked in sterile saline or clean water. If there is massive hemorrhage, the blood clots may block the gas injection channel and cause the closure of the cavity, hence the images in front of the objective lens seem to be blanketed by a red curtain. The method of confirming the blockage is that no emergence of bubbles is observed when the hysteroscope is withdrawn and immersed in water. The gas-injection valve is connected to a syringe and the water is injected under a higher pressure, which can clear out the blocked channels. Sometimes the vision is clear, but under the air pressure, the blood clots may extend to the posterior wall of the uterus and cover

the uterine cornua. If the bleeding points are just located in this site, it might not be detected before the removal of the blood clots. The remedy is to place a catheter into the uterine cavity with its end connected to a syringe, by which the blood clots are sucked out under direct vision. Sometimes when the bubbles are forming, the surgeon should wait patiently for a while because the vision might become clear suddenly and the bubbles might disappear abruptly, the process of which may be accelerated due to the regulation of the air flow pressure (higher or lower). Due to the short period in sustaining a clear view, the surgeon must be ready to make a rapid diagnosis. If the vision is seriously limited, and a comprehensive and reliable diagnosis cannot be made, other uterine-distending techniques should be considered.

2. Hyskon uterine distension: Being a high-viscosity uterine distending medium, Hyskon is not easy to be mixed with blood, so it is suitable to be applied for women with severe bleeding or when uterine distension with CO_2 fails. The intrauterine hematocele should be removed first before it is in use so as to keep a clear view.
3. Low viscosity distending medium: Low viscosity distending media include normal saline, 3% sorbitol, 5% mannitol, 1.5% glycine, Ringer lactate solution, etc., which are convenient for application and safer than high viscosity distending media. In diagnostic hysteroscopy, the operating is short and so the risk of fluid overload is minimal.
4. Contact hysteroscopy: Another alternative technique is the contact hysteroscopy. After the contact of the objective lens with the mucosa, the intrauterine hemorrhage volume is not a problem any longer. The only restriction is that the surgeon must be proficient in this technique and be able to interpret the images correctly. While faced with difficult-to-control bleeding, contact hysteroscope should be replaced by hysteroscope with continuous perfusion. Such hysteroscope is equipped with two channels: inflow channel and outflow channel. After the entry of fluid into the uterine cavity, the intrauterine blood and debris can be washed out while the uterus is distended so that the surgeon can observe the whole uterine cavity clearly.

8.2.1.3 Hysteroscopy for AUB

Barbot reported the hysteroscopic findings in 768 patients who had AUB at different age groups (Table 8.4). In women of childbearing age, uterine myomas, endometrial hyperplasia, and endometrial polyps were the most common findings under diagnostic hysteroscopy, which almost accounted for more than a half (54% of the cases in a group reported by Barbot), followed by the bleeding associated with pregnancy. In menopausal women, endometrial hyperplasia, endometrial polyps and uterine myomas were the most common findings, followed by endometrial atrophy and endometrial carcinoma.

Table 8.4 Hysteroscopic findings in 768 patients who had AUB at different age groups

	In women with child-bearing age	In postmenopausal women
Common findings	Uterine myomas Endometrial hyperplasia Endometrial polyps Placenta polyps Decidua (ectopic pregnancy) Endometrial atrophy Adenomyosis Endocervical cancer	Endometrial hyperplasia Endometrial polyps Endocervical polyps Uterine myomas Endometrial atrophy Endocervical cancer Adenomyosis

8.2.1.4 Roles of Hysteroscopy in the Diagnosis of Non-pregnancy AUB

Most intrauterine benign lesions are endometrial polyps, submucous myomas, and endometrial hyperplasia, which have different features. The initial symptoms of those lesions are often AUB, which cannot be diagnosed by gynecological examinations like speculum examination and bimanual examination. In recent years, it has been fully proved that the standard diagnostic procedures to explore and identify these lesions are not reliable. In the interpretations of HSG abnormal images, 30–50% of them are uncertain or even incorrect. D&C cannot remove the uterine myomas, and often miss endometrial polyps as well. However, accurate diagnosis is required clinically to be able to identify these three kinds of lesions, and also to suggest correct method of treatment. With extensive application of hysteroscopy, diagnostic hysteroscopy has been highly valued and applied in the diagnosis of chronic endometritis recently.

Endometrial Polyps

Diagnosis

Due to the lack of typical and constant symptoms, endometrial polyps are usually difficult to be accurately diagnosed clinically. In diagnosing endometrial polyps, space-occupying lesions like filling defects or an irregular uterine wall might be revealed under HSG, but it is easy to be confused with submucous myoma and bubbles, and excessive injection of contrast media can mask polyps. Sometimes typical polyp can be scraped off by D&C, thus a confirmed diagnosis may be made. However, it is more likely to miss scraping the polyp which is too small or too large. Since it lacks a specific structure, a polyp is hard to be diagnosed pathologically once it is curetted into debris, which may only be reported to be the proliferative endometrium or endometrial hyperplasia. Therefore, there is high rate of false negative results. It can be concluded that both HSG and D&C have limitations in diagnosing endometrial polyps, so if the patients have such clinical symptoms as menorrhagia, prolonged menstruation, continuous dripping, and infertility, especially if HSG is abnormal or cervical or endocervical polyps found during gynecologic examinations, hysteroscopic examination should be considered so as to determine whether there exists any endometrial polyp or not. According to Angioni's report, in diagnosis of endometrial polyps with hysteroscopy, the sensitivity was 100%, the specificity was 97%, and the accuracy was 91%, which were almost absolutely consistent with the postoperative pathologic diagnosis. Spiewankiewicz et al. discovered that, in 65 patients with polyps found in the cervical canals with gynecological examinations, six were diagnosed as endometrial polyps under hysteroscopy. In another 13 patients, cervical polyps were identified by gynecological examination, which were confirmed to be endometrial polyps under hysteroscopy.

Under hysteroscope, endometrial polyps can protrude from any site of the uterine wall and at any angle into the uterine cavity, which may also be found in the cervical canal, or just located in the uterine cornua, causing blockage of the fallopian tubal ostia (Fig. 8.58a). The size of polyps generally ranges from 0.2 cm to 3 cm, which can be single (Fig. 8.58b–d) or multiple (Fig. 8.58e), and one polyp may have two pedicles (Fig. 8.58f). A polyp is soft, shiny, and even floating in appearance, with the color being bright red, which is similar to the surrounding endometrium, but there are also exceptions occasionally. A polyp does neither float in flowing distention fluid as an endometrial debris nor is it as solid and firm as the submucous myoma. The polyps are mostly oval but also triangular, conical, or irregular in shape (Fig. 8.58g, h). They have smooth surface, under which fine microvascular networks can sometimes be seen. Most polyps have pedicles, which are long and thin, or short and wide. Occasionally, the top surface of larger polyps is accompanied by necrosis, which appears to be purple-brown. The morphology of polyps does not change with an increase or decrease in uterine-distending pressure.

Values of Hysteroscopy

Diagnostic hysteroscopy can make a correct diagnosis, and an experienced hysteroscopist can obtain visually guided samples for histopathological examination, after which a final diagnosis can be made by pathologists. The polyps may be scraped into pieces by blind curettage, which may be mixed with endometrial debris, causing difficulty in histopathological examination. During a diagnostic hysteroscopy, a relatively complete polyp may be taken out, and the histopathological examination can reveal any transformation from a benign polyp into endometrial adenocarcinoma. Similarly, a thorough direct inspection of the uterine cavity may reveal other lesions concomitant with endometrial polyps, such as endometrial hyperplasia or submucous myoma. Finally, after selective resection of endometrial polyps, a complete scraping of the endometrium for examination is suggested for women over the age of 40 years, and then the hysteroscope is inserted again to make sure that the uterine cavity has been emptied so as not to miss any early lesions of endometrial carcinoma. In 2007, Timmermans et al. reported 178 patients with postmenopausal bleeding and endometrial thickness >4 mm with ultrasonography examination. Endometrial polyps were found in 90 patients (50%) with hysteroscopy. Burke et al. reported that endometrial pathology was diagnosed in five women when they had been investigated for infertility, with atypical polypoid adenomyoma in three cases, complex endometrial hyperplasia in one and stage 1 endometrial adenocarcinoma in one. Only the last patient had menstrual abnormality. They believed that the possibility of detecting endometrial pathologies increased during fertility investigations, because women in this category are likely to be older and obese. Antunes et al. reported that among 475 cases of perimenopausal and postmenopausal women with endometrial polyps identified, atypical hyperplasia was found in 1.05% of cases, and endometrial polypoid cancer in 2.74%.

Submucosal Myoma

Diagnosis

1. Submucosal myoma: It is usually easy to diagnose. Its typical hysteroscopic appearance is one of a circular mass, which protrudes into the uterine cavity (Fig. 8.59a, b). The endometrium covering the myoma usually appears to be atrophic with its color brighter than its surrounding endometrium. On its surface, a dilated vascular network is visible (Fig. 8.59c). When the myoma is touched with the end of the objective lens, it feels hard in texture, and interferes with the introduction of the telescope, which can only bypass it from its side and goes into the upper cavity. If a submucosal myoma has a pedicle, it may be difficult to be differentiated from endometrial polyps (Fig. 8.59d). When extending to the cervix, the myoma turns flat, and becomes redder in color at its end (Fig. 8.59e, f).
2. Intramural myoma: The endometrium covering the surface of the intramural myoma is the same as the surrounding endometrium in appearance, except that it protrudes slightly into the uterine cavity, so it is easy to be missed in diagnosis by hysteroscopy (Fig. 8.59g, h). The only indication for intramural myoma may be that the symmetry of uterine cavity disappears (Fig. 8.59i) when the hysteroscope is placed at the internal orifice of cervix.

Values of Hysteroscopy

The diagnostic hysteroscopy is of great value in the diagnosis of submucous myoma, especially the small ones which are located in the uterine cavity causing severe bleeding, but cannot be detected by internal examination. When HSG cannot be done due to continuous bleeding, a prompt diagnosis can be made by hysteroscopy, and unnecessary D&C is avoided. Sometimes the existence of submucosal myoma can be suspected by "feeling" a firm bulge accidentally during D&C, but in most cases it would be missed. Due to the friction of myomas in the uterine cavity, the mucosa may ulcerate, thus leading to continuous abnormal bleeding. Even when myoma of uterus is detected during bimanual examination occasionally, myoma cannot be taken lightly as the cause of bleeding. Hysteroscopy can often avoid misdiagnosis due to the presence of intrauterine lesions, such as endometrial hyperplasia, polyps, or cancer. Angioni et al. reported that hysteroscopy demonstrated a sensitivity of 100%, speci-

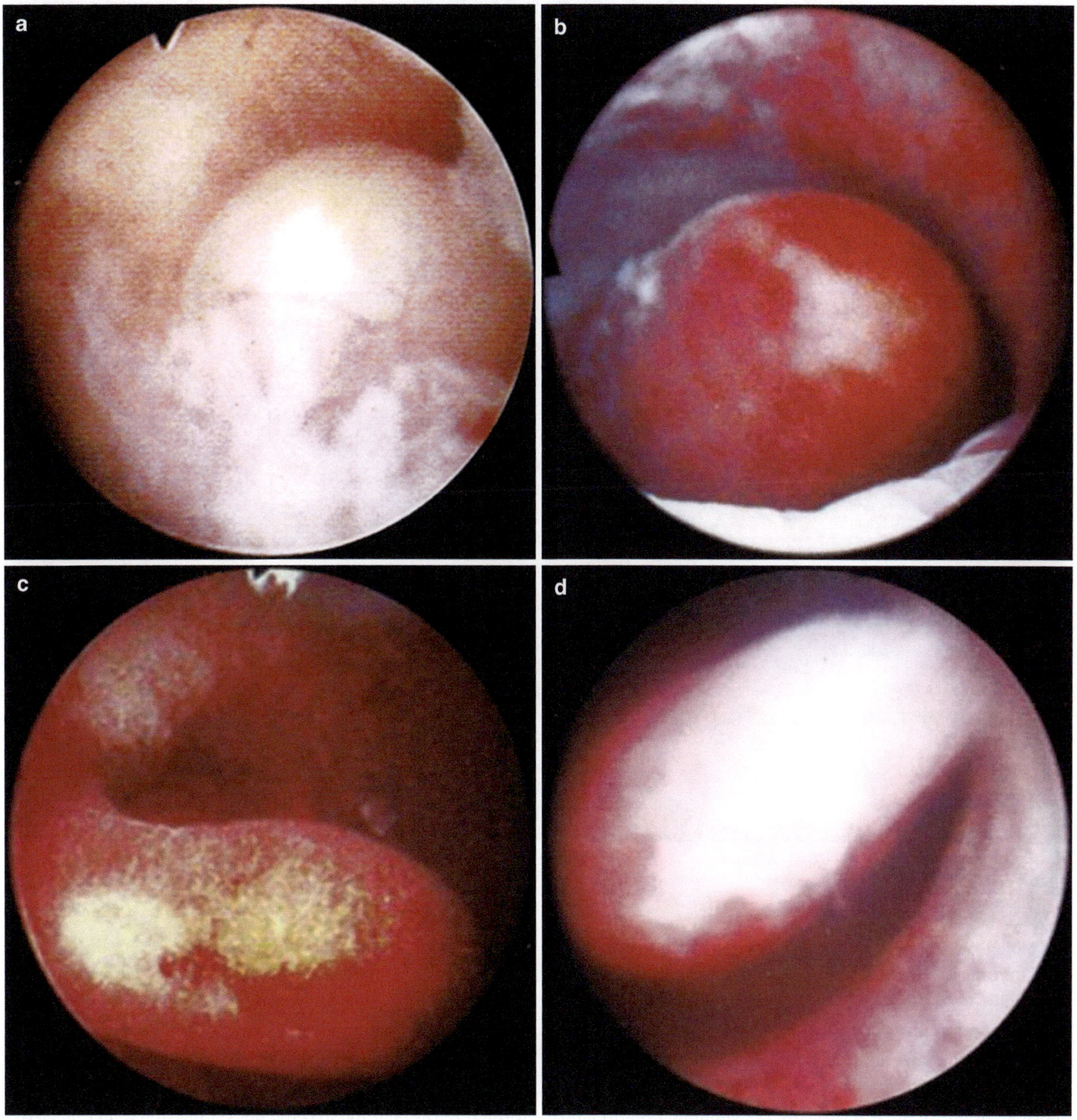

Fig. 8.58 (**a**) Small endometrial polyp in the tubal ostia of left uterine cornua. (**b–d**) Single endometrial polyp. (**e**) Multiple endometrial polyps. (**f**) Endometrial polyp (double pedicles). (**g**) Strawberry-shaped endometrial polyp. (**h**) Endometrial polyp with double pedicles

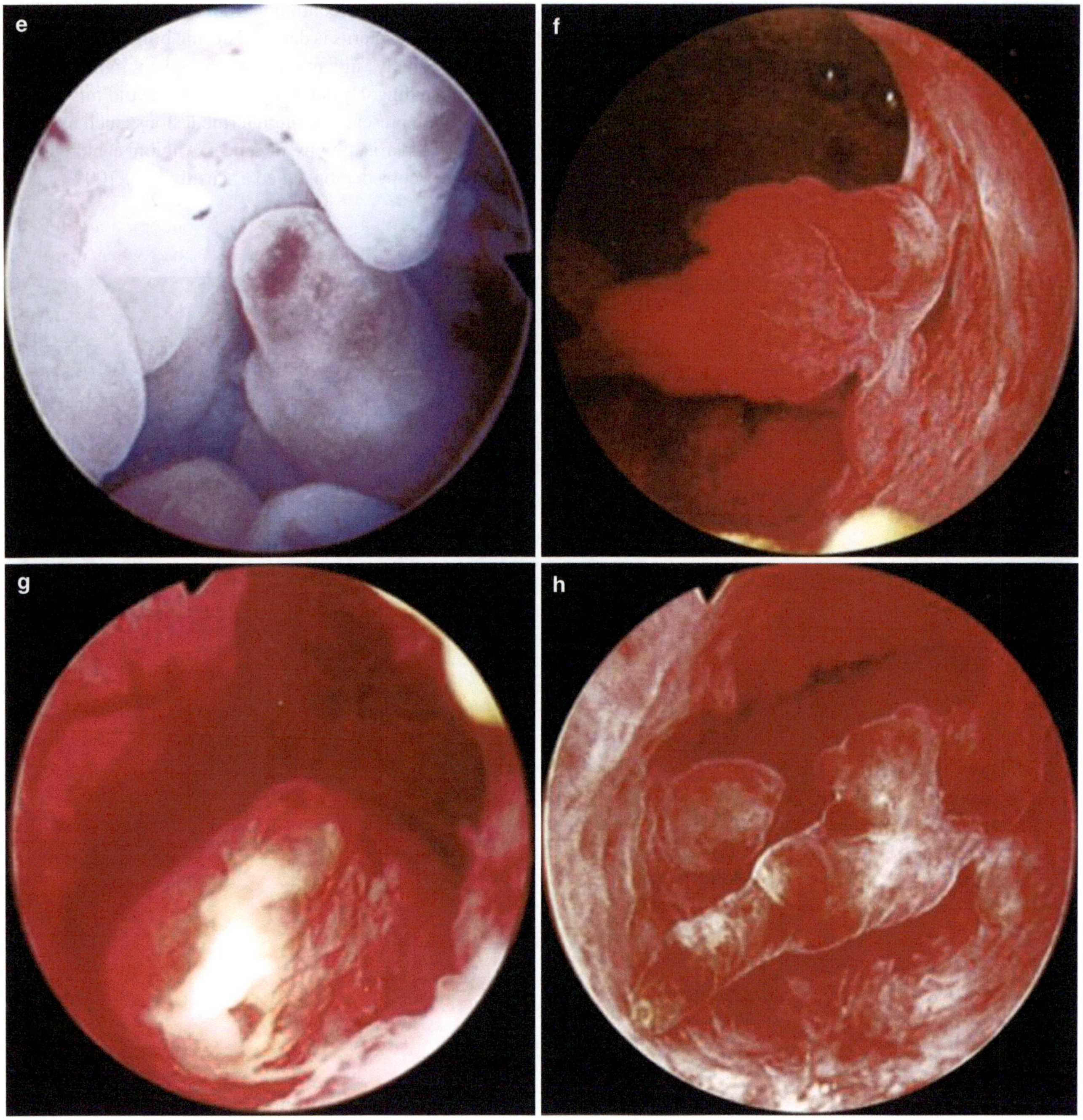

Fig. 8.58 (continued)

ficity of 98%, and a diagnosis accuracy of 99% for submucous myomas. The kappa value was 0.82 for hysteroscopy, which corresponded highly with final pathologic diagnosis.

The hysteroscopy is also extremely useful in the choice of a proper treatment, which can help patients be treated conservatively so as to avoid laparotomy or hysterectomy. An accurate and noninvasive resection of pedunculated submucous myoma can be performed easily by operative hysteroscopy. Hysteroscopic resection of sessile myoma is very difficult, but high-frequency electricity or laser under ultrasonography monitoring can be used to resect safely the sessile submucosal myomas embedded in the uterine wall. Before removal of intramural or subserosal myomas with laparoscopy or conventional laparotomy, preoperative hysteroscopy can be performed to rule out the myoma coexisting in the uterine cavity and avoid a perforation to the uterine cavity during operation.

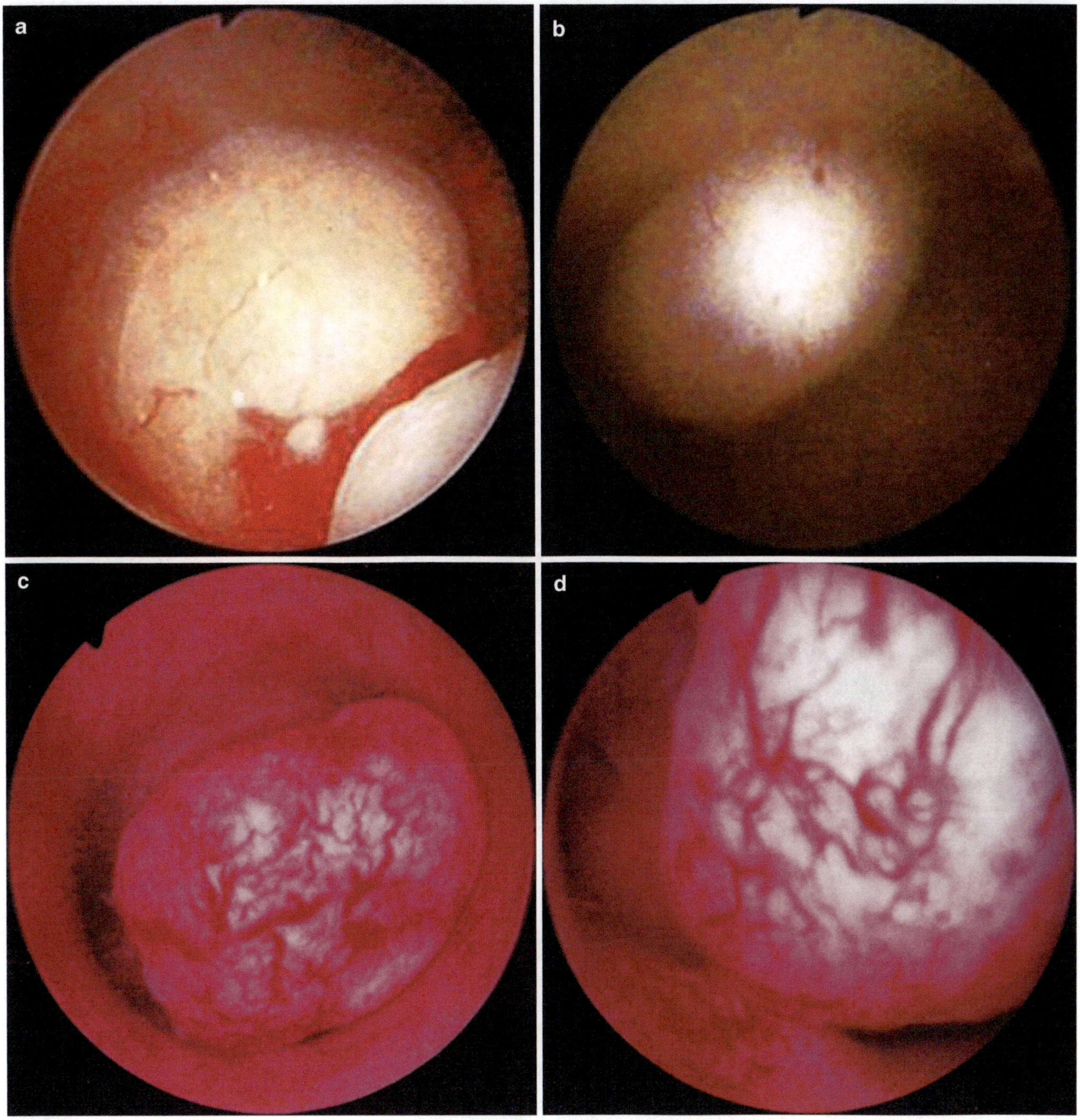

Fig. 8.59 (**a**) Submucosal myoma. (**b**) Submucosal myoma with a pedicle on the anterior wall. (**c**) Submucosal myoma with dilated vascular network visible on its surface. (**d**) Submucosal myoma with pedicles. (**e**) Submucosal myoma which protrudes out of the cervical os. (**f**) Submucosal myoma which protrudes out of the cervical os. (**g**) Intramural myoma which protrudes into the cavity. (**h**) Intramural myoma which protrudes into the cavity. (**i**) Intramural myoma, which protrudes into the cavity, leading to compression and deformation of uterine cavity

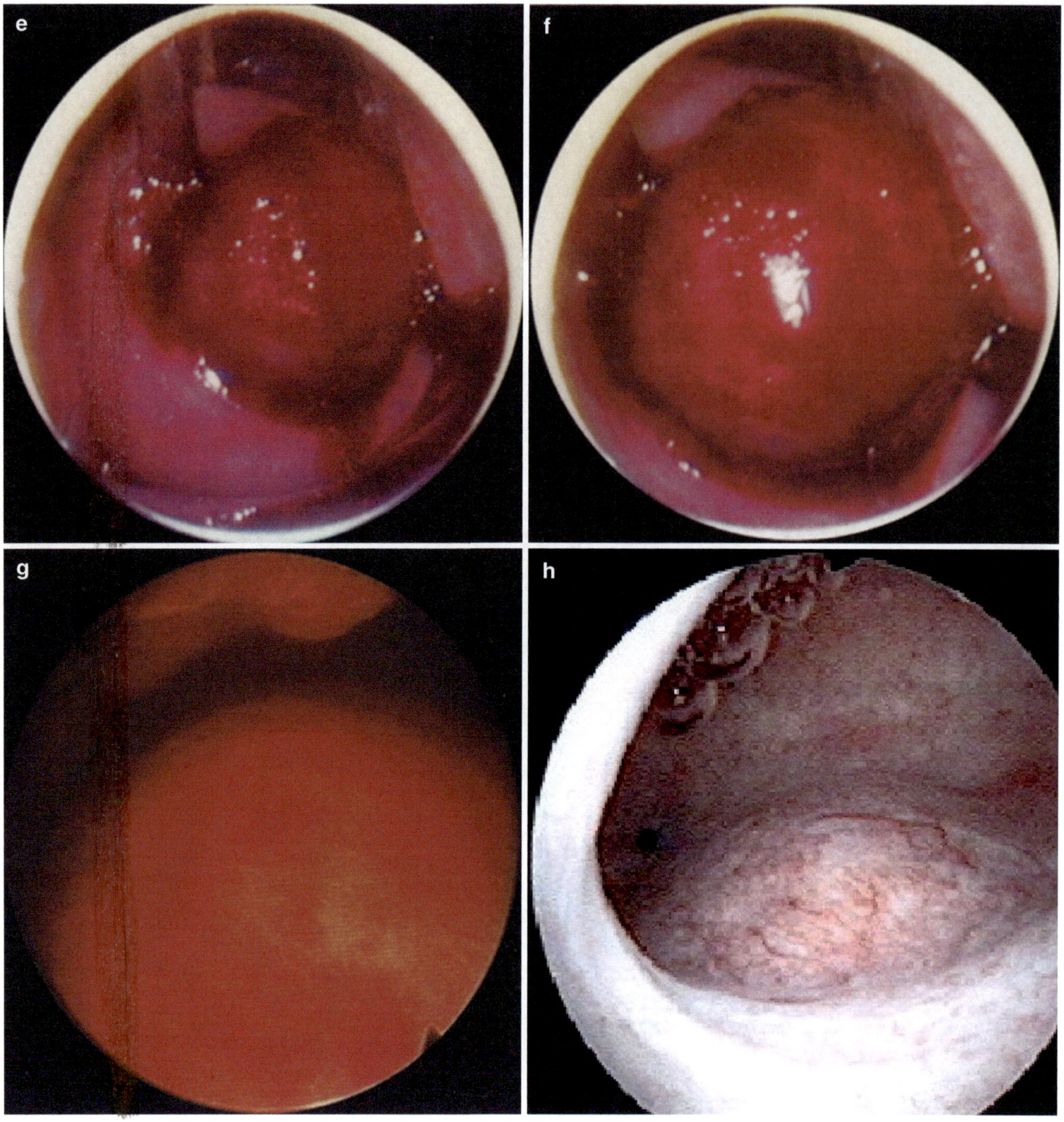

Fig. 8.59 (continued)

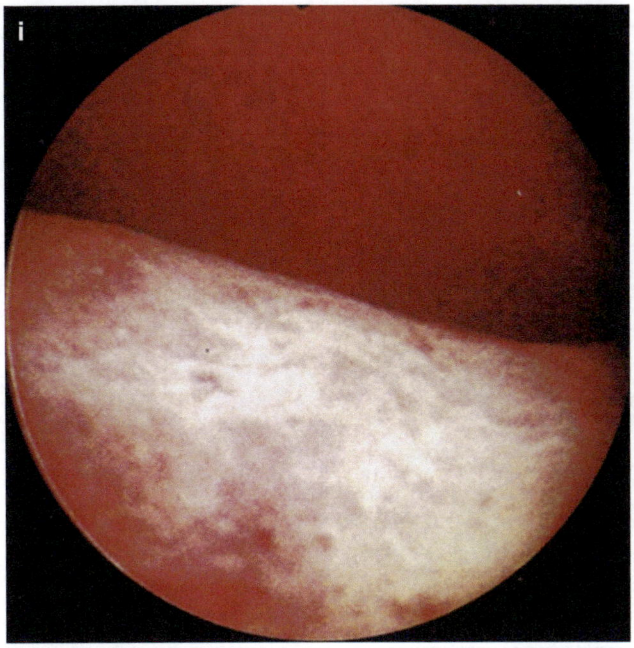

Fig. 8.59 (continued)

Benign Endometrial Hyperplasia

Diagnosis

Benign endometrial hyperplasia is defined as normal endometrium, glands and interstitial cells increased in number and density. However, these increases are well coordinated, which still maintain normal ratios. This is the differentiation point between benign (simple endometrial hyperplasia, Fig. 8.60a) and atypical endometrial hyperplasia or uterine adenomatous hyperplasia (complex endometrial hyperplasia, Fig. 8.60b), in the latter endometrial glands replace the normal supportive interstitial tissues. According to the above definition, benign endometrial hyperplasia can be classified into several types: (1) simple hyperplasia, which manifests as normal endometrium with increase in thickness; (2) polypoid hyperplasia, the mucosal surface of which is wave-shaped (Fig. 8.60c) and resembles polyps; (3) benign cystic hyperplasia, in which the glands are enlarged and expanded, and a "Swiss cheese" form is shown histologically. Endometrial hyperplasia can be diffuse or localized. The latter is isolated and excessive proliferation of endometrial cells can be found in normal endometrium. There is some difficulty in diagnosing endometrial hyperplasia with hysteroscopy. Normal endometrium changes constantly throughout the menstrual cycle, the thickness of the endometrium reaches its peak in late proliferative phase, during which the endometrium is not affected by secretion of progesterone, and the appearance of endometrium is similar to hyperplasia. Therefore, the physicians must be familiar with endometrial images at different phases of the menstrual cycle so as to make appropriate hysteroscopic diagnosis. Although the hysteroscope cannot be compared with the microscope, but it can identify the endometrium in different physiological phases. The methods for identification lie on four conditions: endometrial thickness, color, vessels, and texture. Another difficulty is associated with hysteroscopic techniques. The examination of a normal endometrium on the same day by a contact hysteroscope with gas uterine-distension or liquid uterine-distension may get completely different results. Without any artificial distention of the uterine cavity, contact hysteroscopy may certainly obtain the results closest to the actual condition of the endometrium. In the late proliferative stage, the endometrium is thickened and wavelike, with many wrinkles on its surface. Such a change is not a polypoid hyperplasia and such a feature can be maintained under contact hysteroscopy, but due to the compression of the contact hysteroscope, the endometrium turns into pink-and-white, the blood vessels become less and thinner, and the tissues may be divided or fragmented.

Endometrium at secretory phase (Fig. 8.60d) appears to be thickened and wavy, but light-colored, greyish, and transparent; the vessels are significantly increased in number, with their calibers widened to be sinusoid; and the tissue is dense and cannot be easily crushed. All of these changes are caused by the effect of progesterone. The panoramic hysteroscopy which uses CO_2 as uterine-distending medium may find endometrium flat but its thickness invisible. The pressure of the gas causes the uterine cavity to expand and plicae to disappear. At this time, if panoramic hysteroscopy uses liquid as uterine-distending medium instead, the endometrial plicae might reappear and seems to be larger. In spite of expansion of the uterine cavity, the endometrium still remains like the seaweed, and the outwardly growing shoots are quivering in liquid. An experienced hysteroscopic surgeon must understand these changes so as not to make a false-positive or false-negative diagnosis of endometrial hyperplasia. When contact hysteroscopy is performed, simple endometrial hyperplasia is similar to preovulatory endometrium in color, vessels, and texture, and the abnormally thickened endometrium may form many rugae, accumulating into compound layers. Simple endometrial hyperplasia is very difficult to be diagnosed by panoramic CO_2 hysteroscope, because the endometrium seems to be flat even though it becomes thickened. Porto suggested drawing a furrow in the endometrium with the end of objective lens so as to estimate the thickness of the endometrium. The features of polypoid hyperplasia are obvious, so its diagnosis is relatively easier. Since there is no uterine distention, the polypoid hyperplasia looks like many leaflets piling up together under the contact hysteroscopy, the image of which does not disappear when the uterus is distended, so a panoramic hysteroscope is more suitable. The severity of intrauterine lesions under hysteroscopy is associated with the expansion of the cavity. The more expanding the uterine cavity is, the less obvious are the

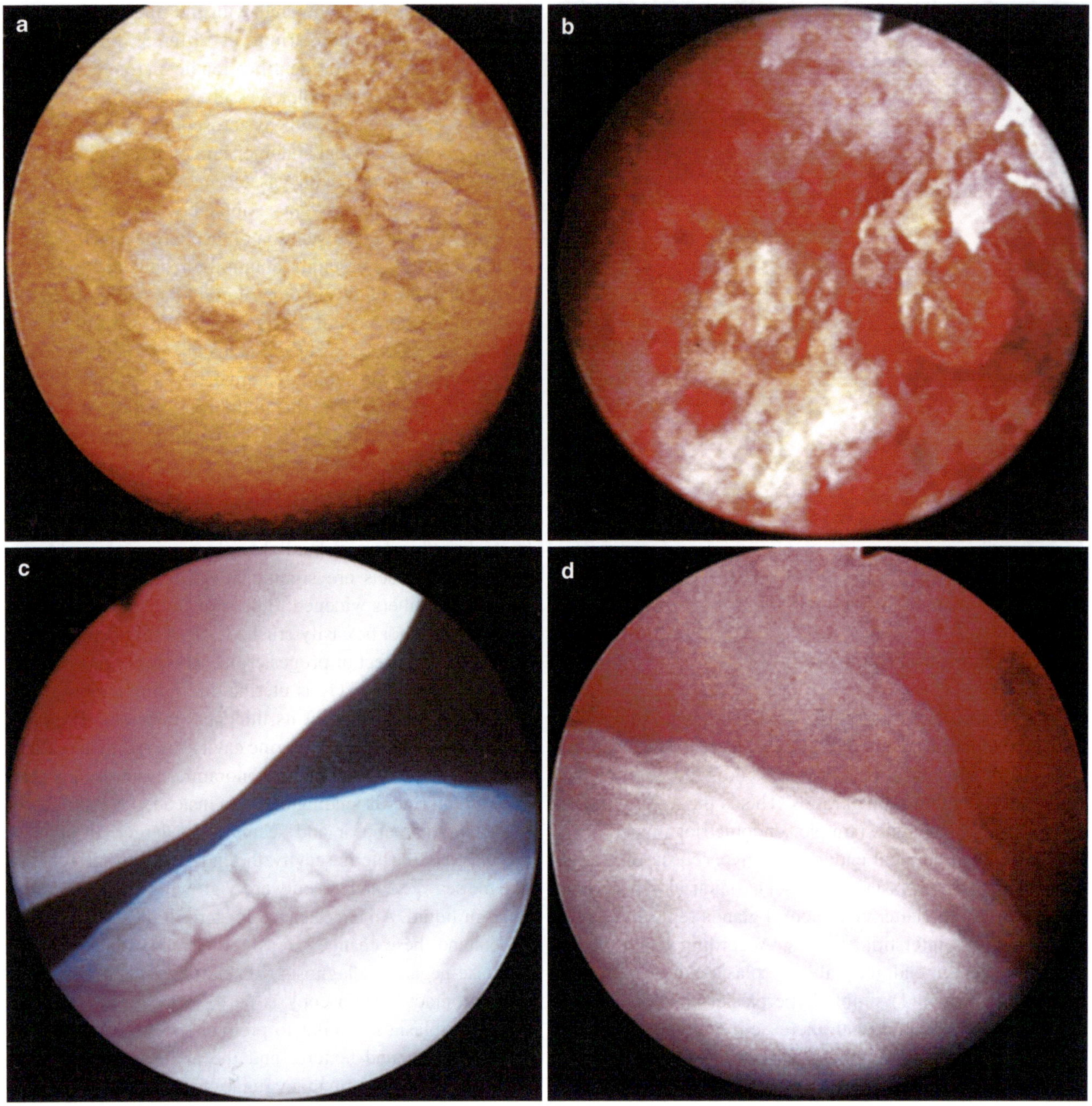

Fig. 8.60 (**a**) Simple endometrial hyperplasia. (**b**) Complex endometrial hyperplasia. (**c**) Mucosal surface of polypoid hyperplasia. (**d**) Endometrium at secretory phase

lesions. The endometrial cystic hyperplasia can be seen clearly under contact hysteroscope.

Values of Hysteroscopy

Compared with HSG and D&C, hysteroscopy is the only way to observe the endometrium in vivo inside the human body. The inferences drawn from an irregular contour and filling defects with HSG are always incomplete. D&C random sampling only offers limited information and blind curettage may destroy the endometrial structure, hence only debris can be taken for pathological examination. HSG often misses the focal endometrial hyperplasia. At the beginning of injecting a contrast agent, nonspecific hidden filling defect may sometimes be seen, which disappears after the continuous injection of the contrast agent. D&C often cannot detect the disorders either. However, with hysteroscopy, it can look directly into the uterine cavity, with the endometrium being flat or polypoid, diffuse or focal. The extent of lesions can be defined and the diagnosis of focal endometrial hyperplasia can be made. When focal endometrial hyperplasia is found in a routine hysteroscopy due to AUB, its relationship with AUB should be carefully considered and other causes for bleeding should also be searched for at the same time. Endometrial hyperplasia is often accompanied by a high estrogen state, so lesions induced by the coexisting estrogen stimulation must be considered. The focal atypical endometrial hyperplasia or early endometrial cancer should not be missed and a biopsy must be taken from the sites with atypical vessels. One of the advantages of hysteroscopy is that the condition of the endometrium can be fully revealed before biopsy sampling or treatment. Focal endometrial hyperplasia is similar to polyps occasionally, and contact hysteroscopy can be performed earlier in case of doubt. The true polyps have pedicles, which are mostly composed of stroma with typical axial feeding vessels. The pedicles are firmly attached to the uterine wall and resist the pressure from the hysteroscope. However, these structures of focal endometrial hyperplasia are not firm and are easy to be penetrated or poked away by hysteroscope. Another advantage of hysteroscopy is follow-up of endometrial hyperplasia therapeutic effect. According to the statistics, in a conventional blind curettage, 25% of the endometrium would not be sampled at all. For severe diffuse endometrial hyperplasia, a repeat curettage should be performed under the hysteroscopic guidance in order to take enough endometrium for histopathology examination. If hormone therapy is administered in the patients, diagnostic hysteroscopy can accurately assess the reaction of endometrium to progestogen after medication.

Atypical Endometrial Hyperplasia and Endometrial Carcinoma

Diagnosis

Atypical endometrial hyperplasia is a precancerous lesion, which may develop into endometrial carcinoma if not treated. It is even difficult for experienced pathologists to distinguish the differences between atypical endometrial hyperplasia, carcinoma in situ, and early invasive carcinoma, so adjunct diagnosis with hysteroscopy is brought forward, which could not only diagnose endometrial carcinoma with obvious malignant appearance but also early carcinoma in situ. Hysteroscopy has the same diagnostic procedures as colposcopy, that is, to identify the most suspicious site for biopsy. However, it is a pity that there is not a single reagent [such as acetic acid and compound iodine solution (Lugol's solution)] that can show atypical endometrial hyperplasia and early endometrial carcinoma. So only when the hysteroscopic physicians have the knowledge about hysteroscopic images of normal endometrium and of various benign endometrial hyperplasia, can the more serious abnormalities be diagnosed. Close attention should be paid to the endometrial tissues which have different colors, fluctuation, and toughness from the surrounding normal endometrium. For a highly suspected neoplasm at the site with atypical vessels, the application of a contact hysteroscopy and the magnification of images may increase the accuracy of diagnosis and provide more detailed information.

Due to the technical and anatomical reasons, early endometrial cancer does not manifest as lumpy structure available for screening, and diagnostic hysteroscopy is usually performed due to AUB. Since hysteroscopic images have distinct characteristics, diagnosis should not be a problem. However, influenced by inspection techniques and equipment, contact hysteroscopy eliminates the reflection of light, making the color of the endometrium more natural and the graphics of the blood vessels displayed, enabling the thickness of lesions to be assessed. Panoramic hysteroscopy is suitable to be used to determine the location of the tumor, to draw an accurate outline of its shape, and to establish its extension. CO_2 used in uterine-distention can have a good illumination, but make the undulant endometrium be flattened, so its surface appears smoother. When fluid is used in uterine-distension endometrial tissue may be extended outward, but the field of vision is made narrower and the color turns white.

Sugimoto described four types of endometrial carcinoma with fluid used in uterine-distension. (1) Polypoid type: It is polypoid-like in appearance, but irregular in shape with enlarged and twisted blood vessels; (2) Nodular type: It has a wide base, coarse surface and atypical blood vessels; (3) Papillary type: It has a polypoid or nodular appearance, but its surface is covered with tiny papillar projections fluttering in the distending fluid; (4) Ulcerated type: All the above types may finally develop ulcers.

Barbot classified endometrial carcinoma into three types through an observation of 87 cases with CO_2 insufflation. (1) Exogenous type: It is the most common, and the carcinoma tissue is white and growing outward, which is equivalent to Sugimoto's type of nodular and papillary types. These projections are difficult to manifest themselves when CO_2 insufflation is used, thus hardly be detected; (2) Polypoid type: It has a feature of the endometrial polyp with a narrow base, but a more distinct shape of cylinder, with its surface coarse and irregular, and vessels enlarged; (3) Medullary type: The lesions are extensive with the neoplasms whitish and irregular, and separated by deep grooves, which are similar to brain tissues.

Any type of endometrial carcinoma mentioned above can develop ulcer, necrosis or hemorrhage, making the surface greyish or yellowish, which may conceal the original lesions and be mistaken for normal images. The contact hysteroscopy may reveal an image of the lesion itself.

Values of Hysteroscopy

Far in 1907, David reported on observation of endometrial cancer with contact hysteroscope. In 1928, Gauss described in detail the findings about neoplasms visible during panoramic hysteroscopy with fluid as uterine distention medium and drew many pictures. However, HSG and fractional D&C were still the only methods in diagnosing endometrial cancer and determining the extent of its invasion. In 1971, Swedish Joelsson recommended hysteroscopy as a routine method in the assessment of endometrial cancer.

AUB is the main symptom for 80% patients with endometrial cancer, so it is more commonly seen in pre-menopausal and post-menopausal women who have undertaken diagnostic hysteroscopy due to AUB, and the detection rate rises along with an increase in patients' age. Sugimoto reported that among 1824 women who were examined with hysteroscopy due to AUB, 53 women had endometrial carcinoma. Barbot reported that in 1400 cases who had AUB, 56 were found to have endometrial carcinoma by hysteroscopy.

Currently, hysteroscopy can provide the most reliable information about the diagnosis of endometrial cancer and the extent of intrauterine invasion. Endometrial cytology smear may provide false negative results, especially for well-differentiated or small tumors. The result of HSG may be suggestive of endometrial carcinoma, but often misleading. Blind D&C is often inaccurate, and small cancer foci may be missed in the deep cornua or the rear of the submucosal myomas during curettage. In most cases, the tumor may be clearly observed under hysteroscopy and its outcomes may be predicted. Hysteroscopic examination may reveal a more obvious outward-extending extent of the tumor than HSG, but the depth of myometrial infiltration cannot be detected. Visual inspection cannot replace the pathological diagnosis, so samples must be taken for histopathological examination.

Diagnostic hysteroscopy can also provide staging for tumors, as tumor may spread to the uterus (stage I) or invade the cervix (stage II), for which the treatment and the prognosis are completely different. Liukko et al. investigated the specimens of the removal of uterus which were diagnosed to be endometrial carcinoma stage I by fractional curettage prior to operation and 16% of which were found to be cervical infiltration postoperatively. Stelmachow reported that among 22 cases with stage I endometrial carcinoma diagnosed by HSG and D&C, 9 were proved to be with stage II by diagnostic hysteroscopy; and among 9 cases who had been diagnosed to be with stage II, 2 were actually with stage I. These data indicated the advantages of hysteroscopy in detecting the infiltration of the cervix. During hysteroscopy, the cervical canal is examined with tissues scraped prior to cervical dilation, thus misdiagnosis is avoided.

Gynecologists are concerned about whether hysteroscopy can cause focal spread or metastasis of the tumor, and the same problem also goes to HSG and D&C. Experimental studies have shown that the uterine-distending medium injected into the uterine cavity during HSG may also flow into the abdominal cavity and blood vessels, causing the spread of cancer. The same danger also exists during curettage. Under laparoscopy, the distending fluid used for panoramic hysteroscopy can be seen spilling into the abdominal cavity. When the intrauterine pressure using CO_2 insufflation is too high, $PaCO_2$ proves that CO_2 enters the vessels. The contact hysteroscopy may have extremely small risk of danger in cell dispersion. The essential problem is whether the disseminated cancer cells may lead to plantation and metastasis of cancer cells or not. Johnson reported that, in a comparison study of the metastasis rate in patients with endometrial carcinoma who were in group of examination with curettage and HSG, and in group with simple curettage, no significant difference was found. In short, regardless of what method for diagnosis, there does exist the possibility of metastasis, but it may not necessarily occur.

Chronic Endometritis

Diagnosis

In 2005, Cicinelli reported that 35% of patients with chronic endometritis suffered from AUB. The sensitivity, specificity, and positive and negative predictive values for diagnosis of chronic endometritis with hysteroscopy for women with endometrial hyperemia and edema were 91.8%, 92.9%, 63.9%, and 98.8%, respectively; with the diagnostic accuracy of 92.7%. If concomitant with micropolyps, the sensitivity, specificity, and positive and negative predictive values were 55.4%, 99.9%, 98.4%, 94.5%, respectively, and a diagnostic accuracy was 93.4%.

Values of Hysteroscopy

Chronic endometritis is a subtle condition that is difficult to be detected, but may lead to abnormal uterine bleeding and infertility. Few data exist about the appearance of chronic endometritis at diagnostic hysteroscopy which uses fluid as distending medium (hereafter referred to as fluid hysteroscopy) and about the value of fluid hysteroscopy in the detection of this condition. In Cicinelli's experience, under fluid hysteroscopy, the characterizations of chronic endometritis was associated with stromal edema and either focal or diffuse hyperemia and micropolyps (<1 mm in size). Among 910 cases in his research, hyperemia and edema were detected in 158 patients (17.4%), including micropolyps in 61 patients (6.7%). Among 158 patients, 101 (63.9%) were confirmed the diagnosis of chronic endometritis was confirmed by histopathological examination in 101 cases (63.9%).

8.2.1.5 Role of Hysteroscopy in Diagnosis of Postmenopausal Bleeding

With the prolonged life span in women and increasingly widespread applications of hormonal replacement therapy (HRT) and tamoxifen (TMX), there are more and more cases with postmenopausal bleeding (PMB). It was reported that at least 60% of postmenopausal women suffered from bleeding. Its etiology is complex, with atrophic endometrium as the most common reason, and hormonal effects as the second, being followed by other reasons such as endometrial polyps, submucous myoma, IUD, endometrial carcinoma, and so on. Its hysteroscopic findings can be classified as atrophic endometrium, irregular endometrial hyperplasia, endometrial polyps, submucous myoma, and suspected endometrial cancer. Due to their potential risk of endometrial cancer, it is very important to investigate the cause of the bleeding.

Currently, the diagnostic methods are D&C, transabdominal ultrasonography, transvaginal sonography (TVS), sonohysterography (SHSG), diagnostic hysteroscopy, computed tomography (CT), and so on. Gimpelson and Rappold carried out a study on 276 women who underwent both hysteroscopy and D&C. More information was revealed in 44 cases with hysteroscopy, and in nine cases with D&C. Hysteroscopy was especially superior to D&C in making an accurate diagnosis of endometrial polyps and submucous myoma. Hysteroscopy revealed the pathological conditions in some of these patients while repeat curettage showed no abnormalities. Usually, 10–35% of the intrauterine lesions may not be detected by D&C, especially endometrial polyps and submucous myoma. Therefore, in the endoscopic era, blind D&C should no longer be a main method. Among the various examination methods, TVS and hysteroscopy, especially biopsy under direct vision of hysteroscope is the most accurate method. From the data reported by Valenzano et al., it was suggested that the sensitivity of detecting intrauterine disorders in women with PMB was 90% with TVS and 93% with hysteroscopy. However, the specificity of TVS was only 30%. Alcazar and Laparte also pointed out that in the diagnosis of PMB, both TVS and hysteroscopy had high sensitivity, but hysteroscopy had a higher specificity than TVS. Therefore, hysteroscopy has the highest diagnostic value to etiology of PMB. Outpatient diagnostic hysteroscopy should become the preferred method of examination for PMB due to its high degree of accuracy and acceptability of the patients. Now patients can receive hysteroscopy in outpatients, and hysteroscopic assessment of PMB has been very popular in some countries. Hysteroscopy can have a direct view of the intrauterine lesions in women with PMB such as endometrial polyps, submucous myoma, focal endometrial pathology including endometrial adenocarcinoma and its precursors. Meanwhile, biopsy of suspected sites can be taken to confirm these pathological conditions so that the sampling error may be avoided. However, hysteroscopy is still an invasive procedure which takes a little longer.

In recent years, the flexible fiber hysteroscope produced by Olympus Corporation in Japan is entirely applicable to PMB, which generally does not require cervical dilation and anesthesia, thus reducing the discomfort of patients with PMB, except for very few menopausal women or women with extreme stenosis of cervical canal due to adhesions. Due to cervical atrophy in postmenopausal women, a hysteroscopy should be small enough and also permit a direct biopsy through its operating channel. For these women, the operators may use fiber hysteroscope to investigate the cervical canal from the squamocolumnar junction above the external orifice of the cervix, to observe the whole uterine cavity without any blind spots, and to take targeted biopsy at any suspected sites. Once the endometrial polyps are discovered, they should be immediately removed. If there is endometrial hyperplasia, biopsy can identify whether there is cellular atypia or not. If endometrial adenocarcinoma is found, staging should be done immediately. The failure rate of a fiber hysteroscopy was reported less than 3%, and that of a rigid hysteroscopy was twice higher. A comparison was made of a series of data on the results following diagnostic hysteroscopy in 286 patients from France, 444 patients from Japan, and 251 patients from Belgium who were in perimenopausal period (age ≥49 years old with amenorrhea <1 year) or post-menopausal period (amenorrhea for 1 year), and with uterine bleeding. It was found that 49–50% of the patients had normal atrophic endometrium, 25–26.9% had polyps, 13.9% had pedunculated, submucosal or intramural myoma, 4.2–8.3% had endometrial hyperplasia, and 2.1–3.8% had adenocarcinoma. There were no differences in the detection rates between these countries, and the lowest failure rate was found with fiber hysteroscopy in France. It was concluded in this paper that fiber hysteroscopy had a higher diagnostic accuracy than that of TVS, as TVS may miss some focal hyperplasia or adenocarcinoma. Even with endometrial findings by TVS and SHSG, direct biopsy under hysteroscope would be required. Therefore, fiber hysteroscopy is superior to TVS in examining lesions from uterine bleeding in perimenopausal and postmenopausal women for the following four reasons. First, taking the thickness of double layers of endometrium without hormone therapy <4 mm as cut-off point, the rate of missed diagnosis of abnormal endometrium is 5.5% by TVS but the accuracy rate of targeted biopsy by fiber hysteroscopy is higher than 94%. Second, both early endometrial hyperplasia and endometrial adenocarcinoma are focal. TVS may easily miss the diagnosis while fiber hysteroscopy can observe and take a biopsy under direct vision. Third, sometimes the determination of the extension of the tumor or lesions requires more than two biopsies, and fiber hysteroscopy can investigate under direct vision and take multiple biopsies. Fourth, abnormal findings of TVS need to be confirmed by pathology and direct biopsy can be performed by fiber hysteroscopy.

Correctly judgment of endometrial lesions under hysteroscope is the key to the improvement on the accuracy of hysteroscopic diagnosis. Generally, the uterine cavity with atrophic endometrium is smaller, with contour and bilateral tubal ostia clearly visualized, and the endometrium appears to be thin and smooth, orange or white, and sometimes the punctiform and patchy blood spots, or capillary network are visible underneath the mucosa (Fig. 8.61a, b). There may be no tissues scraped with curettage after examination. The endometrium at the proliferative phase is red with smooth surface, and the regularly-distributed white-spot glandular openings are visible with fine vascularity. The intrauterine endometrium involving hyperplasia are thickened totally or partially (Fig. 8.61c, d), which seems like pile blanket with

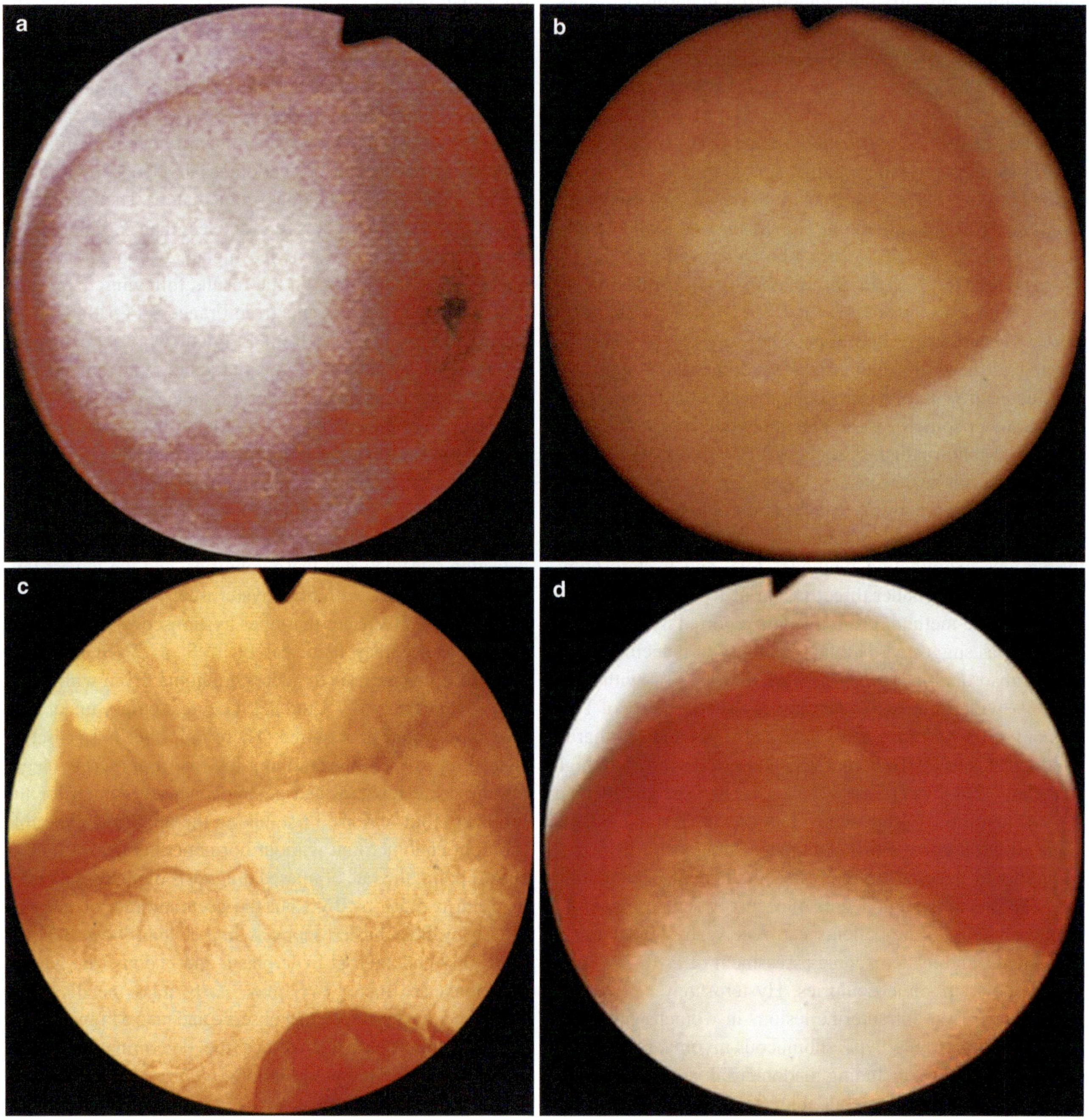

Fig. 8.61 Atrophic endometrium under the flexible hysteroscope. (**a**) A relatively smaller uterine cavity and clear tubal ostia are visible, and the endometrium is filmy and smooth. (**b**) A relatively smaller uterine cavity with a clear contour is visible, and the endometrium is filmy, smooth and yellowish white. Endometrial hyperplasia under the flexible hysteroscope. (**c**) The endometrium is diffusely thickened and seems like a pile blanket, orange colored, and shiny. (**d**) The posterior wall of uterus is seen to be focally thickened, light yellow, and shiny. (**e**) Endometritis under the flexible hysteroscope. The endometrium appears to be dark red with congestion patches visible. (**f**) Endometrial polyps under the flexible hysteroscope. The polyps have papillary protrusions and smooth surface. (**g**) Submucosal myoma under the flexible hysteroscope. The right posterior wall is hemispherically bulged, with its surface pale and blood vessels visible. Endometrial carcinoma under the flexible hysteroscope. (**h**) The thickened and irregularly-run blood vessels are visible. (**i**) Atypical vessels and focal hemorrhage are visible

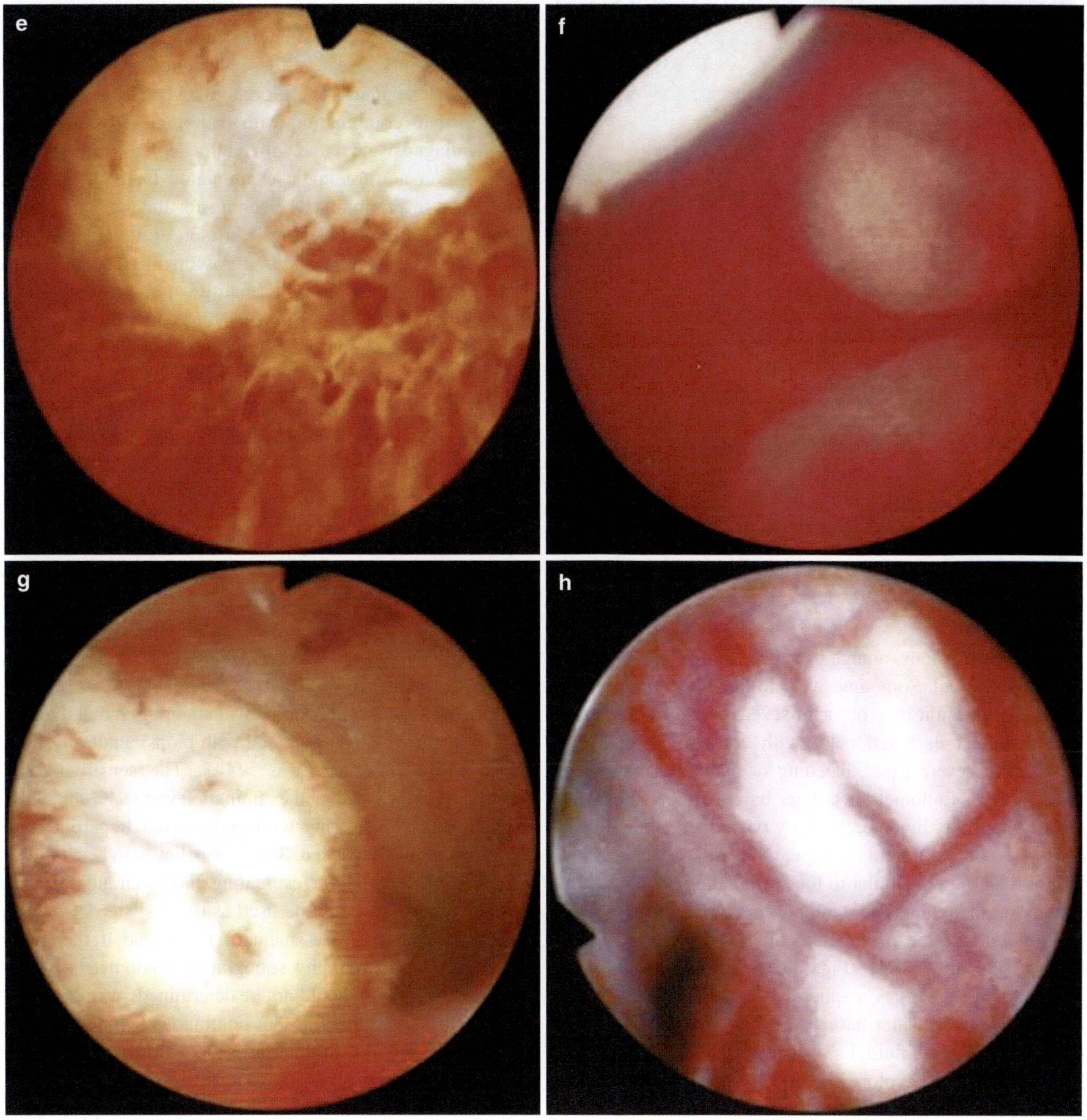

Fig. 8.61 (continued)

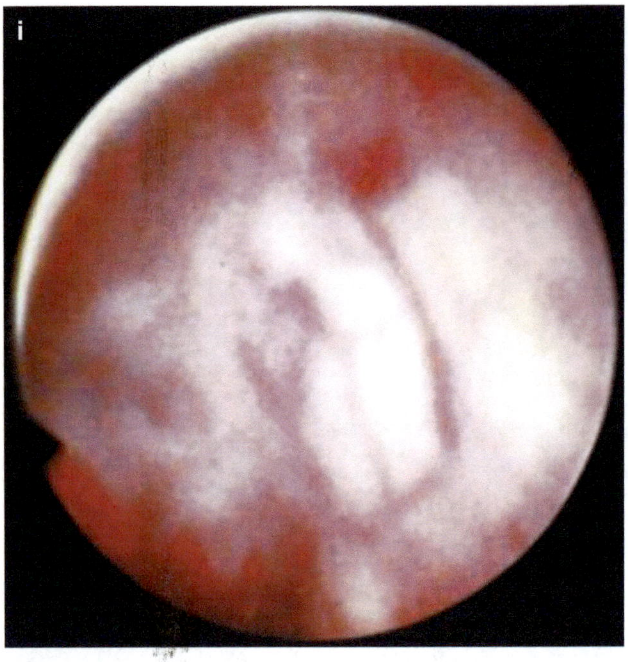

Fig. 8.61 (continued)

villi-like protrusions, orange or yellow, shiny, and relatively more transparent. Sometimes vesicle-like structures are visible, and adhesion may occur in severe cases. Endometritis may manifest dark red color with congestion spots and patches. In severe cases, bleeding or pyometra may occur (Fig. 8.61e). Endometrial polyps have soft pedicles with either fingerlike, ligulate, papillary or mulberry-like protrusions. They are different in shape, with smooth surfaces and bright red colored, similar to the surrounding endometrium, and is soft in texture. The small polyps can exhibit wave-like motion with uterine distention medium and sometimes slender vessels are visible (Fig. 8.61f). Uterine submucous myoma (Fig. 8.61g) is a spherical or hemispherical bulge with a relatively wider base or pedicle, and doesn't move with the distending fluid. Its surface appears to be light pink or pale, and purple colored if there is ulcer or hemorrhage, and sometimes thickened dendritic blood vessels are visible. A large myoma may cause the stenosis and deformation of the cavity, which forms a crescent fissure. The endometrium may appear to be obviously hyperplastic in patients with diagnosed or suspected endometrial carcinoma, which protrudes into the uterine cavity. Its surface is irregular and partly appears to be nodular or polypoid bulges. It is dull, greyish, and somewhat filthy. The endometrial tissues are fragile, whose borders are not clearly distinguished from the surrounding endometrium. The blood vessels become thickened and engorged, and run disorderly, sometimes accompanied by hemorrhage and necrosis (Fig. 8.61h, i). It should be pointed out that hysteroscopy is not omnipotent, and it may also miss the diagnosis of some lesions like atypical endometrial hyperplasia and endometrium influenced by hormones, possibly because they have not caused visually recognizable changes. Therefore, only when hysteroscopy is performed in combination with pathological examination, can the diagnosis be made with a high degree of accuracy.

TVS is a non-traumatic examination method, which is often used in preliminary screening for the causes of postmenopausal uterine bleeding. Karlsson et al. carried out a study on the use of TVS and hysteroscopy in 51 women with PMB. TVS revealed no abnormalities in 12 cases with an endometrial thickness ≤4 mm, among which hysteroscopy revealed small endometrial polyps in 1 case. TVS suggested endometrial abnormalities in 39 cases with an endometrial thickness >4 mm, while a confirmed diagnosis was made by hysteroscopy in 35 cases, and the rest four cases were false positive. There were nine cases with an endometrial thickness ≥8 mm, but hysteroscopy revealed endometrial polyps in eight cases and endometrial polyp or uterine submucous myoma in one case. The pathological findings are set as the final diagnosis. The sensitivity, specificity, positive predictive value, and negative predictive value of TVS were 100%, 75%, 90%, 100%, respectively, while the corresponding results of hysteroscopy were 97%, 88%, 94%, 93%, respectively. So it was believed that TVS screening may be done prior to hysteroscopy. O' Connell et al. reported that the concordance rate of TVS combined with biopsy under hysteroscope and the surgery was >90%. The sensitivity and specificity of the combined examination were 94% and 96%, respectively. No patients with endometrial hyperplasia or cancer were misdiagnosed. So it was believed to be a reliable examination method for evaluating PMB. Granberg et al. declared that TVS could be used as the first step of routine examination in the assessment of PMB, and if there was abnormal ultrasonography sonography (endometrial thickness >4 mm), or if it could not be determined, or if there was normal ultrasonic imaging but continuous symptom in the patient, hysteroscopy and hysteroscopic biopsy must be performed simultaneously in order to rule out or detect pathological conditions. Application of hysteroscopy in the diagnosis of the causes of PMB can be summarized as shown in Fig. 8.62.

Gumus et al. conducted a prospective study of the values in diagnosing the endometrial abnormalities with hysteroscopy or hysterosonography in asymptomatic postmenopausal women. Suspected diagnosis of endometrial lesions with TVS was achieved in 77 asymptomatic postmenopausal women. The most common diagnosed abnormalities were endometrial hyperplasia in TVS (62.33%), endometrial polyps in both hysterosonography (57.14%) and hysteroscopy (51.94%). The sensitivity and specificity were 59.7% and 35.5%, respectively, with TVS, 88.8% and 84.4% with sono-

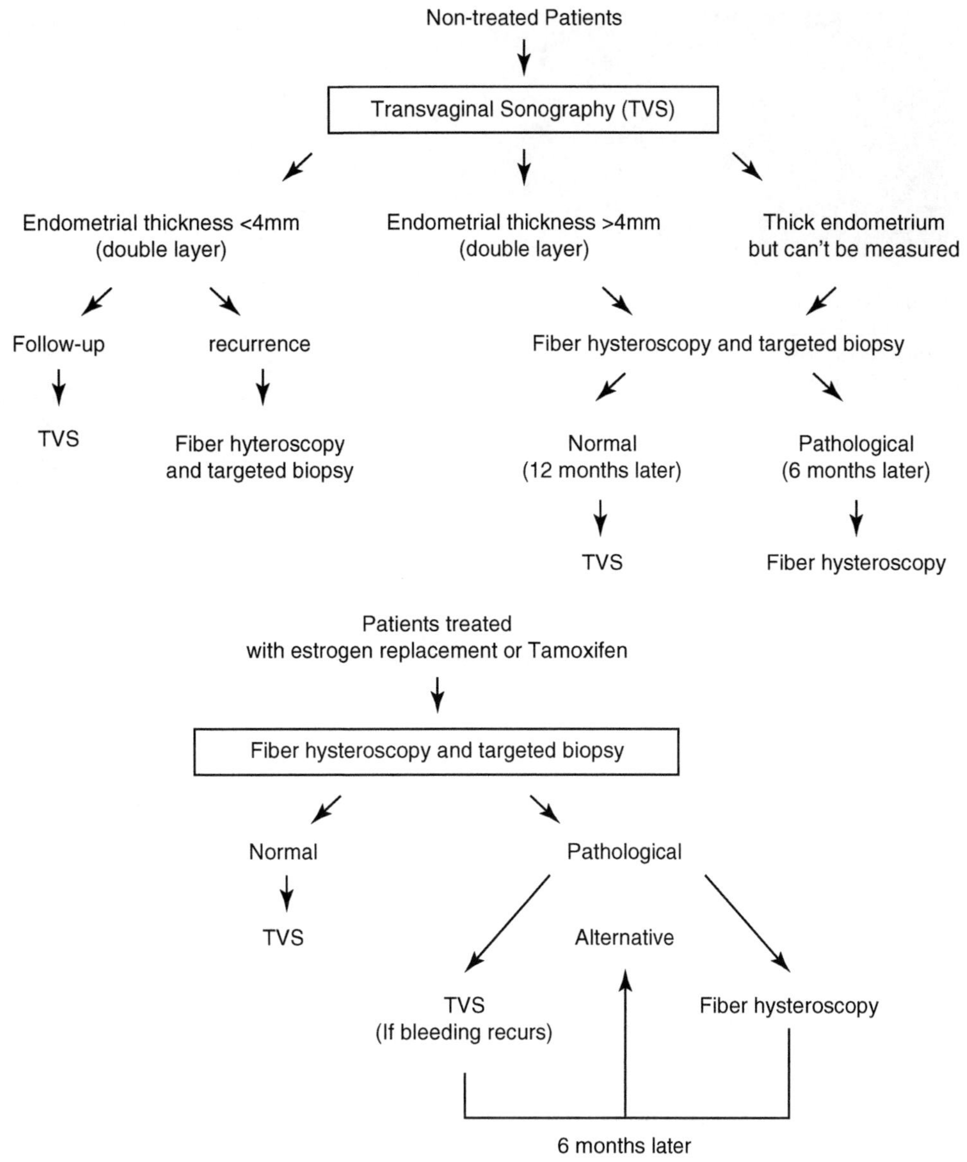

Fig. 8.62 Application of fiber hysteroscopy in etiological diagnosis of PMB

hysterography, and 91% and 82% with diagnostic hysteroscopy. It was suggested to be effective in diagnosis with hysterosonography and hysteroscopy. If the endometrium was suspected to be abnormal with TVS in asymptomatic postmenopausal women, hysterosonography and hysteroscopy should be considered.

8.2.1.6 Other Pathological Conditions Leading to AUB

Other pathological conditions leading to AUB include endometrial polyps, submucous myoma, endometrial hyperplasia, endometrial carcinoma, etc. When patients are of child-bearing age, the causes of bleeding are mainly related to pregnancy. Hysteroscopy can help to find other benign diseases related to the symptoms of AUB, such as endometrial atrophy, anovulatory menstruation, bleeding associated with contraception, and uterine adenomyosis, etc.

Endometrial Atrophy

The elderly women are often seen to have AUB caused by endometrial atrophy. Endometrial cancer should be ruled out in them, but the negative results obtained by both cytological and histopathological examinations are not enough to exclude this disorder. The diagnosis of atrophic endometrium in elderly women is not easy, by HSG or D&C, during which there is always hardly any endometrial tissue. However, simple hysteroscopy can avoid these shortfalls, which can be performed in the outpatient immediately with small diameter telescope under local anesthesia. Tinelli et al. carried out a prospective study of 752 postmenopausal

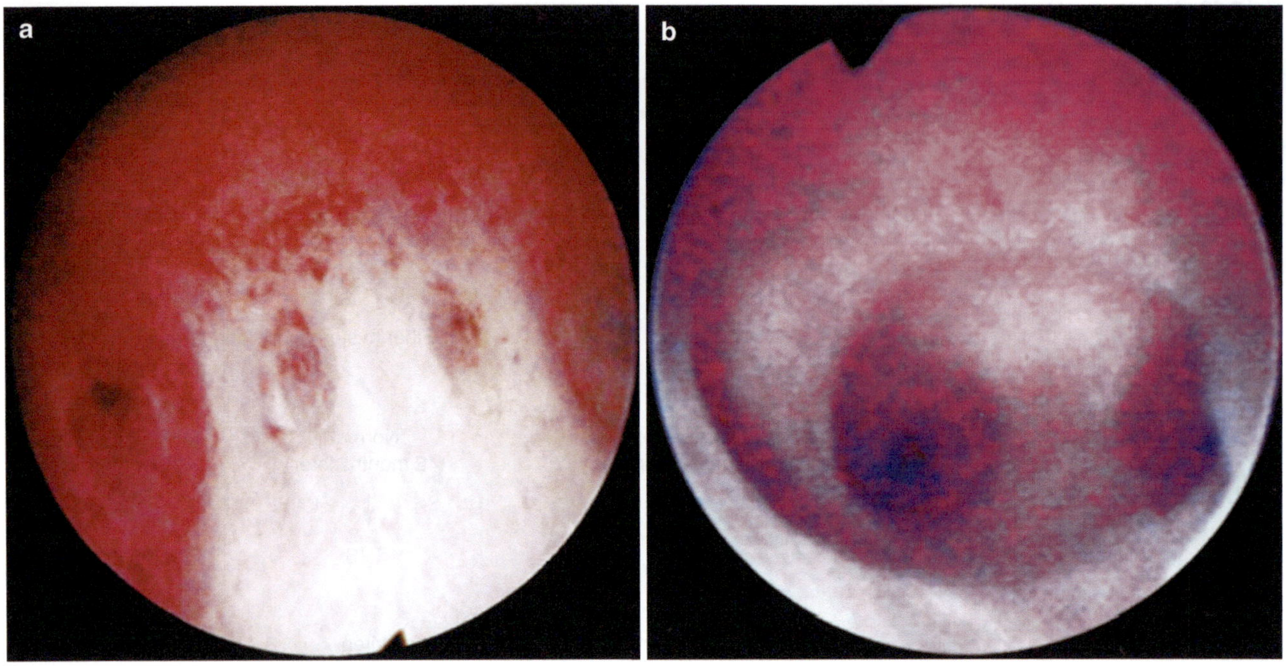

Fig. 8.63 Endometrial atrophy. (**a**) Intrauterine adhesions at the fundus are visible. (**b**) Diverticulum is visible

women with AUB and endometrial atrophy. Only three cases with misdiagnosis of atrophic endometrium under hysteroscopy were revealed to be endometrial carcinoma by histopathological examination. In cases of endometrium <4 mm in thickness, focal abnormalities often cannot be identified by TVS, but can be detected more accurately by hysteroscopy. Hysteroscopy may provide a definite diagnosis of endometrial atrophy, which is characterized by small uterine cavity, difficult uterine distention and possible intrauterine adhesions (Fig. 8.63a). The general manifestation is that there is a decrease in endometrium, which looks like a layer of transparent film, revealing the intertwined muscle bundle underneath, where may exist invagination, sometimes like a true diverticulum (Fig. 8.63b). The presence of ecchymosis indicates its bleeding tendency. The glands of the cystic atrophic endometrium are covered with a superficial atrophic epithelium, and some transparent blue-gray spheres may be detected under hysteroscope. There are no lesions needing biopsy in the uterine cavity, so drug therapy can be administered. The endometrial atrophy is rare in fertile women, which may be caused by hormone therapy and mostly secondary to the long-term use of progesterone or danazol.

Adenomyosis

Adenomyosis is also called internal endometriosis, which is usually accompanied by hypermenorrhea, but rarely with uterine bleeding, and other symptoms include pelvic congestion, dysmenorrhea and enlarged uterus. A pathological feature is the presence of ectopic endometrial island containing stroma and gland in the myometrium, which is surrounded by hyperplastic smooth muscle bundles. The disease was not uncommon in the findings on hysterectomy specimens (frequency 25% to 50%). Cullen pointed out that ectopic endometrium was often related with the endometrium which was on the surface of uterine cavity, and HSG or hysteroscopy was helpful in the diagnosis of adenomyosis. The direct sign in the diagnosis of adenomyosis by HSG is that there are branches outside the contour of the cavity connected to the diverticulum, which appears only when lesions communicate with endometrial cavity (Fig. 8.64a). Hysteroscopy can only reveal that the diverticular openings have an appearance of dark or blue concave of varying sizes. These openings are variable in number and changing in appearance, and large diverticulum and great numbers of small dots can be seen to be distributed on the endometrial surface (Fig. 8.64b). The glandular openings may be covered by thick or hyperplastic endometrium, so the optimal time for examination is just after menstruation. Hysteroscopy can also reveal the focus of adenomyosis which is not connected with the superficial endometrium and not too far from the cavity, being a transparent blue or brown area. Muscle fiber hyperplasia and fibrosis can also lead to the deformation of the uterine cavity, which can also be suspected to be adenomyosis (Fig. 8.64c). During the combined examination with hysteroscopy and ultrasonography, under the intrauterine pressure, the distending fluid and air enter the ectopic endometrial glands via the openings in the uterine cavity, and cloudy strong echo in the uterine wall is visible on ultrasonography, which is most obvious in the anterior wall and also is suggestive of adenomyosis. HSG

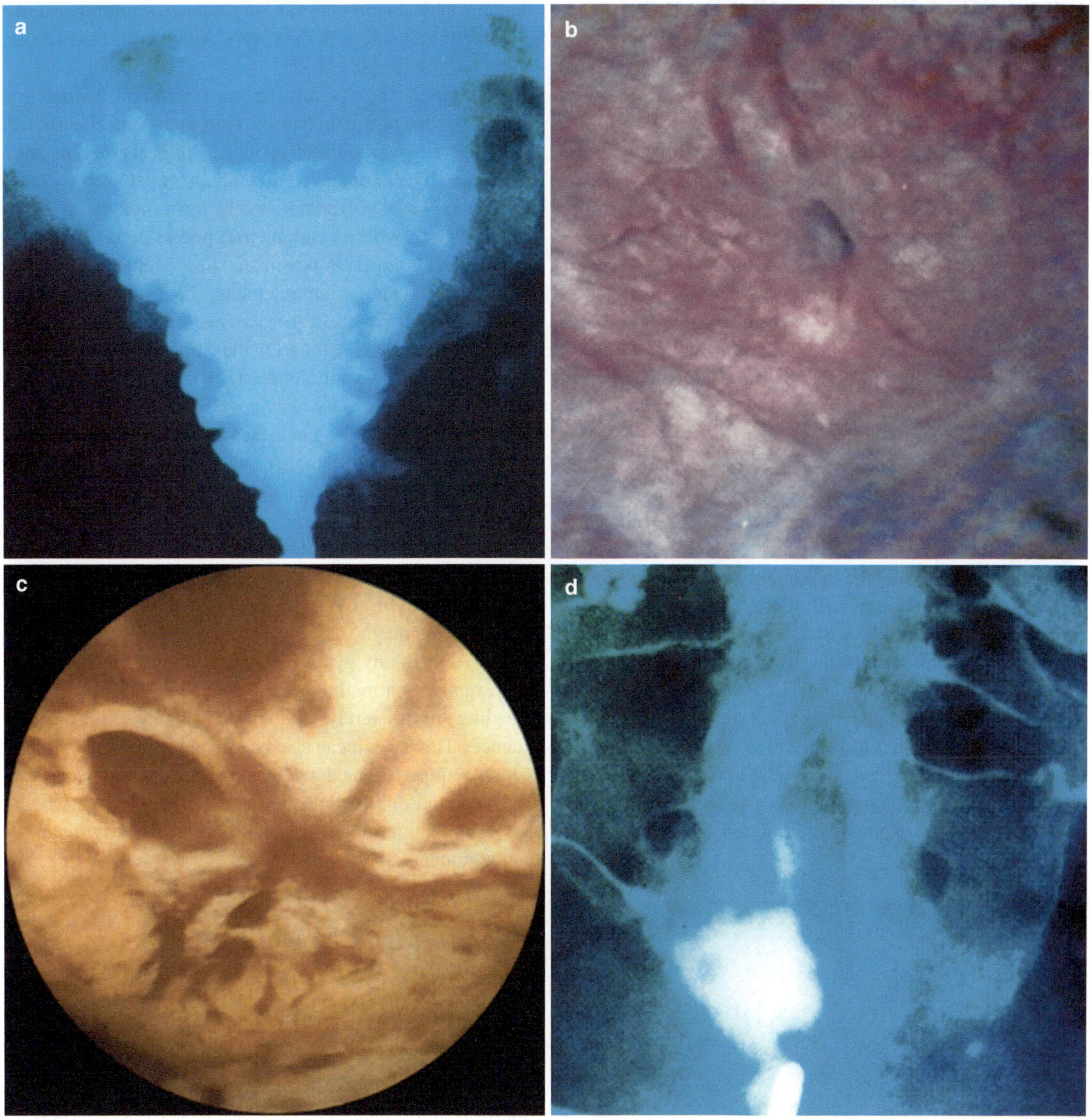

Fig. 8.64 (**a**) Adenomyosis diagnosed by HSG. Diverticulum outside the contour of the cavity can be seen. (**b**) Adenomyosis. The glandular openings are on the surface of endometrium, presenting as small pyriform diverticulum. (**c**) Adenomyosis. The endometrium has an appearance of false endometrium. (**d**) Adenomyosis which is shown as an image of "bullhead" by HSG

reveals that the contour of uterine cavity is stiff and forms angles, with the cornua expanded and the tubes vertical, which forms a "bullhead" image and is characterized as adenomyosis (Fig. 8.64d). Under hysteroscope, tubal ostia are crack-like and the fundus appears to have trabecular structure due to muscle fiber hyperplasia, which is also a sign of adenomyosis. The treatment with ovarian inhibitors of GnRH analogs or danazol may have effects of temporarily restraining its development. Hysteroscopic diagnosis is another alternative, which can only be applied in the cases when adenomyotic lesions are close to the surface of the endometrium. The visible diverticulum can be treated by electrocoagulation or laser vaporization, but a more radical method is to remove the whole endometrium, but lesions in the deep layer cannot be removed, so hysterectomy is still the only option for severe cases.

AUB Caused by Contraception or Hormone Therapy

Insertion of IUD often causes increased menstruation, and also leads to intermenstrual bleeding, excessive menstrual bleeding, and prolonged menstruation, and can induce complications as well (Fig. 8.65). AUB can be a forerunner of organic diseases, which alerts the patient to undergo intrauterine inspection. Prior to diagnostic hysteroscopy, IUD should be left in situ rather than be blindly removed, so that if no organic diseases are found by hysteroscopy, other reasons such as translocation or incarceration of the IUDs could be established. Such diagnosis would be missed if IUD is removed first. The removal of IUD under direct vision can avoid the shortcomings of blind removal including failure in its removal or fracture of the IUD, and even perforation of the uterus. In some cases, IUD is in good place and there are no intrauterine abnormalities.

Patients taking oral contraceptives may have breakthrough bleeding, if AUB still exists after regulation of the dosage, organic lesions should be excluded before other contraceptive measures are taken instead. Hysteroscopy is the most rapid and safe method to rule out any organic lesions.

18–40% of the patients with uterine hemorrhage caused by HRT have focal endometrial lesions. Long-term use of TMX after radical mastectomy may lead to asymptomatic endometrial changes, which increase the risk of endometrial hyperplasia and endometrial polyps, and there are also cases found with endometrial cancer. It was reported by Mourits et al. and Anteby et al. that, Tamoxifen could induce specific endometrial changes consisting of cystically dilated glands with periglandular stroma gathering and overlying epithelium atrophy (Fig. 8.66a). These changes occur either in the endometrium itself or in the polyps which protrude from the endometrium (Fig. 8.66b–f).

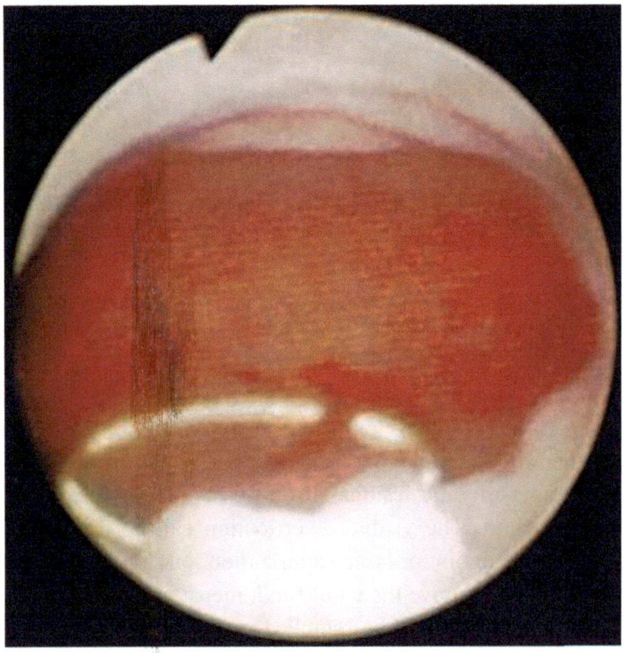

Fig. 8.65 Intrauterine device

Endometrial polyps are the most common endometrial pathology in postmenopausal women taking tamoxifen. Cohen et al. reported that up to 3% of these polyps were malignant. They conducted a comparison between 54 cases with endometrial polyps resected by hysteroscopy (Group I) and 210 cases with no endometrial polyps detected by hysteroscopy (Group II) in postmenopausal women with breast carcinoma and tamoxifen treatment. The results showed that compared with Group II, the patients' ages in group I were significantly older ($P = 0.0162$), the duration of having breast disease was significantly longer ($P = 0.0026$), and the body weight was significantly heavier ($P = 0.0364$). Therefore it was believed that these three factors and a thicker endometrium may contribute to higher risks of development of endometrial carcinoma in these patients.

Dysfunctional Uterine Bleeding (DUB)

DUB may be diagnosed if an IUD is not placed; no contraceptives taken; or no intrauterine lesions found. The confirmation of the diagnosis depends on the patients' age.

For AUB in any gynecological field, hysteroscopy is the key examination method. In a woman's life, abrupt uterine bleeding occurs rarely, and often with no serious consequences. However, it can also be a signal to a serious disease, which requires immediate diagnosis. Regrettably, lack of attention and only simple symptomatic medication without any examination may lose opportunities for early diagnosis and treatment.

8.2.2 Infertility

More than 100 years ago, when hysteroscopy was still at infancy stage, it was an important method to diagnose and treat some diseases causing infertility. The instruments in use include panoramic hysteroscope, contact hysteroscope, micro-hysteroscope, and flexible hysteroscope, each of which has its own advantages and disadvantages.

Hysteroscopic examination conducted in infertile women aims to assess whether anatomies of reproductive organs are normal or not and also to check the patency of fallopian tubes. Hucke et al. reported that different grades of intrauterine abnormalities were detected by hysteroscopy in 20% of infertile patients, with uterine malformations the most common disorder. Pansky et al. reported that intrauterine abnormalities were visible under hysteroscopy in 30% of 221 women who have either primary or secondary infertility, with no significant difference between groups of primary and secondary infertility. Thus diagnostic hysteroscopy should be done as a routine method.

In the diagnosis of infertility, hysteroscopy cannot be a substitute for HSG, and hysteroscopy and HSG are complementary rather than competitive to each other. Firstly, HSG is a relatively cheap method, which can provide important information about the cervical canal, cervical internal os, uterine cavity, and full length of the fallopian tubes. The conditions of fallopian tubes are very important to infertility. Secondly, HSG can outline the contours of the uterine cavity more clearly than hysteroscopy, and is also superior in the detection of adenomyosis. Finally, HSG can provide the information requiring to change the therapy. For example, if a hydrosalpinx is found by HSG to be too large for reconstruction operation, In Vitro Fertilization and Embryo Transfer (IVF/ET) should be considered instead. Moreover, bilateral tubal obstruction caused by pelvic tuberculosis can only be detected by traditional radiology.

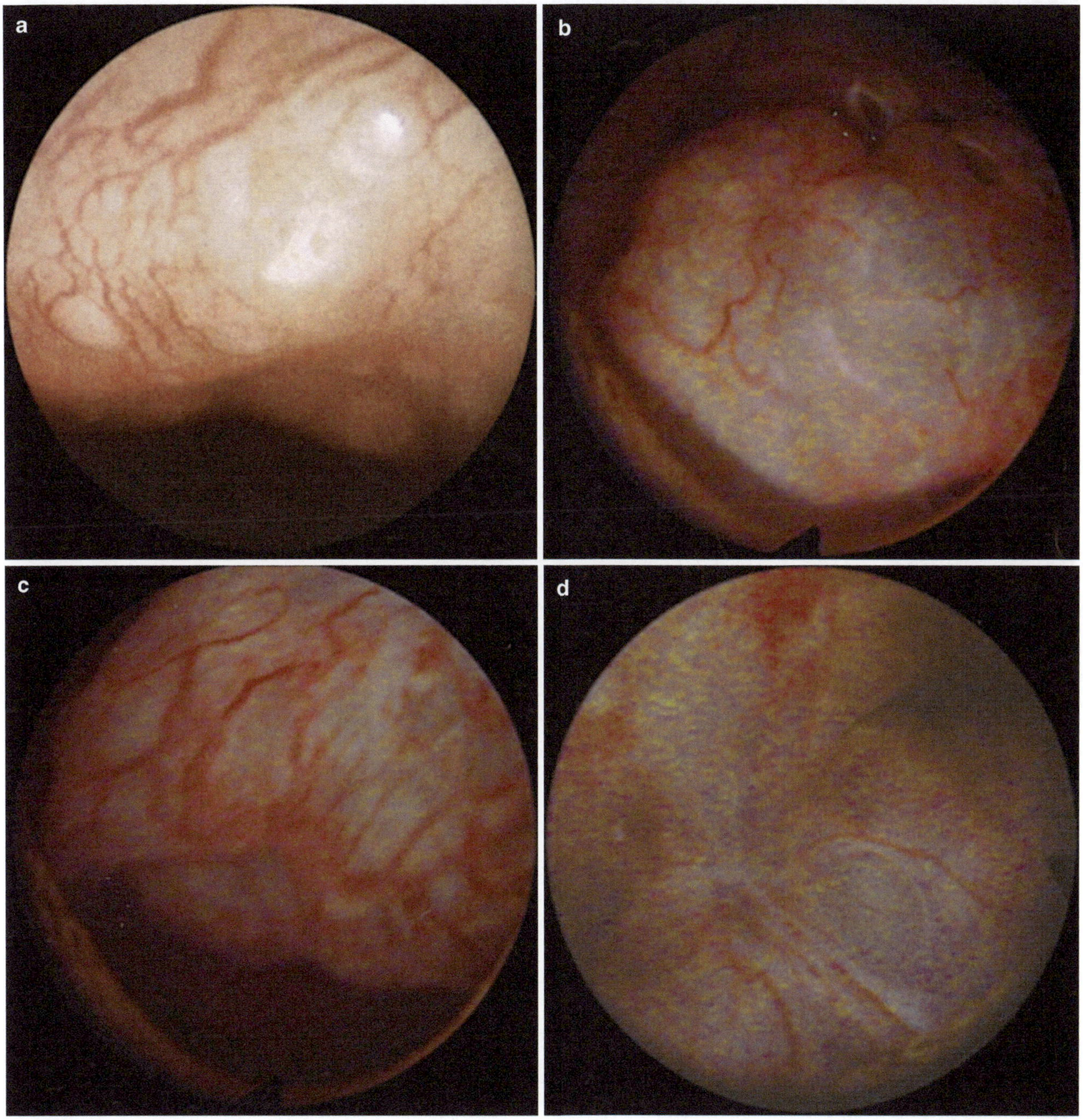

Fig. 8.66 (**a**) Cystic atrophy of the endometrium and hyperplasia in blood vessels are visible in a woman with bleeding after TMX treatment. An endometrial polyp in a woman who has had menopause for 24 years and taken TMX for 2 years after radical correction for right breast cancer. (**b**) An endometrial polyp is seen under hysteroscope. (**c**) The blood vessels on the surface of the polyp. (**d**) The endometrium. (**e**) Electroresection of the endometrium and polyp. (**f**) The resected polyp tissues

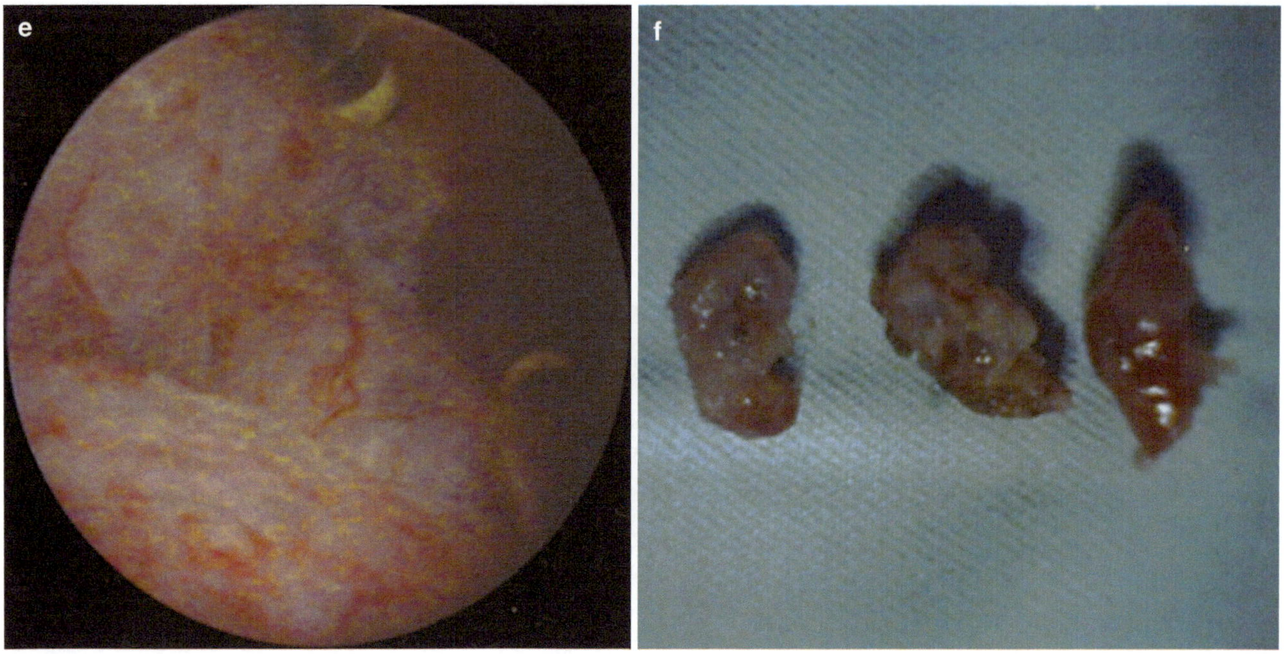

Fig. 8.66 (continued)

Table 8.5 Comparison between hysteroscopy and HSG

Hysteroscopy	HSG
Can directly inspect the uterine cavity	May outline of the uterine cavity with contrast medium
Can confirm the diagnosis of "tumors"	Can only make a provisional diagnosis
Can precisely locate the lesions	Cannot precisely locate the lesion
Can proceed to do the operative hysteroscopy	Unable to treat lesions
Can only examine the uterus	May examine the uterus and fallopian tube as well
Moderate cost	Low cost
No radiation	Small quantity of radiation

A comparison between HSG and hysteroscopy is made in Table 8.5, and it can be concluded from the table that hysteroscopy is significantly superior to HSG. However, as a screening method, HSG is low in cost and can provide some useful information, therefore it should not be given up.

Some authors have suggested that hysteroscopy can detect lesions in infertile patients even with normal HSG. If a recent HSG reveals a normal endometrial cavity (including that in the early filling stage with the uterine axis parallel to the film plane), hysteroscopy may not be needed. If HSG shows intrauterine filling defect, hysteroscopy needs to be done to determine the presence of the lesion and its nature.

Hysteroscopy is an important means in the diagnosis of causes of infertility. Meanwhile, it is also of important therapeutic value, very suitable for checking the cervical canal and uterine cavity so as to discover lesions interfering with embryo implantation and (or) development.

The majority of infertile women are nulliparous, and they have higher incidence of genital malformations and anxiety compared with the normal population, so they often cannot tolerate hysteroscopic operation. With the introduction of miniature hysteroscope or fiber hysteroscope in recent years, noninvasive insertion, fluid uterine distension and no requirement of anesthesia make it possible in an outpatient setting, leading to better compliance of the patients.

Common intrauterine lesions causing infertility are submucosal myoma, intrauterine adhesions, endometrial polyps, congenital uterine malformation, intrauterine foreign body, and obstructed fallopian tubal ostia, etc.

8.2.2.1 Indications of Hysteroscopy for Infertile Women

1. AUB.
2. History of complex surgeries of the uterus or the cavity.
3. Repeated pregnancy failures.
4. TVS reveals intrauterine abnormalities.
5. HSG reveals uterine abnormalities or filling defects.
6. Hysteroscopy has not been previously performed, but it can be done simultaneously with laparoscopy.
7. Unexplained Infertility.
8. Patients who has not previously had hysteroscopy and failed to conceive after IVF-ET.

8.2.2.2 Infertility Factors Revealed by Hysteroscopic Examination

Uterine Myoma

The impact of uterine myomas on infertility is still not very clear, but intrauterine myomas can lead to deformation of uterine cavity, and may interfere with fertility similar to a foreign bodies. Histological studies showed that intramural myomas and submucosal myomas can change the structure of the endometrium and myometrium, but subserosal myomas may not affect fertility, most of which do not have symptoms. Hysteroscopy plays important roles in determining the location of myomas (Fig. 8.67) and the necessity for surgery and choice of surgical modality. The influence of the location of the myomas and increased reactive vessels on infertility which is visible through hysteroscope remains to be studied.

Intrauterine Adhesion

Intrauterine adhesion is a common problem in most patients with secondary infertility. The reason for intrauterine adhesions is trauma and infection, which are more common after missed abortion, D&C, cesarean delivery or intrauterine operation. The patients with complete uterine occlusion may suffer from amenorrhea and secondary infertility. However, the mechanism of secondary infertility in patients with incomplete uterine occlusion is still not clear, and may be caused by decreased area of functional endometrium in uterine cavity or increased functional disorder of endometrial vasculature.

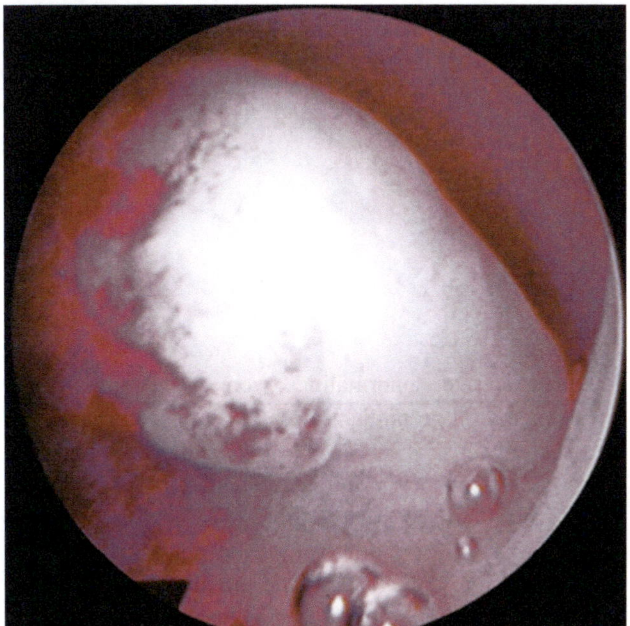

Fig. 8.67 Submucosal myoma in the right uterine cornu

Hysteroscopy is superior in revealing intrauterine adhesions to any other method used in the past but it can only display the uterine cavity below the adhesive level. However, when the joint examination of hysteroscopy and ultrasonography is performed, ultrasonography can also show the conditions of uterine cavity above the adhesive level. Under the guidance of ultrasonography, it is easier for the hysteroscope to go through the narrow adhesive sites so that the inspection of the cavity above the adhesion level can be continued.

Endometrial Polyps

Endometrial polyps may or may not cause infertility or recurrent pregnancy loss, but its exact cause is unknown. Cytogenetics may play an important role. Polyps may induce bleeding during, before and after the menstrual period, but the majority of them are asymptomatic, so it often cannot be diagnosed by HSG (Table 8.6). In addition, a small polyp may not be detected by ultrasonography scanning but hysteroscopy can recognize it clearly, determine its nature, decide on its therapy or remove it at the same time (Fig. 8.68a–c). Compared with curettage, the polyp tissues removed by hysteroscopy is relatively more complete and there is also no trauma to the endometrium.

Congenital Uterine Malformations

The incidence of congenital uterine malformations is difficult to determine, because not all malformations have symptoms or cause infertility. The reported incidence varies substantially, from 0.2% to 10%, the possible reason may be the difference in the subjects studied or the explanations for different lesions given by scholars.

The uterine septum plays an important role in infertility, including complete and incomplete uterine septum. For incomplete septum under hysteroscope, it can be seen that bilateral uterine cornua are completely separated (Fig. 8.69), on top of which the tubal ostia are visible. The septum of a complete septate uterus begins from the fundus, extends directly to the internal os or lower, and divides the uterus into two cavities, but sometimes the septum has an fissure in the cervical canal or the internal os so that both sides of the uterine cavity can communicate. Combined hysteroscopy and laparoscopy can exclude the bicornuate uterus, didelphic

Table 8.6 Detection rate of endometrial polyps with D & C

Research	No. of cases	Diagnosis (%)	Missed diagnosis (%)
Bibbo et al.(1982) (D&C/ hysterectomy)	840	83	17
Burnett (1964) (D&C/ hysterectomy)	1298 (121, 9.3%with polyps)	53	47
Valle (1981) (hysteroscopy /D&C)	553 (179 with polyps)	100/10	0/90

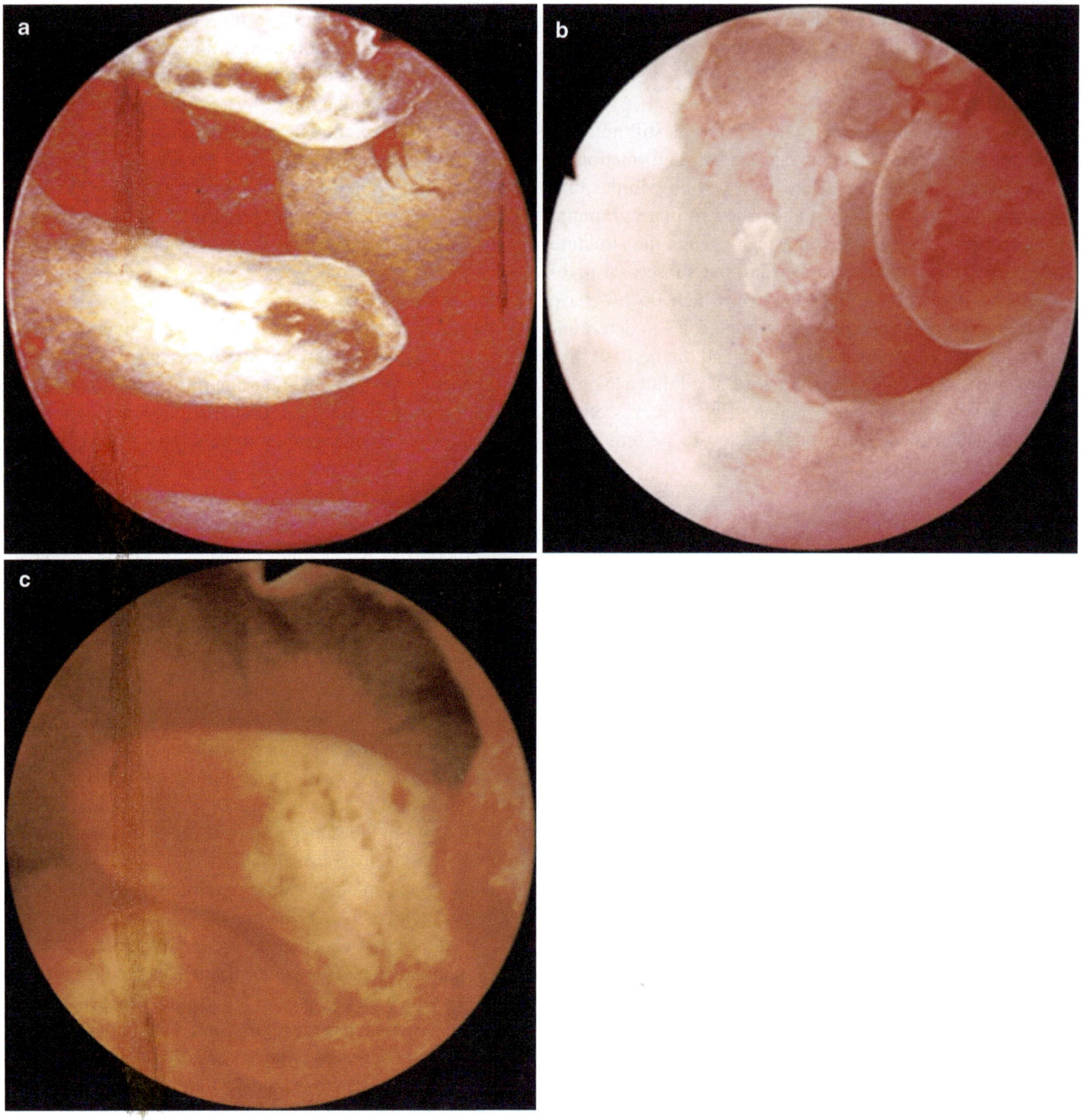

Fig. 8.68 (**a**–**c**) Endometrial polyps

uterus, and unicornuate uterus through laparoscopy. Uterine septum may induce repeated miscarriage more than infertility. Valli et al. analyzed the prevalence of different anatomic abnormalities in women with recurrent pregnancy loss. This study included 344 patients with recurrent pregnancy loss, and 922 women with AUB as control group. In study group, uterine mullerian abnormalities were found significantly more than those in control group (32% and 6%, respectively). Acquired uterine abnormalities were found significantly higher in control group than those in study group (32% and 9%, respectively). There were no significant differences observed in frequency of intrauterine adhesions between the study group and the control group (4% and 2%). It was believed that major mullerian uterine abnormalities were related to recurrent pregnancy loss, and minor uterine abnormalities might increase the risk of recurrent miscarriage.

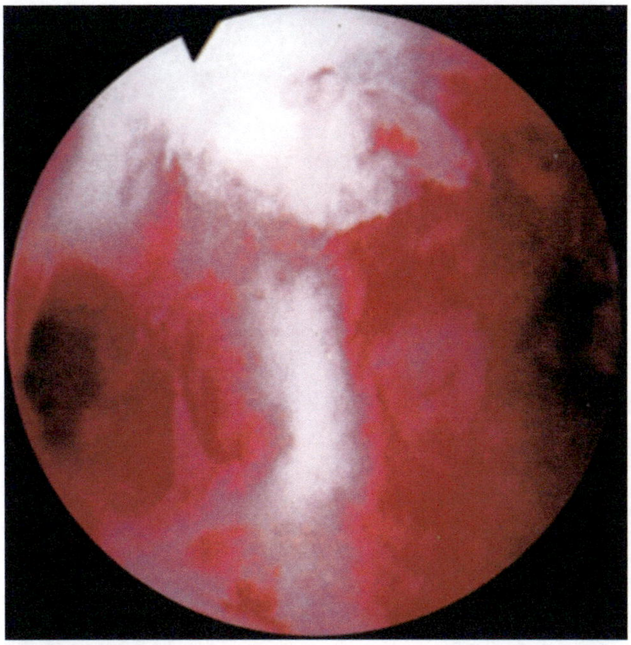

Fig. 8.69 Incomplete uterine septum

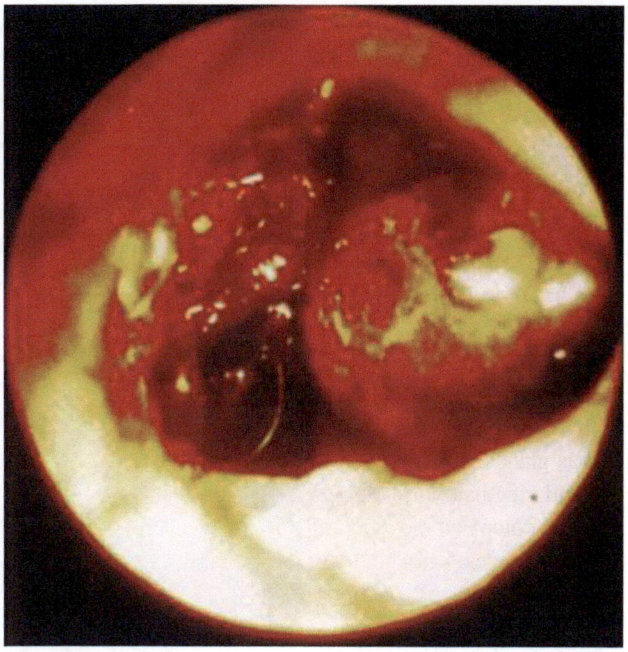

Fig. 8.70 Placental remnants under hysteroscope

Infantile uterus has a normal uterine cavity with a ratio of 1:3 between the uterine body and cervix, which stays in the status of a young girl. Its causes of infertility are the simultaneous presence of functional insufficiency of ovaries instead of uterine anomalies. T-shaped uterus is rare, and it is an offspring deformity induced by diethylstilbestrol which is taken by pregnant women. There were two million to three million pregnant women who took diethylstilbestrol from 1941 to 1971, so it would continue to occur after 2000.

Intrauterine Foreign Bodies

Occasionally, during hysteroscopic examination of the uterine cavity, some intrauterine foreign bodies can be found, and can be removed at the same time. Among these foreign bodies, IUD fragments are the most common, fetal bones and placental remnants are only occasionally seen (Fig. 8.70). Under the guidance and intervention of ultrasonography, it is relatively safe to take them out, and also there are more chances of a complete removal.

Chronic Endometritis

Chronic endometritis has been related to infertility and recurrent pregnancy loss. It is usually asymptomatic, and the diagnosis is rarely clinically suspected. Polisseni et al. performed a prospective study to evaluate the role of diagnostic hysteroscopy for this disease, with sensitivity 16.7%, specificity 93.2%, positive predictive value 25%, and negative predictive value 89.1%.

8.2.2.3 Hysteroscopic Tubal Catheterization and Hydrotubation

Salazar et al. reported that one out of five couples had a transitory problem of infertility at the childbearing age. The most frequent cause is the tubo-ovarian pathological changes, in which proximal obstruction takes up 25–30%. Unfortunately, the conventional method in the examination of tubal patency, such as HSG, often cannot differentiate between an insufficient filling of the tubes, fallopian tubal spasm and tubal obstruction. Catheterization under hysteroscopic guidance (Figs. 8.71a–d and 8.72a–d) and direct observation of dye tubal patency by laparoscopy are extremely useful in the diagnosis of tubal patency or in the determination of partial or total proximal tubal disease, and differentiation can also be made at the same time.

Hysteroscopic tubal catheterization for proximal tubal occlusion is not only diagnostic but also therapeutic, and superior to HSG. Generally, a #3Fr rigid hollow plastic catheter is used and its tip is inserted via the operational channel of hysteroscope into the fallopian tubal ostia and then pushed in so that interstitial regional obstruction may be eliminated. The catheter may be inserted 1–1.5 cm, and then the diluted methylene blue (MB) liquid is injected to the lumen. The degree of tubal patency may be judged according to the pressure and speed of water injection, whether there is liquid overflow, and whether there is return flow after suspension of water injection. In combi-

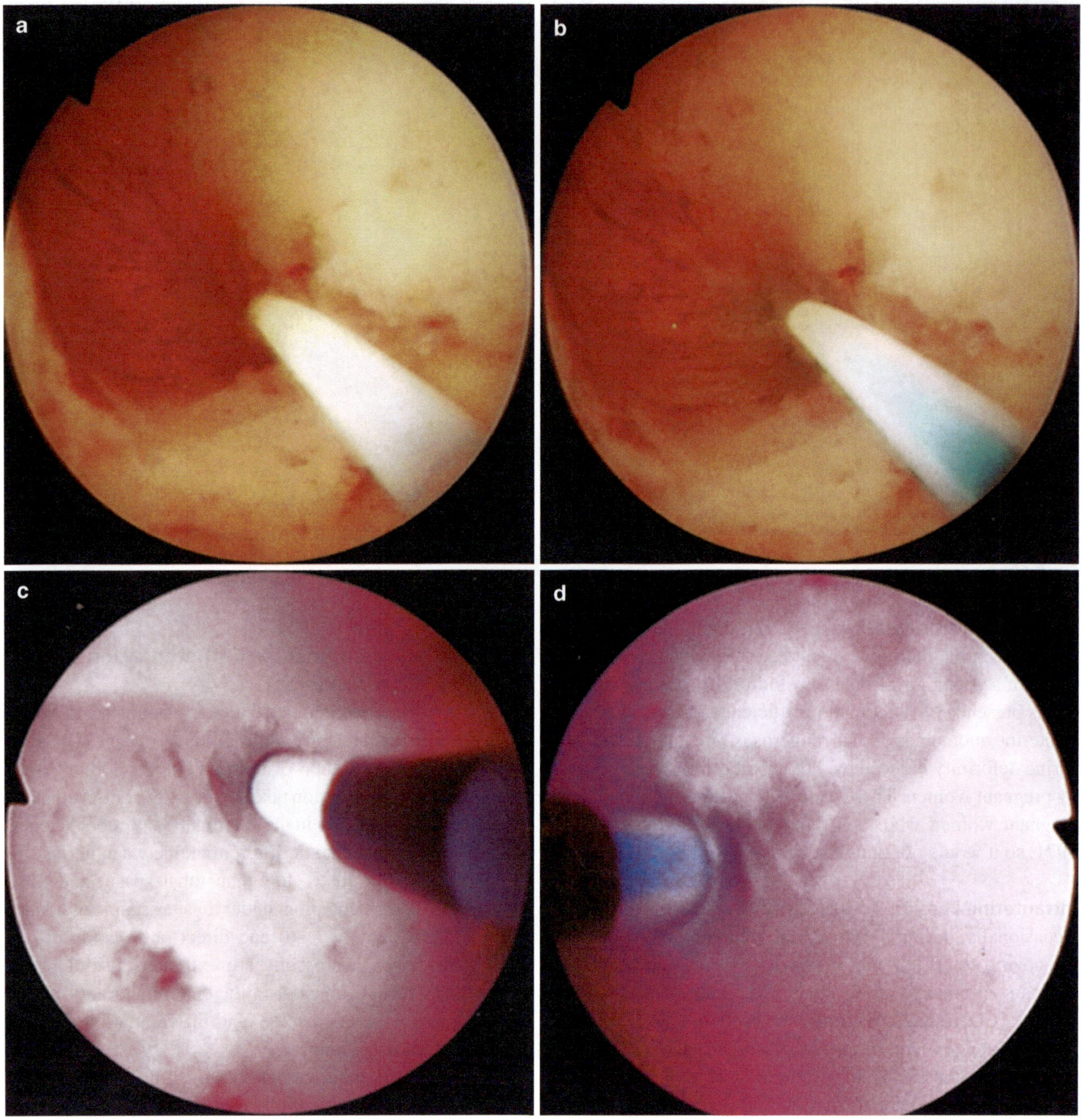

Fig. 8.71 Hysteroscopic tubal catheterization. (**a**) Before the hydrotubation. (**b**) During the hydrotubation. (**c**) Before the hydrotubation. (**d**) During the hydrotubation

nation with laparoscopy, it can be judged according to the flow rate of methylene blue through the tubal fimbria (Fig. 8.73a, b). When the distal end of fallopian tube is being reopened, the stainless steel wire should be placed inside the catheter under laparoscopic monitoring. Kerin's technique is to dilate with balloon after the tubal patency is achieved with guide wire. As the technique of hysteroscopic catheterization for patency is very successful, the transplantation of gametes and embryos under the guidance of hysteroscopy has also been well developed.

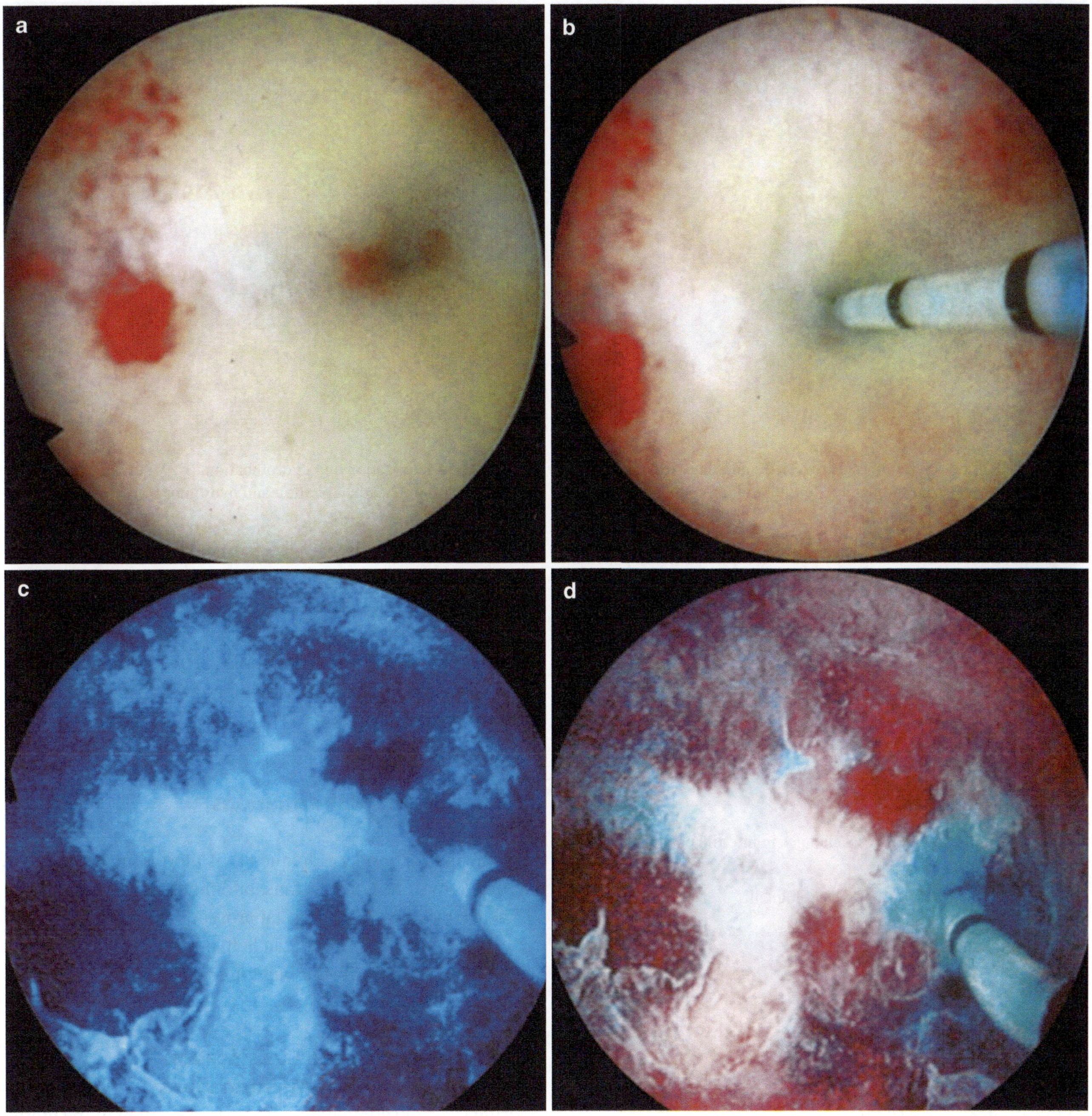

Fig. 8.72 (**a**) Left tubal ostium under hysteroscope. (**b**) Hysteroscopic catheterization under direct vision. (**c**) Instillation of methylene blue liquid. The blue-stained image indicates the tubal impatency. (**d**) Image after being irrigated with distending fluid

8.2.2.4 Endometrial Changes in Patients with Infertility

The endometrial changes in patients with infertility reported by Leuven institute are seen in Table 8.7. Except that hysteroscopy can be performed in the diagnosis of the above obvious major lesions, the miniature hysteroscopy can also often detect some tiny endometrial lesions (Table 8.8), such as moderate and significant endometrial swelling, which may indicate hormonal imbalance.

Vascular structural anomaly is another lesion that can only be seen by hysteroscope, which plays an important role in reproduction. Increased endometrial blood vessels are common in endometritis, submucous myoma, and uterine intramural myomas, but it may exist alone as well. The definition of increased endometrial blood vessels is an obvious increase in the amount of blood vessels at its proliferative phase or that the endometrium grows red, on which the white glandular openings are set, forming a typical strawberry

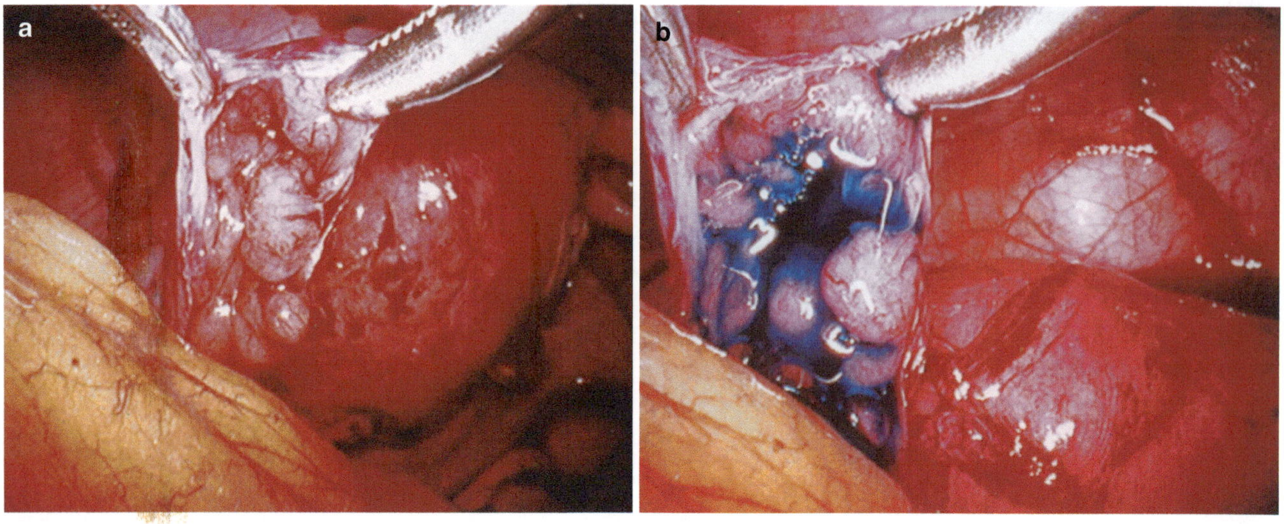

Fig. 8.73 (**a**) Left tubal fimbria is revealed under laparoscope before hysteroscopic catheterization and hydrotubation. (**b**) Methylene blue liquid can be seen flowing out through the left tubal fimbria under laparoscope during hysteroscopic catheterization and hydrotubation

Table 8.7 Endometrial changes by hysteroscopy in infertile patients

Item	No. of gynecological patients (%)	No. of infertile patients (%)
Total cases	4204	530
Abnormal	1189 (28.3)	151 (28.5)
Congenial	70 (1.7)	70 (13.2)
Acquired	455 (10.8)	21 (4.0)
Minimal endometrial lesions	664 (15.8)	60 (11.3)

Table 8.8 Minimal endometrial changes in infertile patients by miniature hysteroscopy

Item	No. of gynecological patients (%)	No. of infertile patients (%)
Minimal endometrial lesions	441 (66.5)	32 (53.3)
Endometrial adhesions	70 (10.5)	14 (23.3)
Increased blood vessels	52 (7.8)	9 (15)
Necrosis	28 (4.2)	4 (6.7)
Diffused polypoid changes	60 (9)	1 (1.7)
Others	13 (2)	0 (0)

image. There is hardly any diagnostic value in either microbiological or histological examinations for such patients. Miniature hysteroscopy plays a key role in evaluating the effects of different treatment modalities in order to maintain a normal intrauterine environment. Hysteroscopy is accurate and effective in the diagnosis of intrauterine lesions in patients with infertility, and can be used as a means of first line screening test for infertile patients. Hysteroscopy has an important practical value for IVF. Herrera found that 38% of cases with failed IVF were found to have intrauterine lesions by hysteroscopy. Feghali et al. conducted a retrospective analysis of the findings of a diagnostic hysteroscopy prior to in vitro fertilization. Intrauterine abnormalities were observed in 45% of hysteroscopies. Hysteroscopy prior to IVF should be performed as a regular investigation that could improve the pregnancy rate.

8.2.3 Uterine Malformations

The means for modern diagnosis of uterine malformations include hysteroscopy, transabdominal ultrasonography, TVS, SHSG, CT, MRI, and laparoscopy, etc. These simple, safe, and effective methods can help physicians to have a better understanding of the anatomical features of uterine malformations.

8.2.3.1 Formation and Classification of the Uterine Malformations

During the embryonic phase, if the development of the uterus is disturbed by some internal or external factors, which leads to the hypoplasia or fuse barriers of Mullerian ducts, various types of congenital uterine malformation would result.

Nowadays, clinically and commonly used classification of congenital uterine malformation is the classification published by American Fertility Society (AFS) in 1988, which included aplasia or dysplasia of Mullerian ducts, unicornuate uterus, uterus duplex, bicornuate uterus, septate uterus, arcuate uterus, T-shaped uterus, etc. (Table 8.9). Recently, European Society of Human Reproduction and Embryology (ESHRE)and European Society for Gynaecological Endoscopy (ESGE)jointly published a new classification of female genital malformations, which was mainly based on

Table 8.9 AFS classification of Mullerian duct anomalies

Class I	Uterine agenesis/ uterine hypoplasia	a. Vaginal b. Cervical c. Fundal d. Tubal e. Combined
Class II	Unicornuate uterus	a. Communicating rudimentary horn b. Non-communicating rudimentary horn c. Rudimentary horn without endometrial cavity d. no horn
Class III	Uterus didelphys	
Class IV	Bicornuate uterus	a. Complete division b. Partial division
Class V	Septate uterus	a. Complete division b. Partial division
Class VI	Arcuate uterus	
Class VII	In utero diethylstilbestrol (DES) exposure (T-shaped uterus)_	

Table 8.10 Scheme for ESHRE/ESGE classification of female genital tract anomalies. Uterus

		Cervix	vagina
U0 normal uterus		C0 normal cervix	V0 normal vagina
U1 dysmorphic Uterus	a. T-shaped b. Infantilis c. Others	C1 septate cervix	V1 longitudinal non-obstructing vaginal septum
U2 septate uterus	a. Partial b. Complete	C2 double cervix	V2 longitudinal obstructing vaginal septum
U3 bicorporeal Uterus	a. Partial b. Complete c. Bicorporeal septate	C3 unilateral Cervical aplasia	V3 transverse vaginal septum and/or imperforate hymen
U4 hemi-uterus	a. With rudimentary cavity (comminicating or not horn) b,. Without rudimentary cavity (horn without cavity/no horn)	C4 cervical aplasia	V4 vaginal aplasia
U5 aplastic	a. With rudimentary cavity (bi- or unilateral horn) b. Without rudimentary cavity (bi- or unilateral uterine aplasia)		
U6 unclassified malformations			

the anatomic characteristics, classified the uterine, cervical, and vaginal anomalies independently and then made a comprehensive evaluation (Table 8.10).

Congenital Uterine Anomalies

U0: normal uterus. For a normal uterus, the interostial line between both tubal orifice is either straight or curved, and the internal indentation at the midline of the fundus is less than 50% of the thickness of the uterine wall.

U1: Dysmorphic Uterus. For a dysmorphic uterus, the uterine outline is normal but the shape of the cavity is abnormal. In addition, septate uterus is not included in this class. Generally the uterus is smaller than a normal uterus, and is further divided into three sub-categories.

U1a: T-shaped uterus. The main characteristic is a narrow cavity with bilateral walls thickening. The ratio of the corpus to the cervix is 2:1.

U1b: infantile uterus. The main characteristic is a narrow cavity without the thickening of bilateral walls. The ratio of the corpus to the cervix is 1:2.

U1c: other dysmorphic uterus. It includes all minor deformities of the uterine cavity with an inner indentation at the midline of the fundus less than 50% of the thickness of the uterine wall.

U2: Septate Uterus. It is caused by failure in absorption of midline septum with normal development and fusion of bilateral Mullerian ducts. The definition of a septate is a normal outline of the uterus with an inner indentation at the midline of the fundus more than 50% of the thickness of the uterine wall. It is subdivided into two categories.

U2a: partial septate uterus. The main characteristic is that the septum extends from the fundus to the cavity which ends above the internal os and divides the uterine cavity partly.

U2b: complete septate uterus. The main characteristic is that the septum extends from the fundus to the internal os and divides the uterine cavity totally. These patients may have or have not cervical and/or vaginal deformities.

U3: bicorporeal uterus. It is caused by fusion defects of bilateral Mullerian ducts and characterized by abnormal fundal outline. The external fundal indentation exceeds 50% of the thickness of the uterine wall, which separate both cornua apart. The inner fundus at the midline protrudes to the cavity and separates the cavity, which is similar to septate uterus. It is further divided into three sub-categories.

U3a: partial bicorporeal uterus. Its characteristic is that the external fundal indentation partly divides the uterus above the internal os.

U3b: complete bicorporeal uterus. Its characteristic is that the external fundal indentation completely divides the uterus up to the level of the cervix.

U3c: bicorporeal septate uterus. It is caused by an absorption defect being combined with a septum fusion defect. The thickness of the fundus at the midline is more than 150% of that of the uterine walls. In these patients, the septum component could be resected by hysteroscopy.

U4: Hemi-uterus. It is caused by normal development of unilateral uterus, and absence or incomplete formation of contralateral uterus. It includes all unilateral formed uterus which fully develops a functional cavity, with the contralateral uterus dysplasia or absent. Hemi-uterus is further divided into two sub-categories.

U4a: hemi-uterus with a rudimentary cavity. Its characteristic is that a rudimentary horn with partial functional cavity lies contralaterally, which does or does not communicate the hemi-uterus. The functional endometrium in contralateral cavity has some clinical values because it can result in hematocele or ectopic pregnancy, which are indications of laparoscopic resection.

U4b: hemi-uterus without a rudimentary cavity. Its characteristic is that the contralateral uterus is absent or a solid horn without any cavity.

U5: Aplastic uterus. It includes all uteri with development defects, and its characteristic is absent of the formation of bilateral or unilateral uterus; in some cases, both or unilateral rudimentary uterine cavity could be found; sometimes a solid uterus remnant without any cavity could be seen. Patients with aplastic uterus can also have co-existent defects such as vaginal aplasia (Mayer-Rokitansky-Küster-Hauser syndrome, MRKH syndrome). Aplastic uterus is subdivided into two categories.

U5a: aplastic uterus with rudimentary cavity. Its characteristic is bilateral or unilateral functional horn.

U5b: aplastic uterus without rudimentary cavity. Its characteristic is uterine remnants or full aplasia.

U6: unclassified uterus. It includes all uteri which could not be allocated to one of above groups, and are caused by formation, fusion or absorption defects occurring during normal embryological development, such as rare uterine malformations, mini anomalies or co-existing deformations.

Co-existent Congenital Cervical Anomalies

C0: normal cervix. It includes all normal developed cervices.

C1: septate cervix. It includes the cervices with septa absorption defects and manifests as a cervical septum in a normal round cervix.

C2: double cervix. It includes the cervices with fusion defects and manifests as two round cervices, which could be fully separated or partially fused. It is classified as U3b/C2 when a double cervix co-exists with a complete bicorporeal uterus.

C3: unilateral cervical aplasia. It includes the cervices with unilateral development and manifests as only unilateral cervical development with the contralateral part aplasia or absent.

C4: complete cervical aplasia. It includes all cases with absolute absence or severe defects of cervical tissues.

Co-existent Congenital Vaginal Anomalies

V0: normal vagina. It includes all normal developed vaginas.

V1: longitudinal non-obstructing vaginal septum.

V2: longitudinal obstructing vaginal septum.

V3: transverse vaginal septum and/or imperforate hymen.

V4: vaginal aplasia. It includes all cases with complete or partial vaginal aplasia.

8.2.3.2 Clinical Manifestations of Uterine Malformation

A patient with congenital absence of uterus or primordial uterus will not have menstruations and has no probability of conception during her whole life. A patient who has aplastic uterus and functional endometrium may have oligomenorrhea, and periodic abdominal pain or hematocele if the outlet for discharging the menstrual blood is obstructed. In patients who have uterine malformations including hemi-uterus, double uterus, bicorporeal uterus and septate uterus, some complications could happen, such as miscarriage and premature delivery, oligomenorrhea and infertility, midtrimester loss, abnormal fetal position, fetal abnormality, premature rupture of fetal membrane, uterine inertia, postpartum hemorrhage, retained placenta, uterine rupture, etc. Patients with uterine malformations may have other co-existing organ aplasia, such as malformation of the urinary system.

8.2.3.3 Diagnosis of Uterine Malformation

Uterine malformation can be presumptively diagnosed via routine gynecological examination, TVS, 3-D ultrasonography, HSG and hystcroscopy, etc. The confirmation of the diagnosis can be achieved by joint investigation of hysteroscopy and laparoscopy in indecisive cases.

1. Routine gynecological examination: It can reveal vaginal septum, double cervix, and uterine malformations with obvious changes in shapes such as double uterus, bicorporeal uterus, and rudimentary uterus.
2. Gynecological ultrasonography: With transabdominal or transvaginal ultrasonography, and 3-D ultrasonography, both the sizes and the outlines of the uterus, and both the

echo and the shapes of the endometrium can be observed, which could achieve a high accuracy for diagnosing uterine malformations. B-mode ultrasonography can deduce the contour of the uterus and the shape of the cavity through transverse and longitudinal scanning, and measure each dimension of the uterus, which is a commonly used investigation for diagnosing the uterine malformations. 3-D ultrasonography can get a three-dimensional image of the uterus, and directly visualize the outline of the uterus, the thickness of the uterine wall and the shape of the cavity, accurately measure the thickness of the fundal wall, the depth of the external indentation of the fundus, and the angles between bilateral endometrium, which have a very high sensitivity and accuracy for diagnosing uterine malformations (Fig. 8.74).

3. HSG: HSG can reveal the location, shape, and size of both the cavity and the tubes. The image of a normal cavity is an inverted triangle. It might be a double uterus or complete septate uterus if HSG reveals two cavities; and might be a unicornuate uterus if it reveals a unilateral long and narrow cavity; and might be a T-shaped uterus if it reveals a "T" shape cavity.
4. Magnetic resonance imaging (MRI): MRI can reveal the shapes of the uterus and the cavity, distinguish different types of uterine malformations, make definite diagnosis and has a high resolution. Furthermore, it can evaluate whether a malformation of urinary system co-exists, which has a high accuracy.
5. Laparoscopic examination: Laparoscopy can identify the shape of the uterine serosa, especially the fundus, and accurately determine the types of the uterine malformation when combined with hysteroscopy (Fig. 8.75a–d).

8.2.3.4 Role of Hysteroscopy in Diagnosis of Uterine Malformation

The hysteroscope can be inserted directly into the cervical canal and the cavity to observe the anatomic changes of the cervix and the cavity, so that it can help to determine the types of uterine malformations. The main observations of hysteroscopy are:

1. The characteristic of the fundus. It can observe the degree of indentation of the fundus to the cavity, and makes measurement under hysteroscope. Taking the connection line between bilateral tubal orifice as the base line, the indentation of the fundus can be measured which can help to diagnose the type of uterine malformation. Generally, it should be a saddle form uterus if the length is less than 1.5 cm, and should be a septate uterus if it is more than 1.5 cm.
2. Intrauterine septum. It should observe the length and the width of the septum, the location of the septum and its ends, the symmetry of bilateral cavities, and measure the length of the septum; identify whether there is a septum in cervical canal, and whether there is communication between two cavities. In complete septate uterus, a communicating of two cavities can always be found above the internal os where the septum is thin. During hysteroscopy, when looking forward, it is like partial septum, but when looking backward, cervical septum can be detected.
3. The shape of the uterus. In septate, bicornuate, unicornuate and Robert uterus, bilateral or unilateral cavity is long and narrow, with the tubal orifice seen at its top. In a T-shaped uterus, the cavity is "T" shaped, with its upper

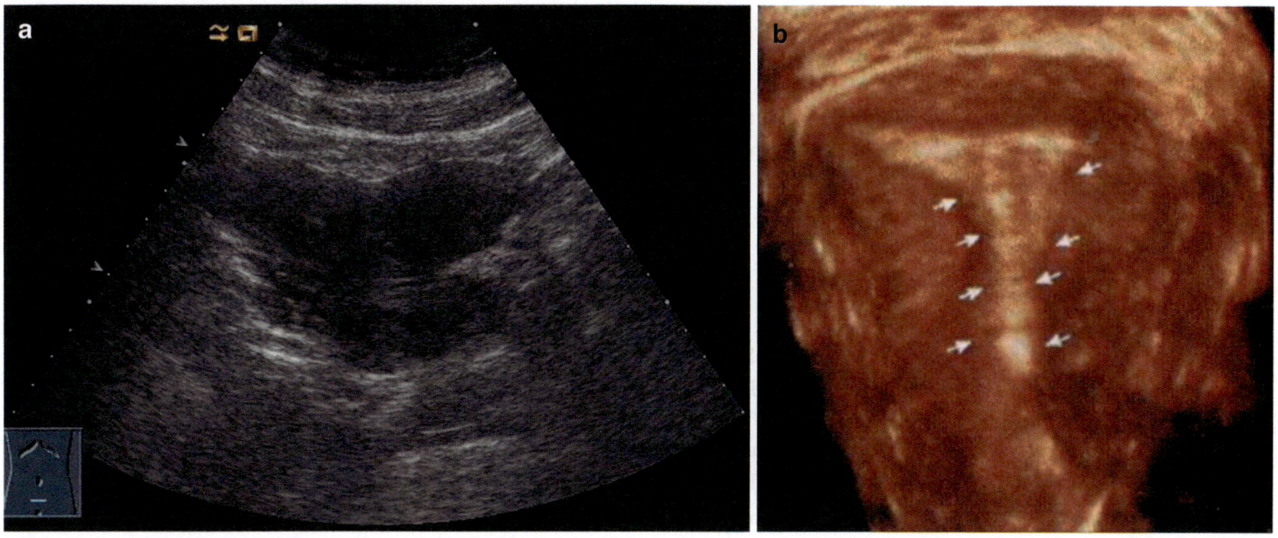

Fig. 8.74 (**a**) Image of bicornuate uterus under B-ultrasonography. (**b**) Under 3-D ultrasonography, the middle and lower parts of the cavity is narrowed with an IUD visible. Suggestion: T-shaped uterus?

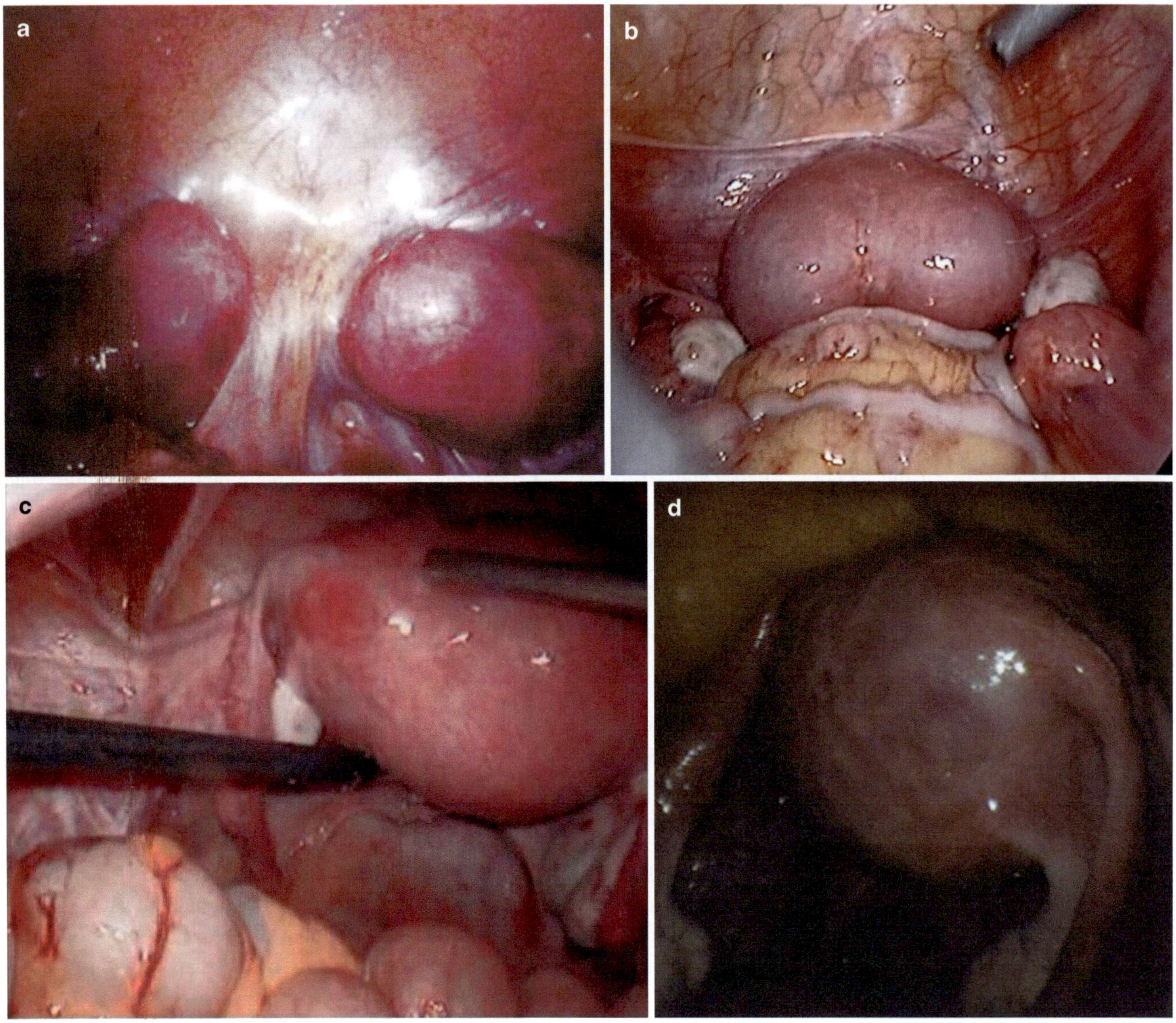

Fig. 8.75 (**a**) Uterus duplex under laparoscope. (**b**) Septate uterus under laparoscope. (**c**) Robert uterus under laparoscope. (**d**) Right unicornuate uterus with left rudimentary horn under laparoscope

part narrow, fundus arched, and bilateral walls thickened at mid and lower parts of the cavity, which forms a cylindrical cavity (Fig. 8.76).

8.2.4 Intrauterine Foreign Bodies

Intrauterine foreign bodies can be detected during ultrasonography scanning or hysteroscopy. Ultrasonography scanning may reveal abnormal echo or space-occupying lesions in the uterine cavity, which can be defined and located by hysteroscopy, and whether they can be removed hysteroscopically can be determined. An attempt can also be made to hook them out under the guidance of hysteroscope (Fig. 8.77a–d).

8.2.4.1 The Embedment or Residual Intrauterine Contraceptive Device (IUD)

IUD embedment (Fig. 8.78a–i), IUD fragments residue (Fig. 8.79a–d), and reversible tubal contraceptive device residual are the most common intrauterine foreign bodies. Olaore et al. reported a case who had adhesiolysis and insertion of IUD due to Asherman's syndrome and was seen with intravesical translocation of the IUD 1 year later, which was removed using bladder biopsy forceps under direct vision of cystoscopy.

8.2.4.2 Residual Fetal Bones or Osseous Metaplasia of the Endometrium

Fetal bone residue after abortion (Fig. 8.80a–c) is a rare complication, which is more common in termination of

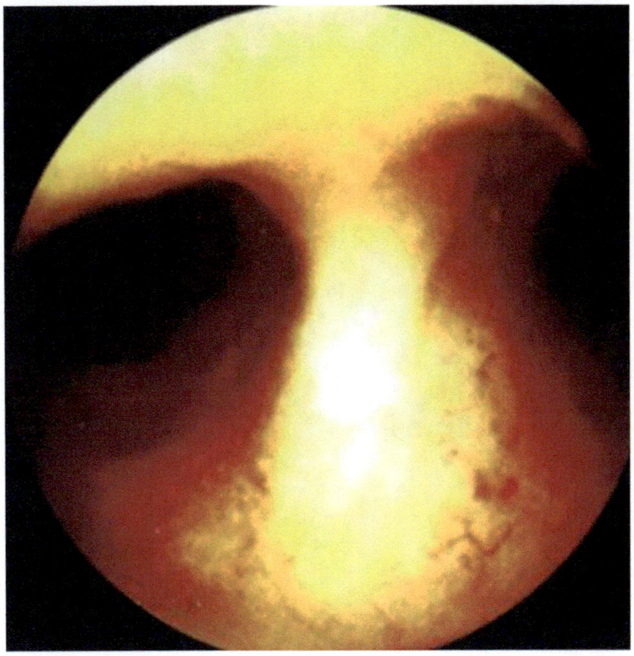

Fig. 8.76 Partial septate uterus under hysteroscope

second-trimester pregnancy, often causes bleeding or secondary infertility, and sometimes may occupy most of the uterine cavity. It is also difficult to be detected by HSG, but more readily by hysteroscopy. Little fetal bone residue needs to be differentiated from osseous metaplasia of the endometrium, and the latter may also cause infertility.

8.2.4.3 Residual Pregnancy Tissue

Placental remnants, induced by delayed miscarriage, incomplete miscarriage, adherent placenta, and placenta percreta, remain inside the uterine cavity, which can cause intrauterine adhesion, amenorrhea or irregular bleeding. If the adhesion is too severe, the residual pregnant tissue may not be detected or completely scraped by D&C. Hysteroscopy can be done not only to make the diagnosis but also in removal or resection of the pregnant tissues with the electric wire loop under the guidance of B-ultrasonography. The tissues removed should be sent for histopathologic examination (Fig. 8.81a, b).

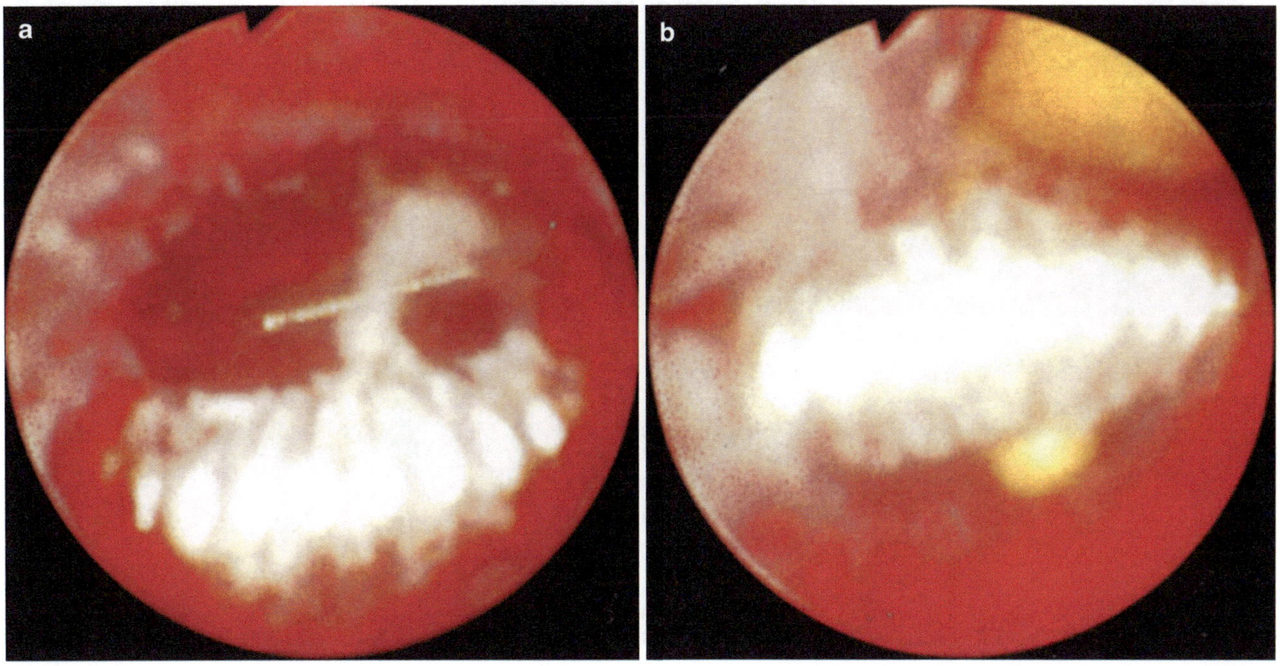

Fig. 8.77 (**a**) A metal ring under hysteroscope, which has been placed in uterine cavity for 16 years in a patient who reached menopause 3 years ago, the IUD could not be removed 1 year ago and the patient has been taking nilestriol for 2 weeks. (**b**) The hook is placed for removal of IUD under hysteroscopic direct vision. (**c**) Removal of IUD. (**d**) Removed IUD

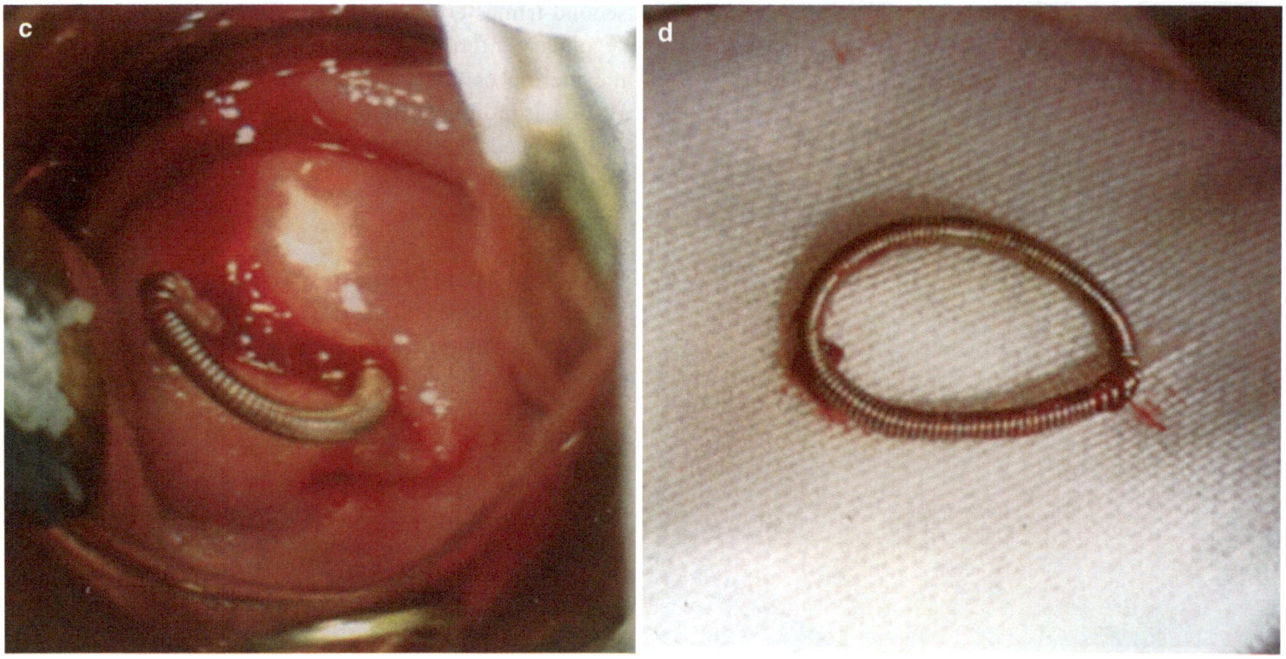

Fig. 8.77 (continued)

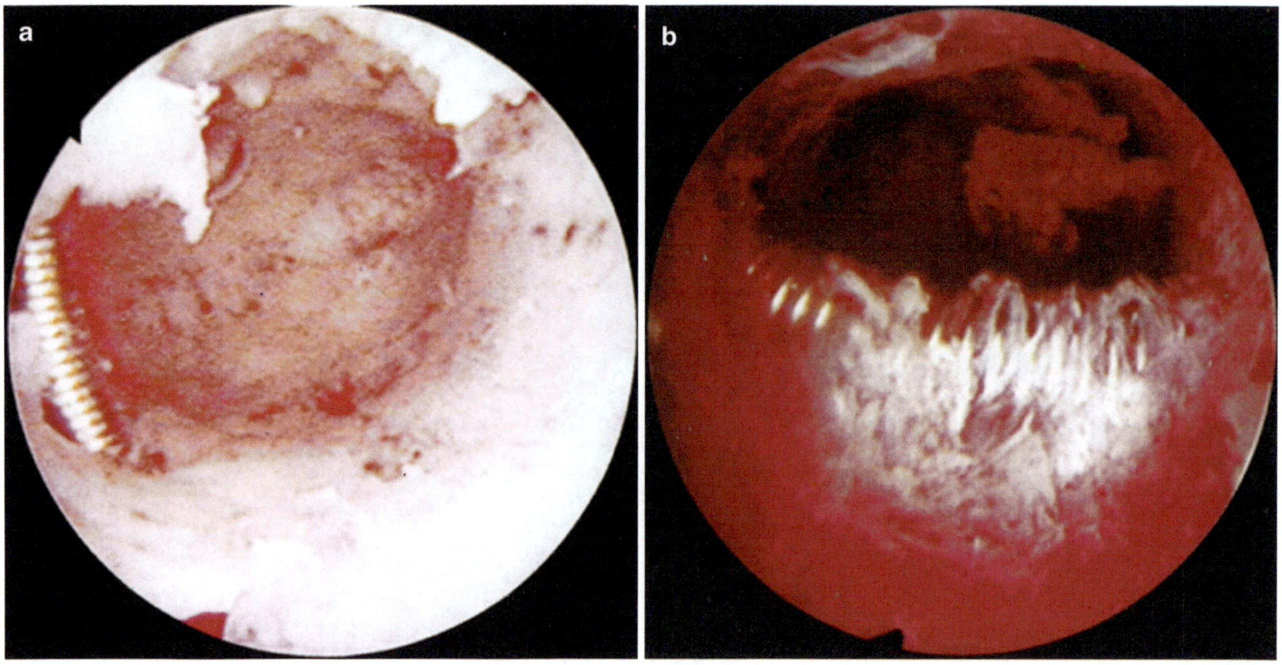

Fig. 8.78 (**a**–**e**) Embedded IUD. (**f**) IUD is put around the myoma. (**g**) A metal ring under hysteroscope, which has been placed in uterine cavity for 22 years in a patient who has been in menopause for 12 years and five earlier attempts to remove the IUD had all failed. (**h**) The left side of IUD is embedded into the left uterine wall. (**i**) The right side of IUD is embedded into the right uterine wall

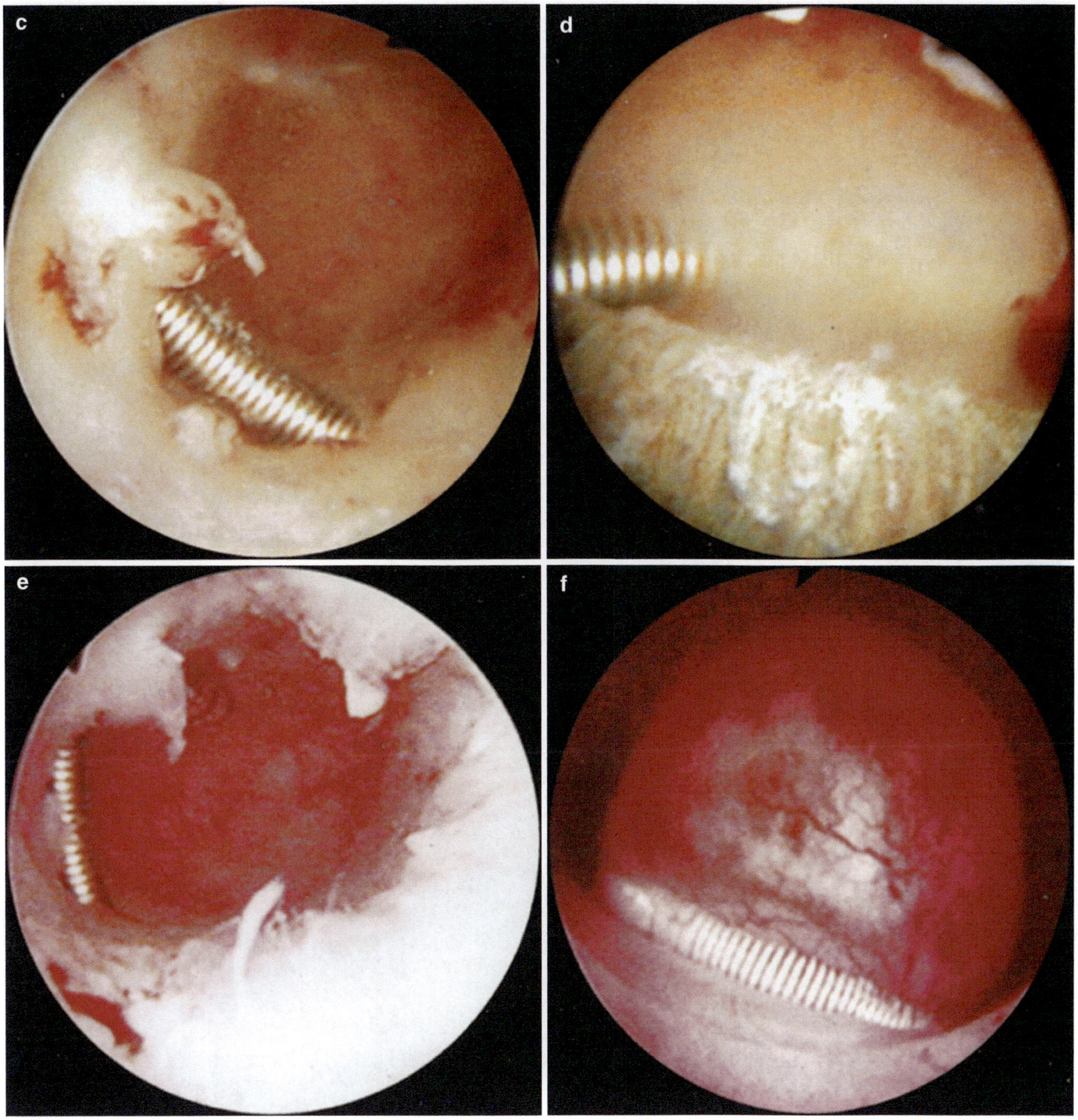

Fig. 8.78 (continued)

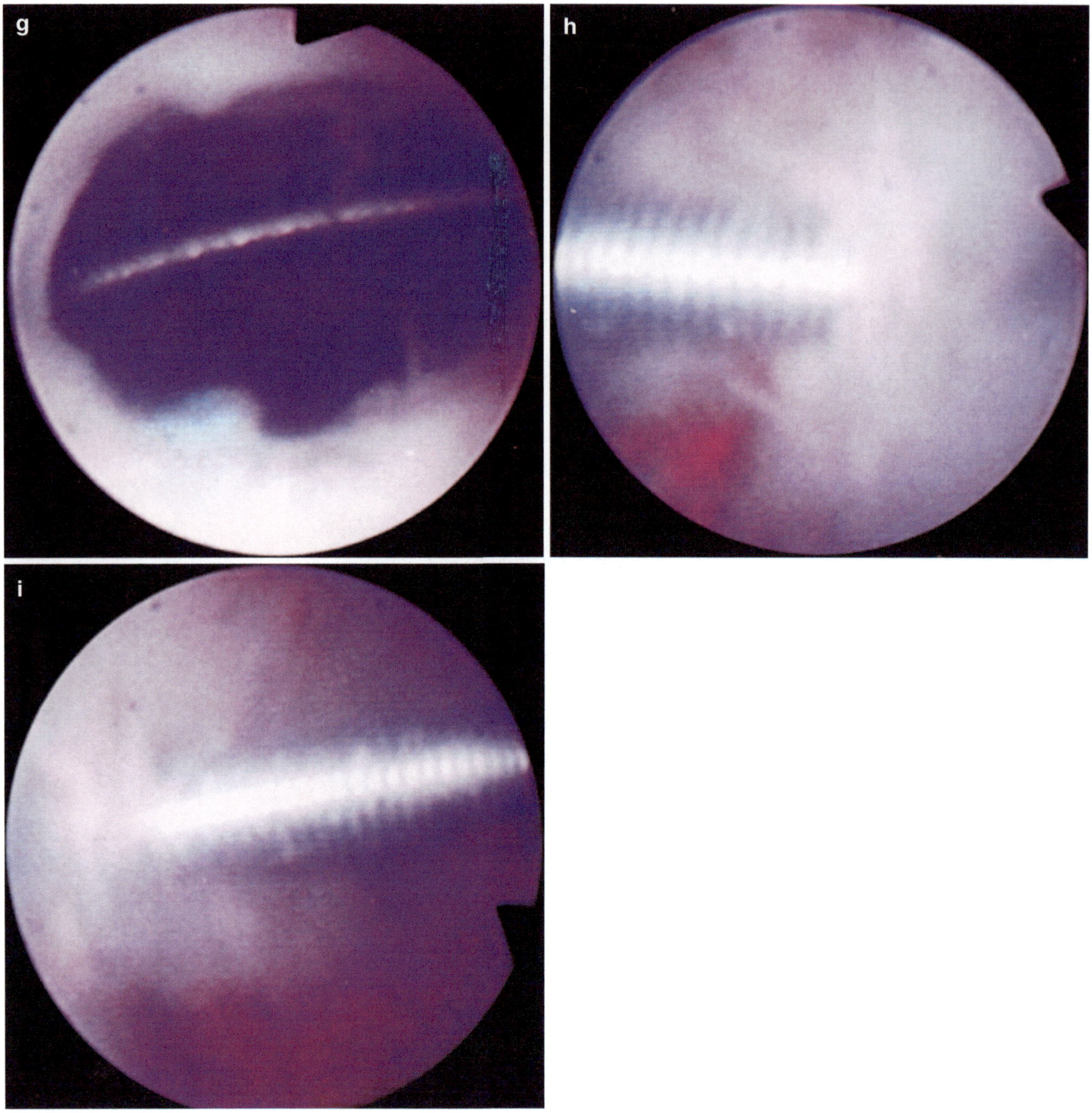

Fig. 8.78 (continued)

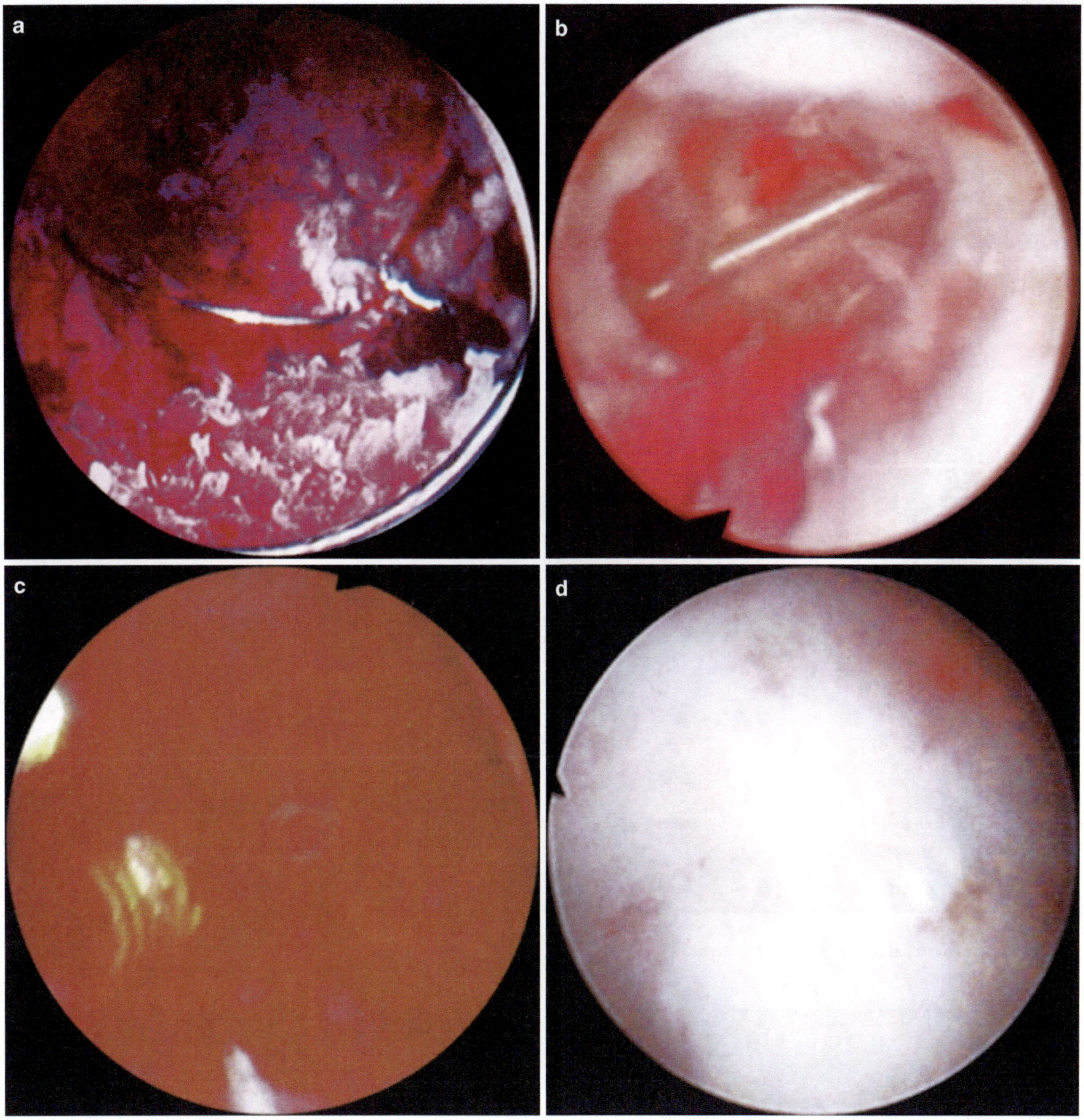

Fig. 8.79 (**a–c**) Residual IUD fragments. (**d**) A hysteroscopic view of a residual IUD, embedded in the left fundus of uterus in a patient with menopause for 1 year and 2 weeks after the removal of IUD

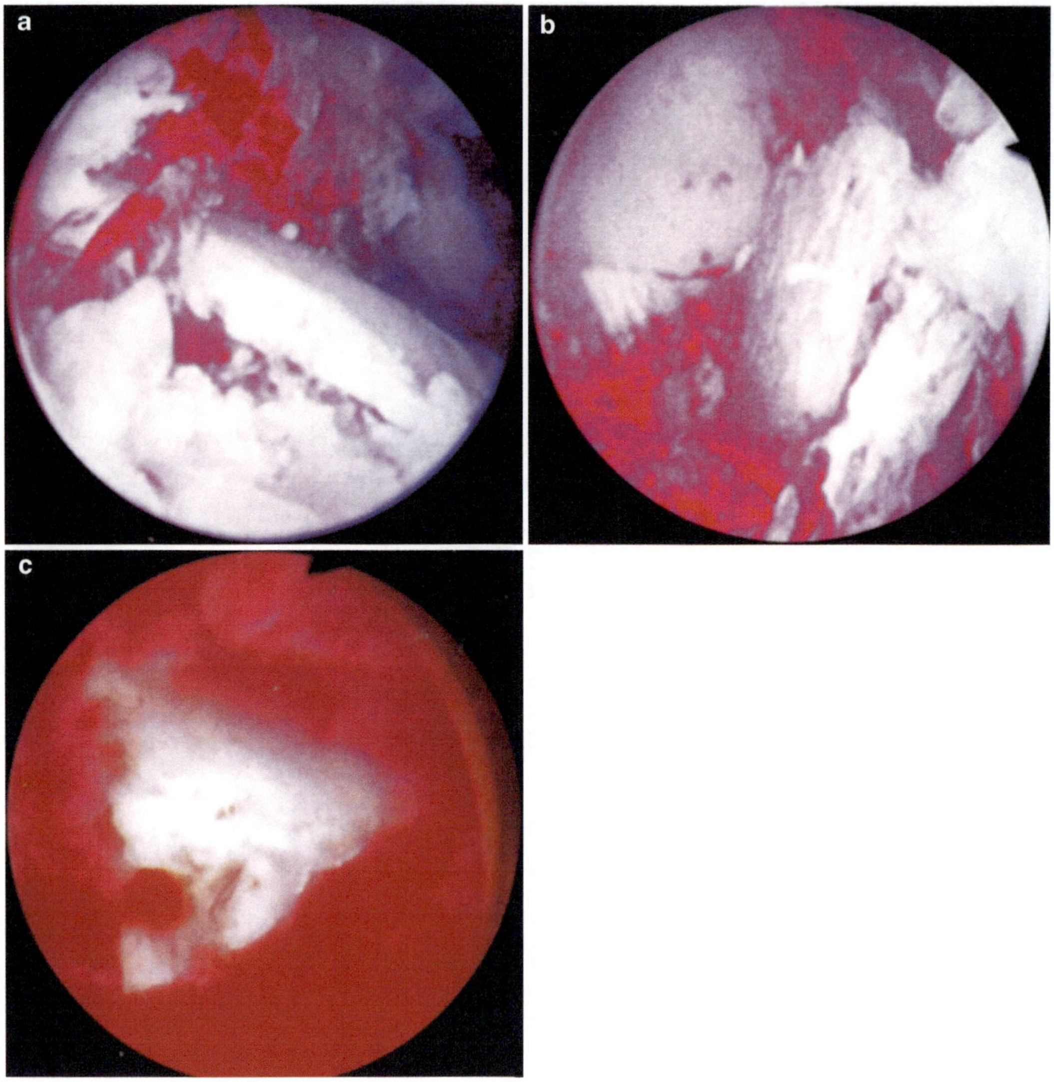

Fig. 8.80 (**a**–**c**) Residual fetal bones under hysteroscope

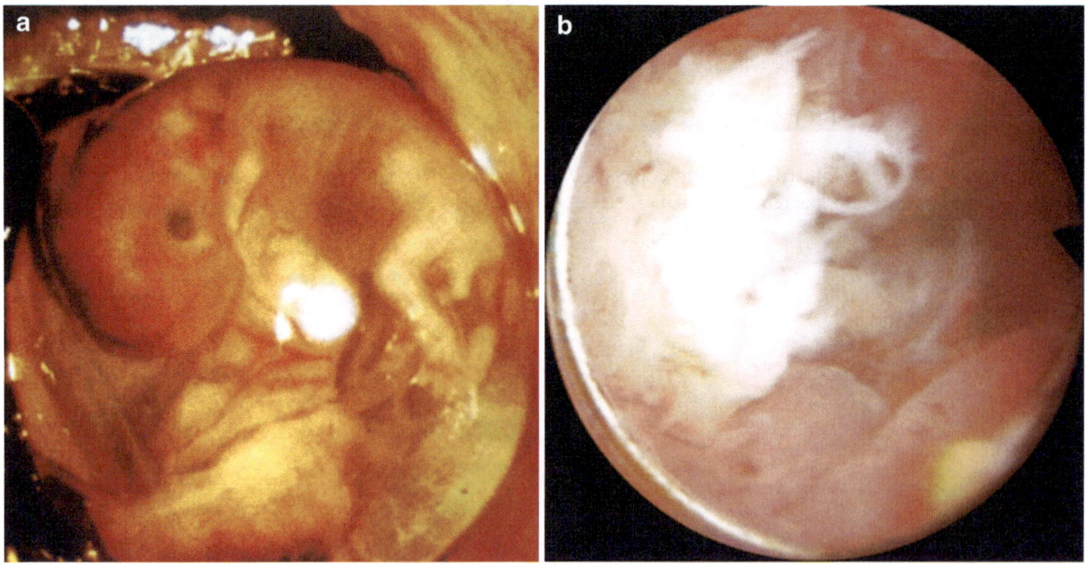

Fig. 8.81 (**a**, **b**) Placental remnants under hysteroscope

8.2.4.4 Ruptured Cervical Dilator or Residual Laminaria Tent

They are quite rare. A cervical dilator or laminaria tent is placed before hysteroscopic surgery or induced abortion in order to soften and dilate the cervix. Sometimes it may be broken inside the cervix when removed, and then fall back into the uterine cavity.

8.2.4.5 Residual Non-absorbable Sutures Following Cesarean Section

The non-absorbable silk thread had been used to suture at Cesarean section previously. Sometimes the residua of thread or thread knot can be seen at the level of internal cervical os during hysteroscopy (Fig. 8.82). These foreign bodies may cause endometrial bleeding or infection.

8.2.5 Intrauterine Adhesions

8.2.5.1 Formation and Classification of Intrauterine Adhesions

Intrauterine adhesion (IUA) is induced by scarring following injury to gravid uterus or uterus shortly after pregnancy, 90% of which is caused by curettage. Salzani et al. studied 109 cases who had been subjected to uterine curettage following abortion and underwent diagnostic hysteroscopy 3 to 12 months later. IUA was found in 37.6% of patients, with 56.1% grade I according to the classification of the European Society of Hysteroscopy, that is, filmy adhesive areas in the uterine cavity.

Usually, injury occurs 1 to 4 weeks after full-term delivery, premature birth, and miscarriages when curettage is needed due to large amounts of vaginal bleeding. At this time, the endometrium is so thin that any injury may be exposed or cause damage to the endometrial basal layer, resulting in fusion of opposite uterine walls and formation of continuously existent trabecula (Fig. 8.83), thus the symmetry of uterine cavity is disrupted. Occasionally transabdominal hysterotomy or metroplasty may lead to intrauterine adhesions, but such kind of adhesions is generally caused by staggered sutures rather than real healing of the denude surface of uterine myometrium after childbirth or suction abortion.

Clinically there were various widely used classification systems for intrauterine adhesions. In 1978, March made the classification of IUA based on the hysteroscopic findings, which is given in Table 8.11. In 1988, according to the observations on HSG and at hysteroscopy, Valle and Sciarra classified intrauterine adhesions into three types (mild, moderate, severe) basing on their severity (Table 8.12). In the same year, AFS produced a classification of IUA basing on HSG findings, hysteroscopic outcomes, and pregnancy prognosis, which is given in Table 8.13. The classification published by ESGE in 1988 is given in Table 8.14.

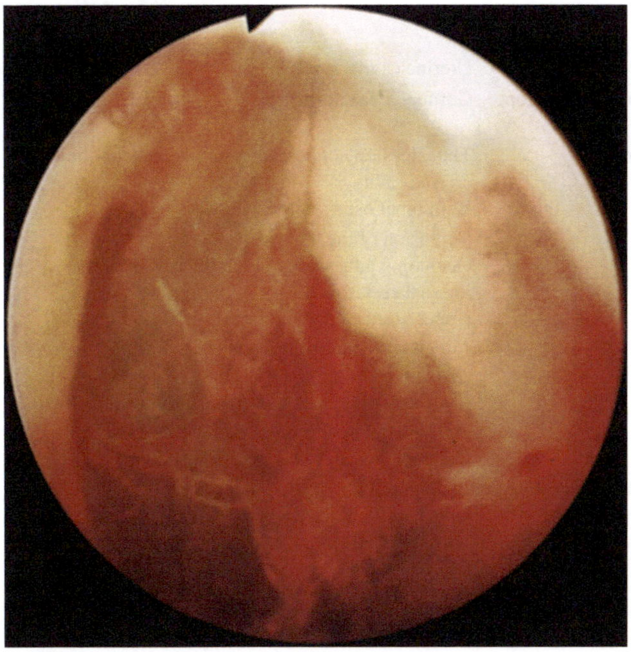

Fig. 8.82 Residual silk thread 15 months after Cesarean section

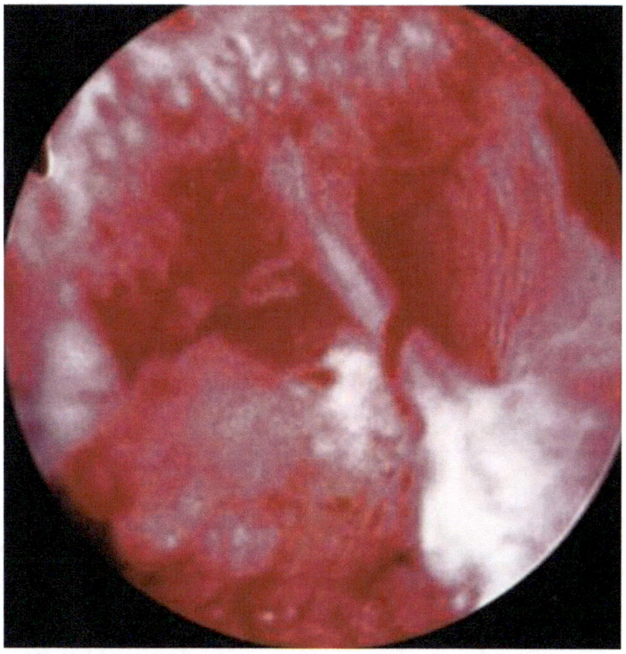

Fig. 8.83 Formation of trabecula in a case with intrauterine adhesions

Table 8.11 March's classification of IUA

Grades	cavity involvement	Adhesions	Tubal ostia and upper segment of the cavity
Mild	<1/4	Filmy or thin	Light or clearly visible
Moderate	1/4 ~ 3/4	No uterine wall adhered	Partly occluded
Severe	>3/4	Uterine wall adhered or adhesive bands thickened	Occluded

Table 8.12 Valle and Sciarra classification of IUA

Grades	Adhesions and endometrium	Cavity
Mild	Filmy adhesions composed of basal layer endometrium, focal or extensive	–
Moderate	Fibromuscular adhesions, thickened and covered with endometrium	Partially or totally occluded
Severe	Connective adhesive tissues with no endometrial tissue	Partially or totally occluded

Table 8.13 AFS prognosis classification of IUA

Characteristics		Score	Hysteroscopy score	HSG score
Cavity involvement	<1/3	1		
	1/3–2/3	2		
	>2/3	4		
Type of adhesions	Filmy	1		0 or 4
	Filmy and dense	2		
	Dense	4		
Menstrual pattern	Normal	0		
	Hypomenorrhea	2		
	Amenorrhea	4		
Total score		/		

Prognostic classification: Stage I (Mild: 1–4 scores); Stage II (Moderate: 5–8 scores); Stage III (Severe: 9–12 scores)

Table 8.14 ESGE classification of IUA.(Under hysteroscope)

Grade	Adhesions	Uterine cavity
I	Thin or filmy adhesions easily ruptured by hysteroscope sheath alone	Cornual areas normal
II	Singular dense adhesion cannot be ruptured by hysteroscope sheath alone	The adhesion connecting separate areas of the uterine cavity Both tubal ostia visible
IIa		Occlusion of the cavity. Occluding adhesions only in the region of the internal cervical os Upper uterine cavity normal
III	Multiple dense adhesions	Adhesions connecting separate areas of the uterine cavity Unilateral obliteration of ostial areas of the tubes
IV	Extensive dense adhesions	Total/partial occlusion of the uterine cavity Both tubal ostial areas (partially) occluded
Va	Extensive endometrial scarring and fibrosis in combination with grade I or grade II adhesions With amenorrhea or pronounced hypomenorrhea	
Vb	Extensive endometrial scarring and fibrosis in combination with grade III or grade IV adhesions With amenorrhea	

8.2.5.2 Clinical Manifestations of Intrauterine Adhesions

1. Abnormal menstruation: Intrauterine adhesions usually lead to menstrual abnormalities, such as hypomenorrhea, or even amenorrhea, depending on the degree of uterine occlusion. Patients who have intrauterine adhesions for a long time may also have dysmenorrhea. More than 75% of patients with moderate or severe adhesions suffer from amenorrhea or hypomenorrhea. When uterine atresia is secondary to intrauterine adhesions, 37% may develop amenorrhea and 31% hypomenorrhea. Patients with small or local adhesion may have no obvious abnormal menstruation, presenting with normal menstruation. March et al. reported 275 cases of intrauterine adhesions, menstrual patterns of whom are given in Table 8.15. The incidence of IUA is unknown, and some patients with IUA are asymptomatic and able to breed normally.
2. Abnormal pregnancy: If the adhesion does not block the whole uterine cavity, patients may have fertility problems and are prone to have pregnancy failures, including miscarriage in early and mid-term pregnancy, delayed miscarriage, ectopic pregnancy, premature labor, and intra-uterine fetus death. In case of a full-term pregnancy, there may be placenta previa, adherent placenta, and placenta accreta. Schenker and Margalioth evaluated 292 patients who had untreated intrauterine adhesions. Of 292 patients, 133 (45%) became pregnant, only 50 (30%) obtained full-term pregnancy, 38 (23%) had premature labor, 66 (40%) had spontaneous abortion, and 21 (13%) had ectopic pregnancy and abnormal placenta implantation.
3. Infertility: Complete amenorrhea or complete uterine occlusion in patients usually manifests as infertility.

8.2.5.3 Diagnosis of Intrauterine Adhesions

Before the advent of hysteroscopy, the diagnosis of IUA depended on the case history, physical examination, laboratory data, and HSG. The patients with hypomenorrhea or amenorrhea after curettage may be suspected to have IUA, and the uterus is more likely to be damaged in patients who are pregnant or shortly after pregnancy than those with a non-gravid uterus. The occurrence of IUA is more likely in women who had curettage 2–4 weeks after delivery or delayed miscarriage. Westendorp et al. prospectively studied 50 women who had their residual placenta removed 24 h after delivery or underwent curettage following incomplete abortions. Diagnostic hysteroscopy was performed 3 months later. Intrauterine adhesions were found in 20 cases (40%), with five patients in grade I, six in grade II, six in grade III, and three in grade IV. The risk of intrauterine adhesions grade II–IV in women with menstrual disorders doubled. Based on these findings, hysteroscopy is recommended only in those patients who develop menstrual disorders or repeated intrauterine manipulations. If the patients have normal ovulation but absence of menstruation, then intrauterine adhesion is highly possible. As intrauterine adhesions and hormone levels are independent, if basal body temperature shows biphasic pattern and progestogen withdrawal in patients with amenorrhea is negative, the diagnosis of intrauterine adhesions can be strengthened. The determination of the ovulation in such patients includes evaluation of basal body temperature and consecutive serum progesterone levels. When the patient has ovulation, the basal temperature should be biphasic but may be atypical. Since the first day of an ovulatory cycle is unknown, the early follicular temperature may not be detected. Endometrial biopsy is done by taking a sample of fibrous tissues, and progesterone level is measured once a week until it exceeds 3 ng/mL. If there is ovulatory cycle but without withdrawal bleeding and if no bleeding occurs after administration of progestogen or sequential application of estrogen and progesterone, the existence of IUA should be suspected. The measurement of the length of uterine cavity can determine whether there is obstruction of the internal cervical os, but this practice had been discarded, because it can increase the probability of uterine perforation and misdiagnosis. HSG had ever been the most meaningful examination in the diagnosis of intrauterine adhesions and could be used to evaluate the internal cervical os and uterine cavity, and describe intrauterine adhesions. If the adhesion does not completely occlude the uterine cavity, the morphology of the rest of the uterine cavity is shown. If HSG displays single or multiple filling defects, the diagnosis of IUA is more reliable. Intrauterine adhesions have been confirmed by HSG in about 1.5% of patients with infertility and 5% of patients with recurrent pregnancy loss. 36% of patients with intrauterine adhesions related history are diagnosed to have IUA by HSG. These adhesions are star-shaped and irregularly star-shaped with strips and dots inside and a rough outside, located in different parts of the uterine cavity. Adhesions are usually located in the central part of uterine cavity, with only a few located in the uterine cornua or lower segment of uterus.

Table 8.15 Menstruation in 275 cases with intrauterine adhesions

Menstrual patterns	Case load
Amenorrhea	183
Hypomenorrhea	50
Oligomenorrhea	5
Normal menstruation	37

8.2.5.4 Role of Hysteroscopy in Diagnosis of Intrauterine Adhesions

HSG is an effective diagnostic method for suspected IUA, which can determine the degree of uterine cavity occlusion, but it cannot assess the toughness and type of adhesions. Therefore, the final diagnosis can only be determined by direct hysteroscopic examination, and diagnostic hysteroscopy is the final arbiter in the diagnosis (Fig. 8.84a–d). Hysteroscopy can rule out 30% of the abnormal results on HSG under direct vision, and is superior to HSG in the determination of the extent and the type of adhesions. Once the final diagnosis is made by hysteroscopy, the corresponding treatment can be administered. Other techniques, such as ultrasonography and MRI, have been used in the diagnosis of IUA, but their accuracy is not clear, and there is not enough experience to prove that these techniques can be the substitutes for HSG, and they are expensive as well.

March reported that HSG and hysteroscopy have a good correlation in the diagnosis of IUA (Table 8.16). HSG often exaggerates the extent of adhesions. There were two most dramatic cases who had endometrial sclerosis but no intrauterine adhesions, in whom complete uterine atresia was diagnosed by HSG. No cases have severe IUA diagnosed by HSG as it is by hysteroscopy.

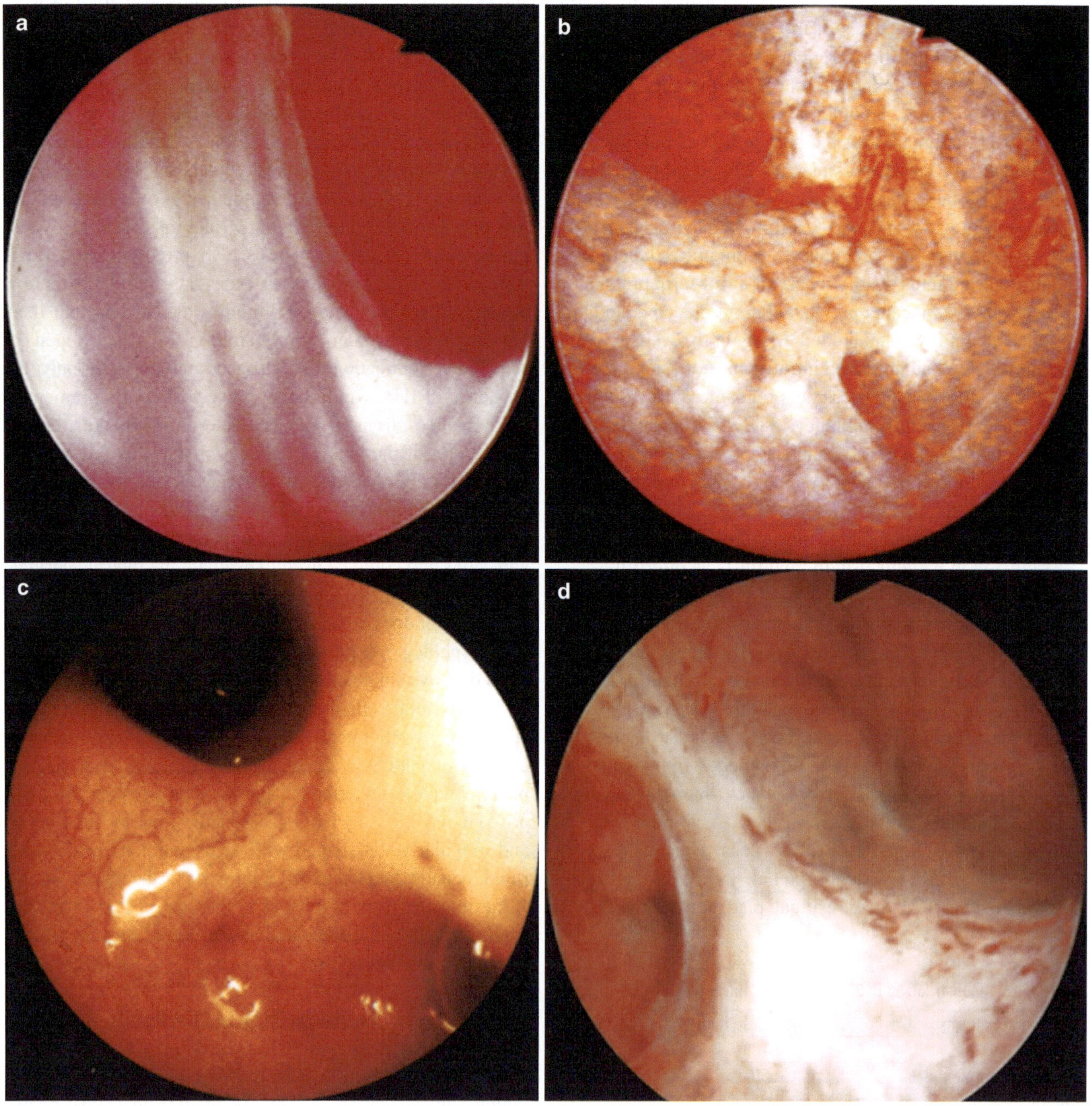

Fig. 8.84 Intrauterine adhesions. (**a**) filmy. (**b**) fibromuscular. (**c**) connective tissue. (**d**) connective tissue

Table 8.16 Severity of IUA diagnosed by HSG and hysteroscopy

		Hysteroscopy		
HSG	Case load	Severe	Moderate	Mild
Severe	124	81	35	8
Moderate	37	0	29	8
Mild	43	0	0	43
Total	204	81	64	59

Table 8.17 Relationship between IUA diagnosed by hysteroscopy and menstruation

		Extent of intrauterine adhesions		
Menstruation	Case load	Severe	Moderate	Mild
Amenorrhea	183	110	49	24
Hypomenorrhea	50	10	24	16
Oligomenorrhea	5	1	1	3
Normal menstruation	37	4	8	25
Total	275	125	82	68

Relationship between hysteroscopic diagnosis of IUA and menstrual patterns reported by March is given in Table 8.17. Most amenorrhea patients suffer from severe or moderate intrauterine adhesions. However, March et al. reported that nine patients with moderate intrauterine adhesions and 5 with severe adhesions had normal menstruation or just hypomenorrhea.

Even if intrauterine adhesions are so severe as to induce amenorrhea, the endometrium with biological activity can still have the potential to develop into cancer. Sandridge et al. reported that a 71-year-old woman who developed post-menopausal bleeding with the use of unopposed estrogen. At TVS a polypoid mass was detected. Extensive intrauterine adhesions were noted during hysteroscopy, and a polypoid lesion was seen around the adhesion, with biopsy confirming endometrial adenocarcinoma.

8.2.6 Endometrial Carcinoma

Endometrial carcinoma is a common malignant tumor of the female genital tract, and its incidence has been slightly on the rise in recent years, and the age of onset has a tendency to be delayed. Direct biopsy under hysteroscopy and pathological examination are the optimal methods in screening high-risk populations for early detection and accurate diagnosis of endometrial carcinoma and precancerous lesions.

In more than 90% of patients with endometrial carcinoma, the first symptom is AUB, and the initial symptom of most benign and malignant endometrial lesions is also bleeding. Zampi et al. made an analysis of the incidence of uterine hemorrhage under various morphological changes of endometrial tissues in a group of 1295 patients who underwent D&C, which is given in Table 8.18.

Table 8.18 Various endometrial histopathology and incidence of uterine bleeding in 1295 cases with D&C

Endometrial histopathology	Incidence of uterine bleeding(%)
Functional or non-synchronous endometrium	66.6
Atrophic endometrium	72.5
Adenomatous hyperplasia	77.4
Endometrial polyps	78.1
Glandular endometrial hyperplasia	79.3
Endometrial carcinoma	97.2
Cystic endometrial hyperplasia	100

The incidence of bleeding caused by cystic glandular endometrial hyperplasia and endometrial carcinoma is extremely high, and the prodromal symptom of other lesions is also hemorrhage. Therefore, hysteroscopy can be considered as a reasonable inspection technique in examining women ≥45 years old with AUB. Biopsy under direct vision is especially useful in discovering endometrial carcinoma earlier and may also make correct diagnosis for benign lesions causing bleeding.

8.2.6.1 Diagnostic Methods of Endometrial Carcinoma

There has always been a lack of simple and accurate methods with minimal invasiveness in the screening and early diagnosis of endometrial carcinoma. In addition to the traditional and the most commonly used D&C and fractional curettage, there are a few reports in the literature on the application of other alternative techniques for detection of the endometrial neoplasm and pre-cancerous conditions including endometrial cytological examination, HSG, TVS, SHSG (SIS), MRI, diagnostic hysteroscopy, and endometrial biopsy, etc. Blind D&C is often inaccurate, and the small cancer foci may be missed at curettage, which may be located in the deep uterine cornua or behind submucosal myomas. Gimpelson et al. reported that 10–35% of the endometrial area could not be scrapped. For the elderly women with the cervix atrophy, the procedure can only be completed after uterine dilatation, which increases trauma to the patients and their pain. Blind diagnostic curettage cannot assess the location and the extent of endometrial cancer. Endometrial cytology smears may provide false negative results, especially in well-differentiated or small tumors. HSG may suggest endometrial carcinoma, but usually misleading. Krample et al. studied the diagnostic accuracy of TVS, SHSG, operative hysteroscopy, and the histological diagnosis. The results showed that the detection rate of intrauterine pathology with hysteroscopy and histological biopsy was 100%, and it was 94.1% with SHSG, but 23.5% with TVS. The endometrial lesions detected by TVS and SHSG still also required direct biopsy through a hysteroscope. Modern hysteroscopic technique makes a gynecologist able to observe the whole uterine cavity directly and closely without blind zones. Its small diameter and multi-purpose design can prompt the implementation of directed biopsy of endometrium, especially the advent of fiber hysteroscopy, which can be applied for the diagnosis of intrauterine diseases in elderly women. Hysteroscopy, being a simple operation providing accurate diagnosis, has become a "gold standard" of modern diagnosis of intrauterine lesions. A great deal of data in recent decades showed that hysteroscopy has been applied in screening of intrauterine lesions for a large number of outpatients and early detection of endometrial cancer with satisfactory results, which has been accepted by the majority of women. Currently, hysteroscopy can provide the most reliable information on the diagnosis of endometrial cancer and the extent of intrauterine invasion. In most cases, hysteroscopy can clearly observe tumors and predict the prognosis. Hysteroscopy can reveal the extent of tumor extending outward more obviously than HSG, but it cannot detect the depth of myometrial invasion. It should be noted that visual inspection cannot replace pathological diagnosis, thus sampling must be taken for histopathological examination.

8.2.6.2 Hysteroscopic Diagnosis of Endometrial Carcinoma

Due to technical and anatomical reasons, endometrial cancer at an early stage does not present nodular structure which is detectable by screening. The diagnostic hysteroscopy is usually performed due to AUB. Therefore, during inspection the hysteroscopist must pay close attention to various aspects of the endometrial tissues including color, undulation and toughness from the surrounding normal endometrium. Neoplasm is highly suspected when there are atypical blood vessels. The findings on endometrial carcinoma at hysteroscopy are very distinct and rarely confused with that of other lesions. The endometrial carcinoma at early stage presents an image of one beginning to overgrow, and the endometrium is irregular and appears to be foliose. The protruding part is fragile and usually necrotic in nature, which bleeds easily. New vessels are irregular and spiral (Figs. 8.85a,b and 8.86a–c). In some cases, the boundary between neoplasm and the normal endometrium is quite clear. Sometimes focal lesions are visible and located in the uterine cornua, which are easily missed in blind sampling. Endometrial cancer can be classified into the focal type and the diffuse type according to the morphology and extent of the lesions. According to the orientation of growth, they can be classified into endogenous and exogenous lesions. The exogenous lesions often develop into the uterine cavity with a higher incidence and special appearance, which can be diagnosed under hysteroscopy. However the diagnosis of the endogenous lesions is more difficult. The basic findings at hysteroscopy include papillary, nodular, and polypoid swellings, which can appear separately, and in mixed forms as well. When the lesions

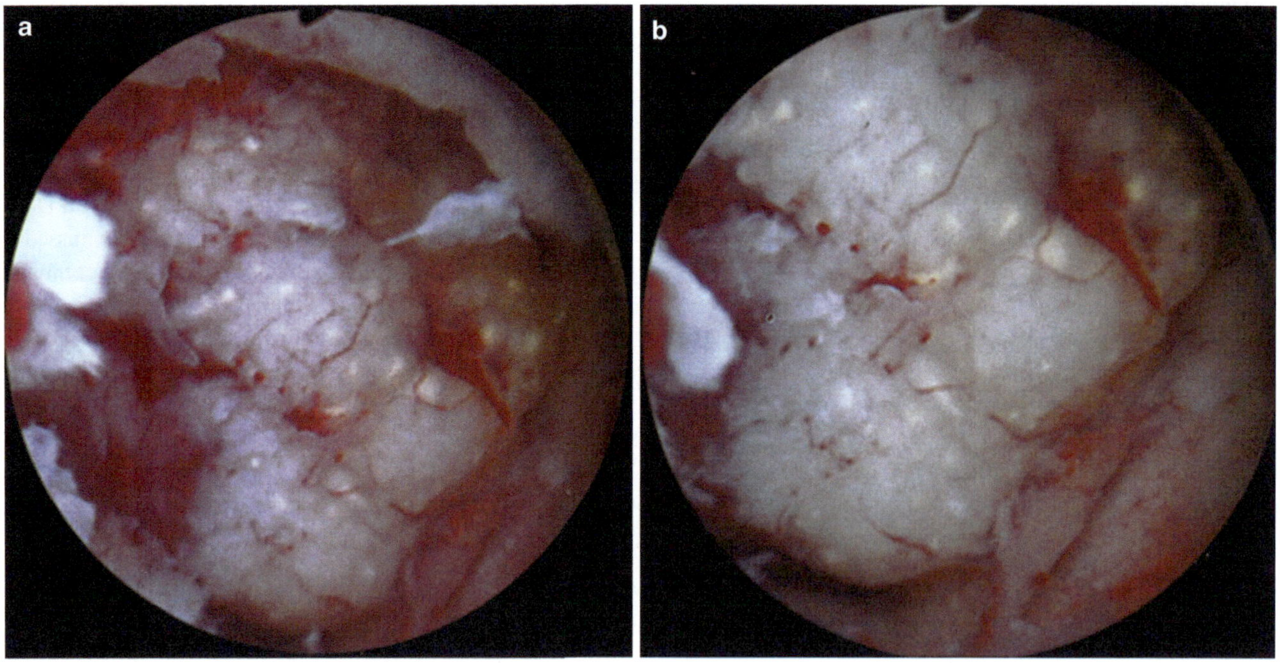

Fig. 8.85 Endometrial carcinoma. This 36-year-old patient has had amenorrhea for 10 years after curettage due to incomplete abortion. Her menses resumed when she received cyclic hormone therapy or progesterone. Four years ago, adenomatous endometrial hyperplasia was diagnosed histopathologically. At that stage, hysteroscopy revealed irregular endometrium with leafy swelling and protrusions, which were greyish white in color and bleeds easily. Endometrial adenocarcinoma (medium to high differentiation) was confirmed histopathologically. (**a**) far view (**b**) close view

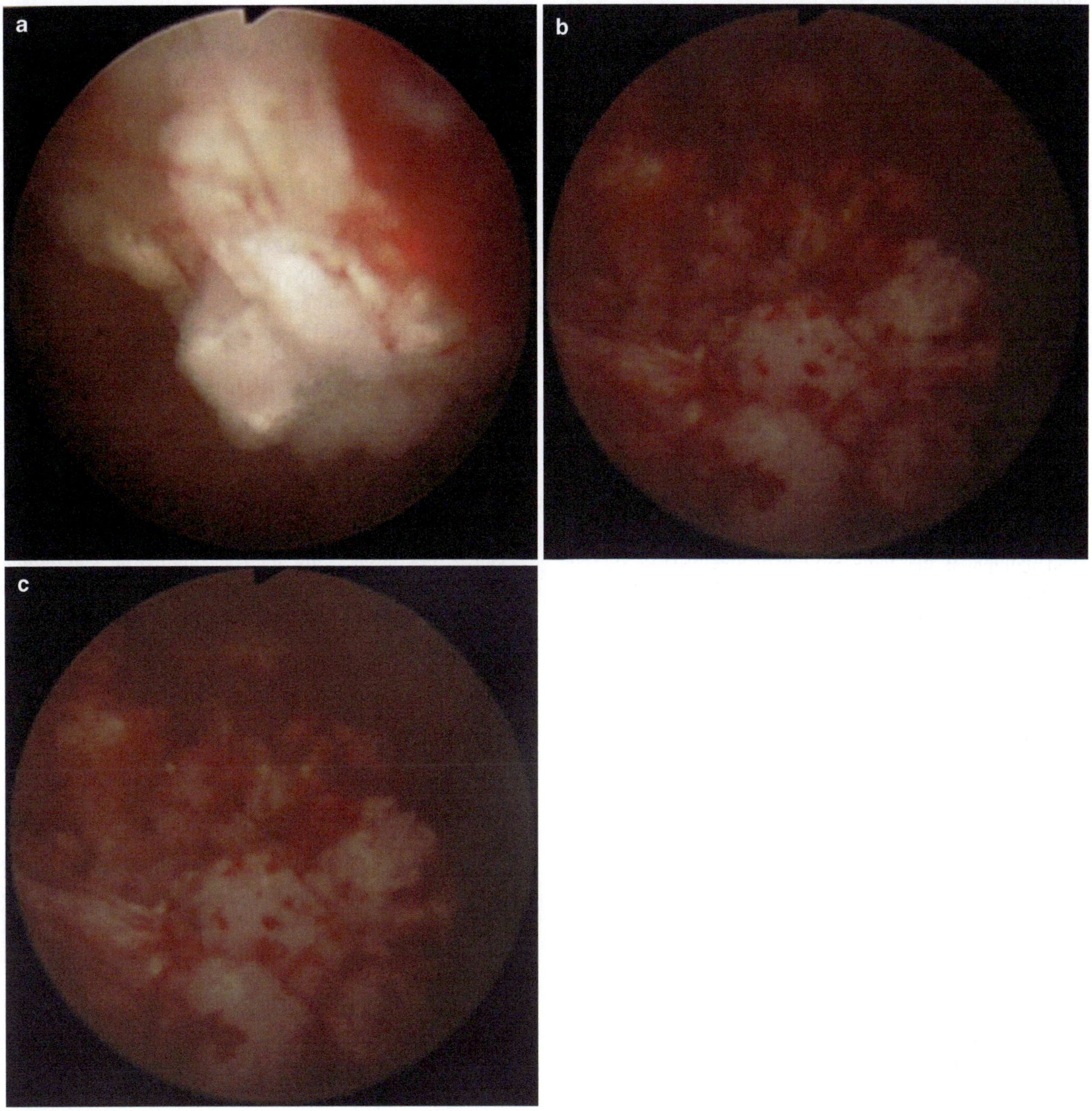

Fig. 8.86 Endometrial carcinoma. This 63-year-old patient has had menopause for 17 years. Intrauterine space-occupying lesions were identified by ultrasonography. Hysteroscopy reveals cauliflower-like swellings on the anterior and posterior walls, over which the blood vessels are disordered and distributed, being fragile, and bleeds easily. (**a**) Nodular swellings on the anterior wall. (**b**) Cauliflower-like swellings on the anterior wall (far view). (**c**) Cauliflower-like swellings on the posterior wall (close view)

develop, the cancer foci may spread from the focal type into a diffuse type, and extensive necrosis, inflammation, and ulcers may also occur. Hysteroscopy may be performed to measure the extent of the endometrial carcinoma involvement in the uterine cavity so as to determine its focal manifestation and images, and is also the only method to guide targeted biopsy.

8.2.6.3 Staging for Endometrial Carcinoma at Hysteroscopy

Liukko et al. investigated with fractional curettage prior to hysteroscopy and the specimens of the removed uterus diagnosed to be endometrial carcinoma stage I, 16% of which were found to spread into the cervix postoperatively. Stelmachow reported that in 22 cases with stage I endometrial carcinoma diagnosed by HSG and D&C, nine cases were proved to have stage II by hysteroscopy; and in nine cases with stage II by HSG and D&C, two cases actually had stage I. These data confirmed the superiority of hysteroscopy in defining whether it had the cervical spread or not. When hysteroscopy is performed, the cervical canal is checked and tissues are scraped before cervical dilation, thus misdiagnosis can be avoided. When the cancer tissues invading the cervix have continuous relations with the intrauterine cancer foci, it can be determined to be infiltrating carcinoma, which is stage II endometrial carcinoma. Single lesions within the cervical canal are more difficult to determine. In addition, there are endometrial carcinoma tissues often hanging from the uterine cavity into the cervical canal. Since such lesions are not true cervical spreading, differentiation between them must be made. The false negative rate of hysteroscopic diagnosis of cervical spread is reported to be 7.9%. Toki et al. conducted a comparison study of endometrial carcinoma for cervical involvement by hysteroscopy, MRI, and endocervical curettage. It was believed that in diagnosis of cervical involvement, MRI was focused on detecting stromal invasion, but hysteroscopy was superior for identifying mucosal involvement, both of which are complementary to each other in evaluating cervical invasion.

8.2.6.4 Screening for High-Risk Population with Endometrial Cancer by Hysteroscopy

Endometrial cancer is closely associated with many high-risk factors such as postmenopausal uterine bleeding, especially in patients with hypertension, diabetes, obesity, high-fat diet, and infertility, and women with hormone replacement therapy (HRT) or taking tamoxifen (TMX) after breast cancer operation, and women suffering from estrogen secreting tumor, etc. Screening for high-risk groups is the focus for prevention and treatment of endometrial cancer.

1. Diagnosis of intrauterine lesions in women with postmenopausal bleeding: Postmenopausal bleeding is a warning signal of endometrial cancer. It has been reported that 10% of those patients were found to have endometrial cancer for the first time. It is generally believed that the possibility of endometrial cancer raised along with the thickening of endometrium. However, it was also pointed out that the endometrial thickness in some patients with endometrial cancer is only 2–3 mm, that is, the so-called thin endometrium. The endometrial thickness is not correlated with endometrial carcinoma, thus hysteroscopy is superior in the diagnosis of endometrial cancer with thin endometrium.
2. Assessment of endometrial lesions in patients receiving TMX therapy after breast cancer operation: The long-term administration of TMX for treatment of breast cancer is a commonly used method clinically to prevent its recurrence. TMX has weak estrogen-like effects, thus the treatment may cause specific and hyperplastic endometrial lesions, including simple hyperplasia and atypical hyperplasia, hyperplasia accompanied with polyp formation, polypoid carcinoma, and adenocarcinoma, etc. After a study on 15 authors' research data, Seoud et al. found that the incidence of endometrial carcinoma in patients taking TMX was 0–8.8%. The endometrial changes in patients taking TMX were associated with their endometrial status before medication. Baldini et al. evaluated patients treated with tamoxifen after surgery of breast cancer for 6–12 months. After 3–4 years of treatment, they observed a higher incidence of atypical endometrial hyperplasia and endometrial polyp lesions in the group of symptomatic patients or patients with endometrial lesions than among the non-treated group and the patients with no endometrial lesions. It has been reported consistently that the administration of TMX after breast cancer operation could induce endometrial carcinoma. Cohen et al. reported that the incidence of endometrial carcinoma in these patients was 1.7–7 times of that in general postmenopausal women. Therefore, when the TVS showed endometrial thickness ≥8 mm, hysteroscopy and targeted biopsy should be performed.

A large number of studies on the assessment of endometrial changes in women treated with HRT have proved the safety of HRT, but epidemiological studies have shown that long-term or un-opposed HRT may increase the risk of endometrial cancer. The incidence of endometrial cancer in women receiving exogenous estrogen therapy increases by 6–12 times. With an increase in the dosage of estrogen and prolonged administration time, the risk increases gradually. The changes in endometrial hyperplasia during the administration of HRT may be focal, thus hysteroscopy with directed curettage is very necessary.

Suggested Reading

Diagnostic Hysteroscopy

1. Abramovici H, Faktor JH, Pascal B. Congenital uterine malformations as indication for cervical suture (cerclage) in habitual abortion and premature delivery. Int J Fertil. 1983;28(3):161–4.
2. Acién P. Incidence of Müllerian defects in fertile and infertile women. Hum Reprod. 1997;12(7):1372–6.
3. Airoldi J, Berghella V, Sehdev H, Ludmir J. Transvaginal ultrasonography of the cervix to predict preterm birth in women with uterine anomalies. Obstet Gynecol. 2005;106(3):553–6.
4. Akar ME, Bayar D, Yildiz S, Ozel M, Yilmaz Z. Reproductive outcome of women with unicornuate uterus. Aust N Z J Obstet Gynaecol. 2005;45(2):148–50.

5. Alborzi S, Asadi N, Zolghadri J, Alborzi S, Alborzi M. Laparoscopic metroplasty in bicornuate and didelphic uteri. Fertil Steril. 2009;92(1):352–5.
6. ASGE TECHNOLOGY COMMITTEE, Song LM, Adler DG, Conway JD, Diehl DL, Farraye FA, Kantsevoy SV, Kwon R, Mamula P, Rodriguez B, Shah RJ, Tierney WM. Narrow band imaging and multiband imaging. Gastrointest Endosc. 2008;67(4):581–9.
7. Aubriot FX, Chapron C, Utérus DES. Polémiques sur l'hystéroplastie d'agrandissement. Arguments pour [Diethylstilbestrol exposure in utero. Polemics about metroplasty. The pros]. Gynecol Obstet Fertil. 2007;35(9):826–31. French.
8. Aubriot FX, Hamou J, Dubuisson JB, Frydman R. Fernandez H. L'hystéroplastie d'agrandissement: à propos des résultats [Hysteroplasty for enlargement: apropos of the results]. Gynecol Obstet Fertil. 2001;29(12):888–93. French.
9. Baggish MS, Barbot J, Valle RF. Diagnositic and operative hysteroscopy. 2nd ed. St Louis: Mosby Inc; 1999. p. 105–6.
10. Barranger E, Gervaise A, Doumerc S, Fernandez H. Reproductive performance after hysteroscopic metroplasty in the hypoplastic uterus: a study of 29 cases. BJOG. 2002;109(12):1331–4.
11. Behnia R, Holley HS, Milad M. Successful early intervention in air embolism during hysteroscopy. J Clin Anesth. 1997;9(3):248–50.
12. Bettocchi S, Nappi L, Ceci O, Di Venere R, Santoro A, Selvaggi L. Vaginoscopic approach in office hysteroscopy-ten years experience. J Am Assoc Gynecol Laparosc. 2004;11(3):S69.
13. Bidziński M, Sobiczewski P. Ocena wartości histeroskopii oraz ultrasonografii dopplerowskiej dla monitorowania efektów leczenia wyłaczna radioterapia u chorych na raka trzonu macicy [evaluation of the value of hysteroscopy or doppler ultrasonography for monitoring treatment effects of radiotherapy in patients with cervix carcinoma]. Ginekol Pol. 2001;72(4):201–6.
14. Blitz MJ, Appelbaum H. Torsion of fallopian tube remnant associated with noncommunicating rudimentary horn in adolescent girl with unicornuate uterus. J Pediatr Adolesc Gynecol. 2014;27(5):e97–9.
15. Bracco PL, Vassallo AM, Armentano G. Complicanze infettive dopo isteroscopia diagnostica [Infectious complications of diagnostic hysteroscopy]. Minerva Ginecol. 1996;48(7–8):293–8. Italian.
16. Braun P, Grau FV, Pons RM, Enguix DP. Is hysterosalpingography able to diagnose all uterine malformations correctly? A retrospective study. Eur J Radiol. 2005;53(2):274–9.
17. Brooks PG, Serden SP. Hysteroscopic finding after unsuccessful dilatation and curettage for abnormal uterine bleeding. Am J Obstet Gynecol. 1988;158(6 Pt 1):1354–7.
18. Brucker SY, Rall K, Campo R, Oppelt P, Isaacson K. Treatment of congenital malformations. Semin Reprod Med. 2011;29(2):101–2.
19. Burke RK. Transcervical tubal catheterization utilizing flexible hysteroscopy is an effective method of treating cornual obstruction: a review of 120 cases. J Am Assoc Gynecol Laparosc. 1994;1:S5.
20. Capito C, Sarnacki S. Menstrual retention in a Robert's uterus. J Pediatr Adolesc Gynecol. 2009;22(5):e104-6.
21. Cicinelli E, Tinelli R, Colafiglio G, Pastore A, Mastrolia S, Lepera A, Clevin L. Reliability of narrow-band imaging (NBI) hysteroscopy: a comparative study. Fertil Steril. 2010;94(6):2303–7.
22. Clark TJ, Voit D, Gupta JK, Hyde C, Song F, Khan KS. Accuracy of hysteroscopy in the diagnosis of endometrial cancer and hyperplasia: a systematic quantitative review. JAMA. 2002;288(13):1610–21.
23. Colgan TJ, Shah R, Leyland N. Post-hysteroscopic ablation reaction: a histopathologic study of the effects of electrosurgical ablation. Int J Gynecol Pathol. 1999;18:325–31.
24. Cravello L, Porcu G, D'Ercole C, Roger V, Blanc B. Reconnaître et traiter une endométrite [Identification and treatment of endometritis]. Contracept Fertil Sex. 1997;25(7–8):585–6. French.
25. Dalal RJ, Pai HD, Palshetkar NP, Takhtani M, Pai RD, Saxena N. Hysteroscopic metroplasty in women with primary infertility and septate uterus: reproductive performance after surgery. J Reprod Med. 2012;57(1–2):13–6.
26. de Kroon CD, Jansen FW, Louwé LA, Dieben SW, van Houwelingen HC, Trimbos JB. Technology assessment of saline contrast hysterosonography. Am J Obstet Gynecol. 2003;188(4):945–9.
27. Deckardt R, Lueken RP, Gallinat A, Möller CP, Busche D, Nugent W, Salfelder A, Dohnke H, Hoffmeister U, Dewitt E, Hennefründ J, Hasskamp T, Krichbaum M, Maucher A, Auweiler U, Brökelmann J, Saks M, Füger T. Comparison of transvaginal ultrasound, hysteroscopy, and dilatation and curettage in the diagnosis of abnormal vaginal bleeding and intrauterine pathology in perimenopausal and postmenopausal women. J Am Assoc Gynecol Laparosc. 2002;9(3):277–82.
28. Descargues G, Lemercier E, David C, Genevois A, Lemoine JP, Marpeau L. Quelle exploration réaliser de première intention face aux méno-métrorragies? A propos d'une série prospective comparant l'hystérographie, l'hystérosonographie et l'hystéroscopie [Which initial tests should be performed to evaluate menometrorrhagias? A comparison of hysterography, transvaginal sonohysterography and hysteroscopy]. J Gynecol Obstet Biol Reprod (Paris). 2001;30(1):59–64. French.
29. Dotto JE, Lema B, Dotto JE Jr, Hamou J. Classification of microhysteroscopic images and their correlation with histologic diagnoses. J Am Assoc Gynecol Laparosc. 2003;10(2):233–46. https://doi.org/10.1016/s1074-3804(05)60305-2.
30. Dueholm M, Lundorf E, Hansen ES, Ledertoug S, Olesen F. Evaluation of the uterine cavity with magnetic resonance imaging, transvaginal sonography, hysterosonographic examination, and diagnostic hysteroscopy. Fertil Steril. 2001;76(2):350–7.
31. Dykes TA, Isler RJ, McLean AC. MR imaging of Asherman syndrome: total endometrial obliteration. J Comput Assist Tomogr. 1991;15(5):858–60.
32. El Saman AM, Shahin AY, Nasr A, Tawfik RM, Saadeldeen HS, Othman ER, Habib DM, Abdel-Aleem MA. Hybrid septate uterus, coexistence of bicornuate and septate varieties: a genuine report. J Obstet Gynaecol Res. 2012;38(11):1308–14.
33. Englund SE, Ingelman-Sundberg A, Westin B. Hysteroscopy in diagnosis and treatment of uterine bleeding. Gynecologia. 1957;143:217–22.
34. Engmann L, Schmidt D, Nulsen J, Maier D, Benadiva C. An unusual anatomic variation of a unicornuate uterus with normal external uterine morphology. Fertil Steril. 2004;82(4):950–3.
35. Epstein E, Ramirez A, Skoog L, Valentin L. Dilatation and curettage fails to detect most focal lesions in the uterine cavity in women with postmenopausal bleeding. Acta Obstet Gynecol Scand. 2001;80(12):1131–6.
36. Ercan CM, Ozturk M, Dede M, Coksuer H, Karasahin KE, Yenen MC. Narrow band imaging hysteroscopy: a new diagnostic technique in recurrent IVF failure? Arch Gynecol Obstet. 2011;283(Suppl 1):135–6.
37. Farrugia M, Nair M, Kontronis K. Narrow band imaging in endometriosis. J Minim Invasive Gynecol. 2007;14:393–4.
38. Feng L, Xia E, Duan H. Diagnosis of uterine diseases by combined hysteroscopy and ultrasonography. Zhonghua Fu Chan Ke Za Zhi. 1996;31(6):334–7. Chinese.
39. Folkman J. Tumor angiogenesis: therapeutic implications. N Engl Med. 1971;285:1182–6.
40. Fujii T, Nakamura M, Kameyama K, Saito M, Nishio H, Ohno A, Hirao N, Iwata T, Tsukazaki K, Aoki D. Digital colposcopy for the

diagnosis of cervical adenocarcinoma using a narrow band imaging system. Int J Gynecol Cancer. 2010;20(4):605–10.
41. Gabriel B, Fischer DC, Sergius G. Unruptured pregnancy in a non-communicating right fallopian tube associated with left unicornuate uterus: evidence for transperitoneal sperm and oocyte migration. Acta Obstet Gynecol Scand. 2002;81(1):91–2.
42. Garbin O, Ohl J, Bettahar-Lebugle K, Dellenbach P. Hysteroscopic metroplasty in diethylstilboestrol-exposed and hypoplastic uterus: a report on 24 cases. Hum Reprod. 1998;13(1O):2751–5.
43. Garuti G, De Giorgi O, Sambruni I, Cellani F, Luerti M. Prognostic significance of hysteroscopic imaging in endometrioid endometrial adenocarcinoma. Gynecol Oncol. 2001;81(3):408–13.
44. Garuti G, Sambruni I, Colonnelli M, Luerti M. Accuracy of hysteroscopy in predicting histopathology of endometrium in 1500 women. J Am Assoc Gynecol Laparosc. 2001;8(2):207–13.
45. Gebauer G, Hafner A, Siebzehnrübl E, Lang N. Role of hysteroscopy in detection and extraction of endometrial polyps: results of a prospective study. Am J Obstet Gynecol. 2001;184(2):59–63.
46. Gergolet M, Campo R, Verdenik I, Kenda Suster N, Gordts S, Gianaroli L. No clinical relevance of the height of fundal indentation in subseptate or arcuate uterus: a prospective study. Reprod Biomed Online. 2012;24(5):576–82.
47. Giacomucci E, Bellavia E, Sandri F, Farina A, Scagliarini G. Term delivery rate after hysteroscopic metroplasty in patients with recurrent spontaneous abortion and T-shaped, arcuate and septate uterus. Gynecol Obstet Investig. 2011;71(3):183–8.
48. Gimes DA. Diagnostic dilatation and curettage: a reappraisal. Am J Obstet Gynecol. 1982;142:1–6.
49. Gimpelson RJ, Rappold HO. A comparative study between panoramic hysteroscopy with directed biopsies and dilation and curettage. Am J Obstet Gynecol. 1988;158:489–92.
50. Golan A, Langer R, Neuman M, Wexler S, Segev E, David MP. Obstetric outcome in women with congenital uterine malformations. J Reprod Med. 1992;37(3):233–6.
51. Granberg S, Wikland M, Karlsson B, Norström A, Friberg LG. Endometrial thickness as measured by endovaginal ultrasonography for identifying endometrial abnormality. Am J Obstet Gynecol. 1991;164(1 Pt 1):47–52.
52. Grimbizis GF, Camus M, Tarlatzis BC, Bontis JN, Devroey P. Clinical implications of uterine malformations and hysteroscopic treatment results. Hum Reprod Update. 2001;7(2):161–74.
53. Gupta N, Mittal S, Dadhwal V, Misra R. A unique congenital mullerian anomaly: Robert's uterus. Arch Gynecol Obstet. 2007;276(6):641–3.
54. Handa Y, Hoshi N, Yamada H, Wada S, Kudo M, Tsuda K, Sagawa T, Fujimoto S. Tubal pregnancy in a unicornuate uterus with rudimentary horn: a case report. Fertil Steril. 1999;72(2):354–6.
55. Haydardedeoglu B, Simsek E, Kilicdag EB, Tarim E, Aslan E, Bagis T. A case of unicornuate uterus with ipsilateral ovarian and renal agenesis. Fertil Steril. 2006;85(3):750.e1–4.
56. Heinonen PK, Pystynen PP. Primary infertility and uterine anomalies. Fertil Steril. 1983;40(3):311–6.
57. Jayasinghe Y, Rane A, Stalewski H, Grover S. The presentation and early diagnosis of the rudimentary uterine horn. Obstet Gynecol. 2005;105(6):1456–67.
58. Katz Z, Ben-Arie A, Lurie S, Manor M, Insler V. Beneficial effect of hysteroscopic metroplasty on the reproductive outcome in a 'T-shaped' uterus. Gynecol Obstet Investig. 1996;41(1):41–3.
59. Kaufman RH. Structural changes of the genital tract associated with in utero exposure to diethylstilbestrol. Obstet Gynecol Annu. 1982;11:187–202.
60. Kobilková J, Kuzel D, Tóth D, Lojda Z. Aspiration cytology from the pouch of Douglas at hysteroscopy. Cytopathology. 2001;12(1):44–7.
61. Krampl E, Bourne T, Hurlen-Solbakken H, Istre O. Transvaginal ultrasonography sonohysterography and operative hysteroscopy for the evaluation of abnormal uterine bleeding. Acta Obstet Gynecol Scand. 2001;80(7):616–22.
62. Kuzel D, Tóth D, Kobilková J, Dohnalová A. Peritoneal washing cytology on fluid hysteroscopy and after curettage in women with endometrial carcinoma. Acta Cytol. 2001;45(6):931–5.
63. Lasmar RB, Barrozo PR, de Oliveira MA, Coutinho ES, Dias R. Validation of hysteroscopic view in cases of endometrial hyperplasia and cancer in patients with abnormal uterine bleeding. J Minim Invasive Gynecol. 2006;13(5):409–12.
64. Wei L, Enlan X. Application value of hysteroscopy in the diagnosis and treatment of infertility. J Pract Obstet Gynecol. 2008;24(1):50–1. Chinese.
65. Liatsikos SA, Tsikouras P, Souftas V, Ammari A, Prassopoulos P, Maroulis G, Liberis V. Diagnosis and laparoscopic management of a rudimentary uterine horn in a teenage girl, presenting with haematometra and severe endometriosis: our experience and review of literature. Minim Invasive Ther Allied Technol. 2010;19(4):241–7.
66. Lin BL, Ishikawa H, Komiyama M. Development of flexible outer sleeve for hystero-fiberscope. Japan J Gynecol Obstet Endosc. 1997;13:169–72. Japanese.
67. Lin BL, Miyamoto N, Tomomatsu M. Development of the scope of new resectoscope for women——application of transcervical resection and endometrial ablation (EA). J Japan Assoc Endos Matern. 1988;4:56–61. Japanese.
68. Lin BL, Miyamoto N, Yukamatsu M. Study and clinical application of flexible hysteroscope. Japan J Gynecol Obstet Endosc. 1987;39:649–54. Japanese.
69. Lin BL, Tomomatsu M, Su L. Development and clinical application of new hystero-fiberscope. Japan J Gynecol Obstet. 1988;40:1733–9. Japanese.
70. Lin BL, Iwata Y, Liu KH, Valle RF. Clinical applications of a new Fujinon operating fiberoptic hysteroscope. J Gynecol Surg. 1990;6(2):81–7.
71. Lin BL, Iwata Y, Valle RF. Clinical applications of Lin's forceps in flexible hysteroscopy. J Am Assoc Gynecol Laparosc. 1994;1(4 Pt 1):383–7.
72. Lin JC, Chen YO, Lin BL, Valle RF. Outcome of removal of intrauterine devices with flexible hysteroscopy in early pregnancy. J Gynecol Surg. 1993;9(4):195–200.
73. Lin PC. Reproductive outcomes in women with uterine anomalies. J Womens Health (Larchmt). 2004;13(1):33–9.
74. Liu X, Hu M, Lu P. Diagnostic criteria of transvaginal three-dimensional ultrasonography in differentiation between incomplete uterus septum and arcuate uterus. J Clin Ultras Med. 2013;15(8):580–1. Chinese.
75. Liu Y, Xia E, Zhang S. Analysis of diagnosis and treatment of 107 uterine septa. Chin J Pract Gynecol Obstet. 2002;18(9):559–60. Chinese.
76. Lolis DE, Paschopoulos M, Makrydimas G, Zikopoulos K, Sotiriadis A, Paraskevaidis E. Reproductive outcome after strassman metroplasty in women with a bicornuate uterus. J Reprod Med. 2005;50(5):297–301.
77. Luo Q, Chen X. Diagnostic value of hysteroscopy for postmenopausal uterine bleeding. Chin J Obstet Gynecol. 1989;24:150–2. Chinese.
78. Markham SM, Waterhouse TB. Structural anomalies of the reproductive tract. Curr Opin Obstet Gynecol. 1992;4(6):867–73.
79. Marty R, Valle RF. Eight year's experience performing procedures with flexible hysteroscopes. J Am Asso Gynecol Laparasc. 1995;3:113–8.
80. Meae J, Fox R. Severe pelvic infection following diagnostic hysteroscopy in women with pre-existing tubal disease. J Obstet Gynaecol. 2005;25(3):317.
81. Mizuno H, Gono K, Takehana S, Nonami T, Nakamura K. Narrow band imaging technique. Tech Gastrointest Endosc. 2003;5:78–81.

82. Moutos DM, Damewood MD, Schlaff WD, Rock JA. A comparison of the reproductive outcome between women with a unicornuate uterus and women with a didelphic uterus. Fertil Steril. 1992;58(1):88–93.
83. Mucowski SJ, Herndon CN, Rosen MP. The arcuate uterine anomaly: a critical appraisal of its diagnostic and clinical relevance. Obstet Gynecol Surv. 2010;65(7):449–54.
84. Murman RJ, Norris HJ. Endometrial carcinoma. In: Blaustein's pathology of the female genital tract. 3rd ed. New York: Springer; 1987. p. 338–9.
85. Nagel TC, Malo JW. Hysteroscopic metroplasty in the diethylstilbestrol exposed uterus and simillar nonfusion anomalies: effects on subsequent reproductive performance: a preliminary report. Fertil Steril. 1993;59(3):502–6.
86. Nagele F, O'Connor H, Davies A, Badawy A, Mohamed H, Magos A. 2500 Outpatient diagnostic hysteroscopies. Obstet Gynecol. 1996;88(1):87–92.
87. Nakhal RS, Cutner AS, Hall-Craggs M, Creighton SM. Remnant functioning cervical tissue after laparoscopic removal of cavitated noncommunicating rudimentary uterine horn. J Minim Invasive Gynecol. 2012;19(6):768–71.
88. Norment WB. The hysteroscope. Am J Obstet Gynecol. 1972;119:696–703.
89. Obermair A, Geramou M, Gucer F, Denison U, Graf AH, Kapshammer E, Neunteufel W, Frech I, Kaider A, Kainz C. Does hysteroscopy facilitate tumor cell dissemination? Incidence of peritoneal cytology from patients with early stage endometrial carcinoma following dilatation and curettage (D & C) versus hysteroscopy and D & C. Cancer. 2000;88(1):139–43.
90. Paschopoulos M, Lolis ED, Alamanos Y, Koliopoulos G, Paraskevaidis E. Vaginoscopic hysteroscopy and transvaginal sonography in the evaluation of patients with abnormal uterine bleeding. J Am Assoc Gynecol Laparosc. 2001;8(4):506–10.
91. Pelosi MA 3rd, Pelosi MA. Laparoscopic-assisted transvaginal metroplasty for the treatment of bicornuate uterus: a case study. Fertil Steril. 1996;65(4):886–90.
92. Porto R. Hysteroscopie. Encycl Med Chir Paris Gynecol. 1974;72:A10.
93. Raju KS. Should outpatient hysteroscopy replace conventional diagnostic dilatation and curettage in gynecologic practice. J Gynecol Surg. 1992;8:225–30.
94. Robert H. Asymmetrical bifidities with unilateral menstrual retention (apropos of 12 cases). Chirurgie. 1970;96(11):796–9.
95. Rogerson L, Bates J, Weston M, Duffy S. A comparison of outpatient hysteroscopy with saline infusion hysterosonography. BJOG. 2002;109(7):800–4.
96. Ross JW. Numerous indications for office flexible minihysteroscopy. J Am Assoc Gynecol Laparoscop. 2000;7:221–6.
97. Sano YK, Hamamoto MY. New diagnostic method based on color imaging using narrow band imaging (NBI) system for gastrointestinal tract. Gastrointest Endosc. 2001;53:AB125.
98. Seamark CJ. The demise of the D&C. Acta Obstet Gynecol Scand. 1997;76:65–8.
99. Sentilhes L, Sergent F, Roman H, Verspyck E, Marpeau L. Late complications of operative hysteroscopy: predicting patients at risk of uterine rupture during subsequent pregnancy. Eur J Obstet Gynecol Reprod Biol. 2005;120(2):134–8.
100. Singhal S, Agarwal U, Sharma D, Sirohiwal D. Pregnancy in asymmetric blind hemicavity of Robert's uterus--a previously unreported phenomenon. Eur J Obstet Gynecol Reprod Biol. 2003;107(1):93–5.
101. Sugaya S. Twin pregnancy after in vitro fertilization in a woman with a unicornuate uterus. Clin Exp Obstet Gynecol. 2010;37(4):317–8.
102. Surico D, Vigone A, Bonvini D, Tinelli R, Leo L, Surico N. Narrow-band imaging in diagnosis of endometrial cancer and hyperplasia: a new option? J Minim Invasive Gynecol. 2010;17(5):620–5.
103. Surico D, Viqone A, Leo L. Narrow band imaging in endometrial lesions. J Mini-Invasive Gynecol. 2009;16(2):9–10.
104. Osamu T, Akira M, Osamu S. Revaluations on diagnostic hysteroscopy prior to operation on endometrial carcinoma. Japan J Gynecol Obstet. 1991;43:622–6.
105. Shahrokh Tehraninejad E, Ghaffari F, Jahangiri N, Oroomiechiha M, Akhoond MR, Aziminekoo E. Reproductive outcome following hysteroscopic monopolar metroplasty: an analysis of 203 cases. Int J Fertil Steril. 2013;7(3):175–80.
106. Tinelli R, Surico D, Leo L, Pinto V, Surico N, Fusco A, Cicinelli MV, Meir YJ, Cicinelli E. Accuracy and efficacy of narrow-band imaging versus white light hysteroscopy for the diagnosis of endometrial cancer and hyperplasia: a multicenter controlled study. Menopause. 2011;18(9):1026–9.
107. Trimble CL, Kauderer J, Zaino R, Silverberg S, Lim PC, Burke JJ 2nd, Alberts D, Curtin J. Concurrent endometrial carcinoma in women with a biopsy diagnosis of atypical endometrial hyperplasia: a Gynecologic Oncology Group study. Cancer. 2006;106(4):812–9.
108. Unfried G, Wieser F, Albrecht A, Kaider A, Nagele F. Flexible versus rigid endoscopes for outpatient hysteroscopy: a prospective randomized clinical trial. Hum Reprod. 2001;16(1):168–71.
109. Valle RF. Office hysteroscopy (panoramic hysteroscopy). In: Baggish M, Barbot J, Valle RF, editors. Diagnostic and operative hysteroscopy. 2nd ed. St Louis: Mosby Inc; 1999. p. 181–2.
110. van Trotsenburg M, Wieser F, Nagele F. Diagnostic hysteroscopy for the investigation of abnormal uterine bleeding in premenopausal patients. Contrib Gynecol Obstet. 2000;20:21–6.
111. Velemir L, Gallot D, Jardon K, Mage G, Pouly JL. Uterine rupture at 26 weeks after metroplasty for uterine enlargement in diethylstilbestrol-exposed uterus: a case report. Eur J Obstet Gynecol Reprod Biol. 2008;138(2):243–4.
112. Wamsteker K, Blok SD. Diagnostic hysteroscopy: technique and documentation. In: Sutton C, Diamond MP, editors. Endoscopic surgery for gynecologists. 2nd ed. London: Wb Saunders Company; 1998. p. 515–6.
113. Xia EL, Duan HL, Feng L. Clinical application of fiber hysteroscope. J Pract Obstet Gynecol. 1998;14:106–7. Chinese.
114. Xia EL, Feng L, Duan HL, Duan H. Analysis of joint inspection of TV fiber hysteroscope and B ultrasound in 2441 patients. Chin J Pract Gynecol Obstet. 1998;14:31–3. Chinese.
115. Xia EL, Liu YH, Huang XW. Hysteroscopic orthomophia combined with laparoscopy for total bicornuate uterus-one case report. Chin J Clinic (Elect Edit). 2009;3(1):135–9. Chinese.
116. Xia EL, Liu YH, Ma N, Peng XB, Li YF, Xiao Y, Qu J. Three successful deliveries after hysteroscopic operations on T-shaped uterus and literatures review. Chin J Obstet Gynecol. 2013;48(6):457–9. Chinese.
117. Xia EL, Peng XB, Ma N, Li YF, Xiao Y, Guo Y, Qu J. Three successful pregnancies following hysteroscopic operations on unicornuate uterus and literatures review. Chin J Obstet Gynecol. 2013;45(9):689–91. Chinese.
118. Xia EL. Application of Idarac and indomethacin suppository in hysteroscopy. Chin J Med. 1993;28:23. Chinese.
119. Xia EL. Hysteroscopy and treatment of adenomyosis. Shand Med J. 2012;52:7–8. Chinese.

120. Zhang D, Luo Q, Duan H. Diagnostic value of abdominal ultrasound and hysteroscopy to postmenopausal uterine bleeding. Chin J Med Imag. 2000;8:30–1. Chinese.
121. Zlopasa G, Skrablin S, Kalafatić D, Banović V, Lesin J. Uterine anomalies and pregnancy outcome following resectoscope metroplasty. Int J Gynaecol Obstet. 2007;98(2):129–33.
122. Zorlu CG, Yalçin H, Ugur M, Ozden S, Kara-Soysal S, Gökmen O. Reproductive outcome after metroplasty. Int J Gynaecol Obstet. 1996;55(1):45–8.

Applications of Hysteroscopy in Gynecological Diseases

123. Alcazar JL, Laparte C. Comparative study of transvaginal ultrasonography and hysteroscopy in postmenopausal bleeding. Gynecol Obstet Investig. 1996;41:47–9.
124. Angioni S, Loddo A, Milano F, Piras B, Minerba L, Melis GB. Detection of benign intracavitary lesions in postmenopausal women with abnormal uterine bleeding: a prospective comparative study on outpatient hysteroscopy and blind biopsy. J Minim Invasive Gynecol. 2008;15(1):87–91.
125. Anteby E, Yagel S, Zacut D. Pseudoendometrial hyperplasia in women treated with tamoxifen. Ultrasound Obstet Gynecol. 1993;2(Suppl 1):64.
126. Antunes A Jr, Costa-Paiva L, Arthuso M, Costa JV, Pinto-Neto AM. Endometrial polyps in pre- and postmenopausal women: factors associated with malignancy. Maturitas. 2007;57(4):415–21.
127. Baldini B, Taddei GL, Tiso E, Visioli CB, Campos KJ, Napolitano AC, Tantini C. Valutazione isteroscopica dell'endometrio in 63 pazienti in post-menopausa trattate con tamoxifene per carcinoma della mammella [Hysteroscopic evaluation of the endometrium in 63 postmenopausal patients treated with tamoxifen for breast cancer]. Minerva Ginecol. 1996;48(6):259–62. Italian.
128. Barbot J, Parent B, Dubuisson JB. Hysteroscopie. Encycl Med Chir Paris Gynecol. 1984;72:A-10. French.
129. Barbot J. Hysteroscopy for abnormal bleeding. In: Baggish MS, Barbot J, Valle RF, editors. Diagnostic and operative hysteroscopy. 2nd ed. St Louis: Mosby Inc; 1999. p. 241–58.
130. Bibbo M, Kluskens L, Azizi F, Bartels PH, Wied GL, Yamauchi K, Herbst AL. Accuracy of three sampling technics for the diagnosis of endometrial cancer and hyperplasias. J Reprod Med. 1982;27(10):622–6.
131. Burke C, Kelehan P, Wingfield M. Unsuspected endometrial pathology in the subfertile woman. Ir Med J. 2007;100(5):466–9.
132. Burnett JE. Hysteroscopy-controlled curettage for endometrial polyps. Obstet Gynecol. 1964;24:621–5.
133. Campo R, Van Belle Y, Rombauts L, Brosens I, Gordts S. Office mini-hysteroscopy. Hum Reprod Update. 1999;5(1):73–81.
134. Carp HJ, Ben-Shlomo I, Mashiach S. What is the minimal uterine cavity needed for a normal pregnancy? An extreme case of Asherman syndrome. Fertil Steril. 1992;58(2):419–21.
135. Cicinelli E, Resta L, Nicoletti R, Tartagni M, Marinaccio M, Bulletti C, Colafiglio G. Detection of chronic endometritis at fluid hysteroscopy. J Minim Invasive Gynecol. 2005;12(6):514–8.
136. Cohen I, Azaria R, Bernheim J, Shapira J, Beyth Y. Risk factors of endometrial polyps resected from postmenopausal patients with breast carcinoma treated with tamoxifen. Cancer. 2001;92(5):1151–5.
137. Dumesic DA, Dhillon SS. A new approach to hysteroscopic cannulation of the follopian tube. J Gynecol Surg. 1991;7:7–9.
138. Féghali J, Bakar J, Mayenga JM, Ségard L, Hamou J, Driguez P, Belaisch-Allart J. Hystéroscopie systématique avant fécondation in vitro [Systematic hysteroscopy prior to in vitro fertilization]. Gynecol Obstet Fertil. 2003;31(2):127–31. French.
139. Feng LM, Xia EL, Duan HL, Zhang M. Joint diagnosis of uterine diseases using hysteroscope and ultrasonic waves. Chin J Obstet Gynecol. 1996;31:334–7. Chinese.
140. Gimpelson RJ, Rappold HO. A comparative study between panoramic hysteroscopy with directed biopsies and dilatation and curettage. Am J Obstet Gynecol. 1988;158:489–92.
141. Gumus II, Keskin EA, Kiliç E, Aker A, Kafali H, Turhan NO. Diagnostic value of hysteroscopy and hysterosonography in endometrial abnormalities in asymptomatic postmenopausal women. Arch Gynecol Obstet. 2008;278(3):241–4.
142. Gupta JK, Wilson S, Desai P, Hau C. How should we investigate women with postmenopausal bleeding? Acta Obstet Gynecol Scand. 1996;75(5):475–9.
143. Hamou J, Salat-Baroux J, Henrion R. Hysteroscopie et micro-hysteroscopie. Encycl Med Chir Paris Gynecol. 1985;72B(10):11–4.
144. Hucke J, De Bruyne F, Balan P. Hysteroscopy in infertility-diagnosis and treatment including falloposcopy. Contrib Gynecol Obstet. 2000;20:13–20.
145. Joelsson I, Levine RU, Moberger G. Hysteroscopy as an adjunct in determining the extent of carcinoma of the endometrium. Am J Obstet Gynecol. 1971;116:696–702.
146. Johnson JE. Hysterography and diagnostic curettage in carcinoma of the uterine body: an evaluation of diagnostic value and therapeutic implications in stage I and II. Acta Radiol. 1973;326(Suppl):1.
147. Karlsson B, Granberg S, Hellberg P, Wikland M. Comparative study of transvaginal sonography and hysteroscopy for the detection of pathologic endometrial lesions in women with postmenopausal bleeding. J Ultrasound Med. 1994;13(10):757–62.
148. Kerin J, Daykhovsky L, Segalowitz J, Surrey E, Anderson R, Stein A, Wade M, Grundfest W. Falloposcopy: a microendoscopic technique for visual exploration of the human fallopian tube from the uterotubal ostium to the fimbria using a transvaginal approach. Fertil Steril. 1990;54(3):390–400.
149. Liukko P, Grönroos M, Punnonen R, Kilkku P. Methods for evaluating the intrauterine location of carcinoma. Acta Obstet Gynecol Scand. 1979;58(3):275–8.
150. March CM, Isreal R, March AD. Hysteroscopic management of intrauterine adhesions. Am J Obstet Gynecol. 1978;130:653–7.
151. Marty R. Diagnostic fibrohysteroscopic evaluation of perimenopausal and postmenopausal uterine bleeding: a comparative study with Belgian and Japanese data. J Am Assoc Gynecol Laparosc. 1998;5:69–73.
152. Mourits MJ, Van der Zee AG, Willemse PH. Discrepancy between ultrasonography and hysteroscopy and histology of endometrium in postmenopausal breast cancer patients using tamoxifen. Gynecol Oncol. 1999;73:21–6.
153. Novy MJ, Thurmond AS, Patton P, Uchida BT, Rosch J. Diagnosis of cannula obstruction by transcervical fallopian tube cannulation. Fertil Steril. 1988;50:434–40.
154. O'Connell LP, Fries MH, Zeringue E, Brehm W. Triage of abnormal postmenopausal bleeding: a comparison of endometrial biopsy and transvaginal sonohysterography versus fractional curettage with hysteroscopy. Am J Obstet Gynecol. 1998;178(5):956–61.
155. Olaore JA, Shittu OB, Adewole IF. Intravesical Lippes loop following insertion for the treatment of Asherman's syndrome: a case report. Afr J Med Med Sci. 1999;28(3–4):207–8.
156. Pace S, Grassi A, Ferrero S, Figliolini N, Catania R, Labi FL, Pachì A, Figliolini M. Diagnostic methods of early detection of endometrial hyperplasia and cancer. Eur J Gynaecol Oncol. 1995;16(5):373–81.
157. Pansky M, Feingold M, Sagi R, Herman A, Schneider D, Halperin R. Diagnostic hysteroscopy as a primary tool in a basic infertility workup. JSLS. 2006;10(2):231–5.

158. Pantaleoni D. On endoscopic examination of the cavity of the womb. Med Press Cir. 1869;8:26–7.
159. Polisseni F, Bambirra EA, Camargos AF. Detection of chronic endometritis by diagnostic hysteroscopy in asymptomatic infertile patients. Gynecol Obstet Investig. 2003;55(4):205–10.
160. Salazar LOC, Mondrogon AHL. Catheterization of the ostium using hysteroscopy under laparoscopic guidance. Ginecol Obstet Mex. 1999;67:64–71.
161. Salzani A, Yela DA, Gabiatti JR, Bedone AJ, Monteiro IM. Prevalence of uterine synechia after abortion evacuation curettage. Sao Paulo Med J. 2007;125(5):261–4.
162. Sandridge DA, Councell RB, Thorp JM. Endometrial carcinoma arising within extensive intrauterine synechiae. Eur J Obstet Gynecol Reprod Biol. 1994;56(2):147–9.
163. Schenker JG, Margalioth EJ. Intrauterine adhesions: an updated appraisal. Fertil Steril. 1982;37:593–610.
164. Schenker JG. Etiology and therapeutic approach to synechia uteri. Eur J Obstet Gynecol Reprod Biol. 1996;65:109–13.
165. Sciarra JJ, Valle RF. Hysteroscopy: a clinical experience with 320 patients. Am J Obstet Gynecol. 1977;127:340–8.
166. Spiewankiewicz B, Stelmachow J, Sawicki W. Hysteroscopy in cases of cervical polyps. Eur J Gynaecol Oncol. 2003;24(1):67–9.
167. Stelmachow J. The role of hysteroscopy in gynecologic oncology. Gynecol Oncol. 1982;14:392.
168. Sugimoto O. Hysteroscopic diagnosis of endometrial carcinoma. A report of fifty-three cases examined at the Women's Clinic of Kyoto University Hospital. Am J Obstet Gynecol. 1975;121:105–13.
169. The American Fertility Society Classification of adnexal adhesions, distal tubal occlusion, tubal occlusion secondary to tubal ligation tubal pregnancies, mullerian anomalies and intrauterine adhesions. Fertil Steril. 1988;48:944.
170. Timmermans A, Gerritse MB, Opmeer BC, Jansen FW, Mol BW, Veersema S. Diagnostic accuracy of endometrial thickness to exclude polyps in women with postmenopausal bleeding. J Clin Ultrasound. 2008;36(5):286–90.
171. Tinelli R, Tinelli FG, Cicinelli E, Malvasi A, Tinelli A. The role of hysteroscopy with eye-directed biopsy in postmenopausal women with uterine bleeding and endometrial atrophy. Menopause. 2008;15(4 Pt 1):737–42.
172. Toki T, Oka K, Nakayama K, Oguchi O, Fujii S. A comparative study of pre-operative procedures to assess cervical invasion by endometrial carcinoma. Br J Obstet Gynaecol. 1998;105(5):512–6.
173. Valenzano M, Costantini S, Cucuccio S, Dugnani MC, Paoletti R, Ragni N. Use of hysterosonography in women with abnormal postmenopausal bleeding. Eur J Gynaecol Oncol. 1999;20(3):217–22.
174. Valle RF, Sciarra JJ. Intrauterine adhesions: hysteroscopic diagnosis, classification, treatment, and reproductive outcome. Am J Obstet Gynecol. 1988;158:1459–70.
175. Valle RF. Hysteroscopic evaluation of patients with abnormal uterine bleeding. Surg Gynecol Obstet. 1981;153:521–6.
176. Valle RF. Office hysteroscopy. Clin Obstet Gynecol. 1999;42:276–89.
177. Valli E, Zupi E, Marconi D, Vaquero E, Giovannini P, Lazzarin N, Romanini C. Hysteroscopic findings in 344 women with recurrent spontaneous abortion. J Am Assoc Gynecol Laparosc. 2001;8(3):398–401.
178. Valli E, Zupi E, Marconi D, Solima E, Nagar G, Romanini C. Outpatient diagnostic hysteroscopy. J Am Assoc Gynecol Laparosc. 1998;5(4):397–402.
179. Westendorp IC, Ankum WM, Mol BW, Vonk J. Prevalence of Asherman's syndrome after secondary removal of placental remnants or a repeat curettage for incomplete abortion. Hum Reprod. 1998;13(12):3347–50.
180. Zampi G, Colafranceschi M, Cucurnia MG, Ambrosi L. La diagnosi istologica delle neoplasie trofoblastiche nel materiale di raschiamento: difficoltà e significato prognostico [Histological diagnosis of trophoblastic neoplasms with curettage material: difficulties and prognostic value]. Arch De Vecchi Anat Patol. 1974;60(2):221–59. Italian.

9 Operative Hysteroscopy

Enlan Xia, Ning Ma, Xuebing Peng, Dan Yu, and Jie Zheng

9.1 An Overview of Hysteroscopic Electroresection Surgery

Enlan Xia

Since the early 1970s, hysteroscopic operation has been introduced in clinical practice. At the very beginning, it was only used for tubal sterilization, which was achieved by electrothermal damage to the interstitial portion of the fallopian tube under direct vision of hysteroscope. Due to its low efficacy and higher risk, it was replaced gradually by other methods of treatment. Thereafter, along with the innovation of technology and constant improvement on operative instruments and energy source, the hysteroscopic operation has also been constantly improved in its safety and efficacy. At present, this minimally invasive approach of hysteroscopy is gradually replacing the traditional traumatic hysterectomy via laparotomy to treat various intrauterine and cervical diseases. Due to its minimal invasiveness and high efficacy, it is recognized as the model of minimally invasive operations.

9.1.1 Facilities of Operating Room and Patient's Body Position

9.1.1.1 Operating Room

An operating room should be spacious, with the operating table put in its center, at the head end of which can be placed the anesthesia machine and monitors used by the anesthetists (Figs. 9.1a, b and 9.2a, b). On one side of the patient, there is a multi-layer cart or a medical crane tower with devices on it including monitor, electricity generator, lighting system, video camera, fluid distending pump, and other equipment. An ultrasound machine is always placed on the other side. In addition, there should be at least three sockets on the wall which can meet the demand of electricity for operation.

9.1.1.2 Gynecologic Operating Table: It Should Have the Following Functions

1. The patient's position can be changed quickly to meet the requirements of operation.
2. There should be enough space in the operating site so as to facilitate electroresection surgery smoothly.
3. There should be a complete distension fluid pump and collecting system so as to adapt to the needs of a large volume of fluid for electroresection surgery.
4. It should be able to support a wide range of gynecological operation in order that the operation can be immediately changed to laparotomy in case of complications.

9.1.1.3 Positioning

The modified lithotomy position is adopted, that is, supporting the legs with the relaxed knees, placing the thigh at an angle of 45° to the horizontal line, abducting legs as much as possible to increase the available space. Compared with full lithotomy position, this position is advantageous as it is associated with low intra-abdominal pressure, and so does not interference with breathing and providing easy access to the tubal ostia. If laparoscopy is performed at the same time, bend the thigh at 30° angle to the horizontal line so as not to affect the laparoscopic procedures. Generally, a slightly low head position is adopted.

9.1.1.4 Prevention of Infection

Prophylactic antibiotics given prior to operation are helpful. Intravenous antibiotics can be given once when operation starts.

9.1.2 Irrigating Methods in Hysteroscopic Operation

There are two kinds of pressure in uterine cavity during operations. One is hydrodynamic pressure, which is generated

E. Xia (✉) · N. Ma · X. Peng · D. Yu · J. Zheng
Hysteroscopy Center, Fuxing Hospital, Capital Medical University, Beijing, China

E. Xia (ed.), *Practical Manual of Hysteroscopy*, https://doi.org/10.1007/978-981-19-1332-7_9

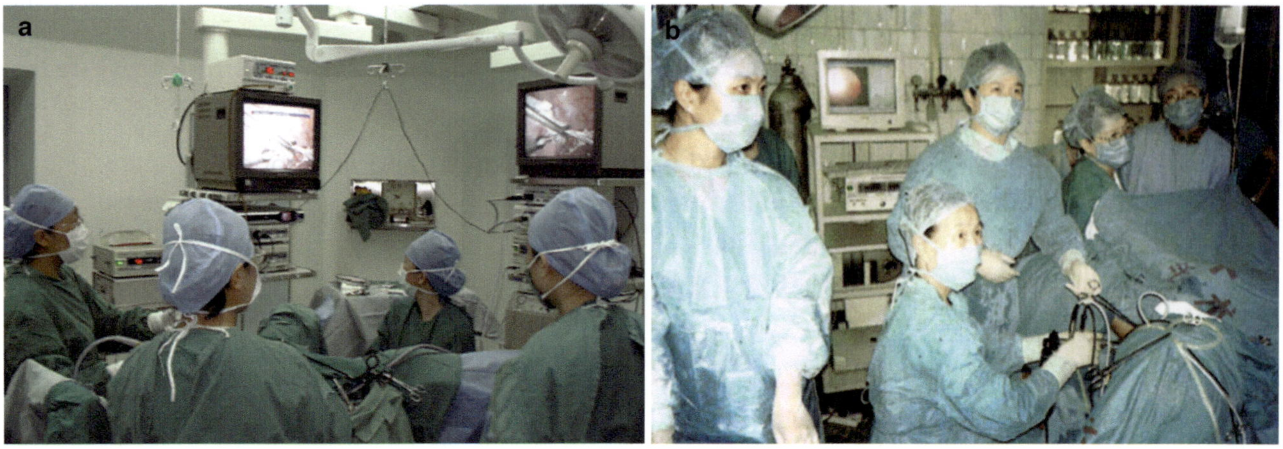

Fig. 9.1 (**a**, **b**) Full view of hysteroscopic operating room

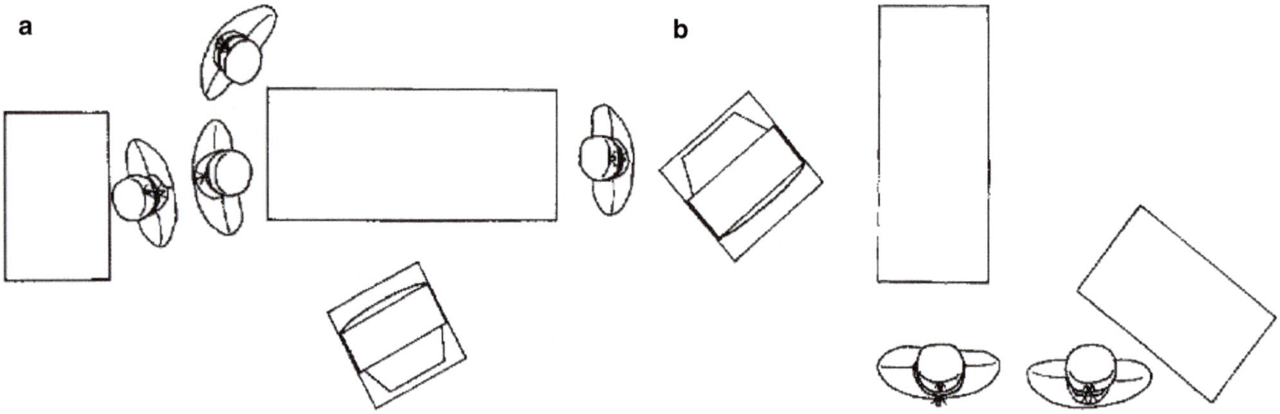

Fig. 9.2 (**a**, **b**) Layout of an operating room

when irrigation fluid is injected in through the endoscope sheath, and determined by the height of irrigation fluid and the hydrostatic pressure of the uterus itself. The other is the hydrostatic pressure, which is intrauterine pressure, and overcome by consuming hydrodynamic pressure.

9.1.2.1 High-Pressure Irrigating

High-pressure irrigating can help to gain clear vision for easier operation, but there might be an increased absorption of the irrigation fluid, hemodilution, and reduced blood sodium. Once uterine perforation occurs, the irrigation fluid may pass quickly through a perforation into the peritoneal cavity. One study on bladder irrigation showed that when the distance between the height of irrigation fluid and the patient's pubic symphysis was 120 cm, the intravesical pressures might be up to 100 cmH_2O (9.8 kPa); when the distance was 80 cm, the intravesical pressure could reach 80 cmH_2O (7.85 kPa) (1 cmH_2O = 98.1 Pa = 0.736 mmHg). If an automatic uterine distending pump is applied, the pressure can be adjusted to the level of mean arterial blood pressure. When operation starts, if thickening endometrium or large submucous myomas occupy the uterine cavity, uterine septum or intrauterine adhesions narrow the cavity, the flow of irrigation fluid into the uterine cavity would be reduced. In cases of obscure vision, the inflow pressure could be increased, but should only be temporary.

9.1.2.2 Low-Pressure Irrigating

The device containing irrigation fluid is placed at a height of 40–60 cm above pubic symphysis. According to the research on the intravesical electroresection, if an aspiration device suctioning irrigation fluid out is used, it indicates that the pressure within the bladder is almost equal to intravenous pressure, thus the volume of fluid that enters into the body via the cutting surface will decrease greatly. But if there is no continuous aspiration, the intravesical pressure is up to 30–60 cmH_2O (2.94–5.88 kPa); if the height of the device is less than 30 cm and there is no aspiration device, the intravesical pressure is up to 30 cmH_2O (2.94 kPa); if there is a continuous suction, the intravesical pressure may be lower than 30 cmH_2O (2.94 kPa), often at 10 cmH_2O (0.98 kPa). Studies on intravesical electroresection suggested that irrigation pressure should be maintained at a level of less than 60 cmH_2O (5.88 kPa), which made it relatively safe.

9.1.2.3 Selection of Irrigation Fluid

Irrigation fluid has distending, irrigating, and cooling effects. The types of irrigation fluid, the intraoperative irrigation pressure and flow rate, and the operation time are all factors affecting the safety of operations. An isotonic nonelectrolyte solution is required for hysteroscopic monopolar electroresection so that the electric current generated when cutting or coagulating may be focused on the contact part of electrode. During operations, the irrigation fluid can be absorbed into the circulation via open veins of the resection surface or into peritoneal cavity via fallopian tubes. Since nonelectrolyte solution is not physiologic fluid, if a great deal of irrigation fluid enters the blood circulation, an increase in blood volume and a change in electrolyte composition would result, which may cause systemic pathophysiological changes and a variety of clinical conditions, such as acute left heart failure, pulmonary edema, water intoxication, and hyponatremia. The typical symptoms are dysphoria, nausea and vomiting, slow response, oliguria and kidney failure, etc. In 1955, Hagstrom named it syndromes of the transurethral resection of the prostate (TURPS). When selecting irrigation fluid, one should take its viscosity, transparency, osmotic pressure, pH, half-life, internal metabolism, and end products into consideration, and also set a reasonable irrigation pressure. The commonly used solutions are 1.5% glycine, 5% mannitol, 3% sorbitol, 5% glucose and Cytol solution, etc.

9.1.3 Cervical Ripening Before Operative Hysteroscopy

Generally, the cervical canal can accommodate an instrument of up to 3–5 mm, but the outer sheath of a resectoscope is 8–9 mm in diameter, so the cervix should be dilated more than the diameter of the resectoscope before hysteroscopic operations. Difficult dilatation often occurs during operative hysteroscopy in cervix without ripening. Inadequate cervical dilatation may lead to cervical laceration, hemorrhage, increased difficulties in operation, prolonged operating time, and increases the risk of uterine perforation and creating a false passage, with a correspondent increase of TURP syndrome. If the cervix is ripened and adequately softened before hysteroscopic operation cervical dilatation to a diameter larger than that of the outer sheath of the hysteroscope could be easily achieved, which could significantly lessen the risk of cervical laceration or uterine perforation, decrease the absorption of distention fluid during operations, and limit the occurrence of TURP syndrome.

So far, commonly used methods for cervical ripening in clinic include osmotic dilators, misoprostol, and phloroglucinol.

9.1.3.1 Osmotic Dilators

Osmotic dilators are used for mechanical pretreatment of cervix, including laminaria tent, silicone rod, and so on, which are generally inserted into the cervical canal at night before the surgical procedures. With a combination of mechanical stimulation, together with the dilator expanding after absorption of water, the cervix is softened and cervical canal is dilated (Fig. 9.3a, b). This method is effective and has been commonly used in clinic.

9.1.3.2 Misoprostol

Misoprostol is a synthetic prostaglandin E1 analog, which promotes both the degradation of the collagenous fibers in cervical connective tissues and the release of collagenase and elastase, so that it can soften, ripen, and expand the cervix in a short period of time. Usually, it is taken orally or is

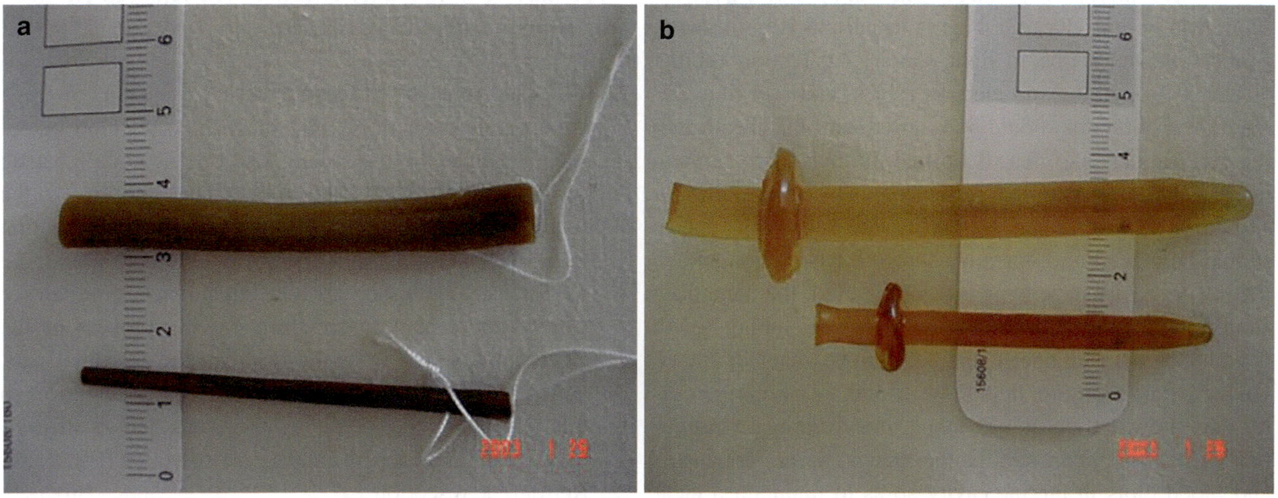

Fig. 9.3 Osmotic dilators. (**a**) Laminaria tent (the one below is of the original size, and the above is of an expanded size after absorption of water). (**b**) Silicone rod (the one below is of the original size, and the above is of an expanded size after absorption of water)

inserted into posterior fornix of the vagina at night or 4 h prior to the operation with a recommended dose of 200–400 μg. This method is applicable for cases with difficult insertion of osmotic dilators.

9.1.3.3 Phloroglucinol

Phloroglucinol is a pro-muscle non-atropine non papaverine class pure smooth muscle antispasmodic agent, which acts on smooth muscles of gastrointestinal and genitourinary tracts. Some research indicated that phloroglucinol was superior to lidocaine and misoprostol in both the analgesic effect during hysteroscopic diagnosis and the degree of cervical distensibility and softness, with side effects less than that of lidocaine and misoprostol. As one of the methods applied for ripening and softening the cervix prior to hysteroscopic operation, phloroglucinol injection is especially useful in long hysteroscopic resections and cases with medical complications such as hypertension and glaucoma, etc. It is applied by intravenous drip 15–30 min prior to operation at a dose of 40–80 mg, which should be finished in 5 min. The duration of action is around 45 min.

9.1.4 Techniques of Hysteroscopic Electroresection

9.1.4.1 Operating Procedures

The patient is put in lithotomy position on the operating table, then the external genitalia is routinely sterilized. If cervical dilator had been inserted, the assistant should wear sterile gloves and remove it from the vagina, which can avoid the likelihood of fracture of cervical dilator caused by other methods or partial retention in the uterine cavity. Then sterilize the vagina and cervix, place vaginal speculum and hold anterior lip of the cervix with a cervical clamp, dilate the cervical internal os gradually until an operative hysteroscope can be introduced, which is usually 9–10 mm. Next, connect the telescope to light sources, distention tubing, electricity generator and electric cables, and working element. The obturator should be inserted with the sheath into the cervical canal so that its tip may further dilate cervical internal os. After entering the uterine cavity, the obturator should be taken out, and then telescope and its handpiece should be placed into operative sheath for operation. When the low viscosity distending medium is used, the handpiece should be connected to two polyethylene tubings with 2.4 mm of outer diameter and 1.6 mm of inner diameter. Under certain pressure, fluid flows in and out of uterine cavity via inflow and outflow channel, thus forming a continuous cycle, which can remove the mucus, tissue fragments, and blood clots in uterine cavity so as to maintain a clear vision in operational field. For discontinuous flow hysteroscope, it has only one channel for both inlet flow and manipulation. The inlet flow tubing must be removed before inserting operative instrument. When camera system is used, the adapter connecting to the camera system should be assembled to the eyepiece of telescope, and the camera focal length, white balance, and focus should be adjusted before the insertion of the hysteroscope. The correct orientation of hysteroscope during insertion is that the fiberoptic cable faces downwards and fore-oblique view faces upwards. After the adapter is connected to the telescope, they should always maintain a certain direction and cannot be rotated, instead the hysteroscope should be rotated clockwise or anticlockwise to observe the lateral wall of uterine cavity. In addition, when using low viscosity distending medium, keep in mind that a plastic collection bag is placed under the patient's hips to collect the intraoperative outflow of liquid, thus the fluid deficit can be accurately measured and the floor will not become wet.

Before placing the endoscopic sheath with its telescope, manipulator handpiece, and active electrode into uterine cavity, be sure to open the inlet and outlet valve, and empty the gas out of inflow tubing. When operation begins, switch on continuous flow system, and then irrigate and flush intrauterine tissue fragments and blood clots. Sometimes, if there is a larger blood clot blocking the sheath and hindering the circulation of irrigation fluid, the hand piece and telescope and the inner sheath must be taken out and cleaned. After achieving a clear vision of the uterine cavity and connecting to the electric cables, the operation can be started. Monopolar circuit is usually used for hysteroscopic resection. Before switching on the power for operation, remember to check the return electrode attached to the patient to ensure a complete current circuit. In this condition, nonelectrolyte solution must be used as distention medium, some active electrodes should be prepared for spare use so that an active electrode can be replaced in time when tissue fragments adhere to the electrode making it no longer effective. The replaced electrode can be reused after being cleaned.

9.1.4.2 Techniques of Resecting

1. Anterograde resection: First push the wire loop out of sheath and extend to a distant position (Fig. 9.4a), then do parallel cutting from distal to proximal according to the requirements on the depth and length of resection (Fig. 9.4b, c). It is one of the most commonly used techniques, easy to master and convenient to use. One can see clearly under hysteroscope the moving process of the electric wire loop from the distal to the proximal part, which means one would not cut other tissues in error, so it is safe. When the sheath is pulled back, longer strips of tissues can be cut out by anterograde resection (Fig. 9.4d).
2. Retrograde resection

   This method is opposite to the above. Place the electric wire loop at proximal site of the tissues to be removed

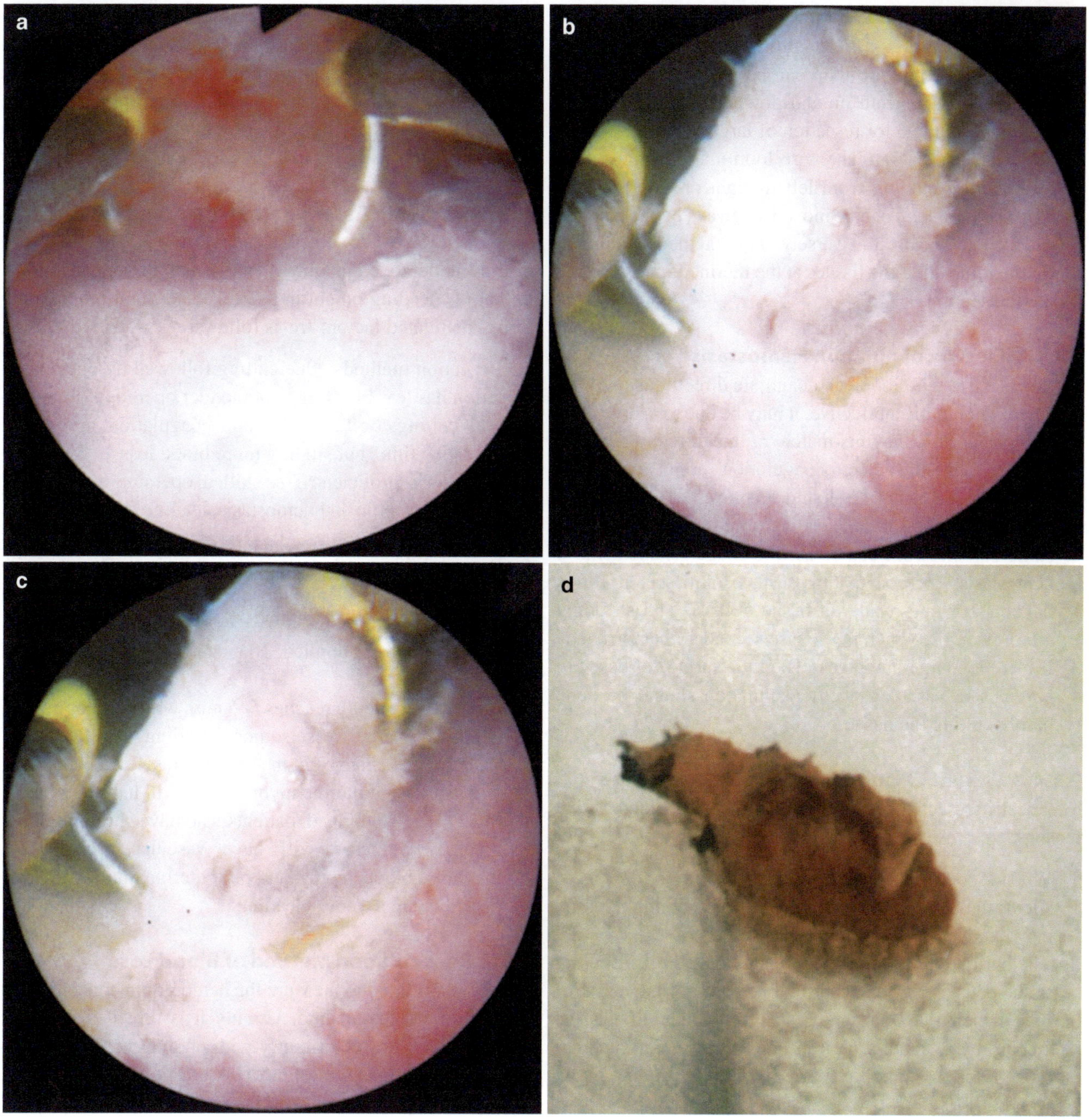

Fig. 9.4 Anterograde resection. (**a**) First push the wire loop out of sheath and extend to the distant position. (**b**) According to the requirements on the cutting depth and length, do parallel cutting from distal to proximal. (**c**) According to the requirements on the cutting depth and length, do parallel cutting from distal to proximal. (**d**) The excised long strips of tissues with wire loop

and then extend it to the distal site gradually while cutting, and cut it off when the electric wire loop reaches the edge of tissues to be resected. Retrograde resection is not easy. Doctors cannot see the distance clearly when electric wire loop moves towards distal end, and carries a higher risk of pushing the wire loop into the uterine wall, even causing perforation. This method is applicable to the following situations.

(a) There are more tissues to be excised, and one cannot see clearly the boundary of distal end.
(b) When the lower border of tissue to be excised is floating and is difficult to resect anterogradely.
(c) If some residual tissues are still connected to the surface and floating, resecting anterogradely would be more difficult and retrograde resection should be applied.

3. Vertical resection: It is cutting by electric wire loop from top to bottom. If vertical cutting method is adopted, movement of the wire loop can be achieved by moving the endoscopic sheath up and down appropriately. This method is suitable for resection of large fibroids.
4. Transverse resection: The wire loop makes a transverse resection by moving from left to right or from right to left. The wire loop can be moved sideways by moving the endoscopic sheath transversely. This method is suitable for the removal of the tissues at the uterine fundus and the uterine septum.

9.1.4.3 Electrocoagulation Hemostasis

1. The electric wire loop can coagulate directly at spraying bleeding point. If ineffective, it may be due to a large arterial bleeder or the mis-match of the direction of the bleeder and the electrocoagulation application site. Therefore the electrode should be moved to coagulate at the adjacent sites of the bleeding point.
2. Rollerball electrode can be used to coagulate and achieve hemostasis. On coagulating surface of tissue, it forms flake eschar and results in tissue necrosis and shedding after operation, which may cause secondary hemorrhage.
3. If there are large blood vessels on the surface of tissue to be excised, vascular electrocoagulation should be done before cutting the tissue.

9.1.4.4 Weight Calculation of the Excised Tissue

The electric resected tissue is light-weighted, which has two reasons.

1. When a complete tissue is cut into a dozen or dozens of slices, the blood, lymph and tissue fluid within the tissue may exude and be lost from its surface.
2. The burning effect caused by coagulating and cutting on tissue cells can cause dehydration of tissue and cell atrophy, which may further reduce the weight of tissues. According to reports on transurethral resection of prostate, different authors reported the reduction of tissue weight differently. It was 20% less in Einarsson's report, but about 30% less in Ruter's report. Yang in China applied electric cutting on isolated prostate, then weighed the tissue, and found that the weight reduced by 23–42.8%, the average being 32.6%.

The weight assessment of the excised tissues is also related to the following factors: (1) resection methods: A thin slice is lighter than a thick slice. (2) current selection: excised tissue is lighter with blended current than that with single cutting. (3) coagulation method: The loss in weight by aimless excessive electrocoagulation is limited, and the excised tissue will be lighter with target electrocoagulation hemostasis.

9.1.4.5 Volume Assessment of Bleeding in Hysteroscopic Resection

The intraoperative bleeding quantity mainly depends on the extent of bleeding on cutting surface and duration of resection. The related factors are as follows:

1. Resection methods: One cutting followed by one coagulation has less bleeding, but a longer operation time; several cuttings followed by one coagulation have short operative time, but slightly more blood loss.
2. Operator's proficiency: A skilled operator may be fast both in resection and hemostasis, leading to the reduction of bleeding.
3. Resected tissue volume and resection time: The more tissue volume excised and the longer resection time it takes, the more bleeding it will have.
4. Types of current applied: Blended current produces less bleeding.
5. If the cutting depth reaches 5–6 mm, which might involve deeper and larger vessels, more bleeding would occur.
6. Pathological changes in the uterine muscles: The patients with fibrosis of uterine myometrium will have less bleeding. On the other hand, patients who have chronic inflammatory in uterus will have vascular proliferation, increased blood supply, and poor uterine muscle contraction, leading to more bleeding.

9.1.4.6 Calculation Method of Blood Loss

It is more accurate to measure the hemoglobin concentration in outflow irrigation fluid. Usually it is direct colorimetry with test tubes, or colorimetry with photoelectric colorimeter. The minimum depth value of general colorimeter is 40%, but the hemoglobin concentrations in outflow irrigation fluid is far below this level, so a special colorimeter is needed for colorimetric determination. A commonly used method is: firstly, measure hemoglobin concentration directly in outflow irrigation fluid (%); then compare the patient's preexisting hemoglobin concentration, and the blood loss volume can be obtained. Calculation formula is as follows.

$$\text{Blood loss volume}(\text{mL}) = \text{the total irrigation volume}(\text{mL}) \times \text{measured hemoglobin}(\text{g}) \times 100 / \text{Original hemoglobin}(\text{g})$$

In recent years, plasma bipolar resectoscope has been introduced. Its cutting and coagulating are consistent with those by monopolar resectoscope mentioned above, except that a second cutting on the cut surface will be more difficult due to the increase in local current impedance. Distention with normal saline is used when bipolar electric cutting is applied, which will reduce the occurrence of hyponatremia. In 2007, Ho et al. made a prospective comparison study of transurethral resection of the prostate among 52 patients in the monopolar group and 48 in the transcervical resection in saline (TCRis) group. The results showed that mean resection time and mean weight of resected tissues were comparable in both groups. The mean postoperative serum Na^+ was reduced, being 3.2 mmol/L in TURis group and 10.7 mmol/L in monopolar group ($p < 0.05$). However, there was no statistical difference in the drop of Hb level following operation between the two groups. It was concluded that it was safer to use bipolar resection.

9.2 Transcervical Resection of Endometrium and Endometrial Ablation

Enlan Xia

Transcervical resection of endometrium (TCRE) is a procedure using high-frequency electricity via hysteroscopic resectoscope with usually monopolar loop electrode to resect functional and basal layers of endometrium as well as underlying 2–3 mm myometrium. Endometrial ablation is a hysteroscopic procedure with high-frequency electricity to coagulate endometrial tissues using monopolar rollerball, or to vaporize endometrial tissues using vaporizing electrode. Both operations lead to postoperative non-regeneration of endometrium, and decreased menstruation or amenorrhea, thus being the preferred surgical treatment for AUB. Before the advent of hysteroscopy, hysterectomy was the treatment for women with intractable uterine bleeding who was irresponsive to the conservative hormonal treatment and D&C. Some information about cases of hysterectomy in the United States from 1975 to 1995 can be seen in Table 9.1. According to data counted by New York State Department of Health, 35,000 cases of hysterectomy were performed each year, among which 10–15% were due to the abnormal menstruation without obvious organic diseases. Hysterectomy is a radical measure to eliminate the symptoms, but it is an open surgery, which requires hospitalization of the patient for days and obviously restricts patients' activities, and the patient may also suffer from complications. Since 1980s, TCRE and EA have reasonably replaced hysterectomy.

In 1981, Goldrath from the United States first applied hysteroscopic endometrial ablation by laser (HEAL; or endometrial laser ablation, ELA), and thereafter, many countries started to carry out this operation. In 1987, De Cherney from the United States used a prostate resectoscope to stop the bleeding successfully in a woman who suffered from intractable uterine bleeding due to hematological diseases, thus creating a precedent in the treatment of endometrial disease by resectoscope. In 1988, Lin from Japan reported on the electrocoagulation of the endometrium by rollerball electrode in the treatment of uterine hemorrhage, which achieved satisfactory results and was named endometrial ablation (EA). Now some scholars called it rollerball endometrial ablation (RBA). In 1989, Magos from the United Kingdom published his preliminary report on hysteroscopic resection of endometrium with loop electrode for treatment of menorrhagia in 16 women who had systemic diseases. After a 6-month follow-up, the effective rate was reported to be 86%, and this procedure was named transcervical resection of endometrium (TCRE). At present, there have been no uniform Chinese translation of TCRE or EA; the commonly used nouns for it are endometrial resection, and endometrial ablation. Other translations for it include endometrial deletion, endometrial dissection, endometrial incision, endometrial coagulation, endometrial destruction, etc. Scholars abroad hold that when the endometrium was resected in this procedure, the partial superficial myometrium was also removed, so it should be called endomyometrial resection. Some scholars performed the procedure of resection to a depth of 4–5 mm beneath the endometrium, resecting deeper in myometrium layer.

Table 9.1 Cases of hysterectomy in the USA from 1975 to 1995

Year	Number of cases	Rate(‰)
1975	724,000	0.6
1976	701,000	8.1
1979	639,000	7.1
1981	674,000	7.3
1983	673,000	6.9
1985	670,000	6.7
1987	653,000	4.6
1988	578,000	4.3
1989	541,000	–
1990	591,000	–
1991	546,000	–
1992	580,000	–
1993	562,000	–
1994	556,000	–
1995	583,000	–

9.2.1 Indications and Contraindications of TCRE or EA

The main indications for TCRE are abnormal uterine bleeding (AUB). Generally, the anovulatory AUB is called dysfunctional uterine bleeding, referred in brief to as DUB; the ovulatory AUB is termed menometrorrhagia. The latter can be divided into menorrhagia and metrorrhagia, the former refers to a heavy bleeding during menstrual period in women with ovulation; the latter refers to irregular bleeding in the ovulatory period. The most common causes for menorrhagia are uterine fibroids, endometrial polyps, and adenomyosis. Moreover, there are some other causes like IUD with no progesterone, hypothyroidism, idiopathic menorrhagia, blood diseases, and other serious medical diseases such as renal failure, liver failure, leukemia, and drug-induced menorrhagia. Any factors resulting in a normal estrogen secretion but anovulation may lead to endometrial hyperplasia manifesting as DUB, which should be regarded as pathological, except for physiological bleeding after menarche or within 1 year of perimenopause. During HEAL in destroying the endometrium, the endometrial polyps and small aggregated submucous myomas can also be removed. EA can be used not only to remove the endometrium, but it can also remove the coexistent endometrial polyps and small fibroids if using vaporizing electrode. The evolution process of TCRE indications can be divided into four stages. Stage 1: In 1987, De cherney used TCRE to treat women who had chronic and intractable bleeding but were reluctant to remove the uterus, or women who couldn't tolerate the removal of uterus due to serious medical problems. Stage 2: Because of its positive effects on hemostasis, in 1989, Magos extended this operation to the patients who had menorrhagia and who voluntarily underwent the operation. A submucous myoma with its size <3 cm can be removed at the time of endometrial surgery if the uterus is not bigger than 8 weeks. Stage 3: In 1990, Shar reported the application of it for sterilization; Garry reported using it to perform partial resection of endometrium for women without AUB, which was intended to reduce the blood loss physiologically and "normalize" the menses. Stage 4: due to the proficient techniques, and improved equipment, in 1991, Magos proposed its operative indications should be extended to the uterus with size <12 weeks, the length of the cavity <14 cm, and submucous myoma with no regard to its size and location. Generally, the operator may grasp the following standards.

9.2.1.1 Indications

1. Intractable abnormal uterine bleeding, excluding malignant diseases
2. Uterus ≤9 weeks of gestational size, uterine cavity ≤12 cm in length
3. Submucous myoma ≤5 cm in diameter
4. No requirements for fertility

9.2.1.2 Contraindications

1. Cervical canal could not be dilated adequately because of cervical scars.
2. The hysteroscope cannot reach the uterine fundus due to extreme bending of the uterus.
3. Acute stage of reproductive tract infection.
4. Acute period of heart, liver, or kidney failure.
5. The patient has no good psychology bearing capacity for the fact that this operation is to relieve symptoms rather than a radical cure.

Recently, Neis and Brandner pointed out that patients with dysmenorrhea plus uterus >10 weeks were highly likely to have adenomyosis. Surgery of TCRE in these patients had an increased failure rate, therefore it should be considered as a relative contraindication of TCRE.

9.2.2 Preoperative Preparations

9.2.2.1 Inquiry of a Detailed History

1. Age: Most patients with dysfunctional uterine bleeding and uterine myoma are over 40 years old, and these patients are selected for TCRE. The younger women should receive treatment with sex hormone in advance for three reasons: (1) DUB are often temporary endocrine disorders, and may recover spontaneously; (2) future fertility problems; (3) high recurrence rate. However, surgery should be considered if a patient has the following conditions: having no response or having too serious side effects to drug therapy; having already been sterilized or bleeding seriously which has obviously affected family life and work; being the only alternative to hysterectomy in young girls with blood diseases. Surgery in women close-to-menopause must be prudent, because it may be possible for them to avoid any surgery. Therefore, all the perimenopausal women must have examinations of the LH/FSH and estrogen level to conclude an appropriate treatment. When postmenopausal women are treated by hormone replacement therapy, most regular withdrawal bleeding is periodic and with less volume. If the bleeding was excessive, hysteroscopic surgery might be considered, but endometrial atypical hyperplasia or malignant diseases should be excluded.
2. Parity: At the beginning of surgery, a cervix shall be dilated at least to Hegar 10 for the placement of the resectoscope. Most patients who underwent TCRE have already given birth to children, thus their cervixes are easy to be dilated. For a woman with no parturition, the cervix may be long and hard to be dilated, thus preoperative insertion of cervical dilator or application of prostaglandins shall be done to soften the cervix.
3. Adaptability of the operation: TCRE requires shorter operating time than hysterectomy, and is advantageous to those with medical complications. The operation can be performed under local anesthesia, but it is still difficult in the lithotomy position for the patient with severe respiratory disease. There are the same situations for patients with bronchitis, emphysema, coronary heart disease, hypertension (especially heart enlargement),

insulin-dependent diabetes mellitus, and chronic kidney disease with impaired renal function. Pathological obesity can cause complications of anesthesia and surgery. The ordinary obese women are more suitable for TCRE than hysterectomy, because the complications of the latter are more serious. The main problems of obese patients are that the size of the uterus and the pelvic lesions are not easy to identify, and circulatory complications resulting from excess absorption of distention fluid must be avoided. Therefore, inflow and outflow volume must be precisely measured, and even if the difference between the inflow and outflow volume (referred to as fluid deficit) is very small, the operator should also be reminded and suspend operation when necessary.

4. Fertility: Successful TCRE can lead to amenorrhea and infertility, which can be accepted by elderly women. But to young women, the operator should explain carefully and make them understand fully the consequences of infertility and ectopic pregnancy. In contrast, patients who have postoperative cyclical bleeding, regardless of the amounts, have the risk of pregnancy. If the embryo is implanted in the residual endometrial island, the pregnancy may continue to full term, but placenta may develop pathological adhesion, even deep implantation, leading to difficulty in the third stage of labor. Such patients should take proper contraceptive measures. It may be more appropriate that TCRE is performed along with laparoscopic sterilization procedures, which can also prevent the irrigation fluid entering into the peritoneal cavity.
5. Bleeding: Prior to operation, to determine whether or not the patient is suitable for operation, the amount of blood loss is crucial, but is very difficult to measure accurately, because it is usually estimated subjectively and may be different monthly. Generally, if the patient has the following conditions, she is obviously to be diagnosed menorrhagia: there are blood clots or blood gushing, which the perineal pad cannot absorb quickly and needs to be changed every hour; one may feel tired and short of breath, or postmenstrual weakness and fatigue, and low hemoglobin with small cell anemia due to blood loss. The periodical menorrhagia may respond well to TCRE, but if the patient has midcycle bleeding, premenstrual or postmenstrual bleeding, or spotting, she should be examined carefully so as to exclude endometrial hyperplasia or endometrial polyp.
6. Pain: Massive bleeding is often accompanied by severe cramps caused by passing blood clots from the uterus. Pain is often confined to lower abdomen, suprapubic and upper thighs, usually bilateral and rarely unilateral, and the lower lumbar pain is rarely seen. The pain can reach a climax when blood clots pass through the cervical canal. The cramp cannot be distinguished from the pain caused by submucous myoma or endometrial polyp. On the contrary, hemorrhage resulting from the endocrine disorders is almost painless, or produces premenstrual abdominal pain possibly due to the pelvic congestion. Patients with endometriosis or adenomyosis can have lower abdominal pain before, during, or after menstruation, often accompanied by severe low lumbar pain. A careful differential diagnosis should be made because TCRE cannot cure these two diseases. After TCRE, the patient may have no menstruation, but if severe dysmenorrhea persists, the only management is to remove the uterus.
7. Past history of uterine operation: If the patient had uterine operations such as repeated curettage or myomectomy, especially opening the cavity or a history of cesarean, it is possible to have intraoperative uterine perforation, so close attention should be paid.

9.2.2.2 Comprehensive Examinations

1. General physical examination: A general physical examination includes blood pressure, pulse, and a complete systemic checkup. If necessary, doctors in relevant departments should be invited for consultation.
2. Gynecologic examination: For a patient with DUB, the uterus is small but movable and the ovaries are not enlarged. If the uterus is retroverted and fixed, or there is a mass in the adnexa, endometriosis should be suspected. The posterior fornix tenderness or nodules may be suspected to be uterine rectovaginal septum endometriosis lesions, and a bulky uterus with tenderness indicates that it may be adenomyosis. Adenomyosis can sometimes proliferate in the local portion of uterus, thus enlarging the uterus, which appears to be fibroids under internal examination. If the uterus is irregular in shape, it could be multiple myomas, which were difficult to be treated with laser or resectoscope. The most suitable operation of hysteroscopy is submucous myoma, which should be suspected when the cervix external os tries to open wide to discharge myoma. The pelvic inflammatory disease can induce abdominal pain, uterine tenderness, and menstrual cycle changes, which cannot be cured by TCRE. One important single index of successful TCRE is the size of the uterus, especially the length of uterine cavity. If the size of the uterus is >12 weeks of gestation or the length of uterine cavity >12 cm, operation would be very difficult, operation time would be prolonged, and the risk of cardiac vascular overload would be increased as well.
3. Laboratory tests: Laboratory tests include hemoglobin, white blood cell counts, platelet, bleeding and coagulation time, blood type; urine routine tests; liver and renal functions; Australia antigen (HBsAg), anti HCV antibody; cervical smear test; vaginal thrush, cleanliness and trichomonas inspection under microscope; if necessary, erythrocyte sedimentation rate, blood glucose, lipids, and sex hormone; thyroid function including T3, T4, TSH, etc.

4. Special examinations: Special examinations include electrocardiogram, chest X-ray and other internal medical diseases are suspected.
5. Ultrasound examinations: Ultrasound examinations help to understand the size, shape, location and echoes of the uterus, the direction of endometrial line, thickness of endometrium, and whether adnexa have mass or not. For those who take drugs to inhibit endometrial hyperplasia, transvaginal ultrasonography can be used to estimate endometrial thickness. An enlarged ovary indicates endometriosis, or benign/malignant tumors.
6. Hysteroscopy: Hysteroscopy can provide accurate information about the size and shape of the uterus, whether there are polyps and submucous myoma, inner bulge and deformation, etc. It can also estimate the possibility and difficulty of operation, and locate the site for biopsy.
7. Endometrial biopsy: 25% of the perimenopausal women with moderate and severe atypical hyperplasia of endometrium may develop into endometrial adenocarcinoma. Therefore, an endometrial biopsy must be taken so as to exclude endometrial atypical hyperplasia and endometrial carcinoma.

9.2.2.3 Consultation

Good consultation is the key to make the patients satisfied, so the operator should explain in detail the infertility, hemorrhage, short-term complications, long-term prognosis, likelihood of recurrence, final demand for hysterectomy, and other issues. The operator should also point out that although abnormal bleeding may be significantly improved post-operation, a small percentage of women will have or develop cyclical abdominal pains, which may be very troublesome. The patients should also be warned that even though there are reports about the postoperative improvement of primary dysmenorrhea and premenstrual tension syndrome, it has no therapeutic effect on the premenstrual tension syndrome because this operation doesn't affect ovarian function. There should be written explanations to guarantee that the patients are fully informed about the operation and a formal consent should be obtained from the patients.

9.2.2.4 Endometrial Pretreatment

The detailed endometrial pretreatment can be seen in Chap. 4.

1. Medical Pretreatment: Medical pretreatment can induce atrophy of the endometrium, decrease the uterine volume, and reduce vascular regeneration, thus leading to a shortened operation time, less bleeding, and an easy operation, and it can be done at any time during the menstrual cycle. The reduction of absorption of intraoperative distending fluid improves the safety and efficacy of the operation. The commonly used drugs are: (1) danazol: 200 mg orally, 2–4 times/day, for 4–12 weeks; (2) nemestran: 2.5 mg orally, 2 times/week, for 4–12 weeks; (3) GnRH analogs: the currently used GnRH analogs are goserelin 3.6 mg, intradermal deposit; triptorelin 3.75 mg, intramuscular injection; leuprorelin 3.75 mg, subcutaneous injection. All of them should be administered once every 28 days, 1–3 times. Among these agents, GnRH analogs are the best but very expensive.

   Donnez et al. reported that after the use of GnRH analogs, both the endometrium and stroma atrophied sharply, which was only 1.6 mm in thickness, but 3.4 mm in those who didn't take it. Romer reported that for those who had preoperative application of GnRH analogs, the postoperative amenorrhea rate was 42%, while only 24% for those who didn't use GnRH analogs. Sowter et al. made a randomized comparison of pretreatment effects of danazol, progesterone, and GnRH analogs on endometrium in intraoperative endometrial thickness, operation time, operation difficulty, irrigating fluid absorption rate and incidence of complications, postoperative amenorrhea rate, menstrual volume, dysmenorrhea, and further treatments. The results were that GnRH analogs had a more lasting effect than danazol in endometrial atrophy, while there was minimal difference in other intraoperative and postoperative outcomes. Steffensen and Hahn (1999) studied the effects of TCRE on the incidence of fluid overload, factors associated with fluid overload, and relationship between the fluid overload and long-term prognosis. The result was that in 265 patients with 1.5% glycine solution as irrigation fluid, fluid absorption was increased after the application of GnRH-a in patients treated with TCRE ($P < 0.007$), and also removal of myoma during the procedure of TCRE ($P < 0.0001$). Rai et al. carried a study investigating whether or not the medical pretreatment of endometrium helped to improve long-term outcome of TCRE. Three endometrial pretreatment agents were used in comparison: danazol, leuprolide, and nafarelin. The cases without pretreatment were included as control group. The measures for determination of prognosis included thickness of the resected endometrium and myometrium; stage of the endometrium at the time of operation; the situation of menstruation and patient satisfaction 1 year after surgery. Of the three pretreatment groups studied, compared with control group, danazol and nafarelin produced significantly endometrial thinner (thin and moderate thickness). Danazol showed the greatest ability to induce atrophy of the endometrial glands and stroma and produced a high amenorrhea rate (no statistical difference). Compared with the control group, there were no significant differences in amenorrhea rate in any pretreatment group, and if the procedure was done at the proliferative phase of the menstrual cycle, there would be no significant improvement in clinical outcome for patients in pretreatment groups.

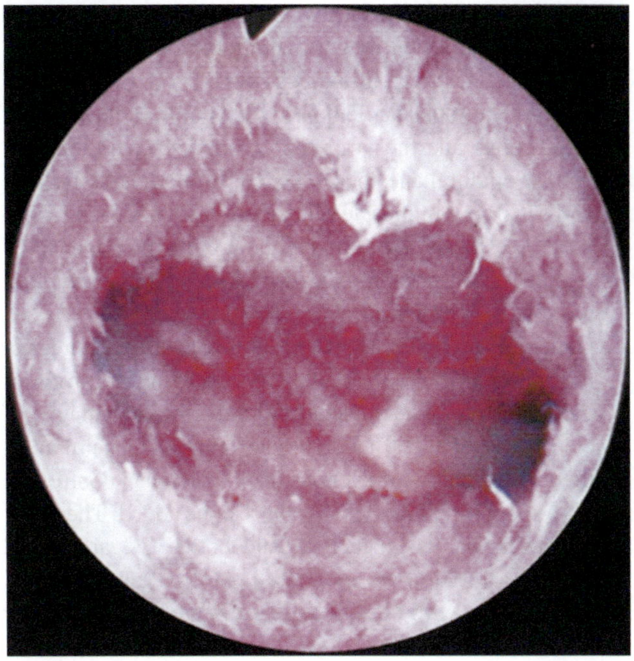

Fig. 9.5 Uterine cavity and endometrium after negative pressure suction

2. Mechanical pretreatment: Prior to TCRE, negative pressure suction can thin the endometrium (Fig. 9.5). Maia reported that the postoperative improvement of menstruation in patients who received endometrial mechanical pretreatment was the same as those who received drug pretreatment.

9.2.2.5 Timing of Surgery

1. After menstruation, the endometrium is at its early proliferative phase and is <4 mm in thickness, which is the ideal time for operation.
2. For those who have had endometrial pretreatment, the endometrium has been thinned or atrophied, operation may also be performed at any phase of nonmenstrual period.
3. If there is an uncontrollable bleeding, emergency operation should be done.

9.2.2.6 Preparation on the Day Before Operation

1. Sterilization of hysteroscope and its equipment.
2. A cervical osmotic dilator or a laminaria tent is inserted into the cervical canal on the night before operation to soften and expand the cervix (Fig. 9.6). When the insertion is difficult, 100 mg rectal indomethacin can be used. Misoprostol 200–400 mg can also be given orally or be inserted into posterior fornix of the vagina at night before or 4 h prior to the operation. Alternatively, phloroglucinol injection can be applied by intravenous drip 30 min prior to operation with a dosage of 80 mg.

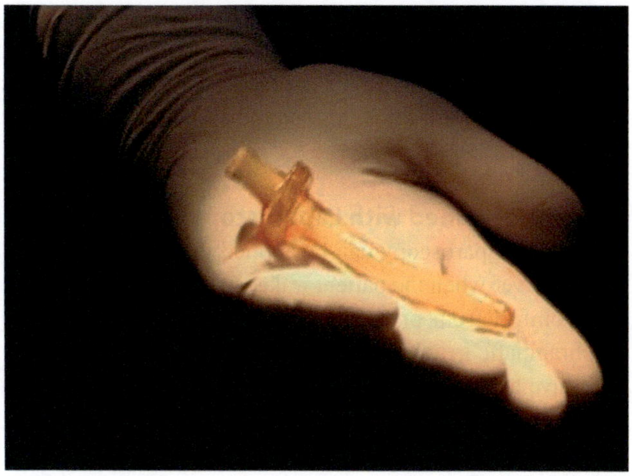

Fig. 9.6 After being inserted into the cervical canal on the night before operation and followed by removal prior to operation, an osmotic dilator is seen expanded and widened

9.2.2.7 Preparation on Operation Day

On the morning of operation, the patient should have fasted and keep a full bladder so as to facilitate ultrasonographic monitoring during operation.

9.2.2.8 Operator's Preparation

Prior to operation, the operator should check all the main devices and their functions, such as transparency of the telescope, flexibility of the operating handle, and whether connectors of current generator, cables, and the electrode plate are loose or not. If there is malfunction with the equipment, it should be repaired timely prior to operation. Meanwhile, there should be a sufficient number of wire loops for spare use.

9.2.3 Anesthesia

The distribution of pelvic nerves is very suitable for local or regional block anesthesia, under which TCRE can be performed. If operation time is short, intravenous anesthesia can be applied (see Chap. 7). When choosing anesthesia, one should take the following points into consideration.

9.2.3.1 Choice of the Patients

Some patients require general anesthesia because they would not like to be conscious in the operating room. Some prefer local anesthesia because they fear general anesthesia or want to see the operating video.

9.2.3.2 Choice of the Operators

It depends on the degree of training, experience of regional anesthesia, and desire of the operators in free talk with the students.

9.2.3.3 Operation Duration

The effect of local anesthesia may last a maximum of 2 h. If the expected operation time lasts over a long period, such as surgery with multiple or large myomas, general anesthesia will be more suitable.

9.2.3.4 Combined with Laparoscopy

Diagnostic laparoscopy can be applied under local anesthesia. However when the patient wakes up, she may experience a discomfort from pneumoperitoneum, shoulder pain from diaphragmatic irritation, and breathing difficulties caused by excessive head-down position. If so, she should choose general anesthesia.

9.2.3.5 Day Surgery

A patient performing TCRE often doesn't need to stay overnight in hospital, especially when the pain and nausea are controlled. She can be discharged from hospital after surgery on the same day. It is suggested that a day surgery should be performed under intravenous anesthesia, and operation time shouldn't exceed more than 30 min.

9.2.3.6 Complications

Epidural anesthesia should not be applied in patients with arrhythmia and hypertension. The commonly used anesthetic methods are as follows.

1. Local anesthesia: The afference of the pain originated from the uterus is transmitted from the cervix into the spinal cord through the second, third, and fourth sacral nerve root. The operator may administer cervical block anesthesia or intrauterine injection with 1% lignocaine containing adrenalin 1:200,000. After the hysteroscope is placed in the uterine cavity through the dilated cervix, a fine needle is inserted under direct vision into the proximal muscle of uterine cornua, and a local anesthetic about 40 mL is injected. Uterus and cervix are rich in blood vessels, so in the process of injection, the operator should always suck back in order to avoid intravascular injection. Although when the above tests are negative, sometimes the patient may also have transient bradycardia, elevated systolic blood pressure, and pale face, so the patient should have ECG and blood pressure monitoring. Patients with mental stress may be given sedatives.
2. Compound intravenous anesthesia: Intravenous anesthetics like ketamine, propofol, and sevoflurane are injected via veins, acting on the central nerve system through blood circulation, and produce general anesthesia. This method is rapid in induction, has no stimulation to the respiratory tract, and can make the patients feel comfortable. But it is poor in muscle relaxation, so it is not suitable for patients with narrow and small uterine cavity and having an expected longer operation time. Hypertension and glaucoma are contraindications.
3. Epidural anesthesia: Patients with contraindications of intravenous anesthesia or more complex operation may choose epidural anesthesia, which is functionally reliable and satisfying in muscle relaxation. With a top-up in epidural anesthesia, the time can be arbitrarily extended. If operation can be completed within 1 h, single epidural anesthesia is preferred.
4. General anesthesia: It is a closed-circuit inhalation anesthesia with tracheal intubation following intravenous induction with succinylcholine, with the advantages of clear airway and sufficient oxygen supply. General anesthetic is given by intravenous drip, which can control the drop speed, and muscle relaxants can be added. The effect of anesthesia is satisfactory, and both ECG and blood oxygen saturation are monitored, so it is relatively safe. The patients with obesity and hernia are not suitable for this anesthesia.

9.2.4 Operative Procedures

9.2.4.1 Transcervical Resection of Endometrium (TCRE)

1. Examine the uterine cavity. If endometrium is found to be thick, suction aspiration can be first used (Fig. 9.7a, b).
2. First, use vertical electric wire loop to resect the uterine fundus (Fig. 9.8). The resecting depth reaches the superficial myometrium beneath the endometrium (Fig. 9.9), with a blended current at the power 80–100 W. Rollerball electrode can also be used to coagulate the endometrium of uterine fundus (Fig. 9.10).
3. A 90° wire loop or band electrode (Figs. 9.11 and 9.12a, b) is used to resect the endometrium and underlying superficial myometrium starting from uterine fundus in a downward direction and clockwise or counterclockwise sequence (Figs. 9.13, 9.14, 9.15, 9.16, and 9.17).
4. The resection of the endometrium and the superficial myometrium usually starts with the posterior wall of the uterus in sequence (Fig. 9.18). If the resection terminates at 1 cm lower to the internal os of the uterus, it is called total resection of endometrium (Fig. 9.19); if it terminates at 1 cm higher above the internal os, it is called partial resection of endometrium (Fig. 9.20).
5. Generally, the moveable distance of electric wire loop is confined within 2.5 cm when resecting. First resect upper 1/3 of the endometrium, then resect middle 1/3. If total endometrial resection is to be done, lower 1/3 of the

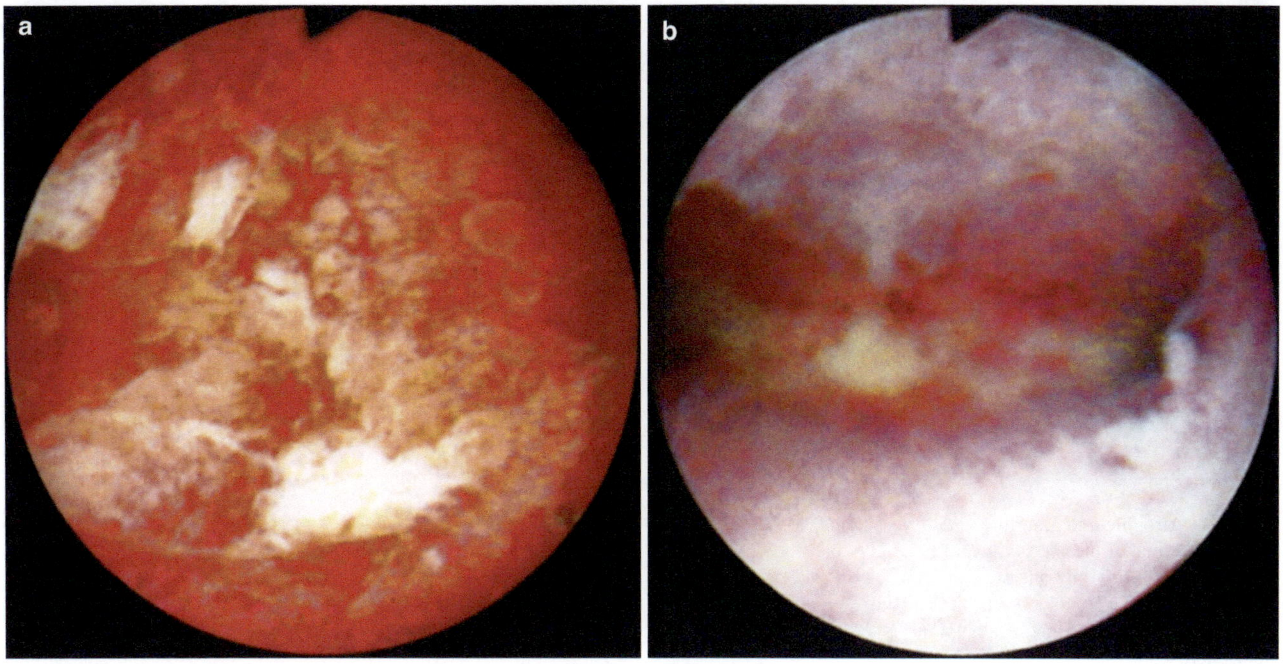

Fig. 9.7 (**a**) Uterine cavity prior to TCRE. (**b**) Uterine cavity after suction aspiration

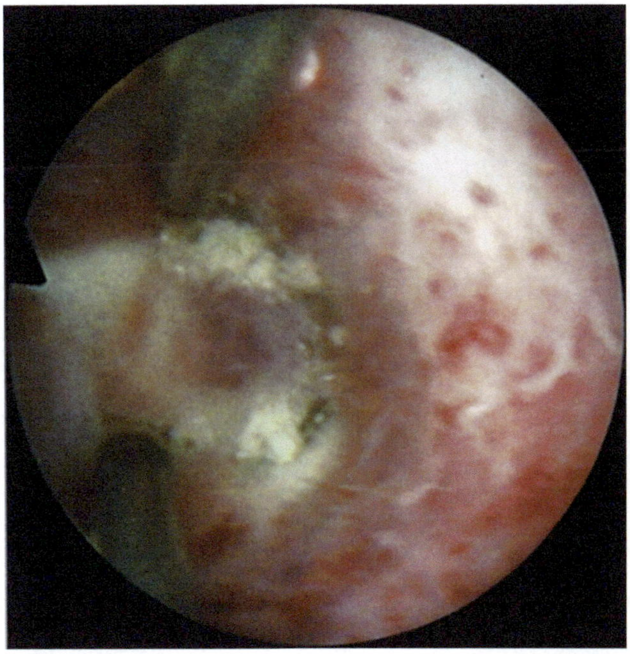

Fig. 9.8 The endometrium at the uterine fundus resected by vertical wire loop

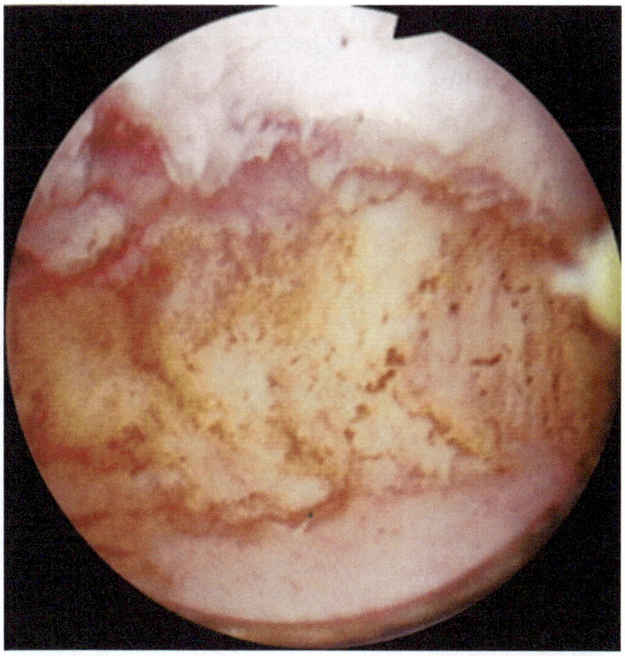

Fig. 9.9 Superficial myometrium visible after resection of the endometrium at the uterine fundus

endometrium shall be resected until the cervical canal. When an oval forceps is used to clamp tissue fragments out of the cavity, the irrigation fluid has to flow out through the cervical canal. Each distension and collapse of uterine cavity may cause uterine bleeding, thus obstructing the hysteroscopic view. A small amount of endometrial fragments can be discharged spontaneously several days after operation. If the operator is skilled and proficient, he can increase the resecting distance through moving the resectoscope from the uterine fundus to the

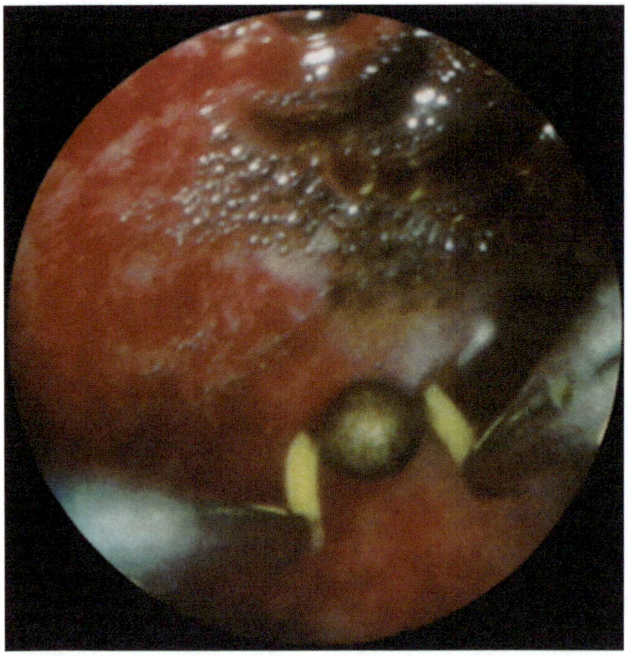

Fig. 9.10 The endometrium at the uterine fundus electrocoagulated by rollerball electrode

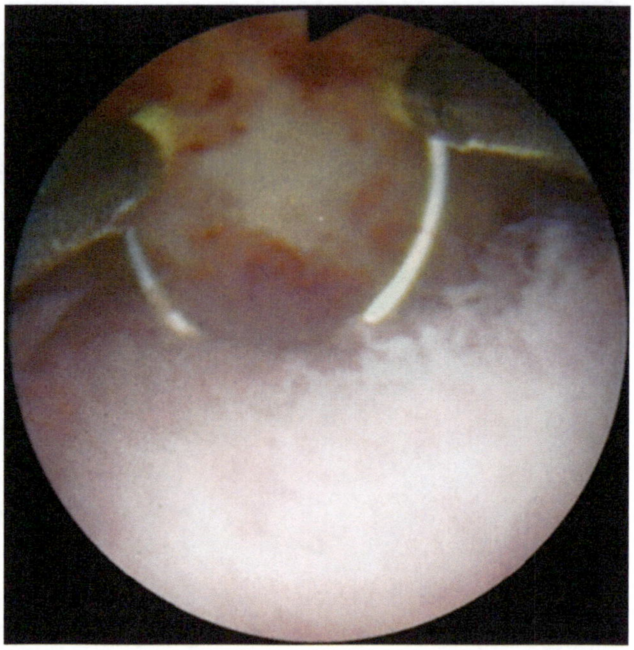

Fig. 9.11 Wire loop electrode

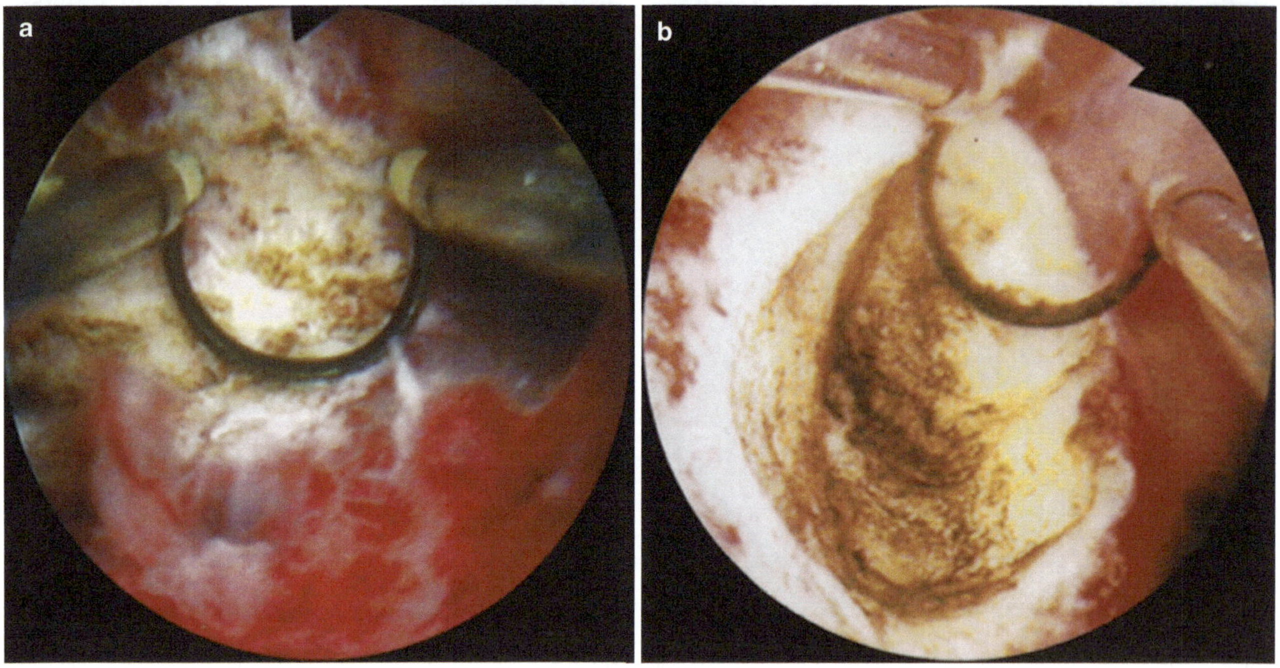

Fig. 9.12 (**a**, **b**) Band electrode

uterine isthmus, and take out the resected tissue strips immediately (Figs. 9.21 and 9.22).

6. After the uterine cavity is made empty, put back resectoscope to check and resect the residual endometrium.
7. When operation ends, reduce the uterine distension pressure, observe the bleeding points (Fig. 9.23), apply electrocoagulation hemostasis (Fig. 9.24), and examine the uterine cavity (Fig. 9.25).
8. After TCRE, a light brown cylinder-shape uterine cavity is formed (Fig. 9.26).
9. Endometrial fragments are sent for histological examination.

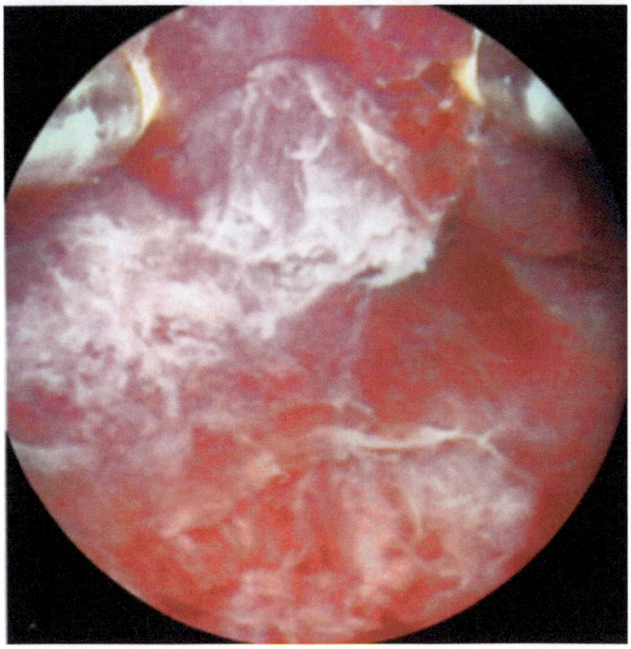

Fig. 9.13 Electric resection of the endometrium and superficial myometrium on the posterior wall

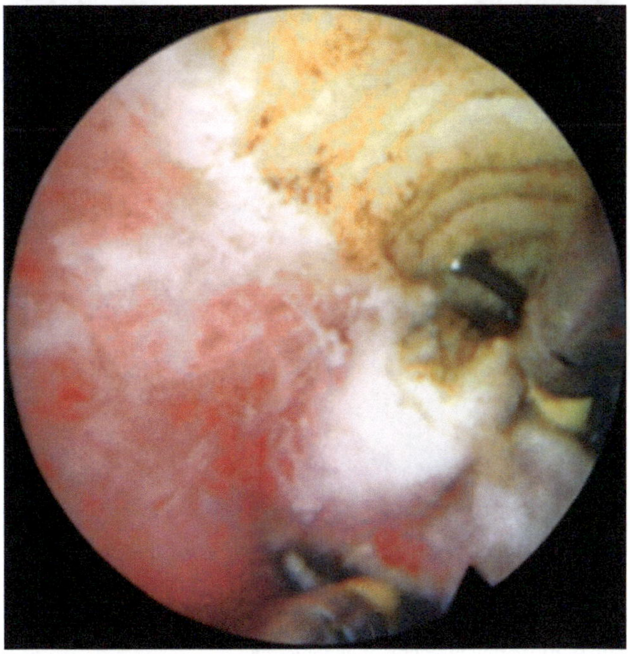

Fig. 9.14 Electric resection on right lateral wall

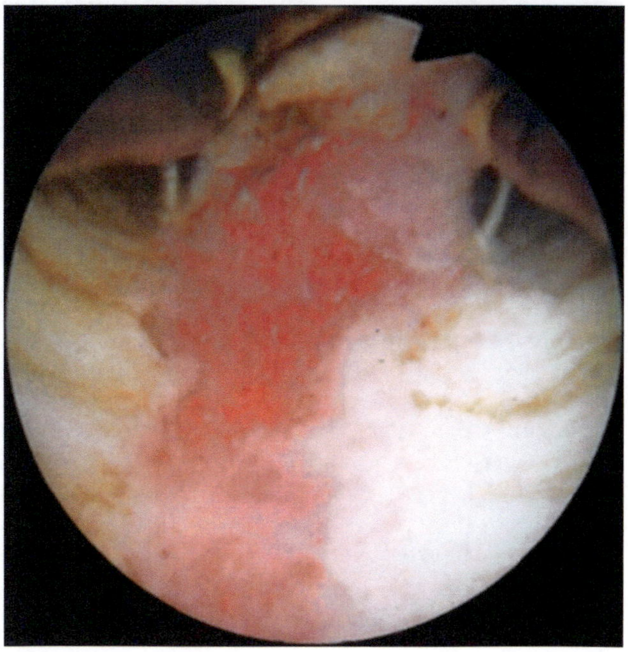

Fig. 9.15 Electric resection on right posterior wall

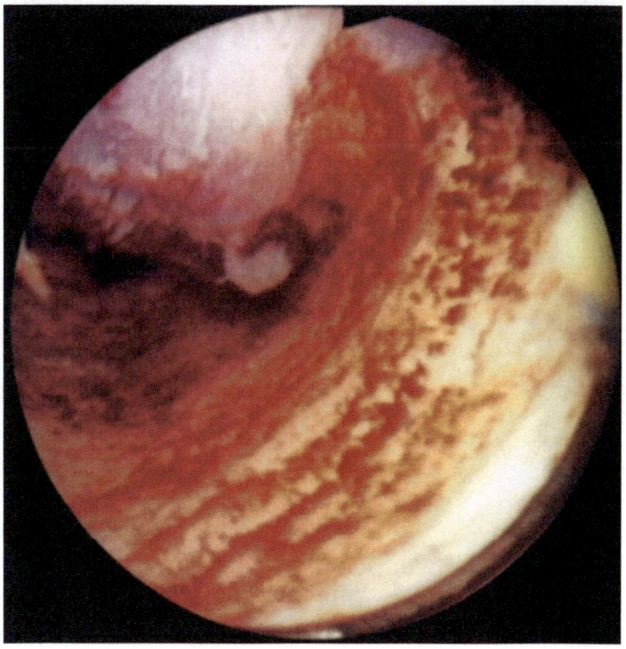

Fig. 9.16 Electric resection from posterior wall to left lateral wall and then anterior wall

10. Precautions
    (a) It is the most difficult to resect and easy to perforate at the fundus, therefore the operator must be very careful not to push the wire loop too far into the myometrium, especially in resecting the endometrium of both cornua, which are the thinnest of myometrial layer. When resecting the endometrium at the uterine cornua, the operator must shave shallow each time until all the endometrium is removed completely, which is at a less risk of perforation than that of a deep cut.

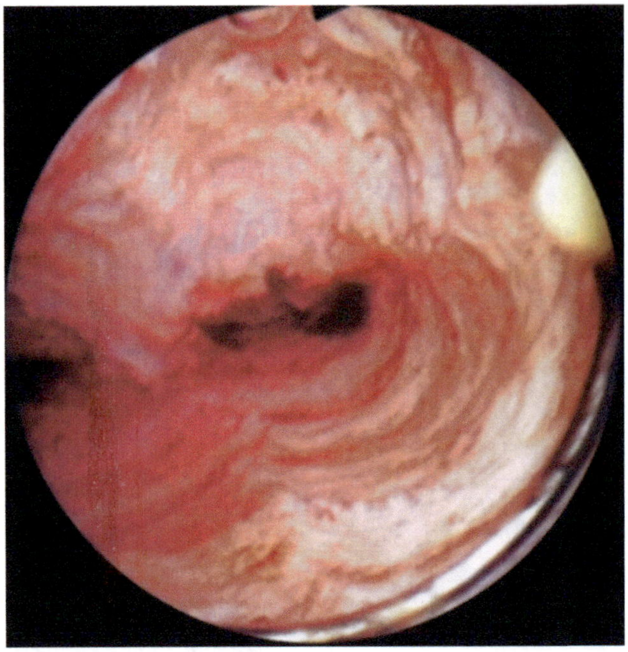

Fig. 9.17 Uterine cavity after a total resection of endometrium

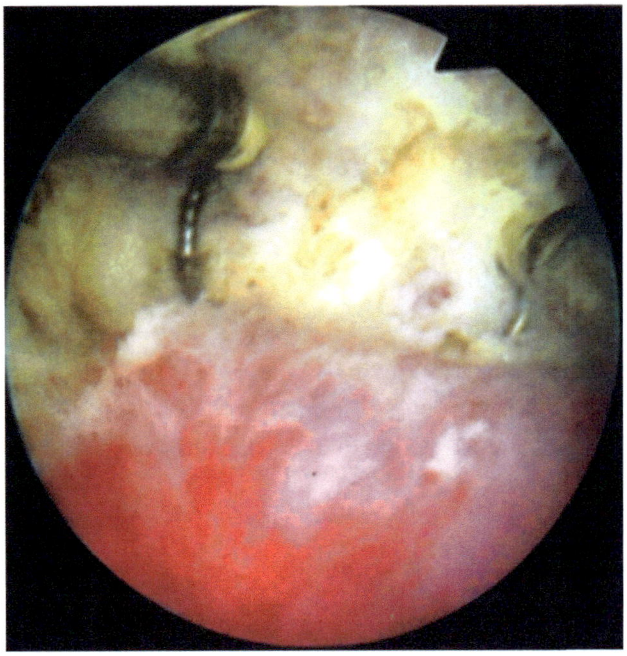

Fig. 9.18 Starting from uterine fundus, resect endometrium of posterior wall, and then resect in a counterclockwise direction

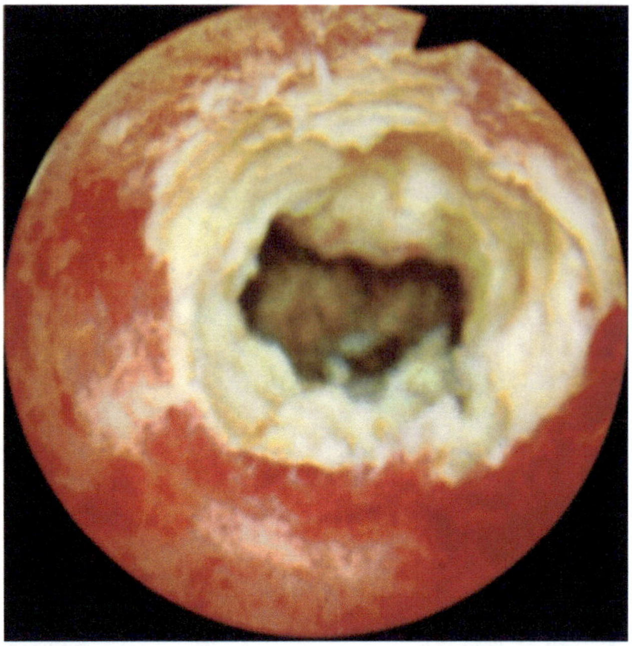

Fig. 9.19 Total resection of endometrium

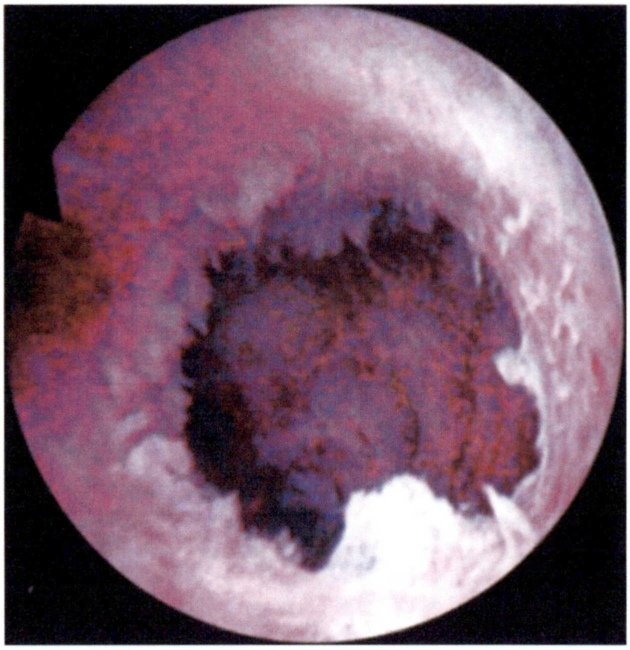

Fig. 9.20 Partial resection of endometrium

(b) The depth of the resection depends on the endometrial thickness, and the aim is to resect endometrium and its 2–3 mm underlying myometrium (Figs. 9.27, 9.28, and 9.29). This depth is sufficient to remove the full layer of endometrium except for the extremely deep endometrium, and superficial myometrium which avoids resecting the large vessels. And if the endometrium has been pretreated, it could reach the desired depth by no more than one resection.

(c) When distending pressure is insufficient, the bilateral walls of uterus can be closed, both sides of the uterine cornua may appear deeper, and often with remnants of the endometrium, so when operation ends, the operator should elevate the distending pressure, inspect and resect the residual endometrial tissue (Fig. 9.30).

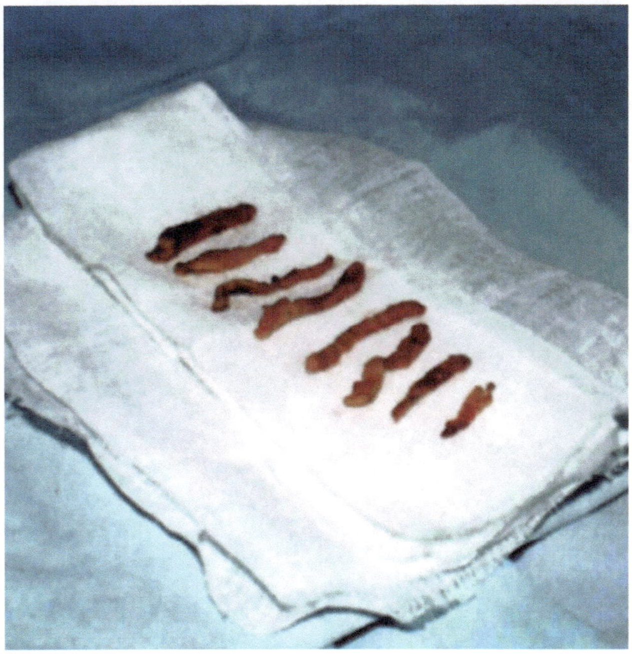

Fig. 9.21 Resected endometrial tissue strips by TCRE

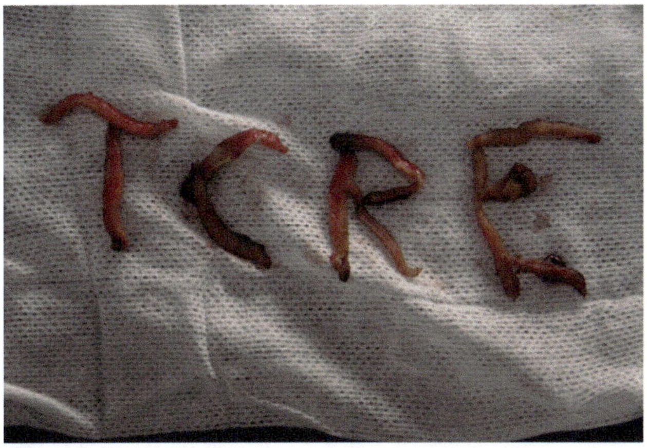

Fig. 9.22 Words formed with the resected endometrial tissue strips by TCRE

(d) After the resection of endometrium and its superficial myometrium, if pink or bright red endometrial tissue in a trumpet-flower shape appears in the resected myometrial surface, it will be the focus of adenomyosis (Fig. 9.31).

(e) If the endometrium is thicker, electrocoagulation can be repeated following the electric resecting, by which the efficacy can be improved (Fig. 9.32).

(f) It has been confirmed by research data that the more extensive the resection is, the bigger proportion of patients achieving postoperative amenorrhea or hypomenorrhea will be. At present, it is rare to have partial resection, and the internal orifice of uterine cervix is regarded as the lower bound of resection by most scholars.

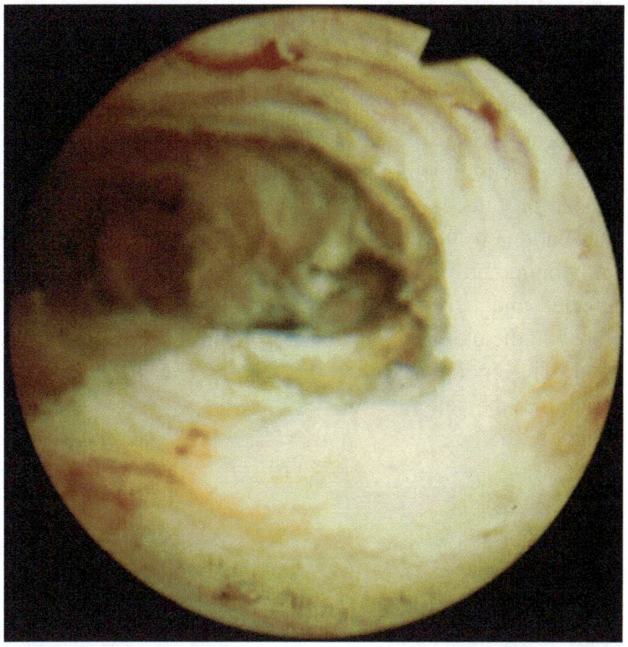

Fig. 9.23 Reduce the uterine distension pressure and observe the bleeding points

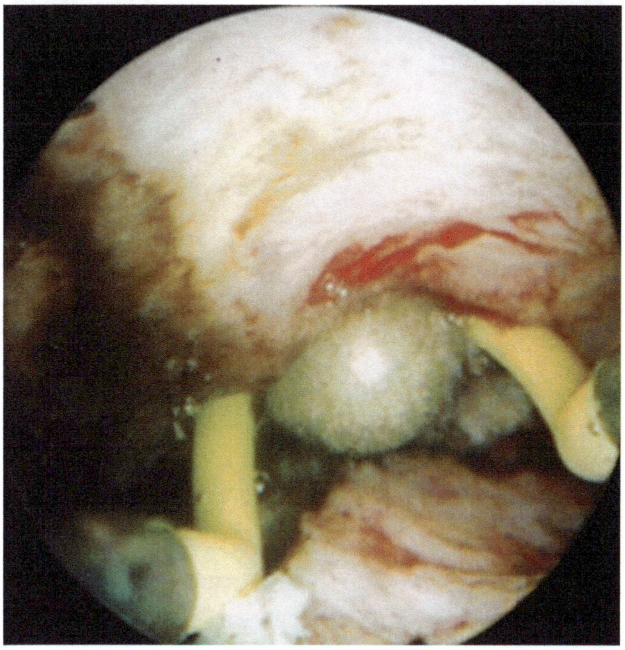

Fig. 9.24 Electrocoagulation of the bleeding point by rollerball electrode

9.2.4.2 Endometrial Ablation (EA)

1. Laser: The preparation before inserting a hysteroscope is the same as TCRE. When it has a clear vision under hysteroscope, insert a quartz laser fiber with a flexible metal protective sheath into its operative channel. There are two kinds of operative modes: dragging and blanching, with power of 55–80 W. During the operation, the color of the endometrium may change from pink to pale,

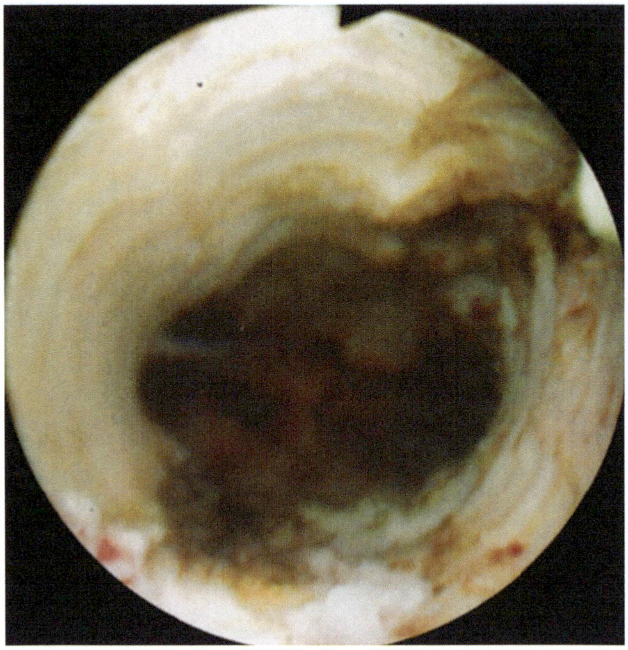

Fig. 9.25 Uterine cavity after TCRE

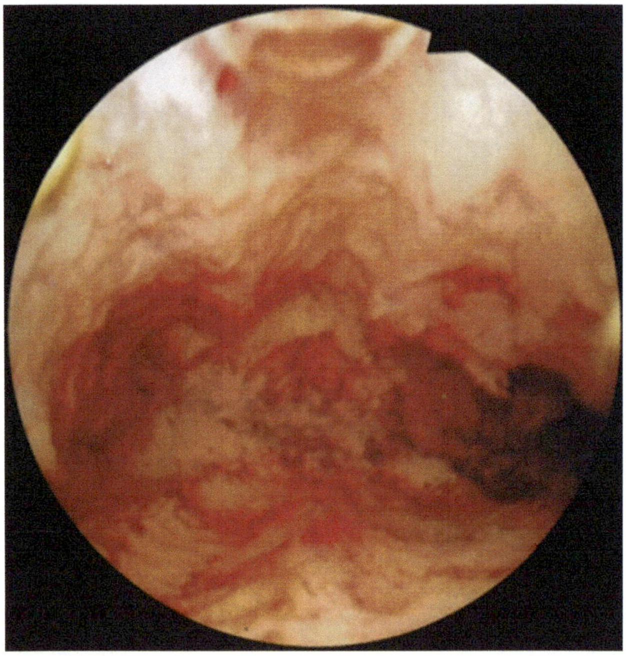

Fig. 9.26 A light brown cylinder-shape uterine cavity after TCRE

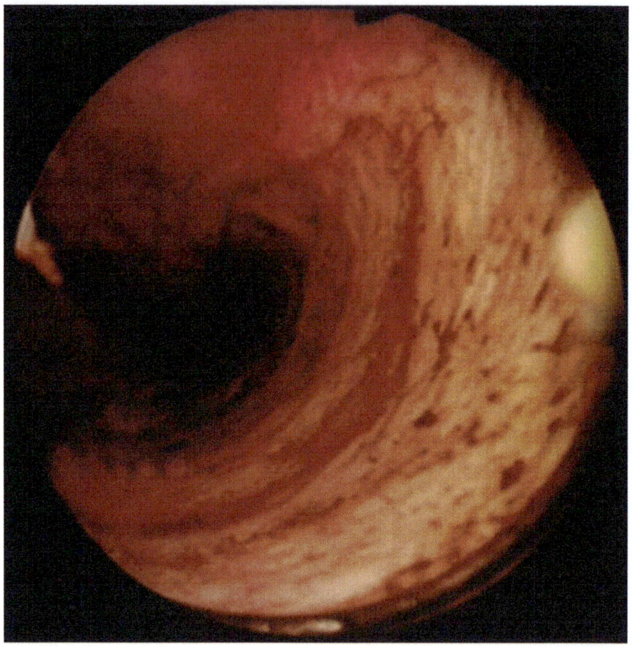

Fig. 9.27 Resection to a depth of 2–3 mm beneath the endometrium

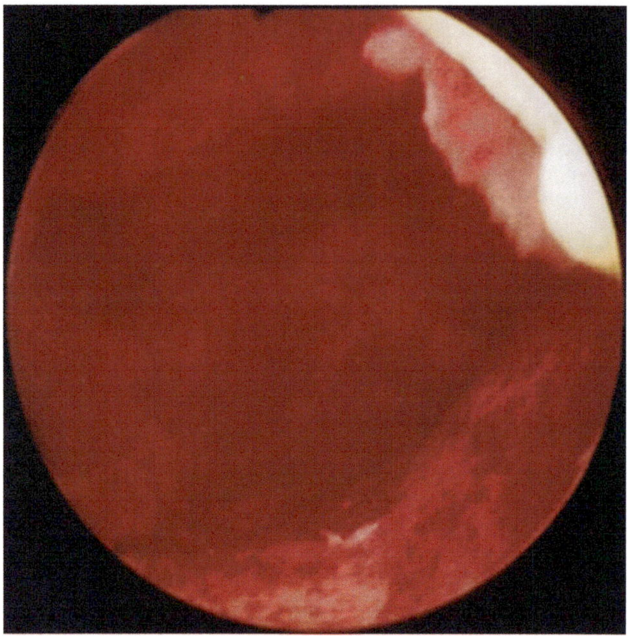

Fig. 9.28 Endometrium lining uterine wall prior to surgery

brown, and then black (carbonization). Tubal ostium is the hardest to visualize, which is also difficult for laser fiber to reach. From the tubal ostium the ablation of endometrium starts, and extends gradually to the uterine fundus, and gets together at the midline. The hysteroscope should always be maintained at the 12 o'clock position, never turning. It is important to keep its direction when an operator performed an operation by watching the monitor. The operator can drag the laser fiber back with right hand, and lift up or push down the proximal end of hysteroscope with left hand so as to control the laser fiber in touching or focusing on the endometrium to be destroyed. After treatment of uterine fundus, ablate the endometrium in the uterine anterior, bilateral and the posterior wall until the internal orifice of uterus. In order to reduce the risk of cervical stenosis, some operators stop the ablation at a few millimeters above

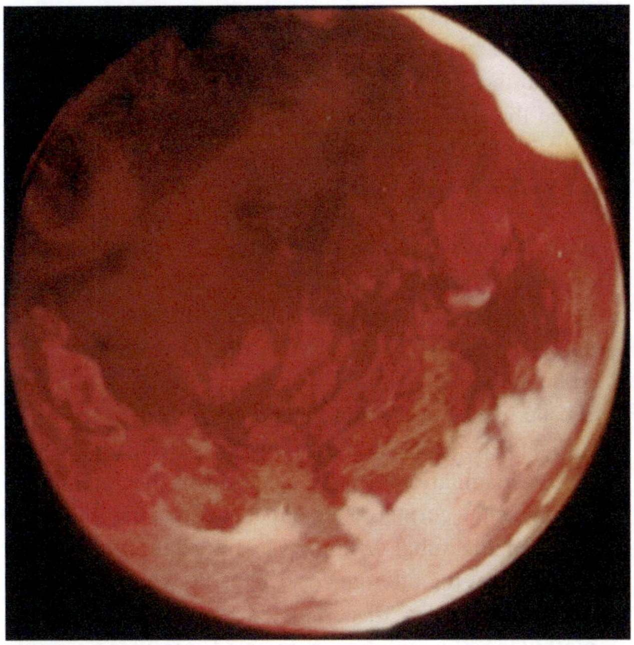

Fig. 9.29 At the end of resection, it removes the full layer of endometrium and superficial myometrium, which reaches the cervical internal orifice

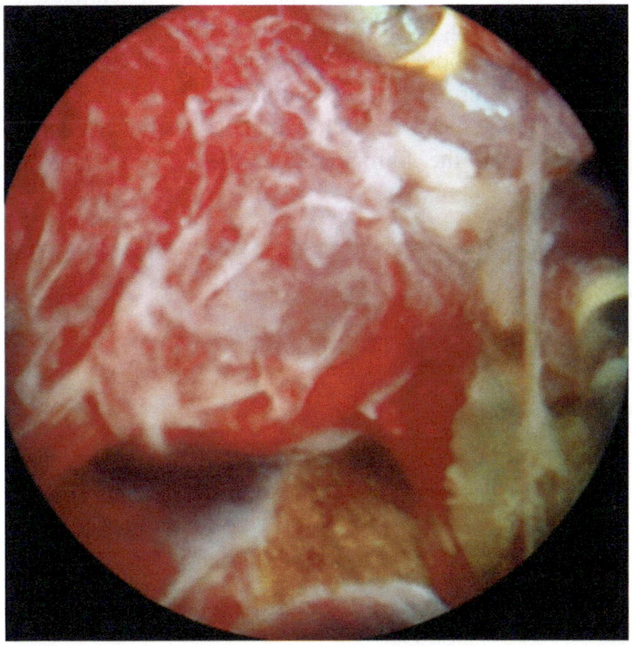

Fig. 9.30 Electric resection of endometrium at right uterine cornu

the internal orifice. There are also operators who do not use hysteroscopy but place the laser fiber directly into the uterine cavity under ultrasonography guidance to destroy the endometrium, which has the same therapeutic effect. The shortcoming of this method is that the endometrium specimens cannot be obtained for histologic examination.

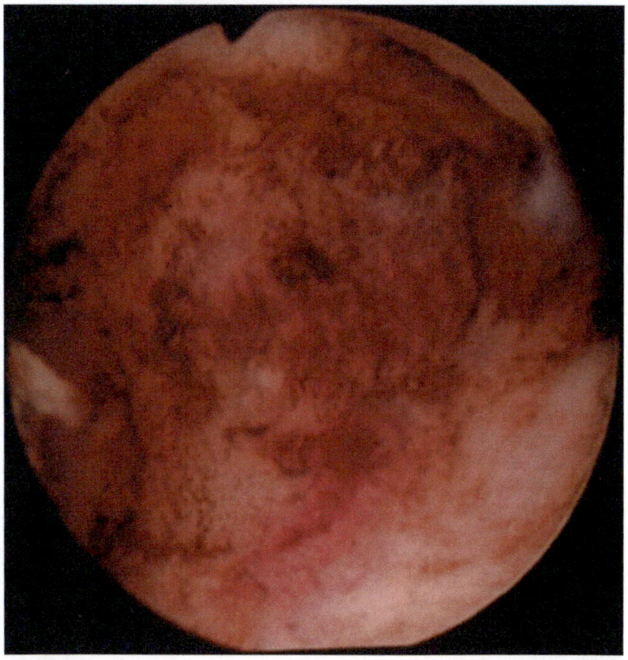

Fig. 9.31 The residual endometrium with bright red color in trumpet-flower shape after endometrial resection is seen in myometrium on posterior wall, which is the foci of adenomyosis

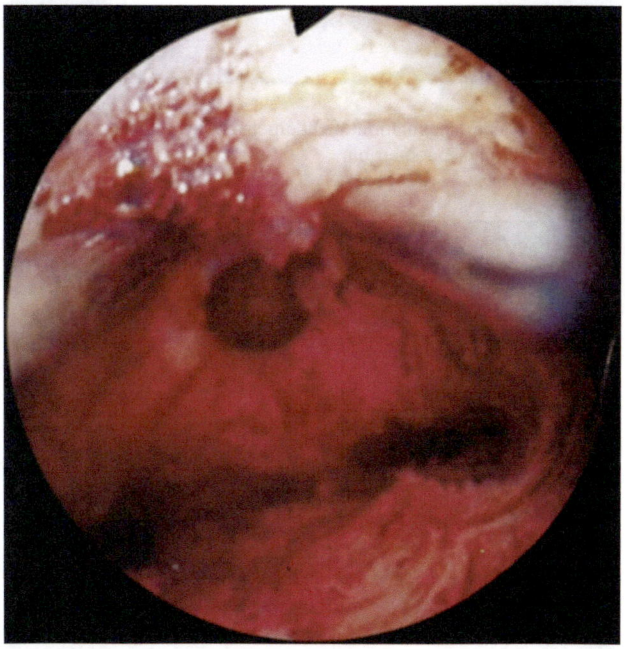

Fig. 9.32 Rollerball coagulation following endometrial resection, with the bubbles caused by tissue vaporization collecting above the rollerball

2. Electrocoagulation: The preparation before inserting a hysteroscope is the same as TCRE. Those who do not have endometrial pretreatment should administer uterine suction aspiration to suck out the functional layer of the endometrium as much as possible, so that a com-

plete ablation could be ensured. Press lightly the rollerball (Fig. 9.33)/roller barrel electrode (Fig. 9.34) in contact with tissues, and step on the electrocoagulation pedal to turn power on, with the power 40–60 W. Due to the amount of thermal damage on tissues by electrode coagulation being relatively high, a short time should be spent at the same point before the electrode is moved. The time required is to wait for the tissues around the electrode to turn white, about less than 1 s. Once the tissues surrounding electrode become white, then move the electrode slowly towards the cervix. When moving, the tissue destruction zone is visible in front of the electrode, and by this way the rolling speed of the electrode is monitored. Electrocoagulation of the endometrium on each wall should be done in a sequence. As it is easy to produce bubbles, usually start from the anterior wall (Fig. 9.35). It is difficult to roll the electrode at the uterine fundus and tubal ostia, so electrode can be placed at a point when doing electric coagulating, and then retract a bit, repeat it several times until electrocoagulation is fully achieved in the fundus and the adjacent cornua. Remember not to push the electrode to the tubal ostium. Electrocoagulation should terminate at the internal cervical ostia, which are sometimes difficult to discern. Hence 10–20 mL diluted methylene blue solution is injected into uterine cavity before dilating the cervix, so that the operator can see the endometrium blue-stain, uterine tubal ostium dark blue spot, and cervical canal blue parallel lines. Because the electric coagulation changes the appearance of endometrium, it is difficult to detect the residual endometrium without coagulation. The shape of endometrial surface after electrocoagulation helps to find adenomyosis. Since the tissue rich with cells has better conductivity than the fibrous tissue, the endometrium has

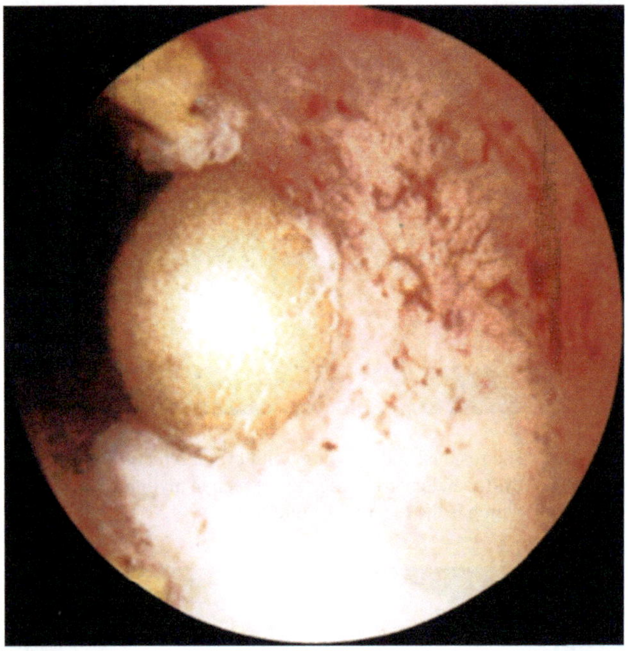

Fig. 9.33 Electrocoagulation of endometrium by contact of rollerball electrode with the endometrium

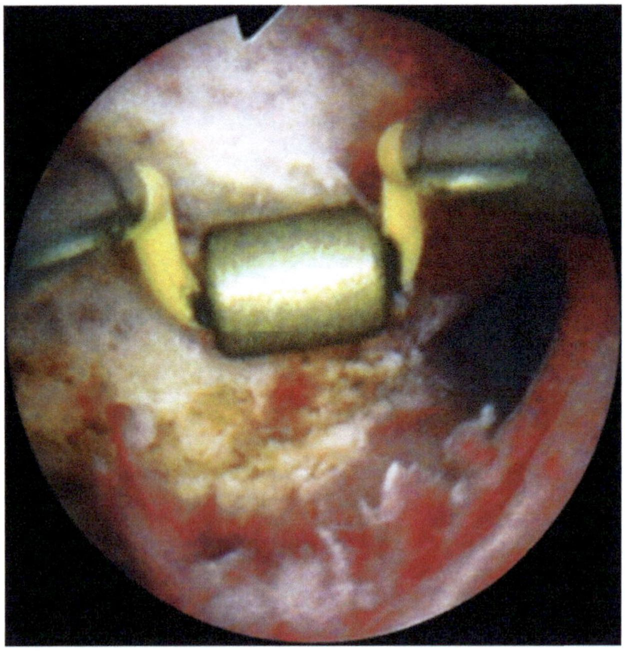

Fig. 9.34 Roller barrel electrode

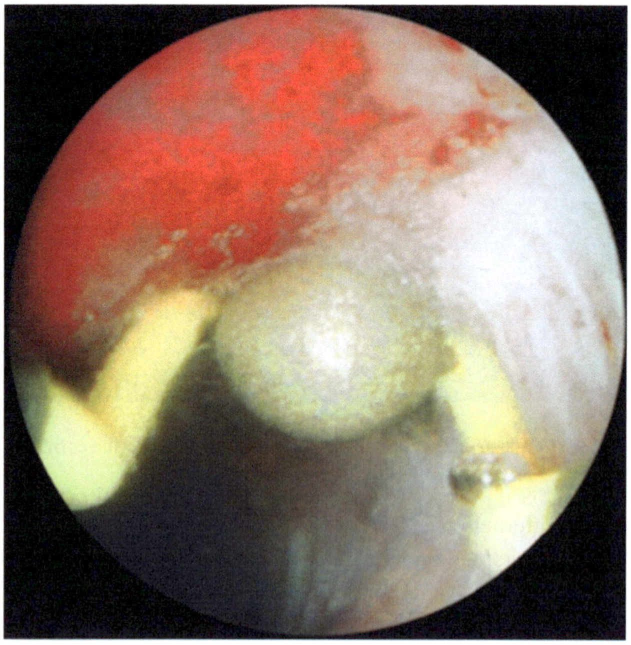

Fig. 9.35 Rollerball coagulation of endometrium at the anterior wall

lower impedance than the uterine myometrial tissue, and is damaged more thoroughly than the surrounding muscle tissue. Therefore, there are transverse slots at locus of adenomyosis and the operator may sense a feeling of collision when the electrode rolls. As the endometrial glands are located deep in the myometrial layer, gland tissues cannot be entirely coagulated, so it needs resection with wire loop at this site.

Vercellini et al. made a comparative study of EA with vaporizing electrode (Fig. 9.36) and TCRE with wire loop. The measures included the absorption of distension fluid, operating time, and the difficulties of surgery. The result was that the mean ± the standard deviation (SD) distension fluid deficit was 109 ± 126 mL in the vaporization group and 367 ± 257 mL in the resection group, $P < 0.001$, and there were no differences in other measures.

Romer and Schwesinger made a retrospective analysis of 40 cases who received pretreatment of the endometrium with gestagen, danazol, or GnRH analog, which were compared with control group. The measurements evaluated by surgeons include the thickness of endometrium and the depth of coagulating damage. The result was that 90% of the cases in danazol group and GnRH-a group had adequate endometrial atrophy. The histological examination revealed atrophic endometrium or a small amount of proliferative endometrium. In a 2-year follow-up of EA, there were higher amenorrhea rates in danazol group and GnRH-a group. It was considered that endometrial pretreatment should be done prior to EA.

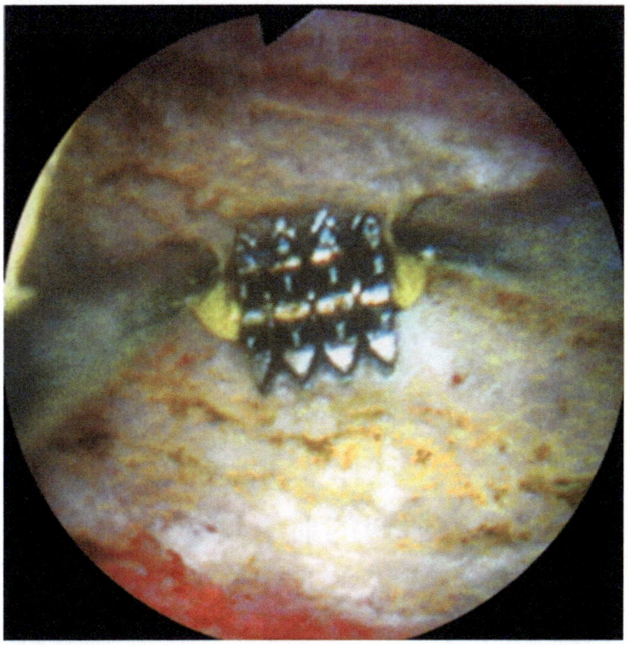

Fig. 9.36 Vaporizing electrode

9.2.5 Intraoperative Complicated Conditions and Managements

9.2.5.1 Inadequate Distension of Uterine Cavity

Inadequate uterine distension is the most common problem, especially those who do not use uterine distending pump. When the uterine cavity is not properly distended, the uterine fundus and tubal ostia are hard to be seen. It is important to adequately expand the uterine cavity with distending fluid to clearly see the whole cavity, and the operation can begin. Otherwise, it may cause insufficient resection and uterine perforation. The common reasons of inadequate uterine distension are cervical incompetence, perforation of the uterus, and low uterine distending pressure. Due to the low intrauterine pressure, the perforation is often accompanied by bleeding. For cervical incompetence, suture or cervical clamp can be applied to occlude the cervix. If uterine perforation is suspected, stop operation immediately and examine abdominal symptoms, and observe whether or not there is free liquid around the uterus and in abdominal cavity by ultrasonography. In cases of low distending pressure, it should be elevated, and if there is no distending pump, it can be solved by using three way pipes, raising the height of irrigating fluid container, or increasing the volume of the irrigating fluid. Sometimes the inadequate uterine distension is caused by uterine contraction, to which intravenous injection of atropine can be applied. Notably, some uterus would not respond to the above managements, the main causes might be too small uterine cavity, uterine fibroids, and adenomyosis. Poor uterine distention might also happen when flow inlet and outlet valves are obstructed, there are blood clots between the inner and outer sheath, the inflow pipe is folded, or air inflow of irrigation container is obstructed.

9.2.5.2 Slow Clearance of the Fragments and Clots Inside the Uterine Cavity

If tissue fragments and blood clots are blocked at the channel between the inner and outer sheaths, the sieve of outer sheath, or inflow valve, or if the outflow suction pressure is insufficient, the fluid cannot flow out smoothly, thus causing irrigation fluid circulation inside the uterine cavity to slow down, and leading to the delay of debris and clots clearance, which affects the field of view and operating process. It can be solved immediately by increasing suction pressure and cleaning the endoscopic sheaths.

9.2.5.3 Insufficient Resection

If the resected tissue is not cut off, the tissue blocks may float like large polyps in the uterine cavity. The most common reason is that the wire loop has not yet returned to the sheath when power is switched off. If so, the operator should check whether the wire loop has broken or deformed. If the deformed wire loop cannot return to the sheath when the resection ends, the operator can use a finger to push inward gently and make it return to the sheath. In addition, if the resecting current intensity is too low, it may also lead to incomplete resection, which can be solved by increasing the current power.

9.2.5.4 Unclear Observation of the Endometrium and Uterine Cavity

In addition to the factors including inadequate uterine distension and slow clearance of intrauterine debris and blood clots, the resected fragments, the bubbles under anterior uterine wall and fibroids protruding into the uterine cavity may all obstruct the vision (Figs. 9.37 and 9.38).The interference of tissue debris is a trouble before the operator learns to push the tissue fragments to gather together at the uterine fundus. The operator can remove the tissue fragments before resecting again, or move the lens body downward to resect along tissue and take it out immediately. Increasing suction pressure or adjusting patients' position may contribute to expel the bubbles under the anterior uterine wall. For intrauterine fibroids interfering with the vision, only total or partial removal can make a clear vision.

9.2.5.5 Too Rapid Absorption of Irrigation Fluid

The causes of it include too high distending pressure and perforation of the uterus. When the fluid overload is detected, the operation should be terminated immediately, and check whether there is perforation of the uterus or not. After the perforation is excluded, operation can be continued. Cervical laceration and incomplete uterine perforation may also increase irrigation fluid absorption. The operation should be completed as quickly as possible if there is no uterine perforation. In addition, attention should also be paid to whether there is leakage of irrigation fluid or not and that the irrigation fluid may not be irrigated into the uterine cavity when uterine distending pressure is too high.

9.2.5.6 Intraoperative Bleeding

The low uterine distending pressure, insufficient electrocoagulating current intensity, too deep of the resection, and the resection of uterine fibroids may all cause bleeding, which hinders the operation. The solution to it is to raise the uterine distending pressure, increase the electrocoagulating power of the blended current and coagulate the bleeding vessels. The vascular layer of uterine myometrium lies 5–6 mm beneath the endometrium, through which there are more vessels passing. Therefore, when the resection reaches into the vascular layer, it can cause massive bleeding. Therefore the depth of resection should be above the vascular layer. If there is myoma bleeding, the vessels can be coagulated around the pseudo-capsule.

9.2.5.7 Postoperative Hemorrhage

Common reasons of postoperative bleeding are too deep resection, infection, and tissue debris remaining in the uterine cavity. The solution is to place balloon catheter in the uterine cavity to stop bleeding by compression, administer antibiotics, and empty the intrauterine residues, and meanwhile, contraction agents and hemostatic agents can be used. The balloon catheter should be taken out after 4–6 h of usage

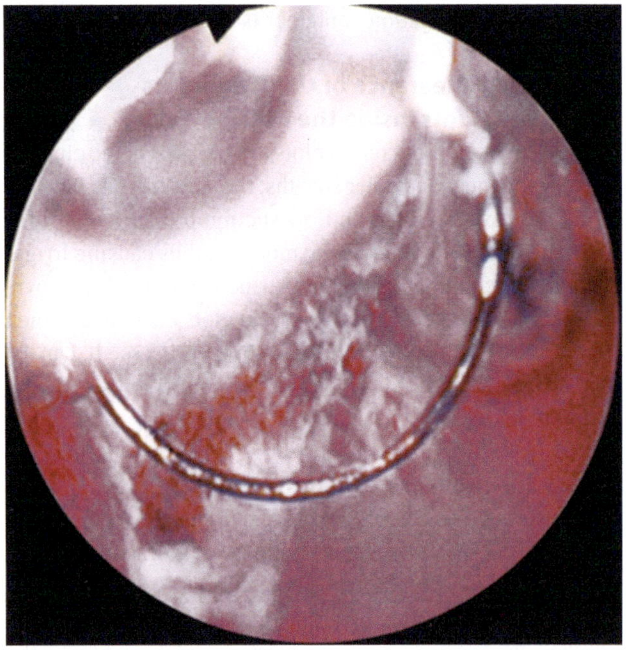

Fig. 9.37 Bubbles under uterine anterior wall interfere with the vision

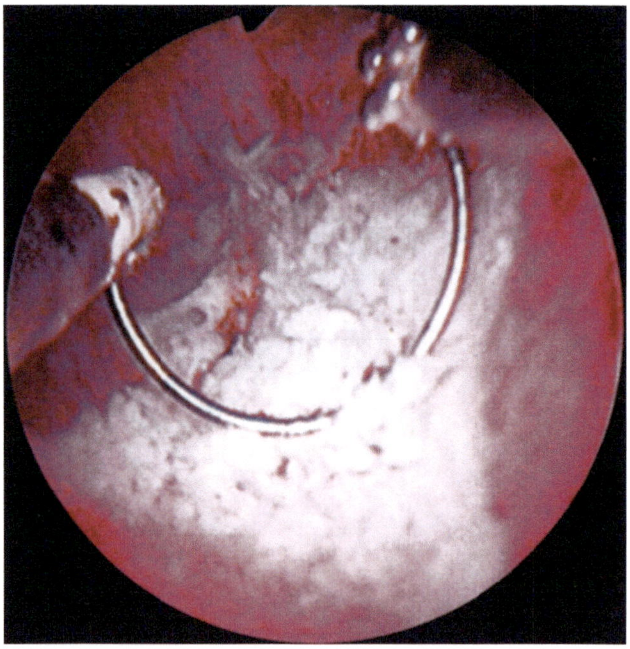

Fig. 9.38 Uterine cavity after the discharge of bubbles

because prolonged placement may lead to necrosis of uterine myometrial wall.

9.2.6 Intraoperative and Postoperative Care

9.2.6.1 Intraoperative Monitoring

Close monitoring during TCRE and EA is mandatory. Considering the operation time, incision, hospitalization time, TCRE, and EA seem to be minor, but are still major operations regarding their potential risks. Operation safety must always be the first consideration, and intensive monitoring is an important component. Operators and other staff should always be alert and warned about two main risks, namely uterine perforation and fluid overload, which may never occur to experienced surgeons under normal circumstances, but are potentially dangerous for beginners.

1. Routine monitorings:
   (a) Symptoms and signs: They include chest discomfort, nausea and vomiting, irritability, lethargy, purple, pale, facial edema, etc.
   (b) Heart rate and blood pressure: The patients who have underlying coronary heart disease and hypertension are likely to develop hypertension and tachycardia before anesthesia, and hypotension may occur during anesthesia and operation. And those having massive blood loss are often accompanied by tachycardia and hypovolemic shock. When there is excessive absorption of irrigation fluid, the systolic blood pressure is on the high side, the heart rate slows down, and pulse pressure is broadened.
   (c) Body temperature: When a large volume of irrigation fluid flows into the uterus, the body temperature will drop, and if the operation time is longer, it is possible to develop chills and shivering.
2. Special monitorings:
   (a) ECG and cardiac function monitoring: It may be applied to those who have cardiac and renal insufficiency.
   (b) Hemoglobin and hematocrit: Due to irrigation fluid absorption and blood loss, the levels of hemoglobin and hematocrit drop, which may take place about 20 min after the start of electric resection.
   (c) Serum potassium and sodium: Irrigation fluid absorption can dilute blood, and also have effects of osmotic diuresis and natriuresis. Operation injury also allows sodium ions to migrate into the cells, thus the intraoperative blood sodium decreases by varying degrees. The degree of hyponatremia is related to the duration of operation, the volume of the irrigating fluid, and the weight of the resected tissues. If the patients develop nausea, vomiting, dizziness, dysphoria, etc., and blood sodium is reduced by 15 mmol/L and above compared to that prior to operation, the operator should be on the alert.
   (d) Plasma osmotic pressure: The absorption of irrigation fluid often leads to a decrease in plasma osmolality.
3. Ultrasonography monitoring: According to Xia et al., when beginners perform TCRE procedure, ultrasonography monitoring (Figs. 9.39, 9.40, 9.41, and 9.42) should be used alongside. Only when the electric resecting technique is proficiently grasped, the depth of resection can be precisely controlled, especially for those with medical pretreatment to thin the endometrium prior to operation, may TCRE surgery be done without monitoring, but mainly through observation under hysteroscope.
4. Laparoscopic monitoring: In order to reduce the irrigating fluid absorption, bilateral fallopian tube may be ligated under laparoscopy. Since laparoscope cannot be used to monitor the posterior wall of the uterus, there are fewer applications at present.

9.2.6.2 Postoperative Care and Managements

1. If antibiotics are not administered during operation, intravenous administration of antibiotics could be given to prevent infection on the first day after operation.

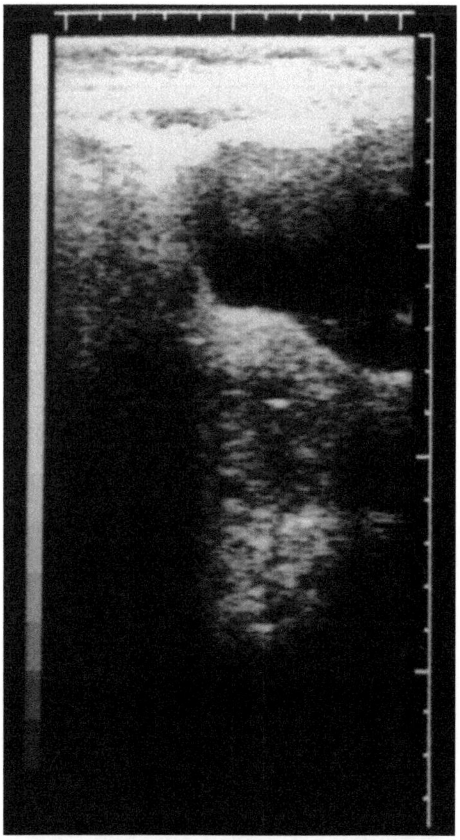

Fig. 9.39 Ultrasonography monitoring (prior to operation)

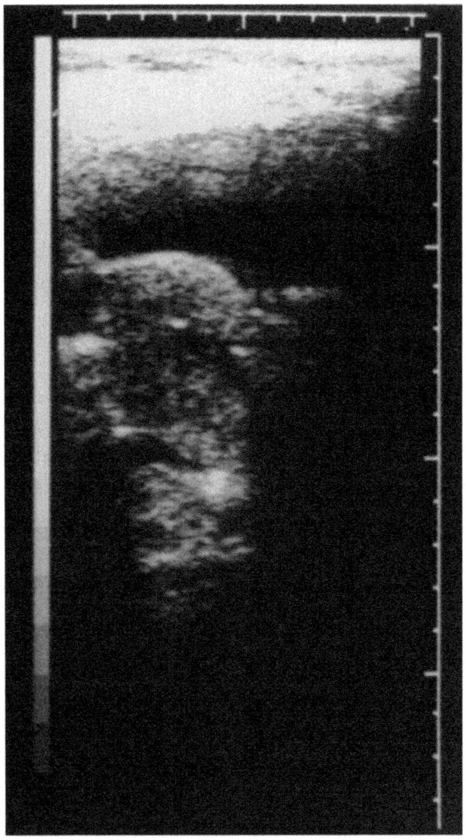

Fig. 9.40 Ultrasonography monitoring (irrigation fluid into the uterine cavity)

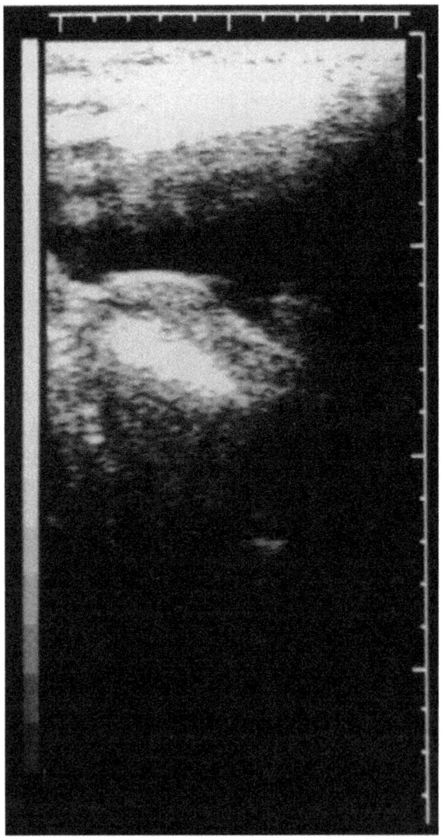

Fig. 9.41 Ultrasonography monitoring (beginning of the resection)

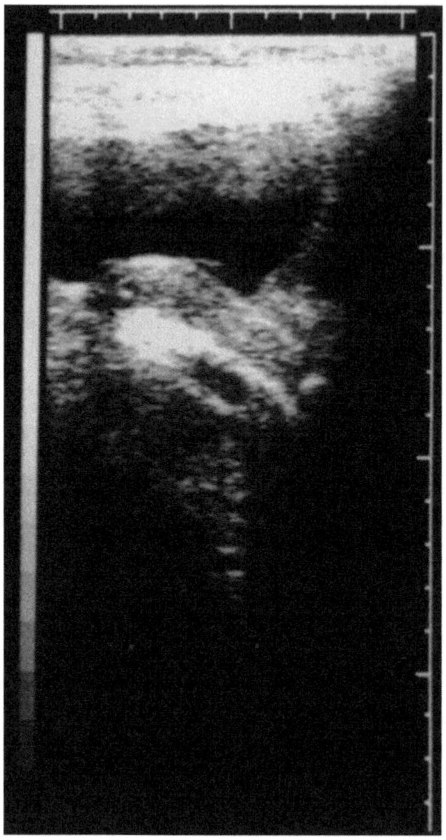

Fig. 9.42 Ultrasonography monitoring (ends of the resection)

2. Observe the body temperature, blood pressure, pulse, heart rate, and reactions during anesthesia recovery period and moving the patients. More intraoperative bleeding and hypovolemia may cause hypotension. If the temperature of distension fluid during operation is too low, the patients may develop hypothermia and shivering after operation, and warm-keeping measures should be taken.
3. Bleeding: Oxytocin and (or) triplet hemostatic agents may be administered: intravenous drip of 5% glucose solution 500 mL + vitamin C 3 g + dicynone 3 g + pamba 0.3 g. If there are cases with acute active hemorrhage, a balloon catheter can be placed into the uterine cavity, and a certain amount of sterile saline is injected into the balloon until the bleeding stops, usually about 8–20 mL. If necessary, electrocoagulation hemostasis should be applied via hysteroscope.
4. Diet: The postoperative reaction to anesthesia often causes nausea, vomiting, etc., thus the patient should fast for 6 h.
5. Attention to electrolyte and acid-base balance: Sodium is the most important cation of extracellular fluid, which accounts for more than 90% of the total number of extracellular fluid cation. If its content is changed, it will have definitive effects on the total cations. If severe hyponatremia occurs during operation, there is often metabolism disorder of hydrogen ion, and acid poison-

ing may occur. Thus much attention should be paid to monitoring and timely correction. According to the urological statistics, more than 80% patients who had the transurethral resection of prostate developed different degrees of hyponatremia, which was TURP syndrome. According to its degree and speed, it can generally be divided into 3°.

(a) Mild degree: The serum sodium is at 137–130 mmol/L, both intracellular and extracellular fluid is hypotonic, and the patients may develop dizziness, headache, fatigue, unresponsiveness, and loss of appetite.
(b) Moderate degree: The serum sodium is at 130–120 mmol/L, the above symptoms may become more severe, and nausea, vomiting, skin relaxation, a decrease in neural reflex, and decline of blood pressure may develop.
(c) Severe degree: The serum sodium is below 120 mmol/L. Both nausea and vomiting may be developed seriously, the patient may also develop dazing, faint, and coma in the end. Its clinical manifestations include lack of muscular tension, disappearance of reflexes, weak pulse, decrease in blood pressure, and even shock.

6. Treatment of hyponatremia:
   (a) Mild: The patient may lack about 0.5 g sodium per kilogram body weight. Intravenous administration of 5% glucose and saline 2000–3000 mL can be used. If the patient's cardiac function is normal, 1000 mL can be given at the first hour, then slow down. Afterwards, the speed of intravenous drip is regulated by checking the serum sodium concentration.
   (b) Moderate and severe: The patient with moderate hyponatremia may lack about 0.5–0.75 g sodium per kilogram body weight, and about 0.75–1.25 g with severe hyponatremia. For patients with moderate and severe hyponatremia, it is proper to use hypertonic saline instead of normal saline. Hypertonic saline may increase the cellular osmotic pressure, transfer the water within the cell to extracellular and reduce cell swelling, thus restoring blood osmotic pressure to normal. The commonly used is 3 or 5% sodium chloride solution.

   Its supply is calculated by the following formula:

$$\text{The sodium content supplemented} = (\text{normal serum sodium values} - \text{measured serum sodium values}) \times 52\%^{*} \times \text{kg of body weight}$$

In which * refers to the total body fluids accounting for 52% of the body weight.

For example: If the patient's body weight is 60 kg, the measured serum sodium is 125 mmol/L. The sodium amount requiring to be supplemented = (142 − 125 mmol/L) x 52% x 60 = 530.4 mmol.

Since the sodium ions in 5% sodium chloride solution of each mL is 0.85 mmol, the required 5% sodium chloride solution = 530.4/0.85 = 624 mL.

On the supply of hypertonic sodium chloride solution, the operator should pay attention to the following points: (1) Give 1/3 or 1/2 of the total at the very beginning, and then the rest of the supplement is determined according to the patient's consciousness, blood pressure, heart rate, rhythm of the heart, pulmonary symptoms and changes of serum sodium, potassium, and chloride. (2) Regarding hyponatremia, be sure not to transfuse a great amount of solution without sodium, and then transfuse with sodium. This is because after a great volume of fluid transfusion, the serum sodium will be made lower, more water moves into the cell from outside and makes them swell, thus worsening the symptoms. (3) The intravenous drip of hypertonic saline is easy to stimulate the local venous intima, causing venous thrombosis. Therefore, a warm compress of the local infusion contributes to the prevention of thrombotic phlebitis.

7. Treatment of hypokalemia

   Generally speaking, if the patient has normal renal function, there is no change in blood potassium during operation. However, if the water intoxication occurs and diuretics is used, one must pay attention to whether there is low potassium levels during operation, and if there is, one must correct it in time.

9.2.6.3 Postoperative Care

In patients suffering from uterine cramps following operation, painkillers or prostaglandin can be taken for pain relief after urinary retention being excluded. A minority of patients may have transient fever, which can be treated by using indomethacin suppositories 100–200 mg per rectum and (or) taking oral liquid of 10 mL Radix Bupleuri with the temperature dropping in 24 h. After operation, the patients may have a little vaginal bleeding, which is known as bloody serous fluid discharge within 2 weeks and simple serous fluid discharge in the following 4–6 weeks. For the patients who have abnormal vaginal discharge, massive or prolonged vaginal bleeding, uterotonic agents, hemostatic agents, and antibiotic medication can be administered. Three months after operation is the time of the return of menstruation, and those who have no bleeding by then have suffered loss of menstruation (amenorrhea).

9.2.7 Detection and Management of Operational Complications

Due to the large operational surface in TCRE or EA, there are more operational complications. Bratshi reported that the incidence of operation complications was 2.5% in 465 cases who had TCRE. Therefore, be sure not to violate patients' will to perform this operation by force.

9.2.7.1 Intraoperative Complications

1. Uterine perforation: The difficulties of TCRE procedures are that if the resection is too shallow and fail to reach the basal layer, subsequent endometrial regeneration will lead to the recurrence of abnormal bleeding, indicating the failure of the treatment. However if the resection is too deep, uterine perforation may occur. Therefore, the principle of TCRE is to give a cut to every location, including endometrial functional layer, basal layer and its underlying 2–3 mm myometrium, and the operator should be very prudent when giving a second cut. When EA is being done with the power on, the rollerball or vaporizing electrode must keep rolling, and its in situ stay can lead to too deep coagulation of myometrial layer, and even coagulation of full layer. If the high heat of electricity spreads to the bowel or bladder adjacent to the uterus, intestinal fistula may develop after operation.
2. TURP syndrome: Due to the large cutting surface of the uterus by TCRE and more open veins, a large amount of irrigation fluid is absorbed into the blood circulation, resulting in a series of systemic symptoms caused by hypervolemia and hyponatremia, and even death in severe cases. The pathways through which the irrigation fluid flows rapidly and abundantly into the circulation are mainly the open veins in the cutting surface, and secondly, fallopian tubes. Some scholars conducted ligation of bilateral fallopian tube under laparoscope prior to electric resection in order to reduce the absorption by the second way. Wood and Roberts, in order to reduce the transtubal absorption, occluded the bilateral fallopian tubes with silastic rings under laparoscope in nine cases prior to TCRE, with the result that mean fluid deficit was 259 mL (0–900 mL), which was lower than 643 mL (100–2030 mL) reported by others.
   (a) Clinical manifestations
      - Hypervolemia: Its consequences are acute left heart failure and pulmonary edema, and if not promptly treated, it can further develop dyspnea and metabolic acidosis, which worsen the heart failure and cause shock or severe ventricular arrhythmias and death.
      - Water intoxication and hyponatremia: The electrolyte components of the extracellular fluid are diluted. Since the main component of electrolyte is sodium, its concentration decreases, thus hyponatremia develops. Water intoxication is the most harmful to the cerebral nerve tissues. When the serum sodium reduces to below 125 mmol/L, water begins to enter the brain cells, which increases the water content within the brain cells, and the patients may present with nausea, vomiting, drowsiness, headache, diminution or loss of tendon reflexes. During coma, some patients may have positive Babinski syndrome, and sometimes develop hemiplegia. When it is severe, the brain cells swell, and intracranial pressure increases, which may cause a variety of neurologic and mental symptoms, such as gaze, aphasia, alienation, directional disorder, drowsiness, dysphoria, muscle twitching, or even convulsions and coma. Severe cerebral edema can develop the foramen magnum herniation or transtentorial herniation, leading to breath-cardiac arrest, and resulting in death.

   (b) Treatment:
      - Diuretic: It is used to relieve the burden of heart, and remove the redundant water out of the body.
      - Treatment of hyponatremia: In emergency circumstances, besides of furosemide being given, intravenous injection of 5% hypertonic saline can be given so as not to delay the rescue time, and there is no need to wait for the report of serum sodium.
      - Treatment of acute left heart failure: Its treatment may be done with digitalis.
      - Treatment of pulmonary edema: Generally, oxygen is given via the nasal tube with defoaming agent, and the use of morphine is forbidden.
      - Treatment of brain edema: Bird et al. used high concentrations of urea. Urea is an osmotic diuretic, and its injection can make the osmotic pressure in intravascular fluid higher than that in tissue fluid, which promote the water moving from the edematous brain tissue into blood vessels, then the cerebral edema can be relieved; corticosteroids can also be used at the same time to stabilize the cell membrane and reduce capillary permeability, thus relieving cerebral edema.
      - Correction of electrolyte and acid-base balance disorders: When a diuretic is used, a large amount of potassium may be passed with the urine, which may cause low serum potassium and arrhythmias.

(c) Prevention:
- Intensive care should be given to cases with high risks such as cases with large myomas, without endometrial pretreatment, and those who have the occurrence of uterine perforation.
- When the fluid deficit is to 1000–2000 mL, mild hyponatremia may occur, and the operation should be terminated as quickly as possible. When the deficit is >2000 mL, the patient may develop severe hyponatremia and acidosis.
- When there is acid-base balance disorder, one should immediately stop the operation. The total operation time should be controlled within 1 h.
- Try to take a low pressure irrigation.
- Operation time can be prolonged if the central venous pressure is measured.
- If a myoma is larger, it can be resected in stages.
- Once TURP syndrome is found, the operation should be stopped as soon as possible.

Bennett et al. studied the methods to prevent TURP syndrome. Twenty women were involved in the study group with the pressure of fluid distention pump set below the mean arterial pressure (MAPs) of the patients. In 20 women of the control group, the pressure was set at random. It was found that both the total volume and deficits of irrigation fluid in study group were significant less than those in control group, supporting the hypothesis that the pressure of fluid infusion pump should be set at or below women's MAPs. Baskett et al. conducted a study to compare two control techniques of irrigating fluid with the risks of fluid overload during operative hysteroscopy. In one group, passive gravity outflow was used, and in another group, direct connection of the outflow to wall suction was used. The result was that the technique of connecting the outflow to wall suction reduced the risk of fluid absorption. It is generally believed that the absorption of irrigation fluid in rollerball electrocoagulation of EA is less than that in wire loop electrode resection of TCRE. In 1999, Klinzing et al. reported a case of a 45-year-old woman, who developed severe hyponatremia after endometrial ablation with rollerball electrode. After irrigating the uterine cavity with 10 L of mixed solution including 2.7% Sorbitol and 0.54% Mannitol for 45 min, she developed pulmonary edema and severe hyponatremia.

3. Bleeding

The vascular layer of the uterine myometrium lies 5–6 mm beneath the endometrium, and is mostly composed of circular muscular fibers with fewer oblique muscle fibers, through which plenty of blood vessels are running. In TCRE, attention should be paid not to injuring the vascular layer. When the operation ends, the bleeding point of pulsatile artery is coagulated. Recently, Robert and Walton reported on a double blind trial under local anesthesia with the paracervical injections of 10 mL of 0.5% bupivacaine and 1:200,000 adrenaline when TCRE began, with the result of significant reduction of intraoperative blood loss ($P < 0.005$) and slight reduction of postoperative bleeding ($P > 0.005$). However, it was not suggested for routine use because the heart rate increased in the drug used group ($P < 0.005$).

4. Venous gas embolism

Among the reported nine cases of gas embolism caused by hysteroscopic operation, five cases underwent TCRE or EA operation (56%), of which 3 survived and 2 died.

9.2.7.2 Postoperative Complications

Complete endometrial ablation appears to be very safe in the short term; however, with the passage of time, some long-term complications may emerge. The problem is the development of postoperative uterine scar and contracture. Any bleeding behind the persistent scar or from regenerated endometrium may lead to problems because of obstruction, such as the intrauterine hematometra, uterine cornua hematometra, PASS (postablation-tubal sterilization syndrome), retrograde menstruation, and delayed diagnosis of endometrial carcinoma.

1. Infection: Among the reported five cases of severe infection following operative hysteroscopy, four cases underwent TCRE or EA, which accounted for 80%. In Loffer's data, the incidence of postoperative infection in TCRE was 0.3%.
2. Bleeding: In the two cases with persistent bleeding in the late postoperative period in the Hysteroscopy Center of Fuxing Hospital, Capital Medical University, both of them were unresponsive to medical treatment, and cured by curettage, the scraped tissue was little, with granulation tissue confirmed by histopathological examination.
3. Uterine necrosis: Up to now, only one case of uterine necrosis has been reported being caused by HEAL.
4. Intrauterine adhesions: After TCRE operation, all surfaces in the uterine cavity is denuded, and its anterior and posterior walls are easy to adhere to each other.
5. Intrauterine hematometra: Turnbull's reported on 59 cases who had magnetic resonance examination after TCRE. It was found that most of patients who had amenorrhea and all of patients who had menses had residual endometrium, and the residual endometrium could not communicate with the uterine cavity, which might lead to hematometra formation, tubal dilatation, and peritoneal cavity effusion.
6. Abdominal pain: Mints et al. reported that 11% of the cases after TCRE developed postoperative abdominal pain, which might be caused by intrauterine adhesions, intrauterine hematometra, and adenomyosis resulting

from the active endometrial cells being squeezed into myometrial layer under intrauterine pressure during TCRE.
7. Post-ablation-tubal sterilization syndrome (PASS): The patients with PASS all had the history of TCRE after sterilization.
8. Adenomyosis: Some scholars proposed that trauma to the uterine myometrium by endometrial ablation might cause this disorder.
9. Pregnancy: There have been reports of postoperative uterine pregnancy or ectopic pregnancy after TCRE. Baumann et al. first reported a successful pregnancy after TCRE and bipolar electrocoagulation of tubal sterilization with good results. Pugh et al. reported one case of successful intrauterine pregnancy after EA. Pinette et al. reported one case of successful pregnancy after YAG laser treatment. The damaged myometrium may cause disastrous consequences in late pregnancy. Therefore, one should minimize the endometrial residues and unnecessary myometrial damages during operation. TCRE/EA has been so widely used in the treatment of AUB that many women of childbearing age choose TCRE/EA, but it may increase obstetric complications significantly, so patients should be informed that desire of fertility is a contraindication. In 2005, Mukul et al. from the United States reported for the first time that a 34-year-old parous woman got intrauterine adhesion and pregnancy after endometrial ablation. She was admitted to hospital after 24 weeks pregnancy because of the shortened cervical canal, multiple intrauterine adhesions, and multiple fetal malformations detected by ultrasonography. Two weeks later, premature rupture of membranes occurred, and the fetal heart appeared to have variable deceleration and classical cesarean section was performed. The fetal multiple malformations were caused by intrauterine adhesion after EA. In a retrospective analysis of 1621 procedures of TCRE from 1990 May to 2005 January in the Hysteroscopy Center made by Xia et al., 32 women with previous TCRE achieved 39 pregnancies, including one case of spontaneous miscarriage, 33 cases of artificial termination of pregnancies, and five ectopic pregnancies. One case developing significant intrauterine adhesion and stenosis after TCRE underwent hysteroscopic adhesiolysis, followed by suction curettage and removal of the gestational sac. One case had heavy bleeding about 700 mL after the gestational sac was aspirated by suction, with general treatment ineffective and bleeding controlled by inserting a Foley balloon to tampon the uterine cavity. One case had right cornual pregnancy and subtotal hysterectomy was performed after a failed artificial suction. One case had left cornual pregnancy and adenomyosis, with hematometra obliterated by adhesions, which was solved by removing the uterus after laparoscopic diagnosis. Cervical pregnancy occurred in one case who developed massive bleeding during suction evacuation. Tubal pregnancy occurred in two. Only one case of intrauterine pregnancy progressed to term and cesarean section was performed, with a small-for-date infant delivered and a subtotal hysterectomy performed because of placenta increta. It indicated that the incidence of postoperative ectopic pregnancy after TCRE was high (12.5%), and the incidence of complications including difficult surgical termination, placental increta, fetal growth restriction, and the abnormalities of the third stage of labor is high. Therefore these women should be regarded as high-risk populations and intensive surveillance should be offered.
10. Malignant lesions of endometrium: TCRE is a new procedure to treat nonmalignant abnormal uterine bleeding, and its data for long-term prognosis are limited and the incidence of endometrial cancer after surgery is unknown. In 2000, Brooks-Carter et al. reported one case of 55-year-old women, to whom EA was applied for the treatment of AUB after the uterine malignant lesion being excluded. Five years later, she developed the same symptoms and was histologically diagnosed as well-differentiated adenocarcinoma (stage 1). It was considered that the endometrial adenocarcinoma was a neoformation because of the intervals and it seems unlikely for high-risk patients with endometrial ablation to obscure the undiscovered malignant or delay the diagnosis. Valle and Baggish reported that the residual endometrium in eight cases after TCRE developed endometrial cancer in later days, and all were detected in time without intrauterine scar concealing the early symptoms of uterine bleeding after TCRE. In 2005, Sagiv et al. from Israel reported that one woman who had EA due to DUB was found to develop endometrial carcinoma 3 years later. Since TCRE/EA cannot remove all layers of the endometrium, even though there was a rigorous screening prior to operation, the patient still has the risk of endometrial cancer after operation, even within 1 year.

9.2.8 Experience and Evaluation of TCRE

After a survey of 5 years' reports from different countries, a successful TCRE and EA is defined as the volume of menstruation is reduced to normal, less, little, or even no menstruation after treatment. Its success rate was from 90 to 95%. With the passage of time after operation, removal of uterus due to recurrence or diseases is on the rise slightly. Among the recurrent cases, excluding those with endometrial carcinoma, a second or a third operation is feasible and

90% of the cases can avoid hysterectomy. As long as the patient selection is proper, the success rate of TCRE will be almost 100%, clinical satisfaction rate after operation decreases slightly every year, and reoperation rate is 6.6%.

9.2.8.1 Effects of Operation

In 2001, Murdoch pointed out that hysteroscopic technique had been applied widely with TCRE usually being regarded as a first-line treatment for DUB, with low mortality. Many researchers pointed out that TCRE is highly effective in the treatment of menorrhagia. Although TCRE has been applied for a shorter time than laser and rollerball electrocoagulation, compared with other hysteroscopic techniques, its advantages are that this operation is faster, is possible to resect the coexisting uterine fibroids, can provide the specimens for histological examination and has lower consumption and operation costs. Liu et al. from the Hysteroscopy Center of Fuxing Hospital, Capital Medical University, explored the influence of TCRE to every grade of uterine artery hematodynamics, and the relationship between TCRE and postoperative effect. They discovered that postoperative outcomes were related to the changes of postoperative uterine hematodynamics with a better outcome in cases with higher resistance of blood after surgery than prior to surgery. As for the long-term prognosis, the worldwide experiences suggested that among TCRE subjects, 70–90% are satisfied with the outcomes of treatment, of which 40–60% have amenorrhea after operation, 30–50% have menstrual reduction, 10–15% have normal menstruation, and the failure rate is 5–12%. The analysis of 5 years of life table after operation indicated that TCRE has made 80% subjects avoid further operation and 91% avoid hysterectomy. Herman et al. reported 270 cases of hysteroscopic operation, with the result that in a 4-year follow-up, only 5.6% of cases who had TCRE needed a second operation, adenomyosis was not a good indication, and only 37% of cases did not require removal of the uterus. Xia reported 366 cases of TCRE with a follow-up from 3 months to 4 years, of which 16 cases underwent hysterectomy due to operation failure, 350 cases had improved menstruation, with the success rate of the operation 95.6%. One hundred forty-six cases (41.7%) had amenorrhea following operation, of which 15 cases had a small amount of menses before amenorrhea; 119 cases (34%) had spotting, of which 22 cases had amenorrhea within 4–18 months after operation; among 85 cases (24.3%) who were found to have adenomyosis during operation, 46 were followed up for more than 3 months, of them 44 cases had menstrual improvement, two cases underwent hysterectomy, with the success rate 95.6%; in 46 cases with original dysmenorrhea, postoperative dysmenorrhea disappeared or were relieved in 36 cases (78.3%). Yin reported 170 cases of EA, of which 70 patients had dysmenorrhea prior to operation, and dysmenorrhea disappeared or reduced in 38 cases (54%) after operation. Tsaltas conducted a postoperative follow-up of 232 cases of TCRE for 6 months to 6 years and 6 months, and found that the satisfaction rate was 78%, 13% had repeat endometrial ablation, and 17% had hysterectomy. Schiotz reported that TCRE had a good effect in short term following the procedure in treatment of menorrhagia, and 20% underwent hysterectomy in the long term. And it was reported in this paper that 324 cases had 348 TCRE procedures, of which 68 cases had fibroids resected simultaneously with a prospective follow-up of 1–8 years (mean 3.8 years), and reoperation including TCRE or hysterectomy was classified as unsatisfied; three cases had uterine perforation (0.9%), with one case solved by laparotomy, 18 cases (5.2%) had hemorrhage, ten cases had fluid overload (2.9%), and five cases (1.4%) had infection. Follow-up results showed 63 cases (19.4%) had hysterectomy, of which 45 cases (67.2%) attributed it to pain partly or wholly. At the late research stage, 246 cases in 260 were satisfied (94.6%). They concluded that TCRE was a safe and effective method in the treatment of menorrhagia. Eighty percent of them might avoid major operations and some patients undergo operation just because of pain, but this pain, being not typical, is difficult to diagnose from uterine origin. El Senoun et al. reported 91 cases of EA from 1992 to 1997 for treatment of menorrhagia in women who were unresponsive to medication. Follow-up was conducted by questionnaire for at least 18 months (6–43), and 88% (80/91) responded. The prognostic indicators included satisfaction rate, symptom relief rate, improvement rate of health and life quality, etc. The results were that 44% of cases (35/80) had amenorrhea, ten cases underwent further treatment, including seven cases (9%) of hysterectomy; 73% of cases had relief in periodic pelvic pain; 65% had improvement in premenstrual tension syndrome; 85% had improved work ability; 96% had improved sexual life; 99% returned to work in 4 weeks. Seventy-nine percent of patients were satisfied with treatment, 91% of patients would like to recommend to friends. The author concluded that EA technique was simple, effective, and an acceptable treatment for the selected cases. And its ultimate effectiveness needed a long-term follow-up. Rosati et al. from Italy reported that in 438 cases of premenopausal women without endometrial pretreatment, the rollerball electrode was used to coagulate the endometrium at the uterine fundus and uterine cornua, and then the wire loop electrode was used to remove the endometrium in the rest of the uterine cavity, and finally the rollerball electrode was used again to burn the uterine cavity with endometrium removed. An average follow-up was 48.2 months, among those who responded, 47.8% had no menstruation, 46% had little menstruation. One case (0.3%) had EA again, 20 patients (5.2%) underwent hysterectomy, of which 15 cases (3.9%) failed in EA, and the other 5 patients were unrelated with EA (endometrial atypical hyperplasia or uterine fibroids). Two hundred ninety-two cases (75.8%)

were very satisfied and 78 cases satisfied (20.3%). There were no major complications. During follow-up, 3 patients (0.8%) had pregnancy. The author believed that EA was a safe and effective method in the treatment of premenopausal menorrhagia and uterine bleeding, and could avoid 95% hysterectomy. However, patients should be informed about the possibility of postoperative pregnancy and could not consider it as a contraceptive method. Munro reported that the therapeutical effect of EA was not so ideal that 25–40% of cases had a second operation within 5 years after EA, which was often hysterectomy. Xia reported that 159 in 1431 cases (10.84%) were treated with drug therapy including hemostasis, analgesics, antibiotics, progesterone, and endometrial inhibitor, of whom 37 cases underwent repeated TCRE (2.59%); 87 cases (6.08%) had ultimately hysterectomy because of recurrence of hemorrhage symptom, dysmenorrhea, or uterine fibroids, of whom one case was found to have early invasive cervical cancer, three cases were endometrial adenocarcinoma, three cases got postablation-sterilization syndrome (PASS), four cases had voluntary removal of the uterus because of continuous dripping for half a year after operation, 31 cases had uterine leiomyoma, which continued to grow, 45 cases had uterine adenomyosis. The cure rate of operation was 93.92%.

1. High-risk factors of TCRE failure: Raiga et al. studied the risk factors associated with failed TCRE and found that when it was followed up for 2–4 years, the results were satisfactory, but there were problems of late recurrence. Both the enlarged uterus and adenomyosis increase the failure rate, so it needs a long-term evaluation. McCausland et al. thought that the deep adenomyosis (invasive depth >2.5 mm) was the main factor of TCRE failure.
2. High-risk factors for hysterectomy after TCRE: Dutton analyzed 240 cases of EA with or without resection of polyps or fibroids for treatment of menorrhagia, with a mean follow-up of 31.2 months. Seventy-one percent didn't have hysterectomy in the first 5 years, ten cases had another EA, of which six cases had the uterus removed finally. After analysis of multiple factors, the conclusion was reached that sterilization was a risk factor for hysterectomy. The women of at least 45 years old had smaller risk for hysterectomy than those below 35 years old. In this report, the duration of the postoperative follow-up of EA was longer than those in previous reports, and a second EA and being young were risk factors for hysterectomy. Boe Engelsen followed up 390 procedures of TCRE in the following 4–10 years, and found that 16.6% had hysterectomy for pain or bleeding; 50% of them were within 2 postoperative years, and 6 were found to have malignant disease. He found that operation prognosis was unrelated to operator's experience. In Munro's study, 25–40% of cases had a second operation within 5 years after EA, most of which were hysterectomy. In 2007, Furst et al. reported a study on follow-up of 61 cases of EA and 59 cases of TCRE for 10 years, with 3% loss of follow-up. There were no differences in prognosis between the two groups. Eleven percent had a second EA, and 11% had a second TCRE; 22% had hysterectomy, mostly in 2 years. The author pointed out that the period of 2 years following EA was risk period for hysterectomy and thereafter, the probability of hysterectomy decreased to 6%.
3. Effect of TCRE and endometrial pretreatment: Donnez et al. reported a prospective randomized double blind study of goserelin pretreatment followed by EA for treatment of DUB with a 3 years follow-up, in which there were 358 premenopausal women over 30 years old from 37 centers of 12 countries. Goserelin was administered 3.6 mg, once per 28 days, for 8 weeks. EA was performed at about the sixth week when the endometrium was the thinnest. The amenorrhea rate of the third year after EA was 21% in goserelin group and 14% in the control group ($P = 0.0571$); 21% of cases in goserelin group had hysterectomy, while there was 15% in the control group; 5.6% of cases in goserelin group and 2.1% in the control group had the second EA. The conclusion was that there was a higher rate of amenorrhea in goserelin group than that in control group. Tiufekchieva and Nikolov reported that GnRH-a could reduce the endometrial thickness. Two doses before TCRE could shorten the operation time and produce a high amenorrhea rate; within 6–12 months after operation, the amenorrhea rate was 62.7% in medication group, while 27.2% in untreated group.
4. Relationship between the outcome of TCRE and the patients' ages: The studies made by Seidman et al. suggested that after TCRE the amenorrhea rate and the complete relief rate of dysmenorrhea were significantly higher in the older women than that in the young. In his postoperative follow-up of 162 cases (95.9%) with the average duration 32 ± 17 months, it was found that postoperative complications were unrelated to age. There were no difference in ratio between a second hysteroscopic operation and hysterectomy. Cravello et al. reported 102 menopausal women aged 47–67 years with postmenopausal bleeding or bleeding due to HRT. By hysteroscopy and ultrasonography, 87 cases were found to have benign intrauterine lesions (51 cases of polyps, 36 cases of leiomyoma), and 15 cases were found without significant lesion; after endometrial ablation with polypectomy or myomectomy, 88 patients (86.27%) were satisfied with the long-term therapeutic effect. They concluded that the therapeutic effect of TCRE depends on the causes of hemorrhage rather than the patient's age.

9.2.8.2 Endometrial Repair After TCRE/EA

Colgan et al. studied the process of endometrial repair after EA. Among 19 cases included, 15 cases were for DUB, and four cases were for endometrial hyperplasia which was discovered by TCRE. The uterus was removed 1–48 months after operation for histological examination. Six specimens were within 3 months post-operation, with myometrial necrosis, red foreign bodies, granulomatous response, thermal damages, and changes of acute inflammation observed. The remaining 13 specimens were obtained 3–16 months post-operation, showing persistent granulomatous response and/or foreign bodies. Most (9/12) had obvious endometrial scar. So, it was thought that the postoperative reaction of EA is granulomatous endometritis. In the Hysteroscopy Center of Fuxing Hospital, Capital Medical University, 26 women were observed hysteroscopically within 3 months to 1 year following TCRE, who were found to have a small amount of endometrium in uterine cavity regardless of menstruation (Figs. 9.43, 9.44, and 9.45), but only those with no period were found to have glandless endometrium.

9.2.8.3 One-Stage TCRE

TCRE usually takes three steps, namely, (1) hysteroscopy and endometrial biopsy; (2) endometrial pretreatment for inhibition of endometrial hyperplasia; (3) resection of endometrium. In 1992, Van Damme tried not to apply endometrial pretreatment with hormone drugs in some cases, but performed (1) and (3) at one operation, thus simplifying the TCRE procedures and reducing the patient's pain, which is one-stage TCRE. The selection conditions for one-stage TCRE are as follows: (1) below 40 years old; (2) even with prolonged bleeding but a regular menstrual cycle; (3) curettage with endometrial pathological results within 6 months; (4) uterus of normal size or slightly larger.

During operation, the procedure begins with diagnostic hysteroscopy. If any suspicion, samples are taken for examination and the procedure may proceed no further; otherwise,

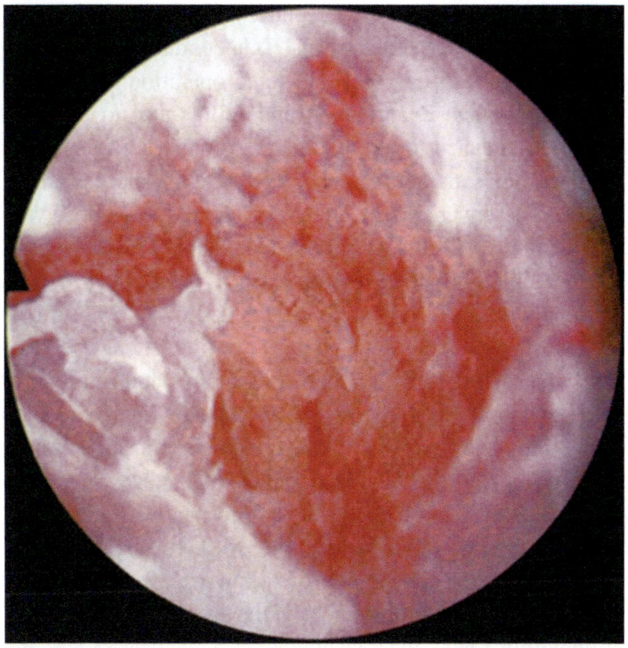

Fig. 9.44 Endometrium and bleeding in uterine cavity after TCRE

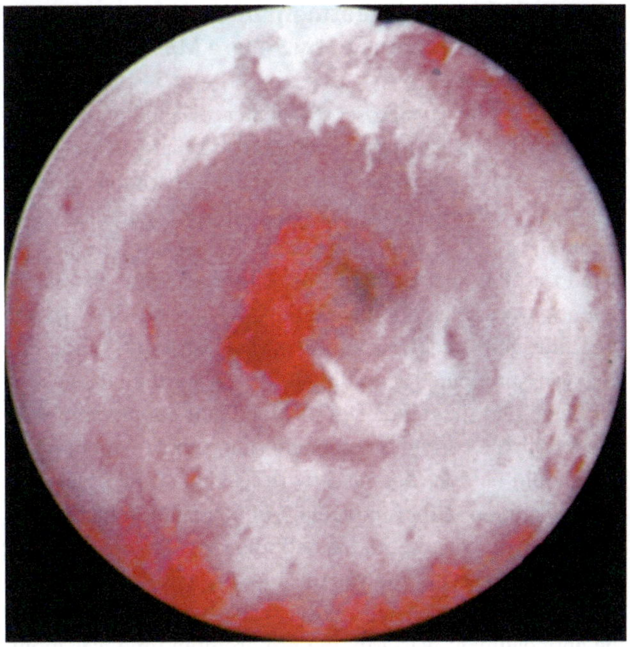

Fig. 9.43 Uterine cavity at 10 months after TCRE

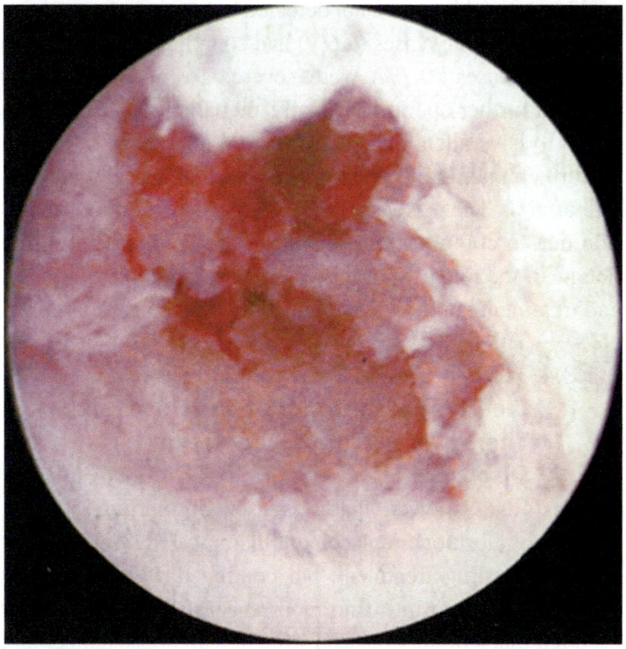

Fig. 9.45 At 14 months after TCRE, the cavity is narrow with tiny amount of endometrium in a woman with little menstruation

dilate the cervix and go on with the operation. If endometrium is thickening, perform curettage first to reduce its thickness, and send the endometrial samples for examination. Then endometrial resection is performed with electric wire loop or endometrial ablation with rollerball electrode. The current power of electric resection is 70 W and the cutting reaches 2–3 mm myometrium beneath endometrium, the resected muscle strips are also sent for histopathological examination; the current power of electrocautery is 60 W and the depth is the site where the endometrial layer disappears, and braided muscle fibers reveal. Xia conducted a prospective study of 125 cases of one-stage operation. Through a histopathological examination and follow-up, no cases of endometrial cancer or premalignant lesions were found with the operation satisfaction rate of 98%, and the success rate of 99.2%. There were no differences compared with those who had the three procedures. It indicated that one stage of TCRE was feasible, safe and effective, and consistent with Van Damme's report of operation satisfaction of 97.5%. To perform one-stage operation, one must pay high attention to two steps: the preoperative selection of patients and intraoperative hysteroscopic diagnosis. Continuously improving and perfecting the ability to evaluate endometrial diseases under hysteroscope is the key to complete one-stage operation. Wortman and Daggett conducted a retrospective study of 304 cases of refractory uterine bleeding, with the average age 41 years and the mean duration of follow-up 32 months after operation. Eighty-three percent of the cases had no menstruation within 1 year, the total amenorrhea rate was 85.5%, and only 0.8% showed no improvement. The histological examination showed that 17 cases (5.6%) had significant endometrial lesions, which were not detected by routine preoperative screening. Twenty cases (6.6%) had complications, of which only two cases (0.7%) were severe. Twenty-seven cases required further operation. Finally, 69 patients (22.7%) were found to have adenomyosis, which did not increase the rate of further operation. They concluded that the amenorrhea rate after TCRE was very high, fewer cases required operation due to complications, histological specimens might be obtained, the rate of morbidity was lower, and the diagnosis and treatment could be completed with one-stage operation.

9.2.8.4 TCRE in the Treatment of Uterine Bleeding Resulting from the Hormone Therapy and Blood Coagulation Disorders

Phillips' data showed that 29 cases of uterine bleeding induced by hormone replacement therapy (HRT) were unresponsive to drug treatment, but continued with HRT after TCRE with the result of no recurrence of bleeding. Romer reported that a premenopausal woman with breast cancer had repeated uterine bleeding after taking tamoxifen and three curettages with no malignant lesion. After undergoing TCRE, she was treated with tamoxifen continuously and had no bleeding in a follow-up of 2 years, and the result of ultrasonography scanning showed no sonographic appearance of endometrium. Goldenberg et al. reported 11 cases of menorrhagia due to blood coagulation disorders who were ineffective to medication. After TCRE, the satisfaction rate was high (10/11) in a postoperative follow-up of 1 year. These patients cannot tolerate the major operations, so the hysteroscopic operation is essential for them. Milad and Valle successfully conducted emergency EA for 3 women with blood coagulation disorders, which eased the sudden severe uterine bleeding resulting from blood disease and reduced the patients' demand for blood products, but could not cure. The use of rollerball electrode in EA is the most simple and safe method to treat severe uterine bleeding. The role of rollerball electrode is to close vessel and cause necrosis. Therefore, it needs low power and high voltage. However, the resection of endometrium or myometrial layer will open new blood vessels and exacerbates bleeding. The uterine bleeding induced by leukemia or drugs can be reduced or stopped by EA.

Romer reported 35 perimenopausal and menopausal women, who underwent EA following hysteroscopy and endometrial biopsy due to HRT induced bleeding with no complications, and continued to use the combined HRT after operation. A follow-up of 12 months showed that 34 cases had amenorrhea and were satisfied with treatment; 1 woman stopped to use HRT for other side effects. It was believed that EA was a minimally invasive approach to treat this disorder without intrauterine lesions, and after operation, HRT can be continued, thus increasing the compliance of HRT in the selected cases.

9.2.8.5 TCRE in the Treatment of Uterine Bleeding Caused by Severe Medical Diseases

Scholars in the Hysteroscopy Center of Fuxing Hospital, Capital Medical University, summarized the experiences of 76 cases with medical diseases, and their operation information can be seen in Table 9.2. In addition to regular TCRE preparation before operation, these 76 cases were also prepared for other medical diseases. The cases with renal insufficiency were treated by hemodialysis, making BUN (blood urea nitrogen) under 80 mmol/L; the cases with blood disease were pretreated according to its causes, with the anemia corrected and the deficiency of blood cell components supplied, both the correction of anemia and supplement of platelets should be done for cases with leukemia; the cases with cirrhosis required the supplement of coagulation factors; the cases with diabetes should take oral hypoglycemic agents or insulin injection to control the blood glucose level below 11 mmol/L; the cases with cardiac valve replacement stopped the anticoagulant warfarin, the prothrombin time was monitored at the same time, and the operation could be done when

Table 9.2 Types of hysteroscopic operations of 76 cases with severe medical complications

Severe medical diseases	Renal failure	Blood diseases	Heart disease	Diabetes mellitus	Hypertension	Cardiac valve replacement	Thoracic deformity	Lupus erythematosus	Cirrhosis	Total
No. of cases	22	18	11	10	9	3	1	1	1	76
TCRE	13	9	5	4	4	2	0	1	1	39
EA	0	5	1	0	0	0	0	0	0	6
TCRM	0	0	4	2	3	1	1	0	0	11
TCRE+P	7	4	0	4	1	0	0	0	0	16
TCRE+M	2	0	1	0	1	0	0	0	0	4

it was normal, and restored taking warfarin in 36–72 h after operation. All 76 patients had successful operations with little intraoperative bleeding, with the average depth of uterine cavity 7.8 cm (6.5–8.2 cm), the average operation time 13.2 min (8–22 min), and the average weight of the removed endometrial tissue 4.6 g (3–7 g). After operation, two cases were complicated with severe anemia and transient fever, one case of cardiac mechanical valve replacement resumed taking warfarin without permission 18 h later after TCRE, which resulted in active arterial bleeding of uterine cavity about 800 mL within 24 h post-operation and shock, then she was sent back to the operating room and bleeding stopped by rollerball electrocoagulation of the bleeding point. Due to the decrease in platelet, the patient was transfused of two units platelet when she was back to the recovery room, and she recovered smoothly. In a follow-up of 6 months to 9 years and 6 months, two cases had irregular bleeding, who were cured with the drug treatment. One case had amenorrhea, and because of the transplanted kidney failure, she died of kidney failure after a year and half of operation; among the rest 75 cases, 36 cases had amenorrhea, 28 cases had dripping bleeding, and 11 cases had obviously reduced menstruation, with the operation satisfaction rate 96%.

Wallwiener et al. reported 34 cases of blood coagulation disorders and refractory to medical treatment. In order to avoid hysterectomy, they underwent EA, with the postoperative result of 64.71% amenorrhea or dripping menstruation. And after a second EA, the amenorrhea or dripping menstrual rate increased to 82.35%, in which the effect of EA on bleeding induced by the use of anticoagulants was obviously superior to those with the endogenous blood coagulation disorders. Therefore, it was considered that EA was a valuable alternative in treating patients who had AUB associated with coagulation and thrombosis disorders. Xia et al. reported 1431 women who underwent TCRE in their Hysteroscopy Center, of them 219 (15.30%) had severe medical complications. After operation, their life qualities were all improved in a short period, and in a long-term follow-up of 88 cases, the satisfactory rate was 100%. It was concluded that TCRE was a good alternative to hysterectomy for AUB patients with severe medical complications.

9.2.8.6 Uterine Malignant Lesions Detected During TCRE/EA

In 2001, Vilos et al. reported three cases of uterine sarcoma which were detected in 2402 cases of TCRE. One of them was low-grade endometrial stromal sarcoma and the other two were carcinosarcoma. Two women underwent hysterectomy and found no residual cancers in the specimen of uterus. The third woman was 82 years old and refused hysterectomy. She had moderate bleeding before surgery and achieved amenorrhea after treatment. The author's experience was that the incidence rate of sarcoma of uterus was about 1/800 of TCRE due to AUB, and that complete endometrial resection may provide a diagnosis and a minimally invasive treatment for patients at high risk for hysterectomy. Agostini et al. assessed the risks of endometrial carcinoma and atypical hyperplasia with postoperative histopathological diagnosis on 325 postmenopausal women who received hysteroscopic endometrial resection or ablation. All of cases had postmenopausal bleeding or HRT related bleeding, and performed diagnostic hysteroscopy with endometrial biopsy, so that endometrial cancer or atypical hyperplasia was excluded. Then 203 cases underwent TCRE (62.5%) and 122 cases received EA (37.5%). Endometrial carcinoma and atypical endometrial hyperplasia were detected in two cases of each group. It was considered that diagnostic hysteroscopy with endometrial biopsy cannot fully exclude endometrial cancer or endometrial atypical hyperplasia, which may be found during hysteroscopic operation.

9.2.8.7 TCRE for Emergency Hemostasis

Franchini et al. underwent emergency TCRE for 25 cases of severe uterine bleeding, of which one case was found to have endometrial carcinoma and received hysterectomy instead, 15 cases had amenorrhea after operation. Therefore, in a follow-up of 19 months, it was found that TCRE could effectively control uterine bleeding, prevent bleeding recurrence and avoid drugs or operation treatment. Osuga et al. underwent successful emergency EA for one postmenopausal woman with cirrhosis and morbid obesity who suffered from severe life-threatening uterine bleeding for invasive operation and had failed uterine artery embolization.

9.2.8.8 Endometrial Adenocarcinoma Found During TCRE

Vilos et al. conducted a retrospective study of 13 women with abnormal bleeding who underwent TCRE and were diagnosed as endometrial cancer by postoperative histopathological examination. All of them failed to take adequate determinable biopsy during diagnostic hysteroscopy and endometrial biopsy before TCRE. Of them 8 women received total resection of endometrium (first group), 5 women received partial resection (second group). By histopathological examination of removed uterus after hysterectomy, two cases in the first group had focal lesions, and no case in the second group had these lesions. There were no recurrences 0.5–9 years after hysterectomy. TCRE/EA are alternatives to hysterectomy in the treatment of DUB. If the existing endometrial cancer is missed for diagnosis prior to EA, it will be difficult to find after operation. In addition, the postoperative residual endometrium may also develop cancerization and its incidence is still unknown. Margolis et al. reported that a 58-year-old woman who had undergone EA 3 years ago was incidentally found to have asymptomatic endometrial adenocarcinoma histopathologically after hysterectomy and Marshall–Marchetti–Krantz operation due to stress urinary incontinence. By histopathological examination of the specimen of the uterus, it showed invasion of the myometrial layer >50%, FIGO stage I_C.

9.2.8.9 A Repeat TCRE/EA

Wortman and Daggett assessed the safety and effectiveness of a second hysteroscopic operation after the failure of EA and TCRE. Twenty-six patients with postoperative pain, bleeding, or asymptomatic hematometra following first endometrial surgery underwent hysteroscopic endomyometrial resection with ultrasonography surveillance. The average time from the start of treatment to the repeated operation was 41.2 ± 47.9 months. Five cases (19.2%) required a simple dilation of the uterus, 21 cases needed cutting the internal cervical os open before entering the uterine cavity. The average operation time was 20.3 ± 9.5 min, the average weight of specimens was 6.7 ± 4.9 g. Fifteen (57.7%) specimens showed adenomyosis. The mean follow-up was 23.2 ± 22.7 months; 23 cases (88.5%) were satisfied and hysterectomy was avoided. Three cases (11.5%) underwent hysterectomy due to postoperative pain or bleeding. It was concluded that a second hysteroscopic operation is effective for those who failed in endometrial resection or ablation, with the result of amenorrhea or pain relief and helping the majority of patients to avoid hysterectomy.

9.2.8.10 Hormone Replacement Therapy After TCRE/EA

Romer reported that more and more patients underwent TCRE when their medication treatment was unresponsive to AUB. Residual endometrial foci could be found in 70% of the patients who had no period after operation. Therefore, they suggested that HRT should be used continuously in peri- or postmenopausal women including progesterone after endometrial resection or ablation. In 2000, Romer et al. reported again that those who needed HRT after EA should be added gestagen. Continuous use of HRT could prevent postoperative bleeding, as well as prevent the residual endometrium from hyperplasia. IUD containing progesterone can be also used as a substitute after operation.

9.2.8.11 TCRE for Infertility

Cravello et al. reported among the patients who underwent EA after ineffective treatment of AUB with progesterone, there were some who had pregnancy after the cure of bleeding and might have a full-term labor.

9.2.8.12 TCRE for Adenomyosis

Xia et al. reported that among 208 patients who underwent TCRE for AUB, 28 were found to have adenomyosis via intraoperative vision under hysteroscope, ultrasonography images of distension fluid penetrating into uterine myometrium, and report of histopathological examinations. After follow-up of 3–34 months, 2 patients underwent hysterectomy, and the other 26 cases were satisfied with the operation, with the operative success rate 92.86%. All of cases achieved improvement of menstruations and cure of anemia. 77.8% of 18 patients with previous dysmenorrhea had elimination of pain, of whom 22.2% achieved relief, with satisfactory outcome in a short term. The improvement of menstruations is caused by failure of functional endometrial generation after the removal of the basal layer of the endometrium. By analyzing the causes of effective treatment for dysmenorrhea, they may have mild lesions with only junctional zone involved and thickened, and most lesions are resected or coagulated. The ectopic endometrial foci are non-existent or reduced, leading to decrease of spasmodic contractions of surrounding leiomyomas, resulting in relief or disappearance of postoperative dysmenorrhea caused by stimulating ectopic endometrial hematocele, edema, and bleeding. For patients who underwent hysterectomy after operation, the lesions of adenomyosis had depth to serosa, which led to the failure of endometrial resection. Keckstein also believed that TCRE/EA could effectively provide the treatment of the symptomatic superficial adenomyosis, and the hysteroscopic operation can cure the selected cases of symptomatic localized adenomyosis. In a study conducted by McCausland V and McCausland A, it was found that the outcome of endometrial ablation will be better in cases with the depth of the penetration of adenomyosis into myometrium <2.5 mm, and be worse in cases with the depth of penetration >2.5 mm. In a retrospective study of success rate in 121 cases with adenomyosis and underwent TCRE due to failure of treatment of AUB with progesterone reported by Quemere et al., with a maximum duration of 8 years follow-up, it showed that the success rate following one operation was 56%, and following one or two operations was 67%. 11% of the cases had repeat resections. 17 cases (19%) had hysterectomy due to the recurrence of bleeding. The result they achieved was similar to those reported by others, and the authors held that adenomyosis was not the failure factor of TCRE/EA, except there is deep adenomyosis difficult to be diagnosed prior to operation. Zheng et al. from Hysteroscopy Center of Fuxing Hospital, Capital Medical University, applied TCRE in combination with LNG-IUS for treating adenomyosis in 20 women who wished to reserve the uterus and without the demand of fertility. A LNG-IUS was inserted into the uterus following the procedure of TCRE. After 12 months of follow-up, all women achieved amenorrhea, which indicated that the combined treatment could effectively avoid the prolonged dripping bleeding caused by the placement of LNG-IUS alone, and prevent the occurrence of the complications including postoperative pregnancy, uterine hematocele, recurrence of bleeding and expulsion of IUD, etc. Furthermore, Dr. Xia held that endometrial resection with the combination of laparoscopic uterine artery blockage, or repeat coagulation of cutting surface with vaporizing electrode following resecting could improve the operative outcomes.

9.2.8.13 TCRE Applied to Larger Uterus

In a retrospective analysis conducted by Eskandar et al., of 42 cases of uterine bleeding, with the uterine volume >12 weeks, the length of uterine cavity >12 cm, and the average age 45.6 ± 6 years, a comparison was made in the application of TCRE and EA of its practicability, safety, prognosis, and irrigation fluid absorption. Twenty-six patients (62%) had endometrial pretreatment, 27 patients (65%) underwent EA surgery, and 27 patients (65%) had TCRE, all of which were done in a day surgery setting. They used multiple regression analysis to explore the correlation between the size of uterus, pretreatment, procedures, operation time, and irrigation fluid absorption, with the result that there was more absorption of irrigation fluid in TCRE than that in EA ($P = 0.04$), and that the absorption volume was related to the type of operation ($R = 0.32$, $P = 0.04$), but unrelated with the operation time, the size of the uterus, and pretreatment. Two women underwent hysterectomy because of uterine fibroids or endometrial cancer. In 39 cases with a follow-up of 12–16 months, amenorrhea was achieved in 30, oligomenorrhea achieved in 6, and normal menses in 3, with the satisfaction rate of 93% (38/39). They held that EA was still a feasible, safe and effective alternative to hysterectomy for treatment of menorrhagia even though the uterus is large.

9.2.8.14 Comparison of TCRE and Drug Therapy for the Treatment of Menorrhagia

Cooper et al. conducted a follow-up of 187 patients with menorrhagia treated by TCRE or medical treatment, respectively. They used a questionnaire to measure the patients' satisfaction, menstruation, health status, and quality of life 5 years after treatment. The follow-up rate was 77% and the results of the fifth year were: in medication group of 94 patients, 7 were still using drugs; 72 finally underwent the surgical treatment, including 17 patients of hysterectomy, with satisfaction rate very low and unwillingness to introduce to friends. In TCRE group, 25 cases had a further operation including 15 patients undergoing hysterectomy. The scores of bleeding and pain were similar between two groups and decreased significantly when compared with preoperation. The health recovery in TCRE group was better than that in medication group. It was thought that in the treatment of severe menorrhagia, the use of TCRE might receive a high satisfaction rate, gain a reduced menstrual flow, improve greatly the patients' health and quality of life, and be safe without additional hysterectomy. Thus it could be introduced to the patients who meet the requirements. Mansour reported that since the development of mirena (levonorgestrel, LNG-IUS), 9 millions of women from the whole world had already used it for contraception and menorrhagia treatment. For women of childbearing age, LNG-IUS is one of the most acceptable drug therapies. Istre and Trolle held that both LNG-IUS and EA have the same therapeutic effects of treating menorrhagia, but LNG-IUS can be reversible and with little operative risk. In 2010, de Souza et al. conducted a randomized prospective study of the application of LNG-IUS or thermal balloon ablation for menorrhagia, and found that the volume of blood loss in both groups was significantly decreased, but no statistic difference was detected between two groups. In another randomized control trial recently reported by Gupta et al., it was found that, when compared with conventional medical treatment, the proportion of the cases changing to other treatment or terminating the treatment in the group of using the LNG-IUS within 2 years was lower, and the satisfactory score achieved in cases using LNG-IUS for menorrhagia was higher. Gupta et al. also compared the effectiveness of LNG-IUS with TCRE in patients with DUB. One year after the treatment, the decrease of the period volume and the rise of hemoglobin levels in LNG-IUS group were nearly the same as those in TCRE group, which indicated that treatment with LNG-IUS had similar effects to surgical treatment in reducing the bleeding and improving anemia. In addition, placement of LNG-IUS required less experience and could provide contraceptive effects.

9.2.8.15 Comparison Between TCRE and Transabdominal or Transvaginal Hysterectomy

From the worldwide literatures reported in cases with TCRE, 70–90% of the subjects were satisfied with the outcome of treatment, of which 40–60% had amenorrhea after operation,

30–50% had oligomenorrhea, and 10–15% had normal menstruation, with a failure rate of 5–12%. It has been found that hysteroscopic surgery has the advantages of shorter operative time, less complications, less requirement for analgesics, quicker postoperative recovery, and sooner return to work compared to hysterectomy. The cost of TCRE abroad is much lower than that of hysterectomy, while they are similar in China. Alexander et al. conducted an important randomized comparative study of the mental factors in cases after hysterectomy and resection of endometrium. The results showed there was a reduction in the mental symptoms following operation in both groups and no differences in sexual life and marriage relationship between the two groups. However, the operator of hysteroscopic procedure requires special training and operative experience; and non-isotonic irrigation fluid and any dangerous energy source can cause complications, while the operator who performs abdominal or vaginal hysterectomy has no such worries. For patients who should undergo hysterectomy due to menorrhagia, Pinion et al. performed hysterectomy in 99 cases and hysteroscopic surgery in 105 cases, of whom TCRE in 52 cases and HEAL in 53 cases. The outcomes observed included complications, postoperative recovery and menstruation, relief of other symptoms, and patients' satisfaction in the two groups. Compared with women who had hysterectomy, women undergoing hysteroscopic surgery had less morbidity in early term postoperatively and had shorter recovery period, with the full recovery period 2–4 weeks, and 2–3 months in women with hysterectomy ($P < 0.001$). With the follow-up of 12 months after hysteroscopic surgery, postoperative outcomes included hysterectomy (17 cases), repeated hysteroscopic surgery (11 cases), menorrhagia or brown discharge (45 cases), and light period (35 cases). Most cases in both groups had a relief in dysmenorrhea or premenstrual symptoms. At 12 months after operations, the satisfaction rates were 89% (79/89) and 78% (85/89) respectively in hysterectomy group and hysteroscopy group ($P < 0.05$), the relief of the symptoms were 95% (85/89) and 90% (86/96) respectively, and the expectation of the patients to recommend their surgery to others were 72% (64/89) and 71% (68/96) respectively. They concluded that hysteroscopic surgery had less complications and shorter recovery time than hysterectomy. Though hysterectomy achieved a higher satisfactory rate, it was between 70 and 90% with hysteroscopic surgery. Hence they insisted that hysteroscopic surgery could be considered as an alternative to hysterectomy for treatment of DUB. Clarke et al. investigated the readmissions of patients within 5 years after TCRE or hysteroscopy, to determine whether TCRE can replace hysterectomy. The results showed that within 5 years following surgery, the readmission rates were 41.7% in women with hysterectomy and 44.6% in women with TCRE. Readmissions for gynecological reasons were 12.6% and 30.3%, respectively. Among women who were readmitted for gynecological reasons, the readmission rates were similar in both groups within postoperative 6 months and were lower in hysterectomy group than that in TCRE group. Therefore it indicated that, within 5 years after hysterectomy or TCRE, the readmission rate in hysterectomy group was lower, especially for those readmitted for gynecological reasons. They concluded that hysterectomy appeared to have more definitive effect. The data presented by Hidlebaugh showed that the cost of transvaginal hysterectomy was the least. Compared with abdominal hysterectomy, the direct cost of laparoscopic-assisted vaginal hysterectomy was higher, while the indirect cost was significantly low. Both direct and indirect costs of TCRE/EA were significantly lower than those of hysterectomy, even including the cost of treatment failures. TCRE/EA avoided major surgery, shortened hospitalization period, rapidly returned to normal activity, and should be the preferred method for patients with AUB.

9.2.8.16 Comparison Between TCRE and Other Methods of Endometrial Ablation

As an alternative to hysterectomy in the treatment of abnormal uterine bleeding caused by benign lesions, endometrial ablation is to use various energy sources or technical design to reduce menstrual blood loss. The rollerball electrocoagulation endometrial ablation and the laser endometrial ablation are two of these minimally invasive techniques, which have the similar therapeutic effects to TCRE. Recently, there are a number of new minimally invasive non-hysteroscopic techniques available in the treatment of menorrhagia, including radiofrequency endometrial ablation, microwave endometrial ablation, bipolar electroresection, uterine balloon thermoablation, cryo-endometrial ablation, photodynamic endometrial ablation, laser beam (laser thermal ablation), hydro thermo-ablation, and so on. Vilos et al. reported an endometrial ablation system with uterine thermal balloon for the treatment of menorrhagia, and the initial results in a postoperative 18-month follow-up indicated that the postoperative improvement in menorrhagia was 77%, which was similar to other techniques of endometrial ablation. However, with the passage of time, the failure rate might be increased, and another endometrial surgery was needed. Since this is a simple operation and just involves the techniques as placement of IUD into the uterine cavity, the chances of severe complications are slim, and thus, it is generally considered as the primary method of treatment for menorrhagia. Nisolle insisted that this non-hysteroscopic EA is only suitable for DUB, and the endometrial biopsy should be done before operation. If biopsy reveals normal endometrium and ultrasonography shows no polyps or fibroids, then it is feasible to administer non-hysteroscopic EA in the treatment of DUB. In 2007, Deb et al. from the United Kingdom collected the data from 610 doctors, of whom 449 (73%) performed TCRE or EA. The most preferred method was thermal balloon ablation (32.1%), then microwave endometrial ablation (29.8%). The orders of other techniques were TCRE alone or combined with roller ball coagulation (18.5%), Novasure (9.8%), hydrotherm ablation (6.9%), rollerball ablation (2%), and laser ablation (0.9%). There were 52.2% of patients applying GnRH analogs as pretreatment medication. Variations in treatment methods have made a challenge of assessment of clinical efficacy. Wamsteker held that the greatest advantage of EA/TCRE under hysteroscope was in completing the treatment under direct vision of uterine cavity from the beginning to the end of operations, while the problems with the other non-hysteroscopic treatments are lack of visualization or control of the procedures. He pointed out that although the above non-hysteroscopic EA operations were often advertised as "day surgery," they were not found suitable for outpatient, at least for now. In addition, the disposable equipment was expensive, and it was useless to operators who were experienced with EA or TCRE. Up to now, a number of studies indicate that the techniques using these devices can produce the same therapeutic effects as the traditional hysteroscopic resection or ablation, but more studies will help to account for the appropriate role of non-hysteroscopic devices for EA in gynecology. In view of the risk and complications of hysteroscopic operation, great care should be taken to prevent the most severe hyponatremia encephalopathy and fluid overload.

It is worth mentioning that recently a large number of retrospective studies were carried out to compare the results of transurethral resection of the prostate (TURP) and open prostatectomy, which indicated that there were only a few cases dying of cardiovascular disease after operation of TURP in an 8-year follow-up of patients, but it was significantly more than that of patients after open prostatectomy. TCRE is similar to TURP in many aspects, but is completely different from TURP in diseased population and operation procedures. Therefore, these findings do not apply to the hysteroscopic operation. However, the research suggests that short-term experience cannot foresee long-term effects, and a proper follow-up is needed when the safety and efficacy of this new technology are evaluated.

9.3 Transcervical Resection of Myoma

Enlan Xia and Ning Ma

Uterine myoma, also named uterine leiomyoma, is the most common solid tumor, and also the most common indication for hysterectomy. It was estimated that 20–25% of women over 35 were suffering from this disease. Its symptoms include menorrhagia and abnormal uterine bleeding, which may lead to anemia, dysmenorrhea and (or) lower abdominal pain, lumbosacral pain, infertility, and premature labor. This is not only common in women of 40–50 years old, but also in young women, and severe bleeding and infertility may be caused. Under normal circumstances, the size of uterine myoma decreases in postmenopausal women. Submucous myoma is often complicated by chronic endometritis, and is at a higher risk of malignancy (leiomyosarcoma) and bleeding tendency. Since the submucous myoma cannot be felt by pelvic examination, and cannot be detected by blind sounding of uterine cavity, only when severe uterine bleeding leads to anemia can it sometimes be found. The commonly used methods in examining uterine myomas include HSG, MRI, ultrasonography (especially transvaginal ultrasonography), and hysteroscopy under direct vison of uterine cavity, etc. The blind dilation and curettage (D&C) may not detect submucosal myomas, and ultrasonography is not accurate in positioning. Thus hysteroscopy is the preferred method in the diagnosis of this disorder. In 1976, Neuwirth and Amin first reported the application of prostatic resectoscope in performing transcervical resection of myoma (TCRM; hysteroscopic myomectomy). Thereafter, with the progress of equipment and technology, operative hysteroscope came out in 1992, which is exclusively applied in gynecologic surgeries. By now, hysteroscopic resection of submucosal myomas and inward-protruding intramural myomas has developed into mature techniques in gynecologic surgery. Compared with hysterectomy and transabdominal myomectomy, hysteroscopic resection of submucosal myomas has many advantages. Firstly, it does not need to open up the abdomen, which significantly reduces postoperative recovery time, and small myomas can be resected at outpatient department. Secondly, there is no surgical incision into the uterus, which greatly reduces the subsequent possibilities of cesarean section. Finally, its prognosis can be comparable with traditional laparotomy.

9.3.1 Classification of Uterine Myomas

Uterine myomas originate from smooth muscle cells, and usually migrate to the site with little resistance in the growing process. If migrating towards the abdominal cavity, it will grow beneath the serosa. If migrating towards the uterine cavity, it will grow beneath the mucosa. According to its location, uterine myomas are divided into three types: (1) submucous myomas: located beneath the endometrium; (2) intramural myomas: located within the myometrial layer; (3) subserous myomas: located directly beneath the serosa. Most of myomas in uterine cavity grow partly in the uterine wall, and partly beneath the endometrium and protrude inwardly, which are named sessile submucosal myomas, and myomas with pedicles are named pedunculated submucosal myomas. The diameter of myoma can be less than 1 cm, or more than 8–9 cm, can be single or multiple. There is always no normal endometrium on the surface of submucous myomas, only covered with a thin and dense capsule. On its surface, the thick blood vessels can be seen easily under hysteroscope. Once the blood vessels rupture, the blood may spurt from blood vessels and fill up the uterine cavity rapidly due to the lack of self-limiting mechanism of hemostasis. Most submucous myomas are located at the corpus of the uterine cavity, attached to the fundus, the anterior, posterior or lateral uterine wall. Small myomas may be located at the uterine cornua, which may interfere with the normal junction of uterus and fallopian tubes. Very few myomas are located at the cervical canal.

According to the relationship between myomas and the myometrium, Haarlem international hysteroscopy training center in the Netherlands classifies the submucous myomas into three types (Fig. 9.46), which has been widely adopted internationally. Type 0 (Fig. 9.47a–d) is pedunculated submucous myomas without intramural extension. Type I (Fig. 9.48a–c) is sessile submucous myomas with intramural extension <50%. Type II (Fig. 9.49a, b) is sessile submucous myomas with intramural extension >50%. Type I can be distinguished from Type II under hysteroscope in that the endometrium migrates from the uterine wall at an acute angle towards the type I myoma while at an obtuse angle towards the type II myoma (Fig. 9.50).

According to the relationship between the myomas and myometrium, and in combination with the operative methods, Lin makes a classification of myomas as follows.

1. Pedunculated submucous myomas: (1) prolapsed myomas; (2) myomas without prolapse.
2. Sessile submucous myomas: (1) 50% $\geq$ the degree of protrusion $\geq$20%; (2) the degree of protrusion <20%.
3. Intramural myomas close to the uterine cavity: (1) intramural myomas protrude into uterine cavity after submucous myomas being excised; (2) the embedded submucous myomas: under irrigating fluid pressure, the sessile submucous myoma may sometimes be embedded into the myometrial layer and turned into intramural myoma.

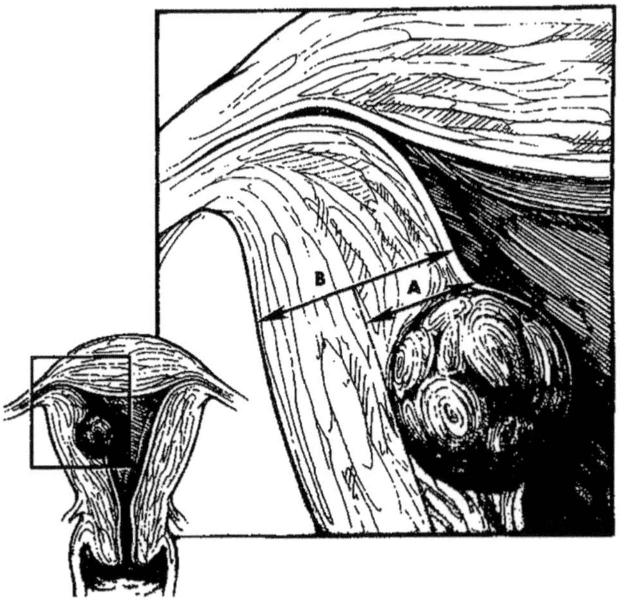

Fig. 9.46 Submucous myoma

Uterine myomas may possibly undergo sarcomatous change, but extremely rare, with its incidence <0.5%. Therefore, the resected tissues of myoma must be sent for histopathological examination.

9.3.2 Indications and Contraindications of TCRM

Any patients with submucous myoma, inward-protruding intramural myomas, and cervical myoma should first consider hysteroscopic operation, although the hysteroscopic surgeries are not applicable to all myomas. In order to have a safe operation and good therapeutic effect, one key point is to select the patients suitable for the operation. The operator must formulate the suitable conditions according to his own experience and surgical techniques, and an improper operation will lead to dangerous consequences. The size of the myoma is generally limited to below 5 cm in diameter, and if skilled, the operator may extend its indications. Sometimes, the operations on the submucous myoma which is embedded deep into the myometrium and inward-protruding intramural myomas need to be performed more than twice. Intramural myomas which don't deform the uterine cavity and subserosal myomas are unsuitable for hysteroscopic operation.

The following conditions should be considered in selecting indications:

1. Menorrhagia or abnormal bleeding.
2. The size of the uterus and the length of the cavity: The size of the uterus is generally confined to 10 weeks of gestation and the uterine cavity is limited to 12 cm in length.
3. The diameter of submucosal or inward-protruding intramural myoma: It is generally restricted to less than 5 cm.
4. The size of a pedunculated submucous myoma: It is generally restricted to less than 5 cm.
5. No cancerous change.

As to the submucosal myoma that has prolapsed into the vagina, its size and the thickness of its pedicle are not restricted.

Its contraindications are similar to that of TCRE.

9.3.3 Preoperative Preparations

9.3.3.1 Case Selection

Before deciding on hysteroscopic operation, a general preoperative examination must be undertaken to determine the

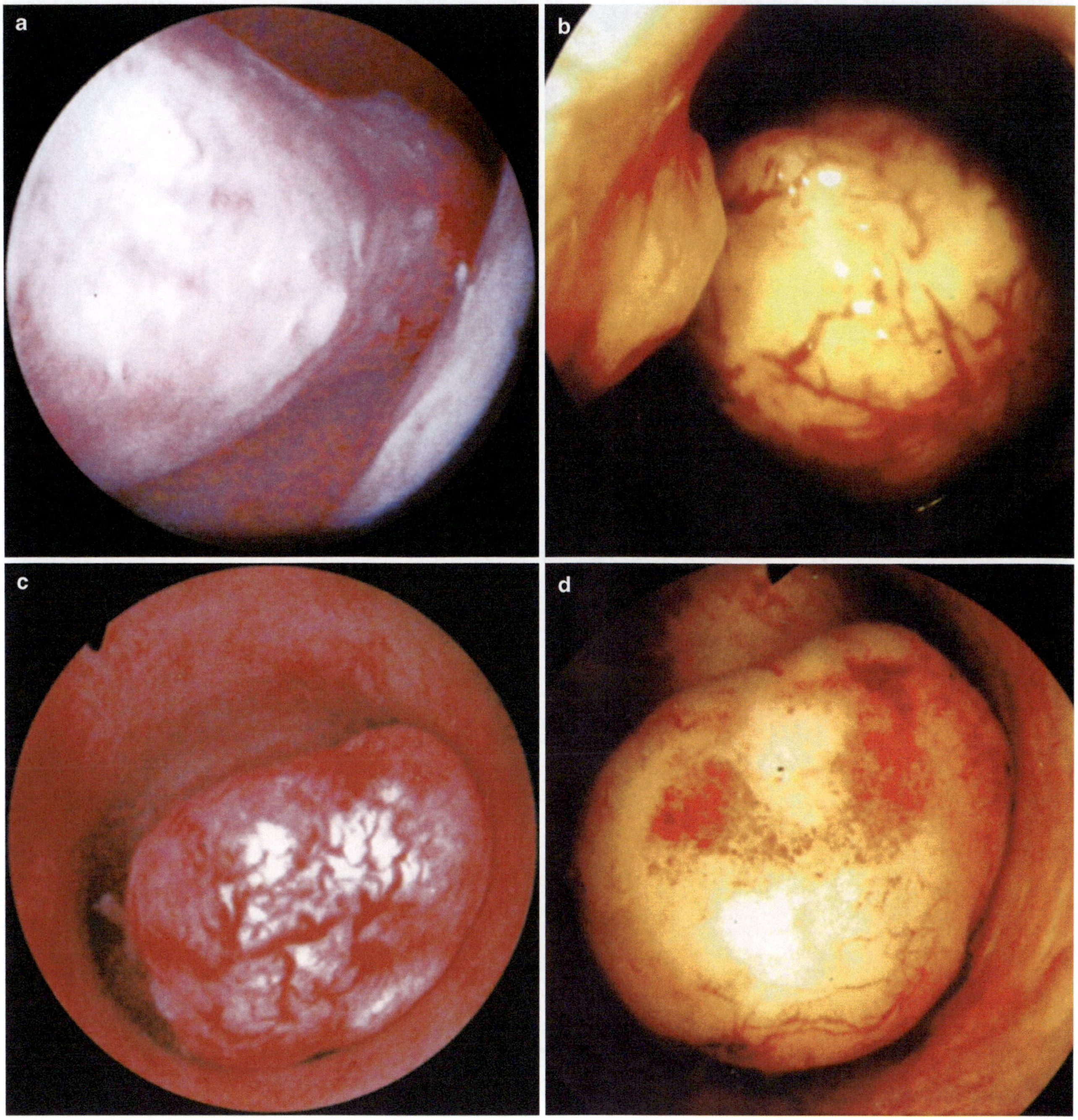

Fig. 9.47 (**a–d**) Type 0 pedunculated submucous myoma

presence of submucous myoma and (or) inward-protruding intramural myomas. The number, size, location, and degeneration or not of myomas are recorded, thus the possibility of hysteroscopic operation is assessed. The common methods for evaluating myomas are as follows:

1. D&C: The uterine cavity may be examined by a sound or explored by a curette, if found uneven, it suggests the possibility of submucosal myoma. Its advantage is that it can take endometrium for histological examination at the same time, but it has a higher false negative rate.
2. HSG: HSG shows intrauterine filling defects, but often misses the small myomas, and may confuse large polyps and bubbles. Its advantages are that it can help to evaluate the fallopian tube patency, and also diagnose adenomyoma with images revealing the multiple channels within myomas being connected with uterine cavity.
3. Ultrasonography: Ultrasonography is used to measure the radial lines of the uterus and submucous myoma with abdominal or vaginal probe. However, myomas may be misdiagnosed with endometrial polyps or thickened endometrium, and it is also not easy to locate myomas.

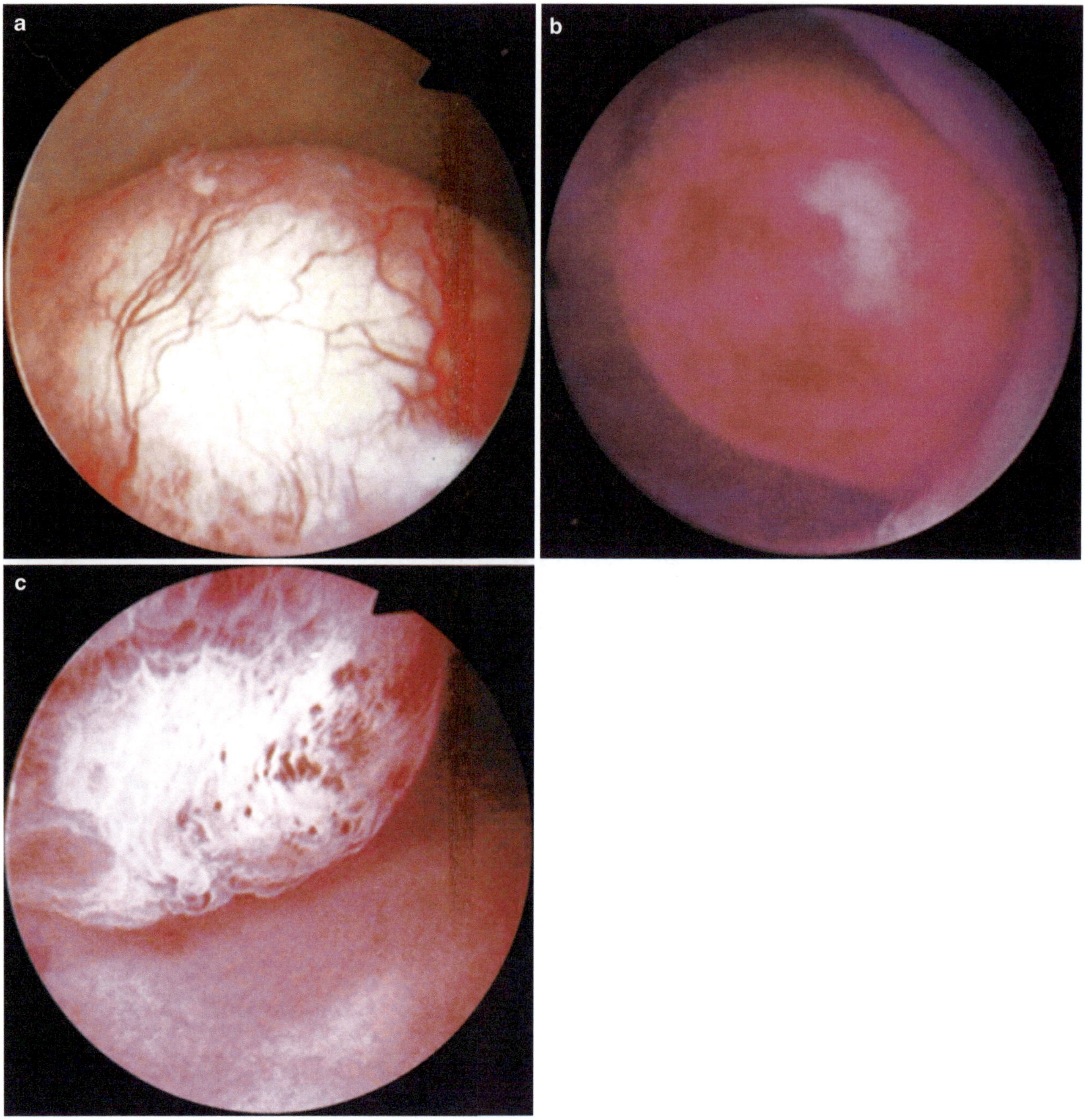

Fig. 9.48 (a–c) Type I sessile submucous myoma

Hysteroscopic examination combined with ultrasonography or saline infusion sonogram (SIS) is convenient for observation and classification of uterine submucous myoma (Fig. 9.51).

4. Hysteroscopy: Hysteroscopy can be used to observe directly the shape, color, and location of submucous myomas, thickness of pedicles, single or multiple, the conditions of the endometrium on their surfaces, and their degree protruding into the uterine cavity, so that a decision might be made as to whether it is suitable for hysteroscopic operation or not. When necessary, in vivo biopsy under direct vision should be done for histological examination to exclude malignant lesions. The deformation or irregularity of the uterine cavity, and asymmetry of bilateral uterine cornua and tubal ostia can be detected in the inward-protruding intramural myoma. However, the hysteroscopy alone cannot help to understand the depth of myomas into uterine wall, the size of myomas, and whether the locations of tubal ostia are involved when the myoma extends to the fallopian tubal ostia.

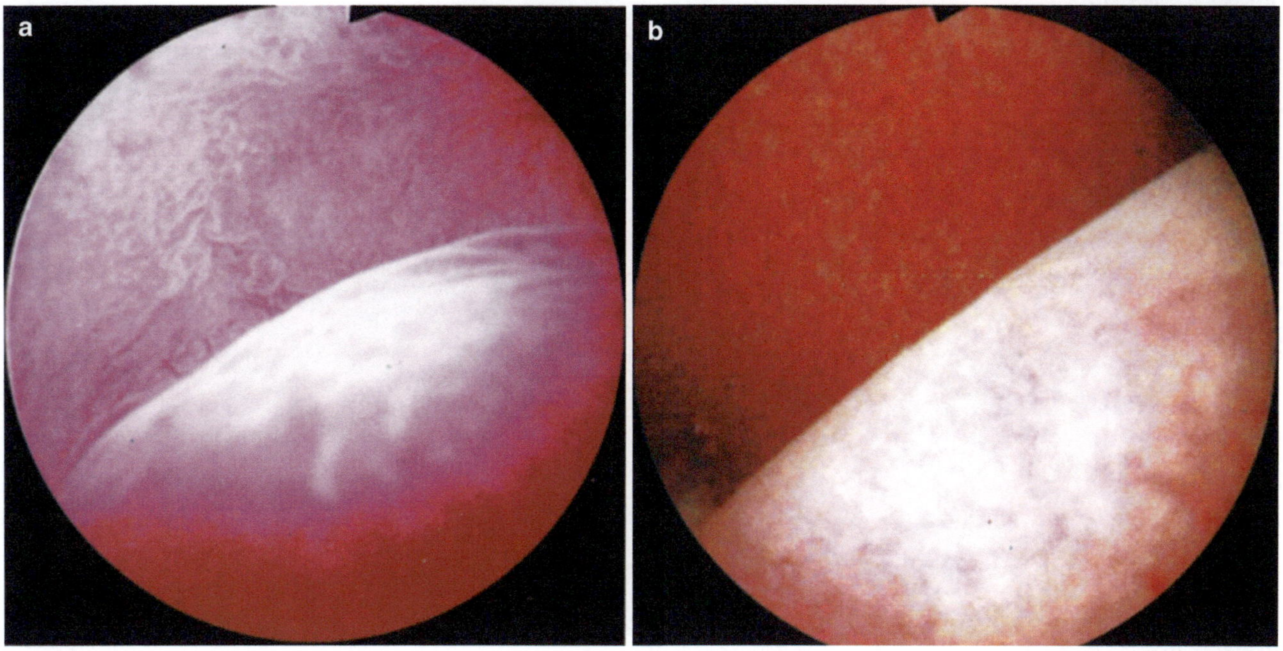

Fig. 9.49 (**a**, **b**) Type II sessile submucous myoma

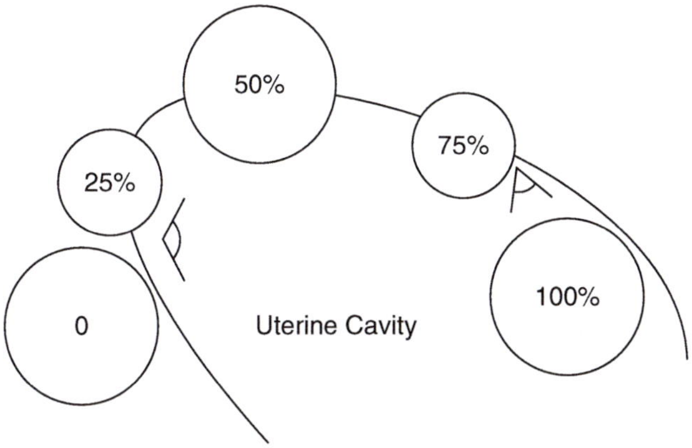

Fig. 9.50 The degree of submucous myomas protruding into the uterine cavity

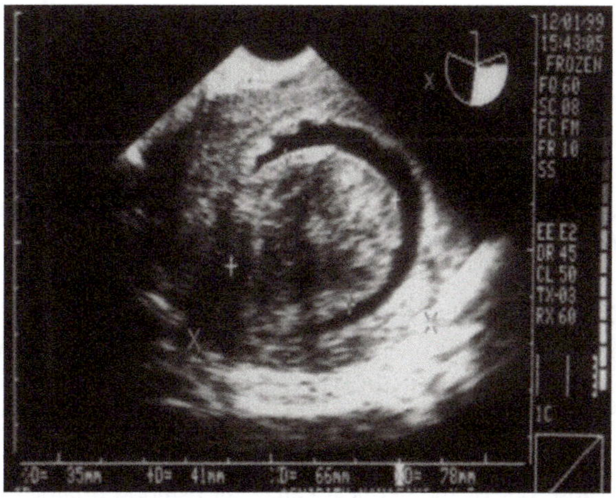

Fig. 9.51 Image of submucous myoma under SIS

5. MRI: MRI can clearly show the soft tissue image and can assess the size of uterine myomas quantitatively.

9.3.3.2 Preoperative Medical Pretreatment

Prior to operation, the patient can be administered danazol, 600–800 mg/day, or gestrinone/nemestran 2.5 mg, twice weekly, for more than 3 weeks, or GnRH analogs for 10–12 weeks, which can reduce the volume of myoma and decrease blood supply. The uterus shrinks faster than myomas, thus it is very beneficial for the myomas to protrude into the uterine cavity, be transformed from the sessile submucous myoma into pedunculated one, and increase the degree of protrusion of intramural myoma into uterine cavity, which facilitates the smooth hysteroscopic operation. Donnez et al. suggested that in reducing the volume of the uterus and submucosal myomas, the effects of GnRH analogs were more obvious than that of other hormones. GnRH analogs can cause the endometrium and uterine vessels to atrophy, making a wide field of vision and less amount of bleeding during operation (Fig. 9.52a, b), while the myoma is fragile and is easy to be clamped out with forceps. Generally, the application of GnRH analogs may lead to amenorrhea and improve the anemia, but one should remember that it must be administered at the early stage of the menstrual cycle. After taking it for the first time, very few patients will have an increased menstrual flow and sometimes need to terminate the administration of GnRH analogs. There have been reports of drug-induced heavy bleeding and emergency rescue required in cases of excessive bleeding.

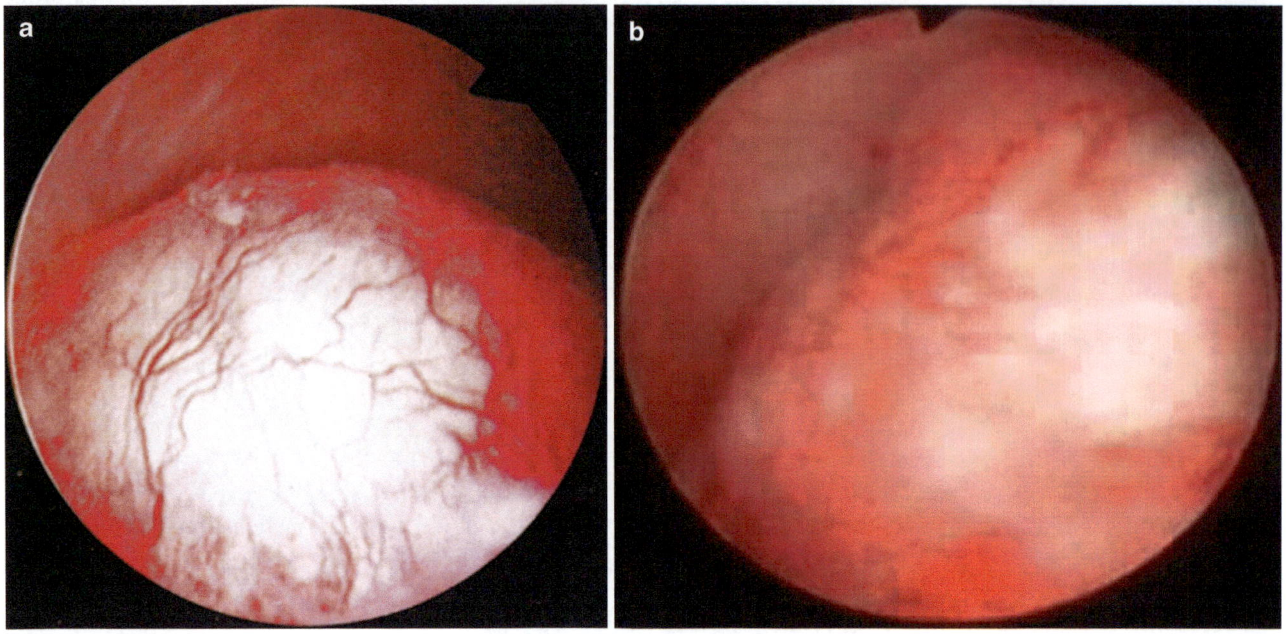

Fig. 9.52 (**a**) The endometrium becomes thin after 2-month application of GnRH analogs. (**b**) The endometrium becomes significantly thin with blood vessels unclear after 3-month application of GnRH analogs

9.3.3.3 Routine Laboratory Examination

Routine laboratory examination includes blood coagulation, electrolytes, liver function, blood type, etc. These results may help to establish a credible base before the operation produces false experimental results, and can be used to make a comparison with all kinds of parameters when fluid overload is suspected during operation.

9.3.3.4 Timing of Surgery

The ideal time for operation is in the first half of menstrual cycle, during which there may be less bleeding at the time of operation. If there is excessive bleeding, the operation must be done even in the secretary phase. If the myoma does not prolapse out of the cervical canal, an osmotic dilator or a laminaria tent can be inserted into the cervical canal on the night before operation.

9.3.4 Anesthesia

The choices of anesthesia can be seen in section of TCRE. All kinds of anesthesia may be administered except for local anesthesia, and general anesthesia should be adopted when laparoscopy is performed at the same time.

9.3.5 Operative Equipment

1. Hystero-resectoscope: A 7 mm hystero-resectoscope with continuous irrigation can be used to cut the thin pedicle of a submucous myoma, or transform sessile submucous myoma into the pedunculated one. When there is a large amount of tissues to be resected, a 9 mm hystero-resectoscope can be used. An 8 mm hystero-resectoscope has the advantages of both 7 and 9 mm resectoscopes.
2. Lin's myoma forceps: If large submucous myomas are resected with hystero-resectoscope alone, there will be a limited amount of tissue resected with wire loop electrode each time, the operation will take a longer time, and the bleeding volume will increase, which may increase the risk for hyponatremia. Lin's myoma forceps has a wider clamping blade, and its inner surface appears to be cross-shaped, hence it can hold and pull out the residual myoma tissues more firmly compared with the oval forceps, and also effectively shorten the operative time.
3. High-frequency current generator: The electric cutting power is set at 80 W, electric coagulating power is set at 40 W, and both can be increased according to the requirements of operation. The blended current with cutting and coagulating is mainly used when resecting tissues. However, the pure electric cutting current may be applied to achieve smooth resection.
4. Irrigation fluid: Since submucous or inward-protruding intramural myomas occupy the partial uterine cavity, if there are more debris of the resected myomas, and if the irrigation fluid cannot distend the uterine cavity adequately during operation, there will be a narrow operative space and poor vision. These may lead to difficulty in cutting myomas, damage to the opposite uterine wall, and even perforation of the uterus. When there is poor irrigation achieved by using the falling pressure of distention fluid and outflow negative suction, an automatic uterine distension pump is needed to distend the uterine cavity mandatorily with a continuous flow.

9.3.6 Operative Procedures

First, examine the location of myoma and the condition of pedicles carefully by ultrasonography. Then, perform operations according to the types of the myomas.

9.3.6.1 Pedunculated Submucous Myomas

1. Prolapsed myomas: The main body of a myoma is located in the cervical canal or in the vagina, but the root of pedicles still remains in the uterine cavity or within the cervical canal, which is the best object of hysteroscopic operation for beginners. During the procedure, the myoma is grasped and pulled outwards first by double hook forceps, rather than being grasped and screwed out roughly. Meanwhile, insert a 7 mm hystero-resectoscope into the uterine cavity to cut off its pedicle. When cutting, in case of difficult positioning of pedicle, move the double hook forceps so the pedicle can be mobile, which makes it distinguishable from the normal tissues. Moreover, as a result of pulling, the normal tissues underlying the pedicle will protrude into the uterine cavity. When hystero-resectoscope is applied to cut off the pedicle, the cutting should be taken at a direction parallel to the normal uterine wall, since the cutting may damage the normal myometrium if it takes the direction of the uterine wall. After removal of myoma, its cutting surface will retract, and an additional resection is not needed generally.
2. Myomas without prolapse: From the external orifice of the cervix, the operator cannot see the site where the pedicle is attached and that the main body of myoma still remains in the uterine cavity or cervical canal. By Lin's method of resection, first use a 7 mm resectoscope to cut the pedicle of myoma into one less than 1 cm, and then use a 9 mm resectoscope to shave the tumor, thus reducing its size, and then screw it out with Lin's myoma forceps (Figs. 9.53, 9.54, 9.55, and 9.56). This is two resectoscopes method, which is very useful.

9.3.6.2 Sessile Submucosal Myoma

The resection of sessile submucous myomas needs highly proficient skills. The operator must first grasp the techniques of resection of pedunculated myomas before performing such more difficult surgeries. The site of myoma is in the uterine cavity or cervical canal. If it is sessile submucosal myoma in the cervical canal, since the cervical wall has become very thin, it is extremely prone to perforation, and the operation is the most difficult. There are two kinds of operating methods according to the protruding degrees of myomas towards the uterine cavity.

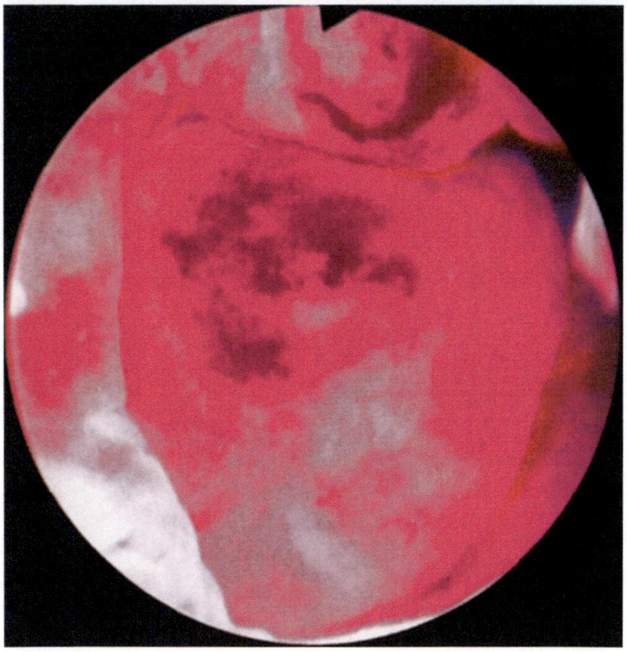

Fig. 9.53 Prior to TCRM

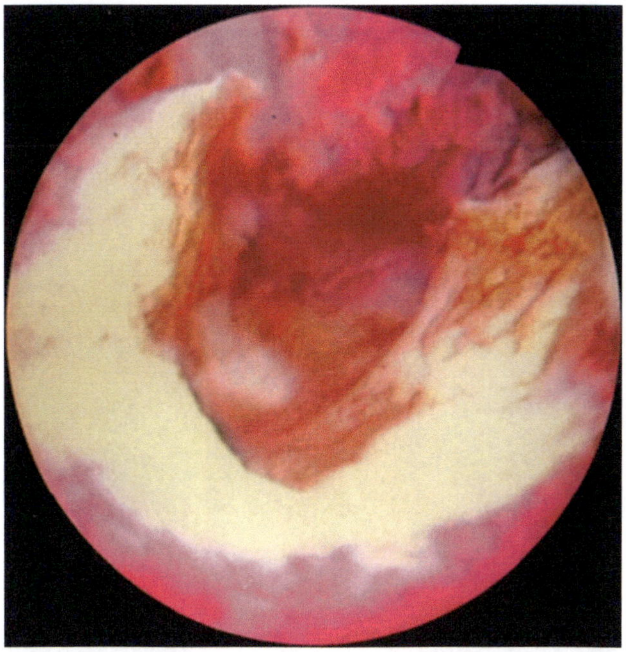

Fig. 9.54 Resection of the right upper portion of a uterine myoma with electric cutting loop

1. 50% ≥ the degree of protrusion ≥20%: To remove such a myoma completely, first of all, one must strive to increase the protruding degree of the submucosal myoma. Under intensive monitoring of ultrasonography, a 7 mm wire loop electrode is used to cut gradually

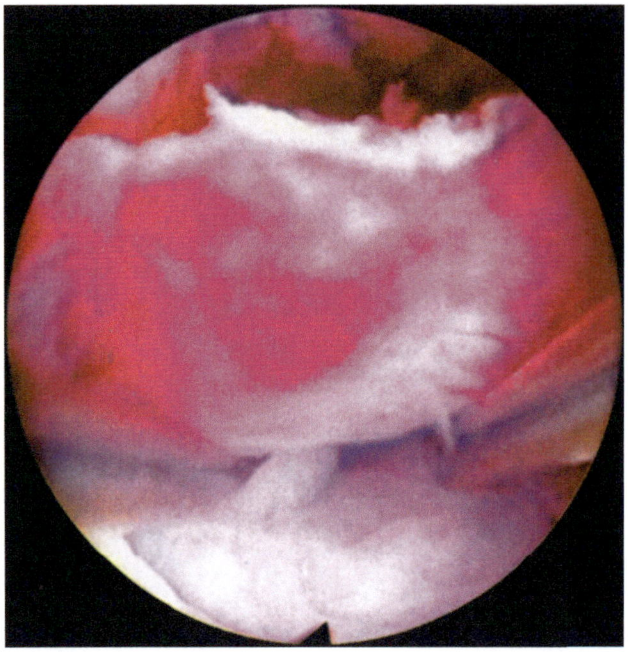

Fig. 9.55 Resection of the left lower portion of a uterine myoma with electric cutting loop

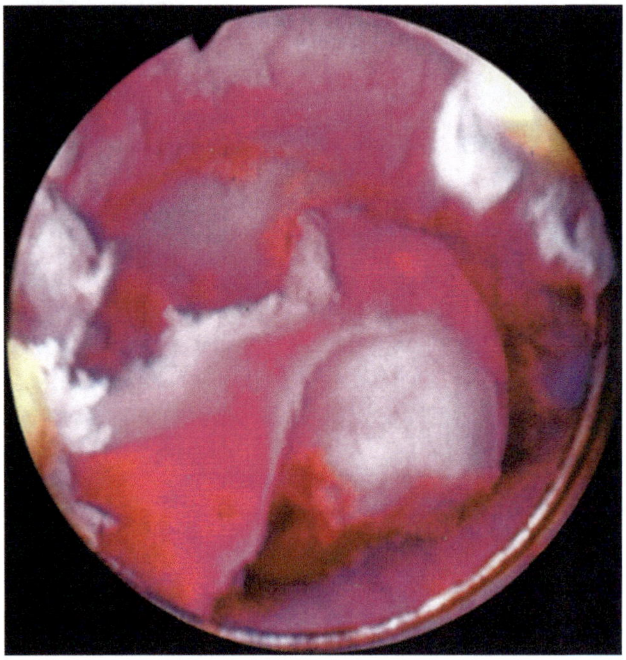

Fig. 9.56 A myoma was resected with incisions from above and below with electric cutting loop so as to be easily clamped out

along the capsule at the bottom of the myoma. Just like abdominal myomectomy, the boundary layer between myoma and myometrium is cut open, and the myoma is dissected bluntly from the muscular layer while using the front tip of the hysteroscope to press myomas. At this moment, the irrigating fluid flowing from the tip of the hysteroscope forms hydro-dissection, which strengthen the dissection effects. The uterine muscle contraction due to the high-frequency electric stimulation and the resectoscopic insertion and extraction may result in a change of pressure in uterine cavity, which further prompts the myoma to protrude into the uterine cavity. When the resection has been undertaken to a certain stage, clamp myomas with myoma forceps, twist and pull under ultrasonography monitoring, which may then develop a pedicle. When a pedicle is formed, the resection is then similar to resection of a pedunculated submucous myoma mentioned above. If it is not possible to screw and twist with forceps, insert a 7 mm resectoscope again to resect the pedicle of myomas, or use a 9 mm resectoscope to make the myoma core smaller. Then use the myoma forceps to screw and twist the myoma or twist the clamped myoma by 360°, pull it out of the uterus and cut it off. However, if the myoma pedicle is too thick and the myoma is seized hastily and pulled roughly, sometimes it will damage the uterine wall and even directly to the serosal layer, resulting in perforation of the uterus. If a laminaria cervical dilator can be inserted to soften the cervix prior to operation, small myoma core may be extracted with myoma forceps (Figs. 9.57, 9.58, 9.59, 9.60, 9.61, and 9.62).

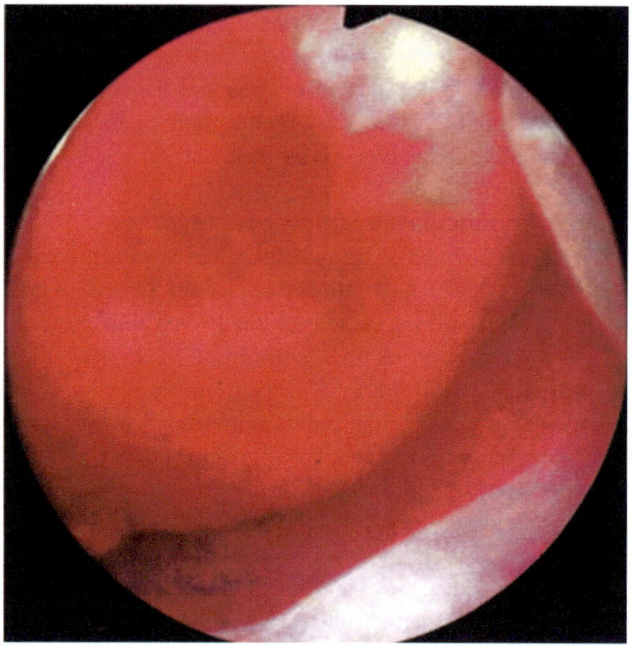

Fig. 9.57 Inward-protruding intramural myoma

2. The degree of protrusion <20%: It is difficult to have a complete resection, thus the operator should consider this sessile submucosal myoma as intramural myoma for treatment. In fact, when resection starts, the myoma begins to protrude into the uterine cavity, thus a complete

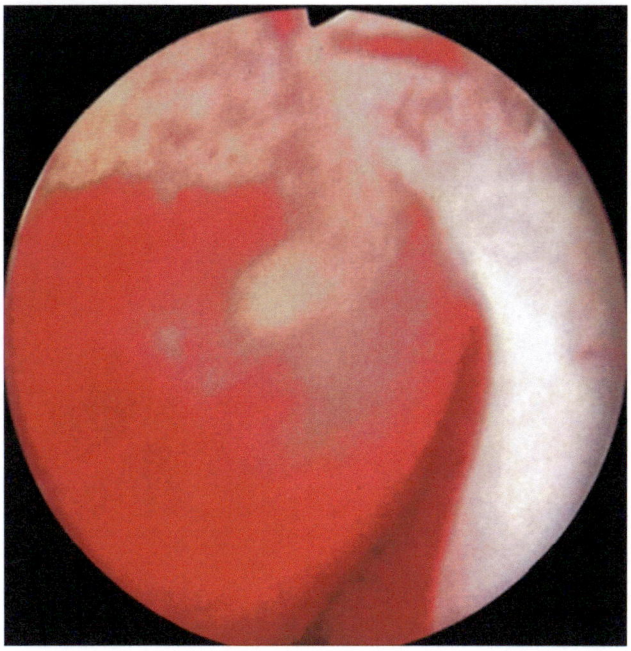

Fig. 9.58 The basal part of myoma

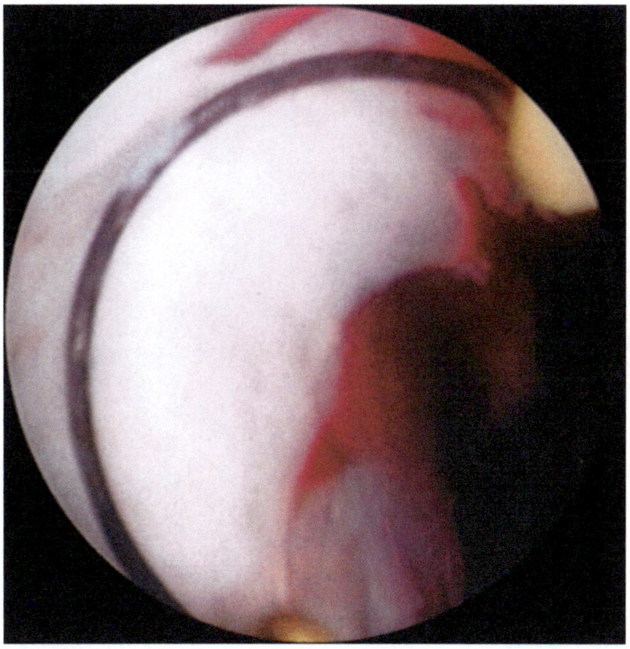

Fig. 9.59 Electric resection of myoma

resection is not uncommon. If it cannot be completely removed, a 9 mm resectoscope can be used to resect the portion of myoma protruding into the uterine cavity and the intramural part of myoma with the cutting depth more than 5 mm. At 2–3 months after operation, a second-look hysteroscopy is conducted, and then TCRM can be performed again to resect the residual myoma completely which has protruded into the uterine cavity, namely, the two-step operation .

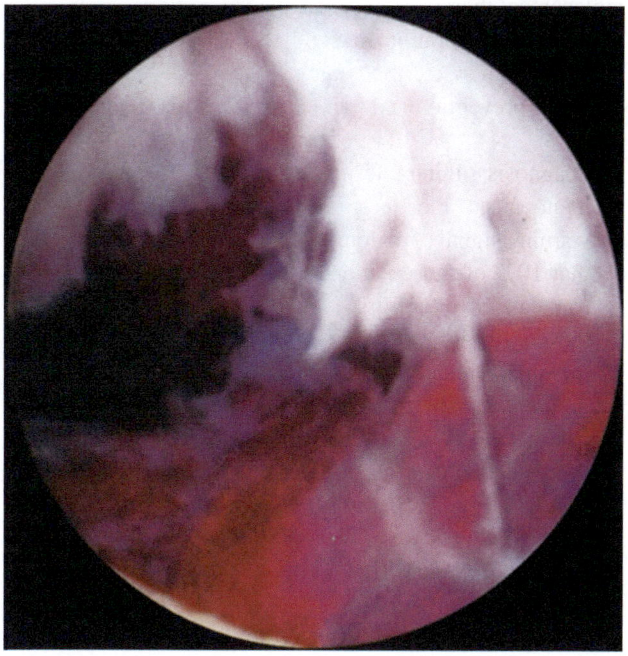

Fig. 9.60 Uterine cavity after TCRM

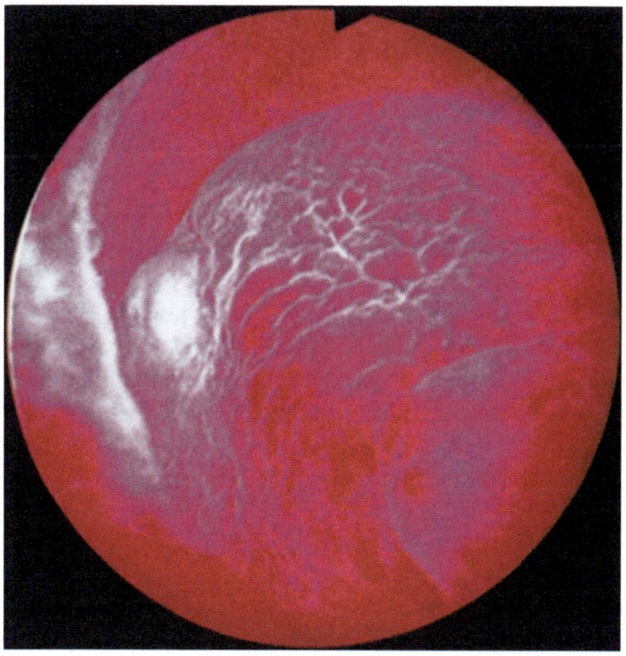

Fig. 9.61 Uterine cavity before TCRM

9.3.6.3 Intramural Myomas with Inward Protrusion or Close to the Uterine Cavity, and Transmural Myomas

1. Intramural myomas protruding into the uterine cavity: Hysteroscopy is available for resection of this type of myomas. Myometrial tissues between the myoma and the endometrium can be seen on the cutting surface. The surgical procedure is in accordance with that of submucous myomas with the protrusion <20% described above.

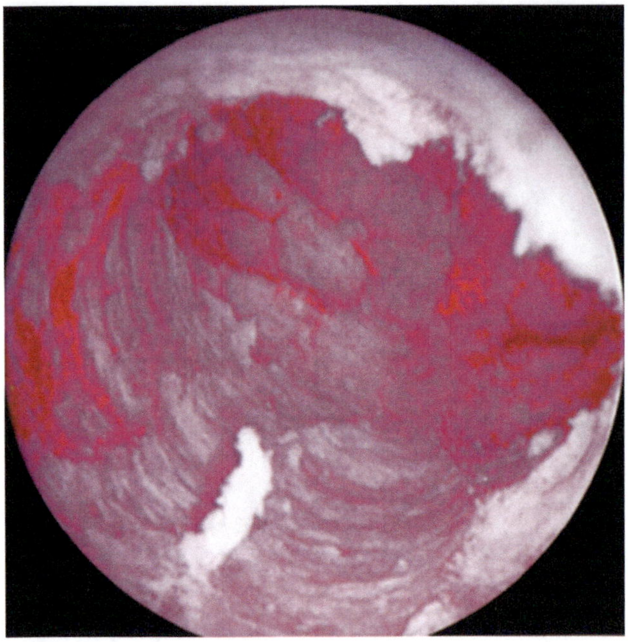

Fig. 9.62 Uterine cavity after TCRM

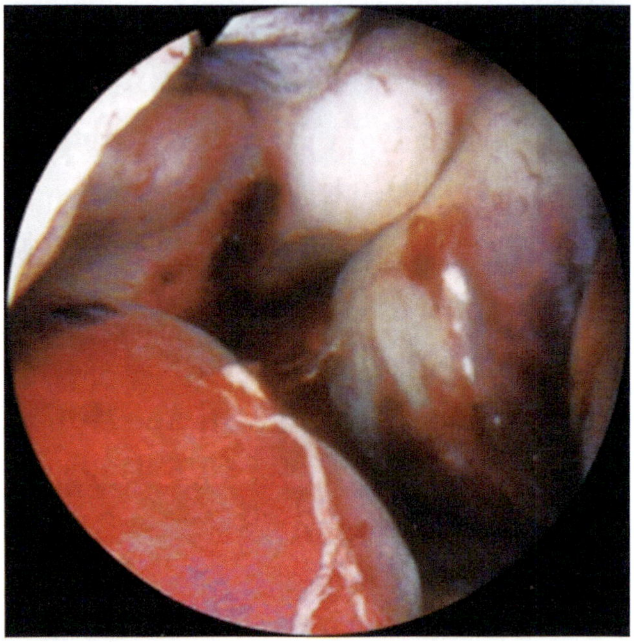

Fig. 9.63 Multiple uterine submucous myoma

2. After resection of submucous myoma, some intramural myomas may protrude into the cavity, then they can be resected according to the procedures of sessile submucous myoma removals.
3. Transmural myoma: It refers to the myoma throughout the full layer of muscle wall, which is compressing on the uterine cavity and protruding to the serosa, and the surgical procedure can be in accordance with sessile submucosal myoma.
4. Embedded submucous myoma: It is caused by pretreatment with GnRH analogs in sessile submucosal myoma, with its normal myometrial tissues becoming brittle and soft. Its resection is very difficult, while there are also successful cases of complete resection under close ultrasonography monitoring.

9.3.6.4 Multiple Submucous and Intramural Myoma

To the women who are suffering from multiple submucous and intramural myomas with infertility, hysteroscopic myomectomy can be applied. The techniques of resection and vaporization are the same as mentioned above, and myomas should be resected as much as possible. When the operation ends, IUD can be placed in the uterine cavity, and taken out 2 months later (Figs. 9.63, 9.64, 9.65, and 9.66).

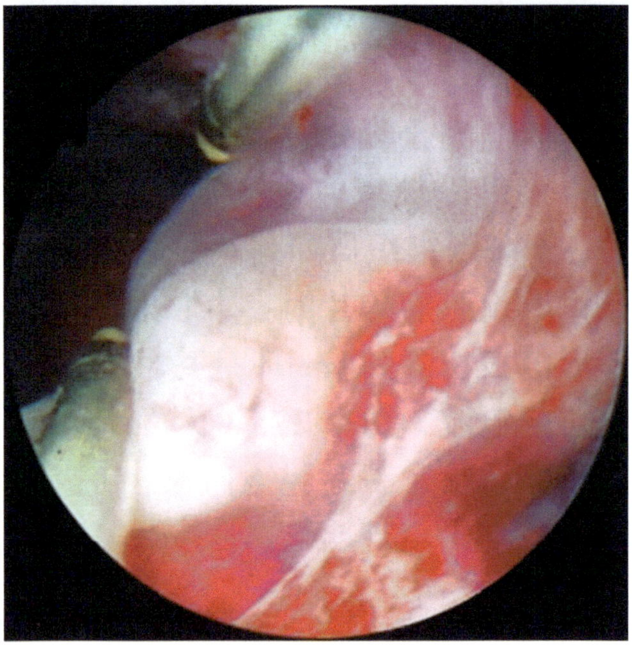

Fig. 9.64 Resection of multiple myomas with wire loop electrode

9.3.6.5 Cervical Myoma

Cervical myomas are all coated. For the cervical myoma prolapsed from the cervical canal, wire loop electrode can be used to cut off the pedicle and remove it completely, or cut open the pseudo-capsule and screw it out. As for the myoma embedded in the cervical walls, as long as its outline is made clear, the wire loop electrode can be used to cut from the thinnest part of the embedded myoma. When cutting reaches the myoma, the incision can be appropriately extended and the myoma can be stripped out from the pseudo-capsules completely. After removal of the myoma, generally its bed does not bleed. If the bed is larger or the outline of cervix is not integrated, the absorbable catgut can be used for suture.

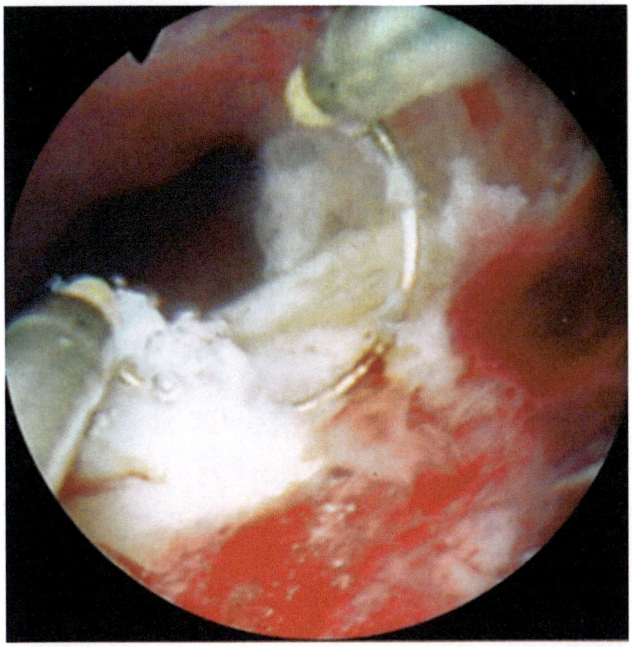

Fig. 9.65 Resection of multiple myomas with wire loop electrode

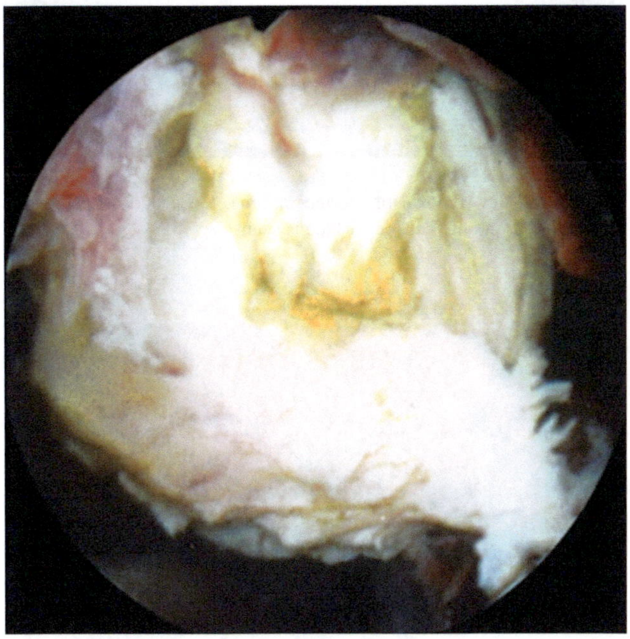

Fig. 9.66 Resection of multiple myomas with wire loop electrode

For sessile submucous myoma in cervical canal, it is extremely prone to perforation since the cervical wall has become very thin.

9.3.6.6 Simultaneous Resection of Endometrium and Myoma

For the women who has severe bleeding and do not require fertility, the operator may consider the simultaneous resection of endometrium and myoma, which can be done with rollerball electrode or Nd-YAG laser. However, there is no report about the comparison on therapeutic effects of two methods.

9.3.6.7 Removal of Adenomyoma

In rare cases, an inward-protruding intramural myoma or a sessile submucous myoma diagnosed clinically or by ultrasonography is really adenomyoma. There are three types of adenomyomas. In type one, the agglomerate structure consists of all adenomyoma tissues, with no clear capsule. And on its section, the clustery endometrium, old blood, and abundant blood vessels are visible. During the resection, the adenomyoma may be deformed along with the contraction of uterus. Therefore, do not overdo it at the time of resection, and remember not to pursue a complete resection of adenomyoma so as to avoid cutting through the uterine wall when the adenomyoma is deformed. Type II is adenomyoma complicated with leiomyoma. Type III is a mixed type of tumor, which is mainly leiomyoma, and at the portion of it close to the cavity, the endometrium invades in and the partial adenomyoma is developed. The second and third types of adenomyomas generally have obvious capsules, and the resection methods are the same as that of the inward-protruding intramural myoma and (or) sessile submucosal myomas.

9.3.6.8 Large Myomas >6 cm in Diameter

Some scholars have conducted special expositions on hysteroscopic resection of large myomas. Lin from Japan used a 7 mm resectoscope to cut the basal part of the myoma, transforming the sessile myoma into the pedunculated one. Then, a 9 mm resectoscope was used to resect the myoma. After the reduction of its size, myoma forceps were used to clamp it out, which greatly reduced the difficulty of operation. Loffer reported 43 women who had large myomas and were given 2 months of danazol or leuprolide before operation. During the operation, the myoma was resected to the level of the surrounding endometrium and the intramural portion of myoma remained inside myometrium. After the myoma fragments in the uterine cavity were cleared out at the end of the resection, the uterus might contract again and the myoma remaining in the myometrium would protrude into the uterine cavity. At this time, the resection should be proceeded immediately so as to avoid the prolapse of myoma, and there were no serious operative complications. Donnez et al. reported 60 cases of laser myomectomy pretreated with GnRH analogs, of which the largest resected myoma was about 4 cm in diameter. His method was to remove myomas as much as possible, destroy the blood supply of the residual myoma by laser, and continue to apply GnRH analogs for 8 weeks after operation. The residual myoma was resected when moving into uterine cavity. Two to three months after treatment, the myomas were not notable and all the patients had normal menstruation. Among 24 women who desired to have babies, 16

(67%) conceived and had full-term delivery of live births (Figs. 9.67, 9.68, 9.69, 9.70, 9.71, 9.72, and 9.73).

9.3.6.9 Diffuse Uterine Leiomyomatosis (DUL)

DUL is a type of leiomyoma with special forms of growth. Its main characteristic is symmetrical enlargement of the uterus, with numerous poor boundary small fibroids involving the whole myometrium, most of which are smaller than 3 cm. Women with DUL usually manifest menorrhagia and infertility. The uterus can be enlarged to 20 weeks of gestation, and total hysterectomy is the traditional treatment of DUL. In recent years, hysteroscopic myomectomy was applied for the treatment of DUL in women who wish to preserve their uteri and expect to achieve good pregnancy

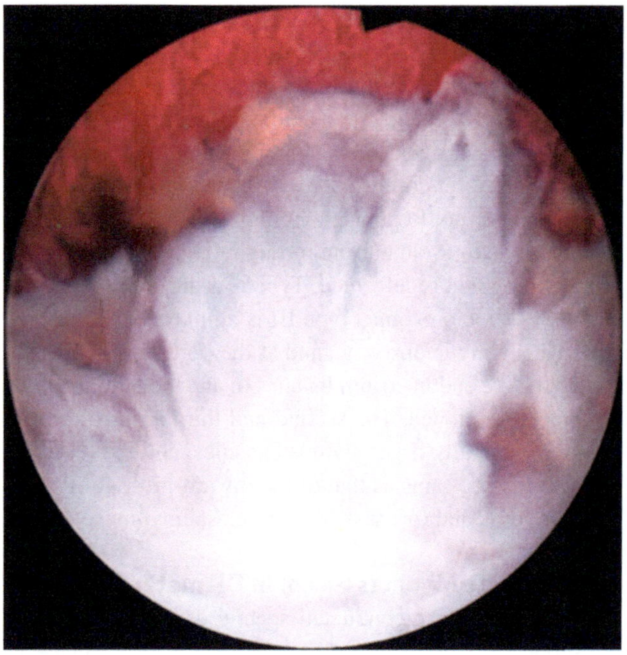

Fig. 9.67 After removal of uterine myoma, pink white pseudo-capsules float in the uterine cavity

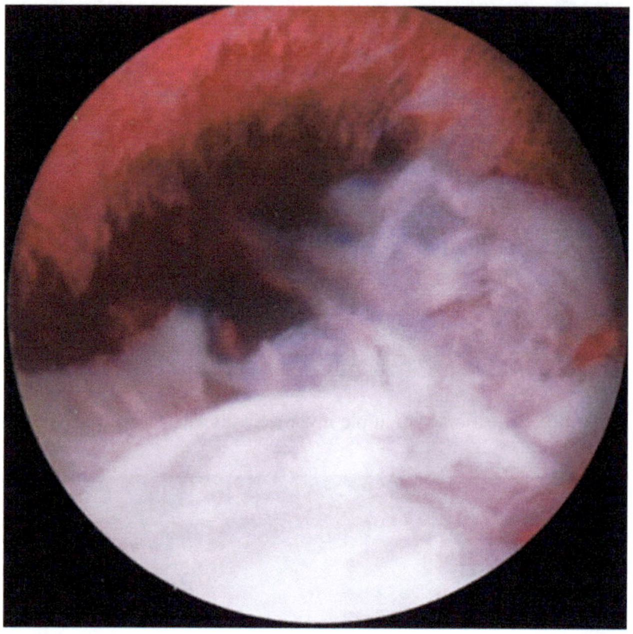

Fig. 9.69 After removal of uterine myoma, the pseudo-capsules are flushed aside and the cutting surface is seen

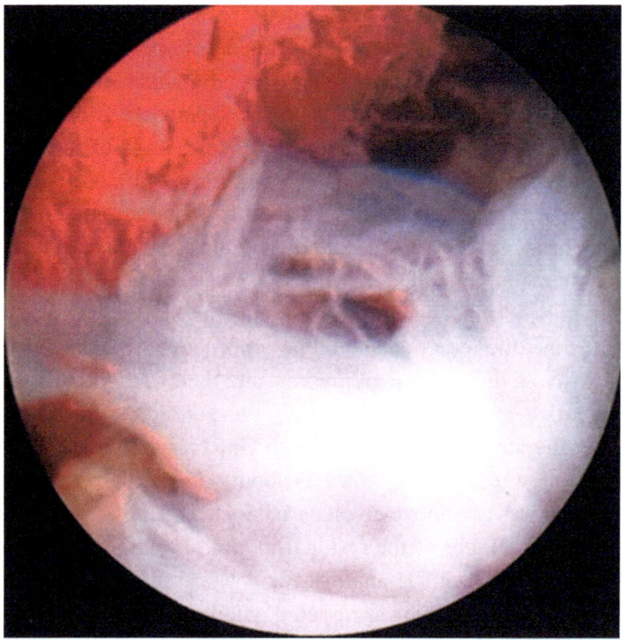

Fig. 9.68 After removal of uterine myoma, the pseudo-capsules shake in the uterine cavity along with the impact of irrigating fluid

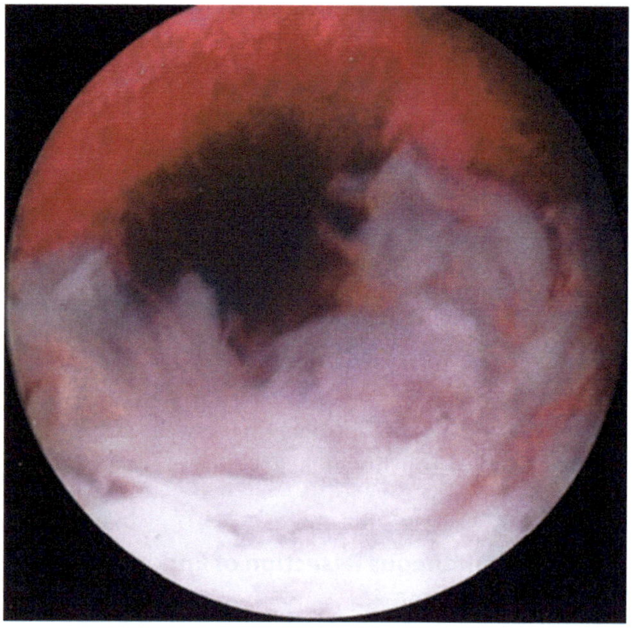

Fig. 9.70 After removal of uterine myoma, the cutting surface is checked without obvious bleeding

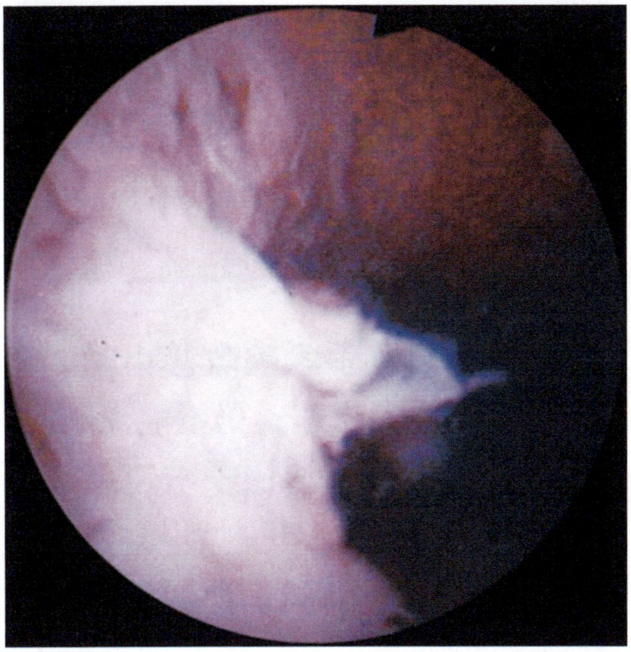

Fig. 9.71 After removal of uterine myoma, there is no bleeding at the base, and the pseudo-capsules do not need further resection

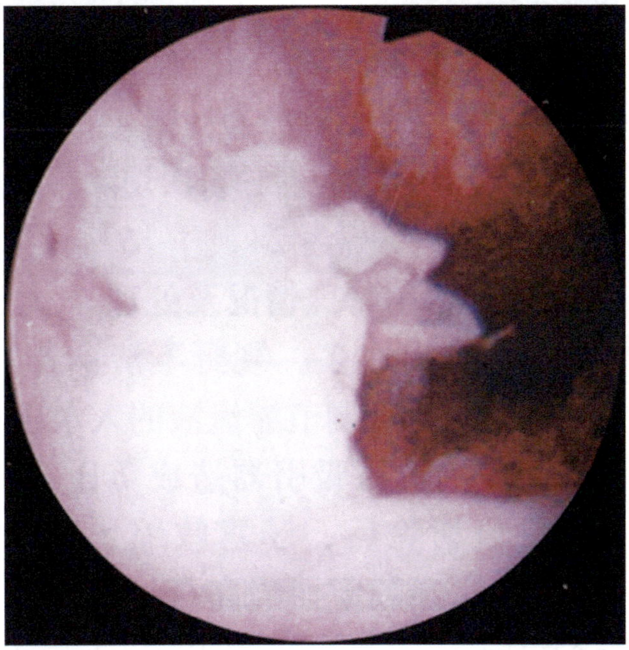

Fig. 9.72 After removal of uterine myoma, there is no bleeding at cutting surface. Decrease intrauterine pressure and retract the hysteroscope to check whether there is bleeding or not

outcomes. The surgical procedures include resection of visible submucous myomas and inward-protruding intramural myomas; simultaneously the measures to stimulate the contraction of the uterus are taken to promote further protrusion of the fibroid into the cavity. During the procedure, the normal endometrium shall be remained as much as possible, and

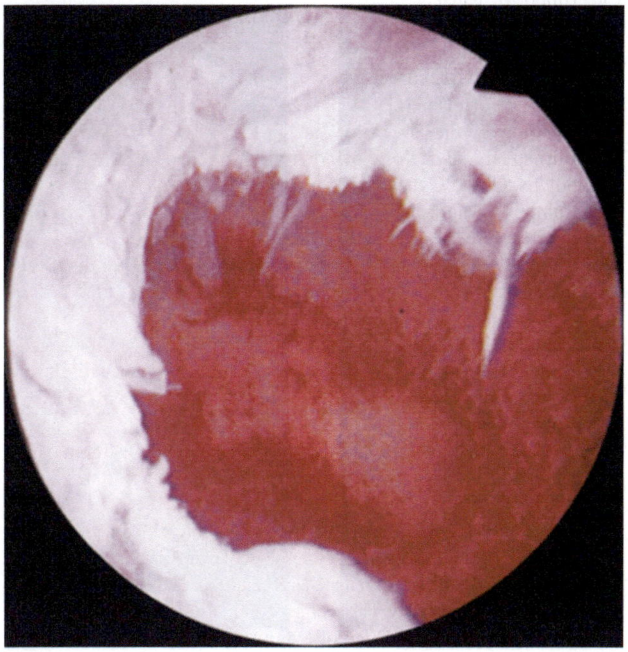

Fig. 9.73 After removal of uterine myoma, the cutting surface is covered by pseudo-capsules. Part of which is resected to reveal the cutting surface and no bleeding is detected

the intramural myoma without inward protruding will not be intervened, so that the shape of the cavity can be restored and the damage to myometrium can be avoided.

9.3.6.10 Operating Techniques of TCRM

1. Xia reported 5-step techniques of TCRM with combination of resection and clamping. (1) Cutting: The wire loop electrode is used to cut antegradely or retrogradely from both ends of the maximum diameter of the free myoma, reduce the size of myoma, and cut out an x-shape wasp-waist dent to fit the clamping of the oval forceps. (2) Clamping: Under the guidance of ultrasonography, the oval forceps is inserted into the uterine cavity to clamp the myoma and pull it backwards. (3) Twisting: the handle of oval forceps is twisted clockwise or anticlockwise to separate the myoma from its base. (4) Pulling: After twisting the myomas for a few circles, pull backwards with force. (5) Expulsion: In the process of pulling backwards, the myoma descends gradually and is expulsed out from the cervix. This method can shorten the operating time effectively and is convenient for a complete removal (Figs. 9.74, 9.75, 9.76, 9.77, 9.78, 9.79, 9.80, 9.81, 9.82, 9.83, 9.84, and 9.85).
2. There are several ways to remove the myoma fragments: (1) the fragments are taken out along with the exit of wire loop; (2) the debris is placed in between the cutting loop and the inner sheath, and taken out along with the exit of the inner sheath, which can reduce the times of the outer sheath into and out of the cervix and uterus; (3) the

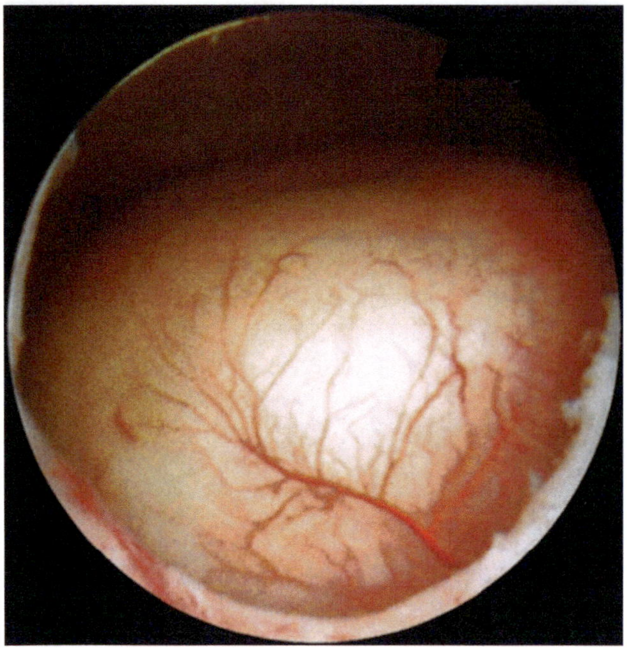

Fig. 9.74 Submucous myoma which is isolated from the surrounding walls

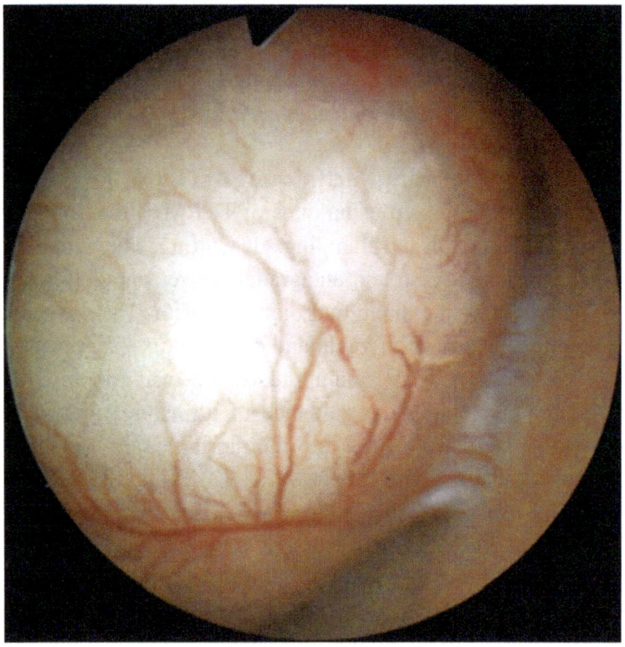

Fig. 9.75 Pedicle of myoma

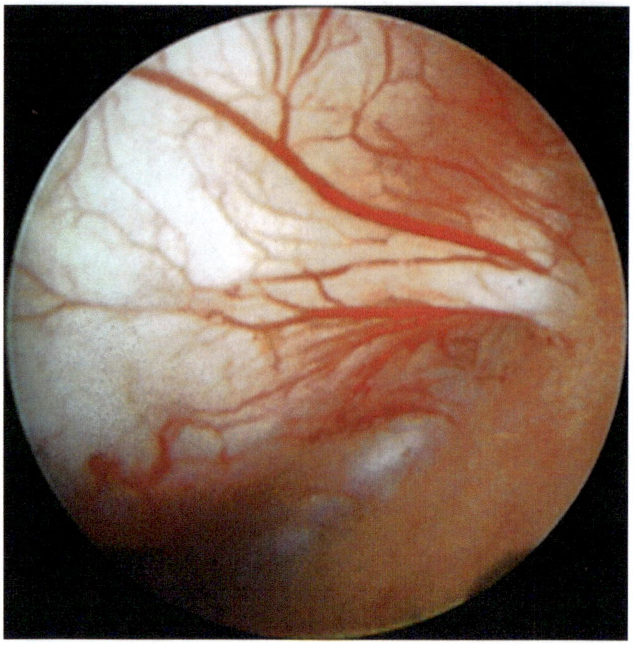

Fig. 9.76 Pedicle of myoma

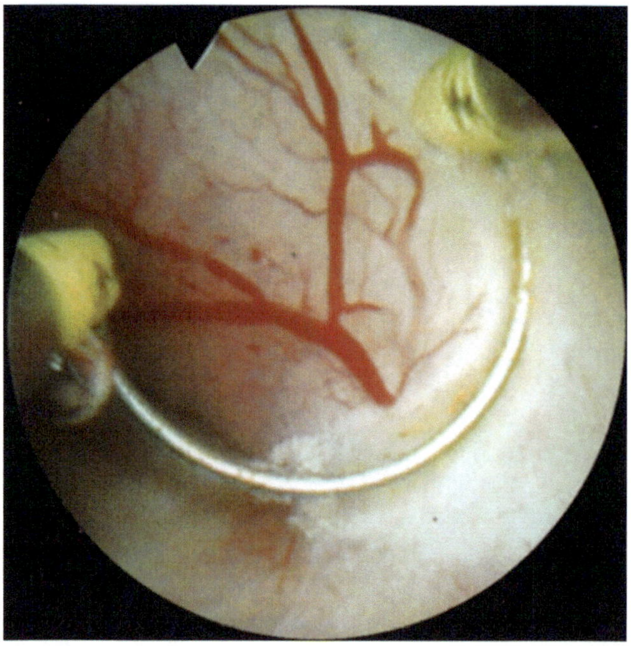

Fig. 9.77 Electrocoagulation of the roots of blood vessels so as to reduce bleeding

myoma fragments may be brought out along with the exit of the hysteroscope together with inner and outer sheath; (4) being clamped out with the oval forceps; (5) being carried out with the myoma forceps; (6) being scraped out with the blunt curette; (7) being sucked out with the suction tube; (8) operative hand bracket is taken out, the inflow pipe is connected to the valve of the outlet pipe, and the irrigation fluid can rinse the tissue fragments out from the inner sheath. In rare cases, myoma fragments could not be removed but remain in situ of the uterus, which will either degenerate gradually, or be discharged at the first postoperative period (Figs. 9.86 and 9.87).

3. The experience of the Hysteroscopy Center of Fuxing Hospital, Capital Medical University, is that in the resection of small submucous myoma it is usually very easy to

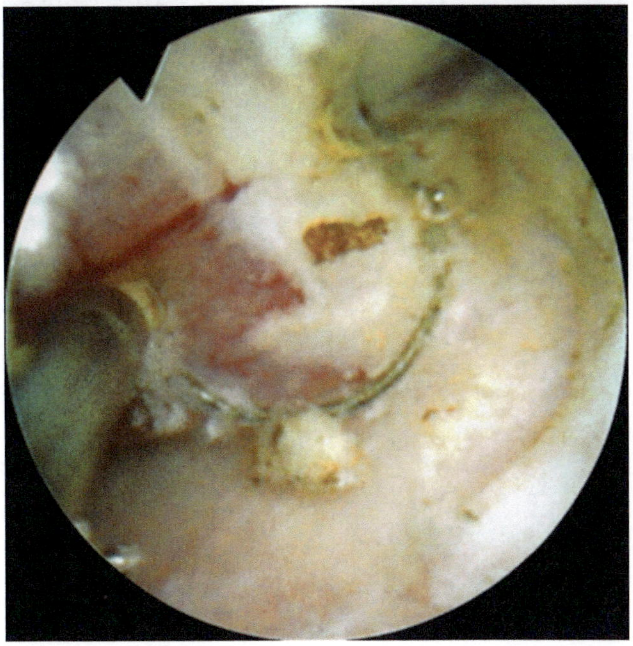

Fig. 9.78 Resection of pedicle of myoma with wire loop electrode (retrograde resection)

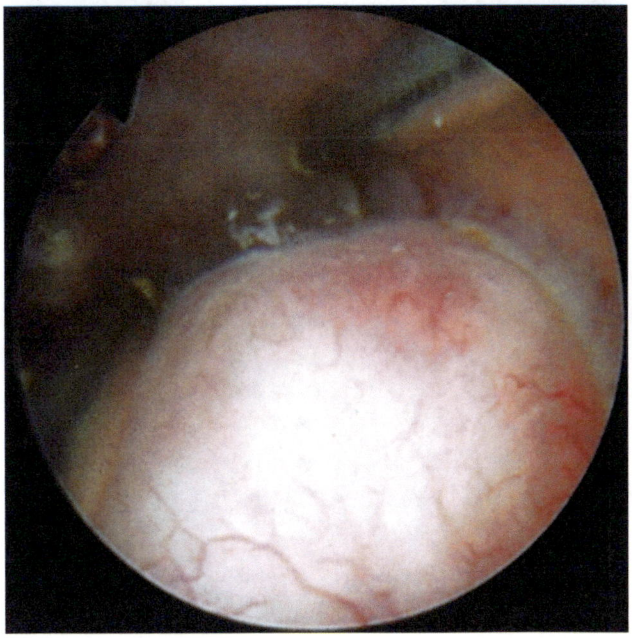

Fig. 9.79 A groove is cut in the upper portion of the myoma

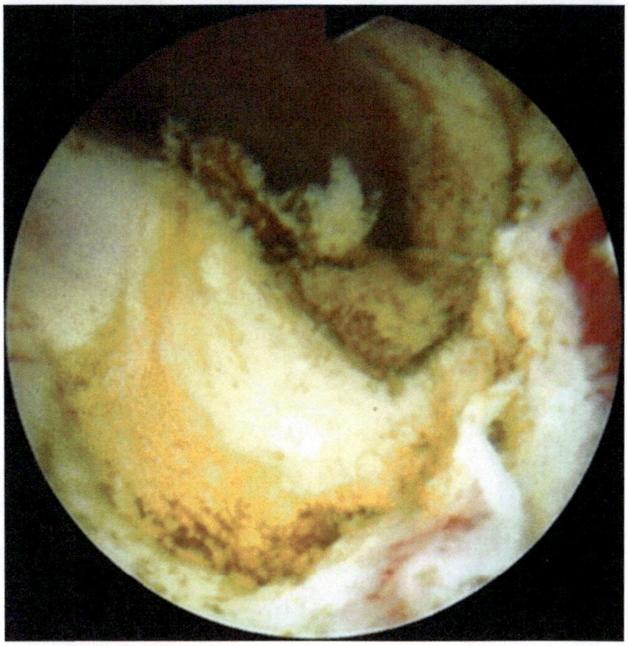

Fig. 9.80 A groove is cut in the upper portion of the myoma

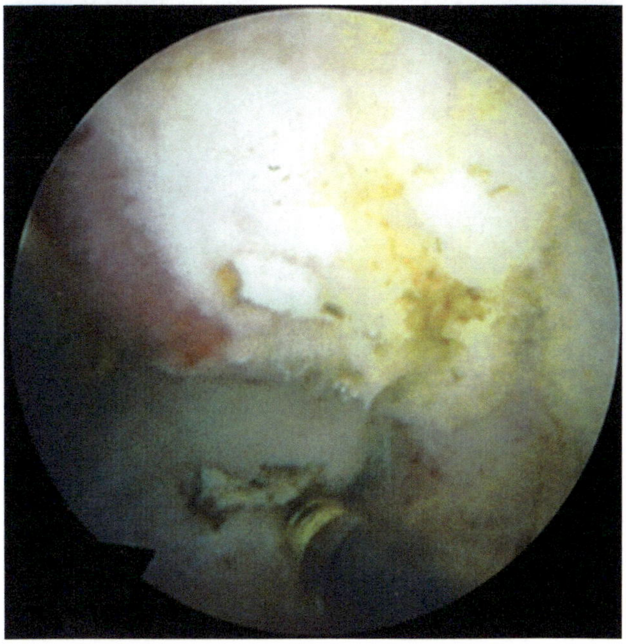

Fig. 9.81 A groove is cut in the lower portion of the myoma

resect with wire loop electrode and vaporizing electrode. The resection of large myoma (usually more than 3 cm in diameter) needs ultrasonography and (or) laparoscopic monitoring. Prior to resection, the operator must identify the anatomical relationship between the myoma and its peripheral myometrial layer, and find the pedicle of myoma. The large vessels on the surface of myoma and blood vessels in the pedicle are coagulated by wire loop or rollerball electrode, which may reduce intraoperative bleeding. Then the myoma is resected into pieces using wire loop electrode, which reduces the size of myoma. Then cut off the pedicle and clamp it out, or resect the myoma completely. During operation, the monopolar blended current is used and produces a certain coagulating effect when cutting, which avoids the intraoperative bleeding. When blended current is used for cutting, it

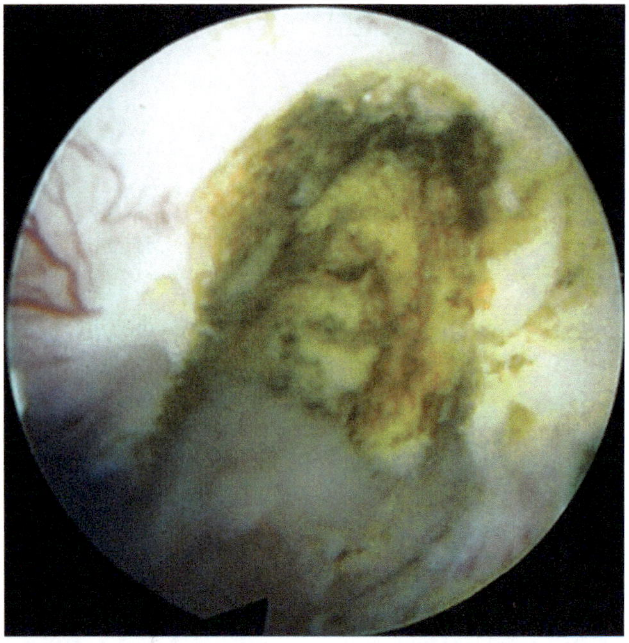

Fig. 9.82 A groove is cut in the lower portion of the myoma

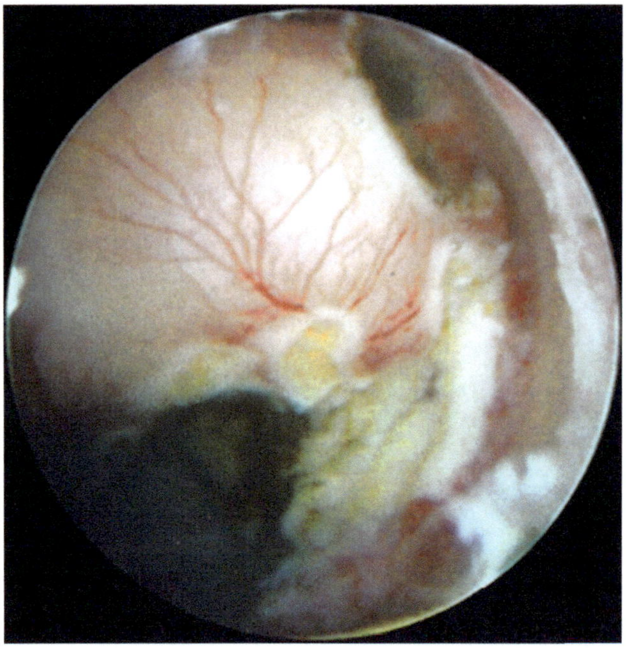

Fig. 9.83 Appearance of myoma after the formation of grooves

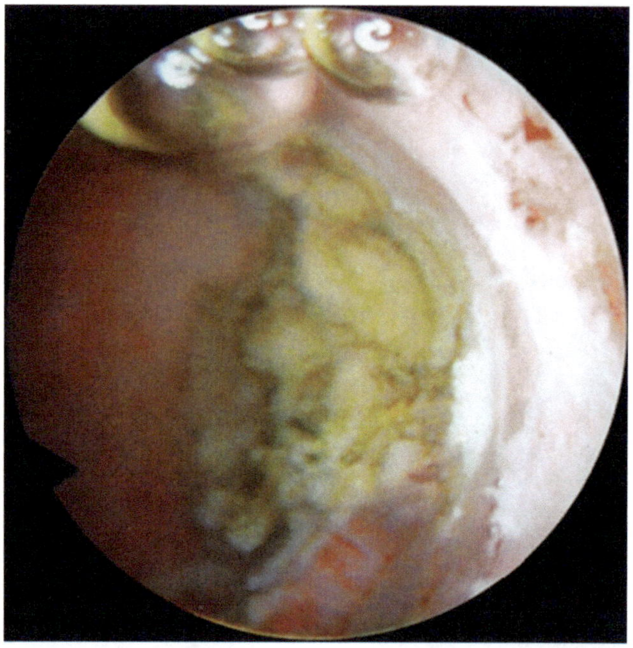

Fig. 9.84 The residual myoma tissues are clamped out with forceps

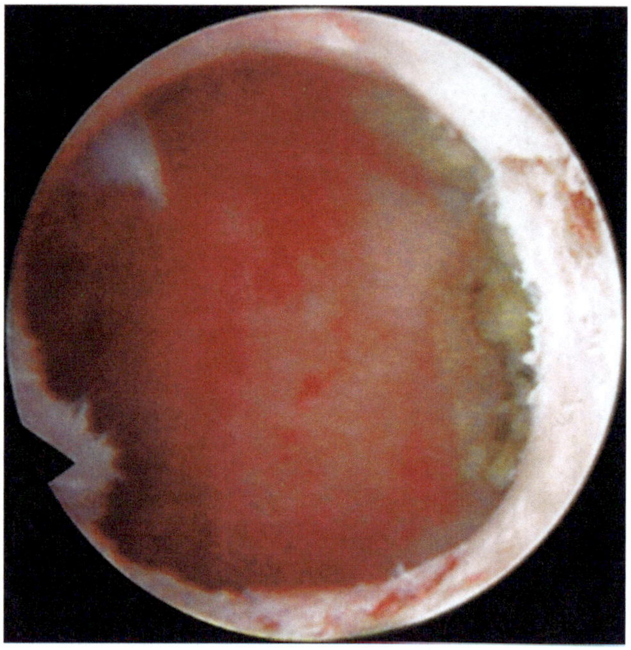

Fig. 9.85 Checkup of the uterine cavity after TCRM

may cause tissue debris to adhere to electric cutting loop. That is why some surgeons prefer the pure monopolar cutting current. When cutting, place the wire loop at the back of the myoma. Then start the cutting power, and retreat the electric wire loop till the resected tissue strip is cut off from the myoma. This method is mostly suitable for the resection of submucous myoma in the center of uterine cavity. When cutting, it is best not to retreat the cutting loop completely into the sheath, instead, let the cutting loop remain a bit outside the sheath, so that the operator can view clearly the relationship between the myoma and uterine wall. This can avoid cutting into the uterine wall and injury of the internal orifice. The operator should be very careful in resecting the base of myoma so as not to damage the surrounding endometrium. If there is bleeding, coagulate the base of myoma, or use tocolytic agents.

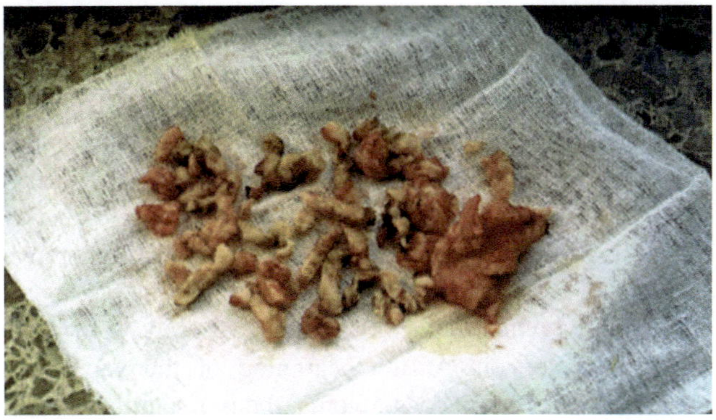

Fig. 9.86 The resected and clamped out myoma tissues (15 g weighed)

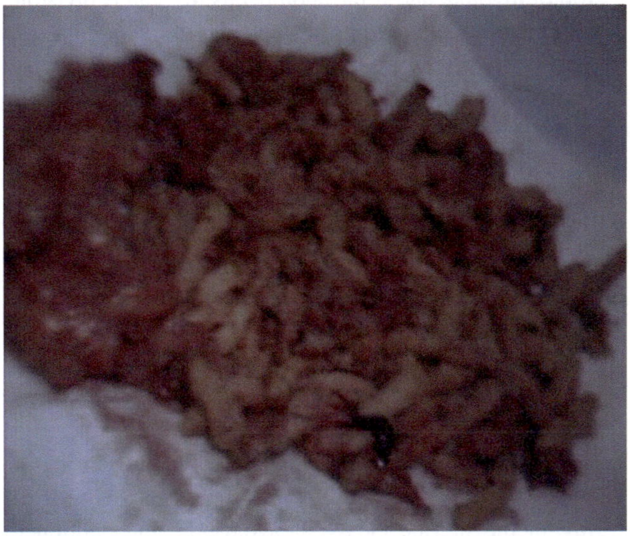

Fig. 9.87 The resected and clamped out myoma tissues (128 g weighed)

4. Osmatic cervical dilator is commonly used for cervical softening prior to TCRM. Generally, after placing the laminaria tent into the cervical canal at the eve of the operation, the cervix will be adequately softened and dilated. It facilitates the insertion and the retraction of resectoscope, as well as the insertion of the oval forceps into the cervical canal at the time of surgery, resulting in the decrease of operative difficulties.
5. For Lin's experience, the intrauterine pressure increases when the hysteroscope is placed in the uterine cavity, and falls suddenly when it is withdrawn. The change in pressure may increase the protruding degree of submucous myoma, and even helps some intramural myomas to protrude into the uterine cavity, which are transformed into the submucous myoma, and are possible to be resected. In addition, it has the feasibility of hysteroscopic resection of embedded submucous myoma. Homou named this phenomenon as "water massage," and Lin calls this mechanical change of the protruding submucous myoma caused by changes in intrauterine pressure "rebound phenomenon." In addition, the electrical stimulation and the clamping of myomas with oval forceps during operation may cause the contraction of the uterus, resulting in the thickening of the uterine muscle wall at the site of the resected myoma, which is very helpful for a smooth operation.
6. A 90° vertical wire loop is generally used to cut antegradely with the current power of 70–120 W, and a 0° horizontal loop is always used to resect retrogradely. For large myomas, under ultrasonography monitoring, when the operator is sure of the cut, he can cut either retrogradely or antegradely immediately after the retrograde cutting. The setting of the current power should start with lower power, and then gradually increase to the point at which the cutting loop is moving without any resistance through the myoma tissues. The setting of the power should be regulated on the basis of easy movement of the loop instead of using a fixed power, which can reduce the possibility of breaking the cutting loop. When the current power is up to 120 W, the operator should drag the wire loop with only very small force and have a clean tissue resection. Only in a clear vision field can the current power be switched on. When resecting the intramural parts of the myoma, the operator must be able to identify the myoma from its pseudo-capsule (Figs. 9.88 and 9.89). The operator can visualize the white fibrous tissues inside the tumor and the glandular crypts in the endometrial tissues under hysteroscope, and decides on the suitable cutting depth according to the identification of the rigid

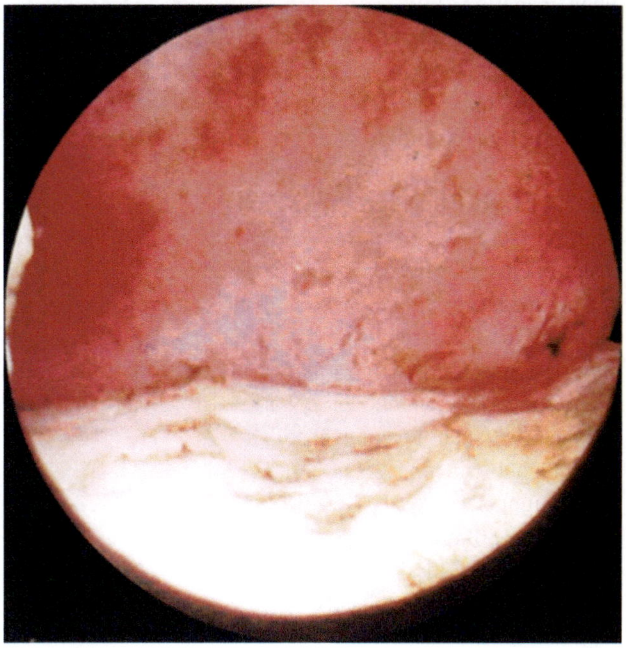

Fig. 9.88 Resection of inward-protruding intramural myoma and identification of its pseudo-capsule

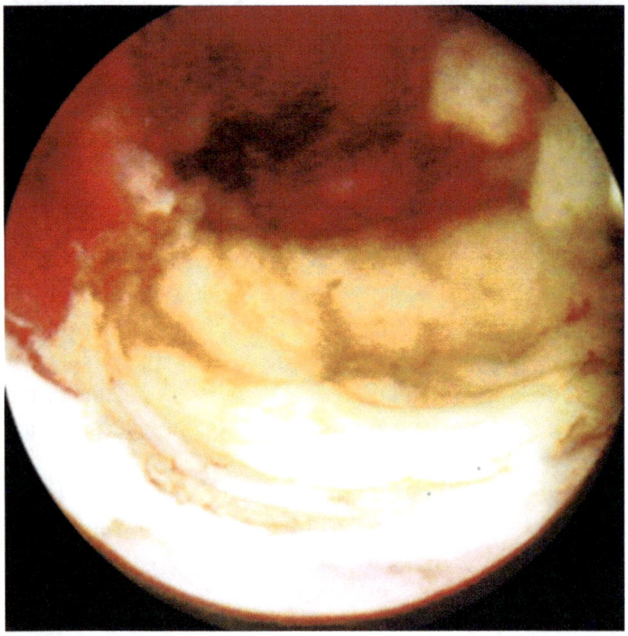

Fig. 9.89 Resection of inward-protruding intramural myoma and identification of its pseudo-capsule

fibrous tissues of the myoma and the surrounding soft myometrium.

7. Nd-YAG laser, argon or KTP-532 laser can also be used for resection of sessile submucous myoma or submucous myoma with a broad pedicle. Nd-YAG laser can be used to smash the large myomas. As for a sessile submucous myoma or a myoma with a broad pedicle, the laser or high-frequency electricity may also destroy the residual myoma tissues in the muscle wall, resulting in necrosis and gradual absorption. There is no comparative study on the resection of myomas by hysteroscopic resectoscope and laser, respectively.
8. A 3 mm bipolar electrocoagulation needle has been used in repeated (20–30 times) poking into the myoma under hysteroscopy, which plays a similar role to laser in producing. Then a 50 W coagulating electrode or 100 W cutting current is used to act on myoma tissues, causing a lot of coagulative necrosis of myoma, interruption of blood supply, tissue shrinkage, and final necrosis.
9. The resection of myoma with wire loop electrode may lead to significant bleeding, which may interfere with the operator's vision. In order to have a clear vision, irrigation fluid needs to be administered under high pressure, and the fragments of myoma needs to be continuously removed, which may result in prolonged operating time, and also significantly increase the risk of irrigation fluid into the blood vessels. Recently, a vaporizing electrode was developed, i.e., VaporTrode, which can vaporize the hyperplastic and hypertrophic prostate, and is seen in the literature of urology. In 1995, Brooks attempted to apply this successful technique and equipment to vaporize submucous myoma. In 1997, Glasser reported his preliminary experience of the application of VaporTrode in vaporizing endometrium and submucous myomas. Compared with the conventional techniques, the operative process is significantly shortened, a large number of myoma debris produced are avoided, intraoperative bleeding and absorption of irrigation fluid decrease significantly, which reduce the dangers caused by hysteroscopic resection. At the beginning of the vaporizing resection of submucous myoma, the pure cutting current should be set at power of 110 W. First, wire loop electrode is used to cut 0.5 cm wedge-shaped tissues from the top of myoma, and if the submucous myoma is invisible, a similar resection with the same depth of the posterior wall is performed from the uterine fundus to the internal orifice of cervix for histopathological examination. Then, apply the vaportrode, and increase the current power by 10 W each time, and gradually up till 200 W. Its current power below 140 W cannot vaporize myomas. The purpose of vaporization of myomas is to reduce its size so that it could be clamped out with a grasping forceps or resected with a cutting loop. In order to obtain some myoma tissues for histopathological examination, the myoma should not be completely vaporized. A 3 mm roller barrel electrode can produce a wider vaporizing channel on myomas, and a 2.5 mm roller barrel electrode can divide the myoma into blocks accurately. During the process of vaporizing the myoma, there is no debris floating in the uterine cavity. It avoids the interruption of vaporizing to remove the debris, which interferes with the vision. It is only when the electrode needs to be changed or when the forceps need to be used to remove myoma debris that the hysteroscope is pulled out. If there is still a small amount of residue in the superficial myometrium, the wire loop electrode can be used for resection. Acc loop is a thick wire loop electrode equipped with a cylinder of five small grooves and with pure cutting current of 275 W, which can vaporize the tissues and stop bleeding of the cutting base. Acc loop may be used to resect the submucous myoma with broad pedicle from the base to the level of the surrounding endometrium. The resected myoma is clamped out with an oval forceps. For large myomas of 3–6 cm in diameter, Acc rod-shaped vaporizing electrode with pure cutting current at power of 275 W is used to resect until the base of myoma. If the base is easy to see, Acc electrode is used to vaporize from periphery to center. Occasionally, when the electrode with a wide surface is used, the myoma can be dissected bluntly from its base, just like a scalpel without the use of electrical current. The myoma fragments should be clamped out with myoma forceps or oval forceps. The myomas embedded in the myometrial layer may continue to protrude into

the uterine cavity during cutting or vaporization, and it should be resected as much as possible. Even if not completely resected, it still has a high success rate. If there are occasionally residue tissues of myomas and persistent menorrhagia, a second resection is required. To women without requirements for fertility, Acc rod-shaped electrode can be applied at the same time in endometrial ablation. Its vaporizing depth is 3–4 mm, similar to that of wire loop electrode resection. If the electrode is covered with eschar or tissue debris, a 70 W electric coagulation current may be powered on, roll rapidly on the vaporized surface of the uterine cavity and it can be cleared. Prior to vaporization, be sure not to apply electrocoagulation of the endometrium, because the inactive tissue on its surface may produce impedance, thus hindering the vaporizing depth. After vaporization, the rollerball electrode at power of 100 W is used to remove the endometrium at the fallopian tubal ostia and coagulate each large bleeding point. The bleeding points can be easily identified when the inflow pipe is shut to lower the intrauterine pressure. The vaportrode uses the pure cutting current at high power of 200–275 W, and this high-power vaporizing current strengthens significantly the blockage of blood vessels and reduces the intraoperative bleeding. Since the vaportrode may divide the myoma into blocks, there are few intraoperative tissue fragments and there is no need to waste time to take out the tissue fragments, thus reducing the risk of excessive irrigation fluid absorption, decreasing the occurrences of complications and increasing the safety of the operation. Some thermal energy may cause coagulation zone of the adjacent tissues. The vaporizing depth depends on the contact time, impedance (caused by the adhesion of debris on the electrode), and the power of the current. The electrode should move slowly on the tissues and can only be powered on when moving towards the operator. If such high-frequency current is acting on a point for a long time, it is easy to cause uterine perforation, so it is only used by the experienced doctors. There have been cases of reports on hysteroscopic operation, the myoma specimens are found to be leiomyosarcoma after histopathological examination. Thus the myoma tissues should not be vaporized completely and part of the tissues should be kept for histopathological examination. Yang and Lin reported 16 cases of submucous myomas which embedded deeply in the myometrium with the thickness between the external boundary of myoma and internal edge of serosa of 5–10 mm. The one-stage hysteroscopic myomectomy was performed, with myoma diameter 3.3 cm and the median weight of myoma 30 g. During the procedure, the myometrial thickness is increased gradually and significantly, from 6.7 mm before operation to 16.1 mm after the removal of myoma. The thickness of the opposite wall was increased from 10.1 mm before operation to 18.8 mm after operation. It is thought that one-stage hysteroscopic myomectomy can remove the deep-set submucosal myoma with a thin (5 mm) myometrial layer.

9.3.7 Intraoperative Special Conditions and Management

1. If there is more intraoperative bleeding, unclear vision of field, and limited operating space due to the uterine cavity being filled with myoma, the use of oxytocin is inappropriate. This can be dealt with by adjusting the inflow pressure of irrigation higher than the arterial pressure and increasing the flow rate. If it still does not work, connect the outflow pipe with a vacuum extractor to produce a negative pressure, which accelerates the irrigation circulation, and quickens the operation speed simultaneously. When most of the myomas are resected, bleeding will naturally decrease along with the contraction of the uterus.
2. After the removal of sessile submucosal myoma, the uterus contracts, the myoma bed closes, and the residual grayish white flocculent pseudo-capsule floats in the uterine cavity. Residual pseudo-capsule does not need a resection since they will dissolve afterwards.

9.3.8 Intra- and Postoperative Monitoring and Management

9.3.8.1 Intraoperative Monitoring

1. Ultrasonography monitoring: It plays a role of guidance in the resection of large myomas, and can also prevent and identify uterine perforation (Fig. 9.90, 9.91, 9.92, 9.93, 9.94, 9.95, 9.96, and 9.97). Recently, there have been reports about the rectal probe for monitoring. Coccia et al. conducted a prospective study of ultrasonography monitoring of TCRS and TCRM in 81 cases, and made a comparison with 45 cases of laparoscopic monitoring. The results were that no complications occurred and there was no need to convert to laparoscopic monitoring just because the ultrasonography cannot see clearly the pelvic structure as laparoscopy. Ultrasonography is very useful in determining the intramural portion of submucous myoma and the boundary of the surrounding muscle walls, and contributes to its complete resection.
2. Laparoscopic monitoring: It depends on the intraoperative specific circumstances. For larger submucosal myomas, especially those that cause the distortion of uterine cavity, if the operator is not sure of the safety of transcervical resection, it will be safer to implement the operation under laparoscopic monitoring. Laparoscopic

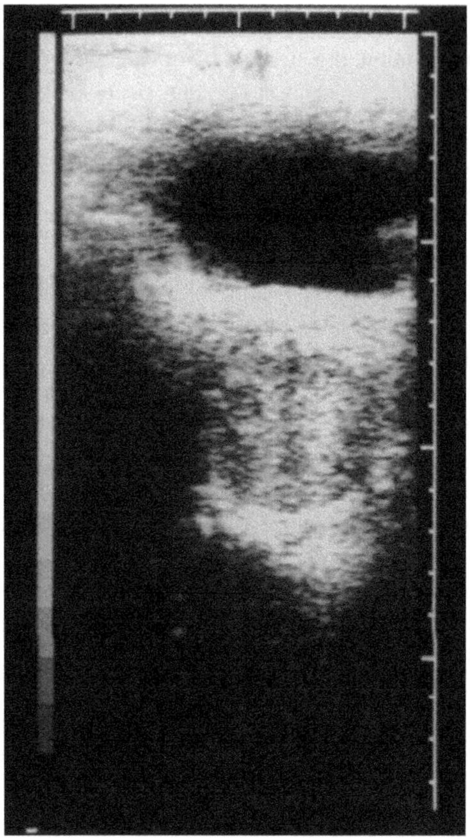

Fig. 9.90 Transabdominal ultrasonography prior to TCRM. Longitudinal scanning shows anterior intramural myoma

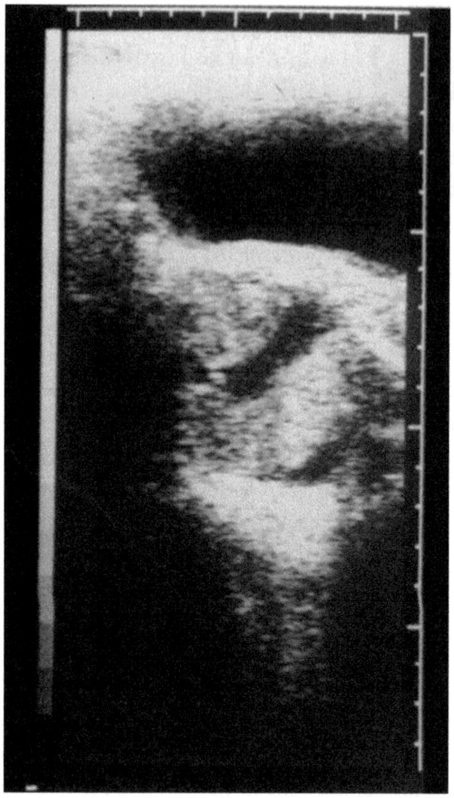

Fig. 9.91 Transabdominal ultrasonography during TCRM. When irrigating the cavity with irrigation fluid, the anterior intramural myoma is protruding into the uterine cavity

monitoring can help to find the complete and incomplete uterine perforation in time, and can deal with it immediately.

9.3.8.2 Postoperative Monitoring and Treatment

1. Application of prophylactic estrogen after operation: To those who wish to conceive later, postoperative application of estrogen can stimulate the growth of endometrium, accelerate re-epithelialization and prevent occurrence of adhesion, especially for those who have larger denude surface in uterus and in vivo low estrogen status induced by preoperative application of GnRH analogs. Second-look hysteroscopy is done 6–8 weeks postoperation. The incidence of the endometrial adhesion after TCRM is unknown, probably very low. Therefore, the advantage of application of prophylactic estrogen is not certain.
2. Transient fever: It is very rare, and the body temperature may increase suddenly up to 40 °C within 24 h after operation. General physical examination and measurement of white cells may find no abnormalities, and symptomatic treatment should be followed, and the temperature mostly return to normal within 24 h. This is commonly seen in patients with severe anemia, and the more serious anemia is, the higher the body temperature will be. There is no consistent view on its cause, and it is mostly agreed that it

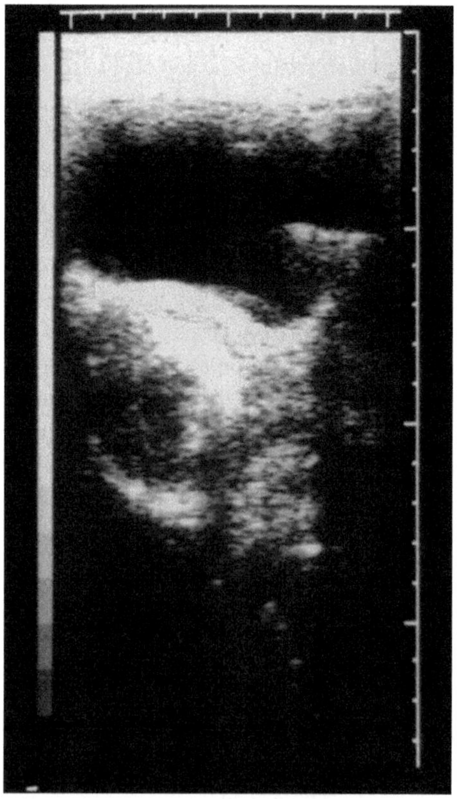

Fig. 9.92 Transabdominal ultrasonography during TCRM. The cutting surface of the myoma appears to show strong echo

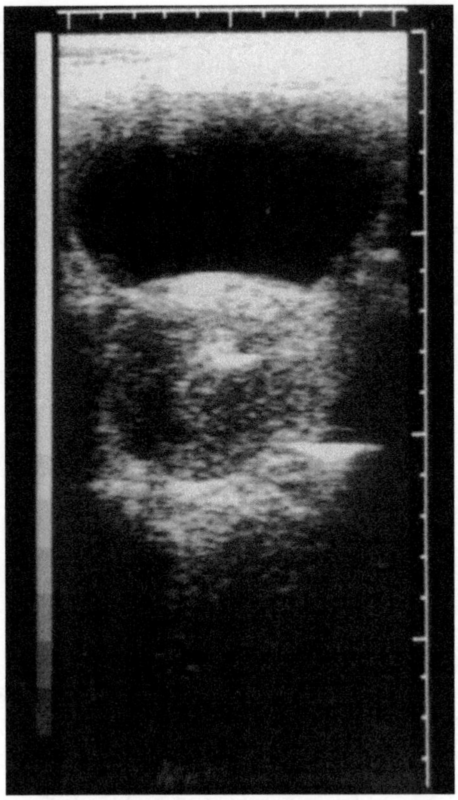

Fig. 9.93 Transabdominal ultrasonography after removal of the myoma. The pedicle appears to show strong echo

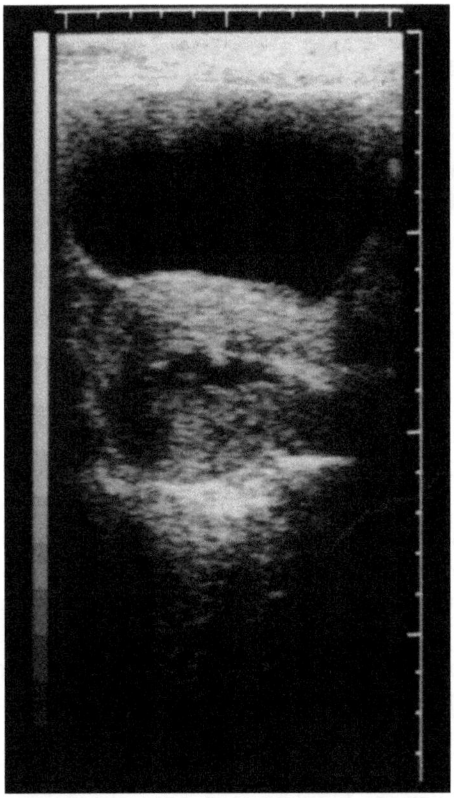

Fig. 9.94 Transabdominal ultrasonography after TCRM. An unobstructed and intact cavity is seen after distending with irrigation fluid

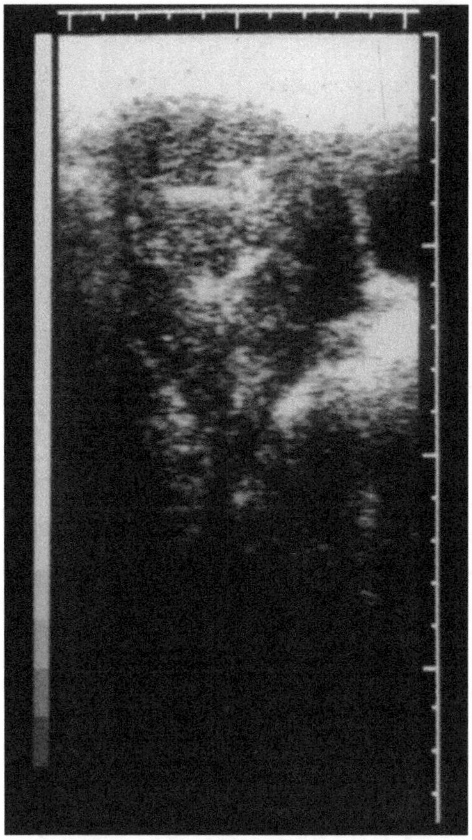

Fig. 9.95 Transabdominal ultrasonography during TCRM. The myoma is separated from the normal myometrium and forms circular strong echo

is due to an allergic reaction caused by the irrigation fluid into the body. But, in transurethral resection of the prostate, the urological explanation given for this complication is transient bacteremia.

3. Abdominal pain: After operation, persistent lower abdominal pain may develop due to uterine spasm contraction. A symptomatic treatment should be given and it should be differentiated from uterine perforation.
4. Vaginal discharge: For those who have large uterine cutting surface, large and deep myoma bed, or resection of endometrium at the same time, before the myoma bed heals or cutting surface is epithelialized, they may have continuous discharge from vagina within 2 months after operation. It may begin with a little blood, then turn gradually to a light red blood water in 1 week, then turn to be pale yellow watery discharge, and finally becomes a colorless watery discharge. If the patient has menstrual bleeding within 2 months after surgery, she should be treated symptomatically and attention should be paid to exclude any prolapse of residual intramural myoma.
5. Since the intrauterine operation has a large cutting surface, IUD should be placed in those who still want to conceive later after operation. If more bleeding occurs

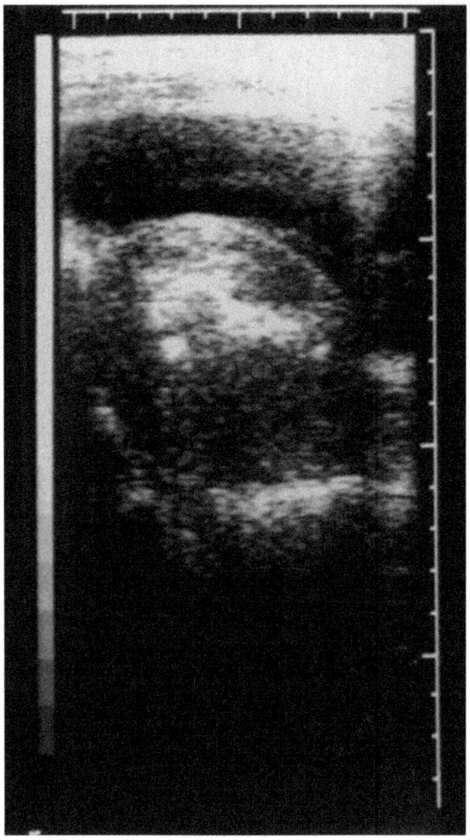

Fig. 9.96 Transabdominal ultrasonography during TCRM. The size of circular strong echo shrinks, suggesting the reduction of the volume of myoma

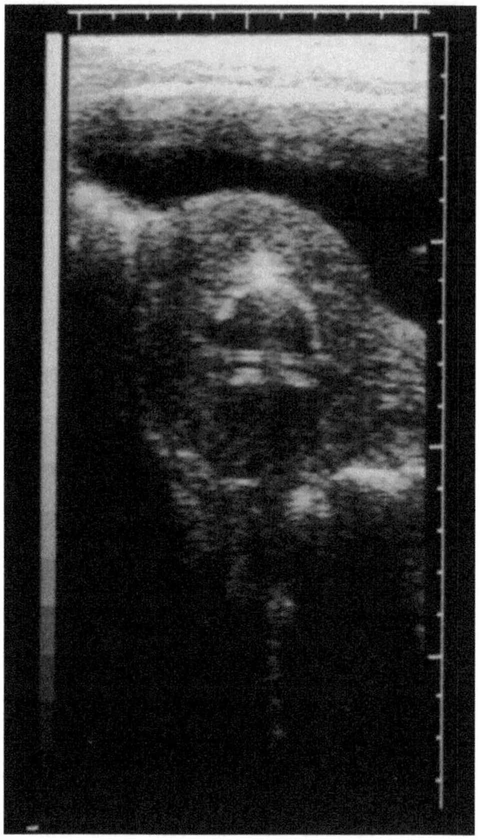

Fig. 9.97 Transabdominal ultrasonography after TCRM. Placement of balloon for hemostasis by compression

following operation, the IUD can be taken out and replaced after the next menstruation. .

6. To those who underwent pretreatment with GnRH analogs, estrogen should be administered postoperatively for 1 week.
7. Few patients may have more menses at the first menstrual cycle after operation.
8. If there are more endometrium resected during the removal of myoma, those who still desire for fertility should undergo hysteroscopy within the second or the third week after operation and have intrauterine adhesion removed, and other patients should have second-look hysteroscopy 4 months after operation to determine its anatomical status.
9. Patients with type I and type II submucous myomas, and patients with inward-protruding intramural myomas who require two-step operation should undergo regular ultrasonography, and decide on the time for operation.

9.3.9 Identification and Treatment of Operative Complications

Loffer reported that the occurrence of complications with TCRM is 0.5%, and 2% for nonexperienced operators.

9.3.9.1 Bleeding

At the resection of type I and type II submucous myomas, and inward-protruding intramural myomas, if the base of the myoma is deep, its hemostasis will be difficult. Electrocoagulation can be conducted for hemostasis on explicit bleeding points, or the intrauterine pressure can be increased through regulating the irrigating fluid pressure to stop the bleeding. If both of them do not work, insertion of a balloon catheter should be considered, its precautions are as follows:

1. The amount of the fluid being injected into the balloon should be less than the volume of the resected specimens.
2. The size of the balloon by ultrasonography scanning should be less than the size of the myoma prior to operation.
3. If the bleeding cannot be stopped by the compression of the balloon, it might be due to insufficient fluid in balloon. Therefore, supplementary injection of fluid into balloon or 8-shaped suture of cervical external orifice with thread can increase intrauterine pressure and stop bleeding. When the balloon catheter is stretched backward, it can stop the bleeding from cervical canal by compression. The sutures can be removed along with the removal of the balloon catheter.

9.3.9.2 Uterine Perforation

The uterine perforation by transcervical resection of uterine myomas often occurs in the normal myometrium adjacent to the myoma. The development and extension of uterine myomas makes the adjacent myometrium stretch to be thinner, where special attention should be paid. A passive operating bracket should be used and the power cannot be turned on when the vision is not clear. Hallez reported one case of uterine perforation in 61 cases of operation. Laparoscopic repair was performed immediately once it was found. Corson and Brooks reported that among 92 cases with hysteroscopic myomectomy, one case of uterine perforation occurred when the resected myoma fragments were taken out. Loffer reported one case of uterine perforation when the resected myoma fragments were taken out. Among 108 cases of TCRM performed by Wamsteker, there was one case of uterine perforation, which was cured after timely treatment. Of 1156 cases of TCRM done by Lin, there was one case of uterine perforation, which occurred when the myoma was clamped out, the oval forceps mistakenly clamped and tore the muscles at the fundus of the uterus, resulting in the perforation.

9.3.9.3 Fluid Overload and Hyponatremia

When type I and type II submucous myoma or inward-protruding intramural myomas were resected, the resection would reach the deep myometrium with rich blood vessels, which is more likely to cause fluid overload and hyponatremia than any other hysteroscopy operation. Therefore, the operator should be highly alert. Loffer reported that 2 of 55 cases, in which the irrigating fluid deficit was above 1000 mL, had transient hyponatremia, and one of them had early pulmonary edema. Among 108 cases of TCRM with 4% sorbitol as irrigation fluid reported by Wamsteker, one case had fluid overload, and developed early pulmonary edema and hyponatremia, in which the anesthesiologist found the oxygen saturation decreased and pulmonary edema. Total hysterectomy and bilateral salpingo-oophorectomy was performed. Of Lin's 1676 patients by hysteroscopic electric resection, one case developed TURP syndrome.

9.3.9.4 Inversion of Uterus

Lin reported a case of removal of 800 g myoma, who developed postoperative uterine inversion, and underwent emergency abdominal hysterectomy.

9.3.9.5 Uterine Fistula

De Iaco et al. reported one case of hysteroscopic resection of intramural myomas, causing uterine fistula. This 38-year-old woman had uterine artery embolization due to uterine myomas, and underwent hysteroscopic resection 6 months later, which resulted in the uterine fistula.

9.3.9.6 Uterine Myoma Malignancy

If there are a few remained myoma tissues at the end of operation, the subsequent incidence of sarcoma of uterus is unchanged, thus its follow-up is necessary. Hansen and Lund reported one case of hysteroscopic myomectomy. Under hysteroscope, the intramural myoma at the uterine fundus protruded into the uterine cavity, with the appearance of fibroma, and there were no other intrauterine pathological findings identified. The tumor was removed from the myometrium with no operative complications, and the patient was discharged on the day of operation. Histopathologic examination suggested mesenchymal tumor cells invading the myometrium with no obvious atypia and mitosis, and no vascular infiltration, which was diagnosed as low-grade malignant stromal sarcoma. The patient was readmitted for total hysterectomy. Low-grade malignant stromal sarcoma is a rare tumor, whose symptoms and clinical manifestations are similar to uterine fibroma. Along with the development and extensive application of TCRM and TCRP, the operator should be alert about this tumor, especially in young women. In addition, it has no special high-risk signs to be identified. Thus it is extremely difficult to make diagnosis only by diagnostic or operative hysteroscopy. In 1995, Marabini et al. reported a case about accidental resection of endometrial stromal sarcoma during hysteroscopic operation. In 1996, Flam and Radestad reported a case of hysteroscopic resection of submucous myoma, with its histopathological examination suggesting uterine endometrial stromal sarcoma.

9.3.10 Experience and Evaluation of TCRM

9.3.10.1 Operating Process and Outcome of TCRM

1. From 1985 to 2000, Dr. Lin totally performed 1137 cases of hysteroscopic resection of submucous myomas. The operation time ranged from 4 to 150 min. Resected specimens varied in weight between 0.5 and 800g. There was one case of uterine perforation, which was repaired under laparoscopy. The recurrence rates of myoma after TCRM were 16.7% (38/228, from 1985 to 1992) and 8.7% (33/378, from 1993 to 1999), respectively. In a long-term follow-up, 26 cases (2.6%) had total hysterectomy, six cases had transabdominal myomectomy, and 23 cases (2.1%) underwent a second TCRM. Eighty-one pregnancies were achieved after operation, including three cases of miscarriage, nine cases of ongoing pregnancy, and 69 cases of full-term deliveries (61 cases of vaginal birth and eight cases of cesarean section). Among 26 cases who had total hysterectomy, the indications were: enlarged intramural myomas (ten cases), uterine sarcoma (eight cases), intramural myoma complicated by endometriosis or ovarian cyst (five cases), sessile submucosal myoma

complicated by menorrhagia (two cases), and ovarian cancer (one case).

2. Vercellini et al. reported the outcomes of TCRM in 108 women over 7 years, which included 54 cases with pedunculated submucous myomas, 30 cases with sessile myomas, and 24 cases with intramural myomas. For women with one operation, the mean operating times were about 18 min, 23 min, and 32 min in resecting pedunculated, sessile, and intramural myomas, respectively; and the fluid deficits were about 204, 278, and 335 mL in resection of those myomas, respectively. For women with more than one procedure, 14 cases were in 54 cases with pedunculated myomas, 8 were in 30 cases with sessile myomas, and 12 in 24 cases with intramural myomas. Twenty-seven women were found to have recurrence of myomas during the follow-up of 41 months, with the recurrent rate of 34% within 3 years. The recurrence of menorrhagia was found in 20 cases (ratio 30% within 3 years). The cumulative postoperative pregnancy rates within 3 years were 49% in pedunculated group, 36% in sessile group, and 33% in intramural group. They suggested that after TCRM, the menstruation may be controlled satisfactorily, with less recurrence of myoma and improvement of pregnancy. For intramural myoma, the operating time and the number of operations required will be influenced, without long-term adverse outcomes.
3. Loffer made a retrospective study about the outcomes of TCRM in 18 postmenopausal women with bleeding and 2 asymptomatic postmenopausal women with abnormal ultrasound findings. Of them, 19 women underwent TCRM, including four cases of concomitant TCRE, and one woman had hysteroscopic biopsy by resection. In a follow-up, it was found that three patients underwent gynecologic surgeries, including one case of hysteroscopy to remove the residual myoma which was found by ultrasonography, and two cases of hysterectomy due to a sarcoma or a cervical carcinoma. It was pointed out that postmenopausal women who have a submucosal myoma might have a higher risk for a sarcoma.
4. Yen et al. reported 5 women who had DUL with multiple numerous myomas (0.5–3 cm in diameters) and massive menorrhagia. Hysteroscopy was used to resect only myomas protruding into the uterine cavity, with intramural myomas being left in place. In total, there were ten procedures performed in 5 women, including one case of hysteroscopic adhesiolysis due to the formation of postoperative adhesion, two cases of repeated TCRM for the recurrence of the fibroids, and one case of two-step TCRM with the administration of GnRH analog following the first procedure. All five cases preserved their uterus and achieved normal menses, with successful pregnancies in 3 women who desired for fertility.
5. In 2007, Bettocchi et al. from Italy proposed a change from "wait-and-see" to "see-and-treat" for women of reproductive age with small (<1.5 cm) submucosal myomas. The reasons are: (1) its surface and volume of endometrium were occupied by myomas; (2) high possibility of small myomas continue to grow at reproductive age, which may cause symptoms or complications; (3) it may have negative effects on spontaneous or assisted pregnancy; (4) the diagnosis related to malignancy with biopsy could not be judged reliably without the direct vision; (5) The hysteroscopic "see-and-treat" is effective.

9.3.10.2 Effects of TCRM

Tulandi and al-Took pointed out that TCRM was the best method to remove the submucous myoma. For the women who suffer from symptomatic myomas and wish to preserve the uterus, retain or improve their fertility, TCRM has three advantages over hysterectomy: (1) the shorter hospitalization and lower cost; (2) the less operative pain and less morbidity rate; (3) if the patient has subsequent pregnancy, it is likely for her to have vaginal delivery, however there is also a risk of rupture of the gravid uterus after TCRM. Yaron reported a woman who underwent hysteroscopic myomectomy for submucosal myoma, with perforation occurred at the uterine fundus, and suturing performed laparoscopically. Later on, when she got pregnant, she suffered from a sudden onset of abdominal pain at 33 weeks of gestation. Uterine rupture with partial placenta protruding to abdominal cavity was identified by laparotomy.

The published literatures confirmed the effectiveness of TCRM, and the results in short-term follow-up indicated that more than 90% of the excessive bleeding was under control in those who had resection of myoma alone or simultaneous removal of endometrium. As to those who had myoma residuals after operation, if they have no severe bleeding and (or) pain, about 50% of myoma residuals degenerate or discharge when following up at 3-month post-operation. If necessary, an "additional resection" should be conducted. In a long-term follow-up of TCRM, 22.3% of resection of submucous myoma alone developed abnormal uterine bleeding, 16.1% required further operation. On the contrary, as for those who had resection of submucous myoma and simultaneous removal of the endometrium, 22.5% developed abnormal uterine bleeding, but only 8.1% required further operation. As for those who used Nd-YAG to remove single myoma and resect the endometrium simultaneously or not, the recurrence rate of menorrhagia and uterine bleeding was 2–4%. However, for those of removal of multiple submucosal myomas and inward-protruding intramural myomas, the recurrence rate was 25%. For the recurrent cases, if they had no fertility desire, the most appropriate method of treatment is hysterectomy. Lin's data showed that the recurrence rate of myoma was 16.7%. From 1993 to April of 1998, of 347cases, 26 cases (7.5%) had recurrent submucous myomas. The results of long-term follow-up were that 23 cases (2.8%) had hysterectomy, three cases had abdominal myomectomy, and 16 cases (2%) had another TCRM. The indications for total hysterectomy were: enlarged myoma within myometrium in ten cases, uterine myomas in six cases, intramural myoma with endometriosis or chocolate cyst in four cases, sessile submucosal myoma with menorrhagia in two cases, and ovarian cancer in one case.

In 1997, Romer reported 70 cases of TCRM in women who had submucous myoma with most portions locating in the uterine wall. GnRH analogs were administrated preoperatively for 2–3 months. With ultrasonography guidance or laparoscopic monitoring applied at the time of operation, TCRM was performed by experienced surgeons. There were no intra- and postoperative complications, except for two cases with large myomas undergoing repeated surgery. Within 5–52 months of follow-up, all patients achieved normal menstruation, without the requirement of hysterectomy. Thus it was thought that when resection of submucous myoma with their largest portion in the uterine wall was performed by experienced surgeons, the complication rate would not be increased. Hallez made a retrospective analysis of the outcomes in 284 cases of TCRM. The patients ranged in age from 25 to 70, and the diameter of myoma varies between 1 and 6.5 cm. There was only one case of complication of uterine perforation, which was immediately repaired. After operation, both good uterine anatomical morphology and better function of the uterus were achieved in 95.6% of patients at 6 months after operation, 94.6% at 1 year, 89.7% at 2 years, 87.8% at 3 years, 83% at 4 years, 76.3% at 5 years, 73.2% at 6 years, and being stable at 67.6% since the seventh year. It was suggested that TCRM could not improve the fertility in women with primary infertility but could increase it in women with secondary infertility. He believed that TCRM was a difficult, but safe procedure, and was a conservative operation worthy to be adopted. In 2000, Romer et al. reported that the cases who had hysteroscopic myomectomy with myoma >3 cm in diameter and (or) intramural myoma, or with secondary anemia were suitable for preoperative application of GnRH-a. The purpose of which was not only to thin the endometrium, but also to reduce the size of myoma and the blood vessels surrounding the myoma. Those who had not been applied GnRH analogs had high failure rates of myomectomy, especially with the large intramural myomas. Polena et al. conducted a retrospective analysis of 235 cases of TCRM, which included the assessment of the effectiveness of TCRM and its relationship with the type and size of myomas. The main reasons for TCRM were AUB and infertility, with 37% of patients having endometrial ablation and 32% having TCRP. Fifty-one percent of all patients were postmenopausal women. 2.6% of cases had intraoperative complications and all were not serious. Among 84% of the patients who were followed up with the median 40 months (18–66 months), 94.4% had successful outcomes. For failure cases, four had repeated operations, three underwent hysterectomy, and four still had AUB. It was believed that, for selected cases, TCRM was a safe and highly effective procedure with long-term satisfying efficacy and fewer complications.

Loffer's studies showed that TCRM along with TCRE contributes to the improvement of bleeding symptoms. There were 177 cases with uterine myoma complicated with menorrhagia, of which only 104 cases underwent TCRM, and the other 73 cases applied TCRM along with TCRE. Among the cases with simultaneous resection of endometrium, 95.9% had menstruation under control, while 80.8% had menstruation under control in those without simultaneous resection of endometrium ($P = 0.003$). The effects of complete resection of uterine myoma were very good ($P = 0.039$), but the effects of simultaneous removal of the endometrium were even better ($P = 0.022$). TCRE might also increase the menstrual improvement rate in those without complete resection of myomas, but there was no significant difference. The rate of hysterectomy was not decreased by TCRE or complete resection of myoma, because the common indications for hysterectomy were pain and dysmenorrhea rather than bleeding.

Yen et al. reported five successful cases with hysteroscopic resection for DUL. The preoperative menorrhagia was significantly improved after TCRM. Huang et al. in the Hysteroscopy Center, Fuxing Hospital, Capital Medical University, reported that 31 infertile women who had DUL, menorrhagia, and anemia underwent TCRM under ultrasound guidance. During the follow-up of mean 31.7 months, 6 women underwent repeated procedures. Three of them had three procedures each. Only one patient experienced laparoscopic subtotal hysterectomy because of postoperative poor improvement of menstruation, and the other 30 patients preserved their uterus. The endometrium was repaired 2–3 months after TCRM, with the improvement rate of menses 93.5% (29/31) and recurrent rate of fibroids 32.3% (10/31).

9.3.10.3 Fertility After TCRM

It is difficult to make a comparison due to different reports. March, Valle, and Hallez reported that the delivery rate of those who had resection of submucous myoma by hysteroscopy or by laser was greater than 50%. It was thought that there was a controversy over the relationship between the uterine myoma and infertility. It was reported in IVF literature that only the deformed uterine cavity needed operation, and the postoperative pregnancy rate of laparotomy, laparoscopy, or hysteroscopy was about 50%. Neuwirth reported that among 26 cases of TCRM, after operation, nine cases required further operations, and 7 patients had hysterectomy.

In view of the fact that some patients following TCRM may have recurrent myomas, it was suggested that the patients who took the treatment with the purpose of pregnancy should try to conceive within 6–8 weeks post-operation. Bernard et al. reported that the postoperative delivery rate was higher in women with resection of one submucous myoma than in women with resection of two or more myomas, which had no relationship with the size and the location of submucous myomas. And in woman without intramural myomas, the delivery rate was higher and the duration between the operation and the delivery was significantly shorter than those with intramural myomas. Giatras et al. made a retrospective analysis of the outcomes of TCRM in 41 infertile women. After TCRM, 25 (60.9%) achieved pregnancy and 20 (48.7%) delivered at term. Among them, 17 women got one baby, 5 got twins including three cases of full-term delivery and two cases of delivery at 33 and 35 weeks of gestation, and one got triplets at 31 weeks. Two women experienced miscarriage at 6 and 8 weeks of gestation, and another woman developed intrauterine adhesions. It was believed that for infertile women, TCRM is an effective treatment for replacement of abdominal submucous myomectomy, and for improvement of pregnancy. In 2008, Caliskan et al. from Turkey first reported a case of myoma which was localized on the intrauterine septum. This 43-year-old woman had uterine septum, double cervix and vaginal septum, who suffered from primary infertility and menorrhagia. The operations were performed in two steps. The first procedures included laparotomy, adhesiolysis, myomectomy, and vaginal septate removal, and the second procedures involved the resection of complete uterine septum hysteroscopically. The length of the cervix postoperatively was measured normal at 26 weeks of gestation.

There are limited data from long-term follow-up. Hallez et al. reported the outcomes of TCRM for sessile submucous myomas in 61 cases. Among them, 93% resumed regular menstruation after operation. Of seven cases who had secondary dysmenorrhea before operation, dysmenorrhea disappeared in six cases after operation. Fifty-four cases had postoperative hysterosalpingography with 49 cases being reported normal. Among 11 cases who had previous infertility, seven cases conceived after operation, including two cases of early spontaneous miscarriage. Brooks et al. reported 52 cases following TCRM and TCRP. In more than 3 months of follow-up, 91% resumed normal menstruation; of 15 infertile women, 33% had pregnancies to full term. Loffer reported 53 women who underwent hysteroscopic resection of intrauterine neoplasms, including 43 patients with pedunculated or sessile submucous myomas and ten patients with large endometrial polyps. Forty-five patients had a long-term follow-up for longer than 12 months. Excessive bleeding was controlled in 93% of the cases. Five patients (9%) underwent hysterectomy, two patients had repeat hysteroscopic myomectomy, and two had laparotomy myomectomy. Seven of 12 patients with previous infertility (58%) delivered live-born infants. Derman summarized the experiences in management of submucous myomas in 94 cases of AUB (94%) and infertility (16%). After TCRM, late postoperative disorders were reported in 24.5% of the patients, and further operations were performed in 15.9%. Within 9 years of follow-up, 83.9% of the patients did not need more surgery. It was suggested that the long-term curative effect after TCRM diminished with time although it still had some effectiveness. After TCRM, in total 21 patients conceived, including two cases of spontaneous miscarriage, five cases of induced abortion, and 14 cases of full-term births. In Lin's report of TCRM in 93 infertile patients, postoperative pregnancy was achieved in 44 cases, with the pregnancy rate 47.3%, of them three cases had spontaneous miscarriage and 41 cases had full-term deliveries, which included nine cases of cesarean section and 32 cases of normal labor, with a full-term delivery rate of 44.1%. Wamsteker reported on 49 cases of TCRM. Of 33 cases with menorrhagia, 30 cases (91%) achieved control of postoperative bleeding. In 16 women who underwent TCRM due to infertility, 9 women (56%) experienced pregnancy after surgery, with full-term delivery in 8 (50%). The improvement of the symptoms was reduced with the increase of the myoma impinging into the myometrium. In order to reduce the failure rate, the operator must determine preoperatively the size, number, and location of the myoma and the degree of extending to the muscle layer by hysteroscopy and (or) ultrasonography so as to determine the feasibility of TCRM. For the myoma buried in the muscle wall >50%, the operation is very difficult, and the myoma can be removed with vaporizing electrode and Nd-YAG laser.

In 1999, Varasteh et al. reported on reproductive outcomes after TCRM in 36 cases who experienced infertility with the ages under 45 years. With the follow-up longer than 18 months, the results showed that the pregnancy and live birth rates in women with resected myoma larger than 2 cm were significantly higher, and the live birth rate achieved statistical significance at a myoma size more than 3 cm. It was believed that TCRM appears to improve the ability of fertility. Although hysteroscopic resection of a large myoma would remove a large area of endometrium, its advantages for fertility were more than the risks. Fernande et al. reported the safety and efficacy of TCRM in 59 cases. After TCRM, the bleeding could be effectively controlled (62%); however, the fertility improvement rate might be limited (with postoperative conception in 27%), and a full-term delivery rate of 10%. The mean age of patients was 36.6 ± 4.6 years, so the advanced age of the patients might be a factor related to infertility. The factor in favor of pregnancy after operation was that myoma was the only etiology (41.6%), and the myoma was ≥5 cm in size.

In Yen et al.'s report of five cases with hysteroscopic treatment for early DUL, four conceptions achieved in 3 patients after TCRM, with three cesarean sections due to breech presentation. Huang et al. in the Hysteroscopy Center of Fuxing Hospital, Capital Medical University, reported 31 cases of TCRM in women with DUL. Among 19 women who had infertility before operation, postoperative conception rate was 52.6% (10/19) and live birth rate was 47.4% (9/19). It was suggested that TCRM could substitute for traditional surgery in treatment of early DUL by improving the menstruation, preserving the uterus and the reproductive ability.

9.3.10.4 Repeat Operation After TCRM

Cravello et al. reported that 49 out of 196 cases following TCRM had a second operation and suggested that with the residual partial myomas remaining in the uterine wall, a subsequent hysterectomy or a second hysteroscopic resection of myoma was possible. Dueholm et al. reported that, in women with myoma residuals, if there were no serious bleeding and (or) sharp pain, 50% of the myoma residuals dissolved or discharged in a 3-month follow-up post-operation, and an "additional resection" might be done if it is necessary. From the observation of the cases of incomplete resection of myomas which embedded in the uterine wall, Valle found the remnants of the myomas might develop necrosis, or have its surface coated with endometrium; in a 12-month follow-up, 75–93% patients had their excessive bleeding under control and did not need further treatment, and 58% who once suffered from infertility had live birth. Fernandez et al. reported hysteroscopic resection of 286 myomas in 200 women. Thirty five women underwent two or three procedures because the myomas were large. Complications were encountered in 12 cases (5%), without any death or seriousness for intense care. Seventy-four percent of the patients achieved improvement of the symptoms. Among women who failed to have improvement after the surgery, the predictive factors included large myomas with the size more than 5 cm, numerous myomas with the number more than 3, bulky uterus with the length longer than 12 cm, and type II myomas, etc. Shokeir evaluated the reproductive outcomes in follow-up of 29 cases with submucous myomas and desire for fertility after TCRM. Among them, 14 cases had primary infertility and 15 women had a history of poor obstetric outcomes. Twenty-five cases had myomas in the uterine cavity (type 0), the other four cases had type 1 myomas, the size of each myoma was <5 cm, with 1.33 cm on average. There were no operative complications, and most uterine anatomical structures returned to normal after operation. There were 30 postoperative pregnancies achieved in 21 women and 13 patients delivered 16 live births. The live birth rate increased from 3.8% before operation to 63.2% after operation, and the miscarriage rate decreased from 61.6% before operation to 26.3% after operation, which indicated the improvement of pregnancy rate and live birth rate in women who had a history of infertility.

The effects of the myomectomy on embryo implantation and pregnancy prior to assisted reproductive treatment are still controversial. In 2007, Vimercati et al. from Italy studied the clinical outcomes of IVF/ICSI in 51 patients (97 treatment cycles) with uterine myomas, 63 cases (127 treatment cycles) who had previous resection of myomas, and 106 cases (215 treatment cycles) without myomas. There were no differences in pregnancy and live birth delivery between groups. Compared with the other two groups, those whose myomas larger than 4 cm needed to increase the treatment cycles. The results suggested that myomectomy prior to IVF was not indicated in women with small or middle size myomas disregarding their location. In 2005, Aziz et al. from the USA reported of one case who had a 6 cm intramural myoma and a normal cavity detected by diagnostic hysteroscopy. When she conceived after IVF, intrauterine growth restriction (IUGR) was found in early pregnancy, which led to termination of pregnancy at 23 weeks of gestation due to its severe disorders, At 6 weeks after delivery, ultrasonography revealed a 1.7 cm intrauterine myoma, which was resected hysteroscopically.

9.3.10.5 Effects of Preoperative Application of GnRH Analogs on the Short- and Long-Term Outcomes Following TCRM

Campo et al. studied 80 consecutive cases of TCRM. In group A, no medication was applied in 42 cases, while in group B, GnRH analogs were given intramuscularly for 2 months in 38 cases. After TCRM, all patients were followed up for 24 months, and assessed for the outcomes including AUB, recurrence of myomas, and repeat surgeries. The operation time in group B was significantly longer than that in group A (57.65 ± 29.61 min versus 40 ± 18.06 min; $P = 0.002$). However, there was no difference in hospitalization between two groups (1.05 ± 0.22 days in group A and 1.15 ± 0.44 days in group B). Only one uterine perforation occurred. Cellular myomas without atypia were found by histopathological examination in three patients of each group. Postoperative abnormal bleeding was found in 36.3% cases of group A, and in 26.6% cases of group B. Three cases in group A and two cases in group B had the recurrence of myomas, with no statistical significance between groups. One patient from each group needed repeat hysteroscopic surgery. The authors concluded that, unless it was used for correction of anemia, the application of GnRH analogs could not improve the short-term and long-term outcomes. The prolonged operation time might be due to difficulty in cervical dilatation, which needs further study to be confirmed. Tiufekchieva et al. conducted a prospective study of 50 women with submucous myomas who underwent hysteroscopic resection. Zoladex was given to ten women for 2 months pretreatments, with a mean decrease of the myoma diameter 10.16 mm, which was very important for myomas more than 30 mm in diameter. The decrease of 10 mm in diameter indicated significant reduction of myoma volume to be resected. Compared to the control group, the mean operation time was decreased by 17.08 min in Zoladex group, and 90% of the procedures were completed without difficulties. They suggested that the administration of Zoladex could reduce the size of the myoma, promote the atrophy of the endometrium, and improve the conditions of uterine cavity, leading to a fast and easy operation with less complication.

9.4 Transcervical Resection of Endometrial Polyps

Enlan Xia and Xuebing Peng

Endometrial polyp is a common cause of abnormal uterine bleeding and infertility. The traditional treatment is blind curettage, but the problem is that it is always difficult to remove it.

Removal of endometrial polyps may be carried out through a variety of devices, including fibroids forceps, curette, specialized polyps resection clamps, etc. However, with the same operative equipment, blind intrauterine operation cannot achieve satisfactory effects. In the past, manual mechanical resection was carried out. If polyps are multiple, even diffused in the uterine cavity, a complete curettage may be administered. If it is a single large polyp and its pedicle is located in the lower portion of uterus, a hysteroscope can be applied to locate it, and then a long curved hemostat or oval forceps can be used to clamp it out. However the endometrial polyps with pedicles are always floating in uterine cavity, so sometimes it is difficult to clamp them out blindly. In 1981, Valle reported that in 179 cases who had endometrial polyps, 150 failed to have polyps removed by blind curettage. Transcervical resection of polyp (TCRP) was performed under direct vision, which can "have a definite object in view," seize and resect the endometrial polyps from the bases of the pedicles (Fig. 9.98). Under hysteroscope, the polyps vary in size from 0.2 to 3 cm, are single or multiple (Fig. 9.99), and one polyp may have two pedicles. The appearance of a polyp is relatively soft, bright, and shiny, with its color similar to that of the surrounding endometrium, a bit bright red, but sometimes there are exceptions. Unlike endometrial debris, polyps do not shift with the flowing of distending fluid, and are not solid and fixed just like the submucous myoma. The shapes of polyps are mostly oval, but also can be triangular, conical, or irregular. Its surface is smooth, on which the fine microvascular networks can sometimes be seen. Most polyps have pedicles, either thin and long or wide and short. Occasionally, the surface of the tip of a larger polyp is accompanied by necrosis and appears to be purple brown. The shape of a polyp does not change with the fluctuation of uterine distention pressure. The sessile polyps are often excised with wire loop electrode, which may not damage the surrounding normal endometrium (Fig. 9.100). No matter which method

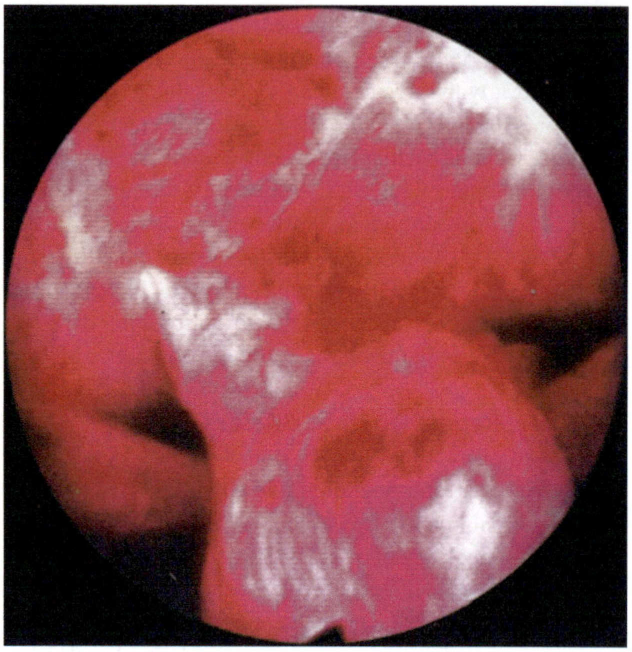

Fig. 9.98 Resection of an endometrial polyp from its base with wire loop electrode

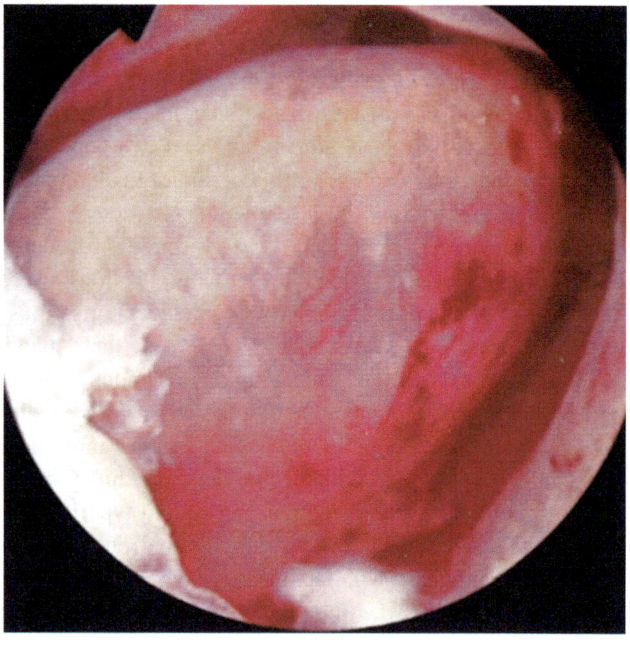

Fig. 9.99 Single endometrial polyp

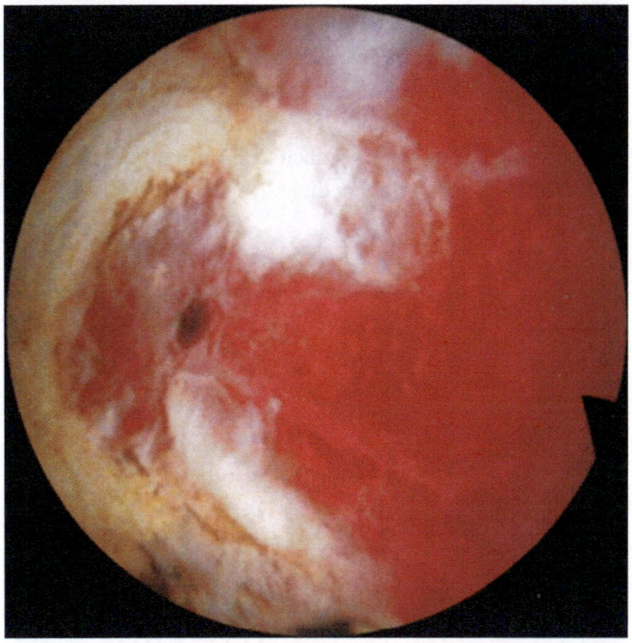

Fig. 9.100 Cutting surface after removal of a polyp, with no damage to surrounding normal endometrium

is used, the pedicle should be removed completely so as to avoid future recurrence.

9.4.1 Histopathological Classification

Endometrial polyps may be located in any position of the cervical canal or uterine cavity. A polyp basically consists of endometrial glandular epithelium and stromal tissues. Morphology is diverse, which depends on the site where the polyp arises and the reaction of polyp tissues to steroid hormones. Polyps are often single, or multiple, and even fill the uterine cavity. Polyps are varied in size, with most having pedicles connecting to the uterine wall, but there are also sessile polyps with wide base. Polyps are conical, oval, or finger-like protrusions, with a smooth, glossy and bright red surface. The surface of the tip of a polyp can develop necrosis, hemorrhage, and superficial ulcer.

9.4.1.1 Originating from Mature Endometrium (Functional Polyp)

The polyps originate from the responses of endometrium to ovarian hormones, and change with the ovarian cycle. Its size is generally small, and may partially or totally shed at the menstrual period. A typical polyp is soft and has a wide base, with its color and vessels similar to that of the surrounding endometrium, therefore it may be misdiagnosed as limited endometrial hyperplasia. Contact hysteroscopy may reveal the central vascular axis of a polyp and tissue cohesion, therefore, the contact hysteroscopy is of great value to the diagnosis of the questionable case.

9.4.1.2 Originating from Immature Endometrium (Nonfunctional Polyp)

The nonfunctional polyp is not sensitive to progesterone but is still reactive to estrogen. Estrogen supports its growth, so it can grow quite large. As the pedicle extends, under compression of both sides of the uterine wall, the polyp may turn flat or triangular. This polyp is yellow red, and sometimes its distal end may be purple red due to ecchymosis. Endometrial polyps have a strong degree of activity, and the pressure of CO_2 gas can oppress it along the uterine wall. When contact hysteroscopy is used, it often slips out of sight. Therefore, it may not be seen sometimes in a hurried hysteroscopy.

9.4.1.3 Adenomyoma Polyp

It is a rare type, and is characterized by the smooth muscle within the polyp tissues, with the endometrium on its surface being atrophy.

9.4.1.4 Postmenopausal Polyp

It is also known as atrophic polyp. After menopause, the hyperplastic or functional polyp degrades, which is similar to the changes of surrounding endometrium. Its histologic features include glandular epithelial atrophy, gland duct dilatation, and stromal fibrosis. Hysteroscopy can reveal a pale-pink and opaque polyp with the vascular dilatation not obvious, but sometimes scattered translucent vesicles and dendritic dilated vessels can be seen.

9.4.2 Indications and Contraindications of TCRP

Indications include removal of symptomatic uterine endometrial polyps, with the exclusion of malignant changes of polyps. Its contraindications are the same as those of TCRE.

9.4.3 Preoperative Preparation and Anesthesia

The preoperative preparation and anesthesia are the same as those of TCRE.

9.4.4 Operative Procedures

9.4.4.1 Clamping Under Hysteroscopy

If a polyp is small, and its pedicle is located in the upper portion of uterus, especially the fallopian tubal ostia, micro biopsy forceps can be used to clamp it out under direct vision of fiber hysteroscope or rigid hysteroscope. If it cannot be removed once, repeat clamping can achieve it.

9.4.4.2 Intercepting Under Hysteroscopy

As for the large polyps with wide pedicles near the uterine fundus, a wire snare can be inserted by passing through the hysteroscopic operating channel into the uterine cavity under direct vision, and then noose the base of the polyp and then rotated, thus the polyp may be removed along with the retrieval of the hysteroscope. Thereafter the hysteroscope is inserted again to confirm complete removal of polyps.

9.4.4.3 Hysteroscopic Electroresection

The polyps with obvious pedicles can be removed by Nd-YAG laser. For those who have wide pedicle or sessile polyps, and those who have persistent symptoms or recurrence of polyps after treatment, the hysteroscopic electroresection is appliable and its operative procedures are as follows.

1. First, an observation is made of the shape and size of the polyp and location of the pedicle (Figs. 9.101 and 9.102), and the relationship between the base of the polyp and its surrounding tissues (Fig. 9.103), then its cutting method is decided.
2. Resection of multiple polyps (Fig. 9.104): If the uterine cavity is filled with polyps, and if there is inadequate filling with irrigation fluid, which obscures its vision, the operator can first use vacuum suction aspirator to suck out the endometrium and polyps. If the endometrium lining the surface of polyps is sucked out, there will only be the interstitial tissue of the polyps left with its size and diameter explicitly shrunk. With the inflow of irrigation fluid, its resection is made easy.
3. At the time of resecting the polyp, a wire loop electrode is placed at its distant end, and then start cutting. The depth of cutting should reach 2–3 mm superficial myometrium beneath the pedicle (Figs. 9.105, 9.106, and 9.107).

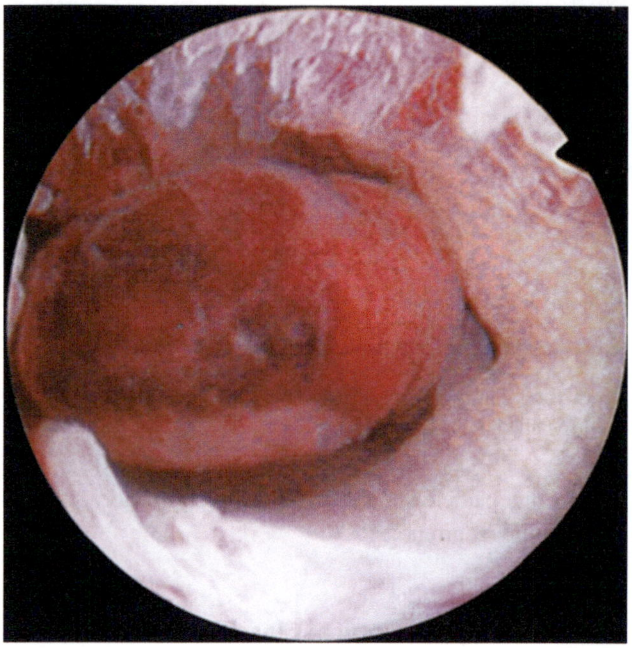

Fig. 9.102 The uterine cavity before surgery

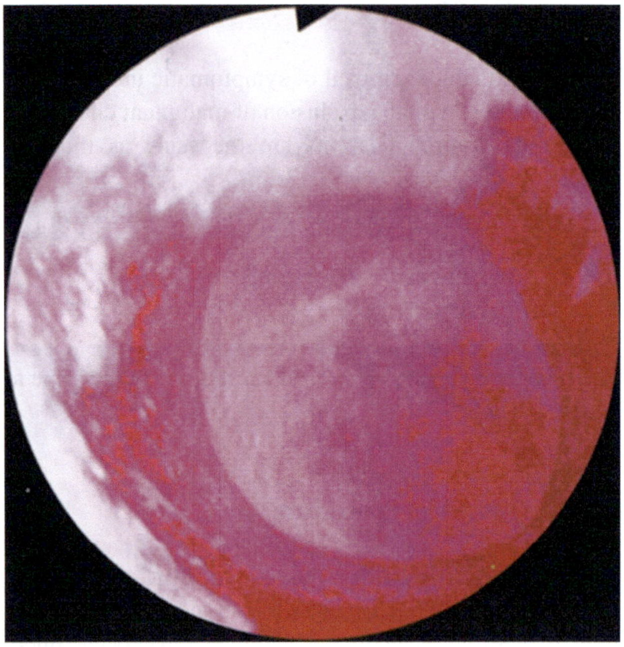

Fig. 9.101 Endometrial polyps before surgery

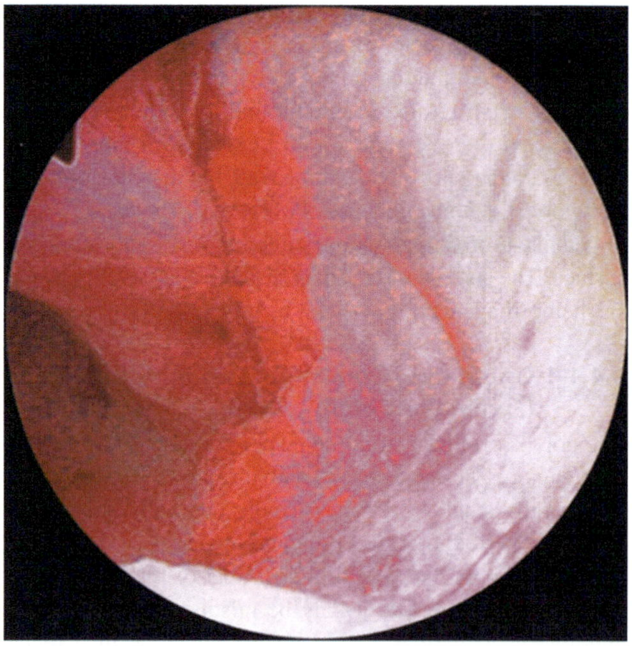

Fig. 9.103 Basal part of a polyp

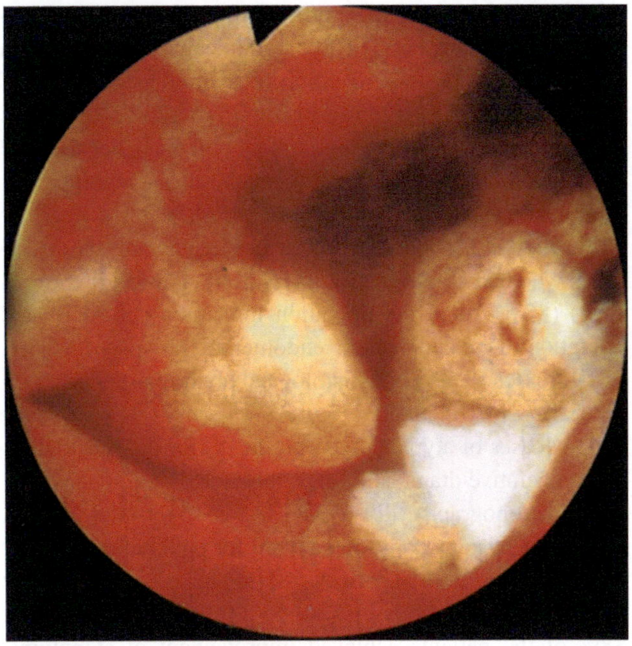

Fig. 9.104 Intrauterine multiple polyps

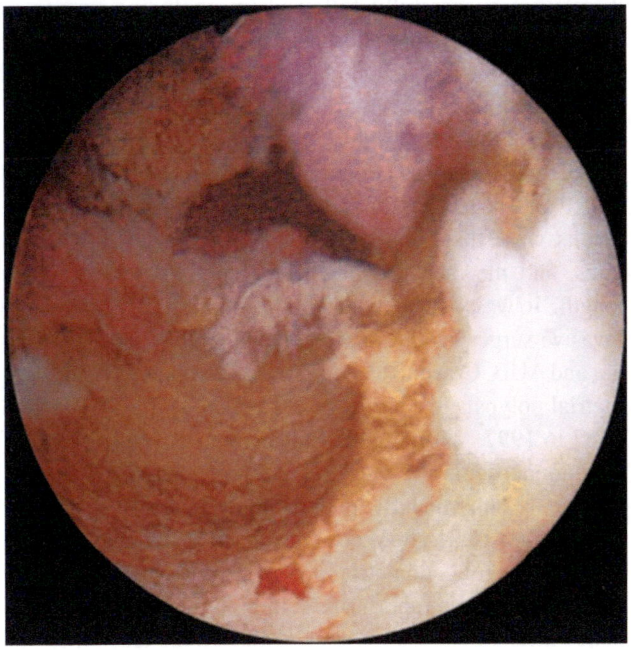

Fig. 9.105 Cutting surface seen in the excised polyp pedicle

9.4.5 Intra- and Postoperative Monitoring and Management

Intra- and postoperative monitoring and management are the same as those of TCRE.

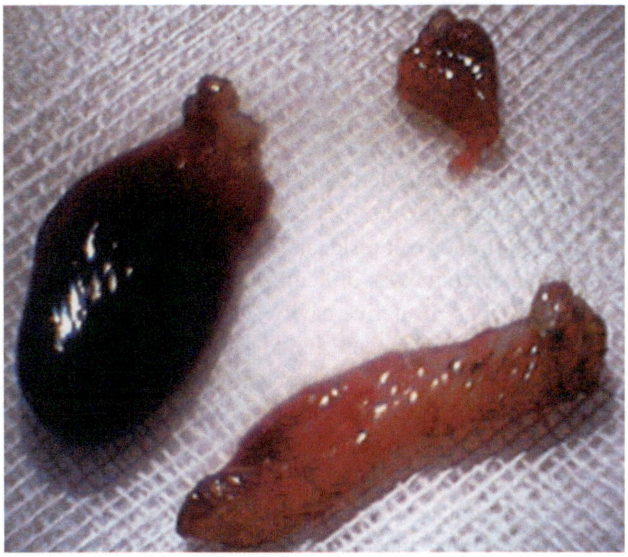

Fig. 9.106 Excised polyps (three pieces)

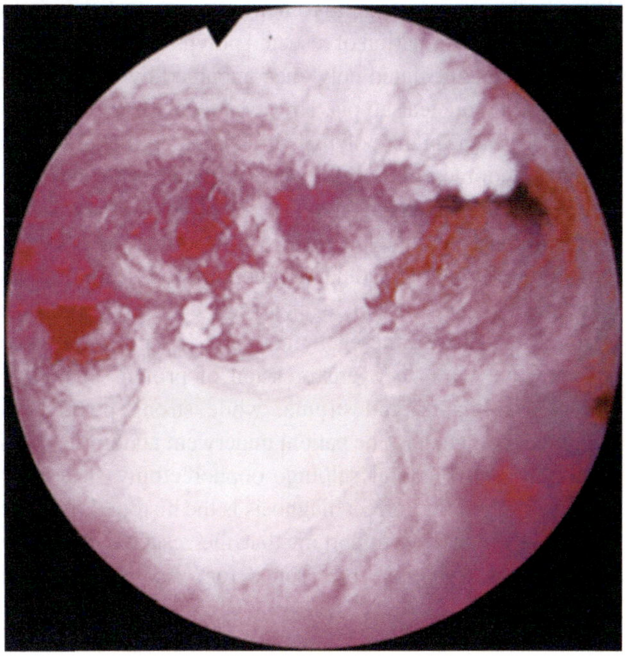

Fig. 9.107 Uterine cavity after removal of polyps

9.4.6 Identification and Management of Operative Complications

Due to the limited cutting range of TCRP and the short operative time, the risks of occurrence of TURP syndrome, intrauterine adhesions, and hematometra are low. In 1995, Marabini et al. reported one case of 26-year-old woman who underwent TCRP for AUB. The polyp had a wide pedicle, was 4 cm in length, and originated from the fundus and posterior wall of the uterus. It had a smooth surface with dilated vessels on it. Histological examination of the resected tissues showed low-grade stromal sarcoma. The patient underwent total abdominal hysterectomy and bilateral salpingo-oophorectomy, with the result of histological examination showing no tumor cell residuals. They insisted that because the stroma sarcoma was difficult to be detected before surgery, all lesions in uterine cavity should be resected completely, and all specimens should be sent for histological examination. Regarding the problem of malignant lesions, Maltez et al. in 1998 reported one case of the focal clear cell carcinoma in a benign endometrial polyp. This patient was 80-year-old and menopaused at 55 years old, without history of hormone replacement therapy. Her main complaint had been little vaginal bleeding for 1 week. The transvaginal ultrasonography examination showed echoluscent areas in uterine cavity, endometrial atrophy, and focal thickening endometrium near the uterine fundus, which did not break through the junction of myometrium and endometrium. Histological examination of resected polyps by hysteroscopy revealed a pedunculated polyp accompanied by dilated cystic glands, no nuclear atypia. However focal clear cell carcinoma was found in the polyps, with benign epithelial tissues around. Endometrial polyps were detected with estrogen receptor and expression of p53 protein for immunohistochemical examination. The results showed that the estrogen receptor in benign glandular epithelium and stromal cells were positive and absent in clear cell carcinoma, but the estrogen receptor of mesenchymal cells of the tumor tissue was positive with no overexpression of protein in benign endometrial glands and stroma, while strong positive in malignant cell nuclei. The patient underwent abdominal hysterectomy and bilateral salpingo-oophorectomy. The only reliable method for correct diagnosis is the histopathological examination, so it is important that the resected tissue by hysteroscopy should be sent for histopathological examination.

9.4.7 Experience and Evaluation of TCRP

TCRP is the only method to visualize clearly the pedicles of polyps and resect them from their roots, as well as make differential diagnosis of the intrauterine occupying lesions.

9.4.7.1 Therapeutic Effect of TCRP

Nathani and Clark conducted a systematic review of the published literatures of MEDLINE (1966–2004) in order to assess the efficacy of TCRP in the treatment of AUB, including menstrual disorders, postmenopausal bleeding with or without hormone replacement and tamoxifen therapy. All TCRP succeeded in a single procedure, with three cases conducting local anesthesia. Three complications occur, which included one uterine perforation. The improvement rate of symptoms after TCRP ranged from 75 to 100%. There was no significant difference in treatment outcomes between the outpatient polypectomy under local anesthesia and inpatient treatment under general anesthesia ($p = 0.7$).

Bradley et al. conducted a retrospective analysis of 201 cases who had TCRP from 1992 to 1998. Among them, 172 cases (85.6%) had the operation indications of AUB, and operations revealed benign endometrial polyps of 91.5%, and 19 cases (9.5%) had histological abnormalities in endometrial polyps, including 13 cases of complex hyperplasia, and six cases of atypical hyperplasia. As for the sensitivities of preoperative diagnostic tools, it was 16.7% for transvaginal ultrasonography (TVS), 83% for sonohysterography, 89.5% for hysteroscopy, and 10.8% for endometrial biopsy. There were no false negative of Saline Infusion Sonography (SIS) and hysteroscopy. A 30-month follow-up showed that 88% of the patients achieved improvement of symptoms. Tjarks et al. reported on the treatment effectiveness of different methods in 78 women with endometrial polyps. Sixty of them were successfully followed up, including two cases being excluded for endometrial adenocarcinoma. The remaining 58 cases included 37 premenopausal women and 21 postmenopausal women, with the mean duration of follow-up 13 months. Twenty-six women underwent TCRP, which was the most common. Other procedures included TCRP and TCRE, TCRP and TCRM, and hysterectomy. The results were that each operation reached high satisfaction rates, and the menstruation decreased to at least half the length. It was believed that both simple TCRP and more invasive surgery could improve the symptoms of menorrhagia and AUB. Cravello et al. reported 195 patients with endometrial polyps and AUB who were treated with TCRP from 1987 to 1997. With a mean follow-up of 5.2 years, 80% of the patients achieved successful outcomes after TCRP. Only 5 patients subsequently underwent hysterectomy, so they insisted that TCRP should be considered as the gold standard for treatment of endometrial polyps. Sentilhes et al. reported that there were no reports about uterine rupture due to pregnancy after TCRP. Garuti et al. evaluated the feasibility of a "see-and-treat" office TCRP. Two hundred thirty-seven patients who underwent either mechanical removal or bipolar resection of endometrial polyps were involved in their study, including 120 cases with paracervical block anesthesia and 117 cases without. Twenty-six patients had to cancel the procedure due to being unsuitable for office operation. Following operations, overall success rate was 81.2%. There were no significant differences found either in success rate or in the visual analog scale (VAS) scores between premenopausal and postmenopausal patients, and no significant differences found either in success rates or in VAS scores between cases with paracervical block and cases without. In parous patients, VAS scores were significantly lower and the rates of polypectomy were significantly higher than those in nulliparous patients. Forty-four patients failed to undergo the procedures, due to the intolerance of pain (18 cases) or large size of the polyp (17 cases). Clinical vasovagal reaction was the only adverse effect (1.7%), except for pain. The author held that the success rate of one-stage polypectomy was 80% and proper selection of cases preoperation might be a reliable option to avoid general anesthesia and TCRP. Stamatellos et al. reported that among patients who have cervical polyps, 25% have coexisting endometrial polyps. Hysteroscopy can be used to make an accurate diagnosis of it and perform resection. In 2005, Persin et al. reported the outcomes of TCRP in 283 cases, with one case (0.35%) of uterine perforation without any intervention, six cases (2.12%) with a second operation to complete the treatment, 3 patients (1.06%) with malignancy of endometrial polyp. 89.05% of all patients did not encounter any long-term complications. For the rest of the cases (10.95%), ultrasonography revealed endometrial pathology, which required further treatment. Two patients were detected to have endometrial cancer. It was thought that vaginal ultrasound was an elementary means for the early detection of the long-term complications following TCRP.

9.4.7.2 Postoperative Recurrence of Endometrial Polyps

Reslova et al. studied the risk factors for polyp recurrence and thought that TCRP could be regarded as an ideal treatment of endometrial polyps and its recurrence could be avoided by resecting the basal layer of the endometrium beneath the polyp. Herman et al. reported about 270 cases of operative hysteroscopy. With a follow-up to 4 years, only 4.6% of TCRP required secondary surgery. Bacsko and Major reported on 163 polyps found during 1900 cases of hysteroscopy. Twenty-two percent of them were found in patients with the first dilatation and curettage (D&C) and 6.6% were found in patients with the second procedures. All of 163 polyps were removed by hysteroscopy, with the indications of hemorrhage in 55%, abnormal ultrasonography images in 25%, and infertility in 15%. There were two perforations (0.89%) occurring in hysteroscopic operations. Histological examination of resected polyps revealed proliferative endometrium in 22 cases, hyperplasia in 17 cases, fibroid and no hormone response in 5 of each, and endometritis, adenomyosis, atrophy, and malignancy in one of each. They held that even though the diagnostic hysteroscopy had a high false positive rate, TCRP is a worthwhile method for minimal invasive and organ saving surgery. Bouda et al. evaluated the recurrence of endometrial polyp after treatment. There were 30 premenopausal and 51 postmenopausal patients undergoing TCRP in group one, with follow-up by diagnostic hysteroscopy 6–12 months after TCRP. There were 36 premenopausal and 64 postmenopausal patients in group two, who underwent fractional curettage and histological diagnosis of endometrial polyp, with second-look hysteroscopy 12 months later. It was found by second-look hysteroscopy that endometrial polyps were found in 11 cases of group one (13.5%), and in 46 cases in group two (46%). Among cases with recurrent endometrial polyps, only one occurred in case with atrophic endometrium, and no recurrence in cases with atrophic endometrial polyp. The conclusion was that TCRP was superior to fractional curettage in the treatment of endometrial polyp, and the recurrence risk factors of endometrial polyp were abnormal proliferation of polyps, or hyperplasia in both the polyp and the surrounding endometrium.

Peng et al. from the Hysteroscopy Center of Fuxing Hospital, Capital Medical University, conducted a laboratory study and confirmed that the expressions of sex hormone receptors and cytokines influencing degeneration of cells and fibrosis of tissues had difference or significant difference with surrounding endometrium. The results of their study on women with endometrial polyps indicated that the expressions of estrogen receptors in endometrial polyps were higher and the expressions of progesterone receptors were lower than those in surrounding endometrium. The expressions of vascular endothelial growth factor (VEGF) in glandular cells of polyps were significantly higher than those of glandular cells of surrounding endometrium, no matter whether it is in proliferative phase or in secretory phase ($p < 0.001$); and the expressions of VEGF in stromal cells of polyps were significantly higher than those of surrounding endometrium in proliferative phase ($p < 0.05$). For transforming growth factor-beta 1 (TGF-β1), its expression in glandular cells of polyps were significantly higher than those of endometrium ($p < 0.05$); and its expression in stromal cells of polyps was significantly higher than those of endometrium, no matter whether it is in proliferation or secretory phase ($p < 0.05$). It was concluded that the expression of VEGF and TGF-β1 was closely related to that of estrogen and progesterone receptors, which might be the correlative factors for the growth and development of endometrial polyps.

9.4.7.3 TCRP Combined with TCRE to Improve Therapeutic Effect

Polena et al. reported on 367 patients that had TCRP 54% of whom had TCRE simultaneously. Minor complications occurred in five cases, 83% of patients were successfully followed up, with the average period of follow-up 40 months (range from 17 to 66 months). The total success rate in all patients was 96.4%. However, when compared with the patients of TCRP group, it was increased in patients of TCRP and TCRE group. Henriquez et al. conducted a retrospective study of TCRP in 78 consecutive premenopausal women. In a 4-year follow-up, nearly 60% of patients required further treatment due to postoperative abnormal bleeding. It was thought that the procedure of TCRP might be combined with TCRE or insertion of a levonorgestrel-releasing intrauterine device to improve the outcome of treatment.

9.4.7.4 TCRP and Infertility

In 2008, Stamatellos et al. reported that 83 women who had AUB and primary or secondary infertility from 2000 to 2005 were diagnosed to have endometrial polyps by transvaginal ultrasonography and diagnostic hysteroscopy. After TCRP, 91.6% of patients had normal menses, 61.4% of patients had spontaneous pregnancy, and 54.2% of them achieved full-term delivery. No statistical differences were obtained between women with the diameter of the polyps up to 1 cm and women with larger (>1 cm) or multiple polyps. Postoperative complication rate was 2.4% and the recurrence rate of polyps was 4.9%. It was believed that TCRP was a safe procedure with low complication rate, improved reproductive prognosis, and increased pregnancy rates in women with infertility which had no definite reasons. The prognosis of pregnancy had no correlation with the size or number of the polyps, and primary or secondary infertility. Most of patients had restoration of normal menses after operation. Gimpelson insisted that TCRP is a simple and effective method for the treatment of endometrial polyps in women with AUB and infertility, which can be completed in an office setting. Xiao et al. from the Hysteroscopy Center of Fuxing Hospital, Capital Medical University, reported that, using cyclooxygenase-2 (COX-2) and VEGF, which were factors evaluating the receptivity of endometrium, during mid-secretory phase, the expression of them in the endometrium from women with endometrial polyps was lower than that in normal endometrium from women without endometrial polyps. It indicated that, in women with endometrial polyps, the receptivity of endometrium to the embryo was changed, which might affect the embryo implantation, leading to infertility in some women. In endometrial polyps and assisted reproductive technique, Isikoglu et al. studied whether the endometrial polyps detected during ovarian stimulation decreased the success rate of intracytoplasmic sperm injection (ICSI) cycles. Patients were divided into three groups: in group one, endometrial polyps were discovered during ovarian stimulation in 15 patients; in group two, TCRP was performed prior to ICSI cycle in 40 patients with endometrial polyps; and in group three, there were 956 patients without polyps. There were no significant difference between the groups in some common characteristics such as age of the patients, age of the husbands, body mass index, total dosage of GnRH-a, length of ovarian stimulation, peak value of estradiol concentrations, endometrial thickness and number of embryos replaced, etc. Only one patient (12.5%) from the first group miscarried at early pregnancy. It indicated that the presence of endometrial polyps with the diameter less than 1.5 cm during ovarian stimulation did not affect the outcomes in ICSI cycles.

Varasteh et al. reported the outcomes after TCRP in 23 women who had infertility for at least 12 months and aged under 45 years old. With the follow-up for at least 18 months, pregnancy and live birth rates in women after TCRP were significantly higher than that in women with normal cavities. It was concluded that TCRP might improve the reproductive ability of infertile women with endometrial polyps. Yanaihara et al. reported that endometrial polyps were mostly located on posterior uterine wall (32.0%), and the pregnancy rate after surgery was the highest (57.4%) after resection of polyps located at the uterotubal junction.

9.4.7.5 Malignancy in Endometrial Polyp

Anastasiadis et al. conducted TVS or sonohysterography, fractional dilatation, and curettage (D&C) to investigate women with AUB. Among 1415 women included, endometrial polyps were found in 126 patients (8.9%), including 94 with benign lesion, 30 (23.8%) with premalignant changes (complex and atypical hyperplasia) and 2 (1.5%) with malignancy, both of whom were menopausal. Bakour et al. pointed out that women with endometrial polyps were more commonly associated with endometrial hyperplasia. They reported that of 62 cases who have endometrial polyps benign lesions were found in 53 (85.5%), hyperplasia in seven (11.3%), and malignancy in two (3.2%). Compared with endometrial specimens without polyps, hyperplasia was quite common in specimens with polyps, with 11.3% in polyp group and 4.3% in control group ($p = 0.04$); however, the incidence of malignancy was the same, with 3.2% in each group. Ben-Arie et al. retrieved 430 consecutive cases with endometrial polyps detected by hysteroscopy. The data reviewed included medical records, TVS, and histopathology findings. Endometrial polyps were identified by hysteroscopy in 95.7% of the cases. Of them, hyperplasia without atypia was found in 11.4%, premalignant conditions were found in 3.3%, and malignancies were found in 3.0%. Although the positive predictive value for malignancy was low, advanced age, menopause period, and polyps larger than 1.5 cm were relevant factors for premalignant or malignant changes. In their study, all the malignant polyps diagnosed were in postmenopausal women, but irregular vaginal bleeding or postmenopausal bleeding was not a predictor of malignancy. Therefore, it was thought that endometrial polyps in postmenopausal women had a higher risk of malignancy, and should be treated by TCRP no matter whether they had symptoms or not. Polyps smaller than 1.5 cm in asymptomatic premenopausal patients can be managed by observation.

Scrimin et al. reported 16 patients who had atypical adenomyomatous endometrial polyps and underwent

TCRP. After 5 years of follow-up, 13 patients were cured, 2 patients removed their uterus because of other reasons, and 1 died due to cardiac disorders. Endometrial adenomatous polyps were a rare type of endometrial polyps, with its stroma containing smooth muscle fibers, and generally smaller polyps. In a report by Liu et al. from the Hysteroscopy Center of Fuxing Hospital, Capital Medical University, there were 1672 cases undergoing TCRP from January of 1997 to February of 2006. Forty-two patients (2.51%) had endometrial adenomatous polyps, of whom the postmenopausal women accounted for 21.43%. Five cases (11.91%) were associated with glandular epithelial atypical hyperplasia (i.e., atypical polypoid adenomyoma), including mild atypical polypoid adenomyoma in three cases, moderate and severe in one case each. The size of endometrial adenomatous polyps was large, with the largest polyps of up to 6cm and the larger polyps ≥3 cm in 47.62% of the patients. All patients were successfully followed up with the duration ranging from 1 year to 10 years. One patient had radical hysterectomy due to cervical cancer 2 years after TCRP, 2 patients had no improvement of AUB, the remaining 39 cases (92.86%) had good prognosis, with no recurrence of polyps. Among six cases of infertility, 1 patient of primary infertility conceived after operation and delivered at term (16.67%). Five cases of atypical polypoid adenomyoma were followed up for 2–7 years, 4 patients didn't receive postoperative assisted medical treatment and hysteroscopy and ultrasound re-examination showed no abnormalities; one case with severe atypical hyperplasia was administered orally large doses of medroxyprogesterone acetate 250 mg q.o.d. for 6 months. After the withdrawal of medication for 5 months, second-look hysteroscopy showed no abnormalities, and the histopathological results of curettage showed an endometrium in proliferative phase.

9.5 Transcervical Resection of Septum

Enlan Xia and Dan Yu

The incidence of uterine malformations in women is approximately 4.3%, with about 3.5% in infertile women and about 13% in women with recurrent pregnancy loss. Uterine septum is the most common malformation (35%), followed by bicornuate uterus (25%) and arcuate uterus (20%). Uterine malformations, especially the septate uterus itself does not seem to be a factor for infertility; however, it can delay pregnancy and is a cause of secondary infertility. In addition, there are adverse outcomes of pregnancy in those who have uterine malformations, even in the early stage of pregnancy. The full-term pregnancy rate in those without any treatment of uterine malformation is only 50%, and the full-term pregnancies are often complicated with obstetric problems. The full-term pregnancy rate is about 45% in untreated women with either unicornuate uterus or bicornuate uterus, and is about 40% in women with untreated septate uterus. The prognosis of pregnancy in women having arcuate uterus is a little better, with the term delivery rate about 65%. Braun et al. reported that the frequency of uterine malformations was 10% in women with infertility. Among these 10% of women, arcuate uterus was the most common (57.6%), followed by partial septate uterus (18.2%), bicornuate uterus with single cervix (10.6%), bicornuate uterus with double cervixes (3.0%), complete septate uterus (6.1%), unicornuate uterus (3.0%), and unicornuate uterus with double vagina (1.5%). Treatments are conducted in symptomatic patients, whose term delivery rates are quite low (5%). After hysteroscopic metroplasty, the term delivery rate was increased to 75% and the live birth rate to 85%.

9.5.1 Embryology and Classification of Uterine Malformations

Uterus and fallopian tubes are all developed from paramesonephric duct (Mullerian duct). In early embryonic period, the distal portions of the paramesonephric ducts fuse. The fused lower portions become the vagina and uterus, and the fused upper portions become the fallopian tube. This process occurs during the fourth to sixth week of embryonic development, and is accomplished by 12th to 14th weeks. When the Mullerian inhibiting factor (MIF) from testis does not exist in the body, the paramesonephric ducts grow normally; during the 19th to 20th week of embryonic development, uterine septum is completely absorbed. If not absorbed or partially absorbed, incomplete septum or complete septum may result. During the process of development and formation of the uterus at embryonic phase, some internal or external interventions may lead to the hypoplasia or fuse barriers of paramesonephric ducts, resulting in the formation of various types of congenital uterine malformations.

The commonly used classifications of congenital uterine malformation are the classification published by AFS in 1988, and a new classification of female genital malformations was jointly published by ESHRE and ESGE in 2013. For details, see Chap. 8, Sect. 8.2. In this section, several feasible treatments of hysteroscopic metroplasty for uterine malformation are elaborated.

9.5.1.1 Septate Uterus

Septate uterus is an anatomical anomaly of uterus which is caused by disruption of fusion, lumen formation, or absorption of the paramesonephric ducts, the extent of which depends on disruption time. Because the uterine fusion is not obstructed, the external contour of the uterus looks intact and need to be distinguished from bicornuate uterus. There are defects in the fusion of bicornuate uterus and the external contour of uterus can be partitioned. The septa that divide the uterine body are different in length and width. Some septa are thin, and some are thick with narrow uterine cavity. Some septa only divide the upper part of the cavity, and some extend to the internal os of the uterus. Some septa extend even to the external os of cervix. Twenty to 25% of patients are complicated with septate vagina. Occasionally, bicornuate uterus is accompanied by uterine septum.

Uterine septum is a very common uterine anomaly. A retrospective statistical analysis conducted by Zabak et al. showed that patients with untreated septate uterus had a poor reproductive outcome, including high rate of early miscarriage, increased rate of recurrent pregnancy loss or missed miscarriage, and increased probability of reproductive failure and obstetric complications. It was found that a septate uterus was not the reason for infertility, but increased the incidence of unexplained secondary infertility (40%). Nowadays, hysteroscopic surgery has replaced conventional laparotomy. Hysteroscopic metroplasty improves the obstetrical prognosis in women with septate uterus. Its advantages lie in easier operation and low morbidity rate, avoiding the consequence of hysterotomy (such as adnexal adhesions). Hysteroscopic resection of uterine septum is suitable for the women with a history of miscarriages (2 or more), which could decrease the miscarriage rate to 15% post-operation. For infertile women, laparoscopy is also required to investigate the pelvis for infertility, determine the type of uterine malformation, and provide an opportunity for treating any coexisting pelvic lesions.

Uterine septum changes the symmetry of uterine cavity, and thus interferes with normal fertility. The traditional treatment for the women who had septum uterus and recurrent pregnancy loss was traumatic surgery. Prior to the advent of hysteroscopy, the symptomatic uterine septum was dealt by either Jones or Tompkins transabdominal metroplasty. Jones procedure involves wedged resection of uterine fundus and septum via transabdominal metroplasty, and the uterine muscle wall is reconstructed, which enables more than 80% pregnancies to continue to survive. Tompkins procedure is to implement incision of uterine body in the uterine midline from the anterior to the posterior, excise the septate tissues transversely and then make sutures. This procedure may involve less bleeding than Jones', and can keep a normal contour of uterine cavity without shrinkage in size. Both these surgeries require laparotomy and incision into uterus, thus the patients may have longer hospitalization and slow postoperative recovery. The patients must use contraception for 3–6 months to allow healing of uterine incisions. Those who have postoperative pregnancy and can maintain pregnancy to full term often require cesarean delivery for the prevention of uterine rupture. Although the postoperative pregnancy rate may be up to 82%, some patients still cannot conceive due to postoperative development of pelvic adhesions, especially ovarian and tubal adhesions. Such patients need another laparotomy and uterine incision, which may cause postoperative adhesions again and a second infertility. Due to the incision in the uterus, patients need more postoperative contraception for 3–6 months, or even longer, and those who have term pregnancy require cesarean delivery. Now there is new minimally invasive surgical therapy for uterine septum, namely transcervical resection of septa (TCRS). Compared with laparotomy, TCRS targets and resects the septum which is the embryonic residual tissue with fewer vessels. Therefore it causes little intraoperative bleeding, has a low postoperative morbidity, and is easily accepted by patients. Since the postoperative epithelialized process of uterine cavity only requires 4–5 weeks, the period for patients waiting for pregnancy after surgery is shortened when compared with laparotomy. In 2007, Lourdel from France pointed out that the septate uterus was the most frequently encountered uterine malformation, which was estimated to be present in approximately 1% of infertile women and in 3.3% of women with recurrent pregnancy losses. They insisted that hysteroscopic resection of septum was the gold standard treatment for the septate uterus. It was concluded that a TCRS was applicable for women who had unidentified infertility and are more than 35 years old with no response to any other technique of reproduction aid, or found a uterine septum when undergoing a combined operation of laparoscopy and hysteroscopy for infertility, needed an assisted reproductive technique (ART), or had a poor obstetrical history. The authors also alerted that although complications of TCRS are not very frequent, it still had the risk of uterine rupture when patients conceived later. TCRS has the advantages of being a simple procedure, less postoperative complications, and improvement of the prognosis of fertility. Nowadays, its application has been extended from the treatment of those with recurrent pregnancy loss and premature delivery to those with infertility, especially women who want to have IVF.

9.5.1.2 Bicornuate Uterus

During the process of embryonic development, after fusion of two paramesonephric ducts, incomplete absorption of the middle part of the plate leads to the formation of one cervix with two uterine cavities. The upper and fundal parts of the cavity present a forked-shape and the end of an unabsorbed plate is blunt and round. Intrauterine plate is similar to uterine septum, with its end reaching the upper, middle or lower part of the cavity, or extending to the level of cervical internal os or cervical canal.

The frequency of bicornuate uterus is about 13.6% of uterine malformations, 40% of which leading to miscarriage, premature delivery, abnormal delivery or infertility, etc.

Traditional treatment of complete bicornuate uterus is Strassman Metroplasty, which is to make a transverse incision along the fundus between two cornua via laparotomy till the cavity is exposed. Then longitudinal sutures of the cutting surface are conducted between the left and right uterine walls to reconstruct a uterus with normal shape. It is not an ideal therapy because of its massive trauma, incision of uterus via laparotomy, prone to developing adhesions and scars, and delay of postoperative recovery. With the development of laparoscopy and hysteroscopy, open metroplasty has been reasonably replaced by endoscopic metroplasty, which is to perform uterine incision and unification via laparoscopy and hysteroscopy. For patients with incomplete bicornuate uterus, the plate in uterine cavity is divided by hysteroscopy, leading to the same thickness of fundus as other uterine walls, which to the greatest extent restores a normal cavity. For incision and unification surgery of bicornuate uterus by laparoscopy combined with hysteroscopy, the first step is to use hysteroscopic resectoscope to resect intrauterine septum, then cut open the myometrium and the serosa of the fundus, causing an artificial perforation. The fundal wall is further incised transversely by laparoscopy till it reaches the cavity. Next, bilateral cutting walls are sutured longitudinally to achieve a normal shape cavity. This surgery may achieve a normal cavity with minimal invasive procedures, and has a good outcome with broad development prospects.

9.5.1.3 T-Shaped Uterus

T-shaped uterus is a developmental anomaly with contraction bands formed in uterine myometrium caused by fetal exposure to diethylstilbestrol (DES) or other external interventions. The upper segment of the cavity is narrow, the fundus is arcuate with the minimal distance between the middle of the fundus and two lateral walls being less than 2 cm, and the middle and lower segment of the cavity is tubular with the lateral myometrium thickening, resulting in a T-shaped cavity. In 1980, Viscomi et al. reported the outcomes of ultrasonography in 18 women who had fetal exposure to DES, and 20 age-matched women in the control group. The results found that the volume of the uterus was 49.4 $cm^3 \pm 25.5$ SD in DES exposure group, and was 90 $cm^3 \pm 22$ SD in control group, which indicated that a T-shaped uterus had the characteristics of uterine dysplasia and a restricted cavity.

Women with T-shaped uterus are always present with primary infertility, miscarriage, ectopic pregnancy and/or cervical incompetence. HSG and diagnostic hysteroscopy can make the diagnosis. The indications of hysteroscopic operation for T-shaped uterus include women with a history of two or more spontaneous miscarriages, women with otherwise unexplained infertility, and infertile women requiring assisted reproductive technique (ART).

Transcervical uterine incision (TCUI) can be conducted for treatment of T-shaped uterus. This involves resecting the excessive myometrial tissues on uterine lateral walls or cutting the myometrium on bilateral walls so as to enlarge the uterine cavity, broaden the endometrial areas, and improve the reproductive outcomes.

9.5.1.4 Unicornuate Uterus

During the process of embryo development, one paramesonephric duct being well developed, but the other side having partial or total lack of development, results in unicornuate uterus. The uterus well developed on one side is unicornuate; the one on the other side with partial development is rudimentary uterus. Total lack of development on the other side leads to absence of rudimentary uterus.

Nearly 65% of unicornuate uterus coexists with rudimentary uterus, with or without communications between them (solid, luminal, or functional cavity). Unicornuate uterus is infrequent with its incidence ranging from 1/4020 to 1/1000, and take up 4.4% of congenital uterine malformations. They have poor reproductive outcomes and 36–40% of them coexist with malformation of urinary system. Occasionally, homolateral ovarian hypogenesis may coexist.

Unicornuate uterus may cause infertility, cervical incompetence, and premature delivery, with the frequency of primary infertility the highest. The poor reproductive outcomes include spontaneous miscarriage or premature delivery, and lower success rate of IVF-ET. The success of fertility lies on multiple factors, such as the blood supply of contralateral uterine artery to the uterus and ovaries, the extent of myometrium defect, the degree of cervical incompetence, other diseases in pelvis such as endometriosis, and the type of the unicornuate uterus. Data from literatures indicated that, in women who had unicornuate uterus, the live birth rate was 15% when there is a communicating horn, 28% when there is a functional non-communicating horn, 35% when there is a non-communicating horn with no cavity, and 0% when there is no rudimentary horn. In conclusion, the live birth rate is the highest in women with unicornuate uterus and non-communicating horn with or without a cavity.

The treatment of a unicornuate uterus may apply a hysteroscopic wire loop to resect the myometrium so as to broaden the cavity, and postoperative pregnancy rate and live birth rate can be increased.

9.5.1.5 Robert Uterus

Robert uterus is an asymmetric obstructional malformation of complete septate uterus. In the classification system of female genital malformations jointly published by ESHRE and ESGE, it is in sub-class U2b. Intrauterine septum locates in one side of the uterus and completely obstructs one cavity, leading to a blind cavity non-communicating with the vagina or contralateral cavity. The obstructed cavity can accumulate secretions or blood (hematometra), which is similar to functional rudimentary uterus in clinical manifestations, including different degrees of primary dysmenorrhea. For adolescent women with severe dysmenorrhea, when Robert uterus is diagnosed, hysteroscopic resection of the septum can be conducted. When intrauterine hematometra increases, the blood clots can retrogradely flow to the pelvis via the fallopian tubes, followed by endometriosis and pelvic adhesions, leading to infertility. Unusual conception in obstructed cavity may occur and can be treated by hysterotomy to remove the embryo. The diagnosis of a Robert uterus is difficult because some routine investigations such as gynecological ultrasonography and HSG always misdiagnose it as unicornuate uterus. A Robert uterus can be confirmed by a combined diagnosis with laparoscopy and hysteroscopy, and effectively treated by hysteroscopic resection of the septum under laparoscopic monitoring.

9.5.1.6 Arcuate Uterus

Arcuate uterus takes up 10% of uterine malformations. Its diagnosis and clinical importance are still controversial. Taking the connecting line between two tubal os as a base line, the diagnosis is determined by measuring the length of the fundal protrusion into the cavity. Arcuate uterus is diagnosed when it is less than 1.5 cm, and septate uterus is diagnosed when it is 1.5 cm or longer. By 3D ultrasonography, if the angle between bilateral endometrium of the septum is acute, a partial septate uterus can be diagnosed; if it is obtuse and blunt round, an arcuate uterus can be diagnosed. Zlopasa et al. reported that the incidence of preterm delivery was high in women with arcuate uterus. Compared with conceptions in women with other malformations, the gestational age and birth weight were low in women with arcuate uterus. The miscarriage rate was reduced and the delivery rate was increased after hysteroscopic metroplasty. Mucowski et al. reviewed the existing literatures and pointed out that there was insufficient evidence to conclude a correlation between an arcuate uterus and poor reproductive outcomes, and so hysteroscopic metroplasty had not been generally accepted. Therefore for symptomatic women, individualized treatment should be considered after excluding other etiology for infertility.

9.5.1.7 Rudimentary Uterus

When the development of two paramesonephric ducts is asymmetric, one paramesonephric duct is dysplasia and forms a luminal or solid horn, which is named rudimentary uterus. Usually the rudimentary uterus does not communicate with the cervix and vagina, and does not communicate or communicate only via a hole with contralateral uterus. The contralateral well-developed uterus is unicornuate uterus.

Most rudimentary uterus (solid, luminal, or functional cavity) coexist with unicornuate uterus with or without communications. Isolated rudimentary uterus with no unicornuate uterus is extremely rare. 3D ultrasonography can obtain integrate coronal images of the uterus, clearly illustrate the characteristic configurations of uterine cavity in rudimentary uterus and unicornuate uterus. Laparoscopy can compensate for the shortage of diagnostic hysteroscopy and make an accurate diagnosis of rudimentary uterus. But occasionally it can be misdiagnosed as a degenerated myoma. As a rudimentary uterus does not communicate or communicate via a small hole with the vagina and contralateral cavity, its clinical symptoms occur early. Usually in puberty, women with rudimentary uterus will present hematocele and periodic abdominal pain because of the obstruction to menstrual flow. With the increase of hematocele and the enlargement of the rudimentary uterus, endometriosis or adenomyosis may develop after the retrograde flow of menstrual blood leading to progressive aggravation of dysmenorrhea and infertility. If the fallopian tube on the side of rudimentary uterus is patent, the fertilized egg can be implanted and grow in the rudimentary uterus, resulting in rudimentary uterine pregnancy. Because the myometrium is hypoplastic in rudimentary uterus and cannot support a bigger fetus, it will rupture spontaneously in second trimester of pregnancy, developing acute abdomen.

Park and Dominguez stated that the risk of rupture in a pregnant rudimentary uterine horn was high (50%), and it mostly occurred in the second trimester. A pregnant rudimentary uterine horn may also develop spontaneous torsion. In order to prevent torsion and rupture of a pregnant rudimentary uterus, Jayasinghe et al. recommended surgical removal of functional rudimentary uteri before conception. Removal of the rudimentary uterus can relieve dysmenorrhea, prevent or lessen endometriosis caused by retrograde flow of menstrual blood, and avoid pregnancy in rudimentary horn or fallopian tube. It has been commonly applied in women with unicornuate uterus coexisting with non-communicating functional rudimentary uterus, especially in symptomatic women. Nakhal et al. reported on a case of surgical removal of functional non-communicating rudimentary horn with remaining of the functional cervix. 2.5–6 years after the operation, the pelvic pain recurred, with large blood-filled mass being detected at the site of previous operations and being confirmed to be remnant functional cervical tissues. Therefore, when removing the rudimentary uterus, the homolateral functional cervix should be excised at the same time. No data has yet suggested that removal of the rudimentary horn can improve the reproductive outcomes. In 1999, Hand et al. first reported a ruptured tubal pregnancy on the side of non-communicating rudimentary horn in a woman with unicornuate uterus. In 2002, Gabriel et al. reported a case of tubal pregnancy on the side of non-communicating rudimentary horn in a woman with unicornuate uterus. They all provided evidence for transperitoneal migration of sperm and oocyte. Therefore, if a rudimentary horn is not removed, the tube on its side should be ligated or excised.

9.5.2 Indications of TCRS

Most women with septate uterus have normal fertility, and only 20–25% have pregnancy failure, which may often present bleeding at the end of the first trimester of pregnancy or at the beginning of the second trimester followed by embryonic death. There is controversy over the relationship between the septate uterus and infertility. However, nowadays, with the advances in the treatment of uterine malformation, primary infertility that requires assisted reproductive technology or intractable infertility should be considered as indications for transcervical resection of septum. Zabak's indications refer to patients with a history of miscarriages (2 or more), patients with an unexplained infertility, and those who require assisted reproductive treatment.

9.5.3 Preoperative Preparation and Anesthesia

9.5.3.1 Preoperative Assessment

There are a lot of techniques to diagnose uterine malformation, including HSG, ultrasonography, hysteroscopy, MRI, etc. Kupesic et al. reported that the sensitivities in the detection of septate uterus were 100% with HSG, 99.3% with transvaginal color Doppler (TVCD), and 95% with TVS. Sheth et al. reported that among 36 women who were diagnosed as bicornuate uterus on HSG, 34 cases were diagnosed to have intrauterine septum by laparoscopy combined with hysteroscopy. Thus there was a big diagnostic error made by HSG, which may be associated with radiologists' experience. MRI is a good method in diagnosing uterine malformation, and its accuracy ranges from 95 to 100% in diagnosing septate uterus. Prior to hysteroscopic metroplasty, other factors leading to pregnancy failure should be evaluated, including: chromosome investigations on couples, midluteal serum progesterone levels, late luteal endometrial biopsy for endometrial maturity, TSH for subclinical hypothyroidism, partial thromboplastin time (PTT), anticardiolipin antibody (ACA) and antinuclear antibody (ANA) for autologous and allogeneic immune conditions, human histocompatibility locus antigen (HLA), and endometrial biopsy to exclude chronic endometritis. As there is close relationship between paramesonephric ducts and mesonephric ducts in the embryonic period, if there is uterine malformation, malformation of urinary system shall be excluded. However, urinary malformation does not often coexist with uterine malformation. It has ever been reported that uterine malformation may be concomitant with double renal calices, nephroptosis, and other similar anomalies. Therefore, these patients should be investigated by intravenous pyelography.

9.5.3.2 Timing of Operation

The operation must be performed during the early days after menstruation, lest the narrow and small uterine cavity may be lined with thick endometrium, which could lead to a poor visibility and difficulty in operative procedures.

9.5.3.3 Operative Preparation

On the eve before operation, a cervical dilator should be inserted. If there is a complete septate uterus, it can be inserted into any one of the uterine cavities in order to achieve the purpose of softening the cervix.

9.5.3.4 Anesthesia

A general anesthesia is administered to the patients under laparoscopic monitoring or an epidural anesthesia under ultrasound monitoring.

9.5.4 Operative Procedures

9.5.4.1 Mechanical Resection with Scissors Under Hysteroscope

It is performed using an operative hysteroscope with the outer sheath 7 or 8 mm. The irrigation fluid may contain electrolyte, but still a continuous irrigation device is needed for monitoring the inflow and outflow fluid in order to prevent the occurrence of body fluid overload. Hysteroscopic scissors can be classified into soft, half-rigid, and rigid scissors. The soft scissors are not easy to control, so the half-rigid scissors are most commonly used (Fig. 9.108), which

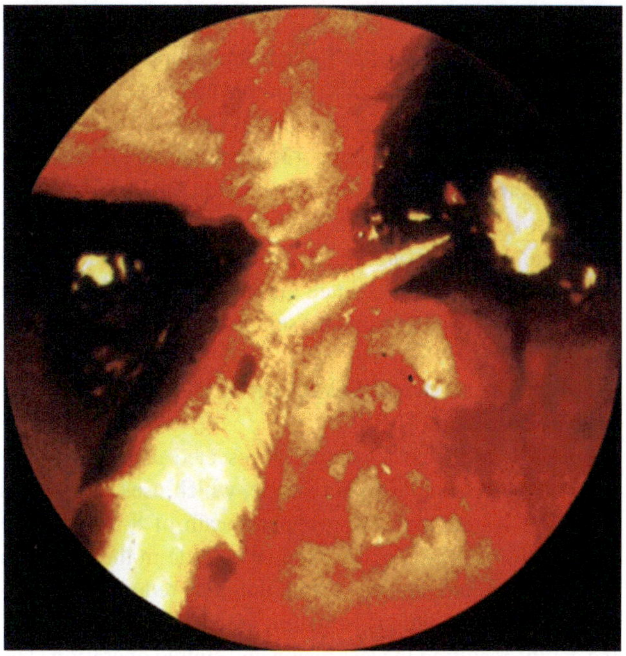

Fig. 9.108 Division of uterine septum with half-rigid scissors

can divide the tissues directly. That is, under conditions of a good panoramic vision, the scissors can selectively divide the tissues that need to be divided and can retreat optionally. The procedures using half-rigid scissors do not need much strength and skills, but it must be kept sharp and strong. The Hook-type scissors are most practical in the resection of intrauterine septa, especially those with wide and large bases, and the residual septate tissues require small and superficial excision so as to avoid deep myometrial perforation. The rigid scissors can be used to divide the fibrous and broad septa. The use of this type of scissors requires excellent panoramic vision. Because these scissors have a sharp tip, when cutting towards the uterine wall with force, it is easy to cause uterine perforation, thus the operator must be very careful.

The application of hysteroscopic scissors in division of uterine septum includes the accurate cutting in the midline of septum where the tissues contain fibrosis and have no blood vessels. Uterine myometrial vessels run from the uterine anterior and posterior walls into the septate tissues. The beginners should avoid cutting the posterior and anterior walls of uterus so as to prevent unnecessary bleeding at the time of operation. The cutting should start from one side gradually towards the opposite side, cutting off a small piece each time. Once the fallopian tube ostia are seen, the cutting should be shallow, and the operator should observe carefully the small blood vessels from the myometrial layer to avoid penetrating the myometrium. After resecting the septum, before the instruments are withdrawn, the fundus should be observed under hysteroscope, and irrigating pressure should be decreased to observe whether there is obvious bleeding. If there is arterial bleeding, target coagulation hemostasis can be carried out.

Scissors have the following advantages in dividing uterine septum: (1) the procedure is simple and fast, and is appliable to all kinds of uterine septum. (2) The scissors are easily placed at the tip of the septum. (3) Since scissors do not consume electric power, the irrigation fluid containing electrolyte can be used so as to reduce the risk of body fluid overload. Its disadvantage is that postoperative adhesion may occur because the septate muscle tissues have not been excised, thus forming acquired septum.

9.5.4.2 Transcervical Resection of Uterine Septum (TCRS)

For TCRS, intrauterine septum is resected using needle or wire loop electrode of hysteroscope, which uses continuous irrigation system and has an outer sheath of 8–9 mm. The advantages of needle or wire loop electrode in the resection of uterine septum are that coagulation may reduce the bleeding, and that continuous irrigation system irrigates the uterine cavity, resulting in clear vision and simple operation. The disadvantage is that the monopolar coagulation may coagulate the adjacent normal endometrial tissues. The operative procedures are as follows:

1. The diagnosis of uterine malformation depends on the shape of uterine fundus, so it is better to perform laparoscopy simultaneously with hysteroscopy for diagnosis (Figs. 9.109, 9.110, 9.111, 9.112, and 9.113) and monitoring.
2. Under hysteroscopy, the observation begins with the sizes and morphological characteristics of the septum and uterine cavity (Figs. 9.114, 9.115, 9.116, 9.117, and 9.118), including the distinction between complete and incomplete septum, the tip width of the septum, the length of the septum from the fundus to its end (longitudinal diameter), the length of the septum from the anterior wall to the posterior wall of the uterus (antero-posterior diameter), and the size and symmetry of two uterine cavities.
3. When ultrasonography is applied for monitoring, the hysteroscopic wire loop may be placed at the end of the sep-

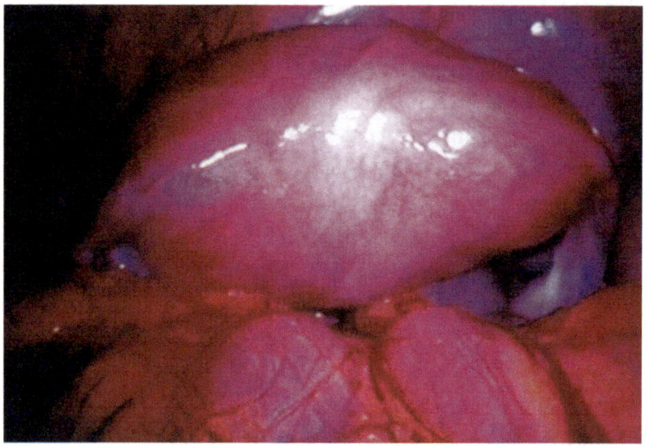

Fig. 9.109 Septate uterus. A broad fundus is seen under laparoscope

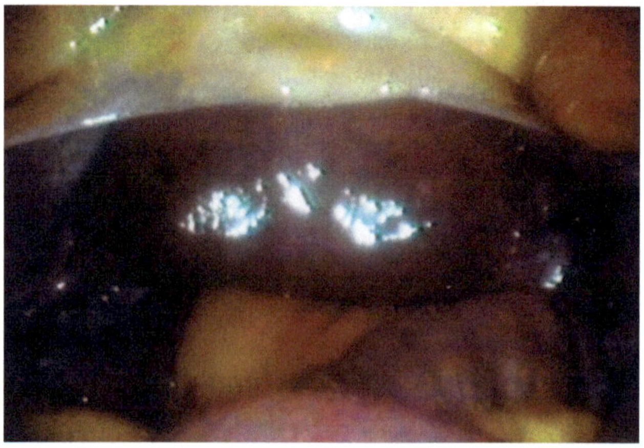

Fig. 9.110 Septate uterus. A concave and broad fundus with slight indentations of anterior and posterior walls is seen under laparoscope

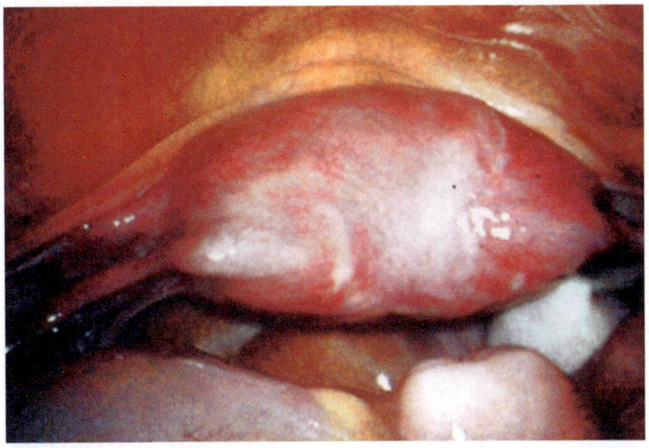

Fig. 9.111 Septate uterus. A slightly concave and broad flat fundus is seen under laparoscope

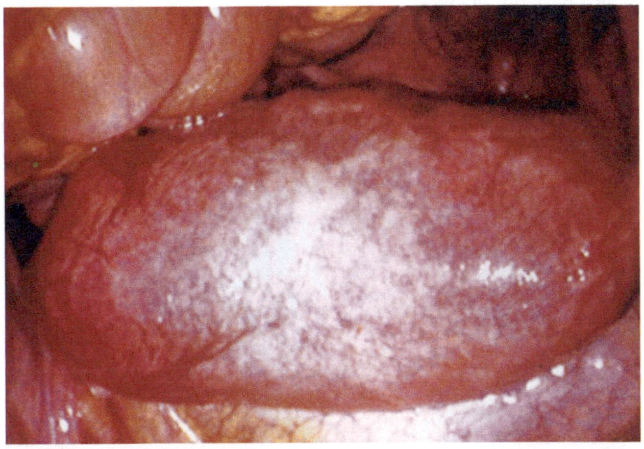

Fig. 9.112 Septate uterus. A broad fundus with flat anterior and posterior walls is seen under laparoscope

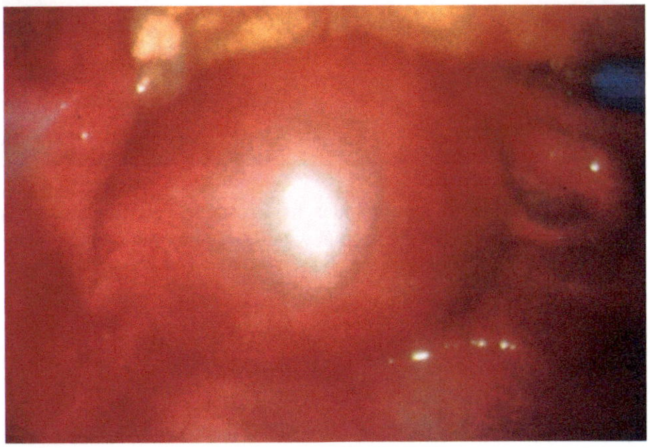

Fig. 9.113 Septate uterus. A normal uterine fundus is seen under laparoscope

tum, its length from the fundus to the end can be measured by ultrasonography scanning (Fig. 9.119).

4. A hysteroscope with the outer sheath 8–9 mm and continuous irrigation system is applied. The septum can be resected

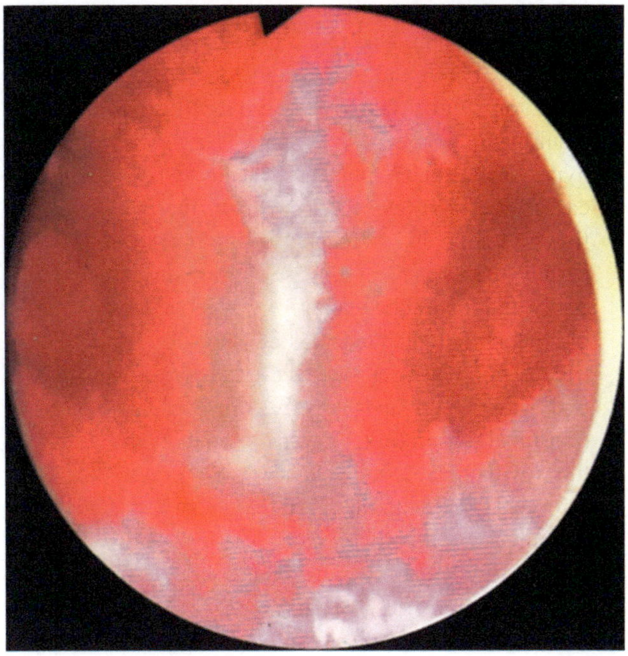

Fig. 9.114 Uterine septum under hysteroscope. A distant view shows a narrow end of the septum and two symmetrical uterine cavities similar in size prior to TCRS

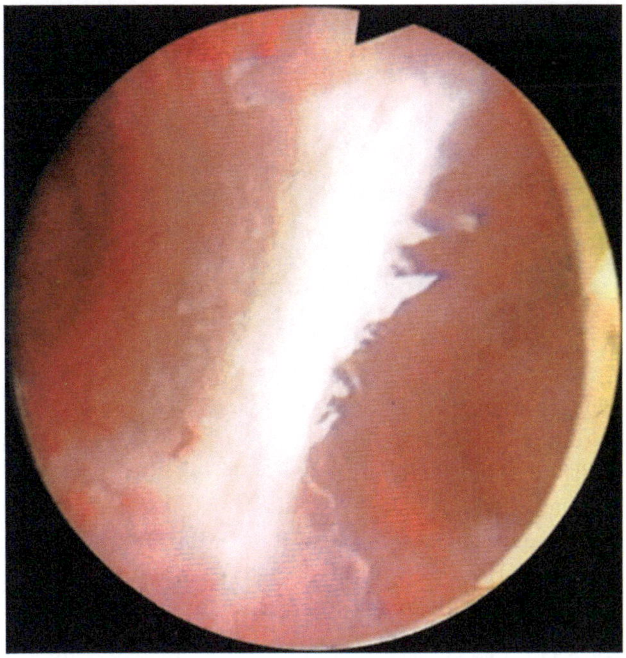

Fig. 9.115 Uterine septum under hysteroscope. A closer look at the septum reveals a longer antero-posterior diameter

by a wire loop (Figs. 9.120 and 9.121) or be divided by a needle electrode (Figs. 9.122, 9.123, 9.124, and 9.125). The base of the septum at the fundus can be gradually trimmed by a needle electrode until it is completely divided (Fig. 9.126). The excessive septate tissues in the anterior or posterior walls at the fundus can be resected by a wire loop

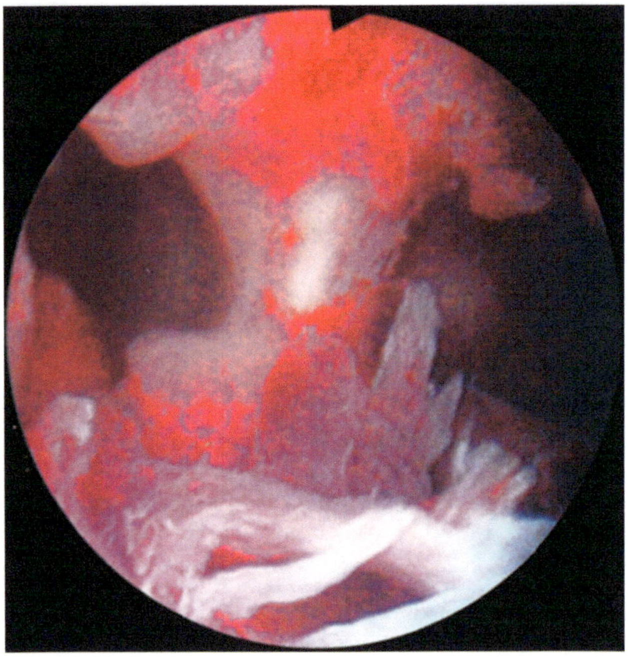

Fig. 9.116 Incomplete uterine septum under hysteroscope. It appears to be short in antero-posterior diameter and broad in its tip

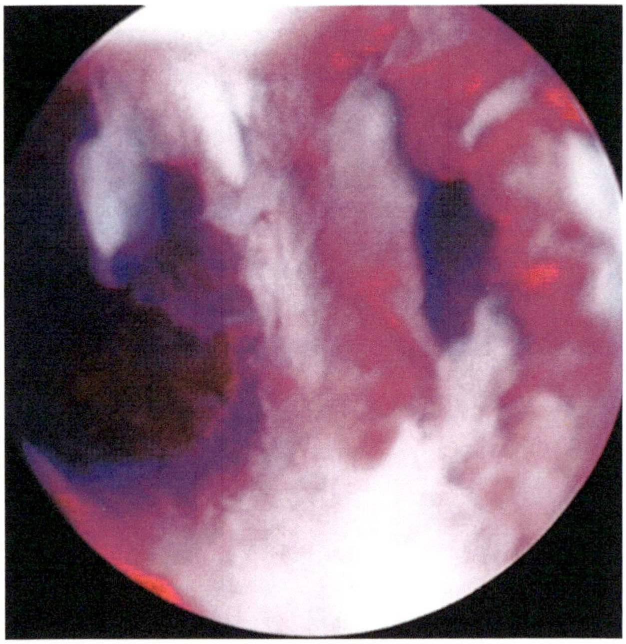

Fig. 9.117 Uterine septum under hysteroscope. Prior to TCRS, two uterine cavities appear to be asymmetrical with right cavity bigger and left cavity smaller, and the antero-posterior diameter of the septum is shorter

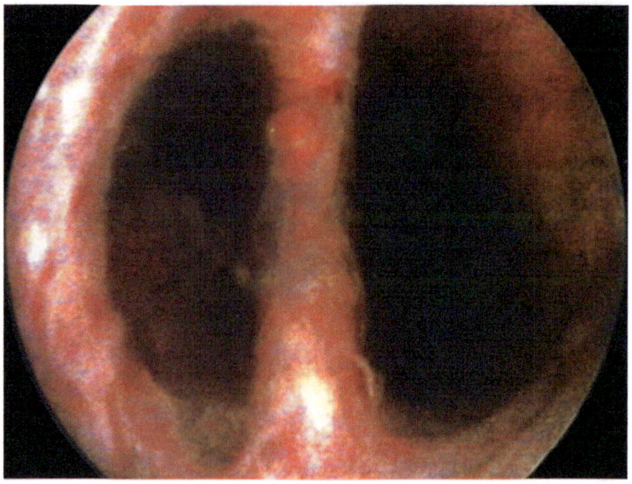

Fig. 9.118 Uterine septum under hysteroscope. It appears to be long in antero-posterior diameter

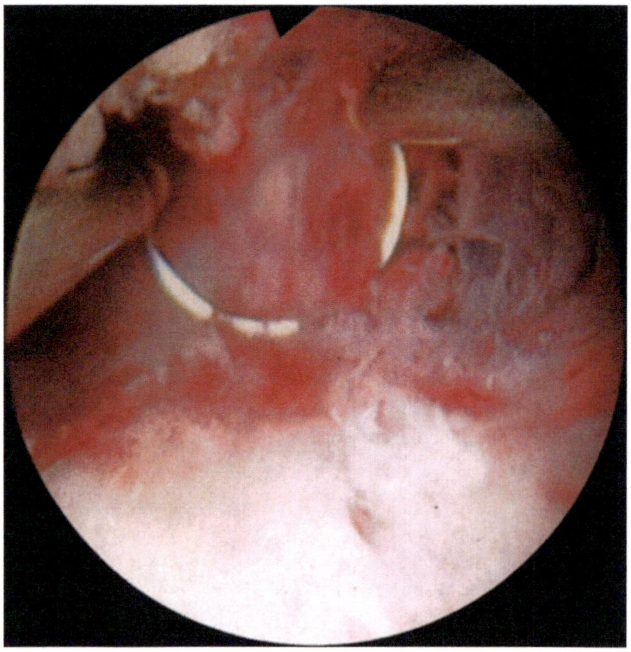

Fig. 9.119 Uterine septum under hysteroscope. The wire loop is placed against the end of the septum with the length of the septum measured by ultrasonography

(Fig. 9.127). Therefore two cavities are made open and form a symmetrical uterine cavity (Fig. 9.128).

5. For correction of arcuate uterus, a needle electrode is applied to divide and trim the inward-protruding fundus (Fig. 9.129) till the bilateral cornua are reached (Fig. 9.130), forming a flat uterine fundus (Fig. 9.131).
6. When cutting, the operator should pay attention to its direction and depth, keeping symmetrical incisions between the left and the right. That is, one cut on each side in turn (Figs. 9.132, 9.133, 9.134, 9.135, 9.136, 9.137, and 9.138). The symmetry of the cavity should be carefully kept to avoid deeper cuttings on one side which deform the cavity.

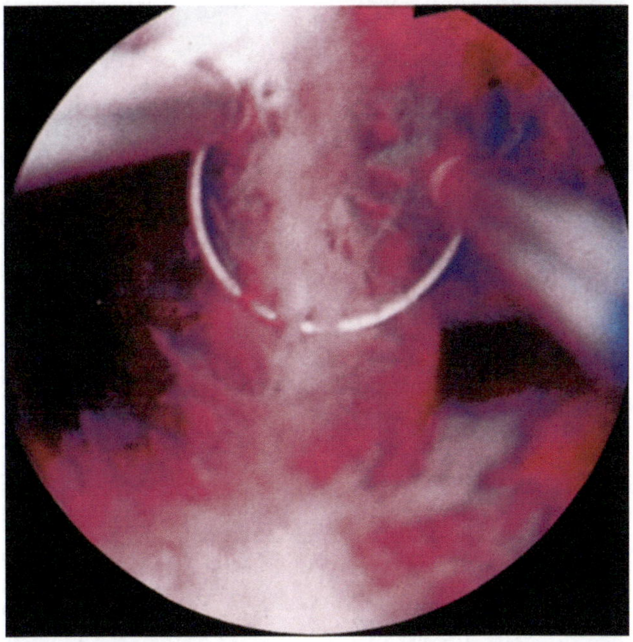

Fig. 9.120 During TCRS, the wire loop is ready for resecting the septum

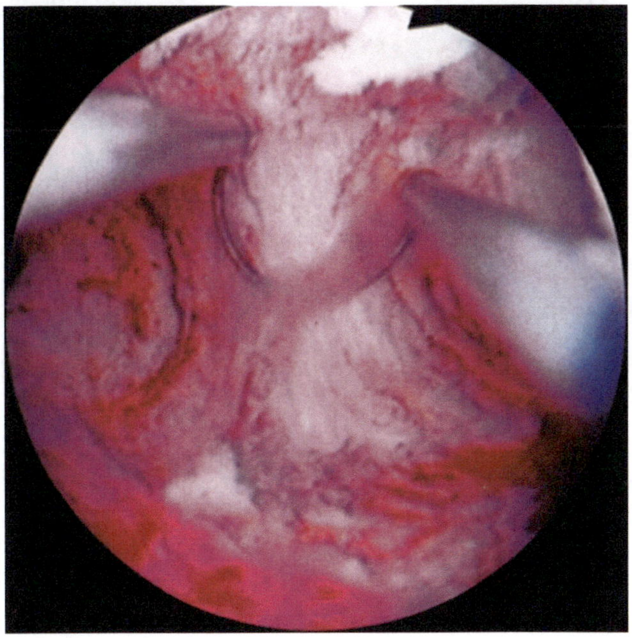

Fig. 9.121 During TCRS, the wire loop is used for resecting the septum

7. When cutting reaches the base of septum, the operator should not cut so deep that it damages the uterine fundus, otherwise it is very easy to cause perforation of uterus.
8. At the end of the operation, IUD is placed in the uterine cavity and taken out 2 months later.

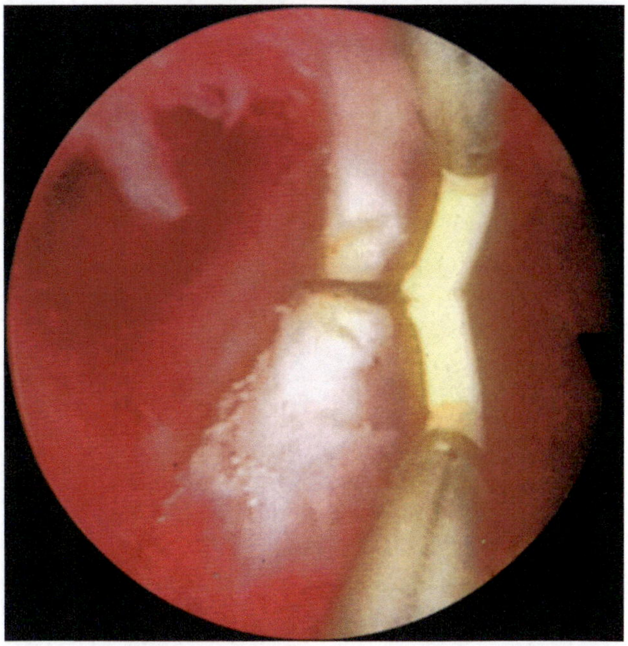

Fig. 9.122 The needle electrode is placed at the end of the septum

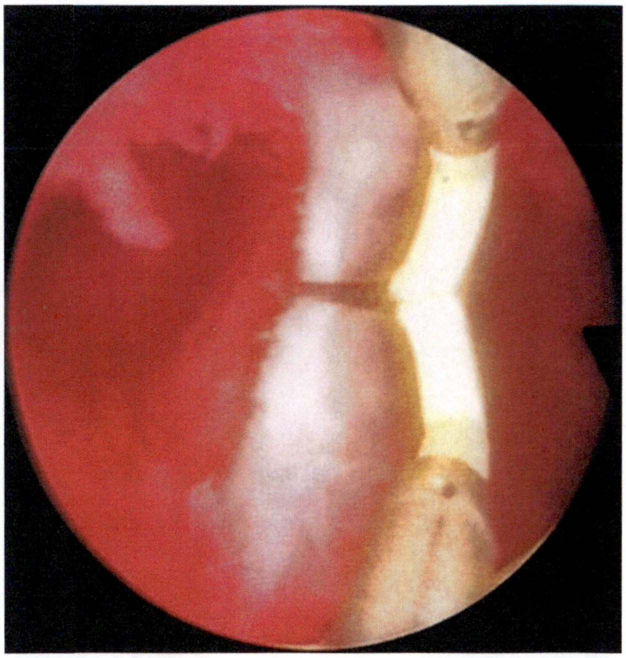

Fig. 9.123 The needle electrode is making incision of the septum

9.5.4.3 Hysteroscopic Resection of Septum by Laser

Uterine septum can be divided by Nd-YAG laser, argon and KTP-532 laser. The laser does not conduct electricity, so the fluid containing electrolyte (e.g., saline, 5% glucose saline solution, lactated Ringer's solution) can be used as irrigation fluid, and may help to improve visibility. The division of

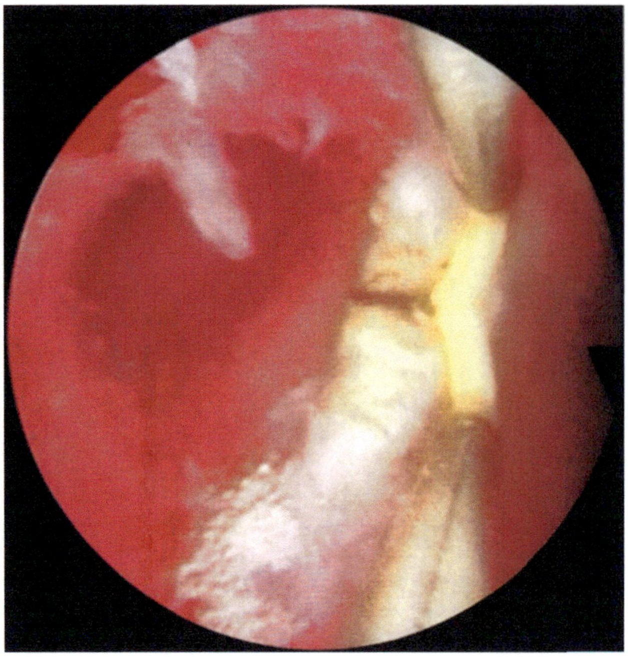

Fig. 9.124 The needle electrode is incising the septum and approaching its base

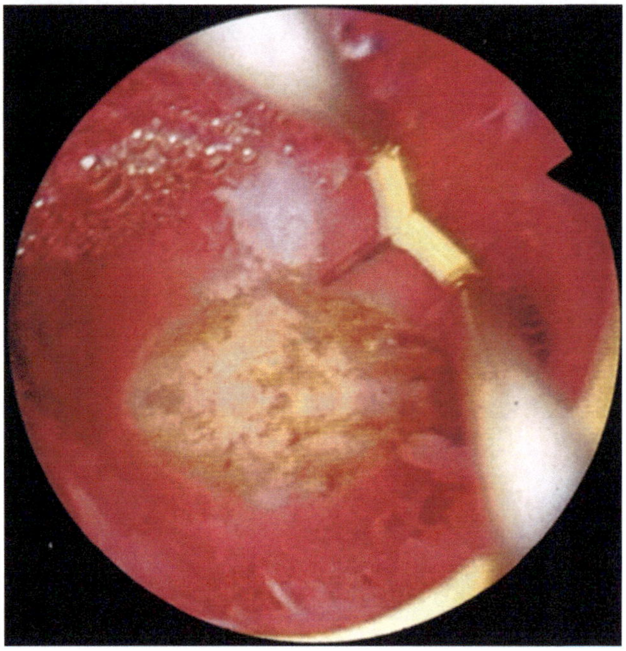

Fig. 9.125 The base of septum is incised by needle electrode

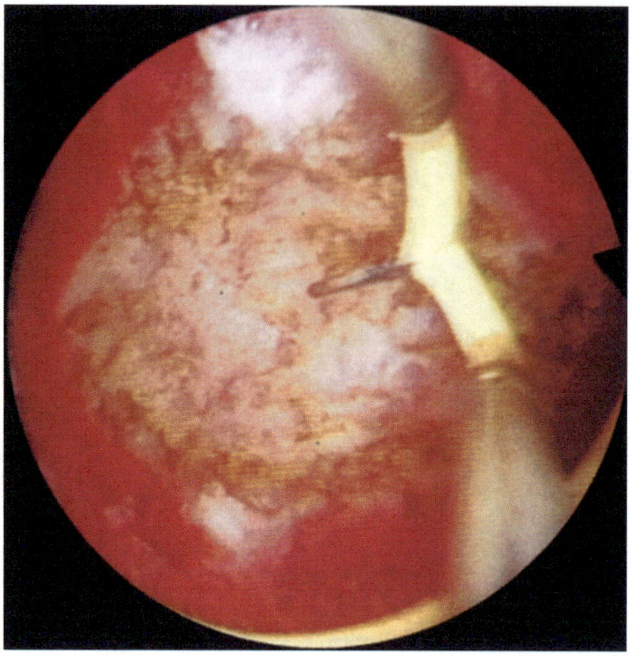

Fig. 9.126 The uterine fundus is trimmed by the needle electrode

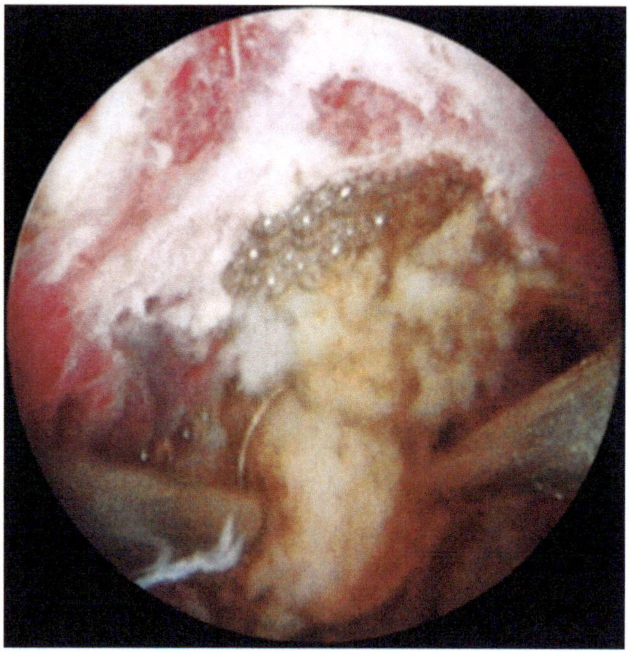

Fig. 9.127 Resection of the excessive tissues in uterine anterior wall

uterine septum by laser should start from the end of septum along the midline and move from one side to the other. Be sure to continually move the optical fiber to avoid the occurrence of uterine perforation. Cho and Baggish suggested that the laser procedure is especially suitable for the patients with wide and thick uterine septum.

Hysteroscopic division of septum by laser has the following advantages: (1) The laser can induce coagulation, so hemorrhage may be avoided. (2) Resection by laser is easy to operate, and easier to master than hysteroscopic resectoscope. (3) There is no electrical energy transmission, so the fluid containing electrolyte can be used as the irrigation fluid. Its disadvantages are as follows: (1) Being expensive. (2)

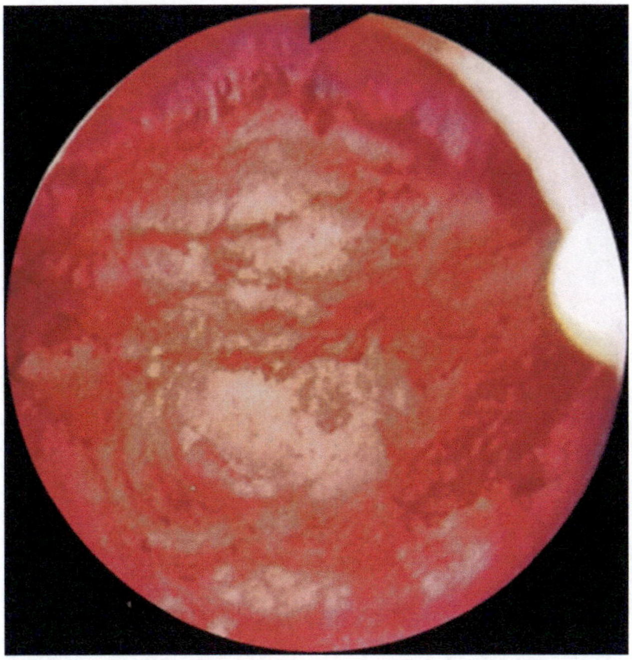

Fig. 9.128 After TCRS, the bilateral uterine cornua is communicated, forming a symmetrical uterine cavity

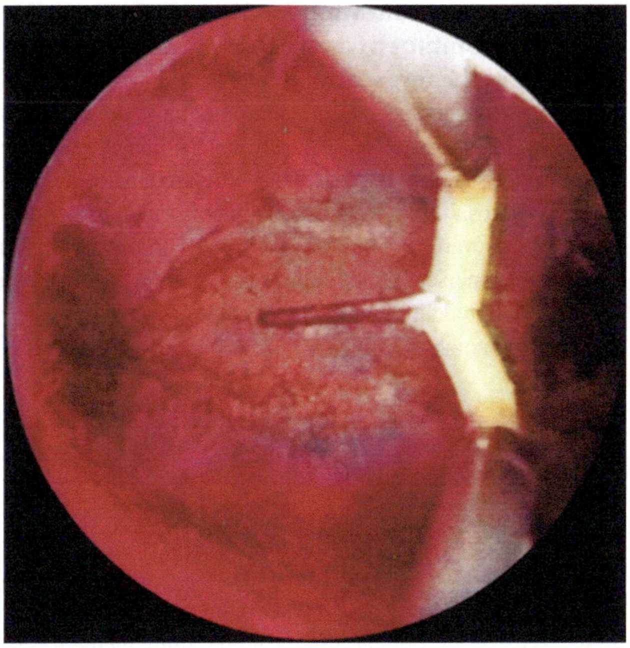

Fig. 9.129 The fundus of an arcuate uterus is incised by a needle electrode

The laser scattered by optical fiber can do damage to the retina of the operator, so special protective glasses need to be worn. (3) The scattered laser can damage the surrounding normal endometrium of septum, leading to slow epithelialization. (4) Longer operation time.

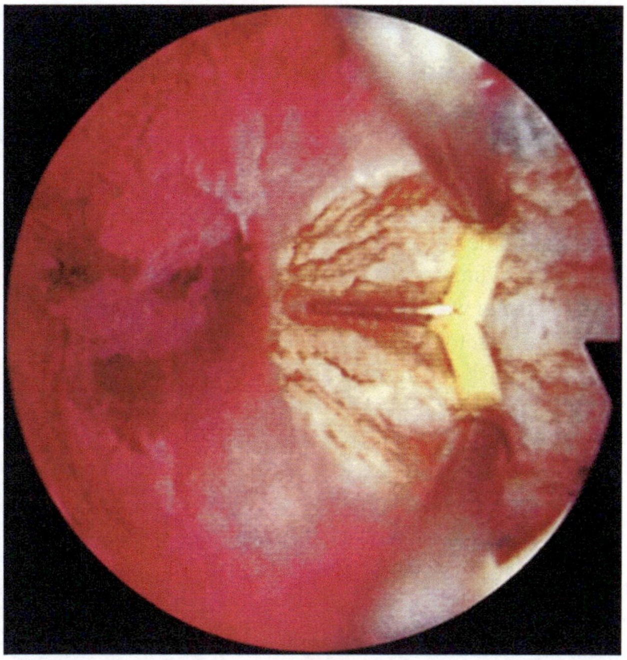

Fig. 9.130 The incision by a needle electrode is approaching right cornu of an arcuate uterus

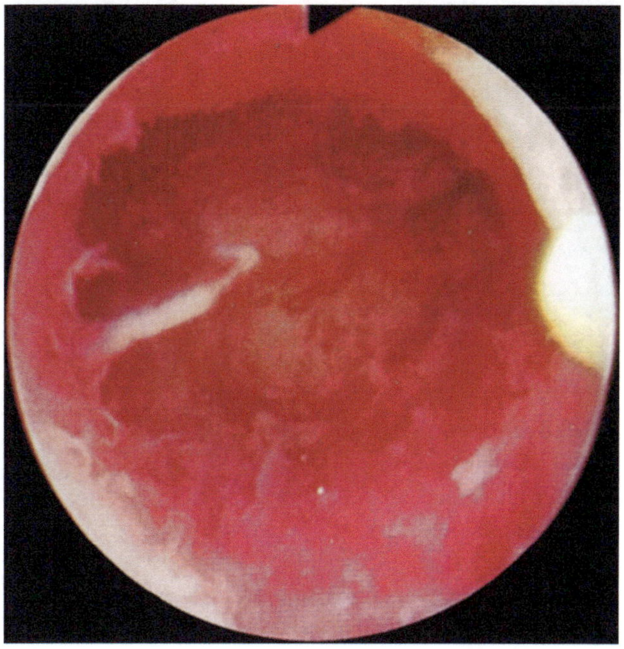

Fig. 9.131 After TCRS in an arcuate uterus, the fundus is flat

9.5.4.4 Transcervical Uterine Incision (TCUI)

Transcervical uterine incision (TCUI) is conducted by excising excessive myometrial tissues on bilateral uterine walls or incising the thickened myometrium on one or two lateral walls to restore a normal cavity, enlarge the endometrial area, relieve the intrauterine pressure, and improve the uter-

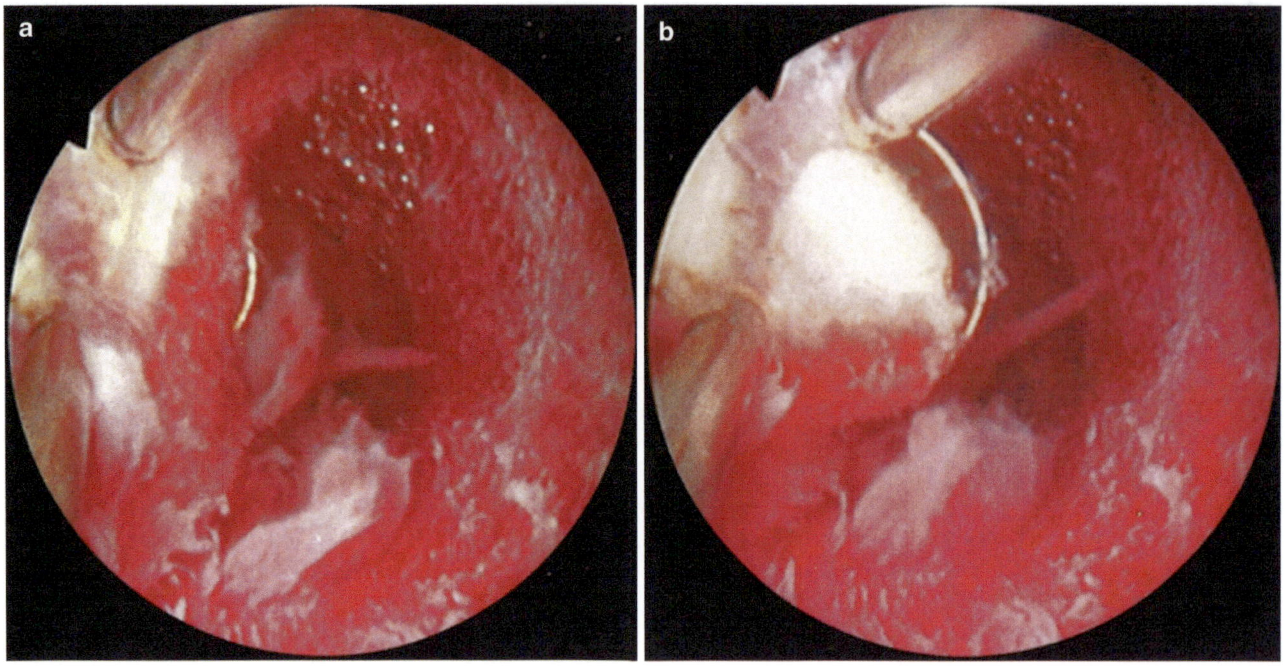

Fig. 9.132 (**a**, **b**) The first cut from right to left with a wire loop

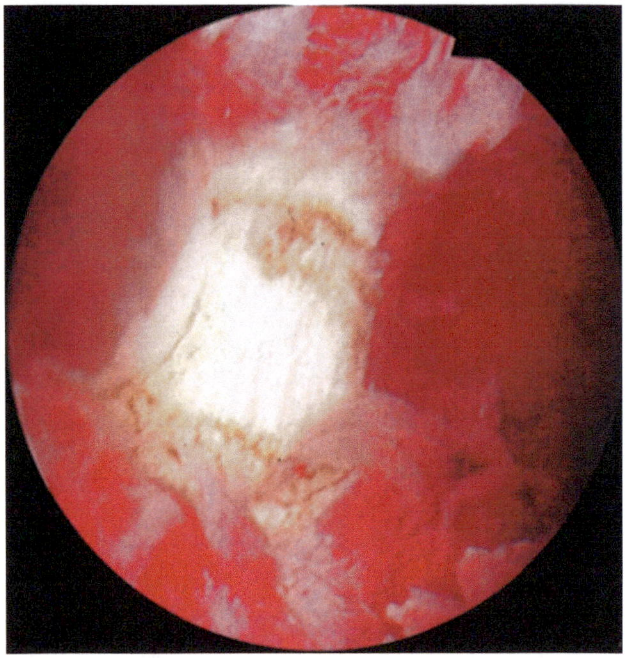

Fig. 9.133 The septum after the first cut

ine blood supply. Therefore, it can facilitate the implantation of the fertilized egg, prevent miscarriage and improve reproductive outcomes. This operation can be applied for treatment of T-shaped uterus, unicornuate uterus, and Robert uterus. For details, see Sect. 9.8.

9.5.4.5 Uterine Unification for Bicornuate Uterus by Combined Laparoscopy and Hysteroscopy

The joint operation of bicornuate uterine unification via laparoscopy and hysteroscopy is performed using hysteroscopic resectoscope to resect intrauterine septum and incise the fundus to its serosa under laparoscopic monitoring, forming an artificial perforation. Then the full layer of the fundus is transversely incised under laparoscopy. Next the incision walls are sutured longitudinally to achieve a normal shape cavity. For details, see Chap. 10.

9.5.5 Intraoperative Complex Conditions and Management

As the broad and large septum may affect the operation of hysteroscopic resectoscope and make the resection of septum difficult, the mechanical resection by microscissors or division by laser optical fiber can be implemented. The resection of a complete uterine septum only requires the resection of septum in uterine corpus. At the time of operation, a 10 mm Hegar dilator can be inserted into one cavity, and the hysteroscope is inserted into another cavity to incise the septum towards the dilator just above the internal os. After cutting through the septum, the dilator is taken out and the operation is continued. Romer reported that a balloon catheter was introduced into one cavity to facilitate the hys-

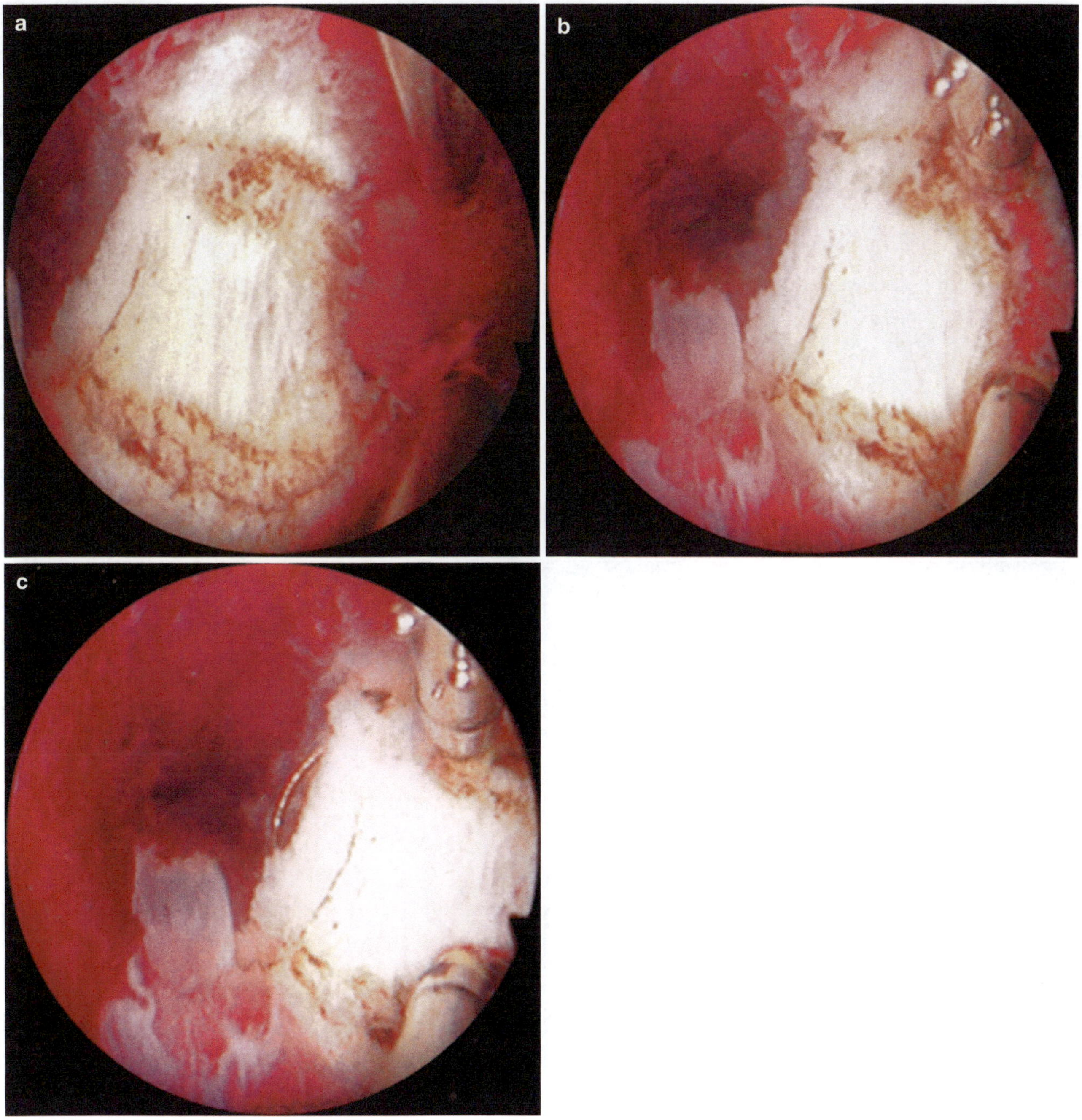

Fig. 9.134 The second cut from left to right. (**a**) A wire loop is placed on the left of the septum. (**b**) The wire loop resects the septum. (**c**) The wire loop resects till the right side of septum

teroscopic resection of complete uterine septum. Rock et al. reported that 21 patients with complete septate uterus were treated between 1985 and 1998 by TCRS with preservation of cervical septum. Among 15 women who attempted to conceive after TCRS, 14 women achieved live birth babies with low morbidity.

9.5.6 Intraoperative and Postoperative Monitoring and Management

Since there is no boundary between the septum and the fundus, uterine cornua are deep, and the serosa of uterine fundus may be concave, TCRS may result in the perforation of uter-

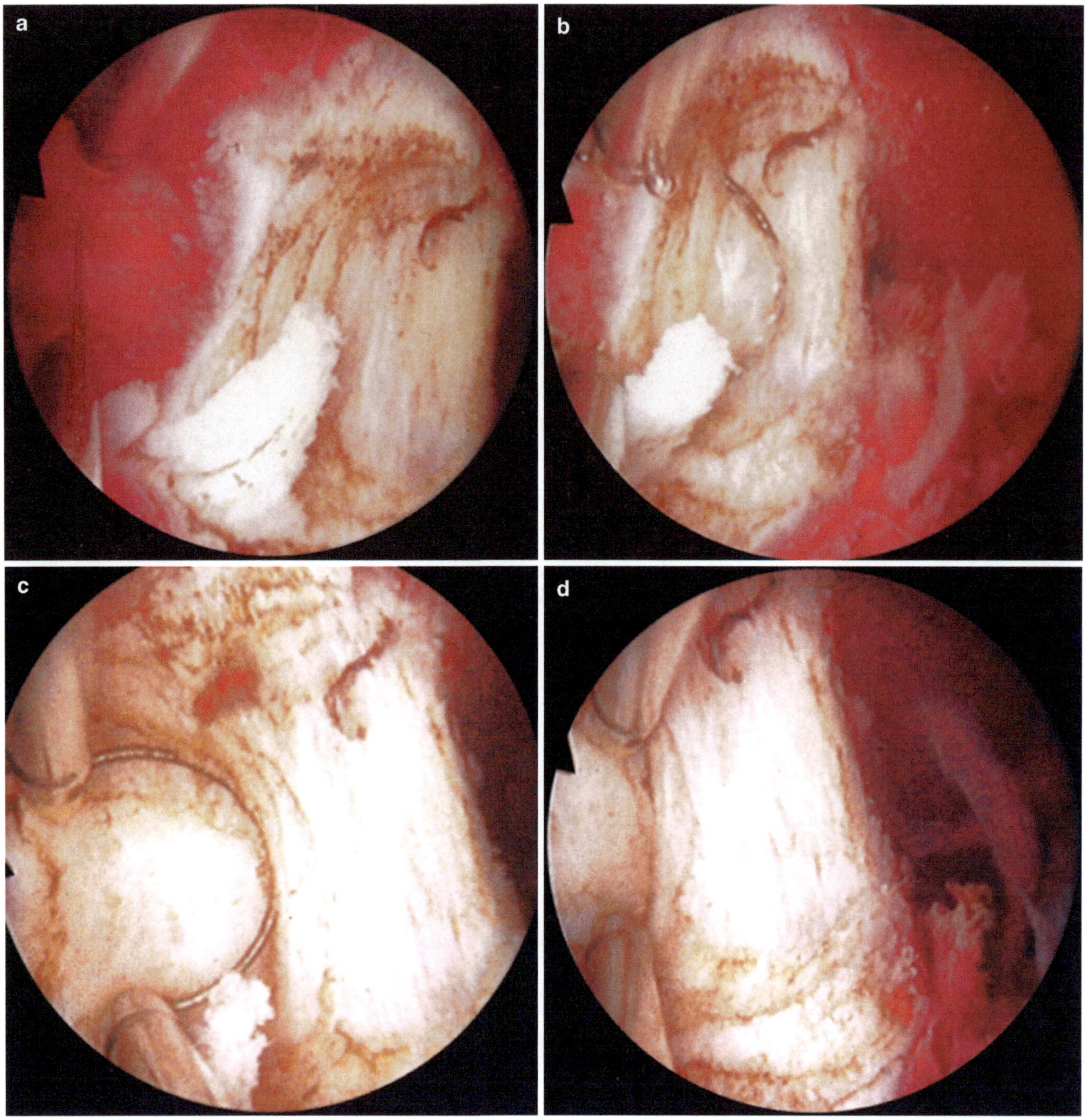

Fig. 9.135 (**a**) A wire loop is placed on the right of the septum and the third cut from right to left is done. (**b**) For the third cut from right to left, the wire loop is going halfway due to the broad septum, with the wire loop seen at the midline of septum. Thus only half of the resection had been finished. (**c**) The fourth additional cut is done from right to left by the wire loop. (**d**) The fourth cut is resecting in the septum

ine fundus. Therefore, it is better to administer laparoscopic and (or) ultrasound monitoring during operation.

9.5.6.1 Ultrasound Surveillance

At the beginning of the operation, ultrasonography scanning is first performed to measure the length of the septum, the broadness of both the end and the base of the septum, and the thickness of the uterine fundus. During procedures, under ultrasonography surveillance, a wire loop electrode is put in place, a suitable direction of cutting is determined and guaranteed, and then the wire loop is activated to resect the septum. Transverse scanning is regularly conducted to observe whether the high echogenic band of the excised tissues is centered or not. After removal of the septum, the cavities are cut through, forming a whole cavity. When the thickness of uterine fundus is 0.7–1.1 cm, it suggests that the operator should stop cutting. Coccia et al. conducted a prospective study of patients who underwent TCRS under ultrasonography guidance as compared to patients under laparoscopic guidance. In cases under ultrasonography guidance, the septum had been resected more extensively with short or without residual septum, and no cases needed a second operation of resection. However in cases under laparoscopic monitoring, 4 of them needed a second operation to resect the residual septum due to initial insufficient resection.

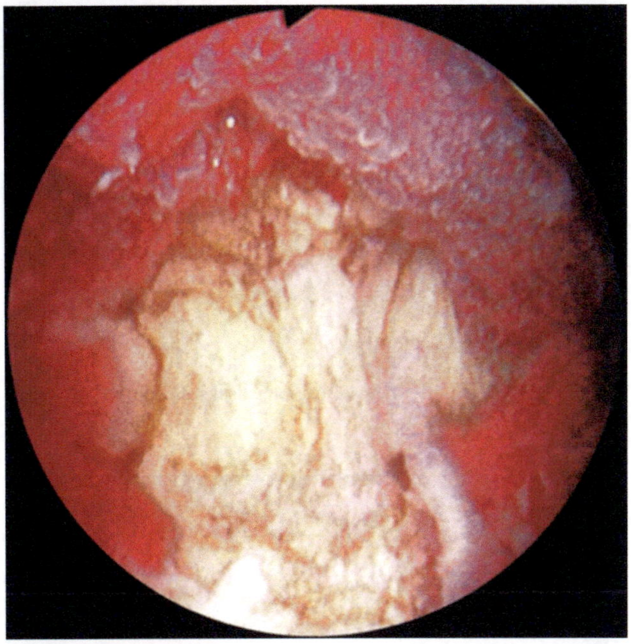

Fig. 9.136 The uterine fundus after resection by a wire loop

9.5.6.2 Laparoscopic Monitoring

Laparoscopy is first performed to observe the external contour of the uterus and exclude bicornuate uterus. During hysteroscopic resection, laparoscopy can monitor the procedure and remind the operator of potential perforation if necessary. . When cutting is approaching the uterine fundus, put the laparoscope in a proper place and dim the light. The transmittance of light through uterine wall from hysteroscope can be seen by laparoscopy. The thinner the uterine wall, when touched with hysteroscopic electrode, the stronger the light seen under laparoscopy. If the light of hysteroscope is obviously seen under laparoscope, it indicates a thin fundus and suggests an impending perforation, which alerts the surgeon to stop the operation.

Since the patients are treated for infertility, the prophylactic use of antibiotics should be strengthened to prevent infections of uterine cavity or fallopian tubes. Intravenous injection of cefotamine 1 g (or kefzol) can be administered half an hour prior to operation, and then cephalosporins is taken orally for 3–4 days after operation.

There is still controversy over the use of large doses of estrogen and the placement of IUD after TCRS. Most experienced surgeons do not prefer the placement of IUD. Since estrogen can accelerate the epithelialization of the denuded zone in uterine cavity, large doses of estrogen may be administered after operation, such as premarin 1.25–2.5 mg, twice per day, 30–40 days for one cycle, and progestin medroxyprogesterone acetate (provera) 10 mg/day is added in the last 10 days. In total, two artificial cycles are always

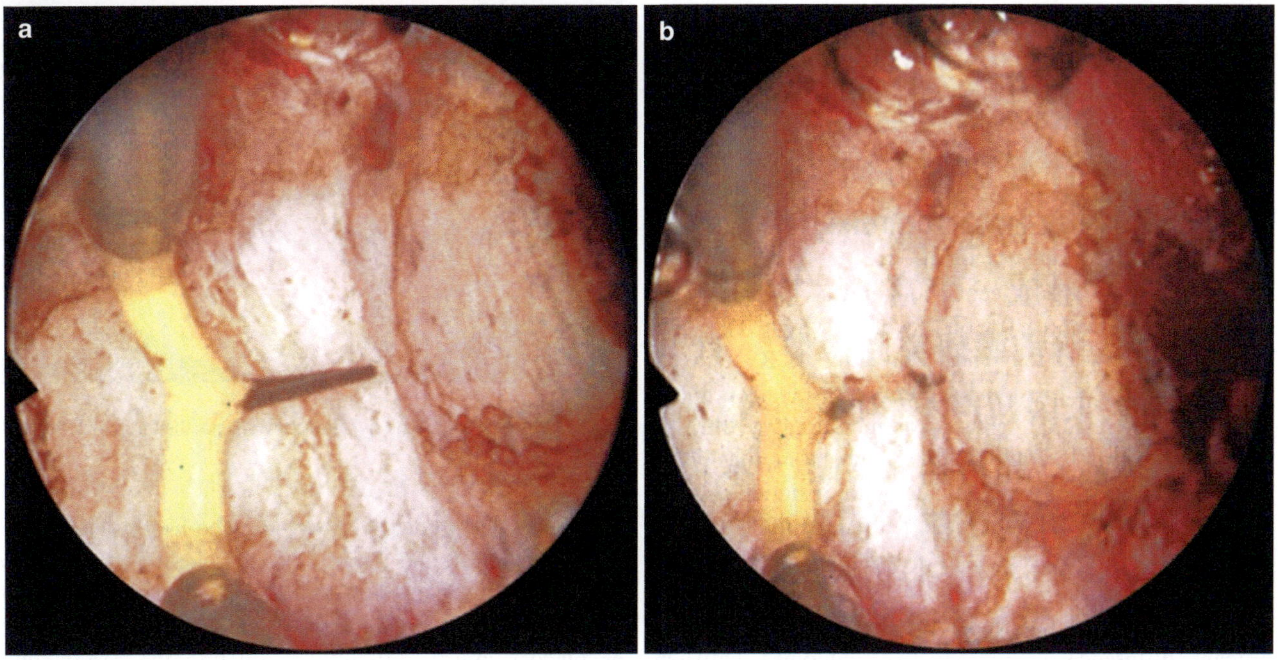

Fig. 9.137 (**a**) The protruding crest-like tissues at uterine fundus are divided from right to left by a needle electrode. (**b**) A needle electrode is incising into the protruding tissues from right to left and then moving backwards to divide it

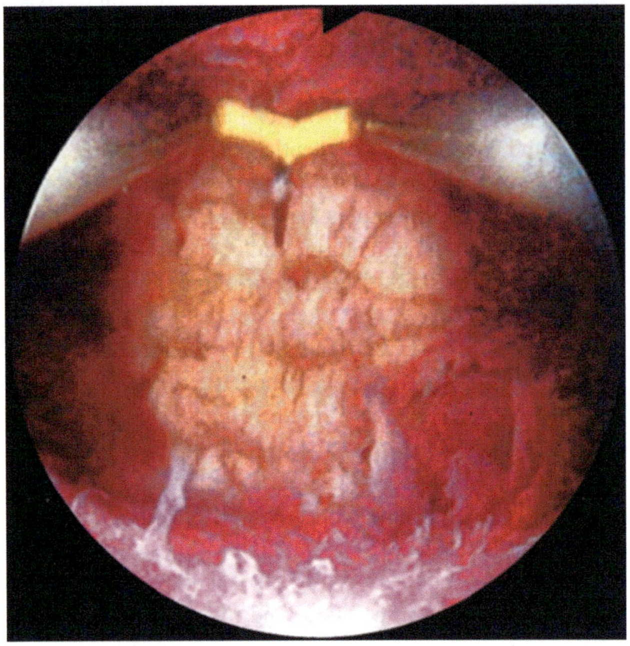

Fig. 9.138 After incision by a needle electrode

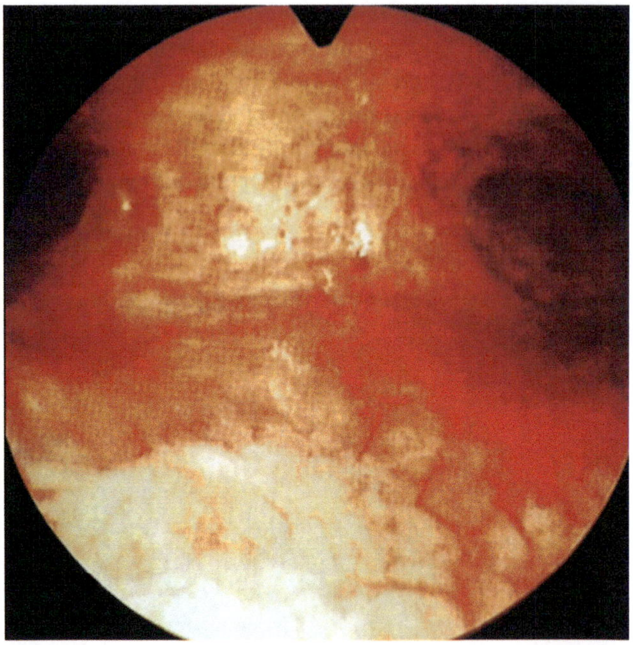

Fig. 9.139 A second-look hysteroscopy checks the uterine cavity at 4 weeks after TCRS

applied. Second-look hysteroscopy should be performed at the fourth and the eighth week post-operation to assess the symmetry of uterine cavity (Figs. 9.139 and 9.140). If a normal cavity achieved, the patient can attempt to conceive.

9.5.7 Identification and Treatment of Operative Complications

The detailed information is described in Chap. 12.

TCRS has become an alternative method for the treatment of uterine septum, but there is a high incidence of uterine perforation in hysteroscopic operations. Roge et al. reported six cases of uterine perforation in 102 women who underwent TCRS (5.8%). Chen et al. reported on two cases of intrauterine adhesions post TCRS. A second operation may be required in patients with incomplete resection of septum found by second-look hysteroscopy. Fedele et al. reported a comparison of 17 women who had a residual septum between 0.5 and 1 cm after TCRS and 51 women who had no residual septum or residual <0.5 cm. The length of residual septum was measured by ultrasonography 1 month after TCRS. Eighteen months after operation, 44.5% of the patients with residual septum (0.5–1.0 cm) and 52.7% of those without residual septum (0 or <0.5 cm) conceived, with no significant difference; the delivery rate was 27.5% and 36% respectively, with no significant difference. It indicated that there was no significant difference in reproductive outcomes between women with a residual septum (0.5–1.0 cm) and women with almost no residual.

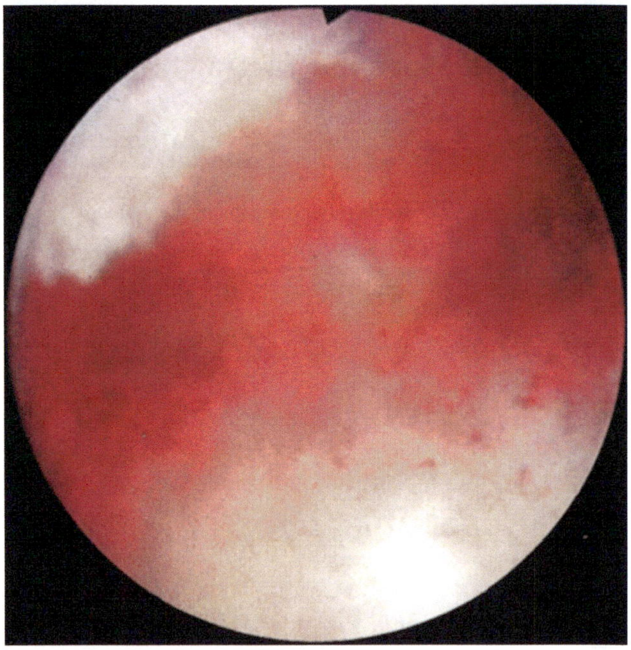

Fig. 9.140 A second-look hysteroscopy checks the uterine cavity at 8 weeks after TCRS

Propst et al. studied 925 women who had hysteroscopic operations and found that the occurrence of complications was 2.7%, which included uterine perforation, fluid overload (≥1 L), hyponatremia, massive bleeding (≥500 mL), bowel or bladder injury, difficulty in dilating the cervix, and procedure-related hospitalization. TCRM and TCRS had the highest odds ratio (OR) (7.4), with fluid absorption overload the most frequent complication. TCRP and TCRE had the lowest OR (0.1).

9.5.8 Experience and Assessment of Hysteroscopic Metroplasty

9.5.8.1 Septate Uterus

1. Therapeutic effects of TCRS: TCRS has equal or better therapeutic effects than traditional laparotomy metroplasty in the treatment of symptomatic uterine septum. Liu et al. from Hysteroscopy Center of Fuxing Hospital, Capital Medical University, made a retrospective analysis of the outcomes of TCRS in 107 patients with uterine septum under ultrasonography surveillance. The mean operation time was 21 min with no complications occurred. In 97 women who were followed up successfully for 5 months to 10 years, the miscarriage rate decreased from preoperative 93.10% to postoperative 29.09%, and the delivery rate increased from 3.45 to 52.73%, both with significant differences. It was believed that the operation of TCRS could greatly improve the reproductive outcome in women with uterine septum. Moreover, it avoided the procedures of laparotomy and hysterotomy, which reduced the formation of pelvic adhesions and consequent pain, thus the patient had no limitation in physical activities. Therefore, hysteroscopy should be considered as the optimal choice when combined with laparoscopy and (or) ultrasonography in treatment of uterine septum. Fedele et al.'s experience suggested that the patients might conceive 4 weeks after TCRS and did not need to undergo elective cesarean section.

   The patients who conceive following TCRS may be at risk of uterine rupture. Creainin and Chen reported that a perforation of the fundus occurred during TCRS in a patient with uterine septum. The patient got a term twin conception after TCRS, and cesarean section revealed a 7 cm defect in the uterine fundus. Howe reported on a 29-year-old woman who had a small fundal perforation during TCRS. When she conceived after TCRS, uterine rupture occurred at 33 weeks of pregnancy which resulted in neonatal mortality and maternal morbidity. Gabriele et al. reported a woman who conceived after complicated TCRS. Uterine rupture during labor induced with prostaglandins E_2 (PGE_2) occurred, which was managed by emergency cesarean section. An ultrasonography scan performed 2 years later revealed a defect of uterine wall which was later verified during cesarean section. The authors hold that PGE_2 is not suitable for induction of labor after complicated TCRS, and ultrasonography can be used for the detection of uterine defects. Sentilhes et al. made a review of English, German, and French literatures about case reports of uterine rupture following hysteroscopic operations, with 14 cases involved. Among them, 12 cases underwent operations for uterine malformations and eight cases encountered uterine perforation. Nine cases of procedures were done by electric resection. All patients conceived between 1 month and 5 years following hysteroscopic operations, with an average interval of 16 months. Postoperative HSG was carried out in six cases with normal reports in five. Ultrasonography scan failed to detect uterine rupture during pregnancy in two cases. Therefore, it was considered that pregnancies following hysteroscopic metroplasty had a high risk of uterine rupture, with which intraoperative uterine perforation and/or the use of electrosurgery was closely correlated but not an independent factor.
2. Different operative procedures and their prognosis: In recent years, a lot of experience has been accumulated in hysteroscopic metroplasty of uterine septum with microscissors in Europe and the United States, and postoperative reproductive outcomes are similar to that with laser. There are also some reports about comparison of electroresection of septum with scissors and laser. It has been reported that the postoperative pregnancy rate after TCRS decreased by 30% because the septum could not be completely removed, especially the broad and large septum. The limited resection might be related to the types of wire loop, especially 90° wire loop. New straight or forward angle wire loop may be suitable for resecting the septum, with the postoperative outcome similar to that with scissors and laser. Which instrument should be selected depends in part on the operator's proficiency and experience in handling various situations. Most doctors prefer resection with hysteroscopic scissors in treatment of uterine septum. Ohl and Bettahar-Lebugle from France reported his experiences in hysteroscopic metroplasty with scissors during a 7-year period in 93 women who had uterine septum. The results of follow-up in patients with previous obstetric history showed that the premature delivery rate decreased from preoperative 13 to 9.4% after operation, the pregnancy loss rate decreased from 78 to 24.5%, and term delivery rate increased from 5.7 to 62.3%. Cararach et al. reported the outcomes of 17 cases of hysteroscopic incision of uterine septum with scissors versus 53 cases of hysteroscopic electroresection of septum in women who had septa and symptoms such as infertility, recurrent pregnancy loss, AUB, and intractable dysmenorrhea. In total, postoperative conceptions were achieved in 51 cases (73%), with the number of spontaneous miscarriage, term pregnancies, and intervals between surgery and conception similar in both groups. For intraoperative complications, uterine perforation occurred in three cases of scissors group and pulmonary edema occurred in one of electroresecting group. The authors

hold that although each technique had their different advantages and more pregnancies were achieved in scissors group, the operator's experience was the most important factor. Vercellini et al. performed TCRS in 23 women, including 12 patients with resectoscope (group 1) and 11 patients with microscissors (group 2). Comparing group 1 and group 2, the mean operating time was 22 ± 6 and 17 ± 5 min ($p = 0.006$), and the mean amount of distension medium used was 890 ± 153 mL and 671 ± 170 mL ($p = 0.003$), respectively. A uterine perforation occurred in one woman with complete uterine septum in group 1 which was managed conservatively. When ultrasonography and hysteroscopy were carried out for follow-up 2 months after operation, residual septa with the depth ≥1 cm were detected and resected repeatedly in four patients of group 1 and two of group 2. It indicated that both methods had the same effectiveness. Assaf indicated that the key points of TCRS were the surgeon's skills and the intraoperative monitoring. Excellent and prudential operation would result in a high postoperative pregnancy rate. In order to avoid the occurrence of cervical insufficiency, the septum in cervical canal was generally preserved during TCRS in women with complete uterine septum. However in 2006, Parsanezhad et al. studied the correlations of resecting the cervical septum during TCRS with intraoperative bleeding, cervical incompetence, and secondary infertility in 28 women who had complete uterine septum and experienced recurrent pregnancy loss or infertility. Patients with resection of intrauterine and cervical septa were included in group A, and patients with preservation of the cervical septum were included in group B. The operating times in two groups were 36.40 ± 10.67 and 73 ± 14.40 min respectively and the irrigation fluid deficit was 456.66 ± 165.68 mL and 673.84 ± 220.36 mL respectively. In group B, pulmonary edema occurred in two cases, excessive bleeding (>150 mL) occurred in 3, and cesarean rate was higher when compared with group A. During follow-up, there was no significant difference in reproductive outcomes between the two groups. The authors insisted that TCRS including the resection of cervical septum was safe and easy, and was worthwhile to recommend in patients with complete uterine septum. Hollett-Caines et al. reported that 26 women who had uterine septum and a history of recurrent pregnancy loss or infertility had hysteroscopic surgery with either bipolar needle or wire loop electrode. Postoperative pregnancy rate was 95% in 19 women who had recurrent pregnancy loss, with the live birth rate 72%. And the pregnancy rate was 43% in seven previous infertile patients, with the live birth rate 29%. It was thought that TCRS using either a monopolar or a bipolar electrode was safe and effective, and could significantly improve the live birth rate. The transcervical uterine incision (TCUI) using a needle electrode can treat the uterine malformations resulting from a narrowed uterine cavity and infertility. Katz et al. reported that T-shaped uteri were diagnosed by HSG and hysteroscopy in eight women with infertility, a history of spontaneous miscarriage, or ectopic pregnancy. All patients were treated by incising bilateral walls hysteroscopically until a normal uterine cavity was achieved without any complications occurred. After operations, four term pregnancies were achieved in 3 women, one ectopic pregnancy was achieved, and no miscarriage happened. The authors pointed out that TCUI could correct a T-shaped uterus, which could improve the reproductive outcome. Serafini et al. performed hysteroscopic metroplasties on two cases for large septate uterus. The first patient performed the operation at the time of oocyte retrieval, and the second at the time of curettage for early spontaneous miscarriage. Both patients had good outcomes and successful pregnancies after hysteroscopic surgery. High level of estrogen was detected in the first case and a history of early miscarriage was in the second case, which would increase intraoperative bleeding and postoperative complications. The authors emphasized that meticulous planning and excellent surgical techniques could obtain success.

3. Treatment of uterine septum coexisting with intrauterine diseases: The intrauterine lesions should be first treated at the time of operation, then the uterine septum is excised, thus a better visual effect of symmetric uterine cavity can be achieved. Sometimes, the uterine septum is first excised, and a single uterine cavity is formed, and then uterine lesions are removed. In 2008, Caliskan et al. first reported a leiomyoma localized in the uterine septum in a 43-year-old woman who experienced primary infertility and menorrhagia, and had uterine septum, double cervix, and a longitudinal vaginal septum. The treatment was arranged into two steps. In the first operation, the patient underwent laparotomy, adhesiolysis, myomectomy, and resection of the vaginal septum, and had TCRS in the second operation. When she conceived after treatment, the cervical length was measured at 26 weeks of gestation and achieved a normal result.

The operator should also pay attention to whether there was the presence of vaginal septum or not when performing TCRS. In 2007, Ziebarth et al. from America reported two cases with delayed diagnosis of partially obstructive Mullerian anomalies. The first 30-year-old woman initially experienced irregular vaginal bleeding, dysmenorrhea, and dyspareunia. On gynecological examination, a bulging mass in vaginal anterior wall with a fistulous duct adjacent to the cervix was recognized. Blood and mucus discharged from the fistulous opening when the speculum compressed the mass. The second 40-year-old nulliparous woman was treated for infertility and dyspareunia, and had a history of transabdominal Strassman's metroplasty. On examination, the vaginal fornix was identified to be bulging, which was diagnosed as oblique vaginal septum by TVS, fistulogram, and HSG.

4. Medical pretreatment prior to TCRS: Romer reported on a comparison of pretreatment with or without a GnRH analog. The results showed no difference in operation time, fluid deficit, the occurrence of complications, the residual of the septum, and the pregnancy outcome. It was suggested that a GnRH-analog pretreatment was not necessary for TCRS, and it could be performed in the proliferative phase of the menstrual cycle.
5. Intraoperative monitoring: Laparoscopy is a good means of monitoring in surgical treatment of symptomatic uterine septum, which can assess accurately the contour of uterine fundus, and clarify the diagnosis of uterine malformations and detect the tubal and peritoneal lesions. Ultrasonography can also be used to monitor the procedure, measure the length and height of septal plate, observe the broadness of the tip and base of septum, and evaluate the uterine fundus at the end of operation.

   Since the uterus is constantly moving during the process of resecting the septum, it is difficult to place the ultrasound scan probe on the same plane with the hysteroscope or resectoscope, and track continuously the operative hysteroscope during the operation. It is also not easy to find certain planes suitable for observation of uterine wall and uterine septum. Nevertheless, when laparoscopy is contraindicated or not suitable for use, the intraoperative ultrasound monitoring can increase the safety of TCRS. Ultrasound can also detect the obviously enlarged ovary or ovarian cysts. But compared with laparoscopy, ultrasound does not have the advantages of simultaneous examination of pelvic structures and management of pelvic lesions.
6. Postoperative treatment of TCRS: Milad and Valle studied whether the postoperative treatment with large dose of estrogen sped up the repair of the endometrium following TCRS. Patients in treatment group were administered postoperative estrogen 5 mg/day for a total of 30 days, while patients in control group were not given any medical treatment. Ultrasonography was conducted every week after operation and the endometrium was assessed in the third week. The results showed that the endometrium was found to be repaired in 2 of 5 cases in treatment group within 1 week after operation, which suggested that the treatment with estrogen after TCRS could accelerate the growth of endometrium. The value of intrauterine placement of an IUD following TCRS is unknown. A second hysteroscopy is done in the second or third month after operation, and the residual septum <1 cm shows no clinical significance.
7. Prophylactic TCRS: Grimbizis et al. believed that TCRS could be applied as a therapeutic procedure to symptomatic women with uterine septum, and it could also be used as a prophylactic procedure in asymptomatic patients, so that it could improve their reproductive outcomes. Patton et al. reported on 16 women who had complete septate uterus, double cervix, and vaginal septum. Of these women, 9 complained of recurrent pregnancy loss and 7 complained of dyspareunia. Procedures were performed hysteroscopically in 11 women and by laparotomy in 5. Before treatment, the rate of pregnancy loss was 81%. After treatment, 17 pregnancies were achieved in 12 women. Three of them miscarriaged in first trimester, with miscarriage rate 18%. Among 12 pregnancies achieved after hysteroscopic surgery, 9 obtained live births (9/12, 75%). Five of 5 women who performed modified Tompkins metroplasty conceived with no miscarriages. Heinonen made a retrospective study and found that septate uterus was not associated with primary infertility, and successful pregnancy may be achieved without surgical treatment.

9.5.8.2 Bicornuate Uterus

In 1996, Pelosi et al. first published a case report on a laparoscopic-assisted transvaginal metroplasty for the treatment of bicornuate uterus. Hysteroscopy was used to illustrate the uterine cavity and reveal both the fundus and the cornua, then laparoscopy was applied by using a monopolar needle to wedge incise the fundus between two cornua. The uterus was taken out through vaginal posterior fornix, integrated by suture and replaced, followed by closure of colpotomy. The patient conceived after operation and achieved a healthy live birth by cesarean section, without any defect detected in uterus. In 2009, Xia et al. first reported in China about uterine metroplasty by combined laparoscopy and hysteroscopy, which could massively restore the contour of the cavity and satisfy the requirement of minimum invasive surgery. Now, the first women who underwent the metroplasty surgery have obtained two healthy girls by two cesarean sections. Another 5 women experienced successful pregnancies and deliveries. Of these women, one underwent cervical cerclage 1 year after metroplasty, followed by successful pregnancy and live birth. In the same year, Alborzi et al. reported on two cases of bicornuate uterus and two cases of duplex uterus who experienced recurrent pregnancy loss. After ascertaining the double cavities hysteroscopically, laparoscopic metroplasty was conducted and good postoperative outcomes were achieved.

9.5.8.3 T-Shaped Uterus

In 1993, Nagel and Malo first reported the outcomes of TCUI in eight cases of uterine malformations who had DES exposure. Postoperative pregnancy and live birth was achieved in

5 women who had initial secondary infertility. However for 3 women who had initial primary infertility, no postoperative conception was obtained. Later, some literatures reported on a decreased miscarriage rate and an increased term delivery rate following TCUI, which reached 87.5% at its highest.

In 2012, Xia et al. from the Hysteroscopy Center of Fuxing Hospital, Capital Medical University first reported the reproductive outcomes of TCUI on 3 women with T-shaped uterus in China, with all women achieving pregnancy and live birth after operation. In varied types of uterine malformations, the term pregnancy rate was the highest following metroplasty of T-shaped uterus (66.7%), followed by complete and partial uterine septum (62.8%), and arcuate uterus (55.6%). These data indicate the effectiveness of hysteroscopic metroplasty of T-shaped uterus. However, TCUI is neither the only treatment for T-shaped uterus, nor the preferred option, and is not recommended to the uterus with the length of cavity less than 4 cm. This is because there may be other factors for infertility, such as implantation, missed miscarriage, preterm delivery, etc. Therefore it is generally recommended to consider cases where uterine constriction ring is the only reason for infertility, failed treatment following diagnosis of infertility, unexplained ART failure, and unexplained recurrent pregnancy loss. There were reports on uterine perforation occurring during TCUI. In 2008, Velemir et al. reported one case of DES intrauterine exposure who experienced uterine rupture at 26 weeks of gestation after TCUI. Moreover, Golan et al. reported that 30% of the patients with uterine malformations had cervical incompetence, with the preterm delivery and late miscarriage decreasing from 50% of cases without cerclage to 21% of cases with cerclage ($P < 0.001$). Kaufman reported that in 537 women who had DES intrauterine exposure, 178 (33%) suffered from cervical disorders. Therefore, in order to improve the effect of treatment, cervical incompetence should be detected following hysteroscopic metroplasty for T-shaped uterus, and prophylactic cerclage or urgent cerclage in symptomatic cases may be conducted. In Xia et al.'s report, 3 women who underwent TCUI for T-shaped uterus did neither apply prophylactic cerclage, nor monitor the changes of cervical internal os during pregnancy. They all achieved pregnancy to term.

9.5.8.4 Unicornuate Uterus

There are few reports on treatment for women with unicornuate uterus and infertility. Markham and Waterhouse indicated that the efficacy of hysteroscopic metroplasty for double uterus, bicornuate uterus, and unicornuate uterus was uncertain in reproductive outcomes, except for septate uterus. Xia et al. from the Hysteroscopy Center of Fuxing Hospital, Capital Medical University, first reported in China successful pregnancies achieved in 3 women who underwent hysteroscopic metroplasty for unicornuate uterus. All women had no other reasons for infertility and conceived at the eighth, fifth, and third month following TCUI respectively under ultrasound/laparoscopic monitoring. One woman was preoperatively misdiagnosed as intrauterine adhesions because diagnostic hysteroscopy just revealed one cornu, and was diagnosed as right unicornuate uterus when undergoing combined operations of laparoscopy and hysteroscopy. She conceived 8 months after operation and miscarriaged at 20 weeks of gestation because of cervical incompetence.

There were several reports indicating that for women with unicornuate uterus and a history of miscarriage in second trimester of pregnancy, cervical cerclage could increase the fetus live birth rate. Golan et al. reported that cervical cerclage could decrease the preterm delivery and late miscarriage rates, with significant difference ($P < 0.001$). Abramovici et al. pointed out that the cervix contained more muscle tissues and less connective tissues in women with uterine malformations, which is inadequate to resist the increased asymmetric intrauterine pressure in the third trimester of pregnancy, leading to miscarriage and preterm delivery. In their study, 15 women who had uterine malformations and experienced recurrent pregnancy loss received cervical suture at the 11th or 12th week of gestation. All women had no clinical or radiological signs of cervical incompetence, and did not undergo any correction surgery for uterine malformations. After cervical operation, 13 women obtained term delivery and two experienced preterm delivery, with all infants alive. The authors suggested that in women who suffered from infertility for uterine malformation, although the evidence of cervical incompetence is absent, before considering the surgical correction, cervical cerclage is recommended to prolong the gestational weeks and increase the fetus live birth rate. Transvaginal ultrasonography had been reported to accurately predict preterm labor, but had not been well studied in women with uterine malformations. Airoldi et al. prospectively applied transvaginal ultrasonography to evaluate the cervix at the 14th to 23rd gestational weeks in women with uterine malformations, with a short cervix defined as the length <2.5 cm. The results showed that the rates of cervical shortening and preterm birth were the highest in pregnant women with unicornuate uterus. So, for treatment of unicornuate uterus, cervical incompetence should also be considered.

9.5.8.5 Robert Uterus

Dr. Xia from the Hysteroscopy Center of Fuxing Hospital, Capital Medical University, had treated a 28-year-old woman with progressive dysmenorrhea after menarche at 14 years old. She married 2 years after left cystectomy for chocolate cyst and salpingectomy and experienced infertility. Investigation by HSG suggested right tubal blockage, with no treatment followed. After two failed IVF treatments, laparoscopic adhesiolysis, diathermy of endometriosis, and patency test were performed with the result being normal contour of uterus and right tubal patency. She conceived 3 months later and underwent curettage for bleeding and inevitable miscarriage at 2 months of gestation, and then had hysteroscopic resection of Robert septum 4 days later. The patient got pregnant again 5 months after hysteroscopic operation, and delivered a healthy girl at 39 weeks and 5 days of gestation by cesarean section, with the weight of newborn 3500 g. This is a typical case of Robert uterus, with left cavity obstruction. From adolescence to fertility age, the patient experienced the symptoms and the process of diagnosis and treatment including dysmenorrhea, left hematosalpinx, left ovarian chocolate cyst, pelvic adhesions, IVF failure, spontaneous pregnancy, and miscarriage. Therefore, hysteroscopic resection of Robert uterus is effective with minimal invasion, has an easy recovery, has no scars, and is in favor of postoperative conception.

9.5.8.6 Arcuate Uterus

Gergolet et al. carried out a prospective study to compare the outcome of hysteroscopic metroplasty on septate uterus and arcuate uterus. Preoperative miscarriage rates in both groups were high, which significantly decreased after operation, and were similar postoperatively between the two groups (14% in septate uterus and 11% in arcuate uterus). Therefore it was concluded that the pre- and postoperative reproductive outcomes of hysteroscopic metroplasty in arcuate uterus were similar to those in septate uterus.

9.6 Transcervical Resection of Intrauterine Adhesions

Dan Yu

Intrauterine adhesion (IUA) refers to the formation of endometrial fibrosis or adhesive band, resulting from the damage to the basal layer of endometrium, which is mostly following the trauma to a gravid or non-gravid uterus. It is known that trauma to a gravid uterine cavity was the main cause of IUA. Such trauma could be induced by uterine curettage due to excessive bleeding 1–4 weeks postpartum or after miscarriage. During this vulnerable phase, the basal layer of endometrium is easily damaged by any trauma, which promotes the uterine walls adhering to each other and leads to the formation of permanent adhesions, the distortion of uterine cavity, and the absence of its symmetry. Secondly, trauma to a non-gravid endometrium can also result in IUA. It was reported that IUAs may occur after diagnostic curettage, abdominal myomectomy, cervical biopsy, endometrial polypectomy, intrauterine placement of IUD, or the treatment with radium. In addition, IUAs may also happen following various hysteroscopic procedures, such as hysteroscopic myomectomy or resection of uterine septum. In rare circumstances, IUAs may be induced by uterine artery embolization or occlusion.

Patients with IUAs are always present with menstrual abnormalities, including hypomenorrhea and amenorrhea. When cervical internal os is mechanically obstructed, secondary amenorrhea will occur, which leads to periodic abdominal discomfort or pain, hematometra, and even hematosalpinx. IUAs may also cause infertility. Pregnancy for these patients may result in spontaneous miscarriage, recurrent pregnancy loss, preterm delivery, placenta accreta, ectopic pregnancy, etc. Moreover, there are few case reports on intrauterine growth restriction (IUGR) in pregnant women with IUA.

IUAs are classified as endometrial adhesions, fibromuscular adhesions, and connective tissue adhesions according to its characteristics, and as central and marginal adhesions according to its location. The severity of IUAs is divided into several grades on the basis of the findings of HSG and diagnostic hysteroscopy (see Chap. 8, Sect. 8.2). At present, the most widely used classification of IUAs in the world is the classification system proposed by American Fertility Society (AFS) in 1988 and the classification system established by European Society of Gynecological Endoscopy (ESGE) in 1995.

Ultrasonography (US), three-dimensional ultrasonography (3D-US), sonohysterography (SHG), hysterosalpingography (HSG), magnetic resonance imaging (MRI), and diagnostic hysteroscopy are commonly used investigations for diagnosis of IUA. Before the advent of hysteroscopy, HSG was the first-line investigation to reveal the contour of the uterine cavity. HSG can illustrate the areas of adhesive occlusion, display the special filling defects, and even provide assessments of uterine cornua, tubal contours, and tubal patency. Ultrasonography has been used to diagnose fibrosis of endometrium or adhesions in uterine cavity, and display the uterine cavity which cannot be detected by HSG or hysteroscopy, so it is now commonly used in preliminary screening of IUAs. MRI has also been used to investigate IUAs, especially in patients who have difficulties to be diagnosed hysteroscopically or have total atresia of the cervical canal. Diagnostic hysteroscopy can reveal the intrauterine adhesions under direct vision, confirming the extent and the degree of adhesions and determining the quality of the endometrium, which permit the diagnosis of IUAs more accurately. Therefore, diagnostic hysteroscopy has been considered as the gold standard for diagnosis of IUAs.

IUAs can be treated by surgical division or resection of adhesions. In the past, blind division of adhesions has been carried out with curettes, probes, or dilators. Such treatment of blind division of adhesions cannot bring about a satisfying clinical result, and the postoperative reproductive outcome is disappointing. Moreover, hysterotomy with division of adhesions under direct vision has been attempted and described. However, this technique has failed to produce acceptable postoperative outcomes and has been mostly abandoned. The current standard method for treatment of IUA is transcervical resection of intrauterine adhesions (TCRA). It can enable dividing or dissecting intrauterine adhesions under direct vision, which helps to restore normal menstruation after treatment, and improves the outcomes of pregnancy and delivery. It involves not only restoring the shape of uterine cavity via hysteroscopic surgery, but also enhancing the repair and regeneration of endometrium by various methods to prevent reformation of adhesions.

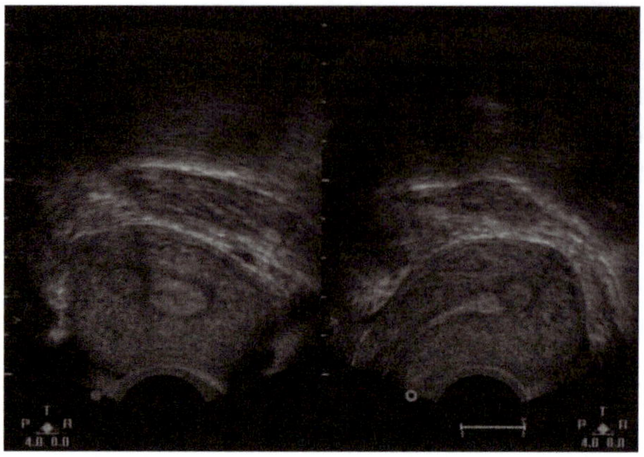

Fig. 9.141 Transvaginal ultrasound scanning of uterus. It shows that the uterus is in a retroverted position and 45 mm × 53 mm × 40 mm in size. The myometrial echotexture is homogeneous. The endometrium is isoechogenic and in midline with its thickness 8 mm and the continuity interrupted. These appearances suggest the diagnosis as intrauterine adhesions

9.6.1 Operative Indications and Contraindications

9.6.1.1 Indications

Any conditions in association with IUA, such as abnormal menstruation, dysmenorrheal, infertility, and pregnancy failure, are operative indications. And the following conditions should be considered as well:

1. Histological examination of endometrial biopsy shows no malignancy.
2. The size of uterus ≤9 weeks of gestation, and the length of cavity ≤12 cm.

9.6.1.2 Contraindications

1. Cervical canal cannot be fully dilated because of cervical scarring.
2. The hysteroscope cannot reach the fundus due to extreme bending of the uterus.
3. The acute stage of genital tract infections.
4. The acute period of organ failure which includes heart, liver, and kidney.

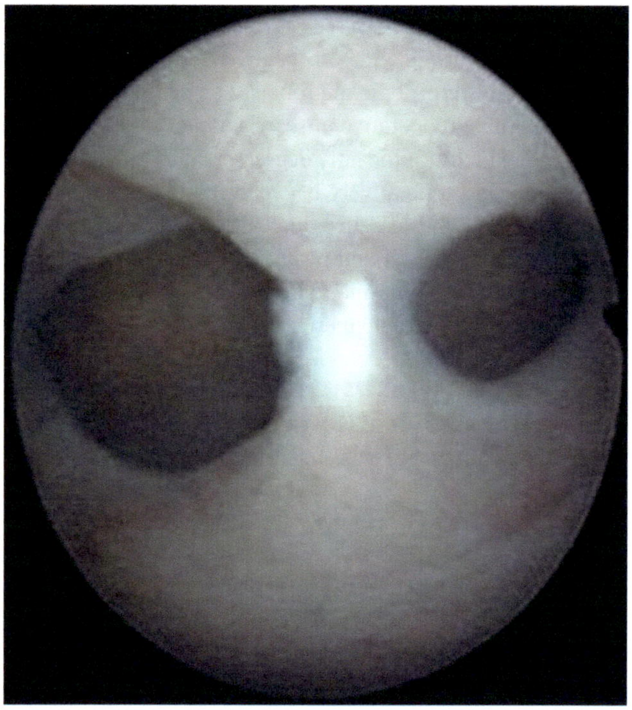

Fig. 9.142 Inspection of uterine cavity under hysteroscopy. It shows an abnormal cavity. An adhesive band is seen in the middle part of the cavity, which is cylindrical, located slightly to the left, and connects the anterior and posterior walls of the uterus. These appearances suggest the diagnosis as intrauterine adhesions (central)

9.6.2 Preoperative Preparations

1. Preoperative preparations include the inquiry of a detailed history and the assessments of comprehensive examinations before hysteroscopic adhesiolysis. Ultrasonography can help to evaluate the size, shape, location, and echoes of the uterus, and to investigate the direction of the uterine lines, thickness of the endometrium, and pelvic masses of adnexa (Fig. 9.141). Diagnostic hysteroscopy permits the inspection of the shape of uterine cavity, the characteristic of endometrium, and the degree of adhesions, as well as any other occupying lesions. Histological biopsy under direct vision can be performed simultaneously to exclude malignant lesions (Fig. 9.142).
2. In general, the ideal time for operation is in the early proliferative phase of the menstrual cycle. A cervical osmotic dilator or a laminaria tent should be inserted into the cervical canal on the night before operation. When insertion of a tent is difficult or the uterine cavity is fully occluded, a 400 μg misoprostol tablet can be inserted into the posterior fornix of the vagina.

3. On the morning of operation, the patient should have fasted and held in urine so as to facilitate ultrasound monitoring during the surgical procedure. Prior to operation, the operator should make ready all instruments and devices which will be used in surgical procedures, and make sure they are in good conditions. The patient is placed in lithotomy position. Operating area is disinfected and the osmotic dilator is removed if it has been used.

9.6.3 Anesthesia

The choice of anesthesia for hysteroscopic adhesiolysis depends on the type and duration of the operation. Hysteroscopic lysis for mild adhesions may apply intravenous anesthesia because of the short operating time. Epidural anesthesia can be considered in patients who have contraindications of intravenous anesthesia or need to have more complex procedures. General anesthesia can be chosen in patients who have to have very difficult procedures resulting in the possibility of pelvic organ injury, or in patients who have laparoscopic monitoring / laparoscopic surgery simultaneously with hysteroscopy.

9.6.4 Surgical Procedures

9.6.4.1 Transcervical Resection of Intrauterine Adhesions (TCRA)

Surgical procedures of TCRA vary on the basis of severity and location of IUAs. Filmy and loose adhesions may be mechanically divided with the sheath of the hysteroscope. Dense and firm adhesions can be dissected hysteroscopically. The principles of the surgery are to restore a normal uterine cavity, to reveal bilateral uterine cornua and fallopian tubal ostia, and to reduce the damage to the residual endometrium. Extensive intrauterine adhesions may not be completely divided by the primary operation, and need multiple procedures. The detailed procedures are as follows:

1. Firstly, fill the bladder moderately, scan the uterus with transabdominal ultrasonography, insert the probe carefully, and then dilate the cervix gradually with Hegar dilators. If the probe cannot approach the fundus due to cervical atresia, or the probe can only reach into the cervical canal, the adhesions could be divided by hysteroscopic surgery afterwards. Alternatively, a probe could be pushed ahead harder along the midline of cervix and uterus to reach the fundus under the guidance of ultrasonography (Fig. 9.143).
2. With ultrasound guidance, the hysteroscope is inserted into uterine cavity through cervical os and cervical canal. The shapes of cervical canal and uterine cavity, the conditions of bilateral uterine cornua and tubal ostia, and the characteristics of adhesions are all observed under direct vision (Figs. 9.144 and 9.145).
3. New and loose endometrial adhesions in either cervical canal or uterine cavity can be divided mechanically by pushing forward the sheath tip of the hysteroscope (Fig. 9.146).

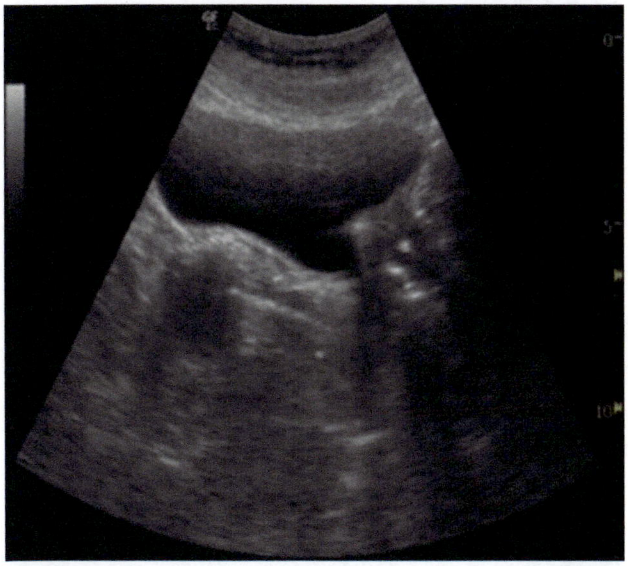

Fig. 9.143 After filling the bladder, sound the cavity using a probe under ultrasound monitoring. When the probe cannot reach the fundus, ultrasonography would guide the probe going forward

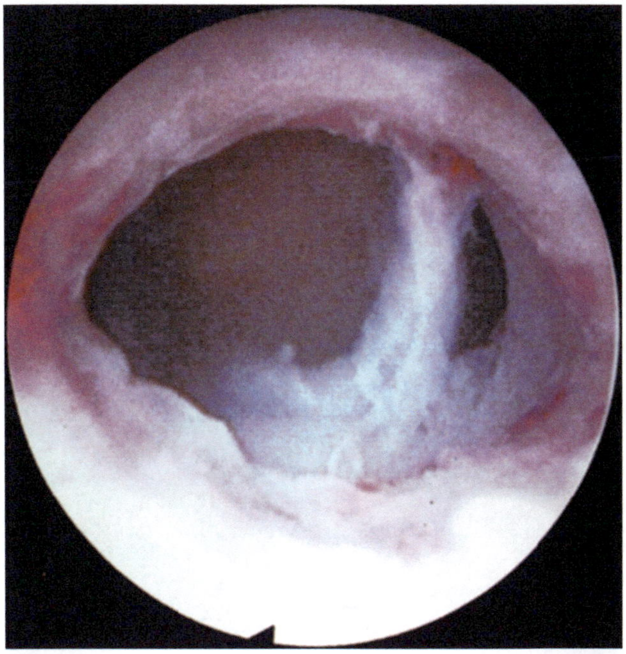

Fig. 9.144 Visualization of intrauterine endometrial adhesive band under hysteroscopy

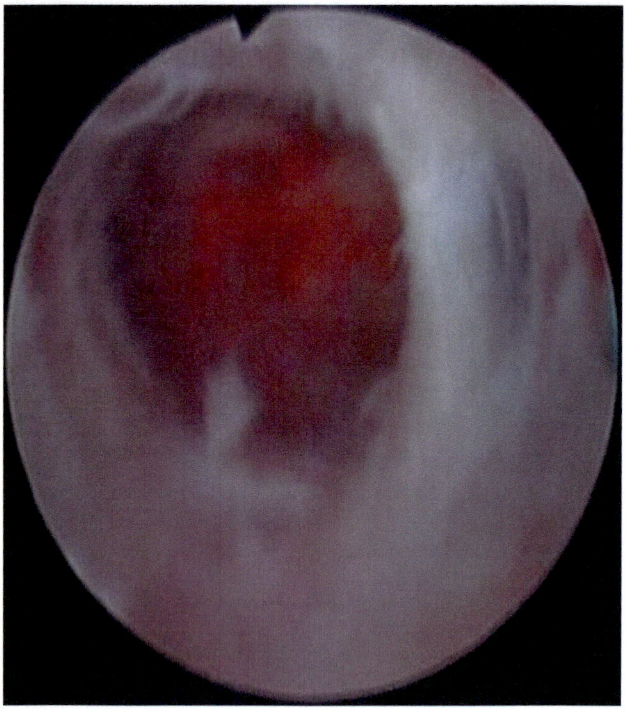

Fig. 9.145 Visualization of intrauterine scar tissues under hysteroscopy

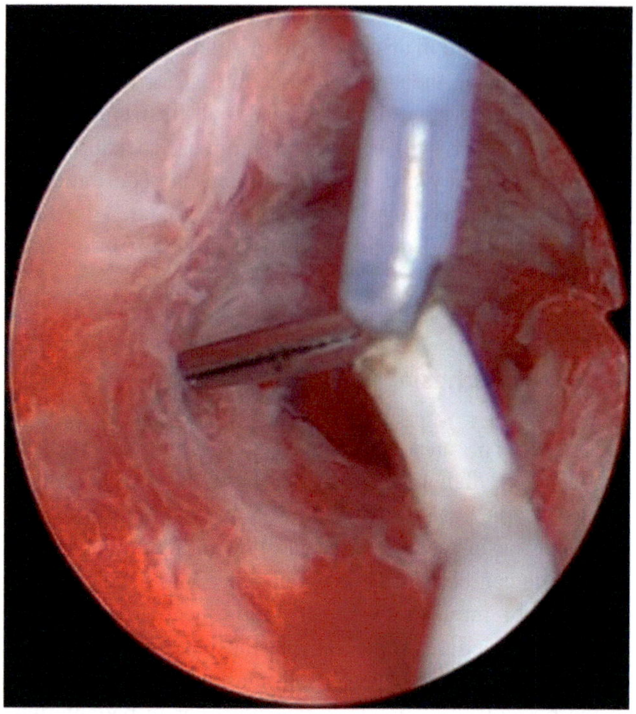

Fig. 9.147 Adhesive scar tissue in cervical canal is divided by hysteroscopic needle electrode

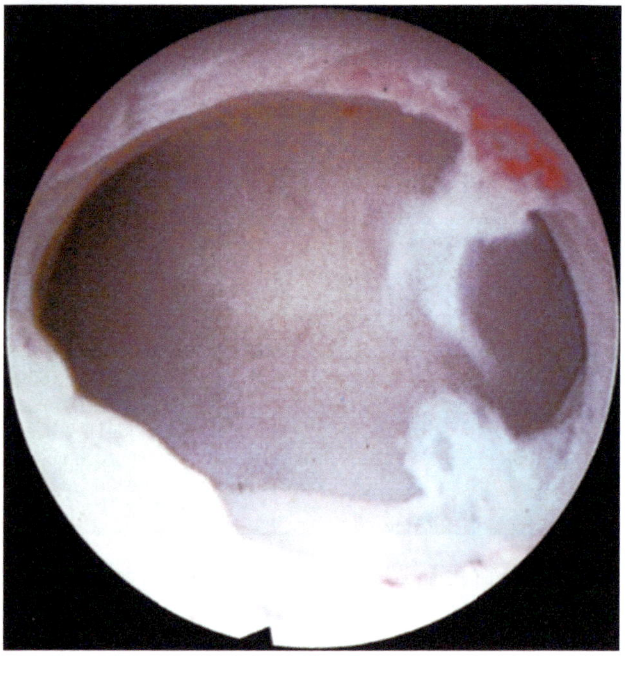

Fig. 9.146 Intrauterine adhesive band is divided mechanically by the sheath tip of the hysteroscope

4. Dense fibrous adhesions in cervical canal can be divided by needle electrode or dissected by wire loop electrode of hysteroscopic resectoscope (Fig. 9.147).
5. Extensive adhesions at fundus can be transversely divided by needle electrode or transversely resected by wire loop electrode, both of which move towards the cornua and completely open the fundus (Fig. 9.148a, b).
6. Procedures of hysteroscopic adhesiolysis try to open bilateral cornua and reveal both tubal ostia. In general, the adhesive bands at cornua are divided by needle electrode under ultrasound monitoring. If it is necessary, cutting loop could be used to resect adhesion tissues as a supplementary method. At the end of procedures, bilateral cornua and both tubal ostia can be seen, and normal shapes of bilateral cornua are restored (Figs. 9.149a–d and 9.150a–d). Moreover, it is important to protect normal endometrium at the area of both cornua.
7. Central fibrous scar tissues in uterine cavity can be excised by hysteroscopic cutting wire loop electrode (Fig. 9.151). Dense central fibrous scar tissues can also be divided by hysteroscopic needle electrode (Fig. 9.152).
8. Scar tissues at anterior, posterior, and bilateral walls of uterine cavity may be incised along longitudinal axis of uterus by needle electrode. They could also be excised by cutting loop if necessary (Figs. 9.153a, b and 9.154a–c).
9. For patients who have a narrowed cavity coming from constricting scars of uterine walls, needle electrode can be used to incise the scar tissues longitudinally 4–5

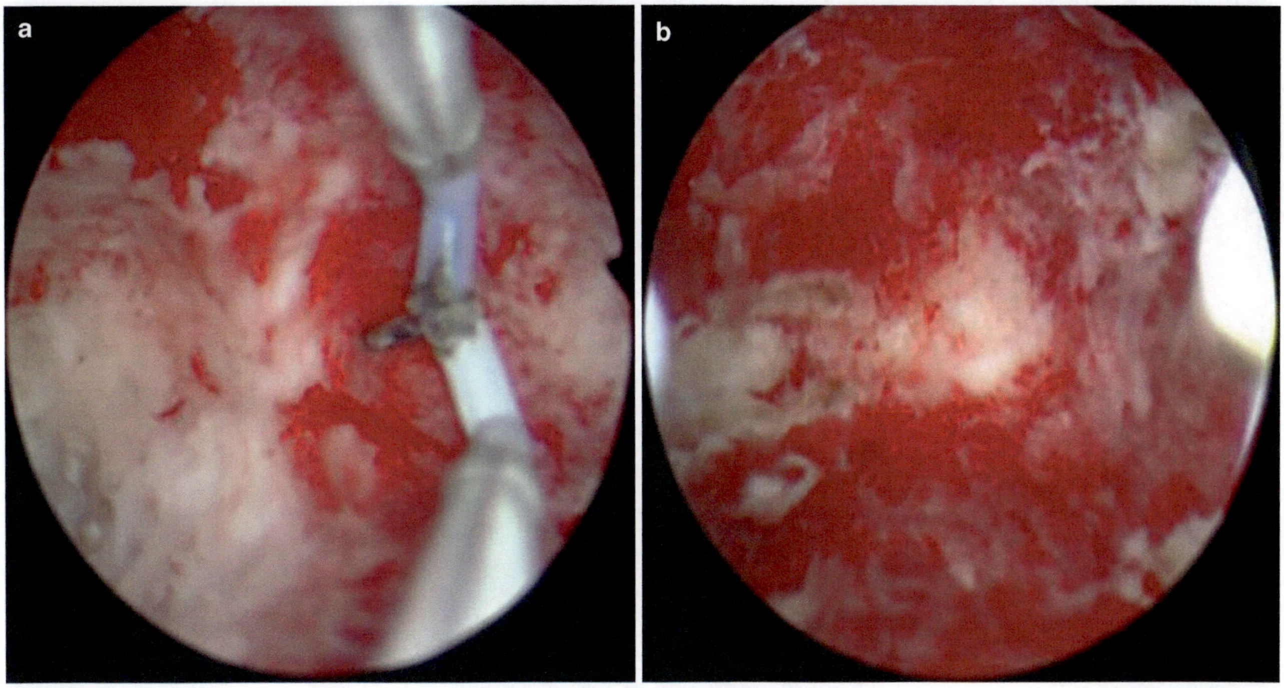

Fig. 9.148 (**a**) Vertical adhesive bands at fundus are transversely divided by hysteroscopic needle electrode. (**b**) All adhesions at fundus are divided by hysteroscopy

times along the long axis of uterus to increase the volume of cavity (Fig. 9.155a–c).

10. In patients with atresia of the uterine cavity, a blind end may be seen in front of the hysteroscope. The operation on these patients should be performed under ultrasound guidance, by pushing gently forwards either the electrified needle electrode or the wire loop electrode along the midline of cervix and uterus. This is to excise some adhesions, cut to open holes, and reveal the uterine cavity (Fig. 9.156a–c). Afterwards, intrauterine adhesions are removed following procedures mentioned above until a normal uterine cavity is achieved (Fig. 9.157).
11. When the procedure is about to end, the resectoscope should be retracted back to the level of cervical internal os and the shape and symmetry of uterine cavity are observed (Fig. 9.158).
12. In patients who take laparoscopic monitoring, methylene blue solution could be injected into the uterine cavity to test the fallopian tubal patency, which can be observed under laparoscope (Fig. 9.159).

9.6.4.2 Hysteroscopic Lysis of Adhesions with Scissors

Many gynecologists like to use hysteroscopic scissors to cut intrauterine adhesions mechanically.

1. The operating method is similar to that of TCRS. The division of adhesions is made from the central of the cavity by using flexible semi-rigid or rigid scissors, so that the cavity can be broadened. In cases of total atresia of uterine cavity, cutting starts at cervical internal os and moves towards the cavity gradually to approach the fundus and bilateral cornua, until a newly formed cavity is achieved (Fig. 9.160a–d).
2. The advantages of hysteroscopic surgery with scissors are:
   (a) It cuts adhesions mechanically, which provides excellent view of adhesions, especially those close to the myometrium. Bleeding might be observed when the cutting reaches the myometrium, which alerts the surgeon to stop further cutting so as to avoid perforation.
   (b) In cases with extensive adhesions, there will be little normal and healthy endometrium, and it will be very important to preserve it. The dissection with scissors may not lead to either the formation of scar tissue or the destruction of normal endometrium produced by resection with electricity or laser. Therefore operations with scissors can maximum preserve the endometrium.
3. The disadvantages of hysteroscopic surgery with scissors are:
   (a) Hysteroscopic lysis of adhesions with scissors may use electrolyte solution as irrigation medium. Wide and denuded surfaces promote the absorption of irrigation medium due to the adhesions being close

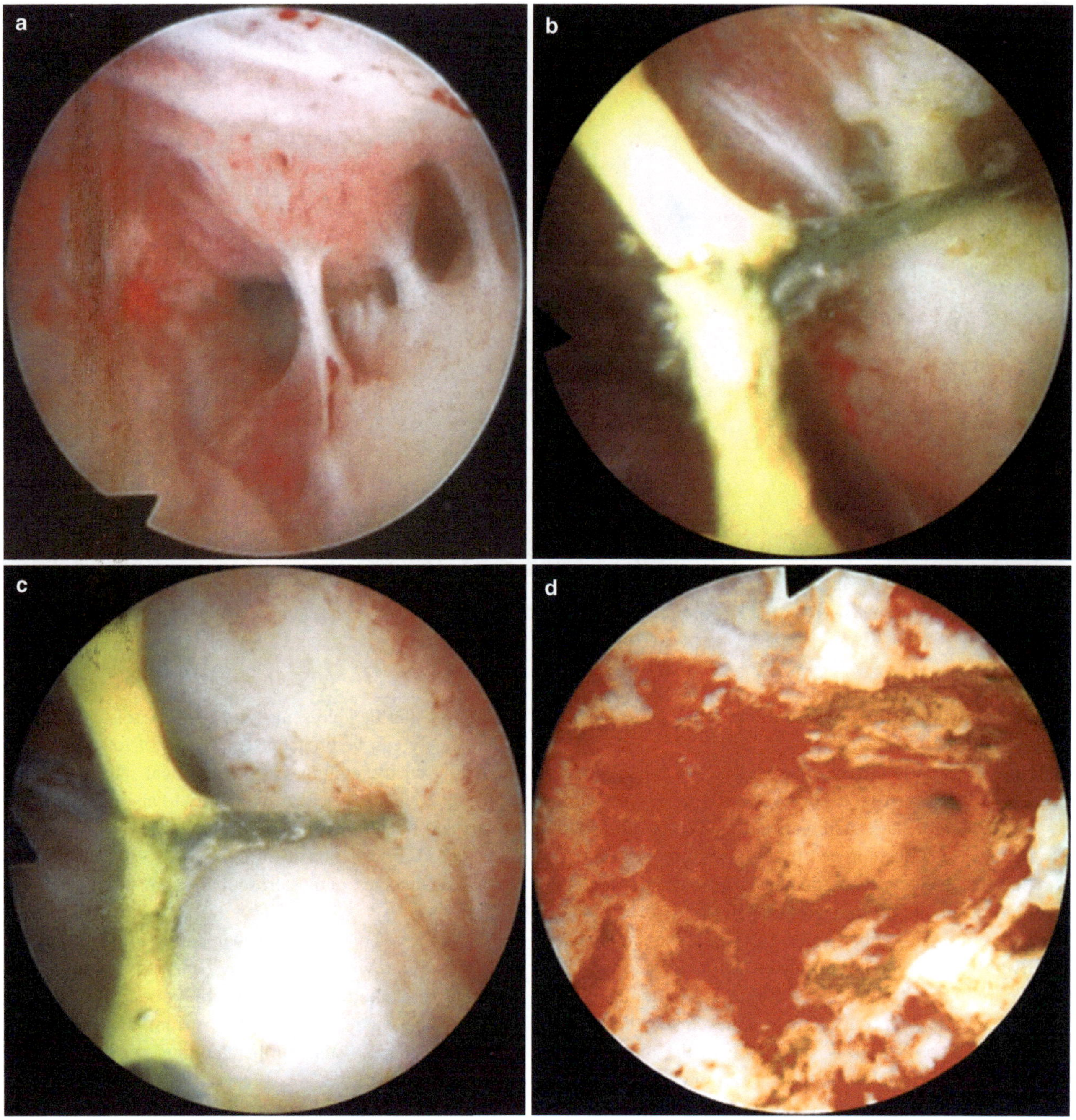

Fig. 9.149 Lysis of adhesions on left cornu. (**a**) Left cornu and uterine wall are visible under hysteroscope, with multiple cylindrical adhesions seen. (**b**) Cylindrical adhesions at left cornu are divided by hysteroscopic needle electrode. (**c**) Scar tissues on the left wall are divided by hysteroscopic needle electrode. (**d**) Left cornu is opened under hysteroscopy, with left tubal ostium visible

to the myometrium. As a result, the probability of fluid overload will increase. Hence distention pressure during operation should be lower than the mean artery pressure (MAP) to avoid fluid overload.

(b) It is sometimes difficult to manipulate the semi-rigid scissors, especially when cutting the adhesions on the posterior walls.

(c) If the scissors are not sharp enough, it would be hard to cut the adhesions.

9.6.4.3 Lysis of Adhesions with Fiber Optic Lasers

Lysis of adhesions with fiber optic lasers is easy to manipulate, but may take longer time than dissection with scissors or resection with electrodes. Furthermore, it is too expensive to be used widely.

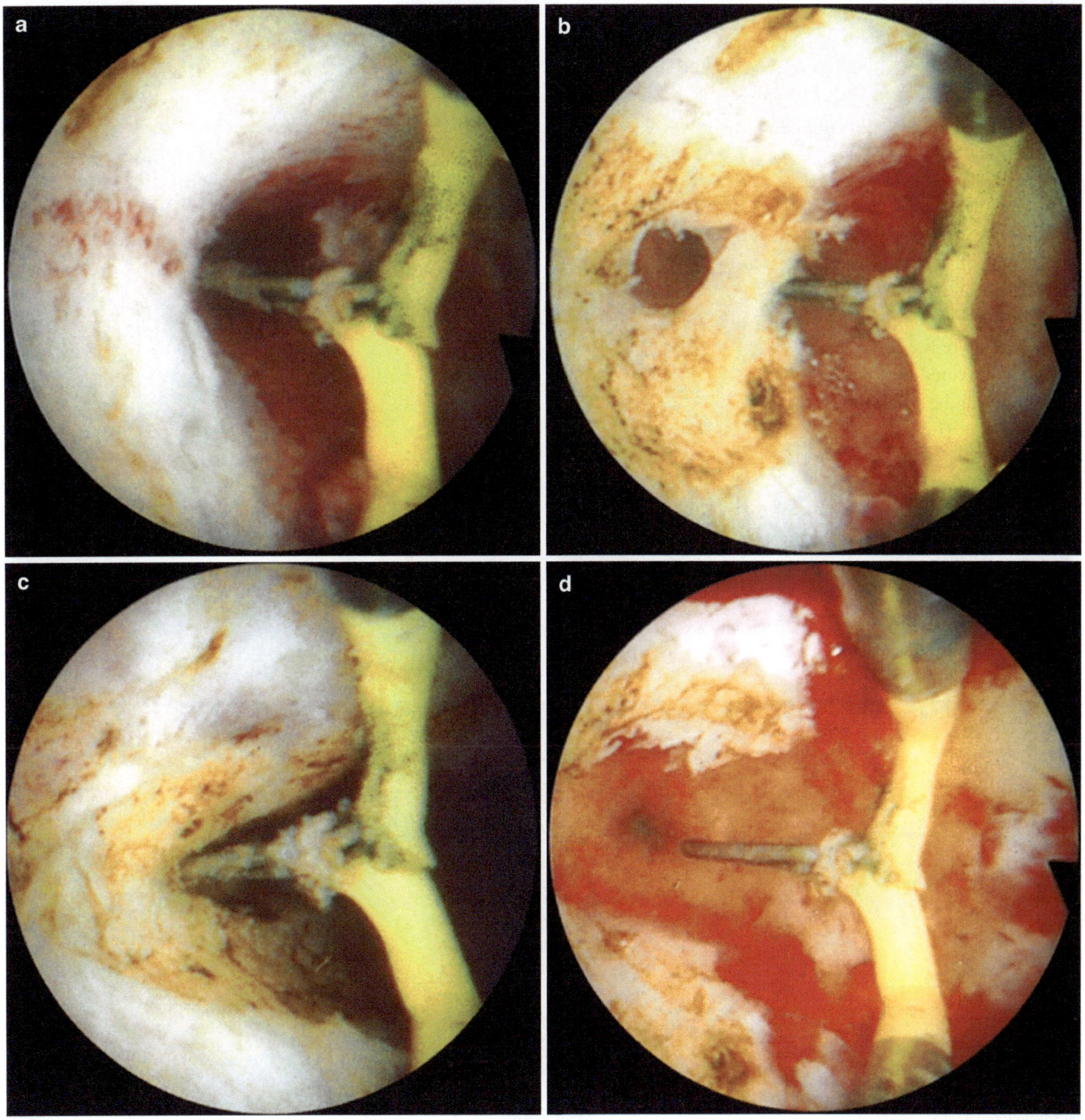

Fig. 9.150 (**a–c**) Adhesions at right cornu are divided by hysteroscopic needle electrode. (**d**) Right cornu is opened under hysteroscopy, with right tubal ostium visible

9.6.5 Intraoperative Complicated Conditions and Cautions

1. Patients with moderate or severe intrauterine adhesions have badly distorted cavities and contracted uterine walls, with the occlusion in cervical canal or middle/lower part of uterine cavity. When hysteroscopic operations are performed in these cases, it is difficult to either distinguish the anatomic structures of cervix and uterine cavity, or determine the direction of resections. Due to difficult procedures, the risks of false passage or uterine perforation during operations are increased. Therefore, monitoring with transabdominal ultrasonography or laparoscopy is necessary in these operations. Under ultrasound guidance, division of adhesions is guided along the midline of cervix and uterus so as to reveal the cavity by hysteroscopic resectoscope. The thicknesses of uterine walls, including fundus, anterior/posterior walls, and bilateral

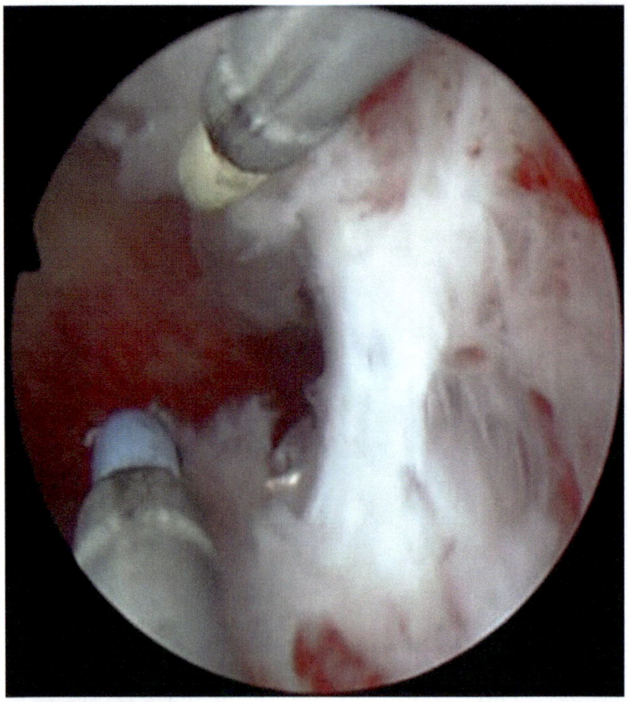

Fig. 9.151 Fibrous scar tissues in uterine cavity are excised by hysteroscopic wire loop electrode

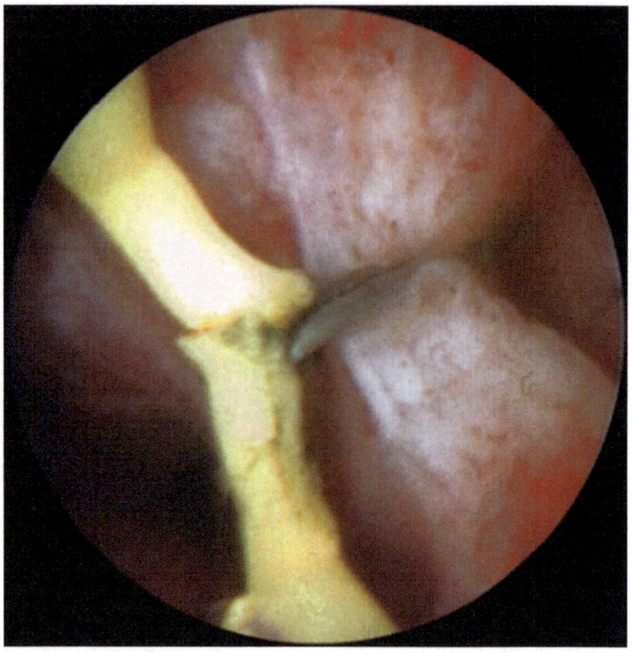

Fig. 9.152 Fibrous scar tissues in uterine cavity are divided by hysteroscopic needle electrode

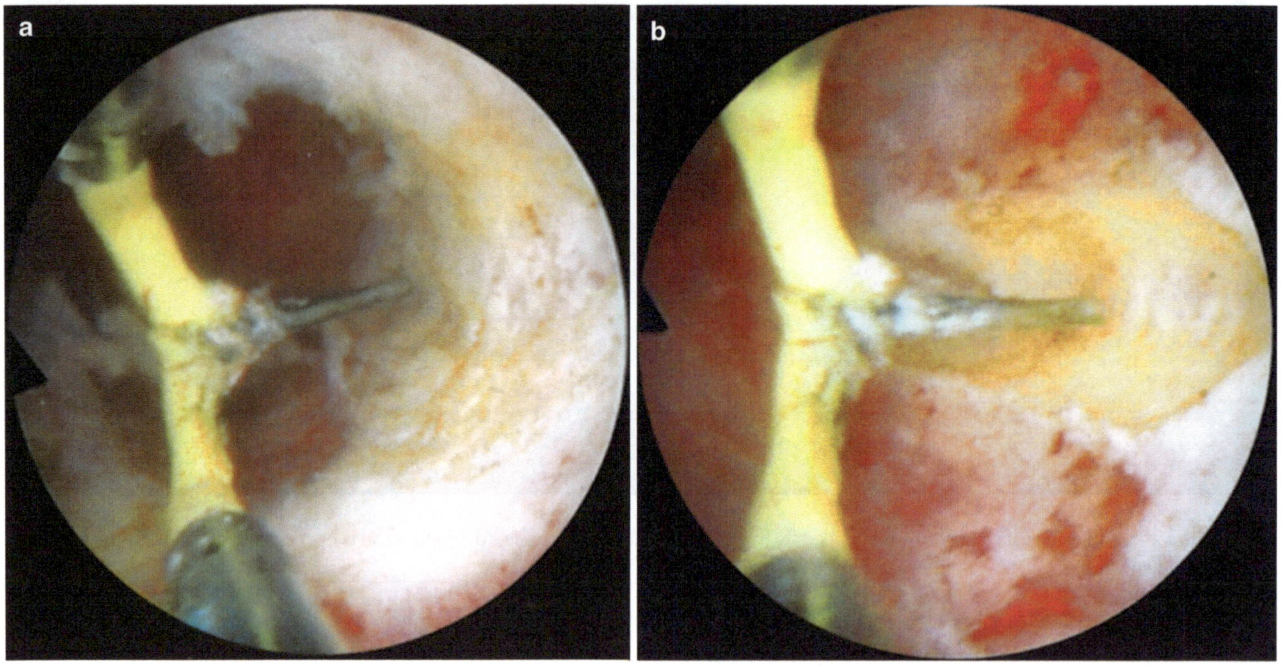

Fig. 9.153 (a, b) Scar tissues on left lateral wall are divided longitudinally by hysteroscopic needle electrode

walls are observed with ultrasonography or laparoscopy to avoid the creation of false passage and occurrence of perforation.

2. In a patient who had a history of multiple operations in uterine cavity, the uterus may have previous false passage or perforation, and the hysteroscope can easily enter into the false passage. Moreover, the possibility of creating a perforation again in this situation is increased because it is difficult to distinguish the anatomic structure in uterine cavity (Figs. 9.161 and 9.162). The procedures of hys-

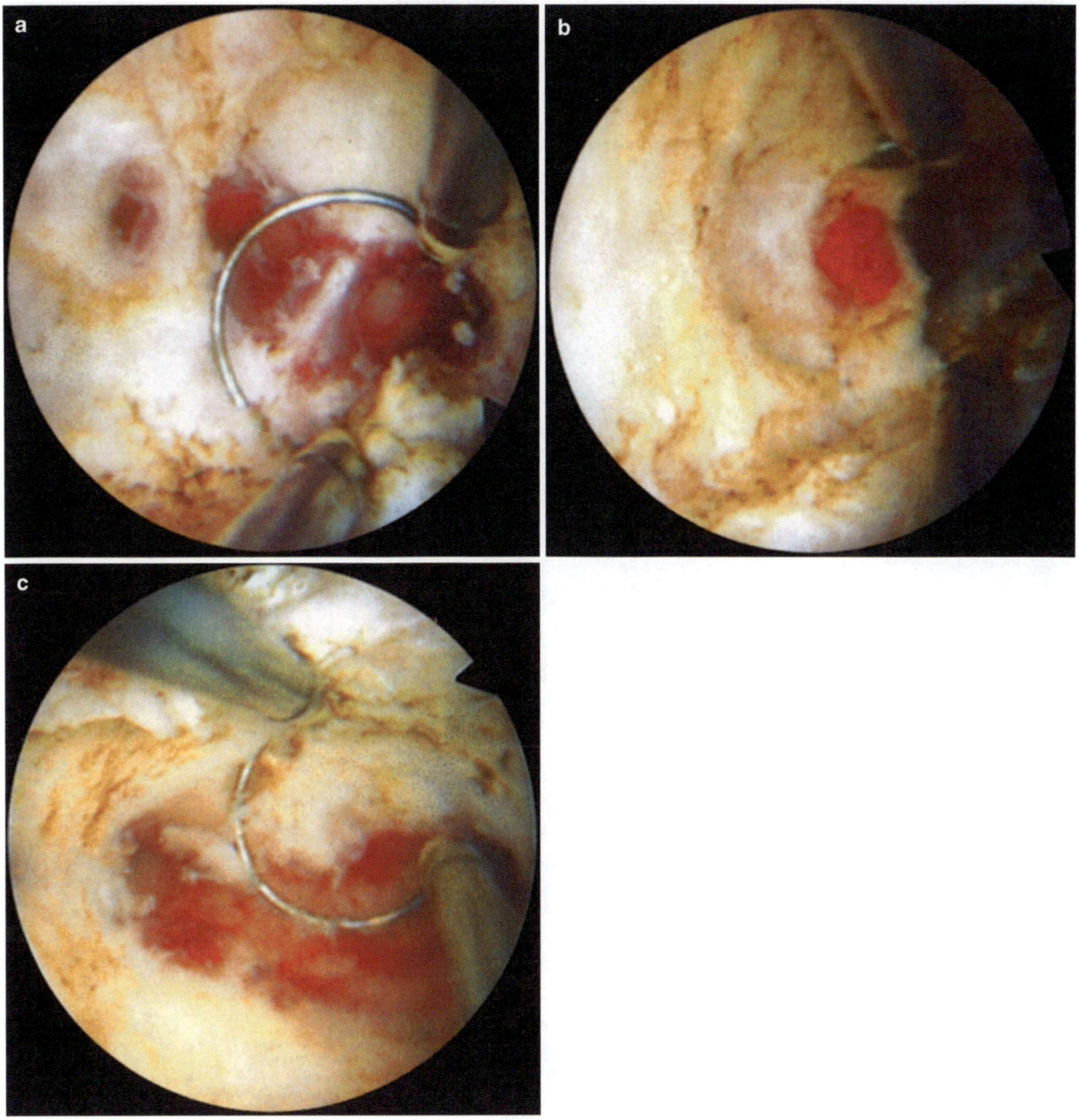

Fig. 9.154 (a–c) Adhesions on right lateral wall are resected by hysteroscopic wire loop electrode

teroscopic lysis of adhesions in these cases need to be monitored by laparoscopy or ultrasonography in order to detect the integrity of uterine serosa and the thickness of uterine walls. This can help to observe the shape of the cavity and to distinguish the scar tissues from normal endometrium or myometrium.

3. Sometimes it is difficult to recognize the borderline between fibromuscular adhesions and uterine myometrium. Therefore we should pay attention to the depth and the extent of incision during procedures to avoid the damage to normal myometrium. In general, intrauterine adhesions are avascular. There might be bleeding from small vessels when cutting approaches the myometrium, which can be stopped by electric coagulation, and should be considered as a warning of stopping resection.
4. It is necessary to protect the normal endometrium during operations, and to avoid the formation of scar tissues and the damage to the adjacent normal endometrium which are caused by energy sources.

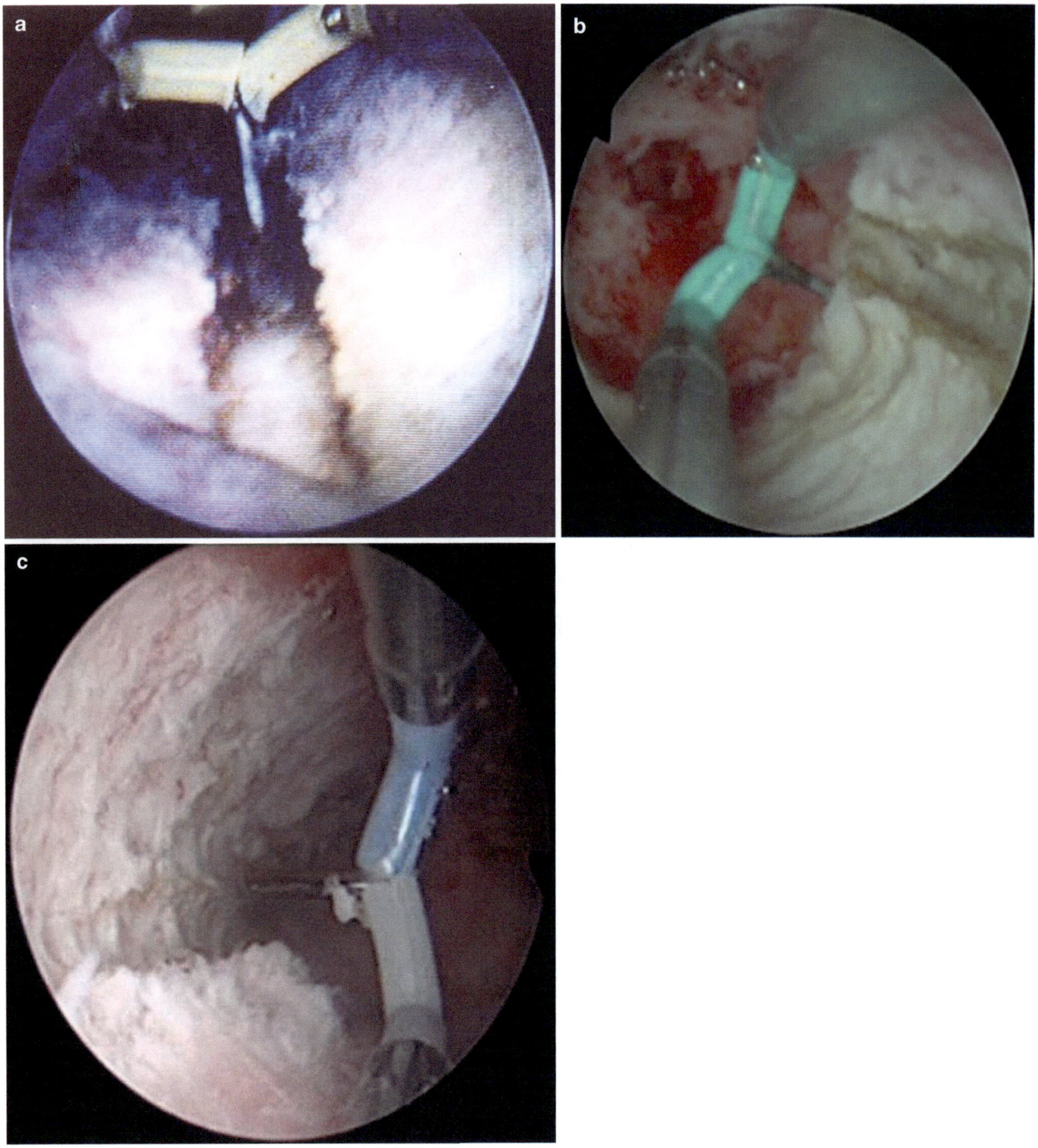

Fig. 9.155 (**a–c**) Scar tissues in uterine walls are incised longitudinally along the long axis of uterus by hysteroscopic needle electrode

9.6.6 Intraoperative Monitoring

The uterine cavity is distorted and narrowed in patients with intrauterine adhesions, especially those with an occluded cavity. It leads to a great difficulty in operations and is prone to uterine perforation, therefore intraoperative monitoring with laparoscopy and ultrasonography should be conducted.

9.6.6.1 Ultrasonography

Compared to other types of hysteroscopic operations, hysteroscopic adhesiolysis is a procedure with a lower rate of success and higher risk of complications, especially in cases with moderate or severe adhesions. Transabdominal ultrasound monitoring can be taken to increase the successful rate and its safety. By a retrospective study, Kresowik et al. found

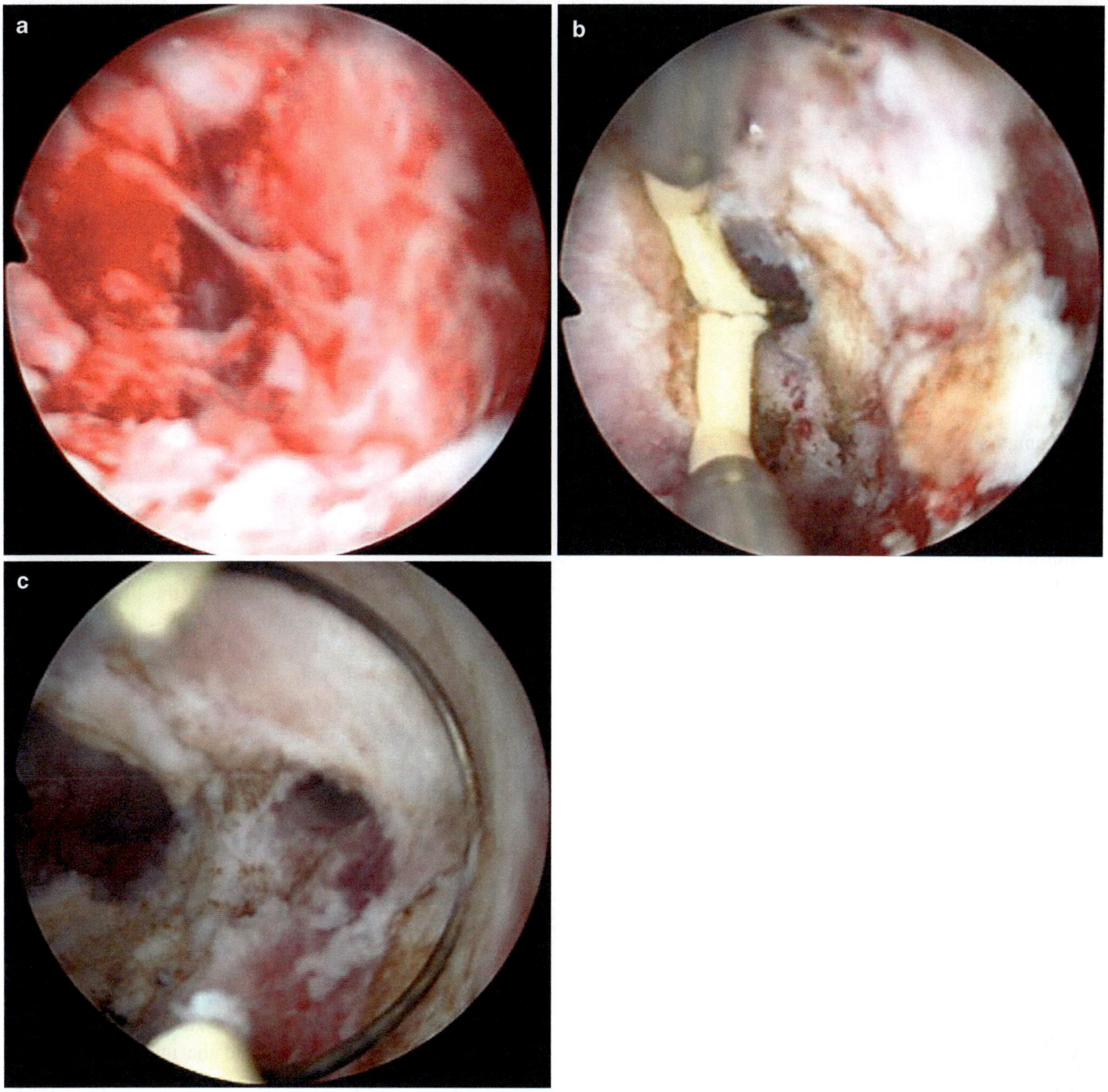

Fig. 9.156 Lysis of adhesions in an atresia uterus. (**a**) A blind end and irregular adhesive bands are visible under hysteroscope. (**b**) Under ultrasound guidance, hysteroscopic needle electrode divides the adhesions along midline of uterus and then a hole is visible. (**c**) Hysteroscopic wire loop electrode is used to excise the adhesions and gradually reveals the cavity

that monitoring with transabdominal ultrasonography could decrease the perforation rate of the uterus and be an ideal method for monitoring the lysis of adhesions.

Transabdominal ultrasound monitoring of hysteroscopic operations may guide the direction of probe or hysteroscope, observe the depth of incision, monitor the process of procedures, alert the surgeon to stop operations, and prevent occurrence of uterine perforations. Thus it can greatly increase the success rate and decrease the complications.

1. At the beginning of the procedure, a comprehensive scan is taken to understand the position and size of uterus, as well as the location of adhesions, with the help of the images under hysteroscope (Fig. 9.163a, b).
2. Under ultrasound monitoring, the wire loop is firstly put in a right place, activated, and then the adhesions are excised after determining the extent of resection and being guaranteed by ultrasonography (Fig. 9.164a, b).
3. During the procedures of hysteroscopy, transverse ultrasound scans are frequently taken to observe whether the

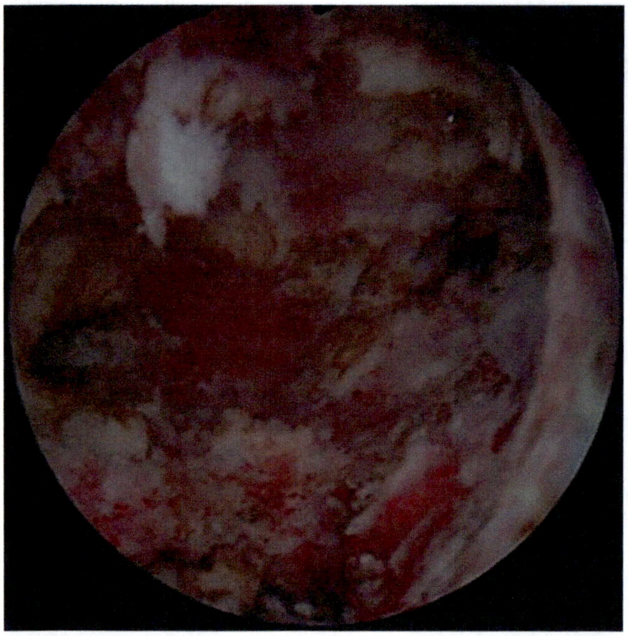

Fig. 9.157 A normal uterine cavity is achieved by hysteroscopic adhesiolysis

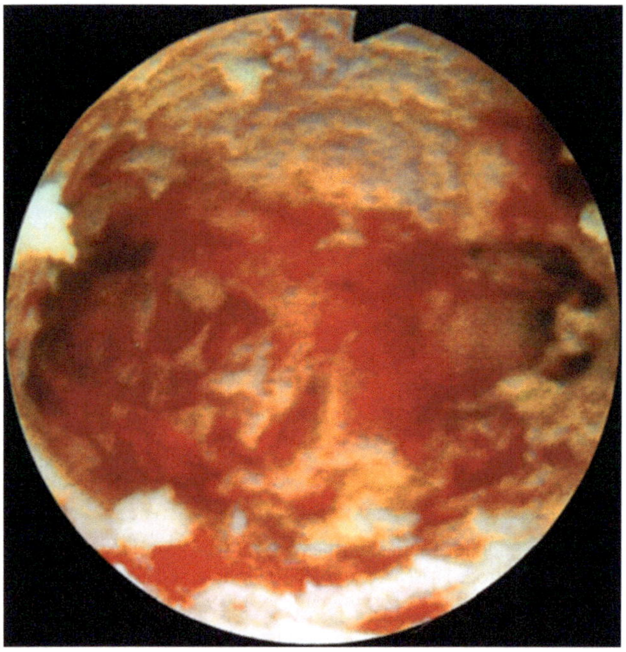

Fig. 9.158 At the end of the procedure, the resectoscope should be retracted back to the level of cervical internal os and the uterine cavity is observed

bright echo caused by electric resection is located in the middle of uterus (Fig. 9.165). After complete removal of the adhesions, the hysteroscope is retracted back to cervical internal os with distention of the uterine cavity. Afterwards, a symmetrical uterine cavity with equal thickness of uterine walls can be observed under transverse or longitudinal ultrasound scanning (Figs. 9.166 and 9.167).

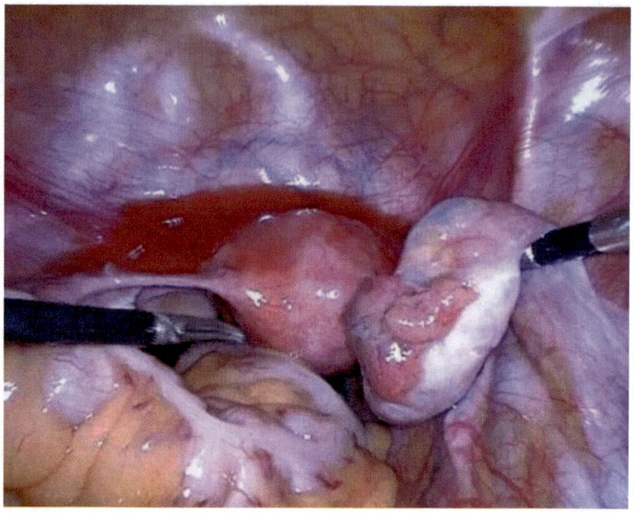

Fig. 9.159 Laparoscopy monitors the procedure of hysteroscopic adhesiolysis. Tubal patency test is taken and the right patent tube is observed under laparoscope

4. In cases with atresia of the uterus, the hysteroscope is inserted through cervical canal under ultrasound guidance. Transverse and longitudinal ultrasound scanning is conducted to guide the resectoscope dividing the adhesions gradually along the long axis of uterus, so that both the cervical canal and uterine cavity are opened.

9.6.6.2 Laparoscopy

Laparoscopic monitoring is performed to inspect the pelvis, to observe bilateral tubal patency, and to reveal the serosal changes of uterus, as well as to find and repair any damage to the uterus. Therefore it is an effective method of monitoring hysteroscopic lysis of adhesions.

1. At the beginning of the operation, laparoscopy is performed to explore the pelvic cavity, including observation of the shape of the uterus and the integrity of uterine serosa, determination of the location of the hysteroscope and the light penetrability of uterine walls, as well as any previous injuries (Fig. 9.168a, b).
2. During hysteroscopic procedures, the changes of the uterine serosal layer should be noticed. If there are small blisters, it suggests an impending perforation of the uterus and the operation is to be stopped immediately (Fig. 9.169a, b).
3. During hysteroscopic procedures, both laparoscopic light transmission test and the reverse test can be taken. The objective lens of laparoscope might be placed close to the serosal layer of uterine fundus, with the light dimmed. If the light inside uterine cavity transmits across the uterine wall and can be seen under laparoscope, it indicates that the uterine wall of the fundus has become thin, which warns the surgeon to stop operation there. It is named light transmission test (Fig. 9.170a, b). When the objective lens of laparoscope is placed close to the serosal layer

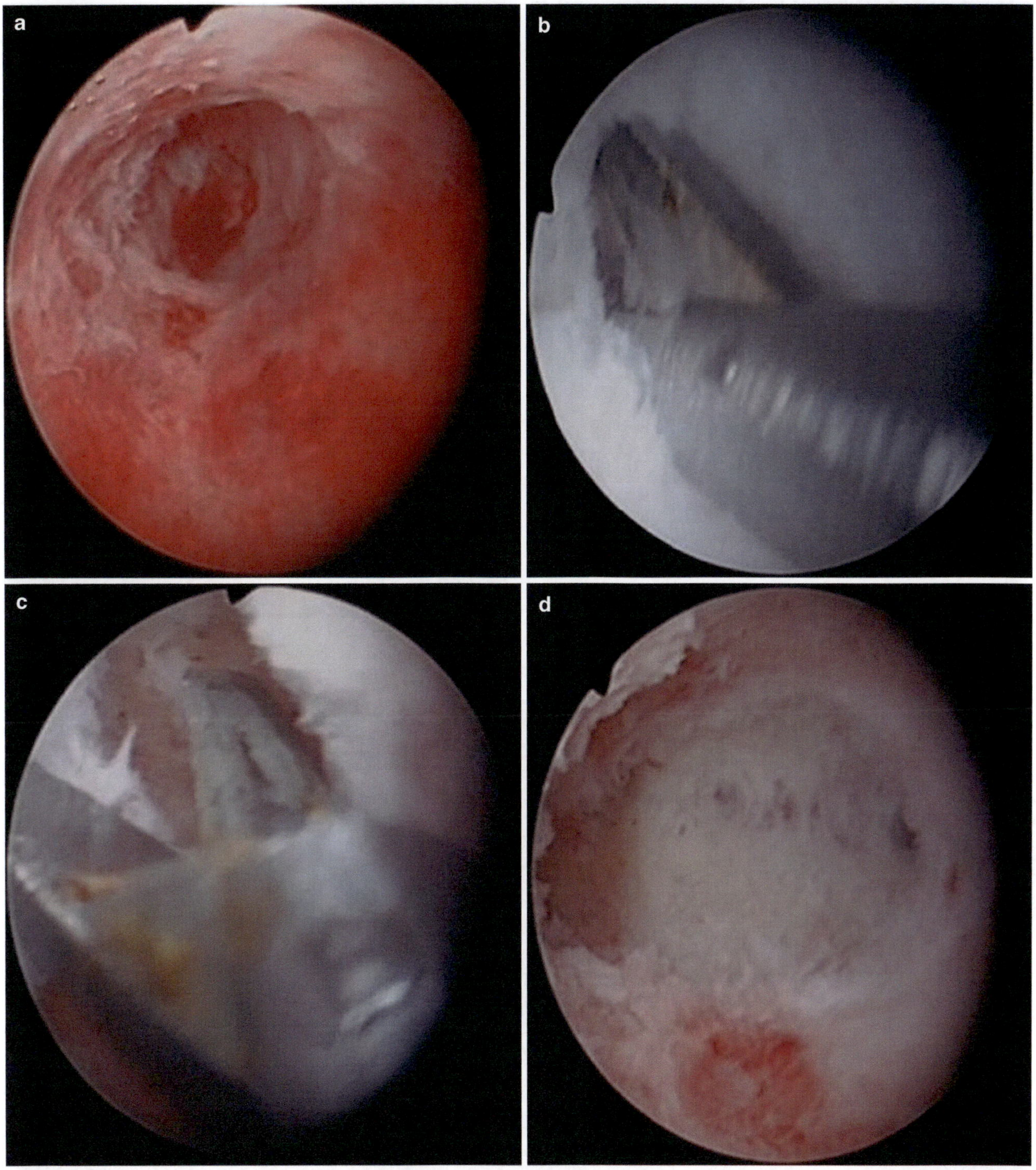

Fig. 9.160 Division of adhesions by hysteroscopic scissors in a patient with atresia of the cavity. (**a**) A blind end is shown in cervical canal in front of the hysteroscope. (**b**, **c**) Intrauterine adhesions are cut by hysteroscopic scissors. (**d**) Uterine cavity is visible after dissection of adhesions

of uterine fundus, and the light from hysteroscope is dimmed, if the light from laparoscope transmits across the uterine wall and can be seen under hysteroscope, it indicates that the uterine wall has become thin, and is named reverse light transmission test (Fig. 9.171a, b).

4. In patients who want to get pregnant, methylene blue solution can be injected into the uterine cavity at the end of the operation so as to observe whether the tubal fimbria has a discharge of methylene blue solution or not via laparoscopy.

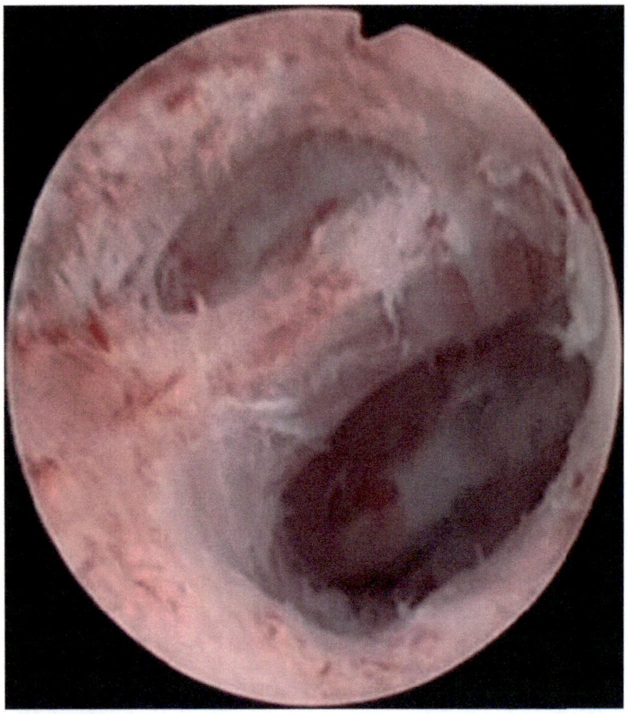

Fig. 9.161 A previous false passage in anterior wall of the uterus is seen under hysteroscope

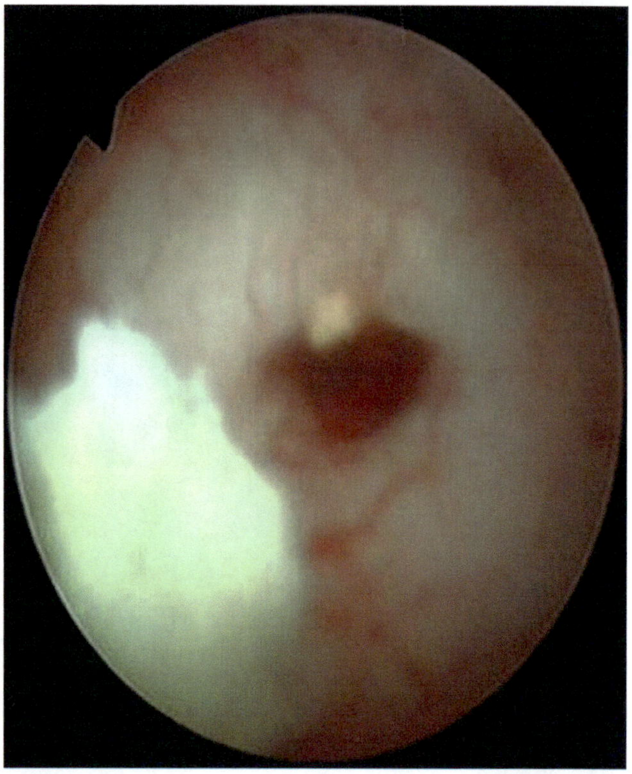

Fig. 9.162 A previous perforation is seen under hysteroscope

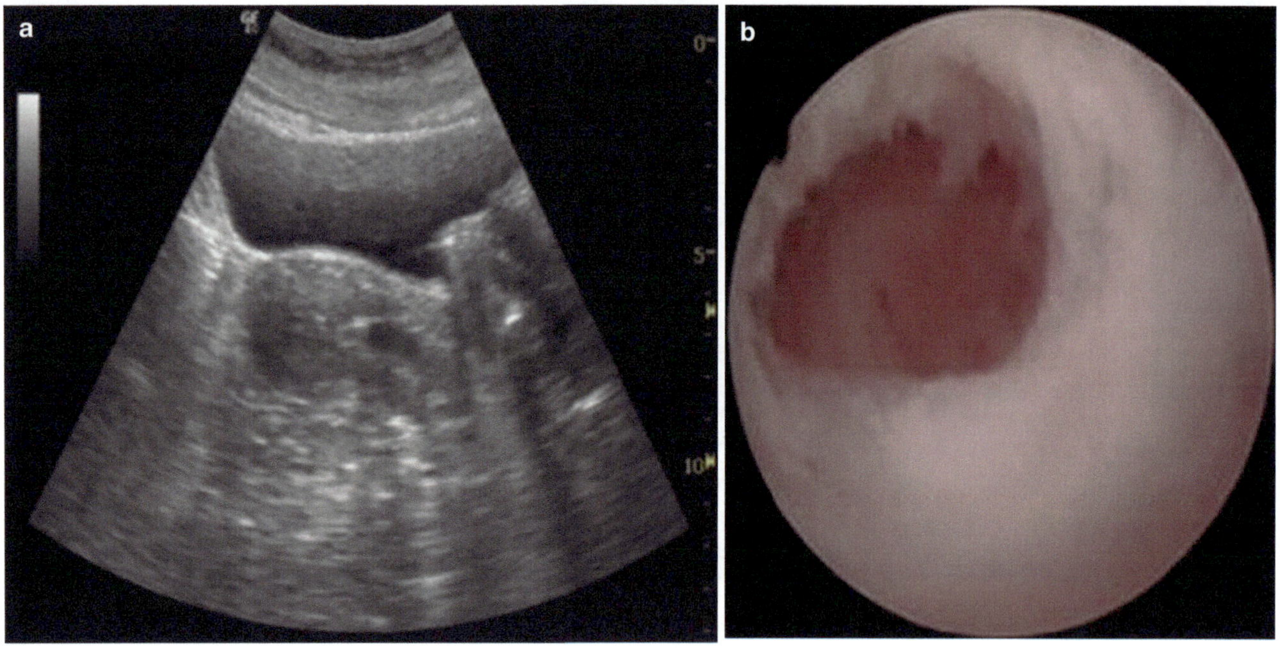

Fig. 9.163 (**a**) Ultrasound scanning of the uterus. The position and size of the uterus are revealed. (**b**) A uterine cavity is seen under hysteroscope. Adhesions occlude the fundus and fibrous scars are seen on uterine walls

9.6.7 Postoperative Management and Adjunctive Therapy

Hysteroscopic adhesiolysis can divide the adhesions and restore a normal cavity. However, in patients with IUA, the endometrium is fibrotic and badly damaged, the injured surface is difficult to heal after operation, and the risk of adhesion recurrence is high. Thus, the treatment of IUA includes not only performing hysteroscopic surgery to restore a normal uterine cavity, but also taking measures to promote the

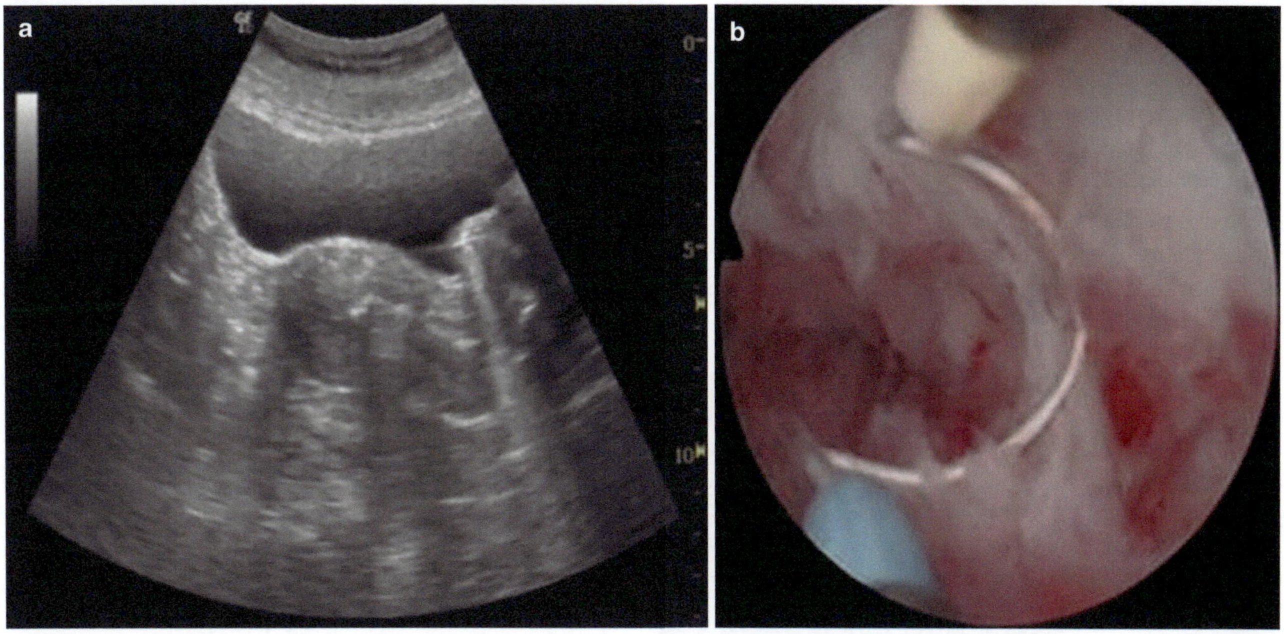

Fig. 9.164 (**a**) Ultrasound scanning guides the cutting direction of hysteroscopic needle electrode. (**b**) Intrauterine scar tissues on left uterine wall are divided by hysteroscopic wire loop electrode

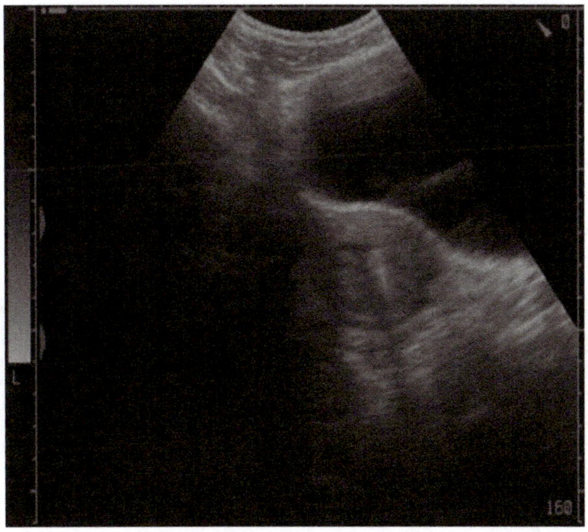

Fig. 9.165 Transverse ultrasound scanning during a hysteroscopic procedure so as to guarantee resection in the middle of uterus

repair of endometrium and prevent the reformation of intrauterine adhesions, so that it can achieve the purpose of restoring the normal reproductive ability of the patients.

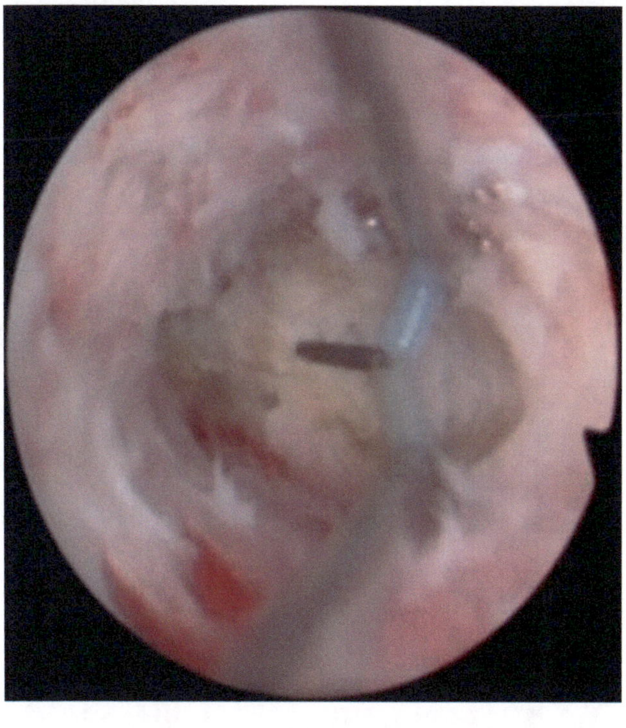

Fig. 9.166 At the end of operation, the hysteroscope is retracted back to cervical internal os and checks the whole cavity

9.6.7.1 Hormone Treatment

Fibrosis of endometrium leads to a diminished ability of endometrial regeneration. Administration of sex hormones with suitable dosage after hysteroscopic operations can stimulate the re-growth of endometrial glands and stroma, and accelerate the repair of endometrium. Therefore, sex hormone treatment stimulating regeneration of endometrium has become a routine adjuvant therapeutic method. A common therapy is the usage of estrogen and progesterone in a consecutive manner for 2 or 3 months, with estrogen 4–9 mg/day for 4 weeks and the addition of progesterone in the last 2 weeks. Chang et al. reported that in cases with cyclic hormone therapy after hysteroscopic adhesiolysis, the thickness of endometrium could increase more than that before operations, but less than that in cases of control group, which could not reach normal in thickness.

Cyclic hormone therapy cannot achieve a satisfied outcome due to poor response of fibrous endometrium to hormone treatment, so some gynecologists attempted to use high dose and long duration of estrogen to enhance the stimulation of endometrial regeneration. Liu et al. from Beijing Fuxing Hospital administrated oral estradiol valerate with a dosage of 10 mg/day for 3 months, and the addition of oral medroxyprogesterone acetate in the last 5 days. Discontinuation of them resulted in withdrawal bleeding. They found that the adjuvant administration of high-dose estrogen following hysteroscopic lysis of moderate and severe adhesions could increase the recovery rate effectively, and continuous usage of synthetic hormone was superior to cyclic hormone therapy. However, it should be noted that high-dose usage of estrogen may result in estrogen-related endometrial pathology. Dr. Ma in Beijing Fuxing Hospital published a case report that a woman with severe intrauterine adhesions developed endometrial atypical hyperplasia resulting from frequent usage of high-dose estrogen. Myers and Hurst studied the response of endometrium to the administration of low-dose estrogen for a prolonged period, and found that, in patients with severe intrauterine adhesions, pre- and postoperative continuous usage of estrogen 4–6 mg/day for 4–10 weeks could achieve some effect.

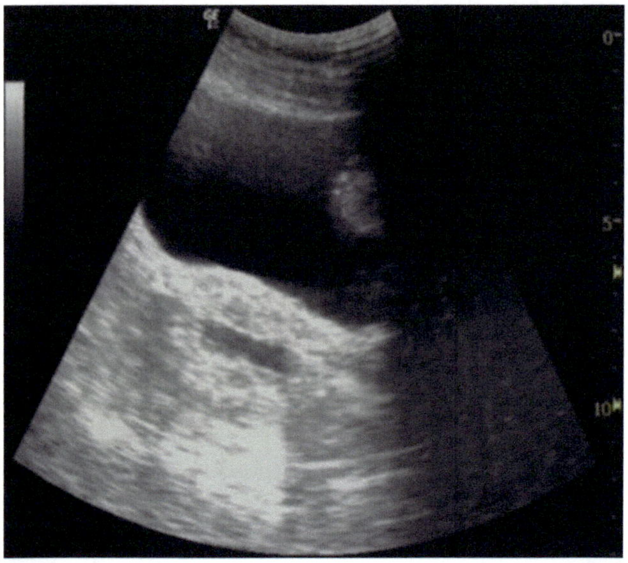

Fig. 9.167 At the end of operation, longitudinal ultrasound scanning checks the uterus and its cavity

9.6.7.2 Intrauterine Placement of Barriers

Intrauterine barriers consist of mechanical barriers and biochemical barriers, such as intrauterine contraceptive device, Foley balloon catheter, Cook balloon, human amnion graft, hyaluronic acid (HA), and seprafilm. During the healing period of intrauterine injured surface, intrauterine barriers keep the uterine cavity separated mechanically and prevent the reformation of adhesions coming from adherence of

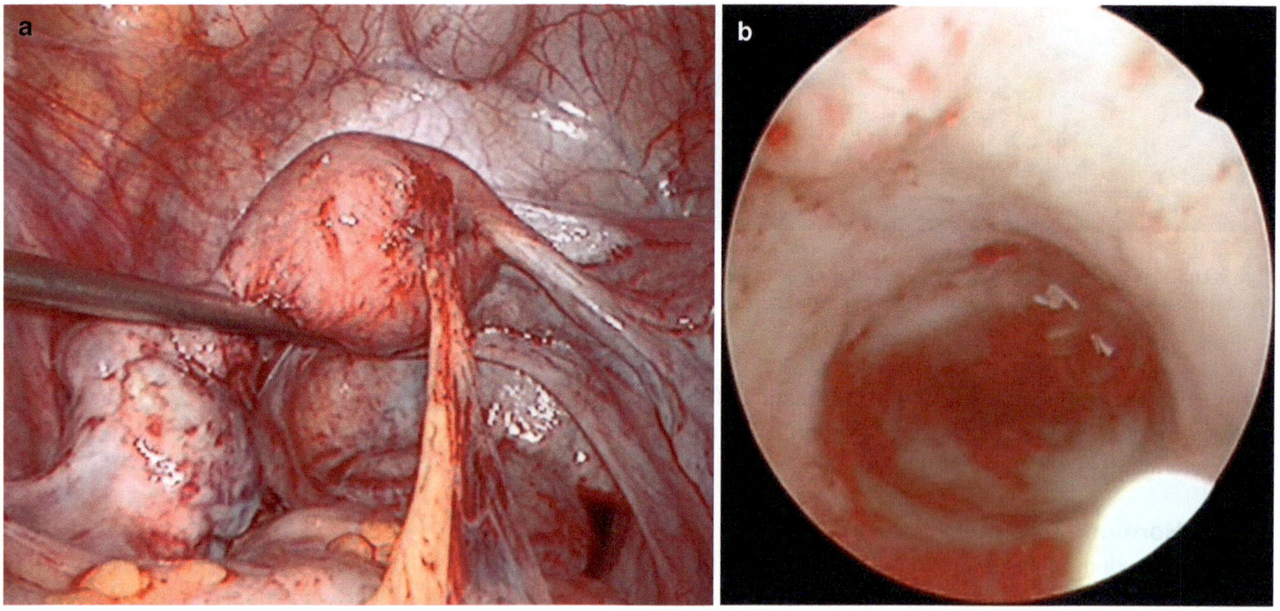

Fig. 9.168 Laparoscopy is conducted during hysteroscopic adhesiolysis. (**a**) Under laparoscope, the uterus is in mid-position, the serosa on right fundus is adherent to omentum, and a previous dent is seen on right posterior wall of the fundus. In addition, the left tube is swollen, twisted, and wrapped by adhesions. (**b**) Under hysteroscope, the uterine cavity is narrowed, with extensive fibrous scars on uterine walls

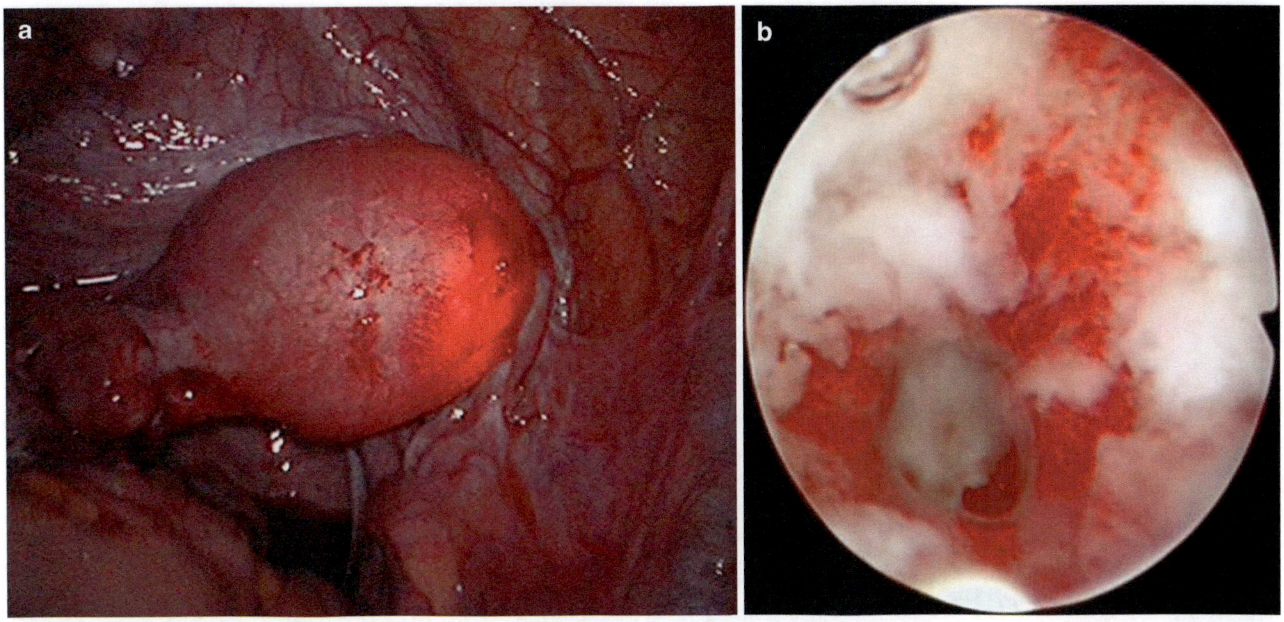

Fig. 9.169 Laparoscopy is done during hysteroscopic procedures. (**a**) Laparoscopy is to observe the light penetrability of uterine walls. It shows a significant light penetration in right posterior walls of fundus, which indicates a very thin uterine wall. (**b**) Hysteroscopy opens the uterine cavity, reveals the right cornua, and shows a scar area of previous perforation

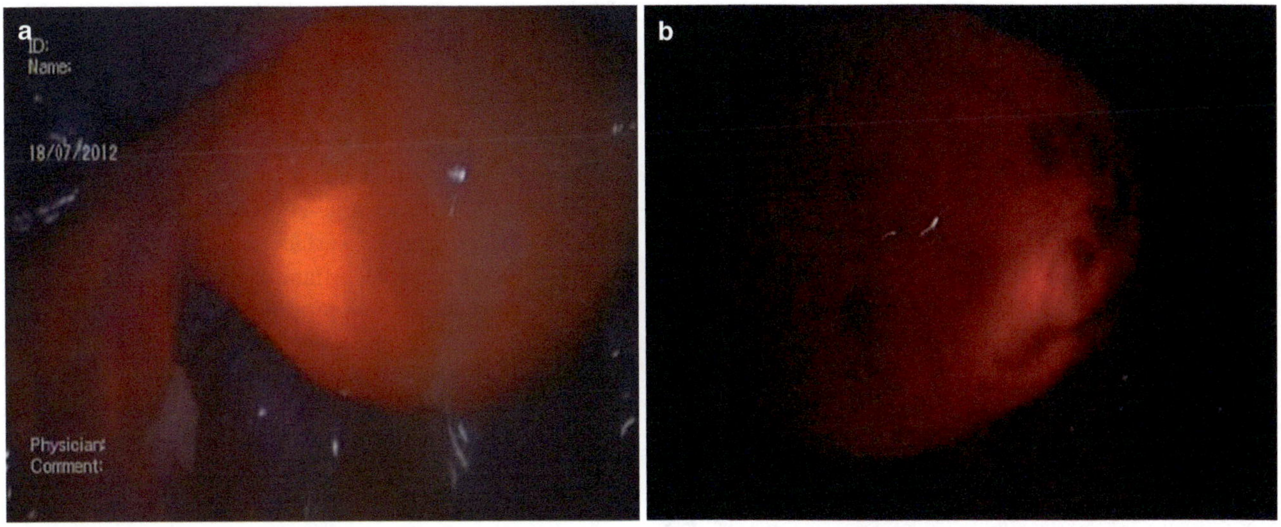

Fig. 9.170 Laparoscopy is performed during hysteroscopic procedures. Place the objective lens of laparoscope close to the serosal layer of uterine fundus, dim the light, and observe the light transmission across the uterine wall. Under laparoscope, the significant penetration of light in uterine wall indicates that the uterine wall in this area is thinner than that in other areas. (**a**) Significant penetration of light in left-posterior wall of uterus. (**b**) Significant penetration of light in right cornua of uterus

denuded surfaces. The combination of hormone therapy is commonly used to accelerate the re-epithelization of the endometrium.

1. Intrauterine contraceptive device (IUD): IUD is often placed into uterine cavity after hysteroscopic surgery, and then removed 1–3 months later, which is a common adjuvant treatment of hysteroscopic lysis of adhesions and always combined with cyclic hormone therapy. IUD is a mechanical barrier, and separates the uterine cavity during healing period of injured surface, so that it can prevent the adherence of denuded surface and formation of adhesions. Frequently used IUDs in clinic include metal loop IUDs, T-shaped IUDs, copper-IUDs, etc. (Fig. 9.172). Lao et al. reported that placement of a T-shaped IUD following hysteroscopic resection was effective in preventing adhesions formed in either uterine cavity or cervical canal. Some scholars from abroad carried out some studies on which type of IUDs being the most suitable

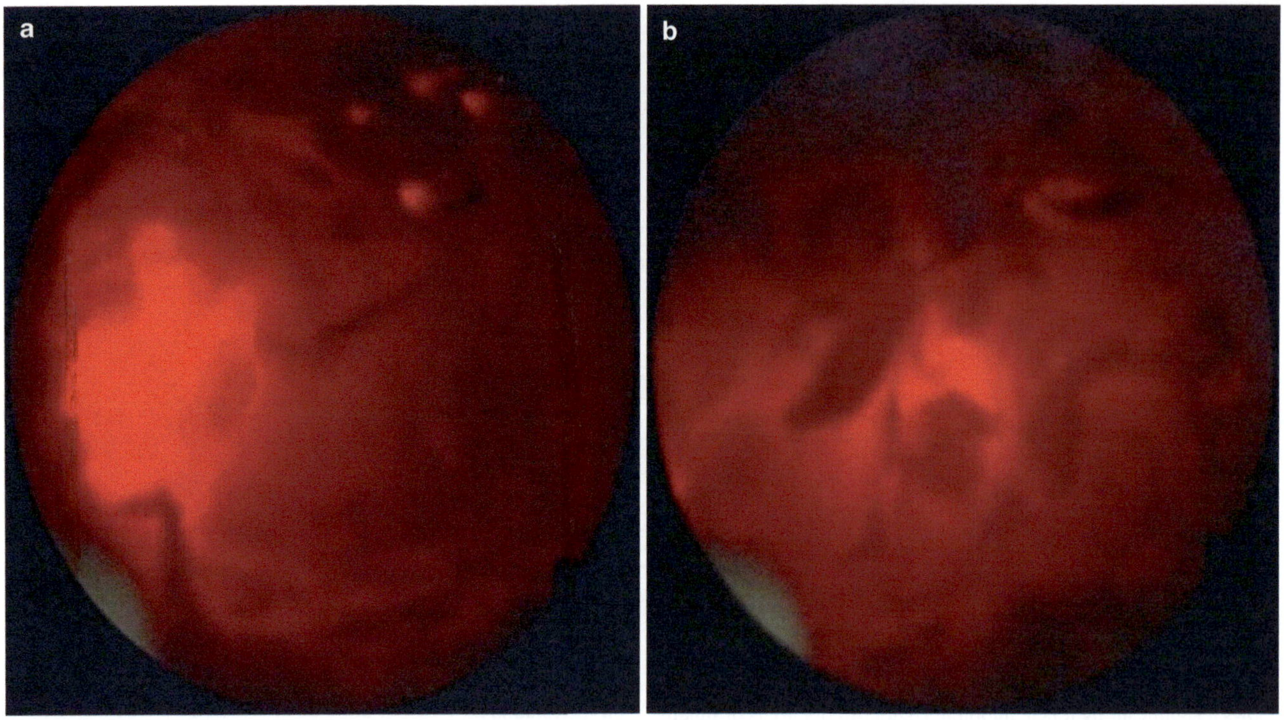

Fig. 9.171 A reverse light transmission test during hysteroscopic procedures. Place the objective lens of laparoscope close to the serosal layer of uterine fundus, dim the light from hysteroscope, and observe the light transmission across the uterine wall under hysteroscope. (**a**) The slight penetration of light in the fundus and significant penetration of light in right cornua are seen under hysteroscope. (**b**) Significant light penetration in the fundus is seen

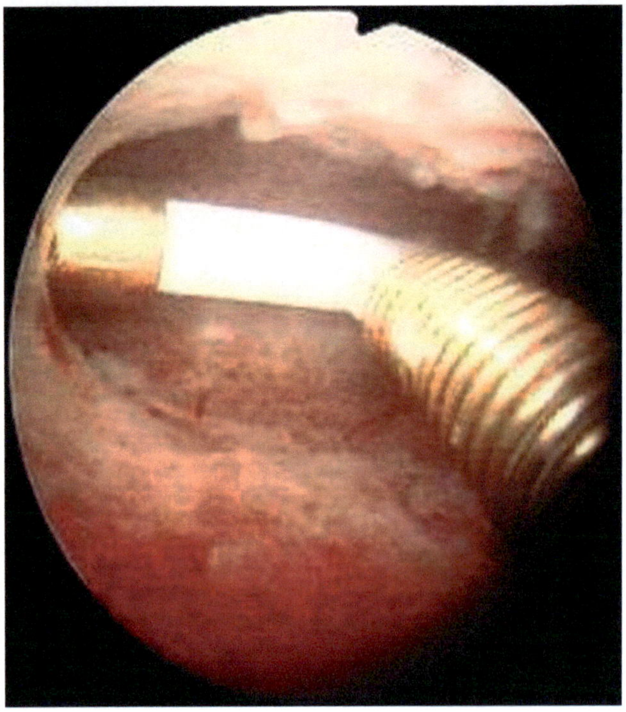

Fig. 9.172 Intrauterine placement of a T-shaped IUD following hysteroscopic surgery (Second-look hysteroscopy on the 15th day after hysteroscopic procedures)

device used after hysteroscopic lysis of adhesions. They concluded that metal loop IUDs should be the best because of the large contact surface. A T-shaped IUD has less contact surface and a copper IUD may induce an excessive inflammatory reaction, so they were considered inappropriate for preventing the adhesions after hysteroscopy.

2. Intrauterine balloon: Aside from IUDs, some scholars also adapted intrauterine use of a Foley balloon catheter or a Cook balloon following operations on IUA to distend the uterine cavity and prevent the recurrence of adhesions. The mechanisms of action are as follows:
   (a) Mechanical barrier. An intrauterine balloon which is inflated with water can effectively keep the uterine walls separate and act as a mechanical barrier.
   (b) Intrauterine stent. Balloon acts as a stent of uterine cavity to promote the regeneration and recovery of endometrium along the balloon surface.
   (c) Drainage. Intrauterine balloon catheter permits the drainage of the clots and liquid out of the uterine cavity to facilitate the repair of endometrium.
   (d) Expansion of the cavity. The balloon inflated with water can expand the uterine cavity and divide the residual adhesions.

The procedures of intrauterine placement of a Foley balloon following hysteroscopic adhesiolysis are as follows:

(a) Firstly, 1 mL of a gas is injected into balloon to indicate the border between the balloon and the catheter, and then the tip of the catheter above the balloon is cut off with scissors (Fig. 9.173).
(b) Secondly, the balloon catheter is inserted into the uterine cavity.
(c) The balloon is inflated with 3–5 mL sterile saline solution, and does not come out when pulled gently.
(d) The balloon catheter is kept in place for 1 week. Simultaneously antibiotics are taken to prevent infections.

A Foley balloon, with its shape a sphere, is often adopted in uterine cavity following the treatment of IUA with hysteroscopy. A Cook balloon, with its shape a triangle, can fit the shape of a uterine cavity to a higher degree, and therefore keep the uterine walls separate effectively. So it was recommended by some scholars.

3. Human amnion graft: Human amnion develops from cytotrophoblast and has a smooth surface and a translucent membrane without nerve, vessels, and lymph. It has been widely used in ophthalmology for ocular surface lesions, burned skin and skin ulcers, and artificial vaginal reconstruction surgeries. In 2006, Amer et al. first reported that human amnion which wrapped around a balloon was placed in uterine cavity following hysteroscopic adhesiolysis as an adjuvant treatment for the management of IUA, and achieved a good result. After that, Amer et al. in 2010 and Peng et al. in 2012 (from Fuxing Hospital, Capital Medical University) reported similar studies on human amnion applied after operations of IUA to prevent recurrence of adhesions and proved its safety and efficacy.

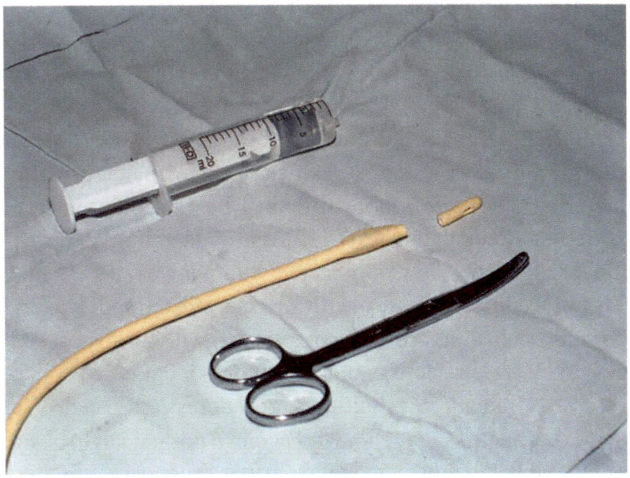

Fig. 9.173 1 mL of gas is injected into Foley balloon to indicate the border of balloon, and then the tip of catheter above the balloon is cut off with scissors

The mechanisms of human amnion on prevention of IUA are as follows:

(a) Biological barrier. Human amnion consists of five layers, i.e., an epithelial layer, a basal layer, a compact layer, a fibroblast layer, and a spongy layer. It is the thickest basement membrane in human body and has enough active surfaces. In addition, it was reported that fresh amnion might remain in the uterine cavity for 21 days, so it could separate the surfaces of uterine cavity effectively for a longer period.
(b) Intrauterine stent. The basal layer of amnion contains both collagen fibers and reticular fibers, and is rich in bioactive substances. It may act as a stent to promote migration and proliferation of surrounding normal endometrium, and therefore facilitate the repair and regeneration of endometrium. So it can prevent the formation of IUA.
(c) Inhibition of inflammatory reactions. Amnion graft adhering firmly to the surface of the cavity can reduce the reproduction of bacteria grown in the cavity. Amnion graft, as a biological membrane, blocks the bacteria passing through. In addition, it contains a variety of protein inhibitors, and therefore inhibits corresponding protease to produce inflammatory reactions.
(d) Anti-fibrosis. Amnion stroma can inhibit the proliferation of fibroblast and differentiation of myofibroblast, and therefore reduce the fibrosis and the formation of scar tissues.
(e) The immune compatibility. Human fresh amnion is a special material with low immunogenicity, and induces minimal immunologic reaction when it is implanted into an alien body.

The procedures of intrauterine placement of human amnion are as follows:

(a) A human amnion graft is cut into a suitable piece, spread on a Foley balloon with the surface of the basement membrane facing outward, and then is introduced into a uterine cavity (Fig. 9.174).
(b) After insertion of the balloon, it is inflated with 3–5 mL of saline solution and fixed in the cavity.
(c) The end of the catheter is connected to a drainage bag, and the balloon is kept in place for 7 days.
(d) Oral antibiotics are given to prevent infections for these 7 days.

4. Hyaluronic acid (HA) gel: Auto-cross-linked HA (ACP) gel, a high concentration gel modified from a biodegradable high molecular biological polymer, has significant effects on prevention of adhesions and repair of soft tissues. Intrauterine injection of ACP gel following hysteroscopic adhesiolysis may play a similar role in mechanical prevention of the adhesions.

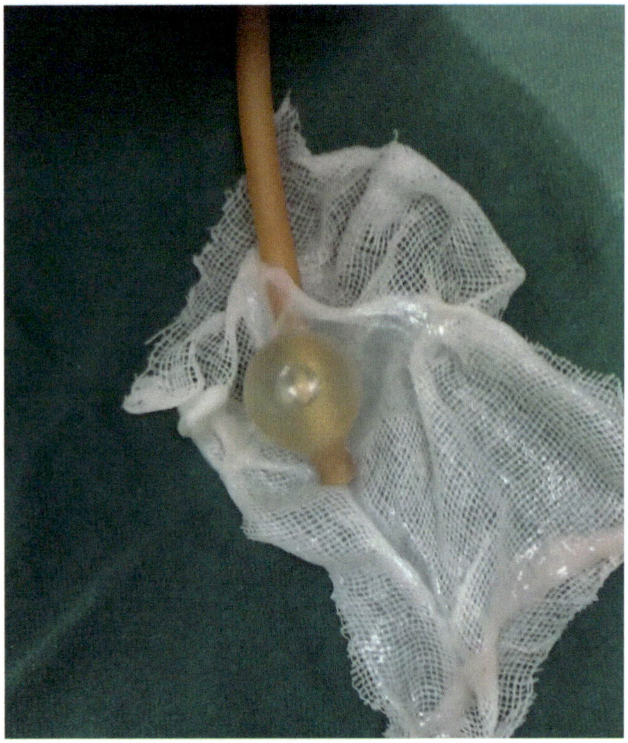

Fig. 9.174 Preparation of human amnion graft. The amnion graft is cut into a suitable size, wraps around a Foley balloon with the basement membrane surface facing outward, and then is inserted into uterine cavity

The frequently used method is to introduce a catheter, which is connected to a gel syringe, into uterine cavity, and then push the gel into the cavity with the dose of 3–5 mL.

9.6.7.3 Prophylactic Antibiotics

Routine administration of antibiotics to prevent infection is not recommended in patients who have hysteroscopic adhesiolysis. However, patients who use IUDs, Foley balloons, human amnion or ACP gel after surgery need to take antibiotics for 3–7 days to prevent infections.

9.6.7.4 Second-Look Hysteroscopy

The crucial period of adhesion formations in uterine cavity after hysteroscopic adhesiolysis is about 1–2 months postoperation. A second-look hysteroscopy may be taken when the withdrawing bleeding stops after hormone treatment for 2 months. The mild endometrial adhesions can be divided mechanically by hysteroscope. Second or multiple operations can be performed in patients for whom moderate or severe adhesions recur. Patients who achieve a normal cavity can try to conceive (Fig. 9.175a–c).

9.6.8 Diagnosis and Management of Operative Complications

Details can be seen in Chap. 12.

In all hysteroscopic surgery involving electroresection, uterine perforation is most prone to occur in TCRA procedures. In Jansen et al.'s study, the risk of complications in TCRA was twelve times higher than that in TCRP. Uterine perforation is the most frequent complications in TCRA. It has been reported that the incidence of uterine perforation was 1.1–2.7% in all cases with intrauterine adhesions, and 3.6–50% in cases with severe adhesions. Bukulmer et al. performed TCRA on the patients with intrauterine adhesions due to endometrial tuberculosis, and found that uterine perforation occurred in 25% of these cases. Furthermore, intra- and postoperative bleeding is also a frequent complication in TCRA, with the occurrence rate reported between 16.7 and 27.3%. In patients who conceive after TCRA, some complications like miscarriage, premature delivery, and placental adhesion may also happen. In addition, recurrence of adhesions in uterine cavity is easily developed after TCRA. It has been reported that the recurrence rate of adhesions after TCRA was 3.1–23.5%, and was 20–62.5% in severe cases. A comprehensive scheme including hysteroscopic adhesiolysis, postoperative adjuvant therapy, and a second-look hysteroscopy in the near future is an effective means for prevention and management.

9.6.9 Experiences and Evaluations of TCRA

9.6.9.1 Success Rate of Operations

The restoration of a normal shape of the uterine cavity is generally considered as a success of TCRA. It was reported in literature that the successful restoration of normal cavity in one procedure was at a rate of 57.8–97.5%.

The central cylindrical intrauterine adhesions caused by adhesion between the anterior and posterior uterine walls can be easily dissected with a high successful rate. The extensive central adhesions are difficult to be removed, but the successful rate of procedures is still high. The management of marginal adhesions is more difficult. The procedures in cases with distorted cavities resulting from both central and marginal scar tissues are complicated with a lower success rate. The procedures in cases with uterine atresia and bilateral cornual occlusions are very complicated with the lowest success rate, which can be guided by ultrasonography or laparoscopy. Sometimes multiple procedures are needed to achieve a success. Patients who achieve normal cavities and both visible tubal ostia may have better prognosis.

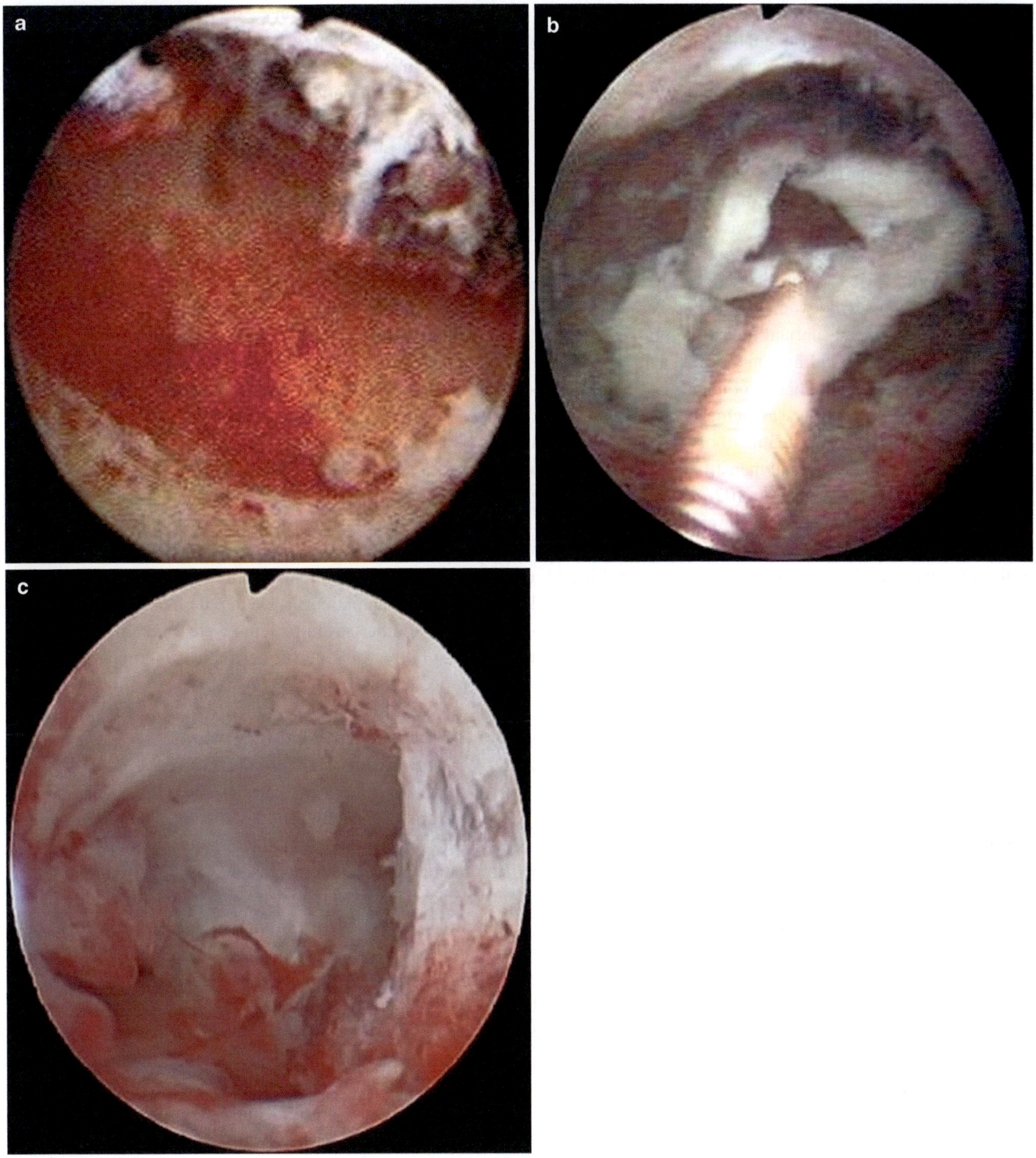

Fig. 9.175 Second-look hysteroscopy is performed. (**a**) One month after hysteroscopic adhesiolysis. The uterine cavity is normal, and the necrotic tissues are seen in the middle of the cavity. (**b**) One month after hysteroscopic adhesiolysis. The uterine cavity is normal, a T-shaped IUD is in right place, and the necrotic tissues are seen in uterine cavity. (**c**) Four months after hysteroscopic adhesiolysis. Fibrous adhesive tissues are shown on left wall of the uterus

9.6.9.2 Postoperative Menstruations

Postoperative menstruation is another target for evaluating the outcomes of hysteroscopic surgeries. However, the procedure only can open a normal cavity and has little influence on the restoration of endometrial functions. Therefore, hormone treatment is often used to help stimulate re-growth of endometrium after hysteroscopic surgery.

It was reported that the rate of menstrual improvement after hysteroscopic adhesiolysis was in the range of 52.4–90.3%. Preutthipan and Linasmita reported that intrauterine adhesions with various degrees were treated by hysteroscopic adhesiolysis. In 44 women who had secondary amenorrhea before treatment, normal menstruation was achieved in 40 women (90.9%) and hypomenorrhea achieved in four (9.1%). In six women who had hypomenorrhea before treatment, normal menstruation was achieved in five (83.3%). Donnez applied laser to the treatment of IUA and found that the rate of restoration of normal menstruation was more than 80%. Roge reported that among 102 cases of intrauterine adhesions, 75% of them achieved improved menstruations. The postoperative rate of menstrual improvement in women with previous amenorrhea was 95.5%. Yu et al. published a review article in 2008 to analyze 625 cases of IUA, and found that 528 cases of them (84.5%) achieved normal menstruation after lysis of adhesions. Then, a further study on infertile women with IUA who had hysteroscopic adhesiolysis was carried out in Fuxing Hospital from 1998 to 2005. Among 64 women who had initial hypomenorrhea or amenorrhea, the postoperative rate of menstrual improvement was 65.6% (42/64).

9.6.9.3 Postoperative Recurrence of Adhesions

The endometrium in cases with IUA develops fibrosis with a poor capacity of regeneration, and the denuded myometrial surfaces in uterine cavity cannot be covered by epithelium, so the possibility of reforming intrauterine adhesions after hysteroscopic procedures is quite high. Furthermore, the recurrence of adhesions is a main obstacle to a successful operation. It was reported in literature that the recurrence rate of adhesions following hysteroscopic adhesiolysis ranged from 3.1 to 23.5%, which was even higher in cases with severe adhesions (20–62.5%).

The recurrence of adhesions is closely related to the degrees of preoperative intrauterine adhesions. The more severe preoperative adhesion is, the higher postoperative recurrence rate will be. Pabuccu et al. studied 40 women with recurrent pregnancy loss or infertility caused by intrauterine adhesions. After hysteroscopic adhesiolysis, all minimal or moderate adhesions were divided successfully. However, in women who had severe preoperative adhesions, 60% of them had postoperative reformation of adhesions. Preutthipan and Linasmita reported that among 65 patients who had hysteroscopic adhesiolysis, before treatment, 29 patients had mild adhesions, 26 had moderate, and 10 had severe adhesions. There was no recurrence of adhesions after treatment in patients with initial mild and moderate adhesions. And in ten patients with initial severe adhesions, the postoperative recurrence of adhesions occurred in two (20%). Yu et al. reported on the outcomes of second-look hysteroscopy performed after TCRA in Hysteroscopy Center of Fuxing Hospital, Capital Medical University. It was found that the recurrence rate of adhesions after treatment was 27.9% (17/61), and it was 41.9% (13/31) in patients with initial severe adhesions.

A repeat operative procedure, or multiple procedures, may be performed in cases with reformation of adhesions. The patients still can achieve satisfying outcomes even after multiple procedures. Roge reported that 148 procedures of adhesiolysis were performed in 102 women who had original adhesions. Among them, four women (3.9%) had three procedures, and five women (4.9%) had four. Capella-Allouc et al. reported on 31 patients who had permanent severe adhesions and underwent hysteroscopic adhesiolysis. All of the patients achieved at least one tubal ostium visible after treatment. Sixteen patients were treated with the primary operation. Seven patients were cured after the second procedure, and another seven patients were cured after three procedures. There was one further patient who was treated by four procedures.

9.6.9.4 Postoperative Conception and Reproductive Outcomes

Hysteroscopic treatment of intrauterine adhesions can increase the pregnancy rate. Pace et al. studied on patients with IUA and found that the pregnancy rate was 28.7% before treatment, and it increased to 53.6% after treatment. It was reported in a study that in patients who had intrauterine adhesions and pregnancy loss more than twice, the live birth rate increased from 18.3% before treatment to 68.6% after treatment. Yu et al. analyzed the data from literature and reported that, in patients who had IUA and wanted to get pregnant, the postoperative pregnancy rate was 74% (468/632), which was much higher than that before operations (46%). In patients who had infertility, the postoperative pregnancy rate was 45.6% (104/228). In patients with IUA and pregnancy failure, the postoperative pregnancy rate was 89.6% (121/135), with the live birth rate 77.0% (104/135). Preutthipan and Linasmita reported that hysteroscopic lysis of intrauterine adhesions was conducted in 45 women who had IUA and infertility. After treatment, 16 women (35.6%) achieved conception.

The pregnancy rate after hysteroscopic adhesiolysis is closely related to the degree of IUA before operations. The more serious the preoperative adhesion is, the worse the improvement of postoperative pregnancy rate will be. It was reported in literature that the pregnancy rate after hysteroscopic operations for IUA in women with infertility was between 34.9 and 62.0%, and was between 20.0 and 43.3% in women with severe adhesions. In a study on hysteroscopic division of adhesions reported by Valle and Sciarra, 43 women with initial mild and filmy adhesions achieved good prognosis after treatment, which included 35 (81%) cases of term pregnancies. In 97 women with moderate or fibromuscular adhesions, 64 (66%) achieved term pregnancies, while in 47 cases with severe connective tissue adhesions, 15 (32%) achieved term pregnancies. In total, after hysteroscopic treatment, the restoration of normal menstruation was achieved in 90% of patients, and term pregnancy was in 79.7%, which were much higher than that with previous blind procedures.

Postoperative complications in women who conceive after TCRA may also occur, which include miscarriage, abnormal placenta implantation, and post-delivery bleeding. Roge reported that 34 conceptions were obtained after treatment in 28 women with IUA, which included ten miscarriages and 24 live births. Baggish collected forty articles and discovered that, in more than 1000 patients who had intrauterine adhesions, the pregnancy rate in women without treatment was 50%. Among them only half of conceptions reached full term. The pregnancy rate after hysteroscopic treatment was 75%, with a lower failure rate of conceptions and fewer complications of delivery. Xu et al. reported that, in thirteen women who wished to conceive after treatment of IUA, nine pregnancies were achieved, including four term deliveries, one placental adhesion, one placenta previa, and three spontaneous miscarriage. Yu et al. carried out a study on 85 women who had TCRA in Beijing Fuxing Hospital. In total, 39 conceptions were obtained after hysteroscopic procedures, with the pregnancy rate 45.9%. Of all cases with pregnancies, 25 (64.1%) got live births, five (12.8%) were ongoing conceptions, eight (20.5%) had spontaneous miscarriage, and one need termination of conception. Of 25 cases with live births, five encountered placenta pathologies, including hysterectomy due to post-delivery bleeding and placenta implantation in two cases. There were two other women who delivered low weight babies at 26–28 pregnancy weeks. Capella-Allouc et al. studied on 31 patients who had severe adhesions and underwent hysteroscopic lysis of adhesions. Among 28 patients who had follow-ups successfully with a mean time of 31 months (from 2 to 84 months), 15 conceptions were obtained in 12 patients. The reproductive outcomes included: 2 patients got missed miscarriage in first trimester, 3 patients had pregnancy losses in second trimester, nine patients got live births, and 1 patient underwent termination of pregnancy in second trimester for multiple fetal abnormalities. In total, the pregnancy rate after treatment was 42.8% (12/28), with the live birth rate 32.1% (9/28). In nine patients who had live births, one underwent hysterectomy for adherent placenta during the procedure of cesarean section, and one had hypogastric arteries ligation due to severe hemorrhage and placenta adhesions.

Consequently, conceptions after hysteroscopic adhesiolysis may be considered as a high-risk pregnancy with an increased risk of miscarriage and placenta pathology. Hence, during the whole period of pregnancy and delivery, the conditions of placenta and uterus should be closely monitored to prevent the occurrence of complications.

9.6.9.5 Factors Affecting Reproductive Prognosis After TCRA

The treatment outcomes and reproductive prognosis in patients who has IUA and infertility have always been an issue of discussion by many scholars. Most specialists believed that the treatment outcomes and reproductive prognosis after treatment of IUA were closely related to the types and the extent of adhesions, as well as the degrees of endometrial injuries. However, the scientific data analyzing the factors influencing reproductive outcomes following TCRA remained insufficient. Yu et al. made a statistical analysis about the possible factors affecting reproductive prognosis following TCRA. Factors evaluated included menstrual pattern before operations, menstrual pattern after operations, the degree of adhesions before operations, and the recurrence of adhesions after operations. In total, 109 procedures of TCRA were performed in 85 women with adhesions who had infertility or recurrent pregnancy loss. The mean follow-up after treatment was 3.9 ± 0.6 years, and 39 conceptions were achieved. In women who had amenorrhea after treatment, two got pregnancy (2/11 = 18.2%), and the pregnancy rate was significantly lower than those who had menstruation after treatment (37/74 = 50%), $p < 0.05$. At second-look hysteroscopy, the pregnancy rate in women who had recurrence of adhesions was significantly lower (2/17 = 11.8%) than those who had no recurrence (26/44 = 59.1%), $P < 0.05$. There were no significant differences of pregnancy rate after treatment in women with amenorrhea, hypomenorrhea, and normal menstruation before operations (39.4%, 48.3%, 52.2%, respectively. $P > 0.05$). The pregnancy rates after treatment in women with initial mild, moderate, or severe adhesions were 64.7% (11/17), 53.6% (15/28), 32.5% (13/40), respectively, with no statistic difference ($P = 0.05$). Thus it can be seen that postoperative menstrual pattern and postoperative recurrence of adhesions are factors affecting pregnancy rate after hysteroscopic operations. Whether the degree of preoperative adhesions being the factor affecting reproductive prognosis after hysteroscopic adhesiolysis or not remains to be investigated by further studies, such as selecting more scientific classification and increasing the number of cases.

Hysteroscopic lysis or removal of intrauterine adhesions can restore a normal cavity, improve the menstruation and increase the pregnancy rate. Hence it has become the most ideal method of treatment in patients with intrauterine adhesions. However, in spite of the wide application of hysteroscopic operations, the postoperative recurrence of adhesions is still very common, and its reproductive prognosis is still unsatisfactory. Comprehensive therapeutic measures including hysteroscopic lysis of intrauterine adhesions, placement of intrauterine barriers, combination with cyclic hormone treatment, and regular postoperative second-look hysteroscopy to explore and divide new-formed adhesions are the best treatment for intrauterine adhesions.

9.7 Transcervical Removal of Uterine Foreign Body

Enlan Xia

Transcervical removal of uterine foreign body (TCRF) is a procedure using hysteroscopic resectoscope to remove the foreign bodies under direct vision. Hysteroscopy can detect and locate accurately the foreign bodies inside the uterus. TCRF procedure has the advantages of safe operation, high success rate, and fewer traumas, which is the best choice for removal of intrauterine foreign body (Figs. 9.176, 9.177, and 9.178).

9.7.1 Intrauterine Device (IUD)

1. The removal of IUD with tail string or the easy removal of IUD can be done without hysteroscope. However, under the circumstances that the tail string is broken, blind removal is difficult, IUD embedment is suspected, only parts of IUD are taken out, fragments of IUDs still remain within the uterus (Fig. 9.179), reversible fallopian tube contraceptive device is deeply embedded in uterine cornua, or in women who are menopausal (the longer the duration of menopause, the more serious the atrophy of

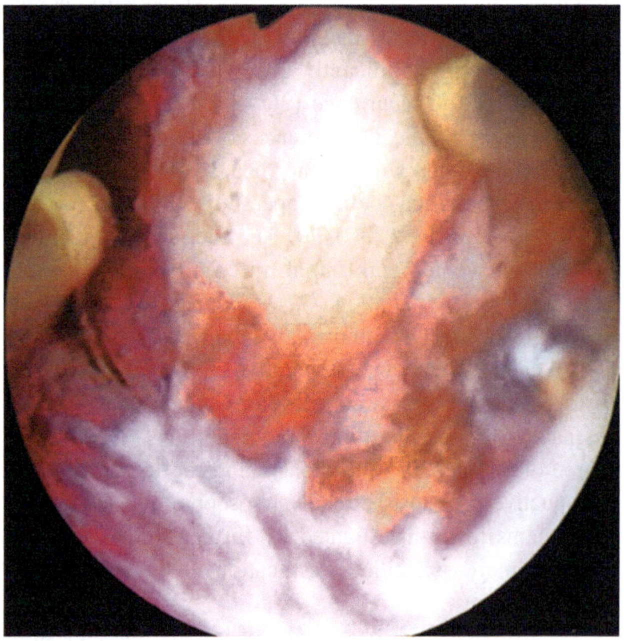

Fig. 9.176 A wire loop electrode is used to remove the broken tip of a hook embedded in the uterine muscle wall

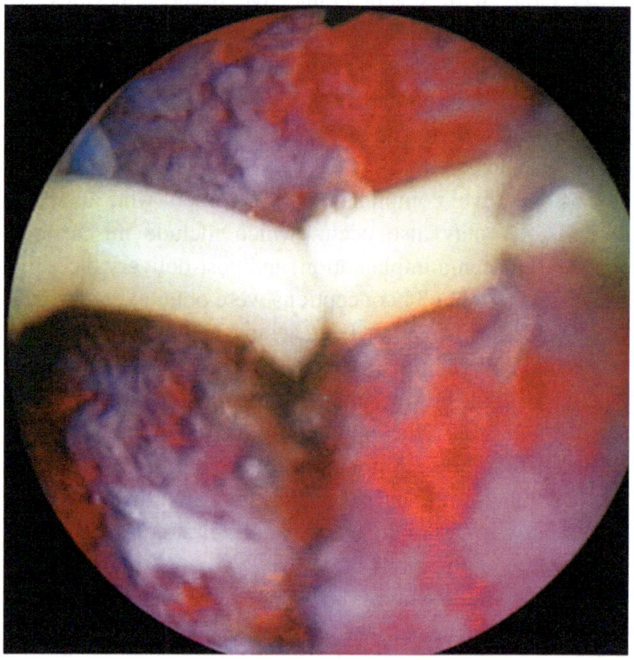

Fig. 9.177 The needle electrode is used to incise the uterine muscle wall and the broken tip of the hook is released

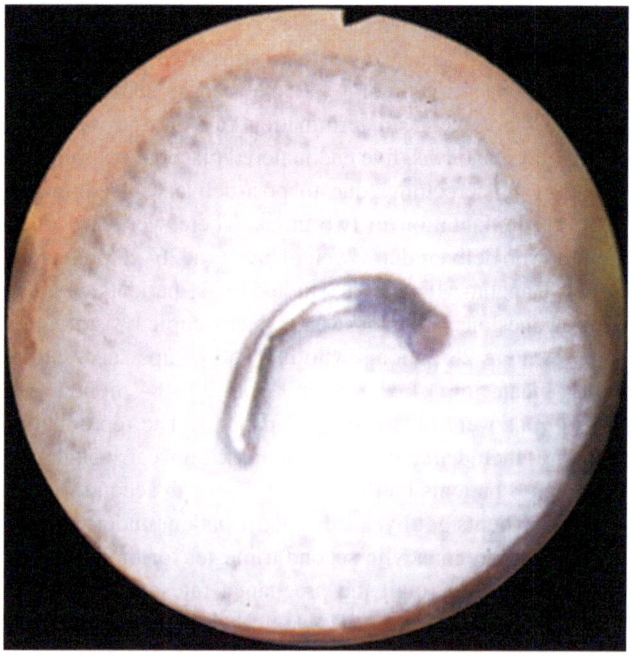

Fig. 9.178 The broken tip of the hook is taken out

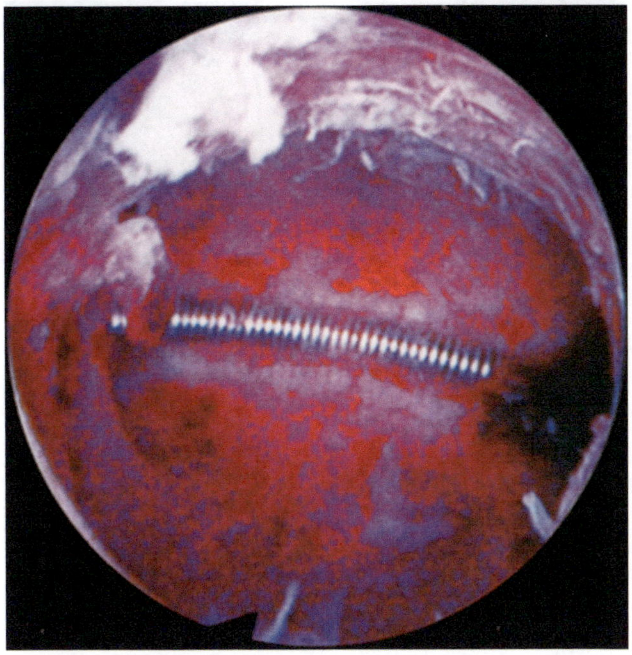

Fig. 9.179 Intrauterine remnants of IUD Fragments. 1/3 of IUD has been taken out and two broken ends are embedded in the bilateral uterine cornua

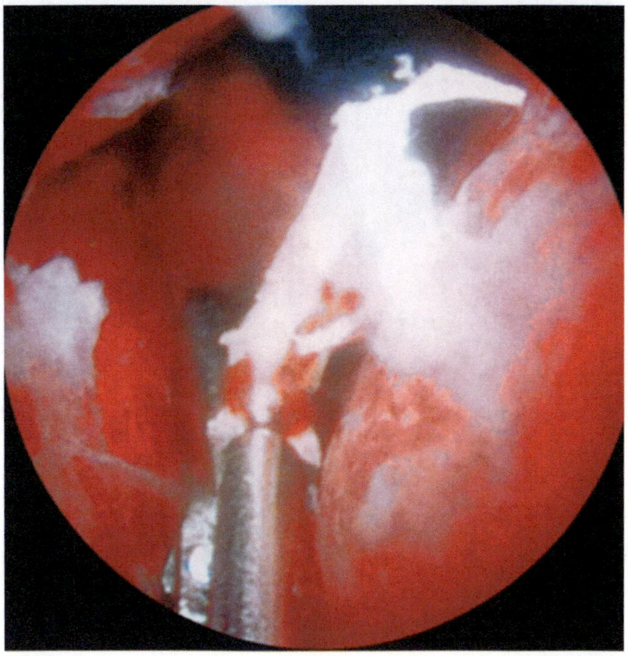

Fig. 9.180 The foreign body is held by a grasping forceps under direct vision

reproductive organ), the removal of IUD will be much more difficult and prone to infection. Hysteroscopic removal of IUD or hysteroscopic removal under ultrasound guidance is required for these situations.

2. The therapeutic hysteroscope is equipped with alligator forceps, foreign body clamps, etc. which can grasp the foreign bodies under direct vision (Figs. 9.180 and 9.181). If it is not powerful enough, or if there is embedment, an operative hysteroscope is needed to replace it.
3. The operative hysteroscope is fit for removal of embedded IUD (Fig. 9.182). A wire loop electrode may be used to hook the residual tip of IUD (Fig. 9.183), and then pull it out (Fig. 9.184). An open semi-circular wire loop can be put into the stainless steel ring and hook it out (Figs. 9.185, 9.186, 9.187, and 9.188). If an IUD is embedded in the uterine wall (Figs. 9.189 and 9.190), passes through the fibroids (Fig. 9.191), or is put around the fibroids (Figs. 9.192, 9.193, and 9.194), the electric wire loop can be used to incise the myometrium around the embedded IUD or resect the fibroid (Figs. 9.195a–c, 9.196a–f, 9.197a–c, and 9.198a–e), and then remove or clamp out the IUD under ultrasound guidance. If the IUD is embedded deeply, the laparoscopic examination shall be performed simultaneously to determine whether the IUD has passed through the uterine serosa (Fig. 9.199) or not.
4. The spring and tail string of the reversible fallopian tube contraceptive device are often embedded in tubal ostia and uterine horns. Once the tail string is broken, IUD will be extremely difficult to remove. In such circumstances, the 21Fr operative hysteroscope and a closed electrode can be used to plow deep into the uterine cornua and take it out. Sometimes, IUD may be discharged automatically during the menstrual period due to the contraction of the uterus, which the patient may not be aware of and it is still thought to be inside the uterus. Therefore it cannot be found during the procedure of removal and its existence

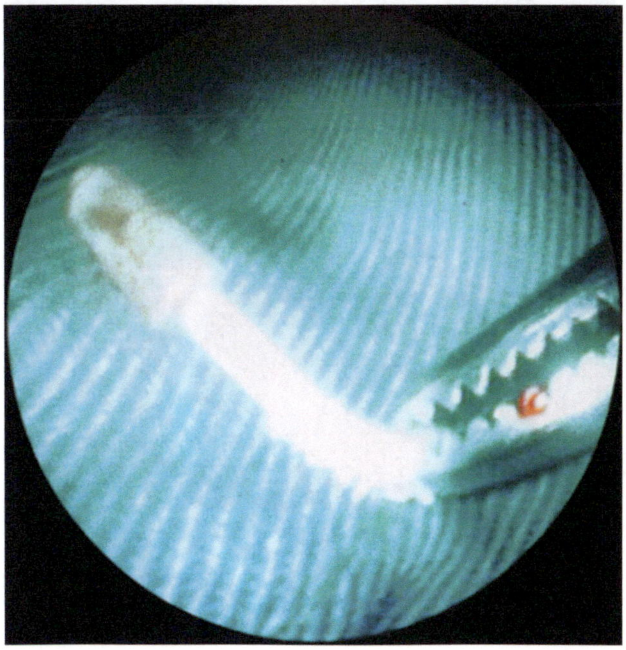

Fig. 9.181 The foreign body is pulled out by a grasping forceps

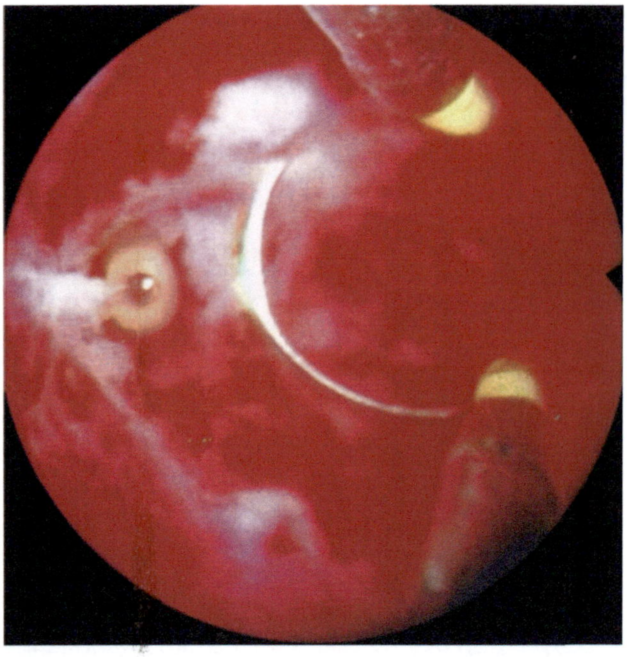

Fig. 9.182 The residual tip of IUD is embedded in the right anterior wall

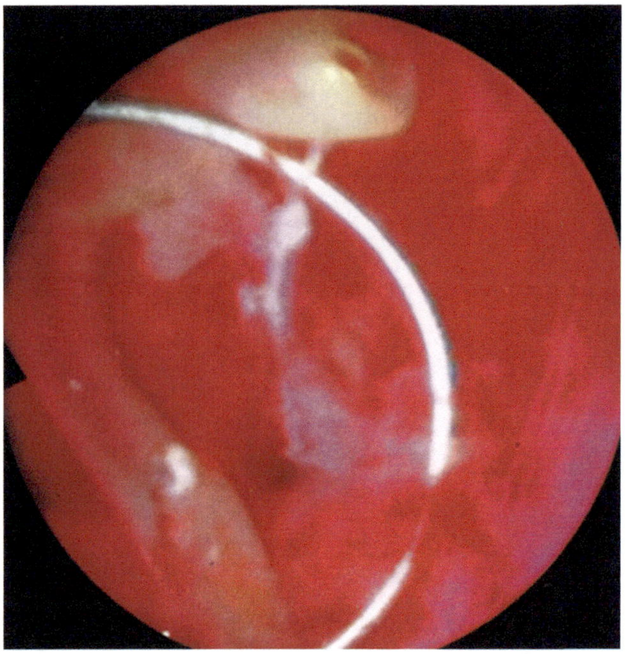

Fig. 9.183 The wire loop electrode is used to hook the residual tip of IUD

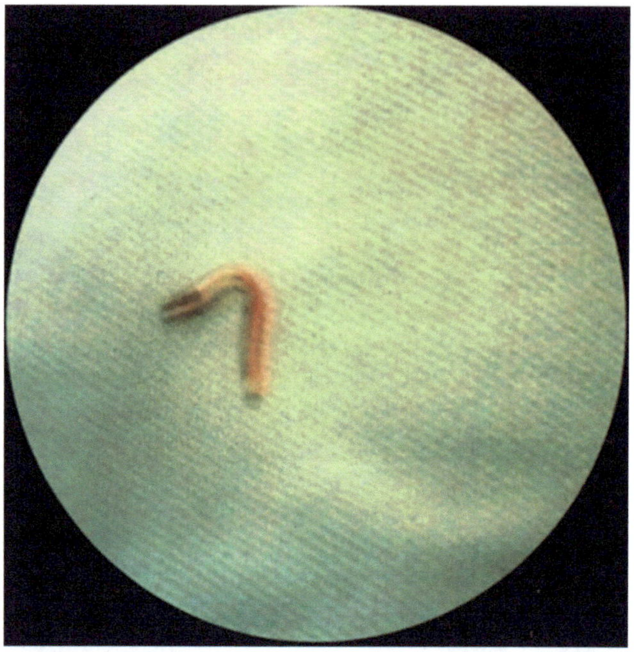

Fig. 9.184 The removed residual tip of IUD

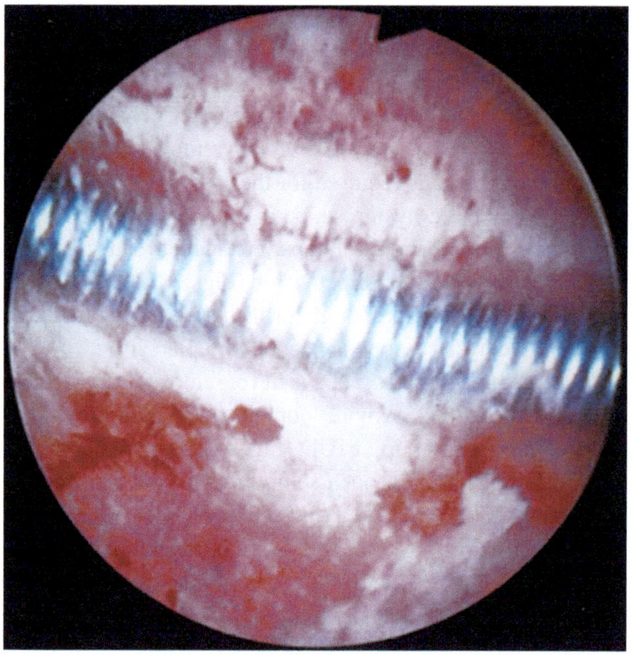

Fig. 9.185 The embedment of IUD in the uterine cavity

is also difficult to be confirmed by ultrasonography. When this is the case, hysteroscopic examination can be done to determine whether there is IUD or not. Valle et al. reported that in 91 patients, IUD was removed successfully in 78 cases under hysteroscopy and no IUD was observed within the uterine cavity in the remaining 13 cases, including six cases of translocated IUD and seven cases of absent IUD. Siegler and Kemmann reported on the hysteroscopic removal of occult IUD in 10 patients, of which two cases had a translocated device (one was buried completely in the uterine muscle wall, and the other was concealed by the amniotic cavity), and one case had the IUD moved out of the lower segment of uterus, only a

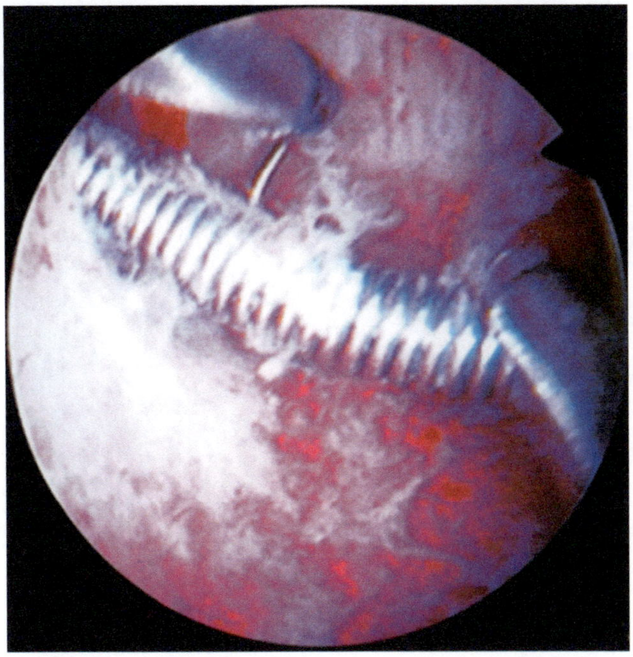

Fig. 9.186 The wire loop electrode can be put into the stainless steel ring and the IUD is hooked out

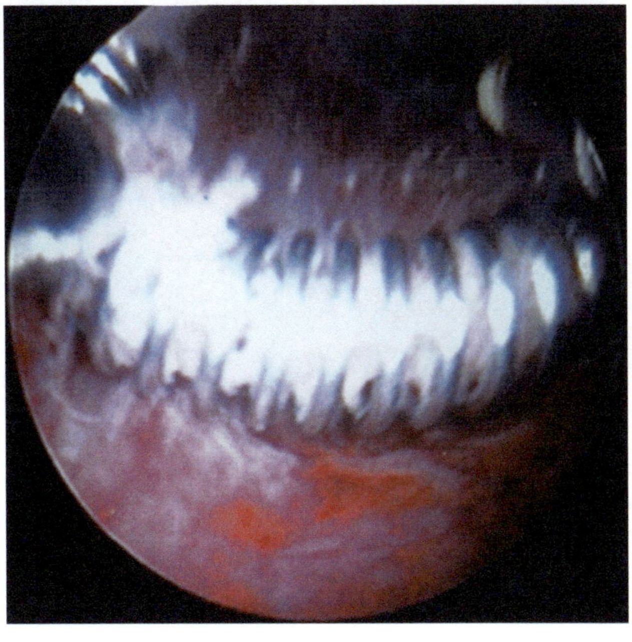

Fig. 9.187 The wire loop electrode can be put into the stainless steel ring and the IUD is hooked out

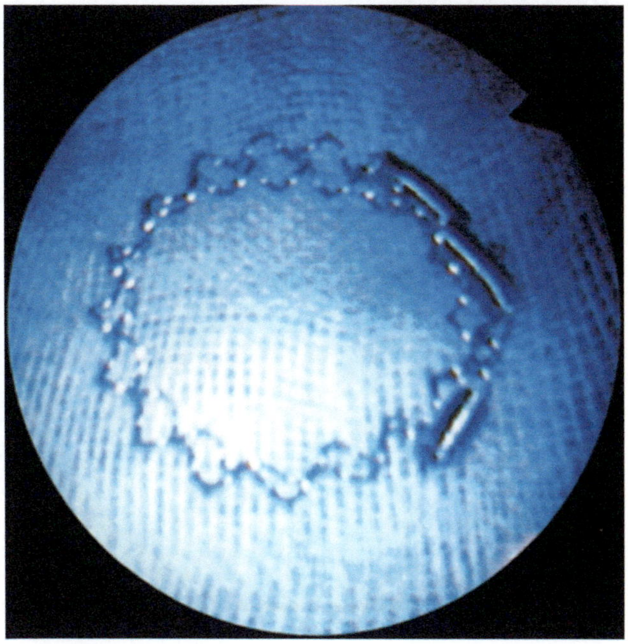

Fig. 9.188 The removed IUD

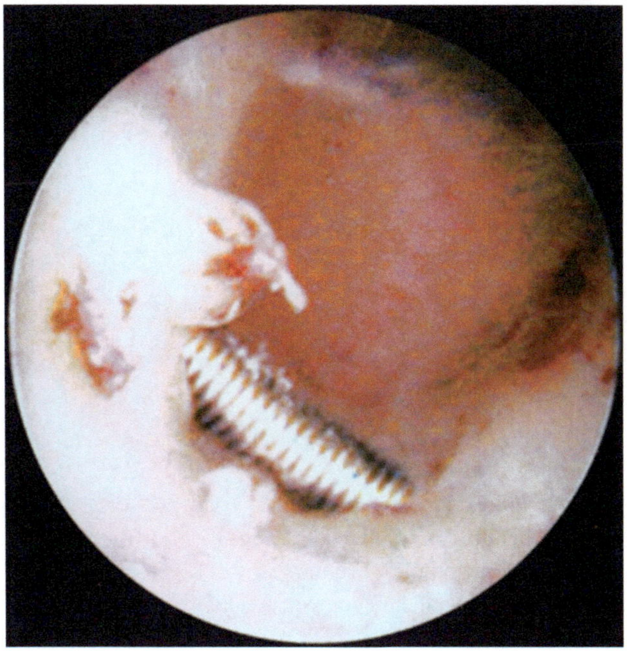

Fig. 9.189 Embedment of IUD in the uterine myometrial layer

very small part of which can be seen by hysteroscopy and was suitable to be removed by laparoscopy. In the Hysteroscopic Center of Fuxing Hospital, Capital Medical University, there was a case, in which the arm of a Tcu IUD penetrated into the bladder, causing the patient to suffer from micturition and hematuria. It was taken out by hysteroscopy under cystoscopic monitoring. An open drainage catheter was placed inside the bladder for 2 weeks and the symptoms disappeared. There was another case, in which only the monofilament tail of Tcu IUD was visible under hysteroscope and IUD was misplaced in pelvic cavity and wrapped by omentum majus, which was removed by laparoscopy.

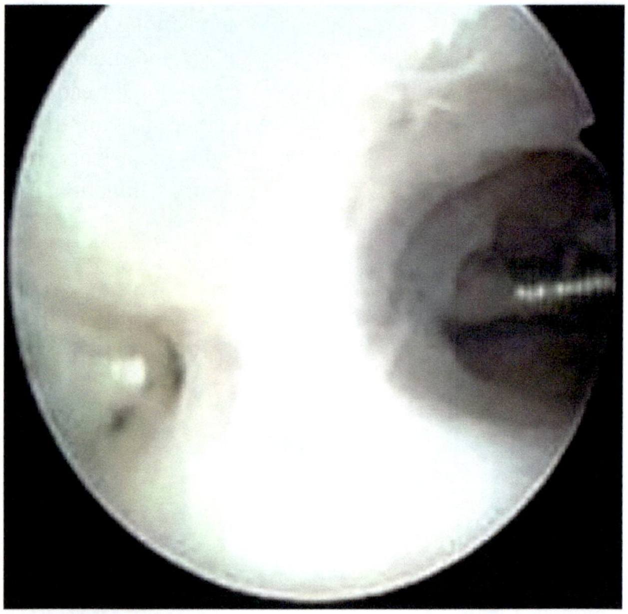

Fig. 9.190 T-shaped IUD is embedded in the myometrium of uterine fundus and lateral uterine wall

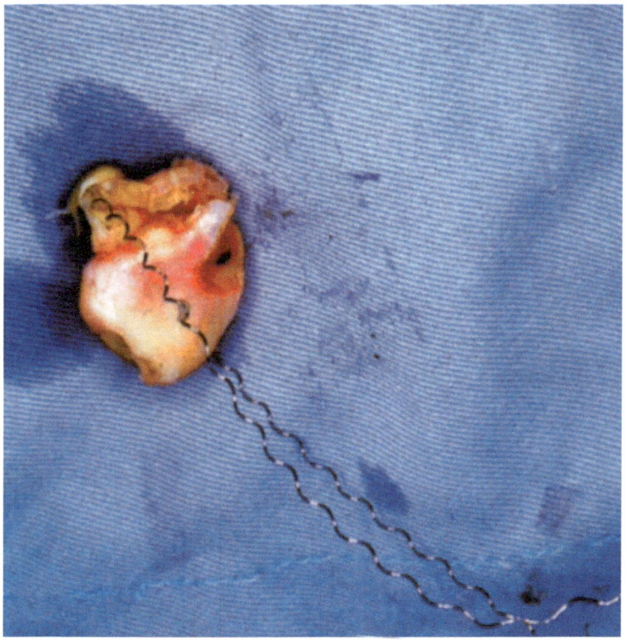

Fig. 9.191 Migration of IUD through the fibroids

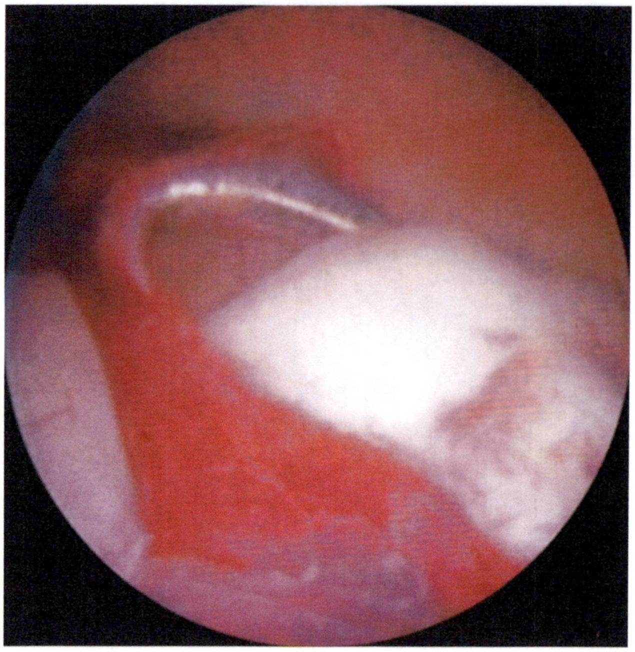

Fig. 9.192 IUD is put around the base of fibroid

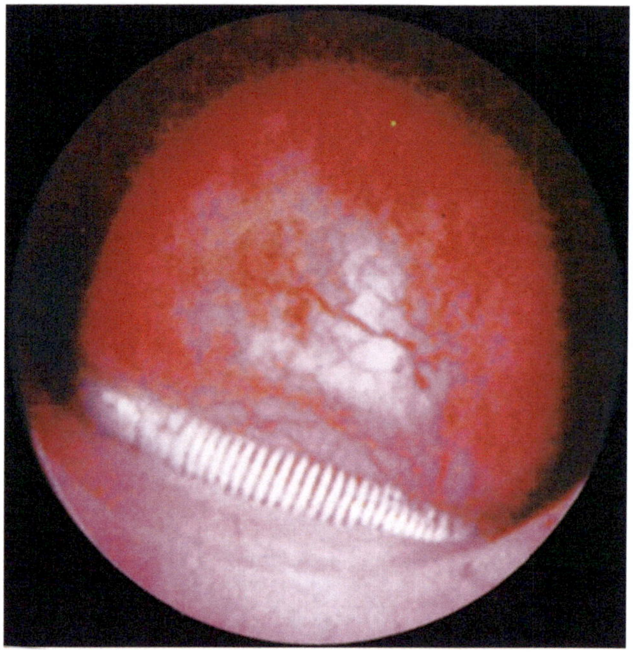

Fig. 9.193 IUD is put around the submucous fibroid

9.7.2 Retention of Fetal Bone

The retention of fetal bone after abortion is a rare complication. Fetal bone remnants may sometimes occur in a late-term induced abortion (Fig. 9.200), which may often cause abnormal uterine bleeding, dyspareunia, and infertility. Elford and Claman reported that a 36-year-old woman had been suffering from secondary infertility for 15 years because of residual intrauterine fetal bones caused by induced abortion. Verma et al. reported a case with chronic pelvic pain resulting from the retention of fetal bones and the patient's pelvic pain was resolved after hysteroscopic removal of fetal bones. Sahinoglu and Kuyumcuoglu reported that a woman experienced persistent postmenopausal bleeding and pelvic pain because of the residual of fetal bones after an induced abortion 17 years ago. Cepni et al. reported a case with a history of 8 years of infertility, hypermenorrhea, and persistent

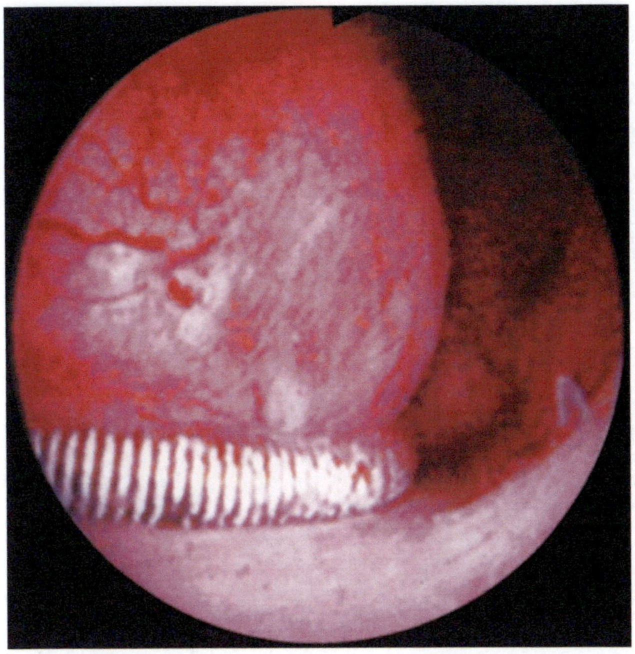

Fig. 9.194 IUD is put around the submucous fibroid

vaginal discharge after termination of a pregnancy. Sometimes the retained fetal bones can take up most of the uterine cavity. HSG generally reveals no findings, but strong intrauterine echoes can be identified by ultrasound and the retained fetal bones can be observed directly under hysteroscope. The traditional management is blind curettage and hysterectomy, which are nearly abandoned today. Letterie and Case reported a successful hysteroscopic surgery using a resectoscope and wire loop under abdominal ultrasonography guidance for removal of retained bones caused by a second-trimester abortion.

The small retained fetal bone should be differentiated from the osseous metaplasia of the endometrium. When the fetal bone is larger or vertical to the long axis of the uterus, a dilator should be inserted into the cervix the night before the operation, and the cervix is dilated to Hegar 12 at the time of operation. After being located by hysteroscopy and under ultrasound guidance, the fetal bones are clamped out by oval forceps or taken out along with the exit of electric wire loop (Figs. 9.201 and 9.202a–e). If it is embedded, the myometrium may be incised and the fetal bone can be clamped out or removed.

9.7.3 Endometrial Ossification and Cervical Ossification

Endometrial ossification and cervical ossification are rare conditions. Most reported cases of endometrial ossification have a previous history of abortion and retention of fetal bones, and only a few cases can be explained by osseous metaplasia. Clinical presentations may include abnormal vaginal bleeding or discharge, dysmenorrhea, pelvic pain, secondary infertility, etc. Hysterectomy or dilation and curettage had been the usual therapeutic methods used. Later, some cases have been treated by means of hysteroscopic resection. Torne et al. reported on a case who had an induced abortion at the sixth week of gestation. Four months later she experienced dysmenorrhea, dyspareunia, and pelvic pain. Ultrasonography revealed a strong echogenic band in uterine cavity and the residual fetal bones were successfully removed with hysteroscopic resectoscope. They pointed out that new residual fetal bones were feasible to be removed by hysteroscopy and were the cause of endometrial ossification. Rodriguez and Adamson reported a case of hysteroscopic removal of osseous metaplasia of the uterus. During the operation, combined examination of laparoscopy and hysteroscopy revealed bony endometrium in the form of spicules which were perpendicular to the endometrium, with most of them located in the posterior wall of the fundus. Firstly, biopsy forceps was applied to remove the bony tissues, and then followed by gentle curettage. Finally, a hysteroscopic resectoscope was introduced into uterine cavity and then the visible remaining spicule bone tissues were resected and removed under direct vision. Intra- and postoperative TVS was applied to identify its existence and confirm its removal. Pathologic examination of removed tissues revealed benign bony tissue. The patient received estrogens for 5 weeks after the procedures. Afterwards, when she got pregnant, ultrasonography at 5–6 weeks of gestation revealed two small calcifications approximately 1 mm each. Finally, she achieved a live birth infant without any recurrence. Garcia and Kably reported a rare case of infertility caused by the osseous metaplasia of the endometrium. The preoperative ultrasonography showed a calcification in uterine cavity. Under laparoscopic monitoring, hysteroscopic removal of osseous metaplasia of the endometrium was done and the calcification was confirmed by histopathologic examination. Postoperative conception was achieved after one spontaneous menstruation cycle. It was concluded that the hysteroscopy was the first choice for treatment of endometrial ossification and should be combined with laparoscopy. In 2007, Nevarez et al. from Mexico reported a rare case of the osseous metaplasia of the endometrium. It was pointed out that its predisposing factor was endometrial metabolic abnormality induced by a history of uterine curettage. Women with endometrial ossification experienced secondary infertility or early pregnancy loss, dysmenorrhea or dyspareunia, with their history and ultrasonography indicating the diagnosis. In the past, D&C and hysterectomy were the choice of therapy, but now, hysteroscopy has become a shortcut of management of this condition.

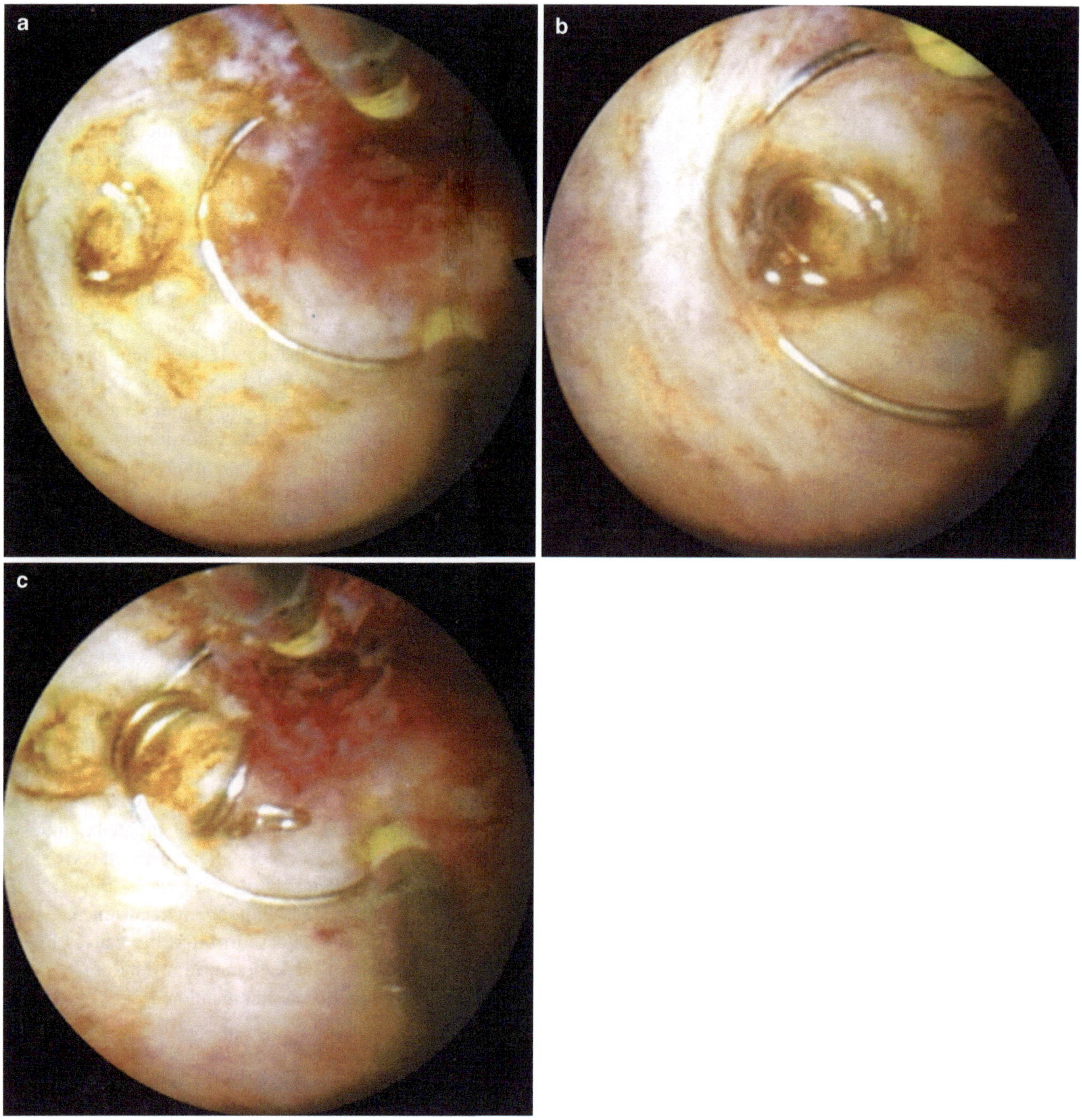

Fig. 9.195 The residual IUD is embedded into the myometrial layer. (**a**, **b**) The surrounding myometrium is incised and IUD exposed. (**c**) The wire loop electrode is used to hook IUD

In addition, chronic cervicitis may cause cervical ossification. Cicinelli et al. reported a 41-year-old woman who had primary infertility, pelvic pain, and chronic endocervicitis. Ossifications were developed in the upper third of the cervical canal. After pretreatment with antibiotics, the bone fragments were removed using grasping forceps under hysteroscopy with no recurrence during 1 year of follow-up. Cepni et al. reported a case with a history of 8 years of infertility, hypermenorrhea, and persistent vaginal discharge after termination of a pregnancy. Fetal bone fragments were removed by curettage with a curette.

9.7.4 Residual Trophoblastic Remnants

The residual trophoblastic remnants in uterine cavity caused by missed abortion, incomplete abortion, adherent placenta, placenta accreta, etc. can lead to intrauterine

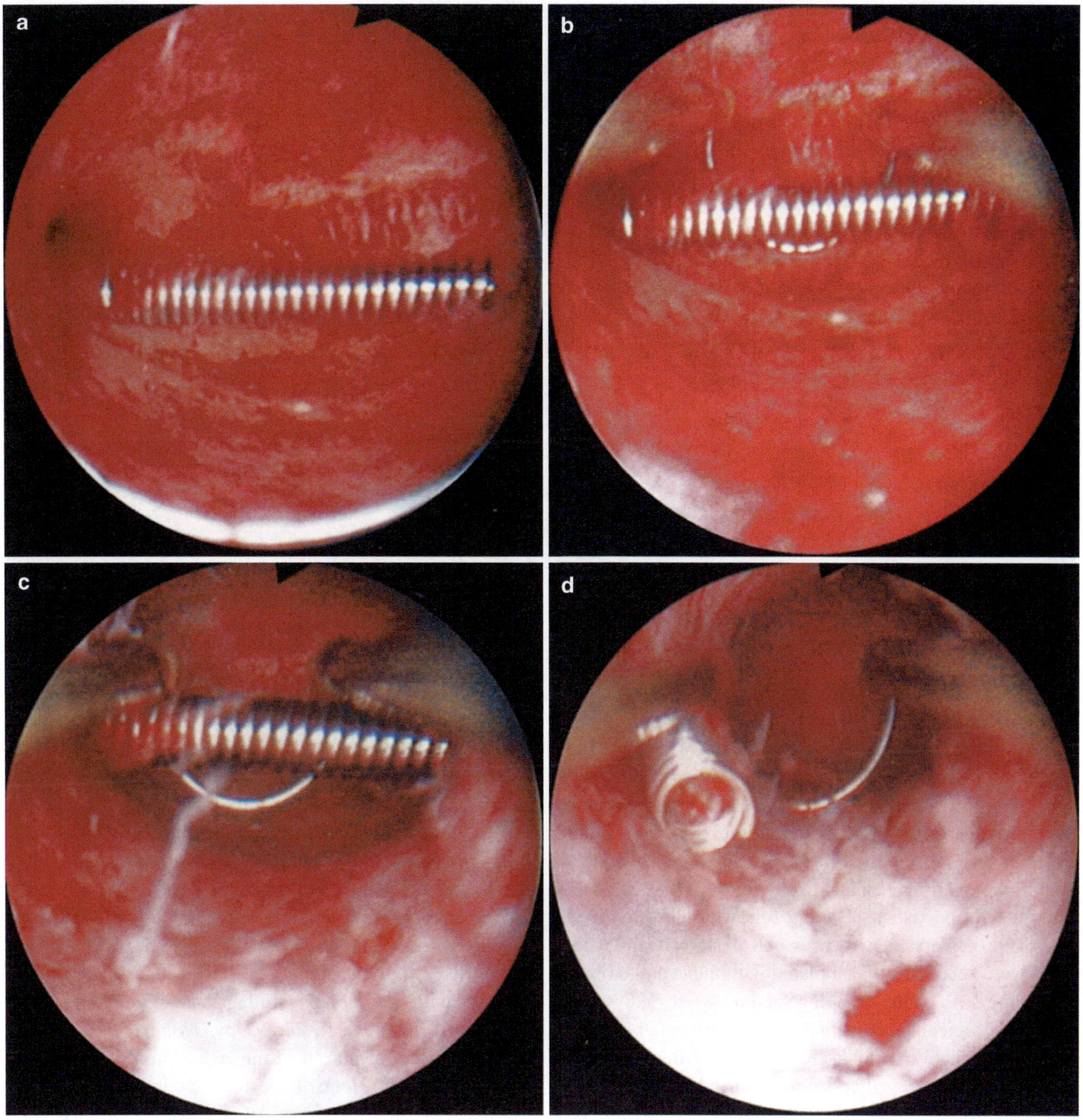

Fig. 9.196 Removal of a residual IUD. (**a**) The residual IUD is located at the uterine fundus. (**b–e**) The wire loop electrode is used to hook IUD. (**f**) The morphology of uterine cavity after removal of IUD

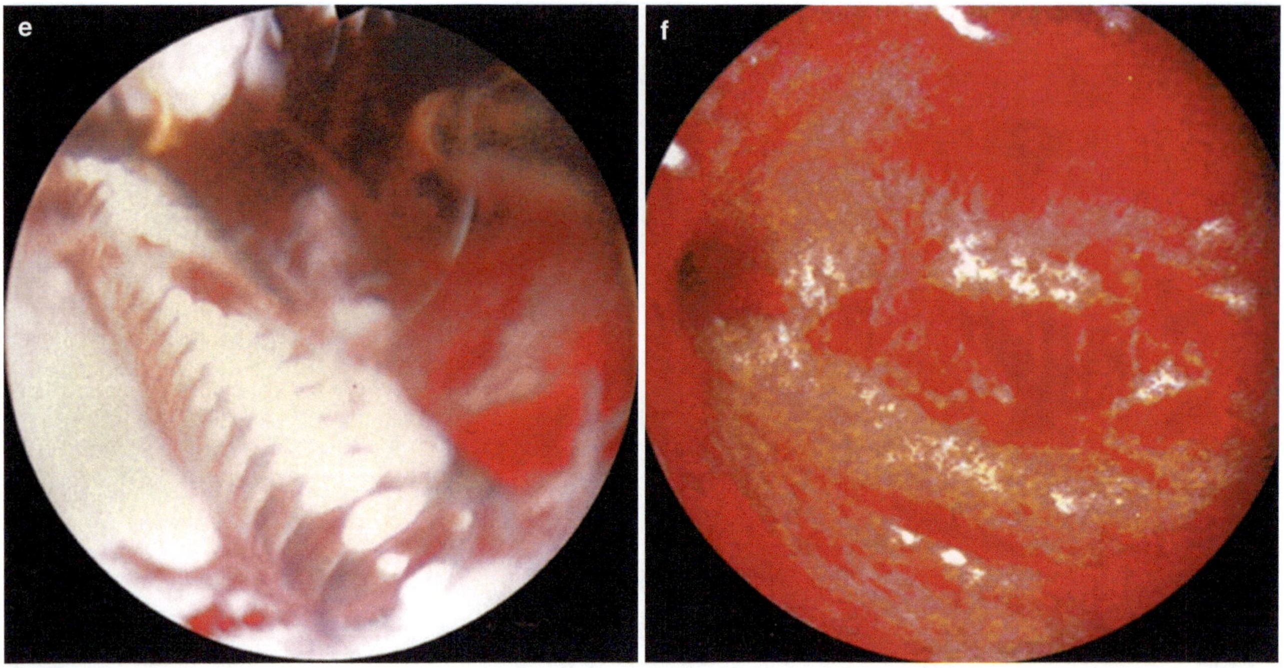

Fig. 9.196 (continued)

adhesions, amenorrhea, or irregular bleeding. If there are severe adhesions, the residual trophoblastic remnants may not be probed and removed completely. Hysteroscopy not only can be used for diagnosis, but also for removal and resection of the trophoblastic remnants using electric wire loop under ultrasound guidance. The excised tissues can be sent for histopathologic examination (Fig. 9.203a–e). Goldenberg et al. reported their experiences with hysteroscopic removal of residual trophoblastic tissues in 18 patients with persistent bleeding following abortion in 16 cases and delivery in two cases. All hysteroscopic procedures were successfully completed with the average operative time 10 min (ranging from 8 to 20 min). Histopathological examination of the suspected residual tissues confirmed trophoblastic remnants. After the procedure, all cases achieved cessation of bleeding and showed no residual tissues by ultrasonography. A second-look hysteroscopy was performed in five patients several weeks later, and confirmed the absence of residuals. It was concluded that operative hysteroscopy was an easy and short procedure to manage residual trophoblastic tissues, made positioning accurate and was superior to routine D&C. There was a case of choriocarcinoma treated in the Hysteroscopy Center of Fuxing Hospital, Capital Medical University, who had induced abortion 80 days ago. Uterine curettage did not stop the persistent vaginal bleeding after abortion. Ultrasonography showed no abnormalities and blood HCG levels were on the rise. A purple blue nodule 3 mm in diameter was identified under hysteroscopy in the middle segment of anterior uterine wall, and was completely excised from its myometrium by an electric wire loop. Histological examination showed choriocarcinoma, which was cured by chemotherapy. Three years later, she got pregnancy and delivered a healthy baby girl by cesarean section. Cohen et al. assessed and compared the effectiveness of curettage of residual trophoblastic tissue between the use of hysteroscopy and conventional, nonselective and blind procedure. In this study, 70 women were suspected of residual trophoblastic tissue clinically or by ultrasonography after abortion or delivery, including 24 cases of traditional curettage and 46 cases of hysteroscopy. Persistence of residual trophoblastic tissue occurred in five (20.8%) patients with traditional curettage and required management with operative hysteroscopy. None of the patients who had selective curettage under hysteroscopy needed a second operation. None of anesthetic complications, perforation of the uterus, fluid overload, or other surgical complications occurred in patients of both groups. It was similar in reproductive outcome of both groups. It seemed that patients in hysteroscopy group tended to conceive earlier, but there was no difference in pregnancy rates. It was believed that hysteroscopic selective curettage of residual trophoblastic tissue should be preferred as an alternative procedure to nonselective, blind curettage.

9.7.5 Cervical Pregnancy

TCRF is applicable to the patients with dead embryo and less bleeding without signs of infection. Hu et al. reported

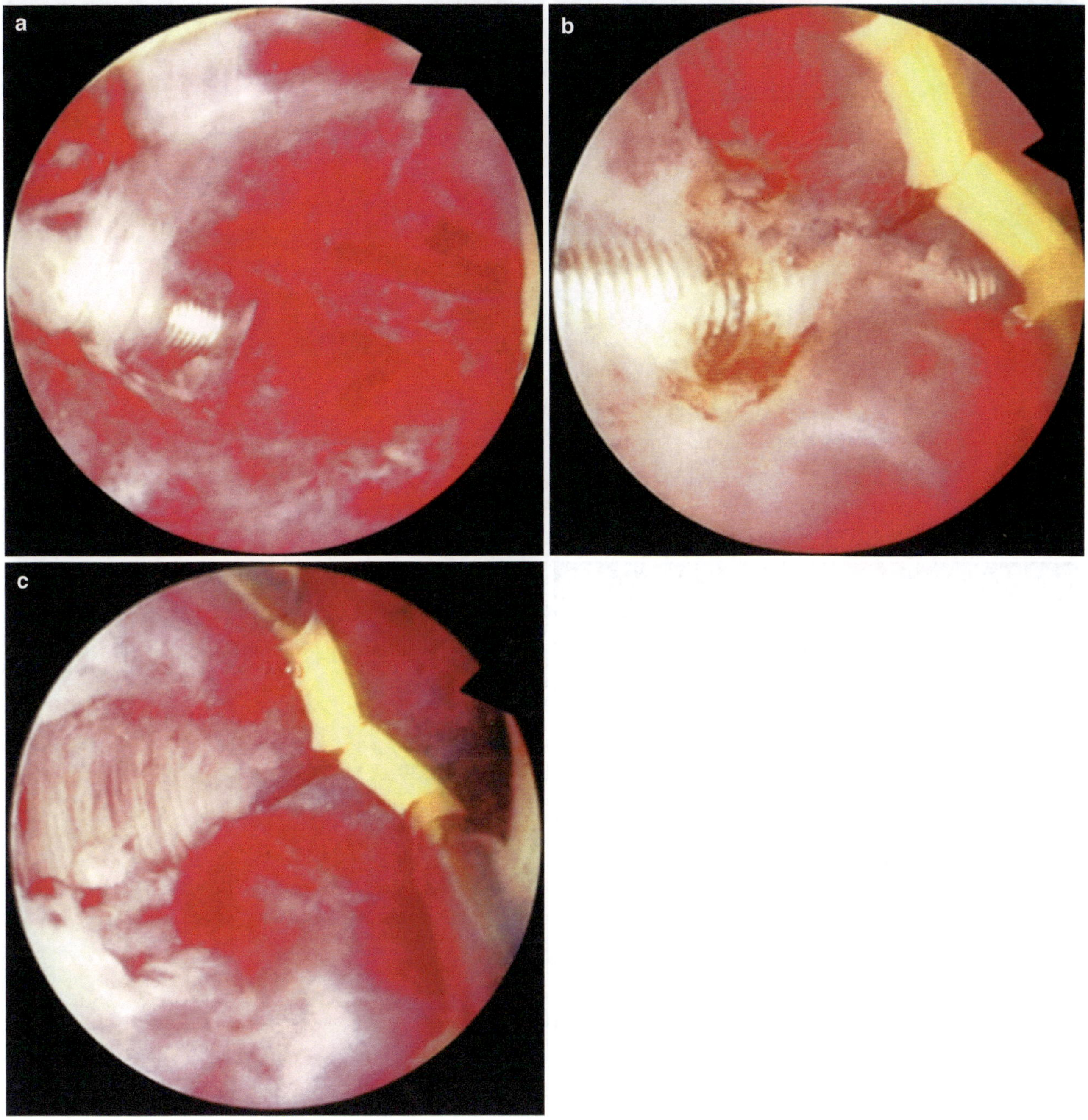

Fig. 9.197 Removal of an embedded IUD. (**a**) The broken tip of IUD is embedded in the myometrial layer. (**b**) The needle electrode is used to incise the surface myometrium of IUD. (**c**) After removal of IUD, the compressing mark on IUD is seen

two cases of cervical pregnancy, which were treated successfully by operative hysteroscopy. The cervical canal cannot hold irrigation fluid, leading to inadequate distention, and hemostasis cannot be achieved to manage bleeding in the cavity. Therefore, excessive hemorrhage should be regarded as a contraindication of this operation (Fig. 9.204a–c).

9.7.6 Cesarean Scar Pregnancy

With the rise in cesarean section rate, the cesarean scar pregnancy increases. Embryo implantation in a scar of a previous cesarean section uterus is a rare but dangerous complication (Fig. 9.205a, b), which may be associated with the poor healing of the uterine incision and wide scar after cesarean sec-

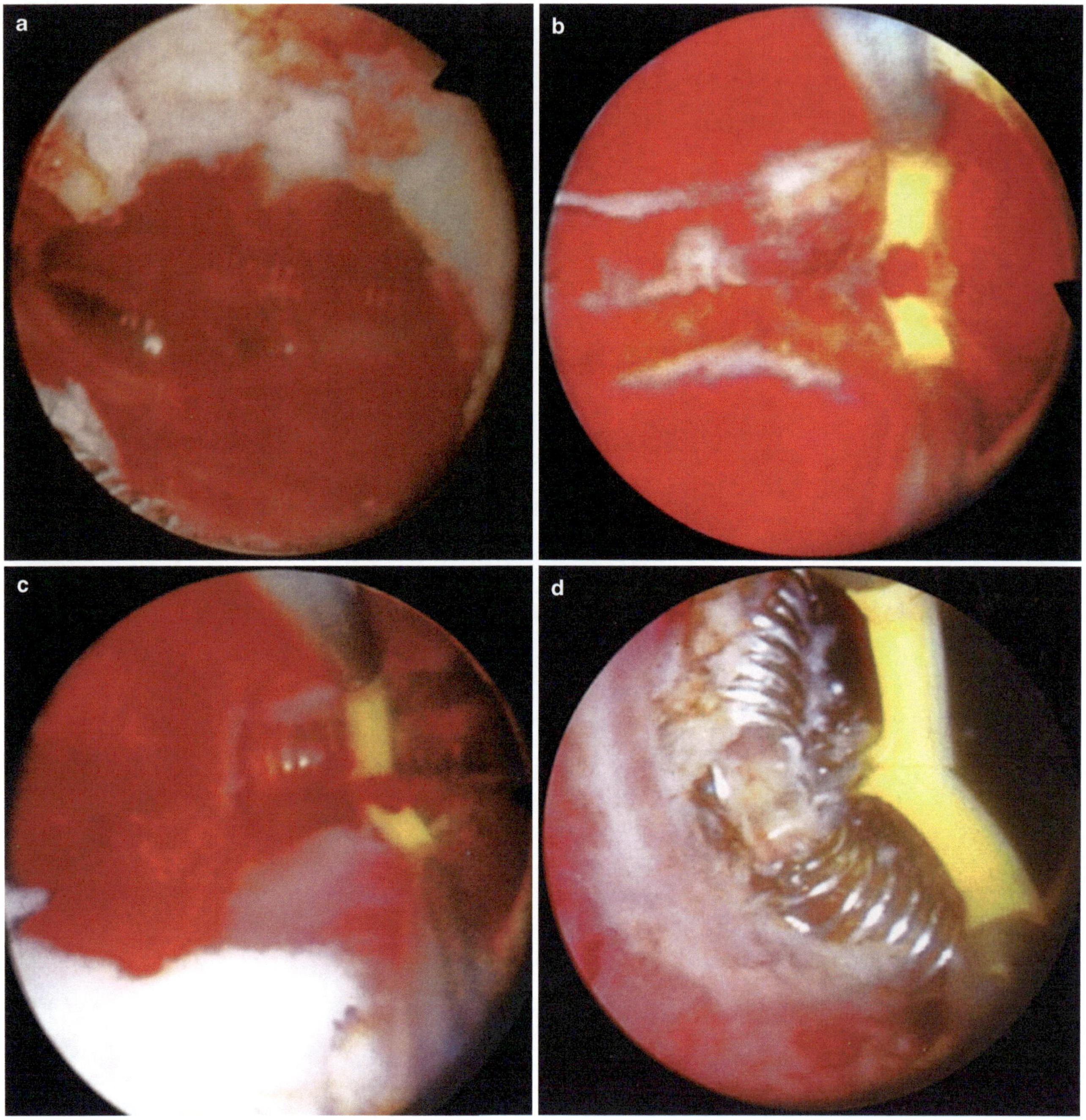

Fig. 9.198 Removal of an embedded IUD. (**a**) After incision of adhesion at the cervical internal os, IUD is found at the uterine fundus and embedded in the myometrial layer. (**b**) After incision of uterine fundal myometrium with needle electrode, IUD is exposed. (**c**) After incision of uterine fundal myometrium with needle electrode, IUD is exposed. (**d**) The needle electrode is used to hook IUD. (**e**) A complete removal of metal ring

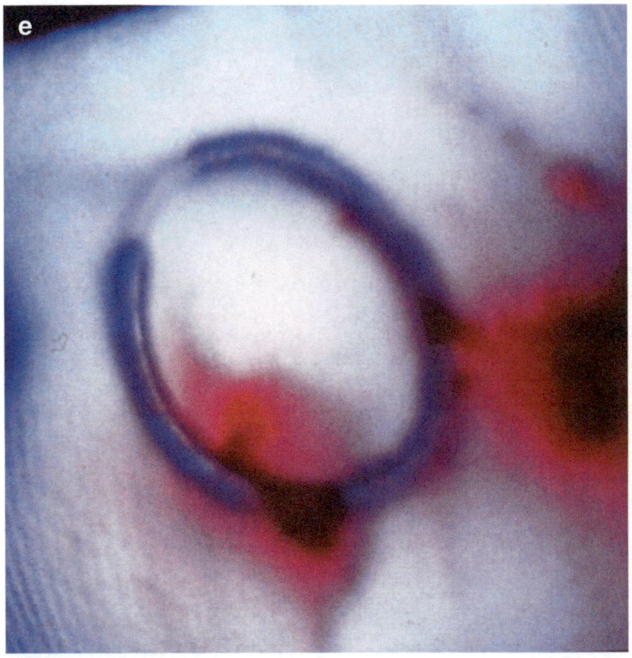

Fig. 9.198 (continued)

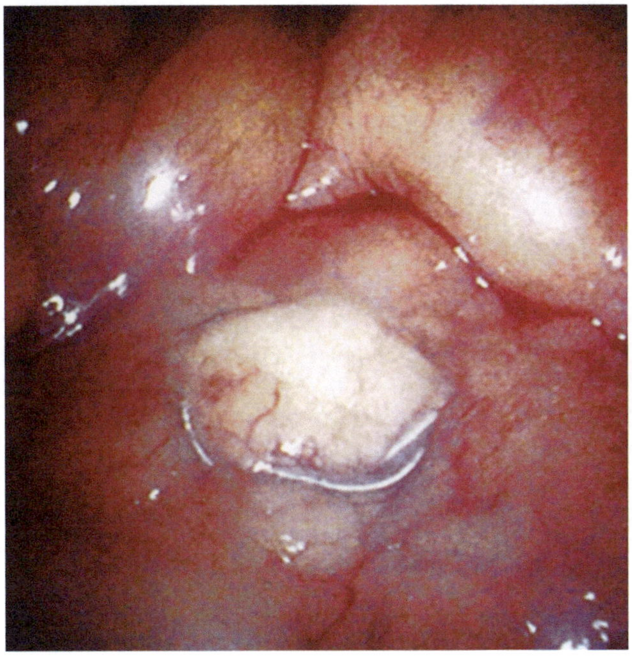

Fig. 9.199 Metal ring is misplaced on the omentum majus in abdominal cavity

tion. The treatment of scar pregnancy should be administered in accordance with that of ectopic pregnancy. The traditional surgical treatment is to undergo curettage under sufficient preoperative preparations. Since the curettage procedure often causes heavy bleeding, ligation of the internal iliac artery and even hysterectomy might have to be done. There are two kinds of possible development of cesarean scar

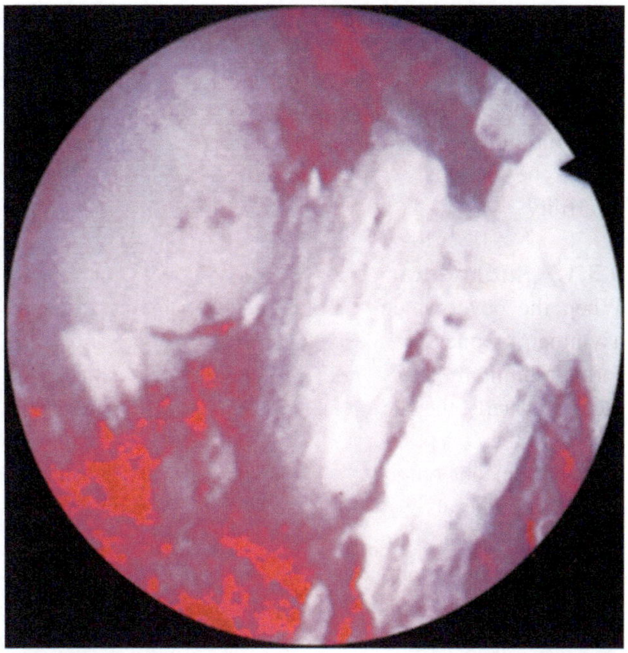

Fig. 9.200 Retention of fetal bones

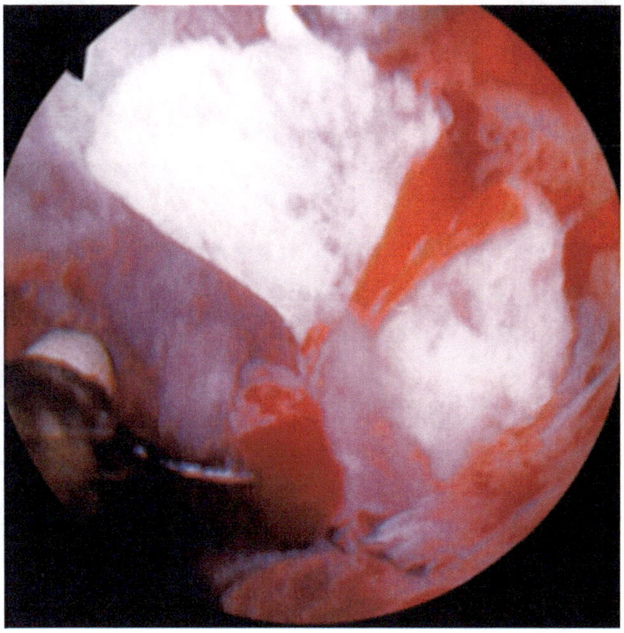

Fig. 9.201 The wire loop electrode is used to hook the fetal bone

pregnancy. One is that the trophoblast may extend into the myometrial layer of the uterus, the other is that the trophoblast may develop into the uterine cavity. The latter may be fit for hysteroscopic operation. Transcervical resection under direct vision can be an alternative surgical treatment, the prognosis is good, and fertility can be preserved. Wang et al. reported that 11 women with cesarean scar pregnancy were treated in their hospital from 1999 to 2004. Cesarean scar pregnancy was diagnosed by TVS and managed with laparo-

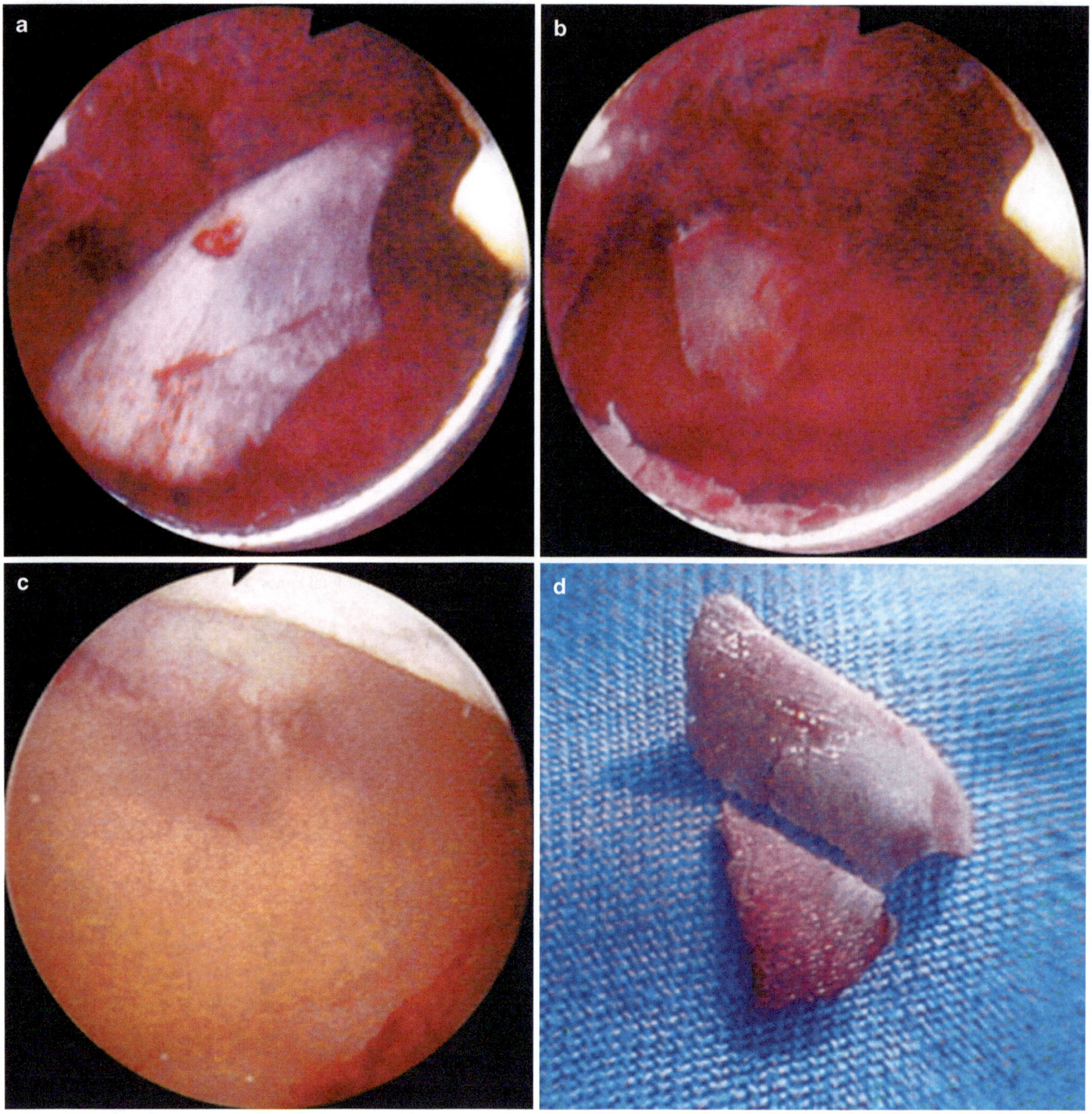

Fig. 9.202 Removal of fetal bones. (**a**) The fetal bones are retained in the uterine cavity after induced abortion 1 year ago. (**b**) After removal of the large bone, a small fetal bone is seen in the uterine cavity. (**c**) The uterine cavity after the removal of fetal bones. (**d**, **e**) The removed fetal bones

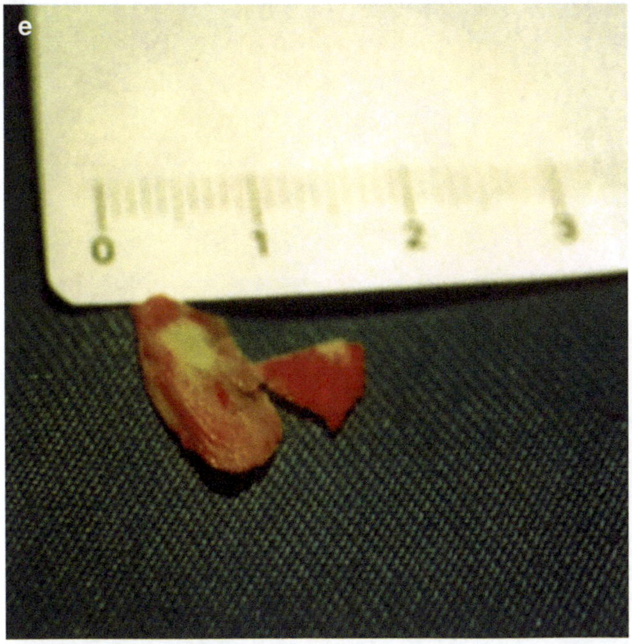

Fig. 9.202 (continued)

scopic and/or hysteroscopic surgery, and the reproductive ability was preserved. The duration of gestation at the time of surgeries ranged from 6 to 11 weeks. The operative procedures included laparoscopy applied in four women, hysteroscopy in six, and hysteroscopy combined with laparoscopy in one, with the average blood loss 110.9 mL (range between 20 and 300 mL) and average hospitalization 1.7 days (range between 0.25 and 3 days). No complications occurred. All of the patients got normal level of serum β-hCG within 4 weeks after operation.

9.7.7 Fragmented Cervical Dilator or Laminaria Tent

It is relatively rare. Before hysteroscopy or induced abortion, a cervical dilator or laminaria tent is inserted to soften the cervix. However, at the time of its removal, some may be found to be broken inside the cervical canal and migrate into the uterine cavity, which can be positioned hysteroscopically and taken out with the electric wire loop. If the fragmented cervical dilator or laminaria is soft and fragile, it can be sucked out with vacuum aspirator. Borgatta and Barad reported on a 32-year-old nulliparous woman, a single laminaria tent was inserted into cervical canal the day before an abortion. Before the procedure, the laminaria was found to be tightly stuck in the cervix. Attempting to remove it led to pushing it into the uterine cavity. On the third day after the abortion, another osmotic dilator was placed to soften the cervix, and then the initial laminaria tent was crushed and removed. However, a small fragment of laminaria was spontaneously discharged 15 months post-operation. Hysteroscopy was conducted and removed about 30 fragments of laminaria.

9.7.8 Surgical Suture Threads

After cesarean section, the silk sutures may be left inside uterine cavity (Fig. 9.206). In the past, the non-absorbable silk suture was used at cesarean section, so the residual thread or thread node may be seen at the internal cervical os under hysteroscopy, and this foreign body may cause endometrial bleeding or inflammation. The residual thread or thread node may be clamped out by alligator forceps or a wire loop electrode under the direct vision of hysteroscope.

Szlyk and Jarrett reported three cases with foreign bodies deeply embedded in the lower urinary tract, with previous failure in attempts of removal by standard cystoscope. However, the 20F hysteroscope was easily introduced into the urethra and successfully removed the foreign bodies.

The removal of intrauterine foreign bodies requires precise positioning, and attention should be paid to preventing uterine perforation, therefore the operation should be performed under ultrasonography and/or laparoscopic monitoring. Laparoscopic ultrasonography (LUS) is higher in resolution than ultrasonography (Fig. 9.207a, b). Its operative procedures are to first establish a pneumoperitoneum, then introduce a laparoscope, instill saline 200–300 mL into the pelvic cavity, and then the laparoscopic ultrasonography probe (Sharplan probe scanning range 180°, frequency of 8 mHz, 10 mm in diameter, probing depth of up to 6 cm) is introduced under direct vision of laparoscopy via the cannula beneath the umbilicus or at lateral side of lower abdomen into the abdominal cavity, allowing for a free scanning of uterus. Both the laparoscopic imaging and ultrasonography imaging are displayed on a monitor via a mixer, which is helpful to accurately understand the shape and the size of the uterus, and identify the extent of the lesions and the resection. For TCRF, laparoscopic ultrasonography can accurately locate the small lesions, discover or rule out invasive intramural lesions and foreign bodies embedded in the uterine muscle wall.

9.8 Other Hysteroscopic Operations

Enlan Xia

9.8.1 Transcervical Uterine Incision (TCUI)

Transcervical uterine incision (TCUI) is using a hysteroscopic needle electrode to incise the uterine wall longitudi-

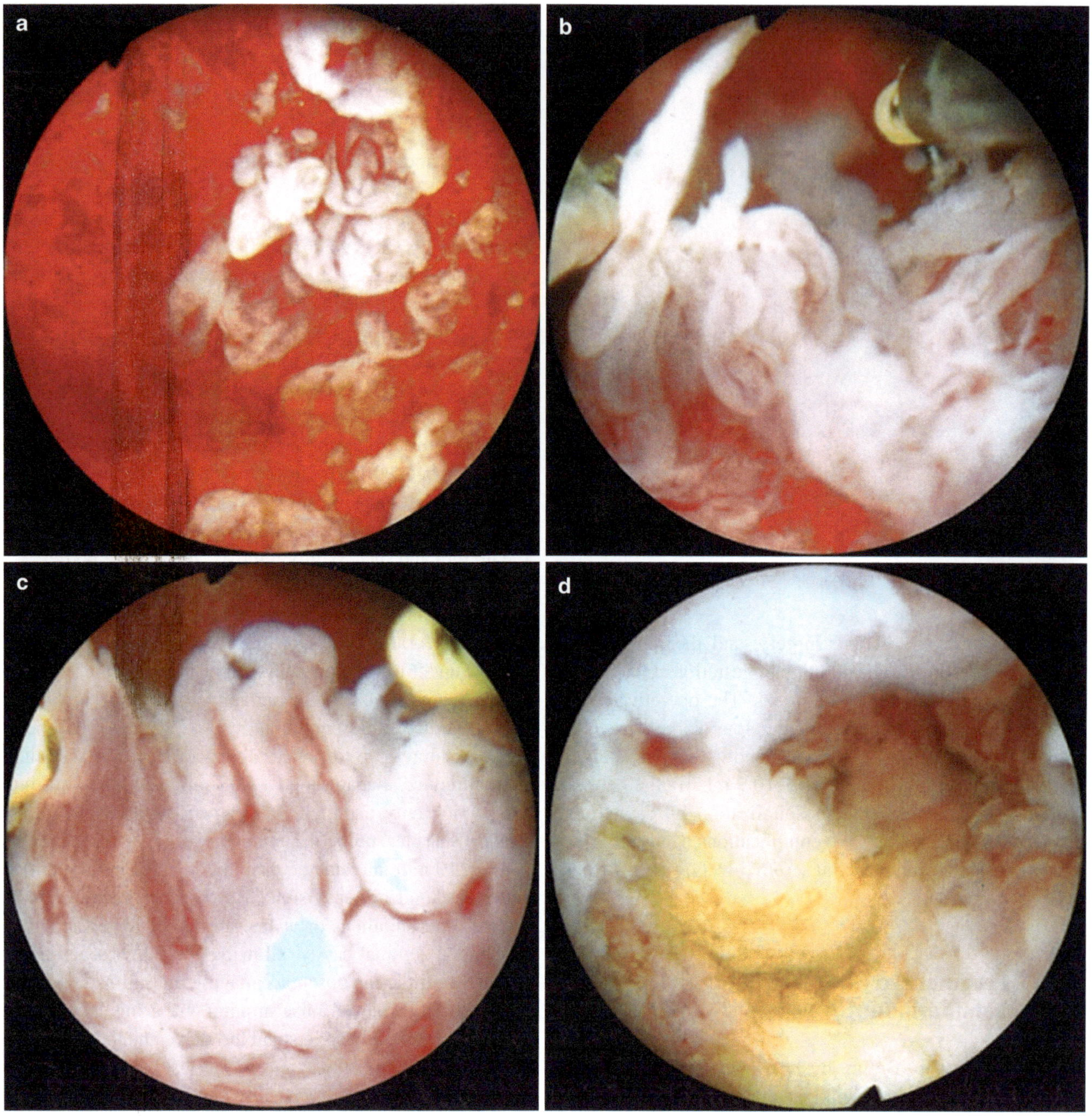

Fig. 9.203 Removal of trophoblastic tissues. (**a**) Trophoblastic remnants with the formation of placenta polyps. (**b**, **c**) Electric resecting of trophoblastic tissues. (**d**) The resected surface. (**e**) Postoperative morphology of uterine cavity

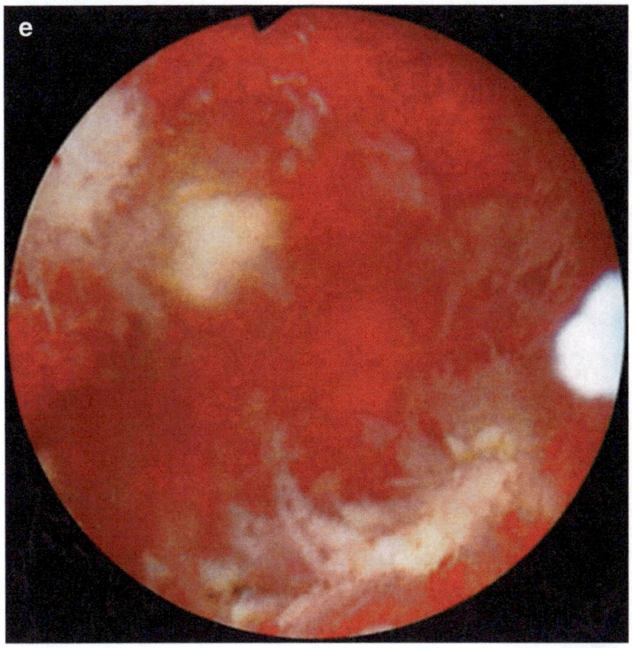

Fig. 9.203 (continued)

nally or using a wire loop electrode to resect the myometrium longitudinally so as to improve the shape of the uterus and broaden the area of the cavity. After the procedure, the decrease of intrauterine pressure and the increase of endometrial blood supply facilitate the implantation of fertilized eggs, prevention of miscarriage, and improvement of reproductive outcomes. This surgery is mainly applicable to narrowed uterine cavity caused by scarred uterine wall resulting from intrauterine adhesions and uterine deformations with narrowed uterine cavity and infertility.

9.8.1.1 Indications

1. Patients who have intrauterine adhesions with scarred uterine wall, a narrowed and small cavity, and amenorrhea.
2. Patients who are diagnosed as T-shaped uterus, unicornuate uterus or Robert uterus, and have one of following conditions:
   (a) two or more spontaneous abortions
   (b) unexplained infertility
   (c) primary infertility requiring assisted reproductive technology

9.8.1.2 Operative Procedures

1. The procedure is to incise the uterine wall with a needle electrode or resect the thickened endometrium with a wire loop electrode along the long axis of the uterus. Generally, 4–5 incisions or resections are conducted to expand the cavity (Figs. 9.208, 9.209, and 9.210).
2. Postoperative hormone therapy is administered to promote the recovery of cutting surface and restoration of menstrual cycle.

9.8.1.3 Experience and Evaluation of the Operation

Katz et al. reported 8 infertile women (aged 27–43) with a history of ten spontaneous miscarriages and one ectopic pregnancy who were diagnosed as having a "T-shaped" uterus by HSG and hysteroscopy. Hysteroscopic incision of uterine lateral walls was performed to obtain a satisfactory cavity. No complications occurred and a normal uterine cavity was achieved in all patients. After the operation, there were four term pregnancies achieved in 3 women, 1 ectopic pregnancy, and no miscarriages. The authors suggested that TCUI could be applied to correct uterine malformations such as T-shaped uterus to improve their reproductive ability. In 2012, Xia et al. from the Hysteroscopy Center of Fuxing Hospital, Capital Medical University first reported three cases of TCUI for T-shaped uterus, with postoperative live birth achieved in all patients.

9.8.2 Transcervical Resection for Biopsy (TCRB)

9.8.2.1 For Diagnosis of Adenomyosis

Adenomyosis is a uterine myometrial disease, and sometimes can be diagnosed by hysteroscopy. Keckstein reported that the transcervical endomyometrial biopsy with punch biopsy forceps or transcervical resection with wire loop could provide more information on adenomyosis and its depth. Endometrial and myometrial coagulation or resection could effectively destroy or remove the superficial adenomyosis, but might result in iatrogenic adenomyosis, which could be managed by a repeated hysteroscopy. Incomplete EA or TCRE might lead to adenomyosis. Therefore, symptomatic focal adenomyosis might be treated by hysteroscopic operation in selected cases. In 1991, McCausland proposed that the hysteroscopic resectoscope could be used to resect the endomyometrial strip of 2 cm in length and 3–5 mm in depth for histopathological examination, which could be used for diagnosis of adenomyosis but not suitable for those who wanted to have a baby. And its accuracy needed to be compared with the routine histological examination of the specimens of the removed uterus. But in 2000, a review article published by Neis and Brandner indicated that hysteroscopic resection of myometrium and histopathological examination of resected specimen could only diagnose some cases of adenomyosis, with the majority of adenomyosis missed in diagnosis. Mercader et al. reported one case of uterine biopsy resulting in a rare complication of vesicouterine fistula, which should be warned about. In 1992,

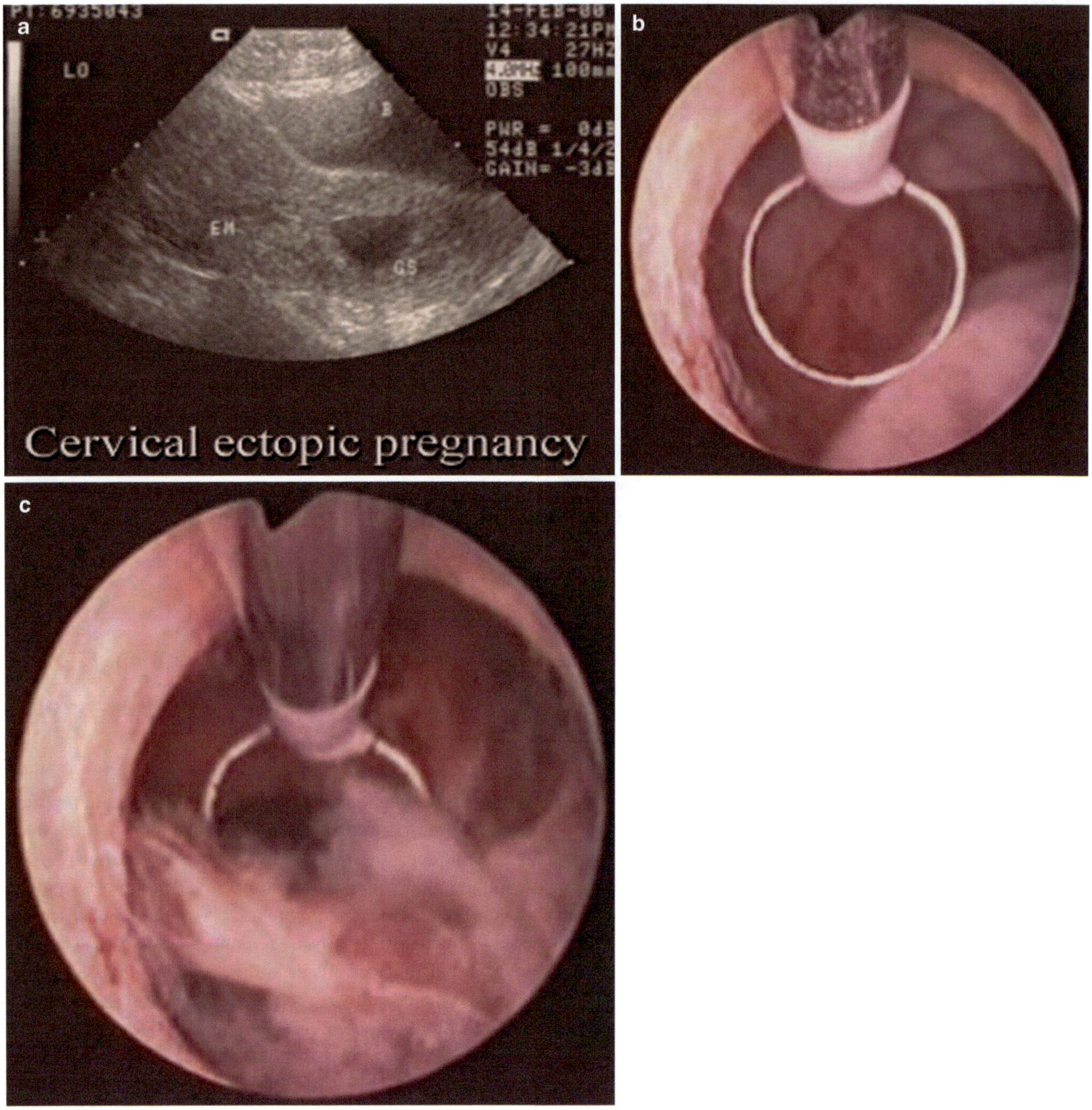

Fig. 9.204 Cervical pregnancy. (**a**) Ultrasonography. (**b**) Embryo sac at right bottom of the screen. (**c**) The removal of trophoblast by hysteroscopy

McCausland reported the depth of adenomyosis seemed to be correlated with the severity of menorrhagia. Patients with superficial adenomyosis might undergo hysteroscopic endomyometrial resection. Patients with deep adenomyosis usually should be offered hysterectomy. Wood et al. conducted hysteroscopic surgery for conservative treatment of adenomyosis, including endometrial resection, myometrial electrocautery, and endomyometrial excision. Improvements of symptoms after treatment with different hysteroscopic surgeries were 4/7, 3/4, and 3/3, respectively, which reduced 30% of the requirement for hysterectomy. McCausland and McCausland's experience was that in patients who had superficial adenomyosis with the endometrial penetration <2.5 mm, hysteroscopic resection could obtain good results. In patients who had deep adenomyosis with the endometrial penetration >2.5 mm, hysteroscopic surgery usually leads to postoperative complications, and in this condition, hysterectomy should be offered rather than a repeat surgery. Neis and Brandner reported that the incidence of adenomyosis varied from 8 to 61% because the definitions used were

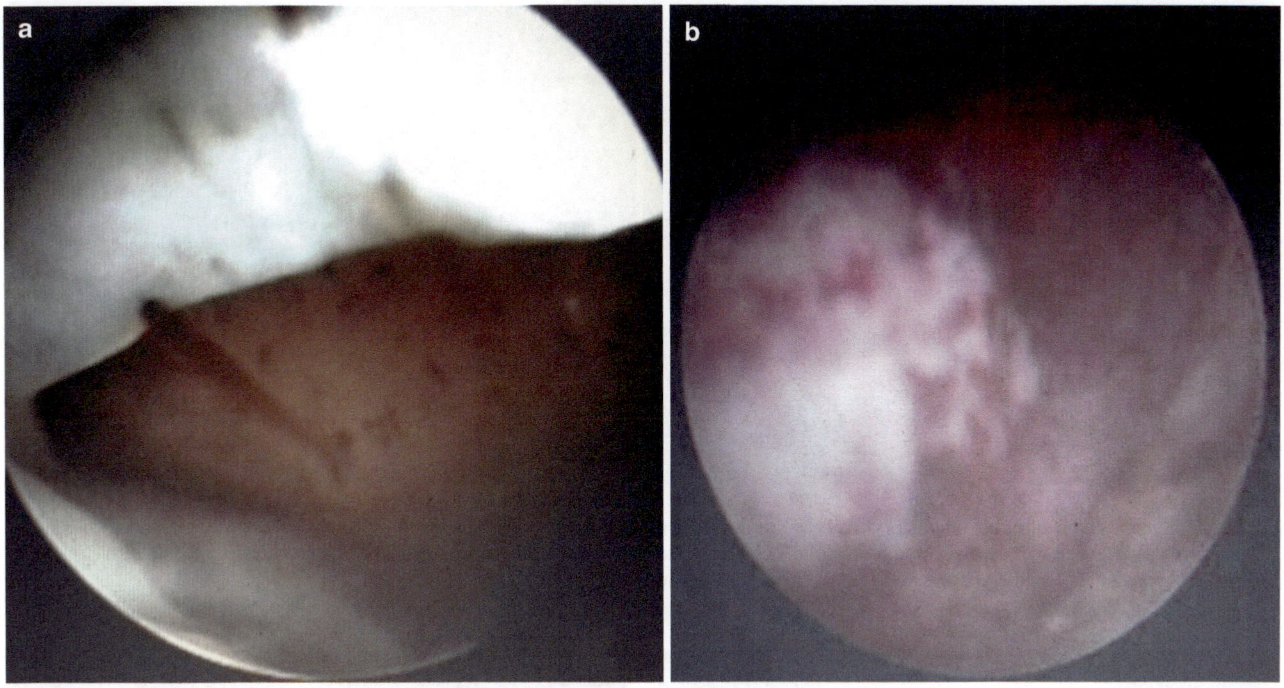

Fig. 9.205 Cesarean scar pregnancy. (**a**) The trophoblast is invading into the uterine myometrial layer. The red line on the left represents vascular bleeding. (**b**) The trophoblast is developing into the uterine cavity

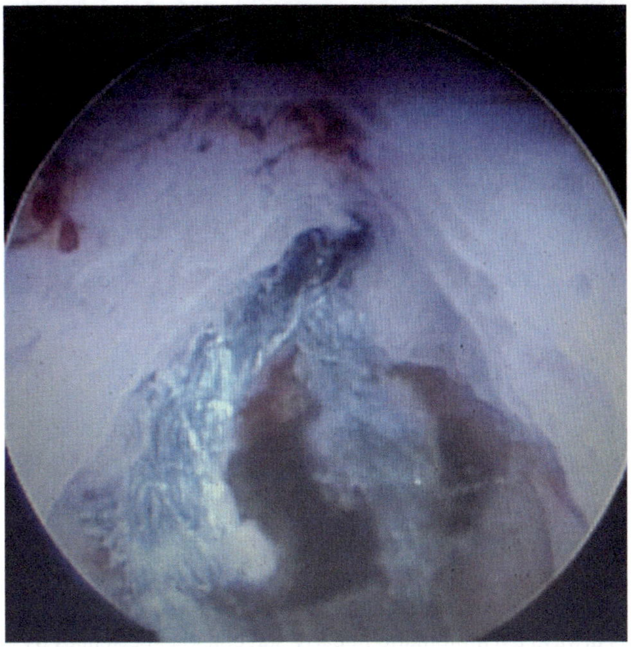

Fig. 9.206 Persistent uterine bleeding 4 months after cesarean section. The residual silk suture is seen under hysteroscope

different. The incidence of adenomyosis diagnosed after hysterectomy for unsuccessful endometrial ablation was between 75 and 100%. It was considered that adenomyosis might be a main reason for failure of hysteroscopic surgery. They suggested that adenomyosis should be highly suspected in patients who experienced dysmenorrhea and had a uterus with the length >10 cm, and should be considered as a relative contraindication of TCRE because of an increased risk of failure.

9.8.2.2 For Diagnosis of Endometrial Tuberculosis

Agboola et al. from UK reported that the tissue biopsy obtained at TCRE confirmed the diagnosis of endometrial tuberculosis for a case. This 62-year-old woman had suffered from primary infertility and experienced unexplained menopause for 30 years. She underwent hormone replacement therapy after failure in various treatments. This time she was admitted to hospital with breakthrough vaginal bleeding. Hysteroscopy revealed a normal uterine cavity, and histological examination of endometrial tissues obtained by biopsy showed benign endometrial polyps, simple endometrial hyperplasia, and chronic granulomatous endometritis with surrounding lymphocytes. Thus tuberculosis was suspected and further investigation was suggested. In a repeat examination 2 months later, hysteroscopy revealed extensive endometrial hyperplasia, which was mostly in the right uterine wall, and scattering endometrial scars, which were subepithelial nodules with the size <5 mm. The small nodules were easily visible under magnifying resectoscope, and were resected with other endometrium for histopathological examination, with the result of tuberculosis endometritis.

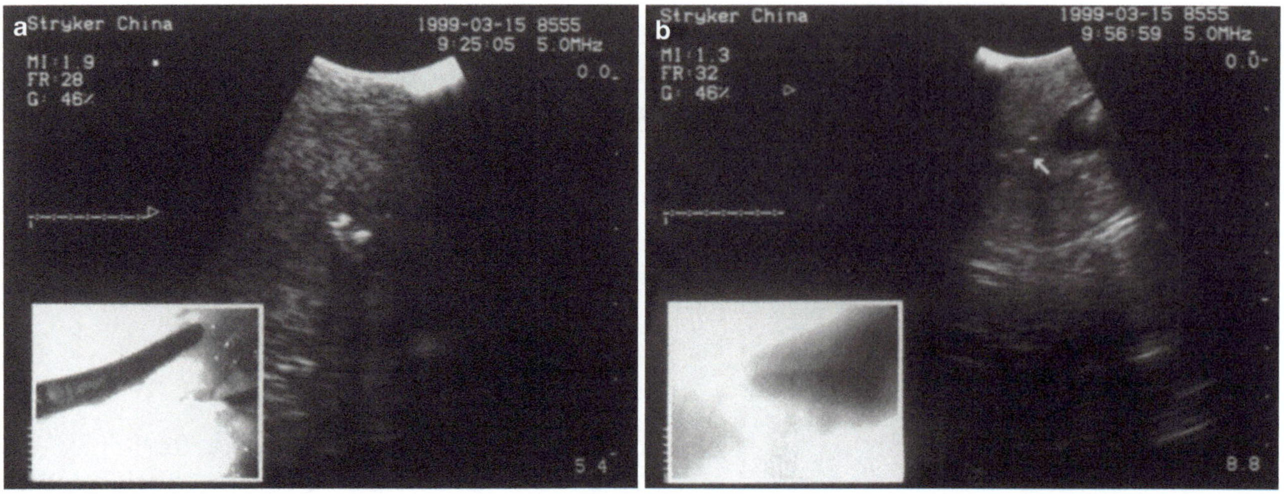

Fig. 9.207 Laparoscopic ultrasonography (LUS). The left lower figure is the laparoscopic image with laparoscopic probe (black color) on the anterior uterine wall. The right upper figure is the LUS image. (**a**) The residual fetal bones in the uterine cavity (white plaque) with acoustic shadow on their back. (**b**) The arrow indicating the adhesive tissues in the uterine cavity

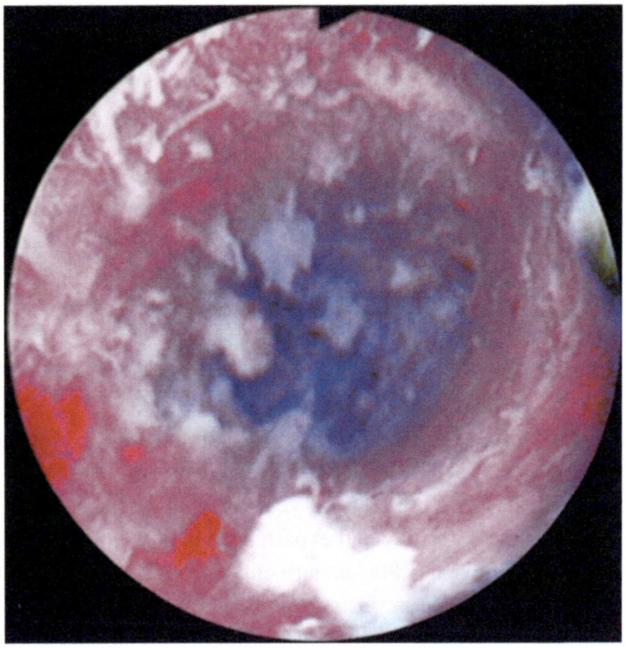

Fig. 9.208 Narrow and cylindrical uterine cavity

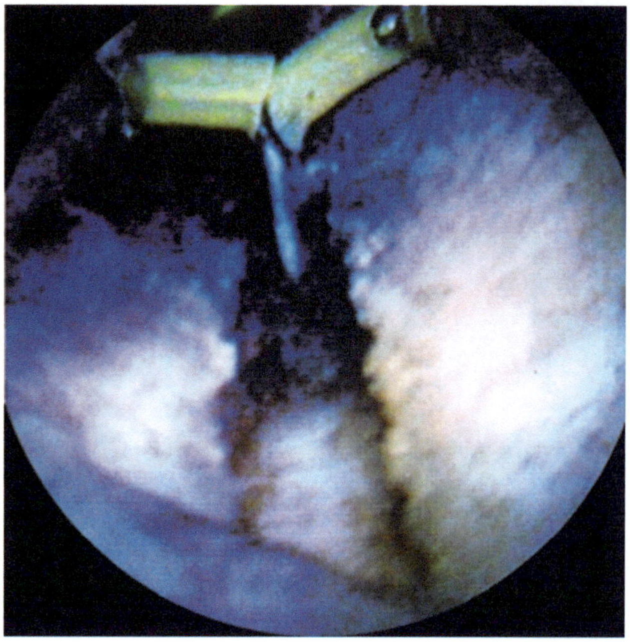

Fig. 9.209 The needle electrode is used to incise along the long axis of uterus

9.8.3 Hysteroscopic Resection of Cystic Adenomyosis

Adenomyosis is developed by the invasion of ectopic glandular tissues and stroma into uterine myometrial layer, forming diffused or focal lesions, and is a common disorder in women of childbearing age. Adenomyosis sometimes presents a cyst containing hemorrhagic material, which is commonly small with the size no more than 0.5 cm. Larger cystic lesions are named cystic adenomyosis, with which the patient is always asymptomatic in early stage, and experiences dysmenorrhea and chronic pelvic pain in severe condition. The occurrence of cystic adenomyosis might relate to previous uterine surgery. By ultrasonography examination, intramural echolucent areas can be detected in patient with cystic adenomyosis, which can be single or multiple cysts of variable size and is the basis of diagnosis. When a cystic lesion locates near the cavity, hysteroscopic operation to incise or resect the lesion is feasible.

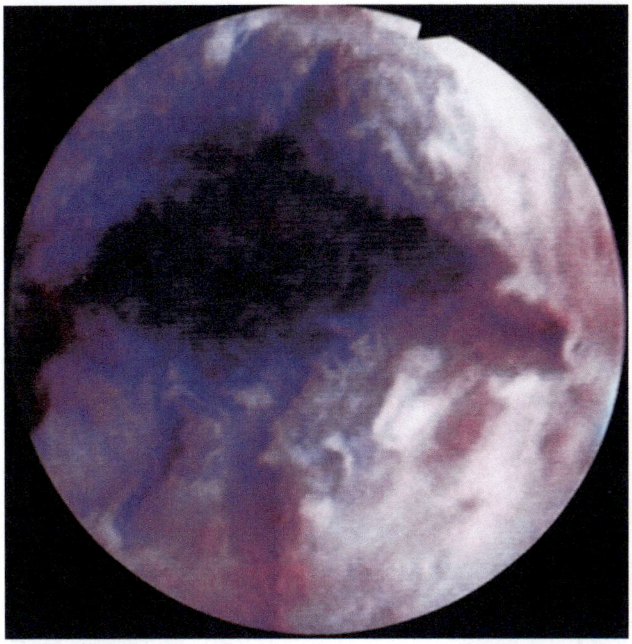

Fig. 9.210 Uterine cavity after TCUI

9.8.3.1 Indications

The indications of hysteroscopic resection of cystic adenomyosis include the symptoms such as dysmenorrhea, chronic pelvic pain, etc., and one of following conditions:

1. The cystic lesions of adenomyosis are close to the uterine cavity.
2. The cystic lesions of adenomyosis do not penetrate the whole layer of the uterine wall.
3. Uterine malignant lesions are excluded.

9.8.3.2 Operative Procedures

1. Diagnostic hysteroscope is applied firstly to observe the uterine cavity and investigate whether there is space-occupying lesions or not. Combined with abdominal ultrasonography monitoring, the size and the site of the cyst, and the distance between the cyst and the uterine serosa can be identified (Fig. 9.211a).
2. Under ultrasonography guidance, hysteroscopic wire loop electrode is used to gradually resect the endometrium and the myometrium on the surface of the cyst so that the cystic wall becomes visible (Fig. 9.211b).
3. After the cyst is opened, effusion of brownish thickened liquid can be seen (Fig. 9.211c). Endometrial-like tissues are visible on the inside surface of the cyst after drainage of the brownish thickened liquid (Fig. 9.211d). Then the endometrial-like tissues and the small cysts in between are excised one by one.
4. In cases with deep cysts, the endometrial-like tissues on the surface of its base may be destroyed by coagulation with hysteroscopic roller ball electrode (Fig. 9.212).

9.8.3.3 Experience and Evaluation of the Operation

Laparoscopic excision is applicable in cases with cystic adenomyosis approaching uterine serosa with a good therapeutic effect. Hysteroscopic resection is suitable for cases with the cyst close to the endometrium, and intraoperative ultrasonography guidance contributes to the positioning of the cyst. Giana et al. published a case report and described that hysteroscopic bipolar loop electrode was used to resect the cystic tissues following TVS suggestion, with the histological examination confirming the existence of typical cystic adenomyosis. Xia et al. from the Hysteroscopy Center of Fuxing Hospital, Capital Medical University, conducted hysteroscopic resection in 3 women with cystic adenomyosis. In the first case with the lesion developed after cesarean section, the cyst is incised by hysteroscopic monopolar electrode under ultrasonography guidance. However, the cyst was too large (5.6 cm × 5.4 cm × 5.8 cm), which led to subsequently hysterectomy. The second woman was treated by hysteroscopic resection of lesions. The wire loop electrode was conducted to cut open the cyst wall in left-posterior myometrium, in which the endometrial-like tissues were visible. The endometrial-like tissues and small cysts with the maximum diameter 2.9 cm in them were excised one by one, and the postoperative prognosis was good. The third woman underwent hysteroscopic adhesiolysis and incision of cysts. The myometrium of posterior wall was cut open by hysteroscopic wire loop electrode and revealed scattered focal endometrium and ectopic lesions inside, with the largest space in the posterior wall and 3 cm in diameter. The distance between the space and uterine serosa was less than 3 mm, which was quite thin. Therefore, hysteroscopic coagulation on the basis of the cyst was conducted and achieved a good outcome.

9.8.4 Transcervical Resection of Cervical Lesion (TCRC)

Cervical benign lesions, including cervical erosion, cervical polypoid hyperplasia (Fig. 9.213), cervical polyps, Nabothian cyst, etc., are common and frequent diseases. Treatment options include cervical electrocautery, cryotherapy, laser, or Loop Electrosurgical Excision Procedure (LEEP) for treatment. Cervical precancerous lesion, also called Cervical Intraepithelial Neoplasia (CIN), is that the cervical epithelial cells are partly or mostly replaced by atypical cells. CIN is classified into three grades: CIN1, CIN2, and CIN3. The

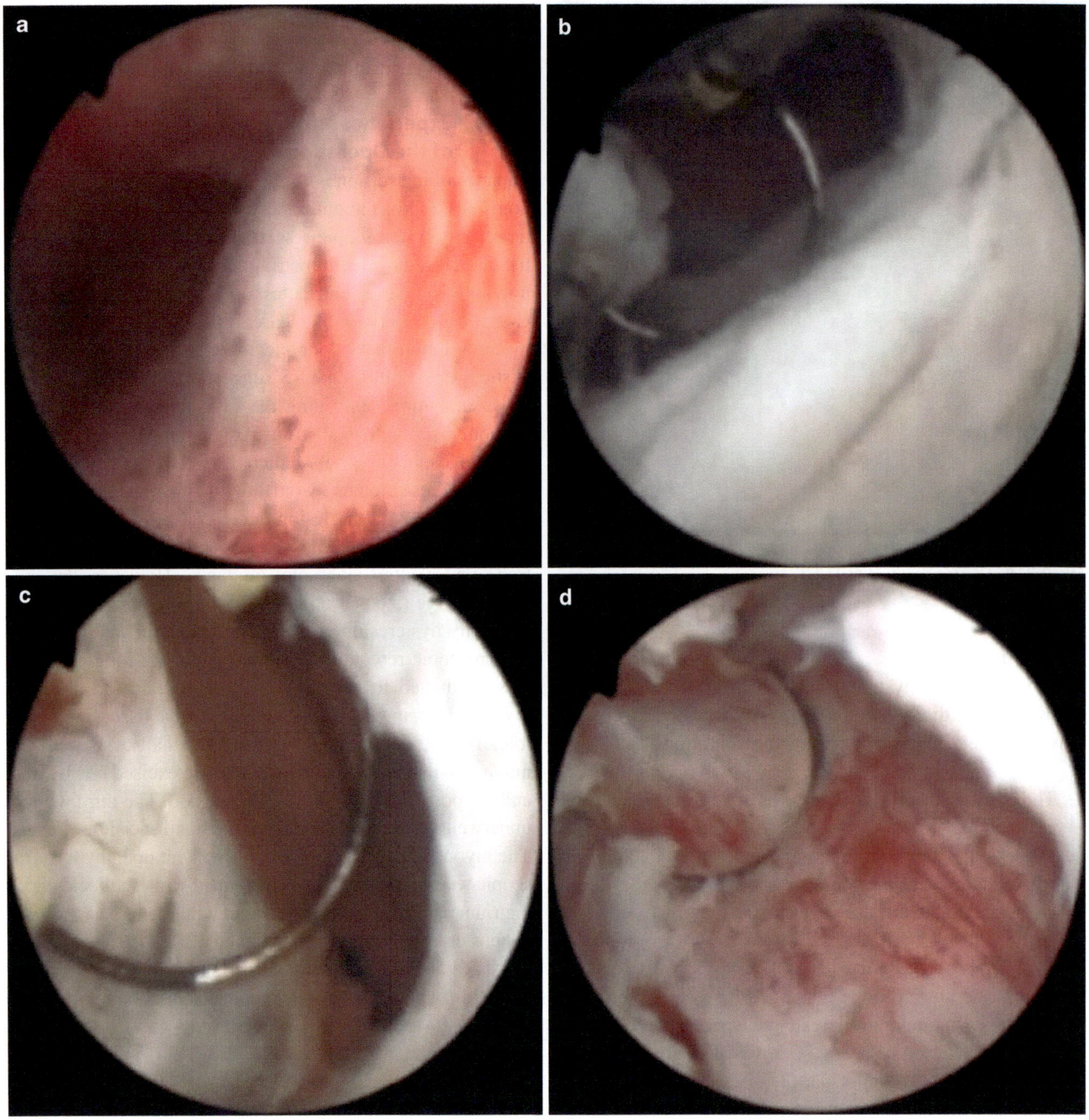

Fig. 9.211 Hysteroscopic resection of cystic adenomyosis. (**a**) Examination of uterine cavity with hysteroscopy. The cystic lesion lies in left-posterior wall of the uterus. (**b**) Hysteroscopic wire loop electrode is used to resect the endometrium and sub-endometrial myometrium surrounding the cyst which locates in left-posterior wall of the uterus. (**c**) The cyst wall is cut open by hysteroscopic resectoscope, with the outflow of brownish thickened liquid. (**d**) The cyst wall is resected by hysteroscopic wire loop electrode, with the endometrial-like tissues on the inside wall of the cyst visible

treatment for CIN includes LEEP, laser conization, cold knife conization, total hysterectomy, etc. Transcervical resection of cervical lesions is performed by using hysteroscopic wire loop electrode to resect the diseased tissues of the cervix, which can not only excise the erosion on the surface of the cervix, but also go deep into the cervical canal, inspect and remove the lesions in cervical canal under the illumination of strong cold light, as well as effective hemostasis.

9.8.4.1 Indications

1. Cervical benign lesions, especially lesions in the cervical canal, such as cervical polypoid hyperplasia, cervical polyps, cervical erosion, cervical Nabothian cyst, etc.

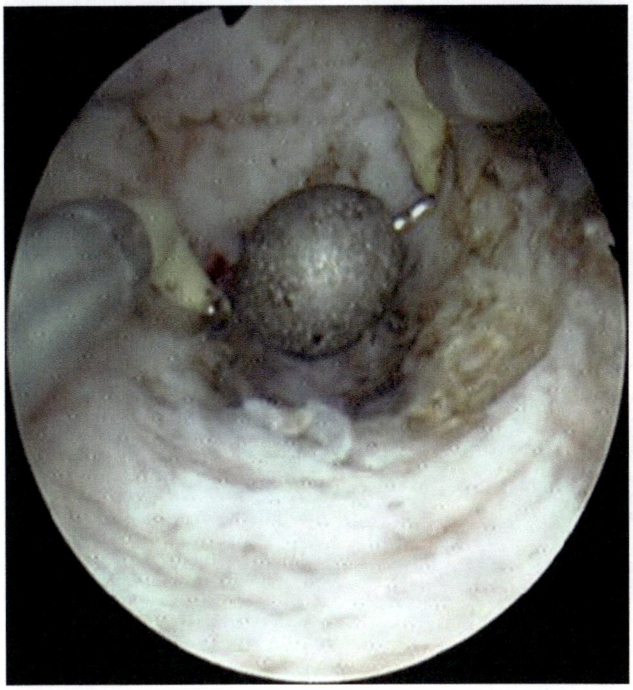

Fig. 9.212 The cyst wall in the posterior myometrium is coagulated by hysteroscopic roller ball electrode

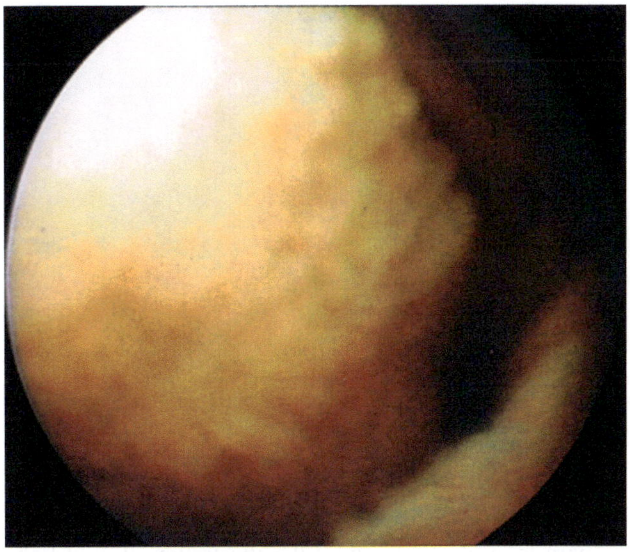

Fig. 9.213 Cervical polypoid hyperplasia

2. CIN grade 1–2 (CIN1, CIN2).
3. Malignant lesions are excluded by cervical cytological examination and/or histological diagnosis.

9.8.4.2 Operative Procedures

1. When monopolar hysteroscope is used, the cutting power is set at 60 W. Coagulating power at 40 W, and the switches of irrigating pump need not to be on. From the beginning, the cervical lesions shall be well inspected and the extent of resection is determined (Fig. 9.214a). In women with CIN, 2.5% iodine tincture is used to swab the tissues of cervix to identify the suspected areas of cervical lesions.
2. The cutting usually starts from the 6 o'clock position. The wire loop electrode is pushed out totally and placed in the cervical canal by touching the cervical posterior tissues gently, with the distance 0.7–0.8 cm to cervical os. After the electricity is activated, the wire loop electrode resects the cervical posterior tissues slowly from the inside to the outside with an "arc" cutting, and stop at 0.1 cm outside the diseased tissues on cervical os (Fig. 9.214b).
3. The cervical tissues are radially resected clockwise or anticlockwise in sequence according to the extent of the cervical lesions, with the cutting surface after resection presenting mushroom-shape in cases with superficial lesions and cone-shape in cases with deep lesions (Fig. 9.214c).
4. The active bleeding on cutting surface can be stopped by coagulating the bleeding points with wire loop electrode, or by switching on the irrigation pump, detecting the bleeding points on cutting surface under the irrigation of the fluid, and then coagulating the bleeding points with wire loop electrode (Fig. 9.215). Hemostasis can be achieved by rollerball electrode coagulation if the cutting surface is oozing.
5. In cases with cervical Nabothian cyst, hysteroscopic wire loop electrode can be used to resect and destroy the cyst. If a cyst is located deeply in the cervix, the procedure shall be performed under ultrasound guidance; if a cyst is large, only a part of the cyst wall can be excised to open the cavity, and then the cyst wall can be coagulated with a rollerball electrode or vaporized with a vaporizing electrode (Fig. 9.216a, b).
6. If cervical polypoid hyperplasia or cervical polyps are coexisting, they can be excised under the irrigation of the fluid and direct vision (Fig. 9.217a, b).
7. All excised tissues should be sent for histological examination. In cases with CIN, the tissues should be sent separately following multiple punch resections.

9.8.4.3 Experience and Evaluation of the Operation

1. Prior to TCRC, cervical cytological examination and/or biopsy histological diagnosis must be obtained. The range of excision during TCRC should be sufficient. The posterior blade of vaginal speculum can be taken for support of the resectoscope when cutting the anterior lip of the cervix. There is always no support when cutting the posterior lip of the cervix.
2. There is still dispute about the treatment of TCRC for CIN. Clinically, it is commonly believed that TCRC can

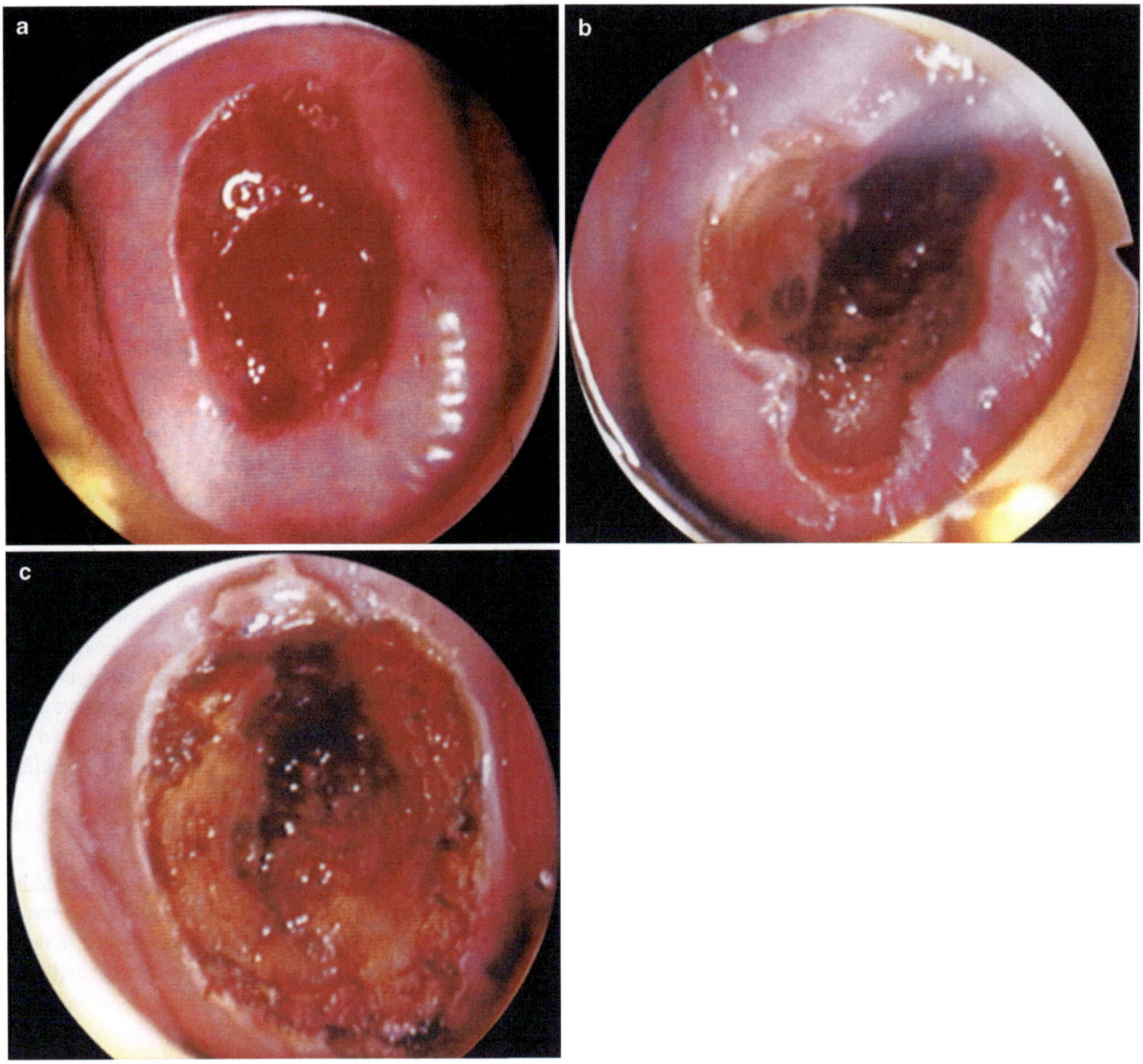

Fig. 9.214 TCRC. (**a**) Prior to TCRC, cervical erosion and polypoid hyperplasia are visible. (**b**) The cervix after several cuttings during TCRC. (**c**) After TCRC, the cervical surface appears to be mushroom-shaped

effectively excise lesions of CIN1 and CIN2, but is not applicable for lesions of CIN3. However, some gynecologists have tried TCRC to treat CIN3 and achieved some effect.

3. Comparison between TCRC and LEEP: With the limitation of the property of the instrument, the extent of treatment with LEEP is often superficial, and the treatment of polypoid hyperplasia, polyps, and Nabothian cysts in cervical canal cannot usually be performed. In addition, bleeding during LEEP resection is always massive and hard to be stopped, which increases the difficulty of the procedure. Hysteroscope can be introduced into cervical canal, and inspect and resect the intracervical lesions with wire loop electrode under the illustration of cold light. The irrigation fluid can flush the cutting surface and permits a prompt and accurate coagulation of active bleeding under direct vision, resulting in effective hemostasis. Zhang Hongwei et al. reported a study that cervical lesions with CIN1 were treated by TCRC in 115 women and by LEEP in 116 women. The results showed that intraoperative bleeding was significantly less in TCRC group than that in LEEP group ($P = 0.000$), and the recovery time of cutting surface was significantly shorter in TCRC group than that in LEEP group ($p = 0.021$).

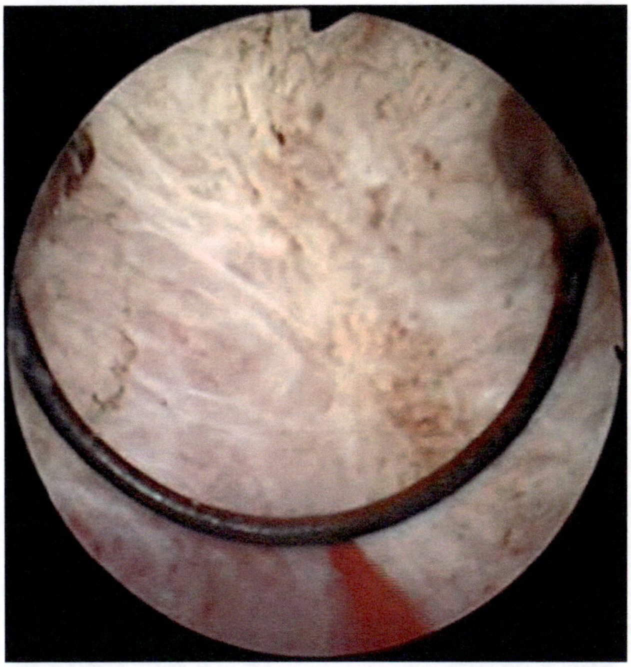

Fig. 9.215 Cervical active bleeding on the cutting surface is coagulated with hysteroscopic wire loop electrode for hemostasis during TCRC

9.9 Other Techniques of Endometrial Ablation

Jie Zheng and Enlan Xia

Endometrial ablation is the greatest advancement in gynecological treatment at the end of the twentieth century. However, hysteroscopic laser or high-frequency electricity endometrial ablation requires proficient surgical skills in hysteroscopy, and serious potential complications may occur. In recent years, a number of non-hysteroscopic devices or procedures for endometrial ablation have been developed, which are also known as the second-generation endometrial ablation. It is characterized by heating rather than direct electrical surgery. Its superiority is simple, rapid and safe operation with some therapeutic effects; its weak points are that there are no specimens obtained for histological examination, the success of the procedure depends on the morphology of uterine cavity, the space-occupying lesion requires further management, and that the equipment cost is very high.

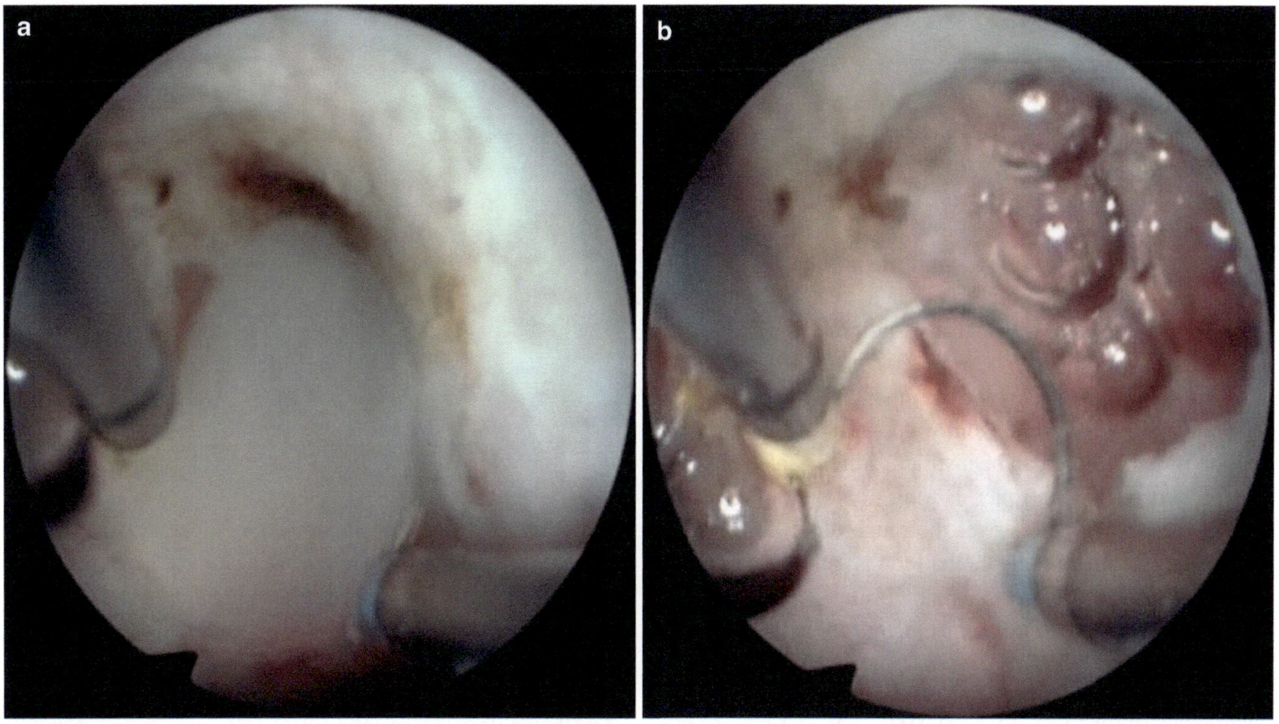

Fig. 9.216 Resection of cervical Nabothian cyst. (**a**) The wall of cervical Nabothian cyst is cut open with hysteroscopic wire loop electrode, with outflow of white thickened fluid visible. (**b**) The base of Nabothian cyst is displayed after the cyst wall is cut open with hysteroscopic wire loop electrode

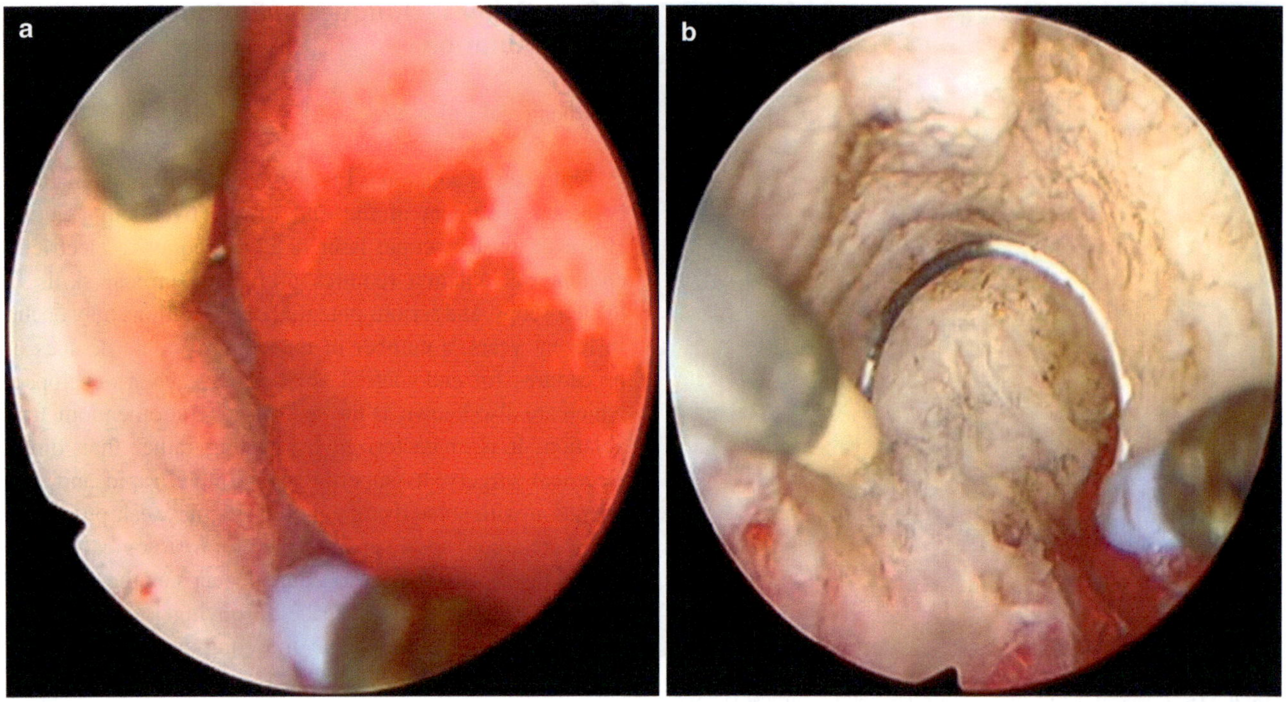

Fig. 9.217 Resection of cervical polypoid hyperplasia tissues. (a) The polypoid hyperplasia tissues on anterior wall of the cervix are resected with hysteroscopic wire loop electrode. (b) The cutting surface after resection of the polypoid hyperplasia tissues with hysteroscopic wire loop electrode

9.9.1 Uterine Balloon Thermo-Ablation (UBT)

The uterine balloon thermo-ablation (UBT) is to use the heated fluid in balloon to destroy the endometrium. The uterine balloon therapeutic system is mainly comprised of a controller and a balloon catheter (Fig. 9.218). The controller can be used to control the temperature inside the balloon and monitor continuously the pressure and treatment duration. The balloon catheter is 16 cm in length and the balloon is 3.5 cm in long diameter. The balloon is made of latex, housing galvanic couple heater, and the other end of balloon catheter is assembled with the inflow port through which the balloon inflating fluid can be instilled, which is also the connection port to the controller. During treatment, if the pressure insidc the balloon is over the range of 45–200 mmHg and the temperature inside the balloon is higher than 92 °C, the controller can automatically shut off the heating element and terminate the treatment. The patients are usually women with menorrhagia who have no desire for future pregnancies. The patients may have curettage prior to operation, or receive pretreatment with danazol or GnRH analogs for a certain period to thin the endometrium and obtain a better efficacy, but endometrial pretreatment may not be administered. The patients may take indomethacin or paracetamol preoperatively to prevent the occurrence of postoperative uterine spasm. The patients can choose general anesthesia, intravenous anesthesia plus local anesthesia, spinal anesthesia, single intravenous anesthesia or single local nerve blocking anesthesia. Some published research showed that local anesthesia is better applied to patients with good tolerance during treatment, which may diminish the complications induced by general anesthesia. The operation should be performed within 3–7 days after menstruation ends. The patient is placed in lithotomy position and intravenous anesthesia is administered. First, connect all the ports of the uterine balloon therapy system, empty the air inside the latex balloon until the negative pressure (−100 to −200 mmHg) is shown on the control unit. Then insert the balloon catheter through the cervix into the uterine cavity with the scale on the balloon catheter equal to the length of uterine cavity. Then inject

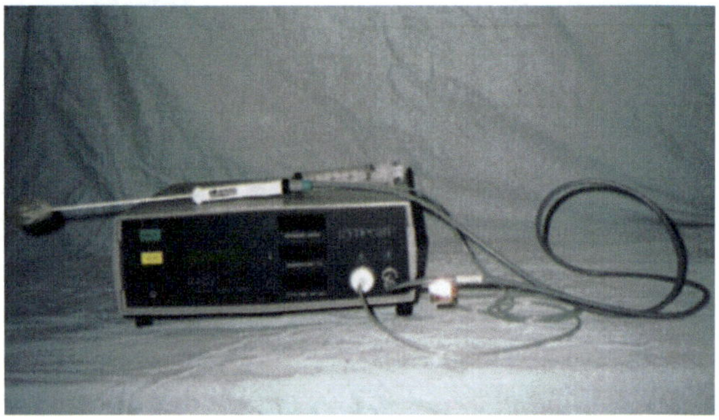

Fig. 9.218 Controller and the balloon catheter

the sterile 5% glucose slowly into the balloon. Heating begins immediately when the pressure becomes stable. When the glucose solution inside the balloon is heated up to 87 ± 5 °C, maintain this temperature for approximately 8 min and then stop heating. When the temperature inside the balloon falls to about 50 °C, pump out the liquid of the balloon and remove the catheter, and then the treatment is completed. Sometimes laparoscopy is performed to monitor the whole procedure. When the uterine cavity is under thermal treatment of 87 ± 5 °C and 170 mmHg, laparoscopy is used to ensure no manifestations of enlargement, apparent expansion and spasm of the uterus, no signs of congestion, hemorrhage or ecchymosis formation and other changes in uterine serosa, no perforation and exudates resulting from thermal balloon rupture, and no surrounding organs affected. After UBT procedure, a hysteroscopy should be followed immediately and can reveal that the endometrium of the anterior, posterior wall and uterine fundus has turned from the previous pink to pale yellow or brownish yellow, there is no flaky congestion or hemorrhage in the endometrial surface, and no perforation or fluid leakage. By histological examination on the uterine section after treatment, the endometrial layer is seen to be edematous, and mostly deciduous; superficial myometrium appears to be pale white or light yellow; there is a pink thermal coagulation zone with a thickness of 3–7 mm in the submucous and superficial myometrial layer approximately 1–2 mm away from the endometrium, the red portions above and beneath turn light red and there is no change in deep myometrial layer. This red thermal coagulation zone is the widest in the uterine fundus and anterior and posterior uterine walls, followed by the junction between the uterine body and cervix, and the narrowest in the uterine cornua, and in some cases there is no thermal coagulation zone in uterine cornua (Fig. 9.219). The vaginal discharges observed after treatment are: pink vaginal discharges within 1–3 days; pink watery drainage within 4–7 days; and watery drainage within 8–14 days, and there may be some shedding of the necrotic mucosa. After operation, the patients may develop different conditions like amenorrhea, dripping menses, normal menstruation, or menorrhagia. The first three of which are indicators of successful treatment, and the postoperative amenorrhea rate is reported to be 20.6%. Gervaise et al. compared the success rate of UBT (73 cases) with that of hysteroscopic endometrial resection (74 cases) in the treatment of dysfunctional uterine bleeding. The overall success rate was 83.0 ± 5% in thermal balloon group and 76.3 ± 6% in endometrial resection group. There were no significant differences between the two groups. The failure factor for the former was the retroverted uterus, and that for the latter was patient's age less than 43 years old. They believed that uterine balloon thermo-ablation was safe, effective, and easy to perform. There were other reports on the overall effective rate of UBT procedure between 83 and 98.3%, which is similar to hysteroscopic endometrial ablation. There are few intraoperative complications, and postoperative complications are 3–4%, including intrauterine adhesions, uterine cavity stenosis, hematometra, persistent pelvic pain, cystitis, etc.

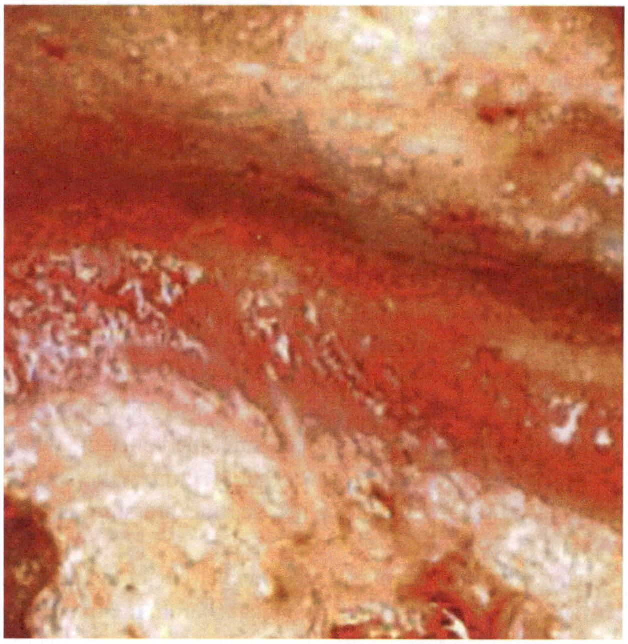

Fig. 9.219 Findings of uterine section

Zheng et al. from the Hysteroscopy Center of Fuxing Hospital, Capital Medical University come to the following conclusions through clinical research:

1. There are no statistically significant differences in therapeutic effects of the patients' parities and uterine positions.
2. There are no significant differences in therapeutic effects of the duration of treatment of 12 or 8 min.
3. The system sometimes presents a gradual decrease in the thermal balloon pressure after the start of treatment, and if the pressure is at a low level, the therapeutic effects will be influenced. When the thermal balloon is at a higher pressure, and if there is a decline in the thermal balloon pressure, a small amount of fluid may be added to the thermal balloon to elevate the pressure and the mean pressure in the process of treatment. If the fluid is added at the early stage of treatment, there is no significant difference in treatment temperature compared with the group without additional fluid, but there is significant difference in the depth of thermal damage. Pathological study has confirmed that different starting pressures taken by the uterine thermal system may cause different depths of damage to the uterine wall. With the intraballoon pressure at 110–180 mmHg, the higher average pressure is, the deeper the damage to the uterine wall. This result is

coherent to the clinical therapeutic effects, that is, the higher starting pressure and final pressure within a certain range will entail a better clinical treatment effect. Aletebi et al. found that when the patients with menorrhagia were treated by UBT at the starting pressure of 80–140 mmHg, 38% still experienced menorrhagia at a 1-year follow-up; if the starting pressure was at 140–180 mmHg, only 13% of the patients after the treatment still experienced menorrhagia. The results suggested that the initial pressure of 140–180 mmHg improved the therapeutic effect. With an increase in the thermal balloon pressure from less than 140 mmHg to more than 140 mmHg, Vilos improved the effective rate in patients from 52 to 89%. This indicates that the higher the starting pressure, the better the therapeutic effects, and also proves that the clinical therapeutic effect is related to the higher starting pressure and the final pressure.

4. The older the patients are, the smaller cavity the patients have, the severer the menorrhagia is before treatment, the better the therapeutic effects will be. Multiple regression analysis of the data demonstrates that only the amount of bleeding before treatment is correlated with the outcome after treatment.
5. The pretreatment by curettage prior to operation increases the failure rate of treatment, and the application of GnRH analogs contributes to the incidence of amenorrhea and hypomenorrhea after treatment.
6. At the early stage of its application, Albert conducted UBT to treat a patient with menorrhagia who was complicated by heart disease and achieved good results. Aletebi reported that the application of UBT in treatment of 46 women with high-risk menorrhagia who were complicated with hematological disease, cardiovascular disease, or post-transplantation of heart or lung achieved an effective rate of 79%. Scholars in China have applied UBT to the treatment of patients with menorrhagia complicated with idiopathic thrombocytopenic purpura. There are also reports on the treatment of the patients who have kidney failure, uremia, cirrhosis of the liver, transplantation of kidney, and aplastic anemia, and they all achieved good results. Therefore the application of uterine thermal balloon system to the treatment of high-risk patients with menorrhagia and severe medical complications can help the patients who are unresponsive to medication and cannot tolerate laparotomy for treatment. This also proves that the uterine thermal system is safe, efficient, and low anesthesia-dependent, thus its application is promising. Gervaise et al. reported that 206 women with DUB were treated by UBT, with three pregnancies (5.2%) achieved in 58 women post-operation, among which two experienced spontaneous miscarriage and one got placenta accreta at 26 weeks. These findings suggested that balloon ablation could not be used as a contraceptive method. Furthermore, UBT can lead to the changes of the endometrium and uterine cavity (for example, synechiae), so it is not suitable for women who want to retain their fertility. Leung and Yuen reported the occurrence of postablation-tubal sterilization syndrome following thermal balloon endometrial ablation.

9.9.2 Hydrothermo Ablation (HTA)

The principle of hydrothermo ablation (HTA) is to instill 0.9% saline solution which is heated to 90 °C through hysteroscope into the uterine cavity to destroy the endometrium. The stimulation from the heated fluid may cause the uterine cornua to retract, which leads to the obliteration of fallopian tubal ostia, thus the heated fluid will not flow into the abdominal cavity and not cause thermal damage to abdominal organs. The procedure begins with hysteroscopic diagnosis using cold saline perfusion for observation of the uterine cavity. The air-insulated outer sheath of hysteroscope can prevent cervical canal from overheating by hot saline, thus the 90 °C hot saline can be injected under direct vision of hysteroscope and continuously flow at 45 mmHg for 10 min. In order to avoid the occurrence of thermal damage caused by the entering of hot fluid into the abdominal cavity via fallopian tube, if the volume deficit between the inflow and outflow is greater than 10 mL, it will be detected automatically and the fluid perfusion is stopped. The thermal damage depth of endometrium reaches 4–5 mm, which has no damage to the basal layer, and the cervical temperature is 42 °C at the time of operation. Guillot et al. reported that HTA technique was applied for treatment in 143 patients with DUB and menorrhagia from six centers, with the average age of patients 48 years (37–67 years). The main complaint of these patients was persistent menorrhagias and 42.4% of the patients had myomas. Intraoperative complications developed in four cases. At follow-up with the mean time 9 months, the postoperative satisfaction rate was 72.7% of the patients, amenorrhea achieved in 44% of the patients, oligomenorrheic in 37% and eumenorrheic in 13%. Seven patients underwent subsequently hysterectomy. Postoperative complications occurred in 13 patients, with the majority being pelvic pain. They concluded that HTA was a simple and effective technique for treatment of menorrhagia and could be applied for cases with uterine fibroids and irregular shaped uterus, and that HTA must be conducted under the inspectation of hysteroscopy to ensure the success of the surgery. Preoperative histopathological examination is compulsory to exclude other conditions.

There was another report on 20 cases with menorrhagia treated by HTA, a 12-month follow-up showed that the postoperative amenorrhea rate was 58%, and the operation success rate was 94.5%.

9.9.3 Multi-Electrode Balloon Ablation (MEBA)

The principle of multi-electrode balloon ablation (MEBA) is to apply the thermal energy coming from monopolar high-frequency current to destroy the endometrium. The device consists of three parts, namely, the multi-electrode balloon guide rod at the front end, the junction part in the middle, and the computer controller behind. There are six electrodes in the front of multi-electrode balloon, and six electrodes behind. The current is powered on after they are being placed in the uterine cavity (pure cutting current of 45–50 W) for 4 min with the intrauterine temperature maintained at 75 °C as well as bilateral cornua at the same temperature. The post-operative amenorrhea rate achieved was 38%.

9.9.4 Microwave Endometrial Ablation (MEA)

The principle of microwave endometrial ablation (MEA) is to use microwave energy to destroy the endometrium. The equipment consists of three parts, namely, the microwave probe at the front end, the junction part in the middle, and a computer controller behind. The intrauterine temperature is displayed on the computer controller as curve line with temperature maintained at 80–95 °C. Move the microwave probe and let its tip make contact with each side of the uterine cavity. The operative time is only 2–3 min and the postoperative amenorrhea rate is 57%. Tawfeek et al. reported on 35 women who underwent MEA either with general or local anesthesia between 1997 and 2005. HSGs were performed intermittently 3 months later and showed that complete occlusion of uterine cavity was found in 30 women (85.7%) and incomplete occlusion of tubes in five cases (14.3%). Lo and Pickersgill reported in a literature review that the incidence of pregnancy after endometrial ablation is 0.7%, and there is a case report of pregnancy after MEA. Cooper et al. carried out a comparison of long-term outcomes following MEA or TCRE. At the follow-up of 5 years after operation, 236 cases (90%) answered the questionnaires. In two groups, the satisfaction rates were 86% and 74%, the acceptance rates were 97% and 91%, and the recommended rates were 97% and 89%, with postoperative bleeding and pain scores significantly reduced, and the amenorrhea rates 65% and 69%, respectively. The hysterectomy rates were 16% and 25% in MEA group and TCRE group, respectively. The results confirmed that both techniques could significantly improve the menstrual disorders and life-related quality, with the rates of satisfaction and acceptability of treatment following MEA being higher than those following TCRE, which indicated that MEA might be a more effective and efficient treatment for menorrhea than TCRE. In 2005, Kanaoka et al. reported that a nulligravida women who was diagnosed as complex endometrial hyperplasia with atypia (CEHA) underwent MEA as a substitute for hysterectomy because of some high-risk complications, with the frequency used at 2.45 GHz. The endometrium at the lower part of the cavity near the internal orifice was preserved to prevent the occurrence of hematometra. Histological examination of endometrial biopsy following operation did not reveal any signs of endometrial hyperplasia. A repeat histological examination of the endometrium 2 years later revealed the recurrence of CEHA. One month after the second MEA, MRI suggested that the endometrial line was totally replaced by avascular area and there were no signs of endometrial regeneration in uterine cavity or cervical internal os. No recurrence was detected 18 months later.

9.9.5 Bipolar Radiofrequency Endometrial Ablation (RFEA)

Bipolar radiofrequency endometrial ablation (RFEA) is also named NovaSure endometrial ablation (NovaSure), which is technique applying bipolar radio frequency energy with precise control of impedance to ablate the endometrium. NovaSure endometrial ablation system consists of a disposable device and a radiofrequency controller, with a radiofrequency of 500 KHz, an output power of 50 W, treatment temperature of 85 °C, and the average treatment time of 90 s. During operation, hysteroscopy is first used to observe the uterine cavity and the endometrium, then the radiofrequency electrode is introduced into the right uterine cornu under abdominal ultrasonography guidance, then the power is switched on. Ultrasonography shows the echo of the action site strengthens gradually, and when the treatment comes to an end, the controller will automatically terminate the energy delivery. The same procedure is conducted for the treatment of the left uterine cornu → the median uterine fundus → the median of the lower segment of the uterine cavity. If the uterine cavity is broader, the corresponding bilateral treatment sites should be added. At the end of operation, when the electrode temperature falls below 60 °C, the electrode can be pulled back. Hysteroscopy is reused to observe the uterine cavity after treatment. Radiofrequency treatment has very small effect on the normal tissues around the targeted tissues. This system can display the real-time temperature, power, and impedance, and is also fitted with an automatic protection device and will automatically terminate RF output in cases of wrong connection, setting or circuit fault, over 110 °C temperature and more than 500 Ω impedance, etc. Therefore, it has a high safety. After comparing the second-generation endometrial ablation of radiofrequency, HTA, thermal balloon and cryoablation, scholars like Thijssen, Sabbah, and Cooper et al. concluded that the radiofrequency endometrial ablation is advantageous in the rates of successful operation, amenorrhea, and patients' satisfaction. In 2005, Baskett et al. reported on 200 cases of menorrhea who were treated by NovaSure. At 1–4 years of follow-up with 146 cases, 43.1% of the patients were amenorrheic, 41.8% were oligomenorrheic, 4.1% were eumenorrheic, and 11% of the patients still had excessive menstrual flow. Twelve (8.2%) out of 146 cases required a second operation, of which ten cases underwent hysterectomy and two cases had a second EA. One of 200 cases who was found uterine perforation on hysteroscopy prior to treatment underwent laparoscopy. Two cases were administered antibiotics for endometritis. After 1–4 years of follow-up, 81.5% of the patients were satisfied with the treatment, and 97.3% would like to recommend it. In 2007, Alperin et al. reported that a 44-year-old woman with a life-threatening uterine bleeding was diagnosed as acute promyelocytic leukemia (APML) by bone marrow biopsy. The control of bleeding was failed when she took hormonal therapy or underwent uterine artery embolization (UAE), but succeeded when NovaSure endometrial ablation was utilized.

9.9.6 Cryo-Endometrial Ablation

Cryo-endometrial ablation is the latest endometrial ablation. This technique applies nitrous oxide to freeze and destroy the endometrium, and postoperative amenorrhea rate reaches 50.3%. Heppard et al. reported that 54% of the patients after cryo-endometrial ablation achieved amenorrhea or only spotting bleeding, and they believed that it was a safe and effective treatment for AUB.

9.9.7 Endometrial Laser Intrauterine Thermotherapy (ELITT)

The laser power per unit in endometrial laser intrauterine thermotherapy (ELITT) is 1000 times lower than that of traditional Nd-YAG laser endometrial ablation. The postoperative amenorrhea rate was reported to be 68%.

9.9.8 Micro-Hysteroscopy Versapoint Bipolar Electrosurgery Intrauterine System (Versapoint)

The energy source for a micro-hysteroscopy versapoint bipolar electrosurgery intrauterine system is bipolar electricity, in which the saline is used to irrigate the uterine cavity to undergo endometrial ablation. This procedure is characterized by safe operation and good effects, and can be performed under local anesthesia. In 2002, Clark et al. reported on the feasibility of versapoint system in the treatment of symptomatic submucous fibroids, which included the safety, efficacy, and cost. The measures for outcomes were menstrual changes, patient satisfaction, time of back work, and use of health service within 6 months after operation. All 37 procedures were successfully completed, with no serious operative complications and the mean amount of uterine bleeding reduced at 6 months after surgeries. Seventy-eight percent of the patients achieved the improvement in bleeding disorders, 92% of the patients were satisfied with the treatment, and no patient required a second hysteroscopic operation. At 6 months follow-up, the cost of treatment using Versapoint system was 40% cheaper than that by hysterectomy or open myomectomy (£1266 vs. £2123). Therefore it was thought that this procedure appeared to be safe, effective, and inexpensive.

Recently, American Isaacson pointed out very definitely that although some new devices were developed to successfully ablate the endometrium, the strong position of hysteroscopic operation was still impregnable.

Suggested Reading

An Overview of Hysteroscopic Electroresection Surgery

1. Brill AI. What is the role of hysteroscopy in the management of abnormal uterine bleeding? Clin Obstet Gynecol. 1995;38:319–45.
2. Chen BH, Giudice LC. Dysfunctional uterine bleeding. West J Med. 1998;169:280–4.
3. Cooper JM, Brady RM. Hysteroscopy in the management of abnormal uterine bleeding. Obstet Gynecol Clin North Am. 1999;26:217–36.
4. Fraser IS. Hysteroscopy and laparoscopy in women with menorrhagia. Am J Obstet Gynecol. 1990;162:1264–9.
5. Ho HS, Yip SK, Lim KB, Fook S, Foo KT, Cheng CW. A prospective randomized study comparing monopolar and bipolar transurethral resection of prostate using transurethral resection in saline (TURIS) system. Eur Urol. 2007;52(2):517–22.
6. Li JH, Yi LD, Peng LB, Cao JH, Lu Q. Pharmacological action and clinical application of phloroglucinol. Chin J New Drugs Clin Remedies. 2011;30(7):494–9. Chinese.
7. Nagele F, Rubinger T, Magos A. Why do women choose endometrial ablation rather than hysterectomy? Fertil Steril. 1998;69:1063–6.
8. Pantaleoni D. On endoscopic examination of the cavity of the womb. Med Press Cir. 1869;8:26–7.
9. Stabinsky SA, Einstein M, Breen JL. Modern treatments of menorrhagia attributable to dysfunctional uterine bleeding. Obstet Gynecol Surv. 1999;54:61–72.
10. Stamatellos I, Stamatopolos P, Bontis J. The role of hysteroscopy in the current management of the cervical polyps. Arch Gynecol. 2007;276(4):299–303.
11. Torrejon R, Fernandez-Alba JJ, Carnicer I, Martin A, Castro C, Garcia-Cabanillas J, Rodriguez-Cornejo J, Moreno LJ, Comino R. The value of hysteroscopic exploration for abnormal uterine bleeding. J Am Assoc Gynecol Laparosc. 1997;4(4):453–6.
12. Wortman M, Daggett A. A hysteroscopic endomyometrial resection: a new technique for the treatment of menorrhagia. Obstet Gynecol. 1994;83:295–8.

Transcervical Resection of Endometrium and Endometrial Ablation

13. Agboola AJ, Walton SM, Hoffman J. Postmenopausal endometrial tuberculosis. Gynaecol Endosc. 2000;9:209–11.
14. Agostini A, Cravello L, Bretelle F, Demaisonneuve AS, Roger V, Blanc B. Risk of discovering endometrial carcinoma or atypical hyperplasia during hysteroscopic surgery in postmenopausal women. J Am Assoc Gynecol Laparosc. 2001;8(4):533–5.
15. Alexander DA, Naji AA, Pinion SB, Mollison J, Kitchener HC, Parkin DE, Abramovich DR, Russell IT. Randomised trial comparing hysterectomy with endometrial ablation for dysfunctional uterine bleeding: psychiatric and psychosocial aspects. BMJ. 1996;312(7026):280–4.
16. Bae IH, Pagedas AC, Perkins HE, Bae DS. Postablation-tubal sterilization syndrome. J Am Assoc Gynecol Laparosc. 1996;3(3):435–8.
17. Baggish MS, Daniell JF. Death caused by air embolism associated with neodymium: Yttriumaluminum-garnet laser surgery and artificial sapphire tips. Am J Obstet Gynecol. 1989;161:877–8.
18. Baskett TF, Farrell SA, Zilbert AW. Uterine fluid irrigation and absorption in hysteroscopic endometrial ablation. Obstet Gynecol. 1998;92:976–8.
19. Baumann R, Owerdieck W, Reck G. Pregnancy following sterilization and endometrium resection. Geburtshilfe Frauenheilkd. 1994;54(4):246–9.
20. Bennett KL, Ohrmundt C, Maloni JA. Preventing intravasation in women undergoing hysteroscopic procedures. AORN J. 1996;64:792–9.
21. Boe Engelsen I, Woie K, Hordnes K. Transcervical endometrial resection: long-term results of 390 procedures. Acta Obstet Gynecol Scand. 2006;85(1):82–7.
22. Bratschi HU. Hysteroscopic endometrial resection. Contrib Gynecol Obstet. 2000;20:121–36.
23. Brook PG. Venous air embolism during operative hysteroscopy. J Am Assoc Gynecol Laparosc. 1997;4:399–402.
24. Brooks-Carter GN, Killackey MA, Neuwirth RS. Adenocarcinoma of the endometrium after endometrial ablation. Obstet Gynecol. 2000;96(5 Pt 2):836–7.
25. Bustos-Lopez HH, Baggish M, Valle RF. Assessment of the safety of intrauterine instillation of heated saline for endometrial ablation. Fertil Steril. 1998;69:155–60.
26. Clarke A, Judge A, Herbert A, McPherson K, Bridgman S, Maresh M, Overton C, Altman D. Readmission to hospital 5 years after hysterectomy or endometrial resection in a national cohort study. Qual Saf Health Care. 2005;14(1):41–7.
27. Colgan TJ, Shah R, Leyland N. Post-hysteroscopic ablation reaction: a histopathologic study of the effects of electrosurgical ablation. Int J Gynecol Pathol. 1999;18:325–31.
28. Cooper JM, Brady RM. Late complications of operative hysteroscopy. Obstet Gynecol Clin North Am. 2000;27(2):367–74.
29. Cooper KG, Jack SA, Parkin DE, Grant AM. Five-year follow up of women randomised to medical management or transcervical resection of the endometrium for heavy menstrual loss: clinical and quality of life outcomes. BJOG. 2001;108(12):1222–8.
30. Cravello L, de Montgolfier R, D'Ercole C, Boubli L, Blanc B. Hysteroscopic surgery in postmenopausal women. Acta Obstet Gynecol Scand. 1996;75(6):563–6.
31. Cravello L, Porcu G, Roger V, D'Ercole C, Blanc B. Hystéroscopie opératoire et fertilité [Hysteroscopic surgery and fertility]. Contracept Fertil Sex. 1998;26(7–8):589–92. French.
32. de Souza SS, Camargos AF, de Rezende CP, Pereira FA, Araújo CA, Silva Filho AL. A randomized prospective trial comparing the levonorgestrel-releasing intrauterine system with thermal balloon ablation for the treatment of heavy menstrual bleeding. Contraception. 2010;81(3):226–31.
33. Deb S, Flora K, Atiomo W. A survey of preferences and practices of endometrial ablation/ resection for menorrhagia in the United Kingdom. Fertil Steril. 2008;90(5):1. 812-7
34. DeCherney AH, Diamond MP, Lavy G, Polan ML. Endometrial ablation for intractable uterine bleeding: hysteroscopic resection. Obstet Gynecol. 1987;70(4):668–70.
35. Donnez J, Nisolle M, Clerckx F, Casanas-Roux F, Saussoy P, Gillerot S. Advanced endoscopic techniques used in dysfunctional bleeding, fibroids and endometriosis, and the role of gonadotrophin-releasing hormone agonist treatment. Br J Obstet Gynaecol. 1994;101(Suppl 10):2–9.
36. Donnez J, Vilos G, Gannon MJ, Maheux R, Emanuel MH, Istre O, AZTEC Study Group. Goserelin acetate (Zoladex) plus endometrial ablation for dysfunctional uterine bleeding: a 3-year follow-up evaluation. Fertil Steril. 2001;75(3):620–2.
37. Donnez J, Vilos G, Gannon MJ, Stampe-Sorensen S, Klinte I, Miller RM. Goserelin acetate (Zoladex) plus endometrial ablation for dysfunctional uterine bleeding: a large randomized, double-blind study. Fertil Steril. 1997;68(1):29–36.
38. Dutton C, Ackerson L, Phelps-Sandall B. Outcomes after rollerball endometrial ablation for menorrhagia. Obstet Gynecol. 2001;98(5 Pt 1):870–5.
39. Dwyer N, Fox R, Mills M, Hutton J. Haematometra caused by hormone replacement therapy after endometrial resection. Lancet. 1991;338(8776):1205.
40. Dwyer N, Hutton J, Stirrat GM. Randomised controlled trial comparing endometrial resection with abdominal hysterectomy for the surgical treatment of menorrhagia. Br J Obstet Gynaecol. 1993;100:237–43.
41. el Senoun GS, Mousa HA, Mahmood TA. Medium-term follow-up of women with menorrhagia treated by rollerball endometrial ablation. Acta Obstet Gynecol Scand. 2000;79(10):879–83.
42. Eskandar MA, Vilos GA, Aletebi FA, Tummon IS. Hysteroscopic endometrial ablation is an effective alternative to hysterectomy in women with menorrhagia and large uteri. J Am Assoc Gynecol Laparosc. 2000;7(3):339–45.
43. Feng LM, Chen RF, Xia EL. Application of hysteroscopic resection in diagnosis of adenomyosis. Chin J Obstet Gynecol. 1998;33:435–6. Chinese.
44. Franchini M, Cianferoni L. Emergency endometrial resection in women with acute, severe uterine bleeding. J Am Assoc Gynecol Laparosc. 2000;7(3):340–50.
45. Furst SN, Philipsen T, Joergensen TC. Ten-year follow-up of endometrial ablation. Acta Obstet Gynecol Scand. 2007;86(3):334–8.
46. Garry R. Hysteroscopic alternative to hysterectomy. Br J Obstet Gynaecol. 1990;97:199–207.
47. Gimpelson RJ, Kaigh J. Mechanical preparation of the endometrium prior to endometrial ablation. J Reprod Med. 1992;37:691–4.
48. Goldenberg M, Zolti M, Hart S, Bider D. Endometrial resectoscopic ablation in patients with menometrorrhagia as a side effect of anticoagulant therapy. Eur J Obstet Gynecol Reprod Biol. 1998;77(1):77–9.
49. Goldrath MH, Fuller T, Segal S. Laser Photovaporization of endometrium for the treatment of menorrhagia. Am J Obstet Gynecol. 1981;140:14–9.
50. Herman P, Gaspard U, Foldart JM. Surgical hysteroscopy or hysterectomy in the treatment of benign uterine lesions. What to choose in 1998? Rev Med Liege. 1998;53:756–61.
51. Hidlebaugh DA. Relative costs of gynecologic endoscopy vs traditional surgery for treatment of abnormal uterine bleeding. Am J Manag Care. 2001;7:31–7.
52. Hill DJ, Maher PJ. Pregnancy following endometrial ablation. Gynaecol Endosc. 1992;1:47.

53. Hoekstra PT, Kahnoski R, McCamish MA, Bergen W, Heetderks DR. Transurethral prostatic resection syndrome--a new perspective: encephalopathy with associated hyperammonemia. J Urol. 1983;130(4):704–7.
54. Istre O, Trolle B. Treatment of menorrhagia with the levonorgestrel intrauterine system versus endometrial resection. Fertil Steril. 2001;76(2):304–9.
55. Gupta J, Kai J, Middleton L, Pattison H, Gray R, Daniels J, ECLIPSE Trial Collaborative Group. Levonorgestrel intrauterine system versus medical therapy for menorrhagia. N Engl J Med. 2013;368(2):128–37.
56. Jeanette SCC, Charles WFM. A case of pelvic and hepatic abscesses following rollerball endometrial ablation. Gynaecol Endosc. 1999;8:183–5.
57. Zheng J, Xia E, Li TC, Sun X. Comparison of combined transcervical resection of the endometrium and levonorgestrel-containing intrauterine system treatment versus levonorgestrel-containing intrauterine system treatment alone in women with adenomyosis: a prospective clinical trial. J Reprod Med. 2013;58(7–8):285–90.
58. Keckstein J. Hysteroscopy and adenomyosis. Contrib Gynecol Obstet. 2000;20:41–50.
59. Klinzing S, Schlensog I, Brauer M, Klein U. Hyponatriämie und Lungenödem bei Endometriumablation mit der Rollerballelektrode [Hyponatremia and lung edema in endometrium ablation with rollerball ablation]. Zentralbl Gynakol. 1999;121(2):98–100.
60. Lam AM, Al-Jumaily RY, Holt EM. Ruptured ectopic pregnancy in an amenorrhoeic woman after transcervical resection of the endometrium. Aust NZ J Obstet Gynaecol. 1992;32:81–2.
61. Letterie GS, Kramer DJ. Intraoperative ultrasound guidance for intrauterine endoscopic surgery. Fertil Steril. 1994;62:654–6.
62. Lewis BV. Guidelines for endometrial ablation. Bri J Obstet Gynecol. 1994;101:470–3.
63. Li PK, Leung CB, Leung AK, Luk WK, Lai KN. Posthysteroscopy fungal peritonitis in a patient on continuous ambulatory peritoneal dialysis. Am J Kidney Dis. 1993;21(4):446–8.
64. Lin BL, Iwata Y, Miyamoto N, Hayashi S. Three-contrasts method: an ultrasound technique for monitoring transcervical operations. Am J Obstet Gynecol. 1987;156(2):469–72.
65. Lin BL, Miyamoto N, Tomomatu M. The development on transcervical resection (TCR) and endometrial ablation (EA). Japan J Gynecol Obstet Endosc. 1988;4:56.
66. Liu YH, Xia EL, Zhang D, Ma Y. Influence of transcervical resection of endometrium on uterine hemodynamics. Chin J Obstet Gynecol. 2004;39:776–7. Chinese.
67. Loffer FD. Complications of hysteroscopy—their cause, prevention, and correction. J Am Assoc Gynecol Laparosc. 1995;3:11–26.
68. Magos AL, Baumann R, Lockwood GM, Turnbull AC. Experience with the first 250 endometrial resections for menorrhagia. Lancet. 1991;337(8749):1074–8.
69. Magos AL, Baumann R, Turnbull AC. Transcervical resection of endometrium in women with menorrhagia. Brit Med J. 1989;298:1209–12.
70. Maia H Jr, Calmon LC, Marques D, Oliveira M, Coutinho E. Endometrial resection after vacuum curettage. Gynaecol Endosc. 1997;6:353–7.
71. Mansour D. Modern management of abnormal uterine bleeding: the levonorgestrel intra-uterine system. Best Pract Res Clin Obstet Gynaecol. 2007;21(6):1007–21.
72. Margolis MT, Thoen LD, Boike GM, Mercer LJ, Keith LG. Asymptomatic endometrial carcinoma after endometrial ablation. Int J Gynaecol Obstet. 1995;51(3):255–8.
73. McCausland AM. Hysteroscopic myometrial biopsy: its use in diagnosing adenomyosis and its clinical application. Am J Obstet Gynecol. 1992;166:1619–26.
74. McCausland V, McCauland A. The response of adenomyosis to endometrial ablation/resection. Hum Reprod Update. 1998;4:350–9.
75. McCausland VM, Fields GA, McCausland AM, Townsend DE. Tuboovarian abscesses after operative hysteroscopy. J Reprod Med. 1993;38(3):198–200.
76. McLucas B, Perrella R. Does endometrial resection cause adenomyosis? J Am Assoc Gynecol Laparosc. 1994;1:S21.
77. Mercader VP, McGuckin JF Jr, Caroline DF. CT of vesicocorporeal fistula with menouria: a complication of uterine biopsy. J Comput Assist Tomogr. 1995;19:324–6.
78. Milad MP, Valle RF. Emergency endometrial ablation for life-threatening uterine bleeding as a result of a coagulopathy. J Am Assoc Gynecol Laparosc. 1998;5:301–3.
79. Mints M, Radestad A, Rylander E. Follow up of hysteroscopic surgery for menorrhagia. Acta Obstet Gynecol Scand. 1998;77:435–8.
80. Mukul LV, Linn JG. Pregnancy complicated by uterine synechiae after endometrial ablation. Obstet Gynecol. 2005;105(5 Pt 2):1179–82.
81. Munro MG. Endometrial ablation: where have we been? Where are we going? Clin Obstet Gynecol. 2006;49(4):736–66.
82. Murdoch JA, Gan TJ. Anesthesia for hysteroscopy. Anesthesiol Clin North America. 2001;19(1):125–40.
83. Nachum Z, Kol S, Adir Y, Melamed Y. Massive air embolism--a possible cause of death after operative hysteroscopy using a 32% dextran-70 pump. Fertil Steril. 1992;58(4):836–8.
84. Neis KJ, Brandner P. Adenomyosis and endometrial ablation. Gynaecol Endosc. 2000;9:141–5.
85. Neuwirth RS. Cost effective management of heavy uterine bleeding: ablative methods versus hysterectomy. Curr Opin Obstet Gynecol. 2001;13(4):407–10.
86. Nisolle M. There is no place for Non-hysteroscopic endometrial ablation. ISGE News. 1999;5:5.
87. O'Connor H, Broadbent JA, Magos AL, McPherson K. Medical Research Council randomised trial of endometrial resection versus hysterectomy in management of menorrhagia. Lancet. 1997;349(9056):897–901.
88. Ostrzenski A. Resectoscopic cervical trauma minimized by inserting Laminaria digitata preoperatively. Int J Fertil. 1994;39:111–3.
89. Osuga Y, Okagaki R, Ozaki S, Matsumi H, Fujii T, Iwase H, Taketani Y. Successful emergency endometrial ablation for intractable uterine bleeding in a postmenopausal woman complicated with liver cirrhosis and morbid obesity. Surg Endosc. 2001;15(8):898.
90. Parkin DE. Prognostic factors for success of endometrial ablation and resection. Lancet. 1998;351:1147–8.
91. Phillips DR. Endometrial ablation for postmenopausal uterine bleeding induced by hormone replacement therapy. J Am Assoc Gynecol Laparosc. 1995;2:389–93.
92. Pinette M, Katz W, Drouin M, Blackstone J, Cartin A. Successful planned pregnancy following endometrial ablation with the YAG laser. Am J Obstet Gynecol. 2001;185(1):242–3.
93. Pinion SB, Parkin DE, Abramovich DR, Naji A, Alexander DA, Russell IT, Kitchener HC. Randomised trial of hysterectomy, endometrial laser ablation, and transcervical endometrial resection for dysfunctional uterine bleeding. BMJ. 1994;309(6960):979–83.
94. Pugh CP, Crane JM, Hogan TG. Successful intrauterine pregnancy after endometrial ablation. J Am Assoc Gynecol Laparosc. 2000;7(3):391.
95. Quemere MP, Cravello L, Roger V, d'Ercole C, Blanc B. Impact de l'adénomyose sur les résultats des endométrectomies [Impact of adenomyosis on results of endometrial ablations]. Contracept Fertil Sex. 1999;27(5):357–63. French.

96. Rai VS, Gillmer MD, Gray W. Is endometrial pre-treatment of value in improving the outcome of transcervical resection of the endometrium? Hum Reprod. 2000;15(9):1, 989-1, 992.
97. Raiga J, Bowen J, Glowaczower E, Canis M, Wattiez A, Déchelotte P, Pouly JL, Mage G, Bruhat MA. Facteurs d'échec d'endométrectomie. A propos d'une série de 196 cas [Failure factors in endometrial resection. 196 cases]. J Gynecol Obstet Biol Reprod (Paris). 1994;23(3):274–8. French.
98. Robert M, Walton SM. The effect of paracervical adrenaline on blood loss in patients undergoing transcervical resection of the endometrium. Gynaecol Endosc. 2000;9:153–6.
99. Romer T, Campo R, Hucke J. Hematometra after hysteroscopic endometrium ablation-a case report. Zentralbl Gynaecol. 1995;117:278–80.
100. Romer T, Muller J, Bojahr B. Hormonal premedication in endometrium ablation-results of a prospective comparative study. Zentralbl Gynakol. 1996;118(5):291–4.
101. Romer T, Schmidt T, Foth D. Pre-and postoperative hormonal treatment in patients with hysteroscopic surgery. Contrib Gynecol Obstet. 2000;20:1–12.
102. Romer T, Schwesinger G. Hormonal inhibition of endometrium for transcervical endometrial ablation—a prospective study with a 2-year follow-up. Eur J Obstet Gynecol Reprod Biol. 1997;74:201–3.
103. Romer T. Benefit of GnRH analogue pretreatment for hysteroscopic surgery in patients with bleeding disorders. Gynecol Obstet Invest. 1998;45(1):12–20.
104. Romer T. Successful treatment of recurrent uterine bleeding during tamoxifen therapy by endometrial ablation. Int J Qynaecol Obstet. 1995;49:51–2.
105. Romer T. Treatment of recurrent bleeding disorders during hormone replacement therapy by transcervical endometrial ablation. Gynecol Obstet Invest. 1999;47(4):255–7.
106. Rosati M, Vigone A, Capobianco F, Surico D, Amoruso E, Surico N. Long-term outcome of hysteroscopic endometrial ablation without endometrial preparation. Eur J Obstet Gynecol Reprod Biol. 2008;138(2):222–5.
107. Rousseau E, Jourdain O, Rabreau M, Cambon D, Dallay D. Nécrose utérine après réduction d'endomètre au laser nd:YAG. A propos d'un cas [Uterine necrosis after Nd-YAG laser ablation of the endometrium. A case report]. J Gynecol Obstet Biol Reprod (Paris). 1996;25(3):264–6. French.
108. Rullo S, Boni T. Broad ligament abscess after operative hysteroscopy. Clin Exp Obstet Gynecol. 1995;22:240–2.
109. Sagiv R, Ben-Shem E, Condrea A, Glezerman M, Golan A. Endometrial carcinoma after endometrial resection for dysfunctional uterine bleeding. Obstet Gynecol. 2005;106(5 Pt 2):1174–6.
110. Schiotz HA. Transcervical resection of the endometrium. Tidsskr Nor Laegeforen. 2001;121(23):2706–9.
111. Serden SP, Brooks PG. Prospective therapy in preparation for endometrial ablation. J. Reprod. Med. 1992;37(8):679–81.
112. Skar OJ. Operative hysteroscopy in the treatment of intrauterine disorders. Acta Obstet Gynecol Scand. 1990;69:565–6.
113. Sorensen SS, Andersen LF, Lose G. Endometriosis by implantation: A complication of endometrial ablation. Lancet. 1994;343:1226.
114. Sowter MG, Singla AA, Lethaby A. Pre-operative endometrial thinning agents before hysteroscopic surgery for heavy menstrual bleeding. Cochrane Database Syst Rev. 2000;(2):CD001124.
115. Steed HL, Scott JZ. Adenocarcinoma diagnosed at endometrial ablation. Obstet Gynecol. 2001;97(5 Ft 2):837–9.
116. Steffensen AJ, Hahn RG. Fluid absorption and the long-term outcome after transcervical resection of the endometrium. Acta Obstet Gynecol Scand. 1999;78(10):919.
117. Steffensen AJ, Schuster M. Endometrial resection and late reoperation in the treatment of menorrhagia. J Am Assoc Gynecol Laparosc. 1997;4:325–9.
118. Sutton GJG, Ewen SP. Thinning the endometrium prior to ablation: is it worthwhile? Br J Obstet Gynecol. 1994;10:10–2.
119. Tapper AM, Heinonen PK. Hysteroscopic endomyometrial resection for the treatment of menorrhagia--follow-up of 86 cases. Eur J Obstet Gynecol Reprod Biol. 1995;62:75–9.
120. Taskin O, Yalcinoglu A, Kucuk S, Burak F, Ozekici U, Wheeler JM. The degree of fluid absorption during hysteroscopic surgery in patients pretreated with goserelin. J Am Assoc Gynecol Laparosc. 1996;3(4):555–9.
121. Tiufekchieva E, Nikolov A. Hysteroscopic ablation of the endometrium in cases of dysfunctional uterine bleeding - advantage of preparations including zoladex. Akush Qinekol (Sofiia). 2002;41(2):30–4.
122. Townsend DE, McCausland V, McCausland A, Fields G, Kauffman K. Post-ablation-tubal sterilization syndrome. Obstet Gynecol. 1993;82(3):422–4.
123. Townsend DE, Richart RM, Paskowitz RA, Woolfork RE. "Rollerball" coagulation of the endometrium. Obstet Gynecol. 1990;76(2):310–3.
124. Tsaltas J, Taylor N, Healey MA. 6-year review of the outcome of endometrial ablation. Aust NZ J Obstet Gynaecol. 1998;38:69–72.
125. Turnbull LW, Jumaa A, Bowsley SJ, Dhawan S, Horsman A, Killick SR. Magnetic resonance imaging of the uterus after endometrial resection. Br J Obstet Gynaecol. 1997;104(8):934–8.
126. Valle RF, Baggish MS. Endometrial carcinoma after endometrial ablation: high-risk factors predicting its occurrence. Am J Obstet Gynecol. 1998;179:569–72.
127. VanDamme JF. One-stage endometrial ablation: results in 200 cases. Eur J Obstet Gynecol Reprod Biol. 1992;43:209–14.
128. Vercellini P, Oldani S, Yaylayan L, Zaina B, De Giorgi O, Crosignani PG. Randomized comparison of vaporizing electrode and cutting loop for endometrial ablation. Obstet Gynecol. 1999;94(4):521–7.
129. Vilos GA, Harding PG, Silcox JA, Sugimoto AK, Carey M, Ettler HC. Endometrial adenocarcinoma encountered at the time of hysteroscopic endometrial ablation. J Am Assoc Gynecol Laparosc. 2002;9(1):40–8.
130. Vilos GA, Vilos BA, RNL P. Endometrial ablation with a thermal balloon for the treatment of menorrhagia. J. Am Assoc Gynecol Laparosc. 1996;3:383–7.
131. Vilos GA, Harding PG, Sugimoto AK, Ettler HC, Bernier MJ. Hysteroscopic endomyometrial resection of three uterine sarcomas. J Am Assoc Gynecol Laparosc. 2001;8(4):545–51.
132. Wallwiener D, Rimbach S, Kaufmann M, Aydeniz B, Sohn C, Bastert G, Conradi R, von Fournier D. Hysteroskopische Endometriumablation in "high-risk"-Situationen und bei haemorrhagischer Diathese [Hysteroscopic endometrium ablation in "high-risk" situations and in hemorrhagic diathesis]. Zentralbl Gynakol. 1995;117(12):652–8. German.
133. Wamsteker K. There is no place for non-hysteroscopic endometrial ablation. 18GE News. 1999;5:4.
134. Wood C, Maher P, Hill D. Biopsy diagnosis and conservative surgical treatment of adenomyosis. Aust N Z J Obstet Gynaecol. 1993;33:319–21.
135. Wood C, Maher P, Hill D. Biopsy diagnosis and conservative surgical treatment of adenomyosis. J Am Assoc Qynecol Laparosc. 1994;1:313–6.
136. Wood SM, Roberts FL. Air embolism during transcervical resection of endometrium. Brit Med J. 1990;300:945.
137. Wortman M, Daggett A. Reoperative hysteroscopic surgery in the management of patients who fail endometrial ablation and resection. J Am Assoc Gynecol Laparosc. 2001;8(2):272–7.

138. Wortman M, Daggett A. Hysteroscopic endomyometrial resection. JSL8. 2000;4(3):197–207.
139. Xia E, Li TC, Yu D, Huang X, Zheng J, Liu Y, Zhang M. The occurrence and outcome of 39 pregnancies after 1621 cases of transcervical resection of endometrium. Hum Reprod. 2006;21(12):3282–6.
140. Xia EL, Duan H, Feng L. Application of B ultrasound and laparoscopic monitoring in hysteroscopic operation. China J Endosc. 1998;4:55–6. Chinese.
141. Xia EL, Duan H, Liu YH, Huang XW, Zheng J, Yu D, Duan HL, Zhang M. Clinical application of hysteroscopic endometrial resection and its evaluative analysis of long-term effects. Chin J Obstet Gynecol. 2004;39(5):296–300. Chinese.
142. Xia EL, Duan HL, Feng L. Stage I transcervical resection of endometrium (analysis of 125 cases enclosed). Chin J Endosc. 1999;5:67–9. Chinese.
143. Xia EL, Zhang M, Duan HL. Endometrial resection for menorrhagia: analysis of 400 cases. Chin J Obstet Gynecol. 1997;32:148–51. Chinese.
144. Xia EL, Zhang M, Duan HL. Endometrial resection for dysfunctional uterine bleeding. Chin J Obstet Gynecol. 1992;27:200–3. Chinese.
145. Xia EL. Application of endometrial ablation in treating dysfunctional uterine bleeding. J Pract Obstet Gynecol. 1998;14:73–4. Chinese.
146. Xia EL. Hysteroscopic diagnosis and treatment of adenomyosis. Shandong Med J. 2012;52:7–8. Chinese.
147. Yin CS, Wei RY, Chao TC, Chan CC. Hysteroscopic endometrial ablation without endometrial preparation. Int J Gynaecol Obstet. 1998;62(2):167–72.
148. Yuen PM. Adenomyosis following endometrial rollerball ablation. Aust N Z J Obstet Gynaecol. 1995;35:335–6.

Transcervical Resection of Myoma

149. Aziz N, Lenzi TA, Milki AA. Severe intrauterine growth restriction associated with the development of a submucosal leiomyoma during pregnancy: a case report. J Reprod Med. 2005;50(7):553–6.
150. Bernard G, Darai E, Poncelet C, Benifla JL, Madelenat P. Fertility after hysteroscopic myomectomy: effect of intramural myomas associated. Eur J Obstet Gynecol Reprod Biol. 2000;88(1):85–90.
151. Bettocchi S, Siristatidis C, Pontrelli G, Di Spiezio SA, Ceci O, Nappi L, Selvaggi L. The destiny of myomas: should we treat small submucous myomas in women of reproductive age? Fertil Steril. 2008;90(4):905–10.
152. Brooks PG, Serden SP, Davos I. Hormonal inhibition of the endometrium for resectoscopic endometrial ablation. Am J Obstet Gynecol. 1991;164:1601–6.
153. Brooks PG. Resectoscopic myoma vaporizer. J Reprod Med. 1995;40:791–5.
154. Caliskan E, Cakiroglu Y, Turkoz E. Leiomyoma on the septum of a septate uterus with double cervix and vaginal septum: a challenge to manage. Fertil Steril. 2008;89(2):456.e3–7.
155. Campo S, Campo V, Gambadauro P. Short-term and long-term results of resectoscopic myomectomy with and without pretreatment with GnRH analogs in premenopausal women. Acta Obstet Gynecol Scand. 2005;84(8):756–60.
156. Coccia ME, Becattini C, Bracco GL, Bargelli G, Scarselli G. Intraoperative ultrasound guidance for operative hysteroscopy. A prospective study. J Reprod Med. 2000;45(5):413–8.
157. Corson SL, Brooks PG. Resectoscopic myomectomy. Fertil Steril. 1991;55:1041–4.
158. Cravello L, Farnarier J, Roger V, D'Ercole C, Blanc B. Myomectomie hystéroscopique. Résultats fonctionnels avec un recul moyen de 6 ans [Hysteroscopic myomectomy. Functional results with an average follow-up of 6 years]. J Gynecol Obstet Biol Reprod (Paris). 1998;27(6):593–7. French.
159. De Iaco P, Golfieri R, Ghi T, Muzzupapa G, Ceccarini M, Bovicelli L. Uterine fistula induced by hysteroscopic resection of an embolized migrated fibroid: a rare complication after embolization of uterine fibroids. Fertil Steril. 2001;75(4):818–20.
160. DeCherney A, Polan ML. Hysteroscopic management of intrauterine lesions and untractable uterine bleeding. Obstet Gynecol. 1983;61:392–7.
161. Derman SG, Rehnstrom J, Neuwirth RS. The long-term effectiveness of hysteroscopic treatment of menorrhagia and leiomyomas. Obstet Gynecol. 1991;77:590–4.
162. Donnez J, Gillerot S, Bourgonjon D. Neodymium-YAG laser hysteroscopy in large submucous myomas. Fertil Steril. 1990;54:999–1003.
163. Donnez J, Nisolle M, Clerckx F, Casanas-Roux F, Saussoy P, Gillerot S. Advanced endoscopic techniques used in dysfunctional bleeding, fibroids and endometriosis, and the role of gonadotrophin-releasing hormone agonist treatment. Br J Obstet Gynaecol. 1994;101(Suppl 10):2–9.
164. Dueholm M, Forman A, Ingerslev J. Regression of residual tissue after incomplete resection of submucous myomas. Gynecol Endos. 1998;7:309–14.
165. Feng LM, Xia EL, Duan HL, Zhang M. Joint diagnosis of uterine diseases using hysteroscope and ultrasonic waves. Chin J Obstet Gynecol. 1996;31(6):334–7. Chinese.
166. Fernandez H, Kadoch O, Capella-Allouc S, Gervaise A, Taylor S, Frydman R. Résection hystéroscopique des myomes sous muqueux: résultats à long-terme [Hysteroscopic resection of submucous myomas: long term results]. Ann Chir. 2001;126(1):58–64.
167. Fernandez H, Sefrioui O, Virelizier C, Gervaise A, Gomel V, Frydman R. Hysteroscopic resection of submucosal myomas in patients with infertility. Hum Reprod. 2001;16(7):1489–92.
168. Flam F, Radestad A. Endometrial stromal sarcoma diagnosed by operative hysteroscopy. Hum Reprod. 1996;11:2797–8.
169. Giatras K, Berkeley AS, Noyes N, Licciardi F, Lolis D, Grifo JA. Fertility after hysteroscopic resection of submucous myomas. J Am Assoc Gynecol Laparosc. 1999;6(2):155–8.
170. Glasser MH. Endometrial ablation and hysteroscopic myomectomy by electrosurgical vaporization. J Am Assoc Gynecol Laparosc. 1997;4:369–74.
171. Hallez JP, Netter A, Cariter R. Methodical intrauterine resection. Am J Obstet Gynecol. 1987;156:1080–4.
172. Hallez JP, Perino A. Endoscopic intrauterine resection principles and technique. Acta Eur Fertil. 1988;19:17–20.
173. Hallez JP. Single-stage total hysteroscopic myomectomies indications, techniques and results. Fertil Steril. 1995;63:703–8.
174. Hanning RV, Harkins PG, Uehling DT. Preservation of fertility by transcervical resection of a benign mesodermal uterine tumor with a resectoscope and glycine distending medium. Fertil Steril. 1980;33:209–10.
175. Hansen UD, Lund CO. Finding of an unsuspected endometrial stromal sarcoma by hysteroscopic endometrial resection. Gynaecol Endosc. 1998;7:279–80.
176. Huang XW, Xia EL, Ma N, Peng XB, Xiao Y. Analysis on the surgical and reproductive outcomes of early diffuse uterine leiomyomatosis with hysteroscopic myomectomy. China J Endosc. 2012;18(6):581–4.
177. Hisayuki K, Tsutomu A. Hysteroscopic submucous myomectomy. Jpn J Gynecol Obstet Endosc. 1995;11:11–26.
178. Kim AH, Keltz MD, Arici A, Rosenberg M, Olive DL. Dilutional hyponatremia during hysteroscopic myomectomy with sorbitol-mannitol distention medium. J Am Assoc Gynecol Laparosc. 1995;2(2):237–42.

179. Lin BL, Iwata Y, Lin KH. Removing a large submucous myoma hysteroscopically with the two-resectoscope method. J Assoc Gynecol Laparosc. 1994;1:259–63.
180. Lin BL, Iwata Y, Miyamoto N, Hayashi S. Three-contrasts method: an ultrasound technique for monitoring transcervical operations. Am J Obstet Gynecol. 1987;156(2):469–72.
181. Lin BL, Iwata Y. Hysteroscopic operation. Clin Obstet Gynecol. 1998;52:1522–5.
182. Lin BL, Iwata Y. Modified laparoscopy for monitoring transcervical surgery. Am J Obstet Gynecol. 1990;163(1 Pt 1):243–4.
183. Lin BL, Miyamoto N, Aoki R, Iwata Y, Iizuka R. Transcervical resection of submucous myoma. Nihon Sanka Fujinka Gakkai Zasshi. 1986;38(9):1647–52.
184. Lin BL, Yuriko Y. Development of hysteroscopic equipment. Jpn J Gynecol Obstet Endosc. 1996;12:60–4. Japanese.
185. Loffer FD. Complications of hysteoscopy—their cause, prevention, and correction. J Am Assoc Gyencol Laparosc. 1995;3:11–26.
186. Loffer FD. Hysteroscopic myomectomy in postmenopausal women. J Minim Invasive Gynecol. 2005;12(4):323–5.
187. Loffer FD. Improving results of hysteroscopic submucosal myomectomy for menorrhagia by concomitant endometrial ablation. J Minim Invasive Gynecol. 2005;12(3):254–60.
188. Loffer FD. Removal of large symptomatic intrauterine growths by the hysteroscopic resectoscope. Obstet Gynecol. 1990;76:836–40.
189. Ma N, Xia EL. Analysis on reproductive outcomes of hysteroscopic myomectomy in 229 infertile women. Shandong Med J. 2012;52(12):31–3. Chinese.
190. Magos AL, Baumann R, Turnbull AC. Transcervical resection of the endometrium in women with menorrhagia. Brit Med J. 1989;298:1209–12.
191. Marabini A, Gubbini G, De Jaco P, Stagnozzi R, Santini D. A case of unsuspected endometrial stromal sarcoma removed by operative hysteroscopy. Gynecol Oncol. 1995;59(3):409–11.
192. Murakami T, Tamura M, Ozawa Y, Suzuki H, Terada Y, Okamura K. Safe techniques in surgery for hysteroscopic myomectomy. J Obstet Gynaecol Res. 2005;31(3):216–23.
193. Neuwirth RS. A new technique for and additional experience with hysteroscopic resection of submucous fibroids. Am J Obstet Gynecol. 1978;131:91–4.
194. Neuwirth RS. Hysteroscopic management of symptomatic submucous fibroids. Obstet Gynecol. 1983;62:509–11.
195. Neuwirth RS. Hysteroscopic resection of submucous leiomyoma. Contemp Obstet Gynecol. 1985;25:103–23.
196. Neuwirth RS, Smin HK. Excision of submucous fibroids with hysteroscopic control. Am J Obstet Gynecol. 1976;126:95–9.
197. Ostrzenski A. Resectoscopic cervical trauma minimized by inserting laminaria digitata preoperatively. Int J Fertil. 1994;39:111–3.
198. Polena V, Mergui JL, Perrot N, Poncelet C, Barranger E, Uzan S. Long-term results of hysteroscopic myomectomy in 235 patients. Eur J Obstet Gynecol Reprod Biol. 2007;130(2):232–7.
199. Romer T, Schmidt T, Foth D. Pre-and postoperative hormonal treatment in patients with hysteroscopic surgery. Contrib Gynecol Obstet. 2000;20:1–12.
200. Romer T. Hysteroscopic myoma resection of submucous myomas with largely intramural components. Zentralbl Gynaekol. 1997;119:374–7.
201. Sanders B. Uterine factors and infertility. J Reprod Med. 2006;51(3):169–76.
202. Serden SP, Brooks PG. Preoperative therapy in preparation for endometrial ablation. J Reprod Med. 1992;37:679–81.
203. Shokeir TA. Hysteroscopic management in submucous fibroids to improve fertility. Arch Gynecol Obstet. 2005;273(1):50–4.
204. Tanaka K, Sato T. Effectiveness of TCRR in endometriosis. Jpn J Gynecol Obstet Endosc. 1995;11:118–22. Japanese.
205. Tiufekchieva E, Nikolov A. Hysteroresection of submucous myomas after treatment with zoladex. Akush Ginekol (Sofiia). 2006;45(1):19–24.
206. Tulandi T, al-Took S. Endoscopic myomectomy. Laparoscopy and hysteroscopy. Obstet Gynecol Olin North Am. 1999;26:135–48. viii
207. Valle RF. Hysteroscopic removal of submucous leiomyomas. J Gynecol Surg. 1990;6:89–96.
208. Varasteh NN, Neuwirth RS, Levin B, Keltz MD. Pregnancy rates after hysteroscopic polypectomy and myomectomy in infertile women. Obstet Gynecol. 1999;94(2):168–71.
209. Vercellini P, Oldani S, De Giorgi O, Milesi M, Merlo D, Crosignani PG. Endometrial ablation with a vaporizing electrode. II. Clinical outcome of a pilot study. Acta Obstet Gynecol Scand. 1998;77(6):688–93.
210. Vercellini P, Oldani S, Milesi M, Rossi M, Carinelli S, Crosignani PG. Endometrial ablation with a vaporizing electrode. I. Evaluation of in vivo effects. Acta Obstet Gynecol Scand. 1998;77(6):683–7.
211. Vercellini P, Zàina B, Yaylayan L, Pisacreta A, De Giorgi O, Crosignani PG. Hysteroscopic myomectomy: long-term effects on menstrual pattern and fertility. Obstet Gynecol. 1999;94(3):341–7.
212. Vimercati A, Scioscia M, Lorusso F, Laera AF, Lamanna G, Coluccia A, Bettocchi S, Selvaggi L, Depalo R. Do uterine fibroids affect IVF outcomes? Reprod Biomed Online. 2007;15(6):686–91.
213. Wamsteker K, Emanuel MH, deKruif JH. Transcervical hysteroscopic resection of submucous fibroids for abnormal uterine bleeding: results regarding degree of intramural extension. Obstet Gynecol. 1993;82:736–40.
214. Xia EL, Duan H, Feng L. Application of B ultrasound and laparoscopic monitoring in hysteroscopic operation. China J Endosc. 1998;4:55–6. Chinese.
215. Xia EL, Duan H, Huang XW, Zheng J, Yu D. Hysteroscopic treatment of uterine myomas: clinical analysis of 962 cases. Chin Med J. 2005;85(3):173–6. Chinese.
216. Yang JH, Lin BL. Changes in myometrial thickness during hysteroscopic resection of deeply invasive submucous myomas. J Am Assoc Gynecol Laparosc. 2001;8(4):501–5.
217. Yaron Y, Shenhav M, Jaffa AJ, Lessing JB, Peyser MR. Uterine rupture at 33 weeks' gestation subsequent to hysteroscopic uterine perforation. Am J Obstet Gynecol. 1994;170(3):786–7.
218. Yen CF, Lee CL, Wang CJ, Soong YK, Arici A. Successful pregnancies in women with diffuse uterine leiomyomatosis after hysteroscopic management. Fertil Steril. 2007;88(6):1667–73.

Transcervical Resection of Endometrial Polyps

219. Anastasiadis PG, Koutlaki NG, Skaphida PG, Galazios GC, Tsikouras PN, Liberis VA. Endometrial polyps: prevalence, detection, and malignant potential in women with abnormal uterine bleeding. Eur J Gynaecol Oncol. 2000;21(2):180–3.
220. Bacsko G, Major T. Hysteroscopic diagnosis and treatment of endometrial polyps. Orv Hetil. 1999;140:2041–5.
221. Baggish MS, Barbot J, Valle RF. Diagnositic and operative hysteroscopy. 2nd ed. St. Louis: Mosby; 1999. p. 274–6.
222. Baggish MS. A new laser hysteroscopic for Nd: YAG endometrial ablation. Lasers Surg Med. 1988;8:99–103.
223. Bakour SH, Khan KS, Gupta JK. The risk of premalignant and malignant pathology in endometrial polyps. Acta Obstet Gynecol Scand. 2000;79:317–20.
224. Ben-Arie A, Goldchmit C, Laviv Y, Levy R, Caspi B, Huszar M, Dgani R, Hagay Z. The malignant potential of endometrial polyps. Eur J Obstet Gynecol Reprod Biol. 2004;115(2):206–10.
225. Bouda J Jr, Hradecky L, Rokyta Z. Hysteroscopic polypectomy versus fractionated curettage in the treatment of corporal polyps—recurrence of corporal polyps. Ceska Gynekol. 2000;65(3):147–51.
226. Bradley LD, Pasqualotto EB, Price LL, Margossian H. Hysteroscopic management of endometrial polyps. Obstet Gynecol. 2000;95(4 Suppl 1):S23.

227. Cravello L, Stolla V, Bretelle F, Roger V, Blanc B. Hysteroscopic resection of endometrial polyps: a study of 195 cases. Eur J Obstet Gynecol Reprod Biol. 2000;93(2):131–4.
228. Garuti G, Cellani F, Colonnelli M. Outpatient hysteroscopic polypectomy in 237 patients: feasibility of a one-stop "see-and-treat" procedure. J Am Assoc Gynecol Laparosc. 2004;11(4):500–4.
229. Gimpelson RJ. Hysteroscopic treatment of the patient with intracavitary pathology (myomectomy/polypectomy). Obstet Gynecol Clin North Am. 2000;27(2):327–37.
230. Henriquez DD, van Dongen H, Wolterbeek R, Jansen FW. Polypectomy in premenopausal women with abnormal uterine bleeding: effectiveness of hysteroscopic removal. J Minim Invasive Gynecol. 2007;14(1):59–63.
231. Herman P, Gaspard U, Foldart JM. Surgical hysteroscopy or hysterectomy in the treatment of benign uterine lesions. What to choose in 1998? Rev Med Liege. 1998;53:756–61.
232. Isikoglu M, Berkkanoglu M, Senturk Z, Coetzee K, Ozgur K. Endometrial polyps smaller than 1.5 cm do not affect ICSI outcome. Reprod Biomed Online. 2006;12(2):199–204.
233. Lin BL, Iwata YY, Valle R. Clinical applications of Lin's forceps in flexible hysteroscopy. J Am.Assoc Gynecol Laparosc. 1994;1:383–7.
234. Liu YH, Xia EL, Lu Y, Peng XB. Analysis of diagnosis and treatment of adenomyomatous endometrial polyp. China J Endosc. 2008;3(14):263–5. Chinese.
235. Maltez A, Maia JRH, Oliveira MC. Clear cell carcinoma arising in an endometrial polyp. Gynaecol Endosc. 1998;7:51–3.
236. Marabini A, Gubbini G, De Jaco P, Stagnozzi R, Santini D. A case of unsuspected endometrial stromal sarcoma removed by operative hysteroscopy. Gynecol Oncol. 1995;59(3):409–11.
237. Nathani F, Clark TJ. Uterine polypectomy in the management of abnormal uterine bleeding: a systematic review. J Minim Invasive Gynecol. 2006;13(4):260–8.
238. Peng XB, Li T, Xia EL, Li J, Huang XW. Is endometrial polyp formation associated with increased expression of vascular endothelial growth factor and transforming growth factor-beta1? Eur J Obstet Gynecol Reprod Biol. 2011;159(1):198–203.
239. Peng XB, Li T, Xia EL, Xia C, Liu Y, Yu D. A comparison of oestrogen receptor and progesterone receptor expression in endometrial polyps and endometrium of premenopausal women. J Obstet Gynaecol. 2009;29(4):340–6.
240. Persin J, Hanousek L, Mrvova V. Results of transcervical surgical therapy on endometrium polyps. Ceska Gynekol. 2005;70(4):273–6.
241. Polena V, Mergui JL, Zérat L, Daraï E, Barranger E, Uzan S. Résultats à long terme de la résection des polypes endométriaux chez 367 patientes. Place de l'endométrectomie associée [Long-term results of hysteroscopic resection of endometrial polyps in 367 patients. Role of associated endometrial resection]. Gynecol Obstet Fertil. 2005;33(6):382–8. French.
242. Reslová T, Tosner J, Resl M, Kugler R, Vávrová I. Endometrial polyps. A clinical study of 245 cases. Arch Gynecol Obstet. 1999;262(3–4):133–9.
243. Sanders B. Uterine factors and infertility. J Reprod Med. 2006;51(3):169–76.
244. Scrimin F, Mangino FP, Wiesenfeld U, Candiotto A, Guaschino S. Is resectoscopic treatment of atypical endometrial polyps a safe option? Am J Obstet Gynecol. 2006;195(5):1328–30.
245. Sentilhes L, Sergent F, Popovic I, Fournet P, Paquet M, Marpeau L. Facteurs prédictifs de rupture utérine obstétricale après hystéroscopie opératoire [Factors predictive of uterine rupture after operative hysteroscopy]. J Gynecol Obstet Biol Reprod (Paris). 2004;33(1 Pt 1):51–5. French.
246. Stamatellos I, Apostolides A, Stamatopoulos P, Bontis J. Pregnancy rates after hysteroscopic polypectomy depending on the size or number of the polyps. Arch Gynecol Obstet. 2008;277(5):395–9.
247. Stamatellos I, Stamatopolos P, Bontis J. The role of hysteroscopy in the current management of the cervical polyps. Arch Gynecol. 2007;276(4):299–303.
248. Tjarks M, Van Voorhis BJ. Treatment of endometrial polyps. Obstet Gynecol. 2000;96(6):886–9.
249. Valle RF. Hysteroscopic evaluation of patients with abnormal uterine bleeding. Surg Gynecol Obstet. 1981;153:521–6.
250. Varasteh NN, Neuwirth RS, Levin B, Keltz MD. Pregnancy rates after hysteroscopic polypectomy and myomectomy in infertile women. Obstet Gynecol. 1999;94(2):168–71.
251. Xiao Y, Peng X, Ma N, Li TC, Xia E. The expression of cyclooxygenase-2 and vascular endothelial growth factor in the endometrium during the peri-implantation period in women with and without polyps. Hum Fertil (Camb). 2014;17(1):67–71.
252. Yanaihara A, Yorimitsu T, Motoyama H, Iwasaki S, Kawamura T. Location of endometrial polyp and pregnancy rate in infertility patients. Fertil Steril. 2008;90(1):180–2.

Transcervical Resection of Septum

253. Abramovici H, Faktor JH, Pascal B. Congenital uterine malformations as indication for cervical suture (cerclage) in habitual abortion and premature delivery. Int J Fertil. 1983;28:161–4.
254. Acien P. Incidence of Mullerian defects in fertile and infertile women. Hum Reprod. 1997;12:1372–6.
255. Airoldi J, Berghella V, Sehdev H, Ludmir J. Transvaginal ultrasonography of the cervix to predict preterm birth in women with uterine anomalies. Obstet Gynecol. 2005;106:553–6.
256. Akar ME, Bayar D, Yildiz S, Ozel M, Yilmaz Z. Reproductive outcome of women with unicornuate uterus. Aust N Z J Obstet Gynaecol. 2005;45(2):148–50.
257. Alborzi S, Asadi N, Zolghadri J. Laparoscopic metroplasty in bicornuate and didelphic uteri. Fertil Steril. 2009;92(1):352–5.
258. Aubriot FX, Chapron C. Diethylstilbestrol exposure in utero. Polemics about metroplasty. The pros. Gynecol Obstet Fertil. 2007;35(9):826–31.
259. Aupriot FX, Hamou J, Dubuisson JB. Hysteroplasty for enlargement: apropos of the results. Gynecol Obestet Fertil. 2001;29(12):888–93.
260. Baggish MS, Barbot J, Valle RF. Diagnositic and operative hysteroscopy. 2nd ed. St. Louis: Mosby; 1999. p. 269–88.
261. Barranger E, Gervaise A, Doumerc S, Fernandez H. Reproductive performance after hysteroscopic metroplasty in the hypoplastic uterus: a study of 29 cases. BJOG. 2002;109(12):1331–4.
262. Blitz MJ, Appelbaum H. Torsion of fallopian tube remnant associated with noncommunicating rudimentary horn in adolescent girl with unicornuate uterus. J Pediatr Adolesc Gynecol. 2014;27(5):e97–9.
263. Braun P, Grau FV, Pons RM, Enguix DP. Is hysterosalpingography able to diagnose all uterine malformations correctly? A retrospective study. Eur J Radiol. 2005;53(2):274–9.
264. Brucker SY, Rall K, Campo R, Oppelt P, Isaacson K. Treatment of congenital malformations. Semin Reprod Med. 2011;29(2):101–12.
265. Caliskan E, Cakiroglu Y, Turkoz E. Leiomyoma on the septum of a septate uterus with double cervix and vaginal septum: a challenge to manage. Fertil Steril. 2008;89(2):456.e3–7.
266. Capito C, Sarnacki S. Menstrual retention in a Robert's uterus. J Pediatr Adolesc Gynecol. 2009;22(5):e104–6.
267. Cararach M, Penella J, Ubeda A, Labastida R. Hysteroscopic incision of the septate uterus: scissors versus resectoscope. Hum Reprod. 1994;9(1):87–9.
268. Chen MY, Edwards VH, Ott DJ, Fayez JA. Hysterosalpingography after hysteroscopic surgery. Abdom Imaging. 1994;19(5):477–80.

269. Chervenak FA, Neuwirth RS. Hysteroscopic resection of the uterine septum. Am J Obstet Gynecol. 1981;141:351–3.
270. Choe JK, Baggish MS. Hysteroscopic treatment of septate uterus with neodymium-YAG laser. Fertil Steril. 1992;57:81–4.
271. Coccia ME, Becattini C, Bracco GL, Bargelli G, Scarselli G. Intraoperative ultrasound guidance for operative hysteroscopy. A prospective study. J Reprod Med. 2000;45(5):413–8.
272. Console D, Tamburrini S, Barresi D, Notarangelo L, Bertucci B, Tamburrini O. Il valore della RM nella valutazione delle anomalie dei dotti di Müller [The value of the MR imaging in the evaluation of Müllerian duct anomalies]. Radiol Med. 2001;102(4):226–32. Italian.
273. Creainin M, Chen M. Uterine defect in a twin pregnancy with a history of hysteroscopic fundal perforation. Obstet Gynecol. 1992;79:879–80.
274. Dalal RJ, Pai HD, Palshetkar NP, Takhtani M, Pai RD, Saxena N. Hysteroscopic metroplasty in women with primary infertility and septate uterus: reproductive performance after surgery. J Reprod Med. 2012;57(1-2):13–6.
275. DeCherney AH. Hysteroscopic management of Müllerian fusion defects. In: Siegler AM, Lindemann HJ, editors. Hysteroscopy principles and pratice. Philadelphia: JB Lippincott; 1984. p. 204–5.
276. El Saman AM, Shahin AY, Nasr A, Tawfik RM, Saadeldeen HS, Othman ER, Habib DM, Abdel-Aleem MA. Hybrid septate uterus, coexistence of bicornuate and septate varieties: a genuine report. J Obstet Gynaecol Res. 2012;38(11):1308–14.
277. Engmann L, Schmidt D, Nulsen J, Maier D, Benadiva C. An unusual anatomic variation of a unicornuate uterus with normal external uterine morphology. Fertil Steril. 2004;82(4):950–3.
278. Fedele L, Arcaini L, Parazzini F, Vercellini P, Di Nola G. Reproductive prognosis after hysteroscopic metroplasty in 102 women: life-table analysis. Fertil Steril. 1993;59(4):768–72.
279. Fedele L, Bianchi S, Marchini M, Mezzopane R, Di Nola G, Tozzi L. Residual uterine septum of less than 1 cm after hysteroscopic metroplasty does not impair reproductive outcome. Hum Reprod. 1996;11(4):727–9.
280. Gabriel B, Fischer DC, Sergius G. Unruptured pregnancy in a non-communicating heterotopic right fallopian tube associated with left unicornuate uterus: evidence for transperitoneal sperm and oocyte migration. Acta Obstet Gynecol Scand. 2002;81(1):91–2.
281. Gabriele A, Zanetta G, Pasta F, Colombo M. Uterine rupture after hysteroscopic metroplasty and labor induction. A case report. J Reprod Med. 1999;44(7):642–4.
282. Garbin O, Ohl J, Bettahar-Lebugle K, Dellenbach P. Hysteroscopic metroplasty in diethylstilboestrol-exposed and hypoplastic uterus: a report on 24 cases. Hum Reprod. 1998;13(10):2751–5.
283. Gergolet M, Campo R, Verdenik I, Kenda Suster N, Gordts S, Gianaroli L. No clinical relevance of the height of fundal indentation in subseptate or arcuate uterus: a prospective study. Reprod Biomed Online. 2012;24(5):576–82.
284. Giacomucci E, Bellavia E, Sandri F, Farina A, Scagliarini G. Term delivery rate after hysteroscopic metroplasty in patients with recurrent spontaneous abortion and T-shaped, arcuate and septate uterus. Gynecol Obstet Invest. 2011;71(3):183–8.
285. Golan A, Langer R, Neuman M, Wexler S, Segev E, David MP. Obstetric outcome in women with congenital uterine malformations. J Reprod Med. 1992;37(3):233–6.
286. Grimbizis GF, Camus M, Tarlatzis BC, Bontis JN, Devroey P. Clinical implications of uterine malformations and hysteroscopic treatment results. Hum Reprod Update. 2001;7(2):161–74.
287. Gupta N, Mittal S, Dadhwal V, Misra R. A unique congenital Mullerian anomaly: Robert's uterus. Arch Gynecol Obstet. 2007;276(6):641–3.
288. Handa Y, Hoshi N, Yamada H, Wada S, Kudo M, Tsuda K, Sagawa T, Fujimoto S. Tubal pregnancy in a unicornuate uterus with rudimentary horn: a case report. Fertil Steril. 1999;72(2):354–6.
289. Hassiakos DK, Zourlas PA. Transcervical division of uterine septa. Obstet Gynecol Surv. 1990;45(3):165–73.
290. Haydardedeoglu B, Simsek E, Kilicdag EB, Tarim E, Aslan E, Bagis T. A case of unicornuate uterus with ipsilateral ovarian and renal agenesis. Fertil Steril. 2006;85(3):750.e1–4.
291. Heinonen PK, Pystynen PP. Primary infertility and uterine anomalies. Fertil Steril. 1983;40(3):311–6.
292. Heinonen PK. Complete septate uterus with longitudinal vaginal septum. Fertil Steril. 2006;85(3):700–5.
293. Hollett-Caines J, Vilos GA, Abu-Rafea B, Ahmad R. Fertility and pregnancy outcomes following hysteroscopic septum division. J Obstet Gynaecol Can. 2006;28(2):156–9.
294. Homer HA, Li TC, Cooke ID. The septate uterus: a review of management and reproductive outcome. Fertil Steril. 2000;73:1–14.
295. Howe RS. Third-trimester uterine rupture following hysteroscopic uterine perforation. Obstet Gynecol. 1993;81:827–9.
296. Jayasinghe Y, Rane A, Stalewski H, Grover S. The presentation and early diagnosis of the rudimentary uterine horn. Obstet Gynecol. 2005;105(6):1456–67.
297. Katz Z, Ben-Arie A, Lurie S, Manor M, Insler V. Beneficial effect of hysteroscopic metroplasty on the reproductive outcome in a 'T-shaped' uterus. Gynecol Obstet Invest. 1996;41(1):41–3.
298. Kaufman RH. Structural changes of the genital tract associated with in utero exposure to diethylstilbestrol. Obstet Gynecol Annu. 1982;11:187–202.
299. Kupesic S, Kurjak A. Diagnosis and treatment outcome of the septate uterus. Croat Med J. 1998;39(2):185–90.
300. Liatsikos SA, Tsikouras P, Souftas V, Ammari A, Prassopoulos P, Maroulis G, Liberis V. Diagnosis and laparoscopic management of a rudimentary uterine horn in a teenage girl, presenting with haematometra and severe endometriosis: our experience and review of literature. Minim Invasive Ther Allied Technol. 2010;19(4):241–7.
301. Lin PC. Reproductive outcomes in women with uterine anomalies. J Womens Health (Larchmt). 2004;13(1):33–9.
302. Liu X, Hu M, Lu P. Diagnostic criteria of transvaginal three-dimensional ultrasonography in differentiation between incomplete uterus septum and arcuate uterus. J Clin Ultrasound in Med. 2013;15(8):580–1.
303. Lolis DE, Paschopoulos M, Makrydimas G, Zikopoulos K, Sotiriadis A, Paraskevaidis E. Reproductive outcome after strassman metroplasty in women with a bicornuate uterus. J Reprod Med. 2005;50(5):297–301.
304. Lourdel E, Cabry-Goubet R, Merviel P, Grenier N, Oliéric MF, Gondry J. Utérus cloisonné: place de la septoplastie hystéroscopique [Septate uterus: role of hysteroscopic metroplasty]. Gynecol Obstet Fertil. 2007;35(9):811–8. French.
305. March CM, Isreal R. Hysteroscopic management of intrauterine adhesions. Am J Obstet Gynecol. 1978;130:65.
306. Markham SM, Waterhouse TB. Structural anomalies of the reproductive tract. Curr Opin Obstet Gynecol. 1992;4(6):867–73.
307. Milad MP, Valle RF. Does hormone therapy after hysteroscopic metroplasty hasten endometrial healing? J Am Assoc Gynecol Laparosc. 1995;2(4 Suppl):S32.
308. Moutos DM, Damewood MD, Schlaff WD, Rock JA. A comparison of the reproductive outcome between women with a unicornuate uterus and women with a didelphic uterus. Fertil Steril. 1992;58(1):88–93.
309. Mucowski SJ, Herndon CN, Rosen MP. The arcuate uterine anomaly: a critical appraisal of its diagnostic and clinical relevance. Obstet Gynecol Surv. 2010;65(7):449–54.
310. Nagel TC, Malo JW. Hysteroscopic metroplasty in the diethylstilbestrol exposed uterus and similar nonfusion anomalies: effects on

subsequent reproductive performance: a preliminary report. Fertil steril. 1993;59(3):502–6.
311. Nakhal RS, Cutner AS, Hall-Craggs M, Creighton SM. Remnant functioning cervical tissue after laparoscopic removal of cavitated noncommunicating rudimentary uterine horn. J Minim Invasive Gynecol. 2012;19(6):768–71.
312. Ohl J, Bettahar-Lebugle K. Ultrasound-guided transcervical resection of uterine septa: 7 years' experience. Ultrasound Obstet Gynecol. 1996;7(5):328–34.
313. Park JK, Dominguez CE. Combined medical and surgical management of rudimentary uterine horn pregnancy. JSLS. 2007;11(1):119–22.
314. Parsanezhad ME, Alborzi S, Zarei A, Dehbashi S, Shirazi LG, Rajaeefard A, Schmidt EH. Hysteroscopic metroplasty of the complete uterine septum, duplicate cervix, and vaginal septum. Fertil Steril. 2006;85(5):1473–7.
315. Patton PE, Novy MJ, Lee DM, Hickok LR. The diagnosis and reproductive outcome after surgical treatment of the complete septate uterus, duplicated cervix and vaginal septum. Am J Obstet Gynecol. 2004;190(6):1669–75.
316. Pellerito JS, McCarthy SM, Doyle MB, Glickman MG, DeCherney AH. Diagnosis of uterine anomalies: relative accuracy of MR imaging, endovaginal sonography, and hysterosalpingography. Radiology. 1992;183(3):795–800.
317. Pelosi MA III, Pelosi MA. Laparoscopic-assisted transvaginal metroplasty for the treatment of bicornuate uterus: a case study. Fertil Steril. 1996;65(4):886–90.
318. Propst AM, Liberman RF, Harlow BL, Ginsburg ES. Complications of hysteroscopic surgery: predicting patients at risk. Obstet Gynecol. 2000;96(4):517–20.
319. Robert H. Asymmetrical bifidities with unilateral menstrual retention (apropos of 12 cases). Chirurgie. 1970;96(11):796–9.
320. Rock JA, Roberts CP, Hesla JS. Hysteroscopic metroplasty of the Class Va uterus with preservation of the cervical septum. Fertil Steril. 1999;72:942–5.
321. Roge P, D'Ercole C, Cravello L, Boubli L, Blanc B. Hysteroscopic management of uterine synechiae: a series of 102 observations. Eur J Obstet Gynecol Reprod Biol. 1996;65(2):189–93.
322. Romer T, Lober R. Hysteroscopic correction of a complete septate uterus using a balloon technique. Hum Reprod. 1997;12:478–9.
323. Romer T. The value of GnRH agonist treatments before hysteroscopic septum dissection. Zentralbl Gynakol. 1998;120:42–4.
324. Sentilhes L, Sergent F, Roman H, Verspyck E, Marpeau L. Late complications of operative hysteroscopy: predicting patients at risk of uterine rupture during subsequent pregnancy. Eur J Obstet Gynecol Reprod Biol. 2005;120(2):134–8.
325. Serafini P, Nelson J, Batzofin J. Resection of large uterine septum during early pregnancy and at the oocyte retrieval--peculiarities of two cases. Hum Reprod. 1994;9:1519–21.
326. Shahrokh Tehraninejad E, Ghaffari F, Jahangiri N, Oroomiechiha M, Akhoond MR, Aziminekoo E. Reproductive outcome following hysteroscopic monopolar metroplasty: an analysis of 203 cases. Int J Fertil Steril. 2013;7(3):175–80.
327. Sheth SS, Sonkawde R. Uterine septum misdiagnosed on hysterosalpingogram. Int J Gynaecol Obstet. 2000;69(3):261–3.
328. Singhal S, Agarwal U, Sharma D, Sirohiwal D. Pregnancy in asymmetric blind hemicavity of Robert's uterus--a previously unreported phenomenon. Eur J Obstet Gynecol Reprod Biol. 2003;107(1):93–5.
329. Sugaya S. Twin pregnancy after in vitro fertilization in a woman with a unicornuate uterus. Clin Exp Obstet Gynecol. 2010;37(4):317–8.
330. Valle RF. Hysteroscopic treatment of partial and complete uterine septum. Int J Fertil Menopausal Stud. 1996;41(3):310–5.
331. Velemir L, Gallot D, Jardon K, Mage G, Pouly JL. Uterine rupture at 26 weeks after metroplasty for uterine enlargement in diethylstilbestrol-exposed uterus: a case report. Eur J Obstet Gynecol Reprod Biol. 2008;138(2):243–4.
332. Vercellini P, Vendola N, Colombo A, Passadore C, Trespidi L, Fedele L. Hysteroscopic metroplasty with resectoscope or microscissors for the correction of septate uterus. Surg Gynecol Obstet. 1993;176(5):439–42.
333. Viscomi GN, Gonzalez R, Taylor KJ. Ultrasound detection of uterine abnormalities after diethylstilbestrol (DES) exposure. Radiology. 1980;136(3):733–5.
334. Xia EL, Liu YH, Huang XW. Hysteroscopic orthomophia combined with laparoscopy for total bicornuate uterus-one case report. Chin J Clin (Electr Ed). 2009;3(1):135–9. Chinese.
335. Xia EL, Liu YH, Ma N, Peng XB, Li YF, Xiao Y, Qu J. Three successful deliveries after hysteroscopic operations on T-shaped uterus and literatures review. Chin J Obstet Gynecol. 2013;48(6):457–9. Chinese.
336. Xia EL, Peng XB, Ma N, Li YF, Xiao Y, Guo Y, Qu J. Three successful pregnancies following hysteroscopic operations on unicornuate uterus and literatures review. Chin J Obstet Gynecol. 2013;45(9):689–91. Chinese.
337. Zabak K, Benifla JL, Uzan S. Septate uterus and reproduction disorders: current results of hysteroscopic septoplasty. Gynecol Obstet Fertil. 2001;29(11):829–40.
338. Ziebarth A, Eyster K, Hansen K. Delayed diagnosis of partially obstructed longitudinal vaginal septa. Fertil Steril. 2007;87(3):697.
339. Zlopasa G, Skrablin S, Kalafatić D, Banović V, Lesin J. Uterine anomalies and pregnancy outcome following resectoscope metroplasty. Int J Gynaecol Obstet. 2007;98(2):129–33.
340. Zorlu CG, Yalçin H, Ugur M, Ozden S, Kara-Soysal S, Gökmen O. Reproductive outcome after metroplasty. Int J Gynaecol Obstet. 1996;55(1):45–8.

Transcervical Resection of Intrauterine Adhesions

341. Acunzo G, Guida M, Pellicano M, Tommaselli GA, Di Spiezio SA, Bifulco G, Cirillo D, Taylor A, Nappi C. Effectiveness of auto-cross-linked hyaluronic acid gel in the prevention of intrauterine adhesions after hysteroscopic adhesiolysis: a prospective, randomized, controlled study. Hum Reprod. 2003;18(9):1918–21.
342. Amer MI, Abd-El-Maeboud KH, Abdelfatah I, Salama FA, Abdallah AS. Human amnion as a temporary biologic barrier after hysteroscopic lysis of severe intrauterine adhesions: pilot study. J Minim Invasive Gynecol. 2010;17(5):605–11.
343. Amer MI, El Nadim A, Hassanein K. The role of intrauterine balloon after operative hysteroscopy in the prevention of intrauterine adhesion: a prospective controlled study. MEFS J. 2005;10:125–9.
344. Amer MI, Abd-El-Maeboud KH. Amnion graft following hysteroscopic lysis of intrauterine adhesions. J Obstet Gynaecol Res. 2006;32:559–66.
345. Baggish MS, Barbot J, Valle RF. Diagnositic and operative hysteroscopy. 2nd ed. St. Louis: Mosby; 1999. p. 277–80.
346. Capella-Allouc S, Morsad F, Rongières-Bertrand C, Taylor S, Fernandez H. Hysteroscopic treatment of severe Asherman's syndrome and subsequent fertility. Hum Reprod. 1999;14(5):1230–3.
347. Chang Y, Zhang Z, Chen Y. Clinical efficacy of severe IUA with transcervical resection and artificial cycle treatment. J Sun Yat-Sen Univ. 2013;1:104–8. Chinese.
348. Cheng J, Xia E, Duan H. Hysteroscopic treatment of tuberculosis caused by severe intrauterine adhesions: an analysis of 14 cases. Chin J Endosc. 2005;2:148–53. Chinese.
349. Coccia ME, Becattini C, Bracco GL, Pampaloni F, Bargelli G, Scarselli G. Pressure lavage under ultrasound guidance: a new approach for outpatient treatment of intrauterine adhesions. Fertil Steril. 2001;75(3):601–6.

350. Colacurci N, Fortunato N, Nasto R, Mele D, Errico G, De Franciscis P, Zarcone R. Outcome riproduttivo dopo sinechiolisi isteroscopica [Reproductive outcome of hysteroscopic lysis of intrauterine adhesions]. Minerva Ginecol. 1997;49(7–8):325–7. Italian.
351. Dawood A, Al-Talib A, Tulandi T. Predisposing factors and treatment outcome of different stages of intrauterine adhesions. J Obstet Gynaecol Can. 2010;32:767–70.
352. Donnez J, Nisolle M. Hysteroscopic lysis of intrauterine adhesions (Asherman's syndrome) an atlas of laser operative laparoscopy and hysteroscopy. New York: Parthenon Publishing; 1994. p. 305–40.
353. Feng ZC, Yang B, Shao J, Liu S. Diagnostic and therapeutic hysteroscopy for traumatic intrauterine adhesions after induced abortions: clinical analysis of 365 cases. Gynaecol Endosc. 1999;8:95–8.
354. Fraser IS, Song JY, Jansen RPS. Hysteroscopic lysis of intrauterine adhesions under ultrasound guidance. Gynaecol Endosc. 1995;4:35.
355. Guida M, Acunzo G, Di Spiezio SA, Bifulco G, Piccoli R, Pellicano M, Cerrota G, Cirillo D, Nappi C. Effectiveness of autocrosslinked hyaluronic acid gel in the prevention of intrauterine adhesions after hysteroscopic surgery: a prospective, randomized, controlled study. Hum Reprod. 2004;19(6):1461–4.
356. Jansen FW, Vredevoogd CB, van Ulzen K, Hermans J, Trimbos JB, Trimbos-Kemper TC. Complications of hysteroscopy: a prospective, multicenter study. Obstet Gynecol. 2000;96(2):266–70.
357. Kresowik JD, Syrop CH, Van Voorhis BJ, Ryan GL. Ultrasound is the optimal choice for guidance in difficult hysteroscopy. Ultrasound Obstet Gynecol. 2012;39(6):715–8.
358. Leung PL, Tam WH, Yuen PM. Hysteroscopic appearance of the endometrial cavity following thermal balloon endometrial ablation. Fertil Steril. 2003;79:1226–8.
359. Lin Y, Li L, Lei L, Hao L, Lei L, Sun W. Study of estradiol valerate for prevention of uterine adhesion after hysteroscopic adhesiolysis. J Chongqing Med Univ. 2011;36:359–61. Chinese.
360. Liu Y, Zhao Y, Jiang D, Xia EL, Liu L, Song D, Zheng J, Peng XB. Effect of high dose estrogen in prognosis of moderate or serious intrauterine adhesion. Shandong Med J. 2012;12:14–6. Chinese.
361. Ma N. A case report on endometrial atypia hyperplasia resulting from repeated application of high dose of estrogen in patients with severe adhesions. Shandong Med J. 2012;12:41–2. Chinese.
362. Mais V, Cirronis MG, Peiretti M, Ferrucci G, Cossu E, Melis GB. Efficacy of auto-crosslinked hyaluronan gel for adhesion prevention in laparoscopy and hysteroscopy: a systematic review and meta-analysis of randomized controlled trials. Eur J Obstet Gynecol Reprod Biol. 2012;160(1):1–5.
363. March CM. Asherman's syndrome. Semin Reprod Med. 2011;29:83–94.
364. Mavrelos D, Ben-Nagi J, Davies A, Lee C, Salim R, Jurkovic D. The value of pre-operative treatment with GnRH analogues in women with submucous fibroids: a double-blind, placebo-controlled randomized trial. Hum Reprod. 2010;25(9):2264–9.
365. Muzii L, Boni T, Bellati F, Marana R, Ruggiero A, Zullo MA, Angioli R, Panici PB. GnRH analogue treatment before hysteroscopic resection of submucous myomas: a prospective, randomized, multicenter study. Fertil Steril. 2010;94(4):1496–9.
366. Myers EM, Hurst BS. Comprehensive management of severe Asherman syndrome and amenorrhea. Fertil Steril. 2012;97:160–4.
367. Nappi L, Di Spiezio SA, Spinelli M, Guida M, Mencaglia L, Greco P, Nappi C, Filippeschi M, Florio P. A multicenter, double-blind, randomized, placebo-controlled study to assess whether antibiotic administration should be recommended during office operative hysteroscopy. Reprod Sci. 2013;20(7):755–61.
368. Newton JR, MacKenzie WE, Emens MJ, Jordan JA. Division of uterine adhesions (Asherman's syndrome) with the Nd-YAG laser. Br J Obstet Gynaecol. 1989;96(1):102–4.
369. Pabuçcu R, Atay V, Orhon E, Urman B, Ergün A. Hysteroscopic treatment of intrauterine adhesions is safe and effective in the restoration of normal menstruation and fertility. Fertil Steril. 1997;68(6):1141–3.
370. Xue-bing P, Enlan X. Safety and efficacy of amnion graft combined with artificial cycle on uterine adhesion. Reprod Contracept. 2012;12:857–61. Chinese.
371. Preutthipan S, Linasmita V. Reproductive outcome following hysteroscopic lysis of intrauterine adhesions: a result of 65 cases at Ramathibodi Hospital. J Med Assoc Thai. 2000;83:42–6.
372. Renier D, Bellato P, Bellini D, Pavesio A, Pressato D, Borrione A. Pharmacokinetic behaviour of ACP gel, an autocrosslinked hyaluronan derivative, after intraperitoneal administration. Biomaterials. 2005;26(26):5368–74.
373. Robinson JK, Colimon LM, Isaacson KB. Postoperative adhesiolysis therapy for intrauterine adhesions (Asherman's syndrome). Fertil Steril. 2008;90:409–14.
374. Roge P, D'Ercole C, Cravello L, Boubli L, Blanc B. Hysteroscopic management of uterine synechiae: a series of 102 observations. Eur J Obstet Gynecol Reprod Biol. 1996;65(2):189–93.
375. Sadrzadeh S, Wamsteker K, Hummel P, Lambalk CB. Secundaire amenorroe door intra-uteriene adhesies: het syndroom van Asherman [Secondary amenorrhea due to intrauterine adhesions: Asherman's syndrome]. Ned Tijdschr Geneeskd. 1998;142(43):2329–32. Dutch.
376. Salat-Baroux J, Pamboo O, Guyot B. Hysteroscopic cure under ultrasonic control of complex and/or recurrent uterine synechaie. Presse Med. 1995;24:811–4.
377. Schenker JG. Etiology of and therapeutic approach to synechia uteri. Eur J Obstet Gynecol Reprod Biol. 1996;65:109–13.
378. Shalev E, Shimoni Y, Peleg D. Ultrasound controlled operative hysteroscopy. J Am Coll Surg. 1994;179:70–1.
379. Taylor PJ, Cumming DC, Hill PJ. Significance of intrauterine adhesions detected hysteroscopically in eumenorrheic infertile women and role of antecedent curettage in their formation. Am J Obstet Gynecol. 1981;139:239–42.
380. Valle RF, Sciarra JJ. Intrauterine adhesions: hysteroscopic diagnosis, classification, treatment, and reproductive outcome. Am J Obstet Gynecol. 1988;158:1459–70.
381. Wamsteker K, Blok SD. Diagnostic hysteroscopy: technique and documentation. In: Sutton C, Diamond MP, editors. Endoscopic surgery for gynecologists. 2nd ed. London: Wb Saunders; 1998. p. 515–6.
382. Xia EL, Duan H, Feng L. Application of B ultrasound and laparoscopic monitoring in hysteroscopic operation. China J Endosc. 1998;4:55–6. Chinese.
383. Xie H. Hysteroscopic lysis of intrauterine adhesions: an analysis of 45 cases. Journal of Practical Obstetrics and Gynecology. 2006;6:353–4. Chinese.
384. Xu Y, Xue F, Wang C. Hysteroscopy in diagnosis and treatment of intrauterine adhesions. China J Endosc. 2005;11:1196–7. Chinese.
385. Yu D, Li TC, Xia E, Huang X, Liu Y, Peng X. Factors affecting reproductive outcome of hysteroscopic adhesiolysis for Asherman's syndrome. Fertil Steril. 2008;89(3):715–22.
386. Yu D, Wong YM, Cheong Y, Xia E, Li TC. Asherman syndrome--one century later. Fertil Steril. 2008;89(4):759–79.
387. Zhang R, Duan H. Applications of amnion graft transplantation in prevention of intrauterine adhesions. Chin J Obstet Gynecol. 2012;47:470–2. Chinese.

Transcervical Removal of Uterine Foreign Body

388. Baggish MS, Barbot J, Valle RF. Diagnositic and operative hysteroscopy. 2nd ed. St. Louis: Mosby; 1999. p. 274–88.
389. Borgatta L, Barad D. Prolonged retention of laminaria fragments: an unusual complication of laminaria usage. Obstet Gynecol. 1991;78:988–90.

390. Cepni I, Kumbak B, Ocal P, Idil M, Aksu F. Infertility due to intrauterine residual fetal bone fragments. J Clin Ultrasound. 2004;32(5):253–5.
391. Cicinelli E, Stanziano A, Parisi C, Marinaccio M, Causio F. Hysteroscopic diagnosis and treatment of endocervical ossification: a case report. J Minim Invasive Gynecol. 2005;12(2):159–61.
392. Cohen SB, Kalter-Ferber A, Weisz BS, Zalel Y, Seidman DS, Mashiach S, Lidor AL, Zolti M, Goldenberg M. Hysteroscopy may be the method of choice for management of residual trophoblastic tissue. J Am Assoc Gynecol Laparosc. 2001;8(2):199–202.
393. Elford K, Claman P. Novel treatment of a patient with secondary infertility due to retained fetal bone. Fertil Steril. 2003;79(4):1028–30.
394. Garcia Leon F, Kably AA. Osseous metaplasia of the endometrium as a cause of infertility. Hysteroscopic approach. Ginecol Obstet Mex. 1999;67:37–41.
395. Goldenberg M, Schiff E, Achiron R, Lipitz S, Mashiach S. Managing residual trophoblastic tissue. Hysteroscopy for directing curettage. J Reprod Med. 1997;42(1):26–8.
396. Graham O, Cheng LC, Parsons JH. The ultrasound diagnosis of retained fetal bones in West African patients complaining of infertility. Br J Obstet Gynecol. 2000;107:122–4.
397. Hu Y, Sun Y, Yang G. Transcervical resection in the treatment of 2 cases of cervical pregnancy. China J Endosc. 1999;5(5):77. Chinese.
398. Letterie GS, Case KJ. Intraoperative ultrasonography guidance for hysteroscopic retrieval of intrauterine foreign bodies. Surg Endosc. 1993;7:182–4.
399. Nevarez Bernal R, Vilchis Nava P, Kably Ambe A. Osificación endometrial: comunicación de cuatro casos y revisión bibliográfica [Endometrial ossification: a report of four cases and literature review]. Ginecol Obstet Mex. 2007;75(3):168–71. Spanish.
400. Puri M, Jain S, Goyal B. Secondary infertility due to retained fetal bones—a diagnostic dilemma. Acta Obstet Gynecol Scand. 2000;79:148.
401. Rodriguez BD, Adamson GD. Hysteroscopic treatment of ectopic intrauterine bone: a case report. J Reprod Med. 1993;38:515–20.
402. Sahinoglu Z, Kuyumcuoglu U. An unusual case of postmenopausal vaginal bleeding: retention bone. Arch Gynecol Obstet. 2003;267(3):160–2.
403. Siegler AM, Kemmann EK. Hysteroscopic removal of occult intrauterine contraceptive device. Obstet Gynecoi. 1975;46:604–6.
404. Szlyk GR, Jarrett TW. Use of rigid hysteroscope for extraction of foreign bodies embedded in lower urinary tract. J Endourol. 1999;13:47–8.
405. Torné A, Jou P, Pagano R, Sanchez I, Ordi J, Vanrell JA. Endometrial ossification successfully treated by hysteroscopic resection. Eur J Obstet Gynecol Reprod Biol. 1996;66(1):75–7.
406. Valle RF, Scjarra JJ, Freeman DW. Hysteroscopic removal of intrauterine devices with missing filaments. Obstet Gynecoi. 1977;49:55–60.
407. Verma U, Chong D, Perez I, Medina C. Fetal bones retained in the uterine cavity as a rare cause of chronic pelvic pain: a case report. J Reprod Med. 2004;49(10):853–5.
408. Wang CJ, Chao AS, Yuen LT, Wang CW, Soong YK, Lee CL. Endoscopic management of cesarean scar pregnancy. Fertil Steril. 2006;85(2):494.e1–4.
409. Xia EL, Duan H, Feng L. Application of B ultrasound and laparoscopic monitoring in hysteroscopic operation. China J Endosc. 1998;4:55–6. Chinese.

Other Hysteroscopic Operations

410. Agboola AJ, Walton SM, Hoffman J. Postmenopausal endometrial tuberculosis. Gynaecol Endosc. 2000;9:209–11.
411. Giana M, Montella F, Surico D, Vigone A, Bozzola C, Ruspa G. Large intramyometrial cystic adenomyosis: a hysteroscopic approach with bipolar resectoscope: case report. Eur J Gynaecol Oncol. 2005;26(4):462–3.
412. Katz Z, Ben-Arie A, Lurie S, Manor M, Insler V. Beneficial effect of hysteroscopic metroplasty on the reproductive outcome in a 'T-shaped' uterus. Gynecol Obstet Invest. 1996;41(1):41–3.
413. Keckstein J. Hysteroscopy and adenomyosis. Contrib Gynecol Obstet. 2000;20:41–50.
414. McCausland AM. Hysteroscopic myometrial biopsy: its use in diagnosing adenomyosis and its clinical application. Am J Obstet Gynecol. 1992;166:1619–26.
415. McCausland V, McCauland A. The response of adenomyosis to endometrial ablation/resection. Hum Reprod Update. 1998;4:350–9.
416. Mercader VP, McGuckin JF Jr, Caroline DF. CT of vesicocorporeal fistula with menouria: a complication of uterine biopsy. J Comput Assist Tomogr. 1995;19:324–6.
417. Neis KJ, Brandner P. Adenomyosis and endometrial ablation. Gynaecol Endosc. 2000;9:141–5.
418. Wood C, Maher P, Hill D. Biopsy diagnosis and conservative surgical treatment of adenomyosis. Aust N Z J Obstet Gynaecol. 1993;33(3):319–21.
419. Wortman M, Daggett A. Hysteroscopic endocervical resection. J Am Assoc Gynecol Laparosc. 1996;4(1):63–8.
420. Zhang H, Liu X, Shen R, Zhang L. Comparison of transcervical resection and loop electrosurgical excision for the treatment of grade I cervical intraepithelial neoplasia. Chin J Minim Invasive Surg. 2008;8(11):1004–6. Chinese.

Other Techniques of Endometrial Ablation

421. Aletebi FA, Vilos GA, Eskandar MA. Effect of intrauterine pressure and duration of thermal balloon ablation. In: Abstract for the global congress of gynecologic endoscopy 28th annual meeting of the American Association of Gynecologic Laparoscopests, Las Vegas; 1999. p. 2.
422. Alperin M, Quaas A, Johnson NR, Hornstein MD. Endometrial ablation in a woman with a persistent uterine hemorrhage due to acute promyelocytic leukemia: a case report. J Reprod Med. 2007;52(6):548–50.
423. Amso NN, Stabinsky SA, McFaul P, Blanc B, Pendley L, Neuwirth R. Uterine thermal balloon therapy for the treatment of menorrhagia: the first 300 patients from a multi-centre study. International Collaborative Uterine Thermal Balloon Working Group. Br J Obstet Gynaecol. 1998;105(5):517–23.
424. Baskett TF, Clough H, Scott TA. NovaSure bipolar radiofrequency endometrial ablation: report of 200 cases. J Obstet Gynaecol Can. 2005;27(5):473–6.
425. Carter JE. Hysteroscopic surgery—avoid the complication of hyponatraemic, encephalopathy. Minim Invas Ther Allied Technol. 1997;6:241–8.
426. Clark TJ, Mahajan D, Sunder P, Gupta JK. Hysteroscopic treatment of symptomatic submucous fibroids using a bipolar intrauterine system: a feasibility study. Eur J Obstet Gynecol Reprod Biol. 2002;100(2):237–42.
427. Cooper J, Gimpelson RJ. Summary of safety and effectiveness data from FDA: a valuable source of information on the performance of global endometrial ablation devices. J Reprod Med. 2004;49(4):267–73.
428. Cooper KG, Bain C, Lawrie L, Parkin DE. A randomised comparison of microwave endometrial ablation with transcervical resection of the endometrium; follow up at a minimum of five years. BJOG. 2005;112(4):470–5.

429. Fernandez H, Capella S, Audibert F. Uterine thermal balloon therapy under local anaesthesia for the treatment of menorrhagia: a pilot study. Eur Soci Human Repro Embry. 1997;12:2511–4.
430. Forin CA, Fulop T, Garza-Leal JG. Long term outcomes of a 3-D bipolar endometrial ablation system. J Am Assoc Gynecol Laparosc. 1999;6:817.
431. Gervaise A, de Tayrac R, Fernandez H. Contraceptive information after endometrial ablation. Fertil Steril. 2005;84(6):1746–7.
432. Gervaise A, Fernandez H, Capella-Allouc S, Taylor S, La Vieille S, Hamou J, Gomel V. Thermal balloon ablation versus endometrial resection for the treatment of abnormal uterine bleeding. Hum Reprod. 1999;14(11):2743–7.
433. Goldrath MH, Barrionuevo M, Husain M. Endometrial ablation for hysteroscopic instillation of hot saline solution. J Am Assoc Gynecol Laparosc. 1997;4:235–40.
434. Goldrath MH. Hysteroscopic endometrial ablation. Obstet Gynecol Clin North Am. 1995;22:559–72.
435. Guillot E, Omnes S, Yazbeck C, Madelenat P, Groupe HTA. Thermodestruction endométriale par la technique HTA (HydroThermAblator): résultats d'une étude multicentrique française [Endometrial ablation using hydrothermablator: results of a French multicenter study]. Gynecol Obstet Fertil. 2008;36(1):45–50. French.
436. Heppard M, Coddington C, Duleba A. Preliminary data from multi-center study using cryogen first option uterine cryoblation therapy in women with abnormal uterine bleeding. Obstet Gynecol. 2000;95:S28.
437. Isaacson K. New developments in operative hysteroscopy. Obstet Gynecol Clin North Am. 2000;27:375–83.
438. Kanaoka Y, Kato M, Tokuyama O, Ishiko O. [A case of complex endometrial hyperplasia with atypia treated by microwave endometrial ablation]. Gan To Kagaku Ryoho. 2005;32(11):1652–3. Japanese.
439. Leung PL, Yuen PM. Postablation-tubal sterilization syndrome following thermal balloon endometrial ablation. Acta Obstet Gynecol Scand. 2006;85(4):504–5.
440. Lissak A, Fruchter O, Mashiach S, Brandes-Klein O, Sharon A, Kogan O, Abramovici H. Immediate versus delayed treatment of perimenopausal bleeding due to benign causes by balloon thermal ablation. J Am Assoc Gynecol Laparosc. 1999;6(2):145–50.
441. Lo JS, Pickersgill A. Pregnancy after endometrial ablation: English literature review and case report. J Minim Invasive Gynecol. 2006;13(2):88–91.
442. Neuwirth RS, Duran AA, Singer A, MacDonald R, Bolduc L. The endometrial ablator: a new instrument. Obstet Gynecol. 1994;83(5 Pt 1):792–6.
443. Pittrof R, Majid S, Murrny A. Initial experience with transcervical cryoablation of endometrium using saline as a uterine distension medium. Minimal Invasive Therapy. 1993;2:69–73.
444. Sabbah R, Desaulniers G. Use of the NovaSure impedance controlled endometrial ablation system in patients with intracavitary disease: 12-month follow-up results of a prospective, single-arm clinical study. J Minim Invasive Gynecol. 2006;13(5):467–71.
445. Sharp NC, Cronin N, Feldberg I, Evans M, Hodgson D, Ellis S. Microwaves for menorrhagia: a new fast technique for endometrial ablation. Lancet. 1995;346(8981):1003–4.
446. Shi Y, Feng Z, Xu L. Thermal balloon used in endometrial ablation for menorrhagia. Chin J Obstet Gynecol. 1999;34:49.
447. Singer A, Almanza R, Gutierrez A, Haber G, Bolduc LR, Neuwirth R. Preliminary clinical experience with a thermal balloon endometrial ablation method to treat menorrhagia. Obstet Gynecol. 1994;83(5 Pt 1):732–4.
448. Soderstrom RM, Brooks PG, Corson SL, Dequesne J, Gallinat A, Garza-Leal JG, Iglesias-Benavides JL, Indman PD, Liu J, van der Pas H, Stern RA, Sutton C, Vancaillie TG, Wamsteker K. Endometrial ablation using a distensible multielectrode balloon. J Am Assoc Gynecol Laparosc. 1996;3(3):403–7.
449. Tawfeek S, Sholapurkar S, Sharp N. Incidence of upper genital tract occlusion following microwave endometrial ablation. BJOG. 2006;113(8):958–60.
450. Thijssen RFA, Rolland R. Radiofrequency endometrial ablation and GnRHa pretreatment. Gynaecol Endosc. 1995;4:49–52.
451. Vilos GA, Fortin CA, Sanders B, Pendley L, Stabinsky SA. Clinical trial of the uterine thermal balloon for treatment of menorrhagia. J Am Assoc Gynecol Laparosc. 1997;4(5):559–65.
452. Vilos GA, Thomas B. A new bipolar system for performing operative hysteroscopy in normal saline. J Am Assoc Gynecol Laparosc. 1999;6(3):331–6.
453. Vilos GA, Vilos EC, Pendley L. Endometrial ablation with a thermal balloon for the treatment of menorrhagia. J Am Assoc Gynecol Laparosc. 1996;3:383–7.
454. Vilos GA. Global endometrial ablation. J Soc Obstet Gynaecol Can. 2000;22:668–75.
455. Vilos GA. Intrauterine surgery using a new coaxial bipolar electrode in normal saline solution (Versapoint): a pilot study. Fertil Steril. 1999;72(4):740–3.
456. Yu S. An efficacy analysis of uterine thermal balloon in the treatment of dysfunctional uterine bleeding. J Wenzhou Med Coll. 1999;29:77–8. Chinese.
457. Zheng J, Xia EL, Feng LM. Thermal balloon in the treatment of menorrhagia complicated by severe internal medical diseases: a report of 4 cases. Chin J Pract Gynecol Obstet. 2000;16:443–4. Chinese.
458. Zurawin RK, Pramanik S. Endometrial balloon ablation as a therapy for intractable uterine bleeding in an adolescent. J Pediatr Adolesc Gynecol. 2001;14(3):119–21.

10 Combined Hysteroscopy and Laparoscopy

Enlan Xia

With the development and improvement of the endoscopic techniques and surgical instruments, the minimally invasive technique has also gained popularity in the gynecological field, and more and more gynecological patients can be treated with minimally invasive techniques. Compared with open surgery, endoscopic surgery has advantages of minimum trauma, less bleeding, less interference with organs, slight postoperative pain or discomfort, and quick recovery. At present, gynecological laparoscopic techniques have been widely used in China, and the treatment of pelvic benign lesions by laparoscopy has shown a tendency to replace the traditional open surgery. Although the development of hysteroscopy comes relatively late, it has been developed very rapidly, and surgical indications have been continuously extended. Moreover, the surgical procedures have been shifted from a simple diagnosis and treatment to complex surgical procedures, such as hysteroscopic resection of large sessile submucosal myomas and inward-protruding intramural myomas; complex surgery of metroplasty, like correction of uterine septum and lysis of severe intrauterine adhesions; hysteroscopic tubal cannulation; and gamete intra-fallopian transplantation transfer. Nevertheless, clinically there are still many intrauterine, intra-abdominal, and intrapelvic disorders requiring urgent concomitant diagnosis and treatment, such as evaluation and treatment of tubal and uterine factors in cases of infertility, concomitant surgery for intrauterine and intra-abdominal lesions, and the monitoring of difficult intrauterine operations. Therefore, combined hysteroscopy and laparoscopy will become a more effective method for clinical diagnosis and treatment.

Combined hysteroscopic and laparoscopic surgery is the simultaneous treatment of more than two kinds of intra-abdominal and intrauterine diseases under a single anesthesia. There have been such reports since 1990s. Compared with a single type of endoscopic therapy, the joint surgery has achieved complementation of their respective advantages of the two minimally invasive surgeries, allowing patients to undergo one operation with one anesthesia, which integrates diagnosis and treatment as a whole and solves the previous problems of inability to simultaneous diagnosis and treat intrauterine and intra-abdominal lesions in a single setting. The dynamic combination of the two procedures will produce positive clinical effects on the correct diagnosis of gynecological diseases and the efficacy of surgical treatment. In 2006, Kaminski et al. reported 724 endoscopic procedures on 636 patients aged 20–41 years old, including 88 cases of combined hysteroscopy and laparoscopy, 476 cases of only laparoscopy, and 72 cases of only hysteroscopy. Compared with women with secondary infertility, women with primary infertility more often had tubal patency, intrauterine malformations, and no visible findings (30%) in pelvis. The remaining 70% of women with primary infertility mostly had polycystic ovarian syndrome and endometriosis. The peritubal adhesions, tubal blockage, and submucosal myomas were more common in the group of secondary infertility than that in the group of primary infertility. All the detected pathologies above were treated. They concluded that laparoscopy and hysteroscopy played an important role in diagnosis and treatment of infertility.

10.1 Indications for Combined Hysteroscopy and Laparoscopy

1. Diagnosis and treatment of infertility;
2. Etiological examination and treatment of chronic pelvic pain;
3. Monitoring of complex hysteroscopic surgery;
4. Endoscopic metroplasty for complete bicornuate uterus;
5. Uterine artery occlusion conducted for hysteroscopic treatment of intrauterine lesions with high risk of bleeding;
6. Diagnosis and treatment of space-occupying lesions in both uterine and pelvic cavities.

E. Xia (✉)
Hysteroscopy Center, Fuxing Hospital, Capital Medical University, Beijing, China

E. Xia (ed.), *Practical Manual of Hysteroscopy*, https://doi.org/10.1007/978-981-19-1332-7_10

10.2 Contraindications for Combined Hysteroscopy and Laparoscopy

Its contraindications include those for hysteroscopy and those for laparoscopy.

10.3 Operative Procedures of Combined Hysteroscopy and Laparoscopy

10.3.1 Step 1: The Joint Examination of Hysteroscopy and Laparoscopy

Disinfect the abdominal skin, perineum, and vagina regularly, place surgical drape sheets under the hips, spread aseptic sleeves over legs, place four surgical towels in diamond shape around the operational field over abdomen and secure them with towel clips, cover the abdomen with large surgical drape, and expose the operational field of abdomen and perineum only. Insert a catheter and empty the bladder. Incise longitudinally the skin below the umbilicus for approximately 1.0 cm to the subcutaneous tissue. After successful puncture of Veress needle, inject CO_2 into the abdominal cavity and when the intra-abdominal pressure is up to 15 mmHg, pull out the Veress needle and introduce a 5 or 10 mm trocar and then a laparoscope. After placement of a uterine manipulator via perineum to lift the uterus, the size and the shape of the uterus, the appearance of ovaries and fallopian tubes on both sides, and other lesions in pelvic cavity are detected laparoscopically. If the exposure of pelvic organ is not sufficient, add a 5 mm trocar in the left or the right lower quadrant of abdomen, insert toothless grasper or retractor to spread the rectum or divide adhesive tissues, thus the pelvic lesions are clarified. At the same time, insert the vaginal speculum, hold and pull the cervix outward with cervical forceps. Under direct vision of laparoscope, dilate the cervix to Hegar 10–12. Choose 5% glucose solution as the distention medium for monopolar surgery (diabetic patients can choose 5% mannitol as distention medium) and 0.9% saline for bipolar surgery, set the distention pressure at 100 mmHg and flow rate at 240–260 mL/min. Insert the hysteroscope and observe the endometrial thickness and intrauterine lesions in sequence from the cervical canal, the fundus, both fallopian tubal ostia, to anterior/posterior and left/right uterine walls. And then, make a contrast with the findings by laparoscopy and determine the treatment protocols (Fig. 10.1a, b).

10.3.2 Step 2: Hysteroscopic Surgery Under Laparoscopic Monitoring

Assemble the hysteroscopic resectoscope, adjust the light source, set the output power at 80–100 W for cutting and 40–60 W for coagulation of the monopolar electrode, and at 300–310 W for cutting and 90–100 W for coagulation of the bipolar electrode, connect and switch on the irrigating systems, and start intrauterine operation under laparoscopic surveillance.

10.3.2.1 Endometrial Resection

The wire loop electrode is used to resect the endometrium, including the functional layer, basal layer and its underlying 2–3 mm of myometrial tissues. In case of active uterine

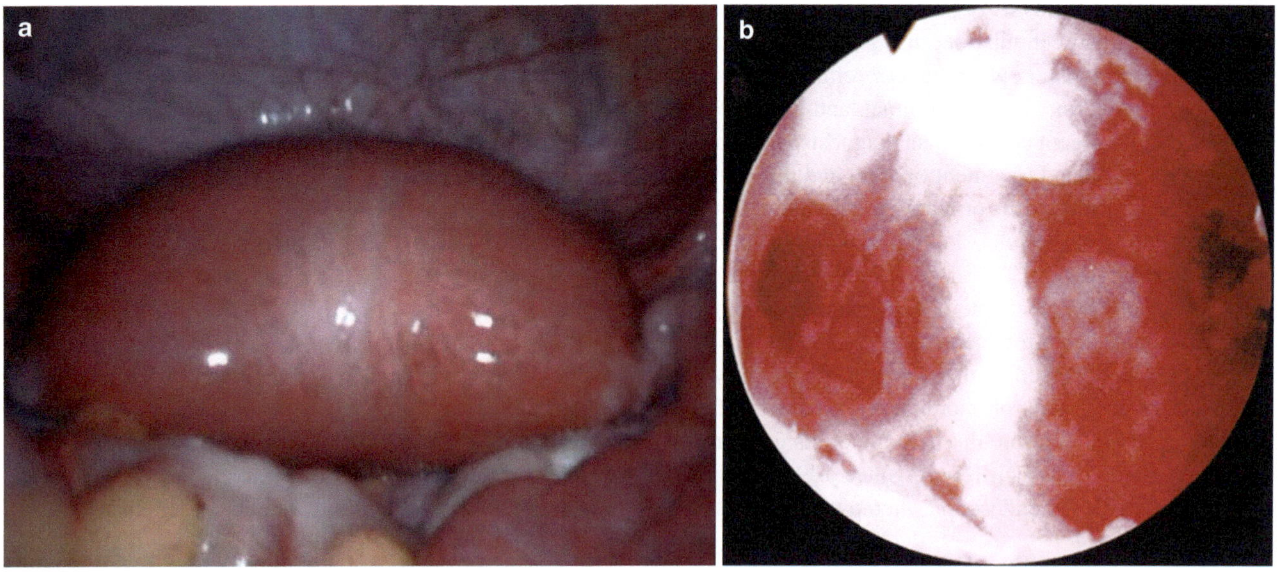

Fig. 10.1 Combined examination of a septate uterus. (**a**) The fundus is transversely broad with slight indentation in the middle under laparoscope. (**b**) Intrauterine partial septum under hysteroscope

bleeding, a rollerball electrode may be used for coagulation hemostasis. As for the adenomyosis tissues detected during the operation, a rollerball electrode or a roller barrel electrode can also be used to destroy the ectopic endometrium in superficial myometrium.

10.3.2.2 Resection of Broad-Based Sessile Submucosal Myomas and Inward-Protruding Intramural Myomas

The sessile submucosal myomas or the inward-protruding intramural myomas all have a broad base in the muscle wall. It should be noted that in the cutting process the border between the myoma and its capsule must be identified and the wire loop could not be used to dig into the uterine muscular wall. The cutting should stop when reaching the myometrial layer. The application of oxytocin can make the uterine wall contraction and squeeze the tumor from myometrium to the uterine cavity. Most of the myoma can be excised with a small amount of myoma tissues remaining in the myometrium, which can develop necrosis and dissolution afterwards. Over-resection of the myoma tissues imbedded in myometrium will cause intraoperative heavy bleeding and uterine perforation. If the remaining myoma tissues in the uterine muscular wall grow and protrude again into the uterine cavity, a second or third hysteroscopic surgery may be needed.

10.3.2.3 Surgical Correction of Uterine Septum

The surgical correction of uterine septum under hysteroscope should start with transverse cutting from the lowest point of septum and left-right alternately till the basal part of the septum (Fig. 10.2a, b). Note that the symmetry of the operation is extremely important during surgery. The closer to the uterine fundus, the more attention should be paid not to damage the uterine myometrial tissues. On the one hand, the uterine tubal ostia may serve as differential markers; on the other hand, with the intervention of laparoscopy, a close monitoring of the uterine fundus should be performed so as to avoid uterine perforation (Fig. 10.3). When hysteroscopic operation reaches the uterine fundus, the operation should be suspended immediately if the small arterial bleeding is visible, which indicates the resection had gone deep into the myometrium. After the septate tissues are completely resected, reduce the uterine distention pressure appropriately, examine the uterine fundus carefully, coagulate any active bleeding areas for hemostasis, and apply balloon tamponade when necessary.

10.3.2.4 Lysis of Severe Intrauterine Adhesions

Operators should be very careful when operating on extensive adhesions with fibromuscular and connective tissues, especially with the high frequency electricity or laser as energy source in surgery. When the surgery is performed to restore a normal uterine cavity, the operator should try their best not to destroy the normal endometrium and submucous myometrial layer. When adhesions approach the uterine cornua, try to avoid deeper resection and damage to the uterine wall so as not to cause perforation. The operation should be

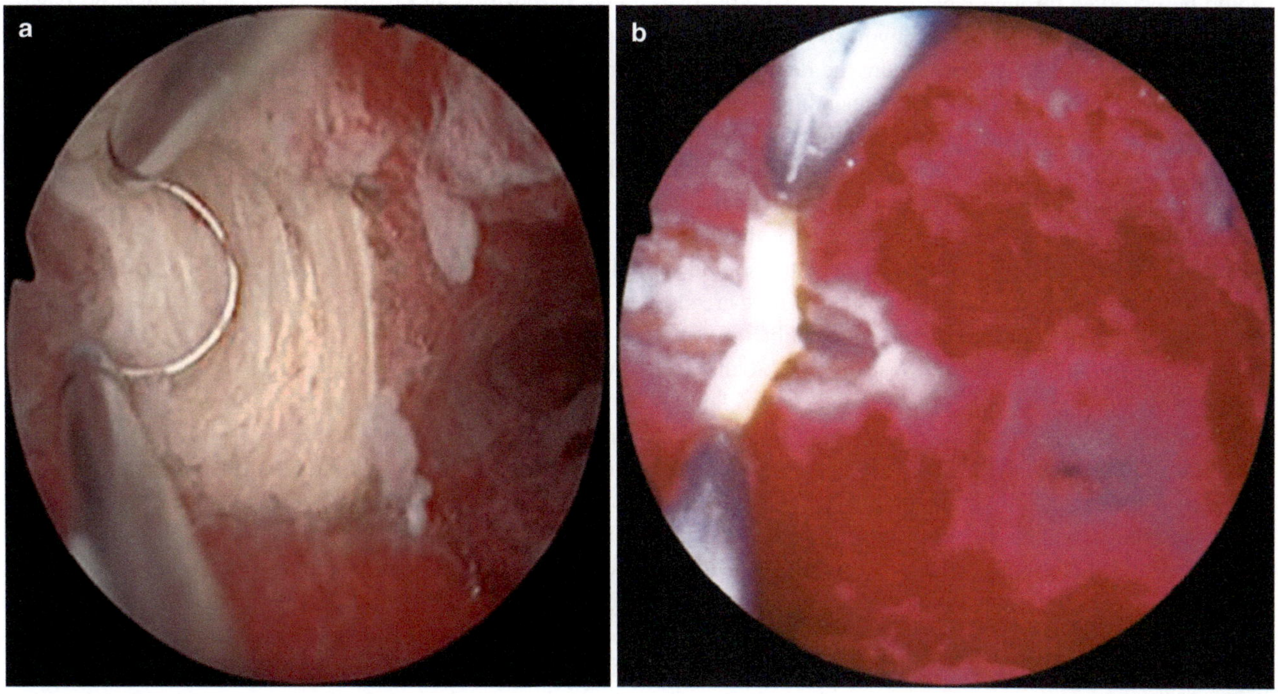

Fig. 10.2 (a) Resection of the septum by hysteroscopic wire loop electrode. (b) Division of the septum by hysteroscopic needle electrode

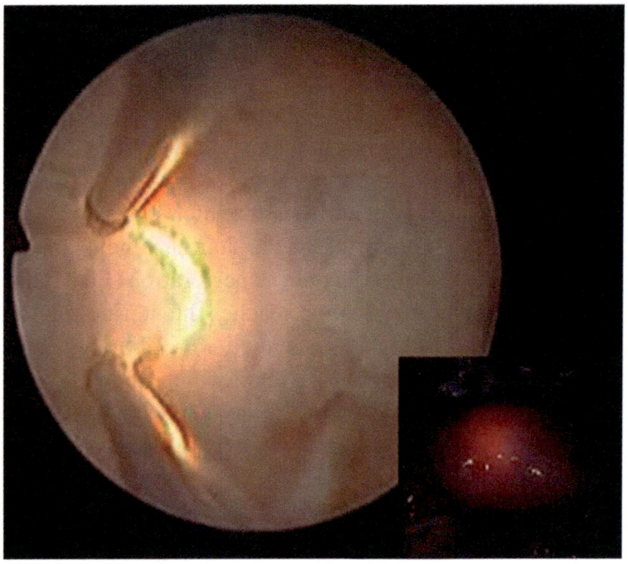

Fig. 10.3 Hysteroscopic resection of uterine septum under laparoscopic monitoring. The hysteroscopic resection reaches the fundus and the light transmittance of the fundal wall is monitored laparoscopically (picture in picture)

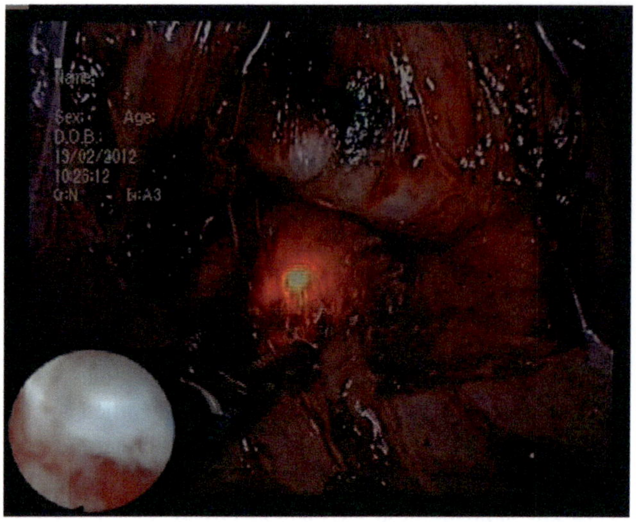

Fig. 10.4 Laparoscopic neoplasty combined with hysteroscopy for cesarean scar diverticulum. After dividing the adhesions at lower section of the uterus under laparoscopy, hysteroscope is placed approaching the site of diverticulum (picture in picture), then the location of the diverticulum and the light transmittance of the diverticulum wall are identified laparoscopically

done under ultrasonography monitoring or laparoscopic surveillance, and the division should not deviate from the midline of uterine cavity. At the end of the surgery, the objective lens should be retracted to the internal os to observe the symmetry of the uterine cavity.

As for the complex intrauterine operations, at the time of hysteroscopic surgery, the focal changes on uterine serosa should be observed through laparoscope. If there are small blisters, local pale changes, or ecchymosis, these indicate that the active electrode is approaching the deeper parts of uterine wall and that perforation is impending, hence the operation must be stopped. During monitoring, the light source for laparoscope may be adjusted dim to observe the uterus, if bright light from the uterine cavity is visible on any site of the uterine surface, this indicates that the part of the uterine wall is unduly thin and the operator should be alerted to terminate the operation on this site. There are also scholars advocating using intra-abdominal light transmission test and intrauterine reversal test on the thickness of uterine wall during hysteroscopic surgery under laparoscopic monitoring. The intra-abdominal light transmission test is carried out as mentioned above. Regarding intrauterine reversal test, the laparoscope is placed close to the serosa of uterine fundus, and the light of hysteroscope is adjusted dim or closed. If light from the laparoscope is visible inside the uterine cavity, the operation on the translucent region should be stopped. This approach not only can suggest to the operator the thickness of remaining uterine wall, but also may help the operator to learn more about the insufficiently resected parts.

10.3.3 Step 3: Laparoscopic Surgery and Hysteroscopic Surveillance

Some laparoscopic surgery needs hysteroscopic surveillance and positioning. For example, in cases of cesarean scar diverticulum, hysteroscopic examination can be conducted before laparoscopy to observe its location and extent, indicate its position and borders, and then followed by laparoscopic neoplasty. During the operation, both light transmission test and reverse test should be applied by observing the light transmittance of diverticulum wall under laparoscopy or hysteroscopy to determine its location (Fig. 10.4).

10.3.4 Step 4: Laparoscopic Exploration and Surgery

After the hysteroscopic operation is accomplished, the hysteroscopic resectoscope is removed. The uterus is lifted again and the pelvic cavity is investigated laparoscopically to see whether there is blister, hematoma, and breach of the uterine serosal surface, and pale trace of tissue denaturation induced by the electrocoagulation, and whether there is hematocele in the lumen of fallopian tubes and blood or fluid in the pelvic cavity. If uterine perforation or active bleeding is detected, electrocoagulation or suture for hemostasis is done under laparoscope. As to the other lesions in the pelvic cavity, if such operations are required like the tubal patency test with methy-

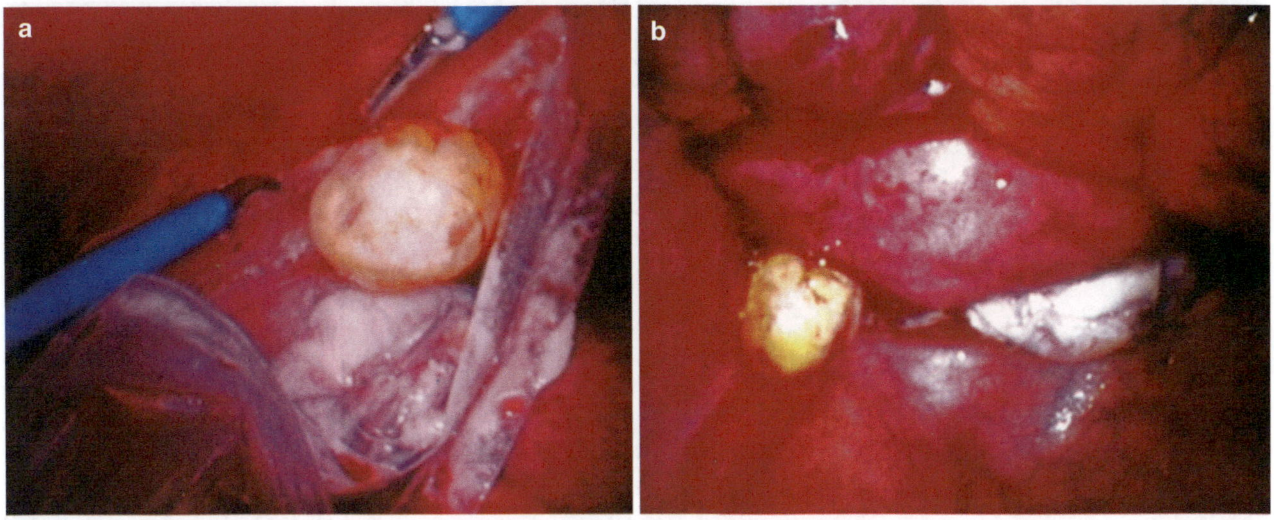

Fig. 10.5 Ovarian teratoma. (**a**) Left ovarian teratoma under laparoscope. (**b**) Laparoscopic removal of ovarian teratoma

lene blue dye, ovarian cyst removal, surgeries for pelvic endometriosis and lysis of pelvic adhesions, proper auxiliary trocars may be added in the lower quadrant of abdomen and the corresponding laparoscopic operation is performed (Fig. 10.5a, b).

10.4 Application of Combined Hysteroscopy and Laparoscopy

10.4.1 Diagnosis and Treatment of Infertility

There are complex factors for female infertility, including tubal factors, uterine and cervical factors, endocrine factors, immune factors, and other factors of unknown origin. Among the factors relating to fallopian tubes, uterus and cervix for infertility, the common factors include tubal atresia, distortion, or adhesion; uterine and cervical myomas; endometrial polyps; endometrial hyperplasia; intrauterine foreign body residues (especially retained fetal bones); intrauterine adhesions and uterine malformation. Nowadays, the combined hysteroscopy and laparoscopy is the optimal means to diagnose and evaluate infertility factors in the uterine cavity, fallopian tubes, and pelvic cavity (Fig. 10.6a, b). Hysteroscopy, characterized by its intuitiveness and accuracy, can be performed to resect the uterine space-occupying lesions, divide intrauterine adhesions, and correct the uterine malformations, thus helping patients to restore normal menstrual cycle and improve pregnancy and delivery outcomes. Therefore, hysteroscopic surgery has become a standard method for treatment of uterine lesions. Laparoscopy combined with hysteroscopy can be performed to diagnose infertility factors inside and outside the uterine cavity.

10.4.1.1 Combined Hysteroscopy and Laparoscopy in Diagnosis and Treatment of Uterine Malformations

A combined examination for uterine malformations was made in 82 cases in the Hysteroscopy Center of Fuxing Hospital, Capital Medical University, from January 1995 to September 2002. Laparoscopy was performed to observe the fundus of the uterus and the diagnosis of septate uterus confirmed in 75 cases, of which incomplete septate uterus was present in 71 cases and complete septate uterus in four cases after hysteroscopic diagnosis. By laparoscopy, four cases were found to have bicornuate uterus, including two complete bicornuate uteri and two incomplete bicornuate uteri confirmed under hysteroscopy. By laparoscopy two cases were diagnosed to have unicornuate uterus with rudimentary horns, which was diagnosed unicornuate uterus by hysteroscopy (Table 10.1).

The treatment of uterine malformations is seen in Sect. 9.5 of Chap. 9. In 2002, Adolph and Gilliland reported that a woman who was found to have a rudimentary horn pregnancy underwent laparoscopic surgery. She conceived later and delivered a live birth infant 15 months after the surgery. They pointed out that the laparoscopic surgery had less operating time, hospitalization, and postoperative adhesions and was thus an optimal option for removal of rudimentary horn. In our study, two cases of rudimentary horns did not undergo removal surgery due to severe bilateral tubal obliteration.

Martinez et al. conducted combined surgeries of laparoscopy and hysteroscopy on 40 patients with Müllerian anomalies and infertility. The results included uterine septum in 23 patients (57.5%), bicornuate uterus in 6 (15%), didelphic uterus in 5 (12.5%), arcuate uterus in 4 (10%), and unicornuate uterus in 2 (5%). Among 23 patients with uterine septum

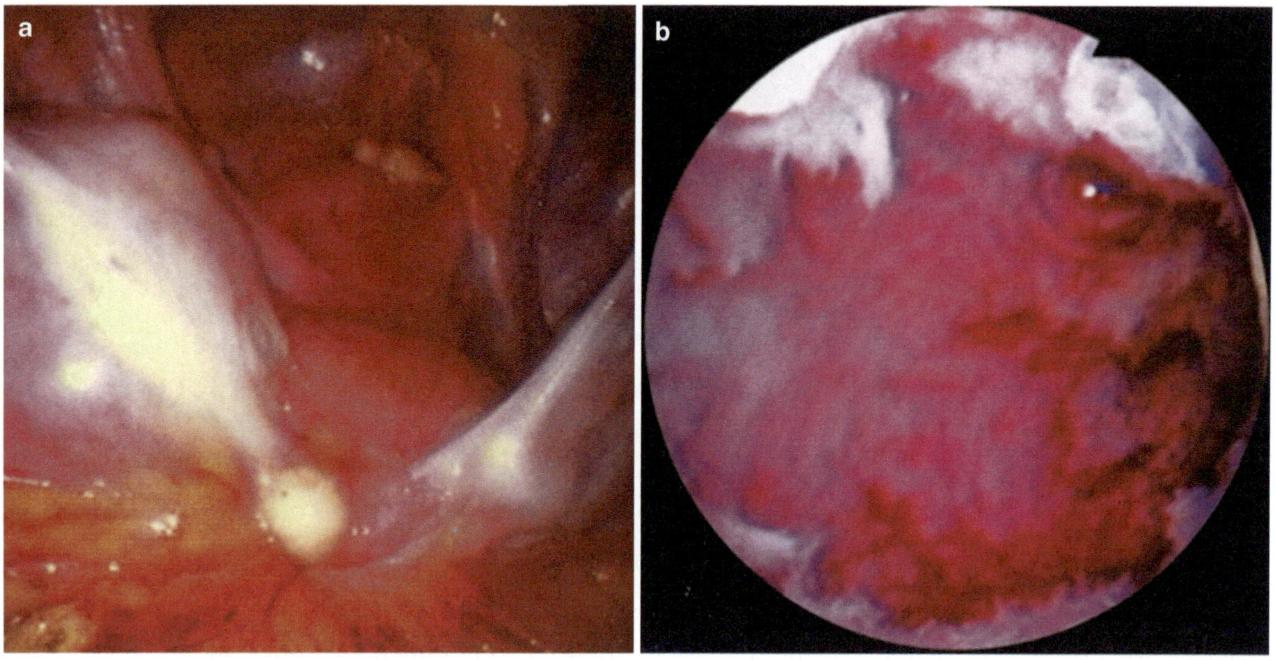

Fig. 10.6 The combined hysteroscopy and laparoscopy. (a) Laparoscopic view of pelvic tuberculosis, with calcification visible. (b) Intrauterine adhesions under hysteroscope

Table 10.1 Combined hysteroscopy and laparoscopy for diagnosis of uterine malformations (no. of cases)

Type of malformations		Hysteroscopic diagnosis	Laparoscopic diagnosis	Joint diagnosis
Didelphic uterus		0	–	1[a]
Bicornuate uterus	Complete bicornuate uterus	–	–	2[a]
	Incomplete bicornuate uterus	–	–	2
Septate uterus	Complete septum	5[b]	–	4
	Incomplete septum	75[c]	–	71
Unicornuate uterus		2	0	0
Unicornuate uterus with rudimentary horns		0	2	2[a]
Total		82	2	82

Notes: – indicates suspicious
[a] Indicates no surgery
[b] Indicates one case of didelphic uterus after combined diagnosis
[c] Indicates complete bicornuate uterus present in two cases and incomplete bicornuate uterus in two cases among 4 patients after combined diagnosis

undergoing TCRS, 13 pregnancies were achieved (56.5%), including two miscarriages, four term deliveries, and seven continued pregnancies with one twin pregnancy. Pregnancies were achieved in two cases after metroplasty in four cases with bicornuate uterus. Of the arcuate uterus, the tissue protruding into uterine cavity was removed. Of the unicornuate uterus, one miscarriage and one term pregnancy were obtained following hysteroscopic surgery. It was thought that the combined endoscopic procedures can not only precisely diagnose the uterine malformations, but also is the best method for improving fertility for women with uterine malformations.

10.4.1.2 Diagnosis and Treatment of Tubal Infertility

Findings of hysterosalpingography performed in infertile patients showed that 10–20% of patients had proximal tubal obstruction, of which 20–30% may be induced by physiological spasm. Presently, it is believed that unblocking the fallopian tubes and treating other pelvic lesions laparoscopically under direct vision is the most effective treatment method. Previously, after laparoscopic diagnosis of proximal tubal occlusion, the treatment was the microsurgical removal of the obliterated part and the tubal anastomosis for reconstruction. However, by observation of the excised diseased portion of fallopian tubes, the findings show that the degree of tubal fibrosis or degree of occlusion is not completely in accordance with the patients' clinical manifestations. Sulak et al. report that the tubal occlusion is caused by the retention of the tissue debris or protein-like substances in most cases, and hysteroscopic cannulation to unblock the tubes is the preferred method of treatment. Under laparoscopic surveillance, the hysteroscopic cannulation can not only relieve the tubal spasm, but also introduce the cannula directly into the interstitial section and accurately into the tubal lumen. Fallopian tube cannulation by combined hysteroscopy and laparoscopy is helpful in understanding the shape of the fallopian tube, evaluating the tubal patency, and also simultaneously diagnosing and treating other pelvic diseases, such as pelvic adhesions, endometriosis and the minimal changes at the fimbrial end of the fallopian tube (Fig. 10.7a–c).

With the improvement of equipment and technique, the curative effect of tubal cannulation is also improved. It was reported that after treatment of tubal cannulation by combined hysteroscopy and laparoscopy, the patency rate was 70–92%. At a 12-month postoperative follow-up, the intrauterine pregnancy rate was 47%, and the ectopic pregnancy rate was 8%. Guo et al. from the Hysteroscopy Center of Fuxing Hospital, Capital Medical University, carried out a retrospective study of laparoscopic diagnosis and treatment on detecting pelvic factors of infertility and its influences on fertility in 324 infertile women from June 2006 to June 2009. The results showed that tubal disease and/or pelvic adhesion were the most common reasons which account for 53.06% (156/294); endometriosis was the second common reason with a proportion of 16.66% (49/294). For postoperative follow-up, 30 women were lost (9.25%) and 294 women succeeded (90.75%). The conception rate following laparoscopy was 41.38% (123/294), including 57 pregnancies achieved in 156 women with initial infertility caused by tubal diseases and/or pelvic adhesions (36.53%), 24 pregnancies in 49 women with initial infertility caused by endometriosis (48.97%), 17 in 29 women with PCOS (58.65%), and 13 in 23 women with uterine myomas (56.52%). One woman got pregnant by IVF after anti-tuberculosis therapy following definite diagnosis by laparoscopic biopsy. One pregnancy was obtained among 7 women following laparoscopic cystectomy. The conception rate was 50% in infertile women

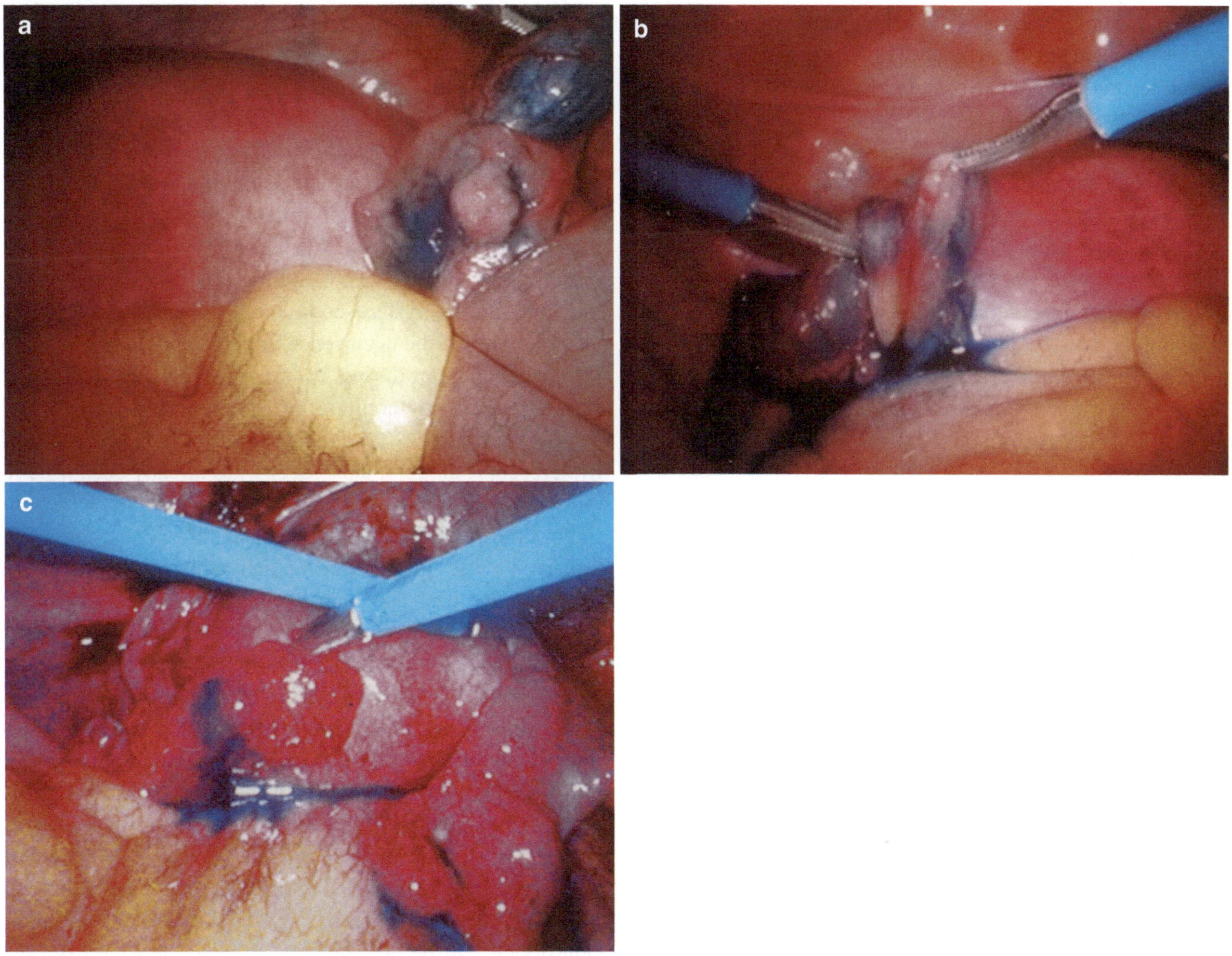

Fig. 10.7 Laparoscopic dye test. (**a**) Laparoscopic view of outflow of methylene blue dye from the right tubal fimbria. (**b**) Laparoscopic view of outflow of methylene blue dye from the left tubal fimbria. (**c**) Laparoscopic view of outflow of methylene blue dye from bilateral tubal fimbria, indicating bilateral tubal patency

with unknown reason following laparoscopic bilateral tubal patency test (10/20). They held that laparoscopic examination can directly identify pelvic lesions and perform surgeries for treatment, and the application of laparoscopic technique had a significant value for diagnosis and treatment of infertility.

10.4.2 Etiological Diagnosis and Treatment of Chronic Pelvic Pain

Chronic pelvic pain is one of the common gynecological symptoms and also a disease more difficult to diagnose clinically. This disease is mostly caused by gynecological disorders or other factors such as genital tract infection, uterine myomas, endometrial polyps, endometriosis, ovarian tumors, reproductive tract abnormalities, cervical lesions, pelvic congestion syndrome, past history of pelvic surgery, and IUD. Due to more complex causes of chronic pelvic pain, it is not easy to make diagnosis and the treatment will be delayed if only traditional gynecological examination or imaging diagnosis is applied. Hysteroscopic and laparoscopic techniques are particularly advantageous in the diagnosis of the intrauterine and pelvic lesions due to its intuitiveness and capacity of amplification (Fig. 10.8). Nezhat et al. studied the causes of chronic pelvic pain in 547 patients. Among them, 48 patients who had previous hysterectomies were excluded, and hysteroscopy combined with laparoscopy were performed in the remaining cases. The results showed that, among 191 women who were diagnosed as endometriosis by laparoscopy, 62 women (32.5%) were found to have intrauterine abnormalities by hysteroscopy; among 105 women diagnosed as single or multiple uterine myomas under laparoscopy, 46 women (43.8%) were found to have intrauterine lesions by hysteroscopy; among 11 women diagnosed as ovarian cyst by laparoscopy, 4 women (40%) were found to have intracervical stenosis by hysteroscopy. Among 118 women with the diagnosis of pelvic adhesions and 96 women with the diagnosis of both endometriosis and pelvic adhesions by laparoscopy, intrauterine disorders were found by hysteroscopy in 24 cases (27%) and 26 cases (28.0%), respectively. In eight cases without abnormal findings by laparoscopy, normal uterine cavity was found in 2 by hysteroscopy. It was concluded that hysteroscopy could provide intrauterine information in diagnosis of chronic pelvic pain. Therefore, laparoscopy combined with hysteroscopy in diagnosis and treatment of chronic pelvic pain was an effective method in improving the postoperative outcome.

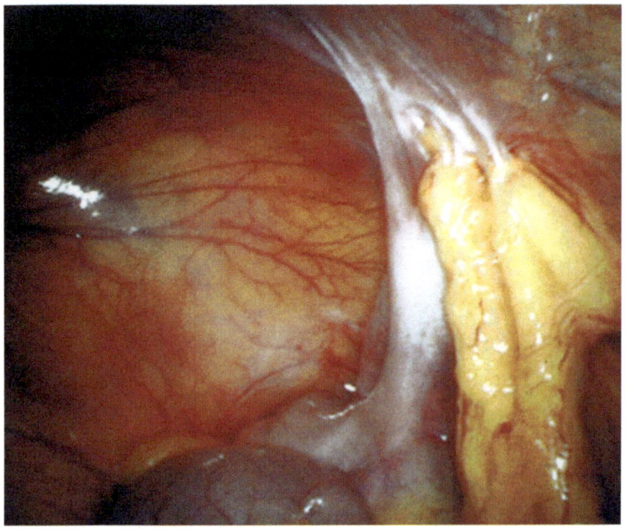

Fig. 10.8 Laparoscopic view of adhesions to the lateral pelvic wall

10.4.3 Monitoring Complicated Hysteroscopic Surgery

Due to the particular structure of the uterus, the strong regenerative ability of endometrium, the limited thickness of the uterine wall, the rich intramural blood supply and other factors, hysteroscopic surgery is very difficult to perform, especially procedures of reconstructive and restorative surgeries of uterine cavity, such as lysis of severe intrauterine adhesions, correction of the uterine septum, and removal of sessile and inward-protruding intramural myomas. It is difficult to avoid uterine perforation during surgery. Loffer and Lewis reported cases with severe bleeding caused by perforation of the uterus during hysteroscopic surgery. Pittrof and Wortman also reported on the occurrence of perforation and trauma to intestine and ureter during hysteroscopic surgery. Therefore, it is necessary to monitor the hysteroscopic surgery and avoid occurrence of complications. At the initial stage of hysteroscopic surgery, laparoscopy has already been used in monitoring hysteroscopic surgery. In recent years, with continuous development and improvement of laparoscopic techniques, its use in monitoring and adjuvant treatment in hysteroscopy has also been well enhanced. Laparoscopic monitoring can be performed to observe directly the changes in the uterine serosal surface. During the process of cutting and coagulating with the active electrode of the hysteroscope, once there is deep cutting or coagulation of the myometrial tissues and imminent uterine perforation, due to heat conduction in local tissues, blisters may occur in uterine serosal surface, or the transmitted light from hysteroscope is visible under laparoscope. At this moment, the operator should be alerted to suspend the hysteroscopic operations. At the same time, under laparoscopy, the intestine or other adjacent organs can be pushed aside to avoid damage from the hysteroscopic active electrode and its thermal conductivity. Compared with the ultrasonography monitoring, laparoscopic monitoring cannot predict the uterine perforation, but can diagnose timely uterine perforation and detect any damage to other organs in pelvic cavity caused by perforation and can be used to repair the perforated organs in time. These advantages are superior to other methods of surveillance.

In the Hysteroscopy Center of Fuxing Hospital, Capital Medical University, 165 cases underwent complex intrauterine operations under laparoscopic monitoring, which included 29 cases of TCRA due to intrauterine adhesions involving more than 1/3 of the uterine cavity or muscular adhesions in both cornua; 52 cases of TCRS; 16 cases of TCRF with the fetal bone residues and IUD fragments embedded in the uterine wall removed; 68 cases of TCRM with multiple or >4.5 cm submucosal myomas resected. During the surgery, incomplete uterine perforations occurred in six cases and uterine perforations in three cases. The incomplete uterine perforations occurred in four cases of TCRM (three cases of myomas greater than 4.5 cm in diameter, one case of multiple submucous and inward-protruding intramural myomas), one case of TCRA, and one case of TCRS, in which the uterine serosal surface appeared to be locally pale white with blister and ecchymosis under laparoscope. Uterine perforation occurred in two cases of TCRA and one case of TCRM, in which a break in the uterine serosal surface was visible under laparoscope, and active bleeding as well. Of two cases of TCRA, one case had uterine perforation in the anterior uterine wall with the diameter about 0.6 cm accompanied with active bleeding, and laparoscopic electrocoagulation was performed for hemostasis immediately. The other case had perforation in the lower segment of posterior uterine wall measuring about 1.5 cm and laparoscopic suturing was done to stop bleeding. The above uterine perforations occurred during the resection of larger submucosal myomas, lysis of severe intrauterine adhesions, and opening occluded uterine cavities. The severely damaged endometrium and deformed uterine cavity, as well as the lost direction of uterine axis, coupled with electrosurgical procedures, all contributed to the active electrode to penetrate the uterine wall, causing perforation. Direct visualization of the changes in the uterine serosal surface under laparoscope solves the problem that ultrasonography monitoring can only suggest but not manage the uterine perforation. At the same time, the intestine or other adjacent organs may be pushed aside under laparoscopy to avoid damage from the hysteroscopic active electrode and its thermal conductivity. The six cases of incomplete uterine perforations mentioned above are all detected by laparoscopy and the hysteroscopic operations were timely terminated, thus avoiding the occurrence of serious complications. Those three cases of uterine perforation are also treated timely by laparoscopy, which eliminate the laparotomy, thus reducing the risk of hysteroscopic complications to a minimum.

The implementation of laparoscopic monitoring in the highly difficult intrauterine surgical procedures can not only detect timely and manage the uterine perforation so as to avoid the occurrence of serious complications, which is of clinical significance. Moreover, it can also diagnose and treat the patients with concomitant pelvic lesions, which avoids the trouble of rehospitalization for another operation, thus reducing the patients' pains and economic burden.

10.4.4 Metroplasty for Complete Bicornuate Uterus

Under laparoscopic monitoring, hysteroscopic wire loop electrode or needle electrode is used to incise transversely on the intrauterine plate and the fundus of bicornuate uterus, causing artificial perforation. Then extend the incision to bilateral uterine cornua, and the full layer of the uterine incision wall is sutured longitudinally by laparoscopy (Figs. 10.9, 10.10a–f, and 10.11a–f).

10.4.5 Laparoscopic Uterine Artery Ligation and Hysteroscopic Surgery for Intrauterine Lesions with High Risk of Hemorrhage

The risk factors for uterine bleeding in hysteroscopic surgery include uterine perforation, placenta accreta, cervical pregnancy, cesarean scar pregnancy, uterine arteriovenous fistula, and coagulation disorders. As early as 1999, Perrotin et al. applied uterine artery ligation to facilitate the surgery for uterine malformation. In 2000, Liu reported that laparoscopic bipolar coagulation was performed to occlude uterine arteries and anastomoses between the ovarian and uterine arteries in three women with symptomatic myomas. All

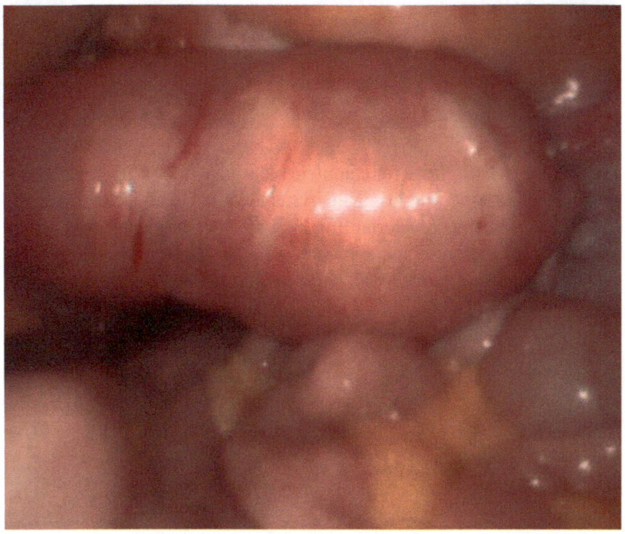

Fig. 10.9 The fundus of bicornuate uterus (prior to metroplasty)

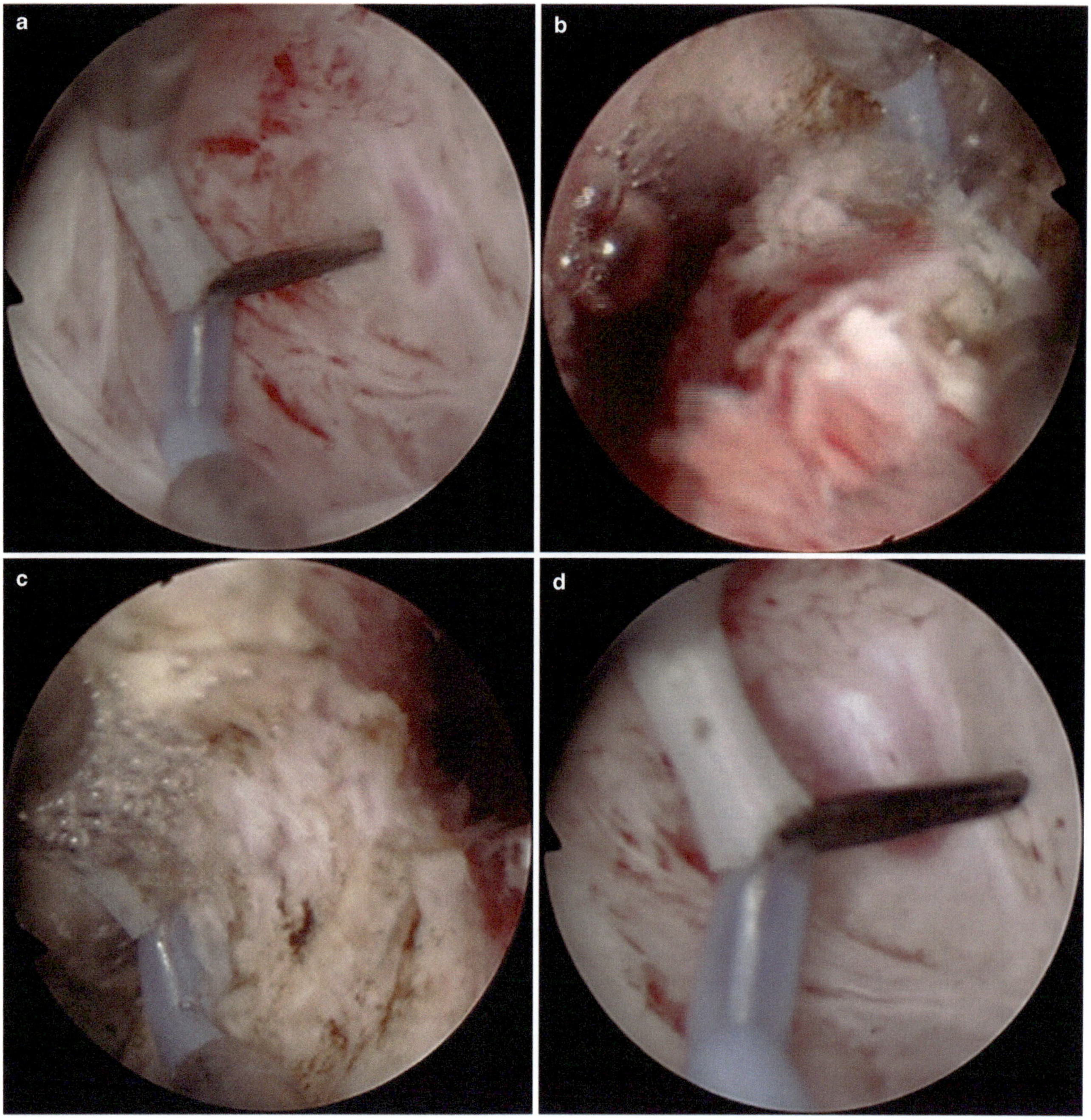

Fig. 10.10 Metroplasty for complete bicornuate uterus. (**a**) Transverse incision of uterine fundus with hysteroscopic needle electrode. (**b**) Transverse incision of uterine fundus with needle electrode to cause artificial perforation which approaches the right cornu. (**c**) Transverse incision of uterine fundus with needle electrode to cause artificial perforation which approaches the left cornu. (**d**) Transverse incision of uterine fundus with needle electrode and perforation is impending. (**e**) Transverse incision of uterine fundus with needle electrode and perforation occurs. (**f**) Transverse incision of uterine fundus with needle electrode and communication between uterine cavity and abdominal cavity

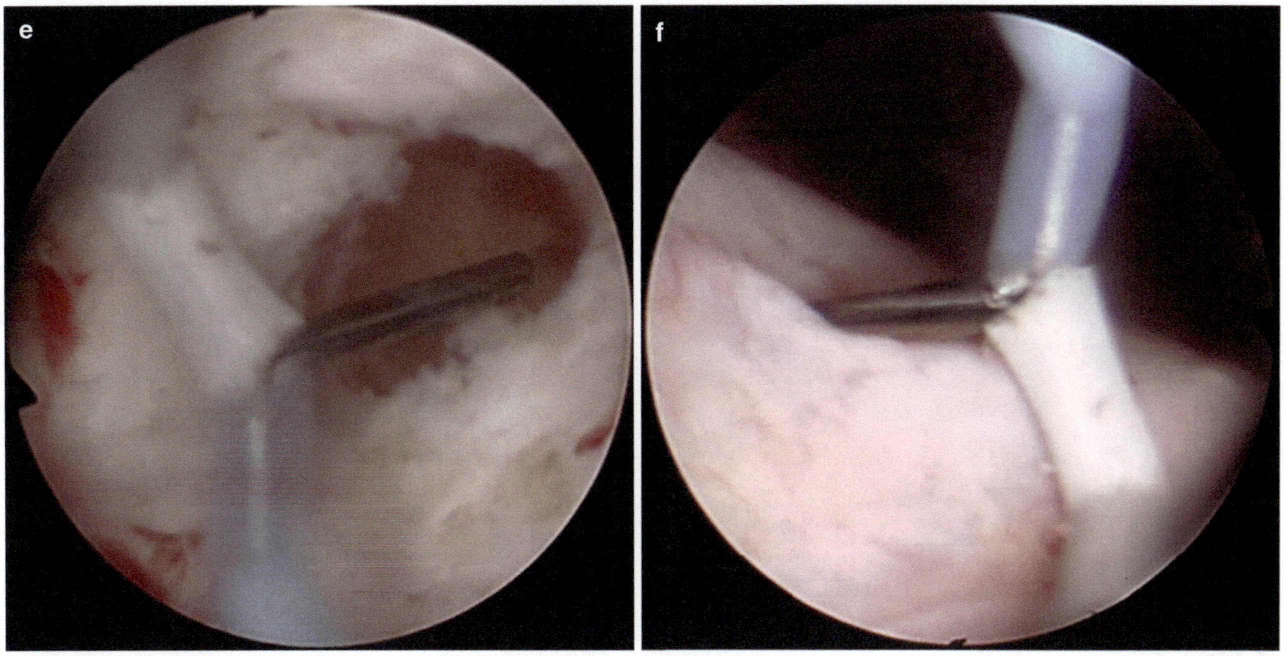

Fig. 10.10 (continued)

women had improvement in menorrhagia and dysmenorrhea symptoms and progressive reduction in size of the uterus and the dominant myoma. Since then, there have been a lot of reports on the application of this technique in the treatment of dysfunctional uterine bleeding, uterine myomas, adenomyosis, or laparoscopic removal of myomas, subtotal hysterectomy, and total hysterectomy. It is not technically difficult to occlude the uterine arteries under laparoscopy on the basis of traditional open surgery. Moreover, there were reports on the occlusion of the uterine vessels using titanium clip, coagulation, suture, ligature, and other various methods, which could achieve the similar effect, and no complications occurred. It has been used in the treatment of uterine arteriovenous fistula and auxiliary treatment of cervical pregnancy with methotrexate. They all indicated that, for hysteroscopic surgeries in patients with high risk factors of hemorrhage, the combined laparoscopy of prophylactic uterine artery ligation was feasible and effective. The methods of uterine artery ligation are shown in Fig. 10.12a–c.

10.4.6 Diagnosis and Treatment of the Coexistent Pelvic and Intrauterine Lesions

The development of gynecological endoscopic techniques prompts the two minimally invasive surgeries of hysteroscopy and laparoscopy combined into clinical use. Any intrauterine lesions concomitant with pelvic disorders can undergo combined hysteroscopic and laparoscopic examination and (or) surgery (Figs. 10.13 and 10.14). In Hysteroscopy Center of Fuxing Hospital, Capital Medical University, 275 patients underwent hysteroscopy, with different types of surgeries in conjunction with laparoscopic diagnosis and intraoperative monitoring. Among them, 108 patients underwent laparoscopic diagnosis and monitoring; 167 underwent one to three types of laparoscopic treatment, and 17 received four or more types of surgeries (Table 10.2). Following the operations, two cases had acute urinary tract infection, one case had upper respiratory tract infection, one

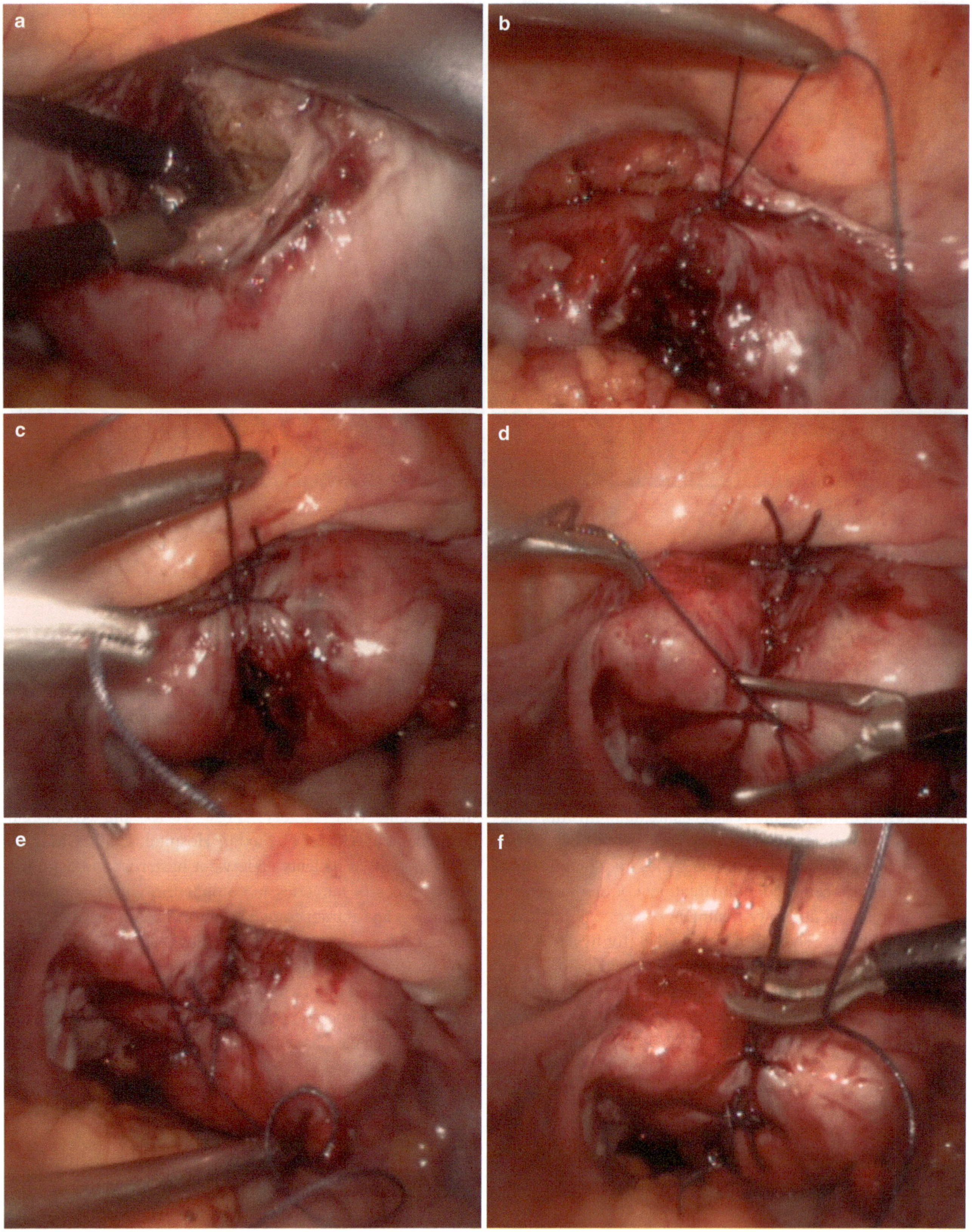

Fig. 10.11 Metroplasty for complete bicornuate uterus. (**a**) The incision of uterine fundus is extended under laparoscopy. (**b**) The first longitudinal suture of uterus under laparoscopy. (**c**) The second longitudinal suture under laparoscopy. (**d**) The third longitudinal suture under laparoscopy. (**e**) The fourth longitudinal suture under laparoscopy. (**f**) The fifth longitudinal suture under laparoscopy and the fundal reconstruction completed

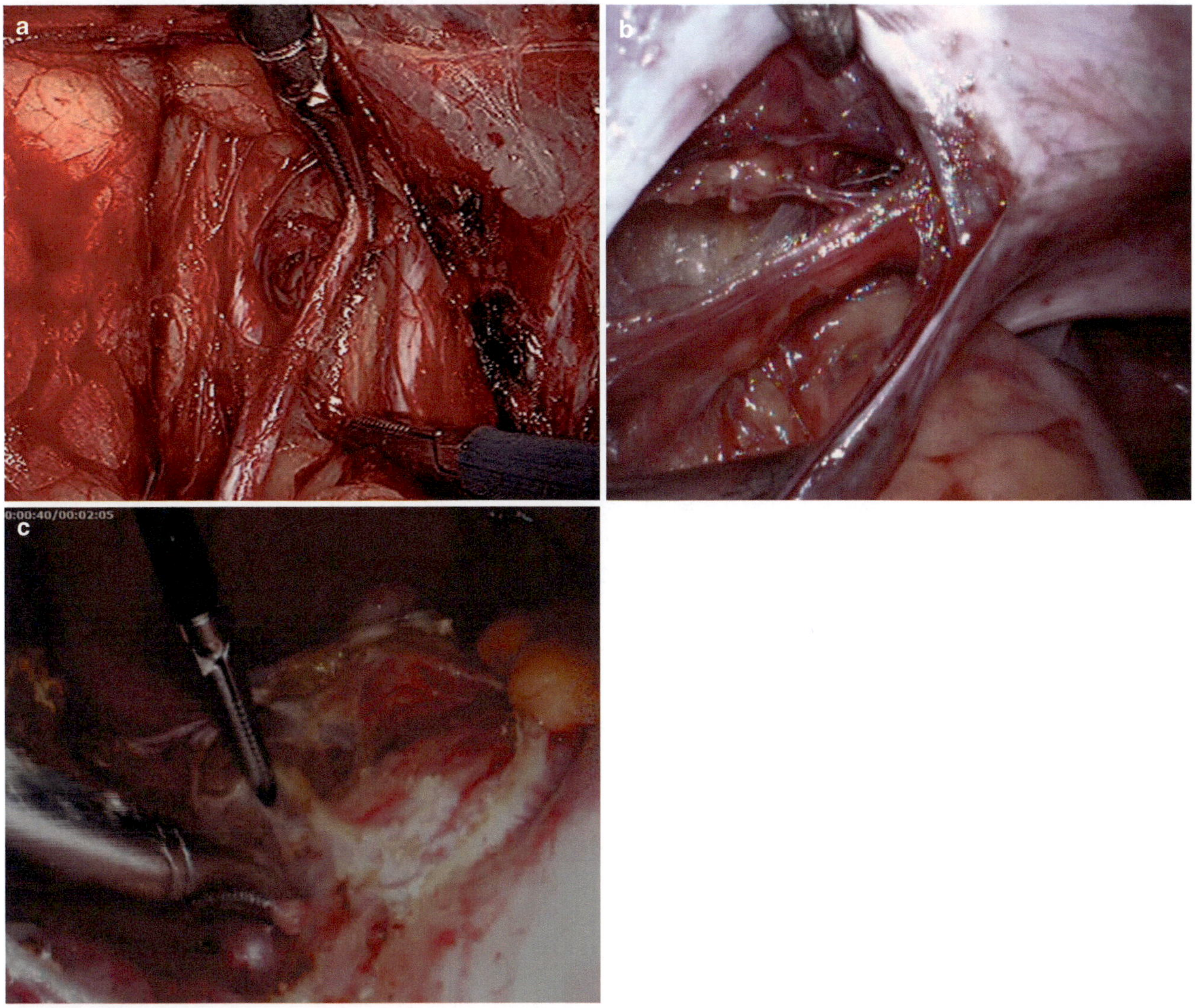

Fig. 10.12 (**a**) Isolation of uterine artery at its origin. The upper clamped artery is the trunk of left uterine artery. The tubular tissue on its left is the obliterated left superior vesical artery, and the tubular tissue on its right is the left ureter. (**b**) Posterior isolation of uterine artery. The left uterine artery is isolated from opened posterior leaf of the broad ligament over left uterosacral ligament. (**c**) Anterior isolation of ascending uterine artery. The lower clamped artery is the left ascending branch of uterine artery

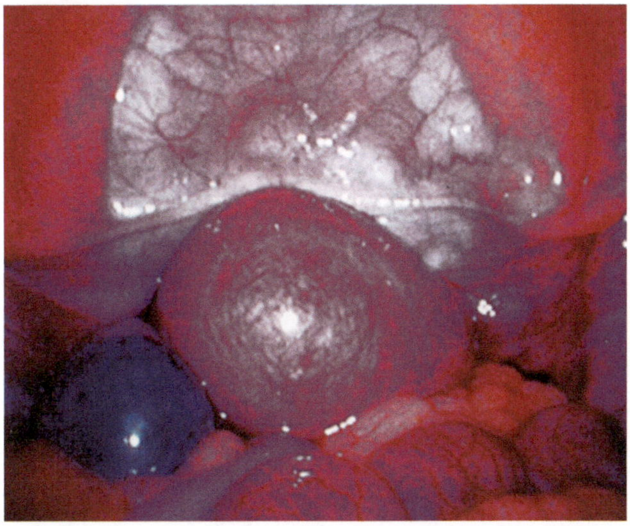

Fig. 10.13 Uterine myoma combined with ovarian cysts

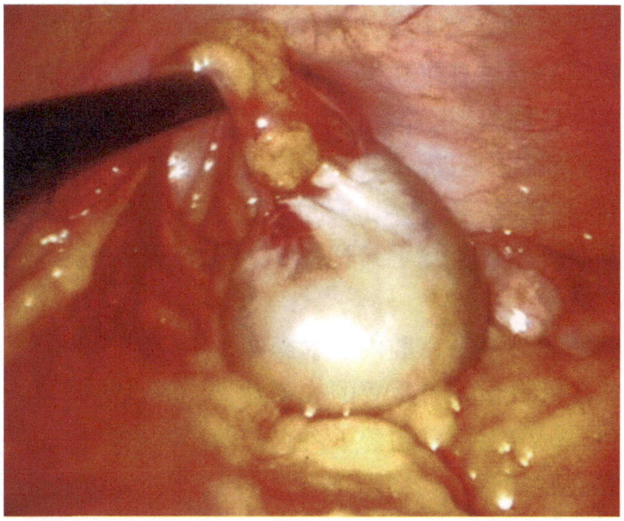

Fig. 10.14 Uterine submucous myomas combined with an omental tumor

Table 10.2 275 cases of combined hysteroscopy and laparoscopy (cases)

Laparoscopy		EMS									
Hysteroscopy		Cytoreductive surgery	Cystectomy	Ovarian cystectomy	Polycystic ovarian drilling	Lysis of adhesions	Salpingostomy	Myomectomy	Hydrotubation	Unilateral salpingectomy	Excision of adnexa
TCRS	77	7	1	5	2	10	1	2	20	0	0
TCRA	33	6	1	4	1	8	1	2	13	0	0
TCRM	70	6	2	4	0	12	0	14	5	1	0
TCRE	43	11	3	23	1	6	0	9	0	2	1
TCRF	18	2	1	0	0	5	0	0	3	0	1
TCRP	29	9	4	4	3	4	1	1	8	0	1
No surgery	5	0	0	0	0	1	0	0	0	0	0
Total	275	40	12	40	7	45	3	28	49	3	3

Note: Each case may undergo laparoscopic treatment of multiple lesions case was converted to laparotomy, and the remaining 271 cases recovered smoothly. The joint surgery does not worsen the patients' sufferings or postpone discharge from hospital. The conversion to open abdominal hysterectomy due to intraoperative bleeding was a complication of hysteroscopic surgery, which was not induced by joint surgery. Postoperative infection is not a unique complication of joint surgery, and there is a good prognosis after symptomatic treatment. Those with multiple uterine myomas who desire to preserve uterus may undergo laparoscopic removal of subserosal, intramural, and penetrating myomas, and hysteroscopic resection of submucous and inward-protruding intramural myomas.

The effective combination of joint surgery makes a better use of the advantages of hysteroscopy and laparoscopy and broadens the scope and variety of endoscopic diagnosis and treatment. The joint surgery can diagnose and treat various disorders in the pelvic and abdominal cavity, without worsening the patient's trauma and pains, and the advantages of minimally invasive surgery are fully exhibited.

Suggested Reading

1. Adelusi B, al-Nuaim L, Makanjuola D, Khashoggi T, Chowdhury N, Kangave D. Accuracy of hysterosalpingography and laparoscopic hydrotubation in diagnosis of tubal patency. Fertil Steril. 1995;63(5):1016–20.
2. Adolph AJ, Gilliland GB. Fertility following laparoscopic removal of rudimentary horn with an ectopic pregnancy. J Obstet Gynaecol Can. 2002;24(7):575–6.
3. Castaing N, Darai E, Chuong T, Benifla JL, Bernard G, Meneux E, Tardif D, Batallan A, Madelenat P. Complications mécaniques et métaboliques de l'hystéroscopie opératoire: à propos d'une étude rétrospective de 352 interventions [Mechanical and metabolic complications of hysteroscopic surgery: report of a retrospective study of 352 procedures]. Contracept Fertil Sex. 1999;27(3):210–5. French.
4. Choe JK, Baggish MS. Hysteroscopic treatment of septate uterus with Neodymium-YAG laser. Fertil Steril. 1992;57:81–4.
5. Cravello L, Porcu G, Roger V, D'Ercole C, Blanc B. Hystéroscopie opératoire et fertilité [Hysteroscopic surgery and fertility]. Contracept Fertil Sex. 1998;26(7–8):589–92. French.
6. Ding P. 50 cases of uterine artery ligation during laparoscopic hysterectomy. J Luzhou Med College. 2005;28(7):64. Chinese.
7. Duan H, Xia EL, Duan H. TV hystero-laparoscopic joint surgery: a report of 85 cases. China J Endosc. 1997;3(5):36–9. Chinese.
8. Feng Z, Huang Y, Cao F. Application of hystero-laparoscopic joint examination in ovulatory infertility. Fertil Contracept. 1990;10:57–60. Chinese.
9. Guo Y, Xia EL, Xiao Y. Analysis of etiology and reproductive prognosis of laparoscopic diagnosis and treatment in 294 infertile women. China J Endosc. 2013;19(10):1115–7. Chinese.
10. Holub Z, Lukác J, Kliment L, Urbánek S. Minimálně invazivní operacní lécba symptomatických myomů pomocí LDUV (laparoskopická disekce dělozních cév): klinická prospektivní studie (cást I) [Minimally invasive surgical treatment of symptomatic myomas using laparoscopic dissection of uterine vessels: prospective clinical study (part I)]. Ceska Gynekol. 2003;68(3):147–52. Czech.
11. Homer HA, Li TC, Cooke ID. The septate uterus: a review of management and reproductive outcome. Fertil Steril. 2000;73(1):1–14.
12. Kaminski P, Gajewska M, Wielgos M, Szymusik I, Ziolkowska K, Bartkowiak R. The usefulness of laparoscopy and hysteroscopy in the diagnostics and treatment of infertility. Neuro Endocrinol Lett. 2006;27(6):813–7.
13. Kivnick S, Kanter M. Bowel injury from roll-ball ablation of the endometrium. Obstet Gynecol. 1992;79:833–5.
14. Li C, Guo Y, Liu Y, Cheng J, Zhang W. Hysteroscopic and laparoscopic management of uterine defects on previous cesarean delivery scars. J Perinat Med. 2014;42(3):363–70.
15. Lichtinger M, Hallson L, Calvo P, Adeboyejo G. Laparoscopic uterine artery occlusion for symptomatic leiomyomas. J Am Assoc Gynecol Laparosc. 2002;9(2):191–8.
16. Lin H, Kung FT. Combination of laparoscopic bilateral uterine artery ligation and intraamniotic methotrexate injection for conservative management of cervical pregnancy. J Am Assoc Gynecol Laparosc. 2003;10(2):215–8.
17. Liu WM. Laparoscopic bipolar coagulation of uterine vessels to treat symptomatic leiomyomas. J Am Gynecol Laparosc. 2000;7(1):125–9.
18. Loffer FD. Complications of hysteroscopy-their cause, prevention, and correction. J Am Assoc Gynecol Laparosc. 1995;3(1):11–26.
19. Loffer FD. Removal of large symptomatic intrauterine growths by the hysteroscopic resectoscope. Obstet Gynecol. 1990;76:836.
20. Martínez Reveles M, Salazar López-Ortíz CG, Gaviño Gaviño F, Castro López JL, Mondragón Alcocer HL. Laparoscopia e histeroscopia en malformaciones müllerianas: utilidad y resultados reproductivos [Laparoscopy and hysteroscopy in Müllerian duct malformations: usefulness and reproductive results]. Ginecol Obstet Mex. 1999;67:4–8. Spanish.
21. McComb PF, Wagner BL. Simplified therapy for Asherman's syndrome. Fertil Steril. 1997;68(6):1047–50.
22. Mittal S, Kumar S, Roy KK. Role of endoscopy in retrieval of misplaced intrauterine device. Aust N Z J Obstet Gynaecol. 1996;36(1):49–51.
23. Nezhat F, Nezhat C, Nezhat CH, Levy JS, Smith E, Katz L. Use of hysteroscopy in addition to laparoscopy for evaluating chronic pelvic pain. J Reprod Med. 1995;40(6):431–4.
24. Perrotin F, Bertrand J, Body G. Case report: laparoscopic surgery of unicornuate uterus with rudimentary uterine horn. Hum Reprod. 1999;14(4):931–3.
25. Phillips DR, Milim SJ, Nathanson HG. Experience with laparoscopic leiomyoma coagulation and concomitant operative hysteroscopy. J Am Assoc Gynecol Laparosc. 1997;4(4):425–33.
26. Pittrof R, Darwish DH, Shabib G. Near-fatal uterine perforation during transcervical endometrial resection. Lancet. 1991;338:197–8.
27. Propst AM, Liberman RF, Harlow BL, Ginsburg ES. Complications of hysteroscopic surgery: predicting patients at risk. Obstet Gynecol. 2000;96(4):517–20.
28. Schenk LM, Coddington CC. Laparoscopy and hysteroscopy. Obstet Gynecol Clin North Am. 1999;26(1):1–22.
29. Sinha RY, Hegde A, Warty N, Jain R. Laparoscopic devascularization of uterine myomata followed by enucleation of the myomas by direct morcellation. J Am Assoc Gynecol Laparosc. 2004;11(1):99–102.
30. Sulak PJ, Letterie GS, Hayslip CC, et al. Hysteroscopic cannulation and lavage in the treatment of proximal tubasl occlusion. Fertil Steril. 1987;48:493–4.
31. Valle RF. Hysteroscopic treatment of partial and complete uterine septum. Int J Fertil Menopausal Stud. 1996;41:310–5.
32. Valle RF. Tubal cannulation. Obstet Gynecol Clin North Am. 1995;22(3):519–40.
33. Wang CJ, Yen CF, Lee CL, Soong YK. Laparoscopic uterine artery ligation for treatment of symptomatic adenomyosis. J Am Assoc Gynecol Laparosc. 2002;9(3):293–6.

34. Wortman M, Daggett A. Hysteroscopic management of intractable uterine bleeding. J Reprod Med. 1993;38:505–9.
35. Wu YC, Liu WM, Yuan CC, Ng HT. Successful treatment of symptomatic arteriovenous malformation of the uterus using laparoscopic bipolar coagulation of uterine vessels. Fertil Steril. 2001;76(6):1270–1.
36. Xia EL, Duan H, Feng L. Application of B ultrasound and laparoscopic monitoring in hysteroscopic operation. China J Endosc. 1998;4:55–6. Chinese.
37. Xia EL. Hystero-laparoscopy combined treatment of intrauterine lesions with high risk factors of bleeding. Chin J Pract Gynecol Obstetr. 2007;23(8):592–4. Chinese.
38. Yen YK, Liu WM, Yuan CC, Ng HT. Laparoscopic bipolar coagulation of uterine vessels to treat symptomatic myomas in women with elevated Ca 125. J Am Assoc Gynecol Laparosc. 2001;8(2):241–6.
39. Zabak K, Bmonifla JL, Uzan S. Septate uterus and reproduction disorders: current results of hysteroscopic septoplasty. Gynecol Obstet Fertil. 2001;29(11):829–40.

Ultrasonography Monitoring During Hysteroscopic Surgery

11

Dan Zhang

Operative hysteroscopy is a surgical procedure implemented using hysteroscopic resectoscope, which belongs to intrauterine gynecology and includes TCRE, TCRM, TCRS, TCRA, and TCRF using wire loop electrode, and EA using rollerball electrode.

Two-dimensional (2D) ultrasonography is done by scanning the uterus longitudinally and transversely to visualize the contour of uterus, the echoes of uterine wall, and the shape of uterine cavity, as well as measuring various lines of the cavity, the wall, the outline, and the cervix. It can diagnose most of uterine abnormalities and has been a routine method of examination to screen for occupying lesions and morphological abnormalities.

Transabdominal ultrasonography is one of the methods in guiding hysteroscopic surgery. Through observation of the intrauterine procedures on 2D imaging and guidance for complex surgical process, the occurrence of complications can be reduced and the surgical safety can be improved. By observation of two contrasted acoustic windows formed by fluid-distension uterine cavity and fluid-filled bladder, ultrasonography scan can clearly visualize the contour of uterus and the shape of cavity, display the location and the condition of intrauterine operating instrument in real-time, indicate the extent and the depth of the incision, and timely suggest for the operator to terminate the operation so as to avoid uterine perforation, ensure successful procedures, and guarantee the operational safety.

11.1 Techniques of Ultrasonography Guidance

The patient is placed in bladder lithotomy position. The bladder is filled, and its amount varies from person to person. For those who have no history of pelvic surgery, the upper section of the uterine corpus needs to be visualized. During hysteroscopy, a cervical forceps is used to pull the cervix outwards to expose the uterine fundus, so that it will not affect the surgeon's operation due to the overfilled bladder. For those who have a history of pelvic surgeries, if there are pelvic adhesions, when the cervical forceps is pulled outwards, the movability of the uterus will be small. Therefore, there will be a slightly more amount of filling fluid in the bladder than those with no pelvic surgery, which makes it appropriate to expose the uterine fundus.

On ultrasonography, the probe entering the uterine cavity can be observed, and the direction of the probe reaching the fundus is determined. Under ultrasonography guidance, the hysteroscope is introduced into the cervical canal to internal os (Fig. 11.1), and the distention medium is irrigated into the uterine cavity. The distention medium injected into the uterine cavity and the fillings in bladder form acoustic windows for double contrast (Fig. 11.2).

From the beginning of surgery to end, the two-dimensional double-contrast ultrasonography imaging is performed to continuously monitor the surgical process. The following contents should be included in observation.

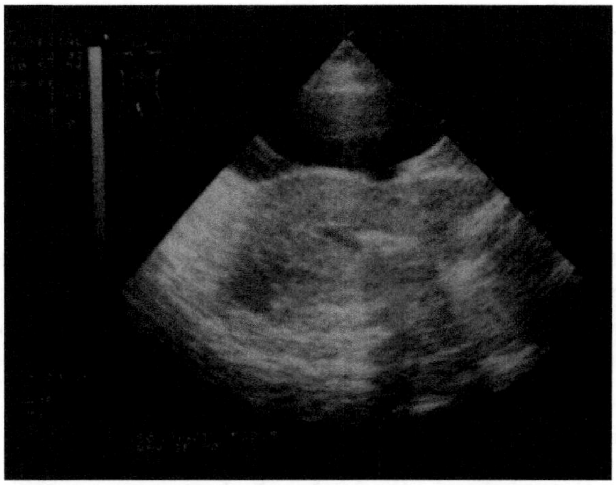

Fig. 11.1 Under ultrasonography guidance, the hysteroscope is introduced into the cervical canal to internal os

D. Zhang (✉)
Department of Ultrasound, Fuxing Hospital, Capital Medical University, Beijing, China
e-mail: dan.zhang@263.net

E. Xia (ed.), *Practical Manual of Hysteroscopy*, https://doi.org/10.1007/978-981-19-1332-7_11

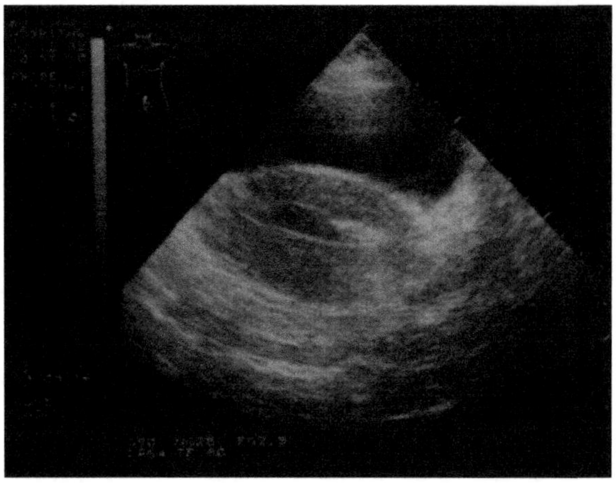

Fig. 11.2 The distention medium injected into the uterine cavity and the fillings in bladder form acoustic windows for double contrast

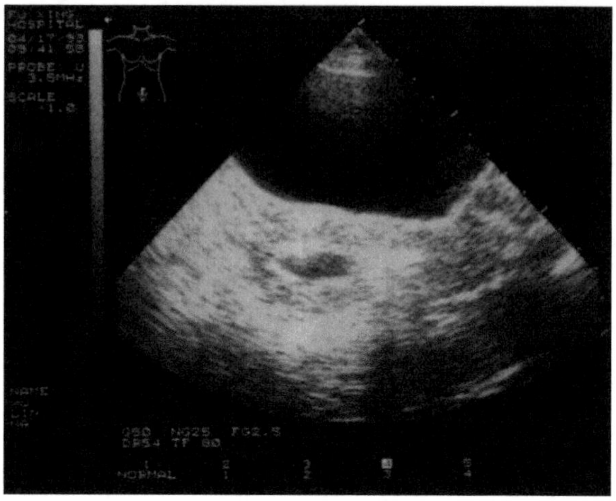

Fig. 11.3 The lining of uterus after resection appears to be strong echogenic band of 3–4 mm in width

1. To observe the changes in the thickness of uterine wall and the location of resectoscope in order to prevent uterine perforation.
2. To identify the signs that suggest changes in the echoes under the electrical thermal effects on the inner uterine lining and the muscle wall so as to determine the depth and extent of resection and intramural lesions.
3. To determine the location and the size of the intrauterine lesions, the relationship between the intrauterine lesions and the uterine cavity, and to monitor the resection of intrauterine and intramural lesions.
4. To explore whether there are uterine malformations and old injuries which are difficult to diagnose or not and make further diagnosis.
5. To observe the effect of intraoperative medication.
6. To observe intrauterine distending pressure: Whether there is irrigation fluid flowing via the fallopian tubal ostia into abdominal cavity or not, and how much has flown into the abdominal cavity.

11.2 Ultrasonography Guidance for Intraoperative Operation

11.2.1 Ultrasonography Guidance for TCRE

Transcervical resection of endometrium (TCRE) is a procedure to resect the endometrial functional layer, the basal layer, and underlying 2–3 mm myometrial layer with the hysteroscopic wire loop, so as to reduce the menstrual flow, relieve dysmenorrhea, and achieve the purpose of artificial menopause. The resected uterine wall may dehydrate and shrink due to heat produced by the high-frequency thermal effect of the wire loop during surgery. The linear echoes in the inner lining of the uterus turn into strong echogenic band of 3–4 mm in breadth (Fig. 11.3). When the cutting reaches myometrium, the strong echogenic band may fade away after 15–40 min of resection. When the cutting depth is confined to the endometrial layer, the strong echogenic band formed may disappear rapidly. During operation, after the uterus shrinks due to the electrical resection, the effect of uterine distension is poor, the inner lining of uterus may become ruffled, leading to missed resection. The important indication for preventing missed resection is the strong echogenic band being intact by ultrasonography. The duration of the strong echogenic band is an ultrasonic indication suggesting the cutting depth. The location of resectoscope can be closely monitored to prevent the wire loop from pushing tight against or penetrating the uterine wall. When the outer edge of the strong echogenic band reaches the deep myometrium, it suggests that the operator should stop the cutting on this site, which may prevent uterine perforation effectively.

11.2.2 Ultrasonography Guidance for Endometrial Ablation

Endometrial ablation (EA) is a procedure performed by rollerball electrode of hysteroscope to destroy endometrium in order to achieve the purpose of reducing menses and treat the dysfunctional uterine bleeding. During EA, when the rollerball electrode is used to destroy the endometrium, the lining of uterus may dehydrate and shrink due to the electric thermal effect and form a strong echogenic band similar to TCRE. However, the strong echogenic band formed after EA may disappear quickly and the duration time is approximately 5 min. Since the thermal effect of the rollerball electrode is enhanced with a prolonged coagulation and is decreased with an increased power, too long local coagulation can cause too deep electric thermal damage to the uterine wall when the power is constant, which is the main cause of uterine perforation during EA. During the operation, when the strong echo developing at the uterine wall reaches the deep myometrium and approaches the serosal layer, this is an important indication to stop local coagulation. Compared with that of TCRE, the indications for ultrasonography guidance during EA are observation of the depth of strong echo developed in the lining of uterus, rather than the duration of the strong echogenic band.

11.2.3 Ultrasonography Guidance for TCRM

Transcervical resection of myoma (TCRM) includes transcervical resection of submucous myoma and transcervical resection of inward-protruding intramural myoma.

Submucous myomas are classified into three types, namely submucous myoma with a narrow pedicle, submucous myoma with a broad pedicle, and sessile submucous myoma. During the growth of the submucous myoma with a narrow pedicle (Fig. 11.4), the pedicle may grow long and narrow with the enlargement of the tumor. The tumor inside the uterine cavity may elicit foreign-body-like stimulation to the uterus, causing uterine contraction and prompting the tumor to prolapse into the cervical canal or vagina with its pedicle remaining in the uterine cavity. Sometimes it can be concomitant with the introversion of uterine wall at the site of tumor pedicle. During the operation, the role of the ultrasonography is to suggest the depth of resection on pedicle and is to guide the surgeon in cutting at the edge of pedicle so as to avoid damage to the introverted uterine wall. As for submucous myoma with a broad pedicle or without a pedicle, the location of its base should be first determined. If the base is lower and the tumor is <3.0 cm in diameter, the operator may start resection from its base under ultrasonography guidance. If the base of the myoma is in upper portion of cavity, or the cavity is fully filled by a large myoma, the operation should start with the lower edge of the tumor or one side. During the operation, ultrasonography should suggest the location of endoscope and the direction of resection and guide the operator to cut the myoma thinner or into oblate spheroid shape so that it can be clamped with oval forceps and screwed out. Larger myomas tend to need multiple cutting and clamping before complete removal. Intraoperative ultrasonography shows that the resected surface appears to be with strong echogenicity (Fig. 11.5). After surgery, myomas are totally removed, the uterine cavity is empty, and the resected surface appears to be with strong echogenicity (Fig. 11.6).

Since 1/2 to 2/3 of an uterine inward-protruding intramural myoma lies in the uterine wall, the normal myometrium outside the tumor is squeezed thin and the 1/3 to 1/2 of the myoma protrudes into the uterine cavity (Fig. 11.7). Under

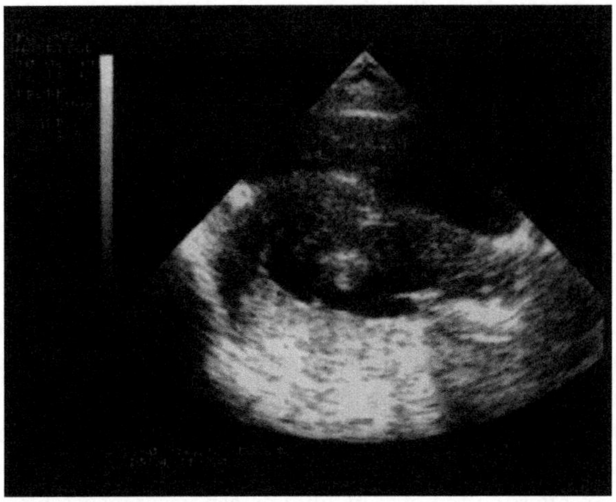

Fig. 11.4 The narrow pedicle submucous fibroid in the anterior wall is visible before operation

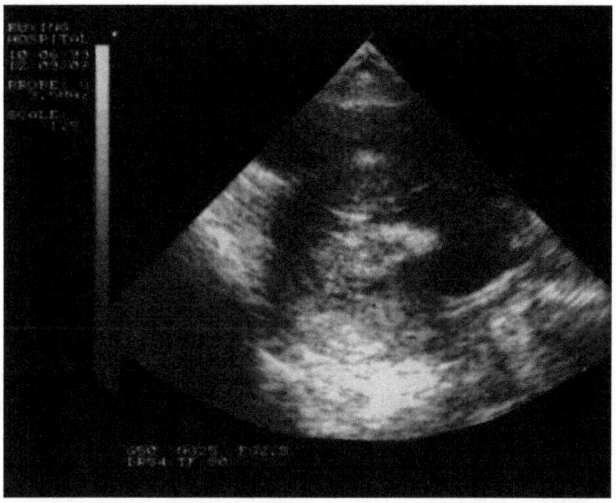

Fig. 11.5 During operation, the narrow pedicle submucous fibroid in the anterior wall is partly resected, and the resected surface appears to be with strong echoes

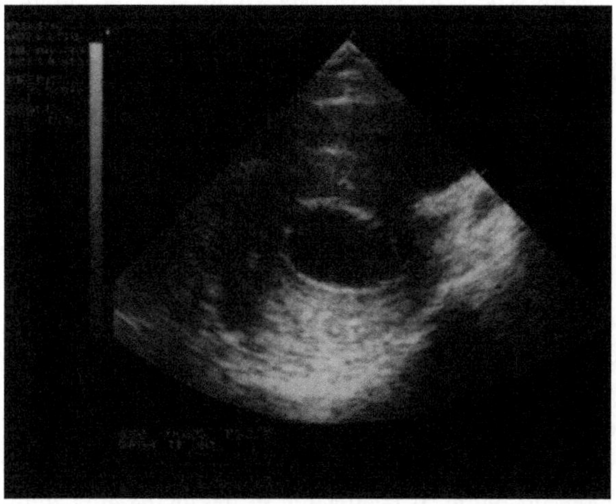

Fig. 11.6 After operation, the narrow pedicle submucous fibroid in the anterior wall is totally resected, and the resected surface appears to be with strong echoes

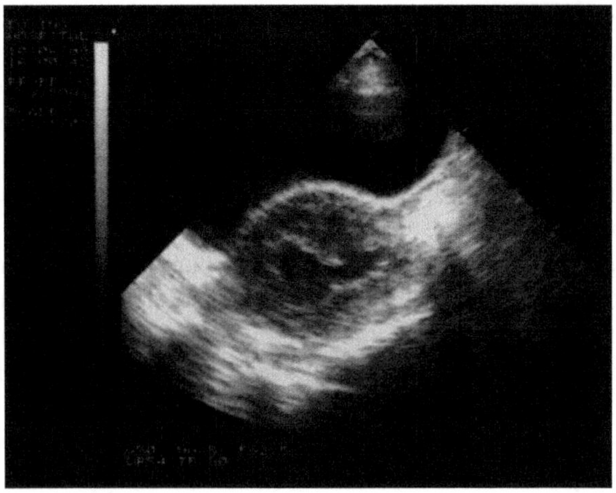

Fig. 11.7 Inward-protruding intramural myoma before resection

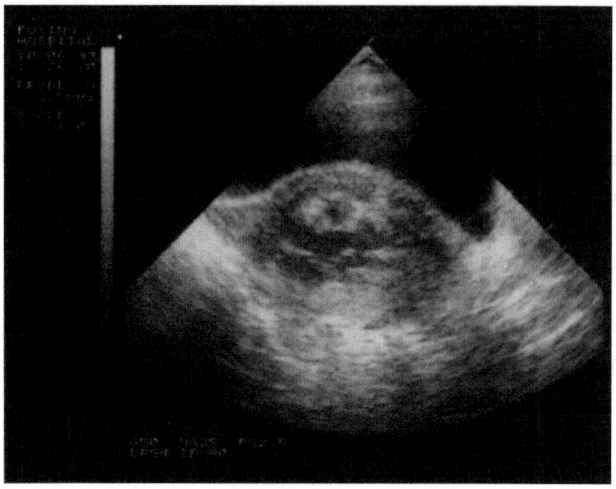

Fig. 11.8 An arc-shaped strong echogenic band between the myoma and the myometrial wall is formed during operation

ultrasonography monitoring, the resection of myoma is firstly performed till parallel to the lining of the uterus. At this moment, intraoperative ultrasonography scan may reveal, due to the uterine contraction induced by cutting with electric wire loop, the myoma within the uterine wall is squeezed into the uterine cavity. Then, the extruded uterine wall at the outer edge of the myoma may gradually restore, the border between the myoma and the uterine wall becomes clear, and the intramural myoma is protruding gradually into the uterine cavity, which suggest that the operator may continue cutting and clamping the myoma. The repeated cutting and clamping may isolate the myoma gradually from the normal myometrial wall. The irrigation fluid and the gas produced from vaporization may infiltrate into the tissue between the myoma and the myometrial wall, where an arc-shaped strong echogenic band is formed (Fig. 11.8). This sign indicates that the myoma may be all squeezed into the uterine cavity and removed by a hysteroscopic resection. If the contraction of the uterus is poor, the sonography will find that the intramural myoma cannot be squeezed into the uterine cavity, in that case intravenous injection of oxytocin 10 IU should be given so as to promote uterine contraction. After intravenous injection of oxytocin, the focus of ultrasonography monitoring is to observe whether there is arc-shaped strong echogenic band between the residual myoma and the uterine wall or not, whether the myoma moves gradually towards the uterine cavity and whether the extruded uterine wall thickens gradually. The extrusion of the intramural myoma and the recovery of the squeezed uterine wall are completed along with the process of the surgery, so the ultrasonography guidance has to provide continuously the information about the resection of myoma and the restoration of the uterus so as to ensure a smooth operation. If contraction of the uterus after intravenous injection of oxytocin is not obvious, oxytocin can be used repeatedly. The maximum amount of application of oxytocin by the author in monitoring transcervical resection of myomas is 30 IU. After the total removal of the myoma, ultrasonography shows that the myoma bed and the surrounding normal uterine wall are almost parallel or concaved. After repeated intravenous injection of oxytocin, if the residual myoma in the uterine wall has not been squeezed into the uterine cavity or isolated from the uterine wall, it indicates that the myoma cannot be removed at one time, and a second surgery may be required. After total removal of intramural fibroids, the uterine cavity is empty and the resected surface appears to show strong echogenicity (Fig. 11.9).

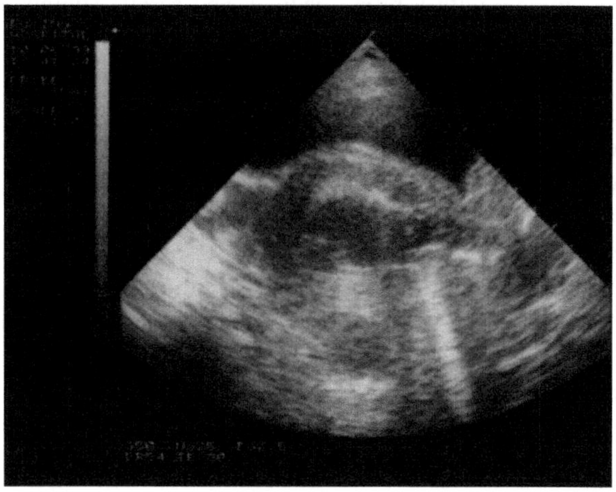

Fig. 11.9 After operation, the uterine cavity is empty and the resected surface appears to be with strong echogenicity

For initial cases, the removal of myomas is always concomitant with the resection of endometrium. Recent studies have found that patients with submucous or inward-protruding intramural fibroids usually have an expanded uterine cavity and thin uterine wall. Therefore, the resection of endometrium after the removal of fibroids can easily cause uterine perforation. Patho-anatomically, the uterine submucous myoma and inward-protruding intramural fibroids may increase the endometrial line, which is one of the causes of menorrhagia. If other causes are ruled out, simple removal of the myoma can be effective in reducing menstrual flow and the surgical success rate is almost 100%. In addition, the uterine submucosal fibroids account for 5% of female infertility and inward-protruding intramural fibroids may cause miscarriage. Application of hysteroscopic removal of myomas may eliminate laparotomy and avoid rupture of scarred uterus after pregnancy. Therefore, hysteroscopic removal of uterine myomas is more suitable for those who want to preserve fertility.

11.2.4 Ultrasonography Guidance for TCRS

The uterus is formed by fusion of the two paramesonephric ducts. During the development process of the uterus, if two paramesonephric ducts are fused completely, but the septum is not absorbed, complete septate uterus is formed. The ultrasonography shows that the uterus has a normal appearance and the uterine cavity is isolated into two parts except that uterine fundus has a wider transverse diameter. If the septum is not completely absorbed, incomplete septate uterus is formed. A typical malformation of septate uterus is that the uterine cavity has two compartments in the corpus of the uterus, and the transverse scanning of the ultrasonography reveals that the uterus has a wider transverse diameter and two cavity echoes, and there is a longitudinal boundary (Fig. 11.10) in the center. On the longitudinal plane, the septate tissues become thickened at the uterine fundus (Fig. 11.11). After irrigation of distention medium, the ultrasonography scan in transverse plane shows the equally tiny dense bright spots echoes formed by muscular tissues at the center of uterine cavity, which are consistent with myometrial echoes. The uterus with bilateral fluid filling cavities forms a "cat's eye sign" (Fig. 11.12).

Prior to transcervical resection of the septum (TCRS), on the two-dimensional ultrasonography, the length of the septum, the widths of its base, and its distal end are measured.

Step one, the septum is resected. Under the double-contrast ultrasonography guidance, the hysteroscopic wire loop or needle electrode is used to resect or divide the septum from the distal end towards the basal portion. Intraoperative cutting depth and direction are monitored by ultrasonography. If the septum is long, its distal end may generally be narrow, and the septum is usually resected with wire loop between left and right interchangeably; if the septum is short and flat, its distal end is generally wider, and the needle electrode can be used to divide and incise the septum longitudinally. No matter which method is taken, when cutting reaches the uterine fundus, the fundal portion appears to be tapered or irregular (Fig. 11.13).

Step two, the uterine fundus takes shape. On ultrasonography, the thickness in diameter of the anterior and the poste-

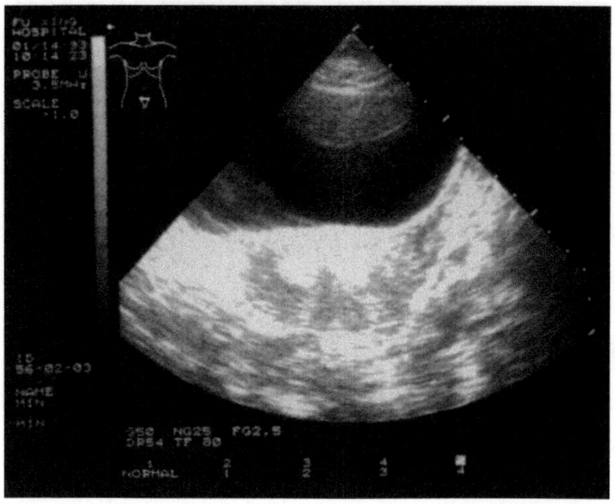

Fig. 11.10 On transverse scan of the uterus, two cavity echoes with a longitudinal boundary in the center are visible

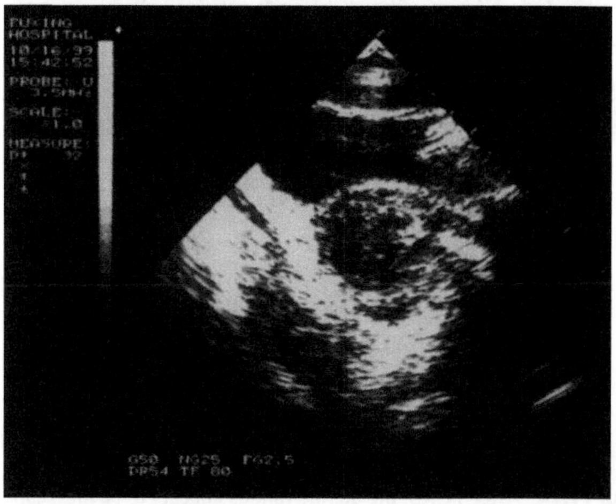

Fig. 11.11 On longitudinal scan of the uterus, the thickened uterine fundus is partial septate tissues

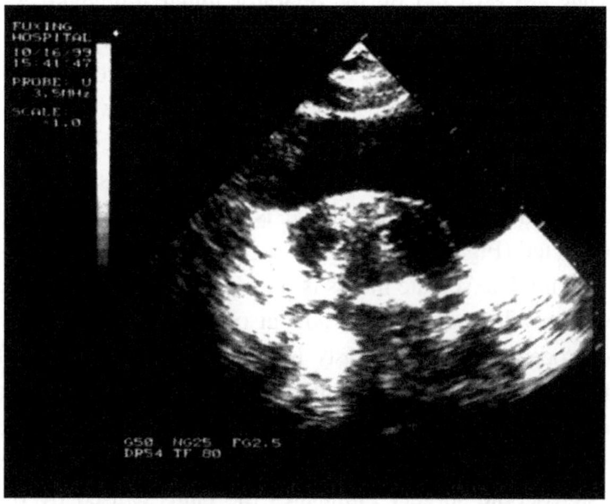

Fig. 11.12 On transverse scan of the uterus, the uterus with cavities on both sides of septum filled with fluid forms a "cat's eye sign"

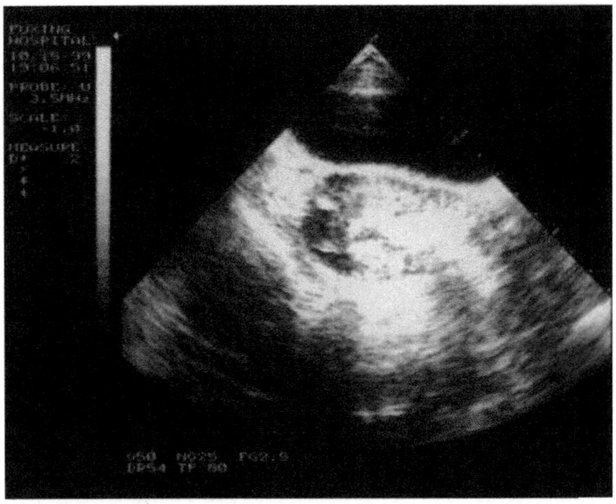

Fig. 11.13 During operation, the fundus appears to be tapered

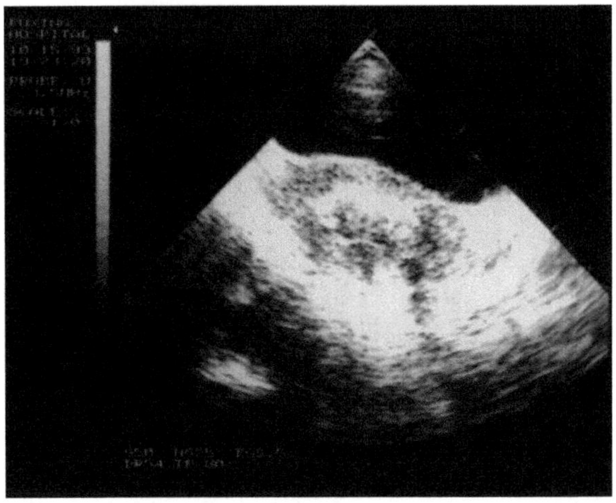

Fig. 11.14 After TCRS, the uterine fundus appears to be arc-shaped

rior walls of the fundus is measured, and then the excess tissues are resected by the operator under guidance. After each cutting, the cavity should be distended by irrigation fluid and the morphology of the uterus should be observed by ultrasonography. When ultrasonography shows that the thickness of the fundus is consistent with that of the anterior and posterior walls, the uterine fundus appears to be arc-shaped and the cutting surface is flat, then the surgery is completed (Fig. 11.14).

Incomplete septate uterus is one of the causes of recurrent pregnancy loss. Before the advent of hysteroscopic surgery, the procedure of metroplasty is to remove the septum after transabdominal incision of uterus. Compared with hysteroscopy, transabdominal surgery has greater trauma, slows recovery, and delays pregnancy for 1–2 years postoperatively. Hysteroscopic surgery eliminates the pains caused by open surgery and avoids the rupture of scarred uterus after pregnancy and pelvic adhesions. Due to the quick recovery after hysteroscopic surgery, the patients may have pregnancy after 2–3 months. Therefore, hysteroscopic resection of septum is easier to operate, with fewer complications and easily accepted by patients, as compared to transabdominal surgery.

11.2.5 Ultrasonography Guidance for TCRA

Transcervical resection of adhesion (TCRA) is a procedure applicable to any uterine adhesion and hematocele for a variety of reasons. The patients present with recurrent abdominal pain, hypomenorrhea, amenorrhea, and infertility. Sometimes menstrual blood may flow into the abdominal cavity and cause severe abdominal pain similar to the ectopic pregnancy, and if not promptly treated, endometriosis may occur. The traditional treatment of the intrauterine adhesions is to swing a cervical dilator or a probe from one side to the other in the uterine cavity to release adhesions. This method is effective for mild, membranous, and some fibrous adhesions. But for the severe, muscular, and some fibrous adhesions and even uterine occlusion, the blind lysis of the adhesion may easily cause damage to the uterine wall and even uterine perforation in severe cases. If hysteroscopic resectoscope is used to divide the adhesions, ultrasonography guidance may indicate the direction of the probe, and the direction and the depth of electric cutting, which may not only ensure an accurate incision of adhesions and guarantee the surgical effects, but also can prevent effectively the occurrence of uterine perforation.

As for mild intrauterine adhesions concomitant with hematocele, under ultrasonography monitoring, a probe or a cervical dilator is used to detect the uterine cavity, if they can penetrate the adhesive zone and drain the hematocele, there will be a clear visual field under hysteroscope. Then the adhesive band adherent to the uterine wall is resected under ultrasonography guidance. If a probe or a cervical dilator cannot penetrate the adhesive zone, or there is severe adhesion or complete uterine cavity occlusion, the probe or cervical dilator should not be inserted with force into the uterine cavity to avoid uterine perforation. Under ultrasonography guidance, the hysteroscopic resectoscope is introduced via the cervix into the lower portion of the adhesions, and the adhesions are resected along the uterine mid axis. After lysis of adhesions, the irrigation fluid is injected into the uterine cavity. When the ultrasonography reveals a good uterine distension and intact lining, it suggests that the surgery is completed (Figs. 11.15 and 11.16). In order to prevent reformation of intrauterine adhesions, IUD is placed in the uterine cavity after surgery and removed 3 months later.

11.2.6 Ultrasonography Guidance for TCRF

Transcervical removal of foreign body (TCRF) is applicable to embedded IUD, fragmented IUD residual, and placental

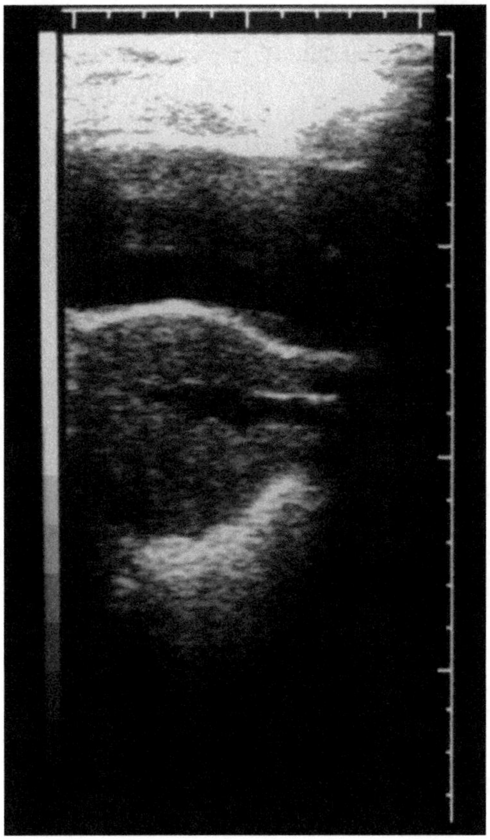

Fig. 11.15 Prior to surgery of peripheral intrauterine adhesions, adhesions are seen at the lining of uterus with an irregular morphology of uterine cavity

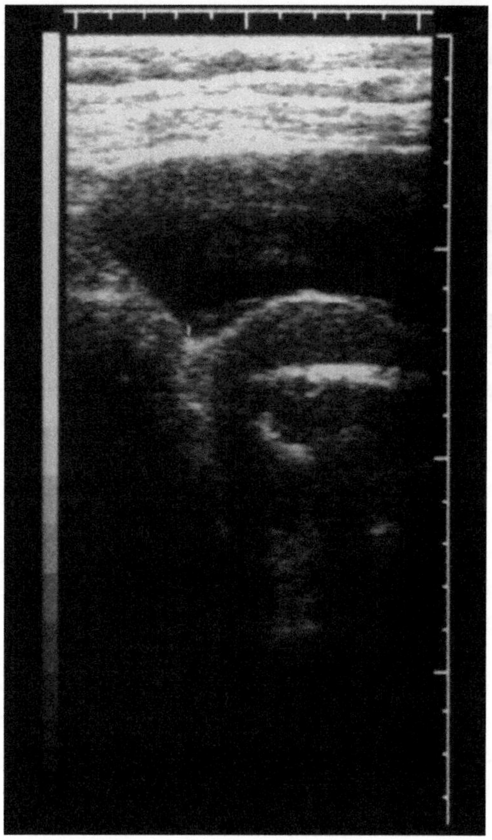

Fig. 11.16 After resection of intrauterine adhesions, the uterine cavity has a good distention

or embryonic retention in the uterine cavity. Since the foreign body can elicit varied degrees of clinical symptoms and different features of ultrasonography imaging, the corresponding surgical approach should be adopted according to different causes.

11.2.6.1 Removal of the Residual IUD

First to determine the location of the residual IUD under ultrasonography. If part of the residual IUD is embedded in the uterine wall, hysteroscopy can reveal its location and ultrasonography can indicate the distance from the embedded end to the serosal layer. If concomitant with uterine or cervical adhesions, or if the intrauterine device is fully embedded in the muscle wall (Fig. 11.17), the residual IUD cannot be seen under hysteroscope. If so, the operator may apply the ultrasonography monitoring to locate the residual IUD by measuring the distance between it and the endometrial line and can resect or divide the adhesions, the endometrium, and myometrial tissues in the surface of residual IUD, so that the fragmented end of it is exposed. Then the hysteroscopic wire loop or oval forceps is used for its removal.

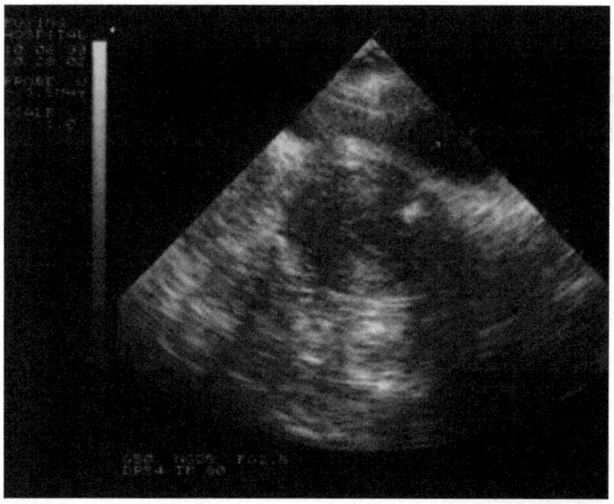

Fig. 11.17 The residual IUD is embedded in the anterior wall of uterus, which presents as strong echoes under ultrasonography scan

11.2.6.2 Removal of Complete or Broken Metal Ring

It is difficult to remove the embedded metal rings in the muscle wall. First, under ultrasonography guidance, determine the location of the embedment. Then the hysteroscopic wire loop is used to incise the embedded tissues. Finally, the hook or oval forceps is used to take out the metal ring. During the clamping process, the metal wire of IUD may be twisted or broken. Therefore, the entire process of removing the metal ring must be monitored continuously by ultrasonography. If there is a twisted or broken ring, ultrasonography shall indicate whether the metal ring has been removed completely or not and locate the fragmented residual ring in the myometrium.

11.2.6.3 Removal of Fetal Bones

Fetal bone retention in the uterine cavity presents as strong echogenic mass with acoustic shadowing under ultrasonography. If fetal bone is visible under hysteroscope, it can be removed directly by hysteroscopy. If the fetal bone is large, ultrasonography can indicate the relationship between the long axis of fetal bone and the long axis of uterine cavity, which is helpful to its removal under hysteroscope. If fetal bone retention is embedded in the myometrial wall or concomitant with uterine adhesions, ultrasonography can reveal if the strong echogenic mass lies in the uterine wall or if there is irregular echo-free zone around the strong echogenic mass, which is a sign of uterine adhesion concomitant with uterine hematocele or hydrohystera. Under ultrasonography surveillance, the hysteroscopic wire loop can be used to resect the adhesions and remove the residual fetal bones or to incise the muscle tissues in the embedded portion for the removal of the fetal bones.

11.2.6.4 Removal of Residual Placental Tissues

Uterine wall adhesions, implantation, and (or) organized tissues may develop due to the placenta residue. The ultrasonography reveals inhomogeneous echogenic mass in the uterine cavity, which shows an unclear border with the uterine wall (Fig. 11.18). Under ultrasonography guidance, the placenta residue, and adhesive or organized tissues in uterine cavity are resected hysteroscopically, followed by the resection of tissues adhered to or implanted in the muscle wall. When ultrasonography indicates that the implanted or organized tissues are in the deep myometrium or serosal layer, the resection should be performed according to the depth indicated by ultrasonography to prevent cutting too deep and causing uterine perforation.

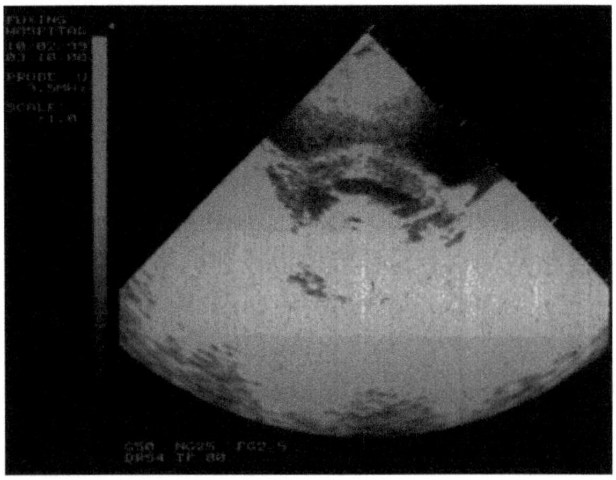

Fig. 11.18 The residual placenta tissues lie in the posterior wall of uterus, showing strong echoes, and concomitant with intrauterine adhesions and hydrohystera

11.3 Ultrasonography Guidance and Uterine Perforation

Hysteroscopic operation is all implemented in the uterine cavity. Due to a narrow field of vision and hard to estimate conduction of electricity, uterine perforation occurs sometimes, and its incidence can be as high as 2%. Therefore, the preoperative knowledge about high-risk diseases and intraoperative timely detection of uterine perforation are very important.

11.3.1 Causes of Uterine Perforation

11.3.1.1 Intrauterine Myomas

As for a submucous myoma with broad pedicle or without pedicle, its base is often deep into myometrium. As for inward-protruding intramural myoma, of which 1/2 to 2/3 locating in the uterine wall, the myometrium at the outer edge of myoma is squeezed to be very thin. Under ultrasonography monitoring, the simple removal of these two kinds of fibroids by hysteroscopy rarely results in uterine perforation. After resection of myomas, the lining of uterus may appear concaved, inward-protruding, or irregular. The excessive traction from the surrounding normal uterine muscle fibers of the large myomas may cause poor contraction of uterus. After removal of myomas, if TCRE is performed in the irregular and poorly contractile uterine wall, uterine perforation may occur easily.

11.3.1.2 Adenomyosis

Adenomyosis is developed by growth of the endometrium from the basal layer to myometrium, within which the ectopic endometrium is embedded. Endometrium in the myometrium is distributed diffusely or focally, causing reactive hyperplasia of muscle fibers and fibrous tissues, which makes the uterus enlarged evenly or unevenly. On ultrasonography, the uneven enlargement is often seen to be significantly thicker in posterior wall than in anterior wall, and it can also be significantly thicker in anterior wall than in posterior wall. If the lesion is intensified locally, the contour of uterus will be irregular, and its image on ultrasonography is similar to that of uterine fibroids, but no clear capsule, which is the difference between adenomyosis and myomas. On routine ultrasonography scan, there are always no abnormalities revealed in atypical adenomyosis. When the cutting depth of TCRE reaches myometrium, the strong echogenic band formed by the electrical thermal effect on muscular fibers may last 15 min. When endometrium invades diffusely or focally into myometrium, forming adenomyosis, even though the cutting depth has arrived at myometrium, different durations of strong echogenic band produced by the electrical thermal effect on the muscular fibers and endometrial tissues may disappear rapidly or intermittently due to the invasive endometrial tissues in the myometrium (Fig. 11.19). This ultrasonography is different from the strong echogenic band formed after TCRE in patients without adenomyosis and is easy for monitoring physician to mistakenly believe that excision is not deep enough. At the same time, if the operator discovers the endometrial tissues reappear in the resected myometrial surface and there is old bleeding and a honeycomb structure, he will also believe that the resection has not reached the desired depth. During the operation, when adenomyosis is encountered, repeated cutting may very easily cause uterine perforation. In addition, the uneven distribution of lesions within the myometrium may cause the uterus to contract unevenly and change under the electrical thermal effect. The ultrasonography shows that the local thickening of the uterine wall may transfer from one uterine side wall to another along with the surgical process. If the operator sees the uterine wall locally swelling but ignores the uneven and changing features of uterine contraction and repeats cutting on the swelling site, uterine perforation may occur easily.

11.3.1.3 Placenta Residues

When decidua is poorly developed, the residual placenta may adhere to the uterine wall and cannot shed by itself, thus placenta adhesion is formed. If uterine decidual layer is developed poorly or missing, the placental villi may be directly implanted into the myometrium, forming placenta accreta. Either partial placental adhesions or partial placental implantation can affect the normal contraction and restoration of the uterus. Old placental adhesions and implantation may cause irregular vaginal bleeding after delivery or miscarriage. The ultrasonography shows residual placenta as uneven echogenic mass protrudes into uterine cavity. At the site of uterine wall where adhesion or implantation occurs, inflammatory cells are infiltrated, granulation tissue grows, and the fibrous scar is finally formed. Under ultrasonography, it shows locally strengthened echoes. The adhered or implanted uterine wall is hard while the surrounding normal wall is relatively soft. When hysteroscopic wire loop is used to resect the old adhesive tissues or implanted placental tissues in the uneven hardness muscle wall, it is likely to cause uterine perforation. If the placenta is implanted into deep muscle wall, when deep lesion is resected, there is higher probability of uterine perforation.

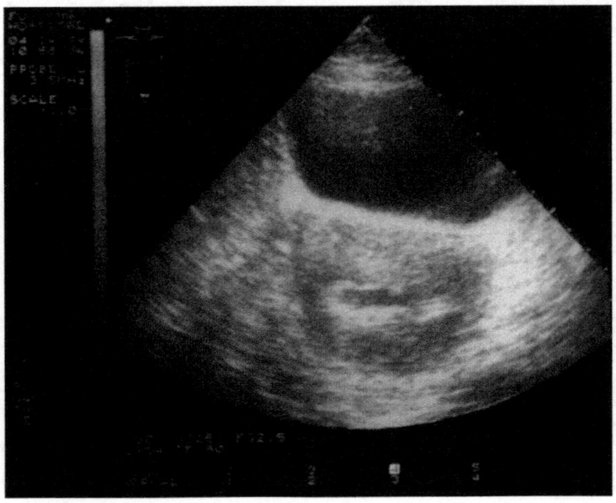

Fig. 11.19 The strong echogenic band formed in the lining of uterus appears to disappear intermittently

11.3.1.4 Intrauterine Retention and Embedment of Fetal Bones

Intrauterine retention of large fetal bone may lead to infertility, but generally may not cause changes in the structure of the uterine wall. If a fetal bone fragment is embedded in the uterine wall, a rejection reaction in local uterine wall will develop, followed by the inflammatory cell infiltration, wrapping of fibrous tissues, and finally hyaline change of the surrounding tissues, which leads to hard texture and poor elasticity of local tissues. Ultrasonography reveals spotty or patchy high echoes within the muscle wall, and heterogeneous moderate echoes in its surrounding tissues. If the fetal bone is embedded deep in the uterine wall, hysteroscopic resection with wire loop will be prone to cause perforation. If multiple fetal bone fragments are more intensively embedded in one side of uterine wall, this may cause local uterine wall to be soft and hard staggered structure. After hysteroscopic wire loop is used to incise the endometrium and the myometrium to expose the fetal bone, even the curette used to scrape off the fetal bone in the muscle wall will be prone to cause uterine perforation.

11.3.1.5 Severe Intrauterine Adhesions

Severe intrauterine adhesions may cause extensive adhesions and stenosis of uterine cavity, even atresia. The synechia tissue has a hard texture, while normal myometrial tissue is relatively soft. When the probe or cervical dilator penetrates the obliterated uterine cavity, if too much force is used or the direction of introduction deviates from the uterine cavity, the probe or cervical dilator may penetrate the softer myometrial tissues after passing through the synechia tissues, leading to uterine perforation or partial perforation. If it is a partial perforation, a false passage may be created in the uterine wall. If both the ultrasonography physician and the hysteroscopic operator do not detect the trauma to the uterine wall and continue to operate in the false passage, uterine perforation will result.

11.3.1.6 Old Injuries in the Uterine Wall

Different kinds of intrauterine procedures such as curettage, induced abortion, and diagnostic curettage may cause uterine perforation or partial perforation in cases of improper operation. If uterine perforation occurs, its clinical symptoms will be significant; therefore, it can be managed in time after clinical or ultrasonographic diagnosis. If it is partial perforation or smaller perforation, clinical symptoms may not be typical and difficult to find clinically. When ultrasonography in combination with hysteroscopy is performed in examining the old injuries induced by partial uterine perforation, the ultrasonography reveals a wedge-shaped defect in the local uterine wall. The muscle wall where old injuries occur is different from the surrounding normal uterine wall in thickness, hardness, elasticity, which constitutes one of the factors of uterine perforation in hysteroscopic surgery. If it is an old uterine perforation and the injured muscle wall was not repaired, any intrauterine procedures such as preoperative exploration of the uterine cavity with a probe and dilatation of the cervix with cervical dilators, or intraoperative hysteroscopic resection of endometrium or lesions with wire loop, are prone to cause perforation.

11.3.1.7 The Position of the Uterus

The best position for hysteroscopic operation is horizontal position (median). Most anterior or posterior uterus may turn to a horizontal position at surgery due to the traction on cervical forceps. As for a small number of uteri which are anteverted, anteflexed, or extremely retroverted, and concomitant with pelvic adhesions, the position of uterus is more fixed and the traction on the cervical forceps cannot change its position. At surgery, the detection of uterine depth with a probe, dilation of cervix with cervical dilator, and the insertion of hysteroscope may cause trauma to the uterine wall due to the introduction of instruments into uterine cavity at an improper angle, and uterine perforation may occur in serious cases. In particular, among the patients who have undergone hysteroscopic surgery due to intrauterine adhesions, the anteverted or retroverted uterus increases the difficulty and dangers in the intrauterine operations. Therefore, the position of the uterus is also one of the reasons affecting the safe intrauterine operation.

11.3.2 Sonographic Features of Uterine Perforation

If uterine perforation is caused by improper operation of the probe, the trauma area is small. If there is no irrigation fluid infiltration, ultrasonogram shows no characteristic change. If uterine perforation is caused by cervical dilator, the trauma area is large and ultrasonogram shows the interrupted echoes in the uterine serosal layer. The uterine perforation caused by electrical thermal damage is displayed on ultrasonogram as strong echoes formed by electrical thermal effect throughout the uterine myometrium with interrupted echoes in the local serosal layer (Fig. 11.20). During operation, uterine perforation caused by electrical thermal damage may lead to the irrigation fluid flowing into the pelvic and abdominal cavity through the perforated site, which presents as irregular liquid echo-lucent area on ultrasonographic imaging. If neither the ultrasonography physician nor the operator detects the perforation timely and stops the infusion of irrigation fluid, ultrasonography can only reveal liquid echo-lucent area in pelvic cavity. If the introduction of irrigation fluid is not stopped timely, liquid echo-lucent area between liver and kidney and even between the intestine canals can be visualized.

11.3.3 Intraoperative Monitoring and Uterine Perforation

In order to improve the safety of operation, the doctors who perform hysteroscopy will apply ultrasonography or laparoscopy, or even laparoscopic ultrasonography to preventing uterine perforation. Ultrasonography scan can guide the operation according to the thickness of uterine wall; laparoscopy may prevent the occurrence of uterine perforation according to the change in uterine serosal surface; laparoscopic ultrasonography can combine both advantages, but the equipment has not yet been popularized, so its application is limited. It should be emphasized that hysteroscopic operation relates to many kinds of diseases, so intrauterine and uterine wall abnormalities are often unexpected. The degrees of surgical

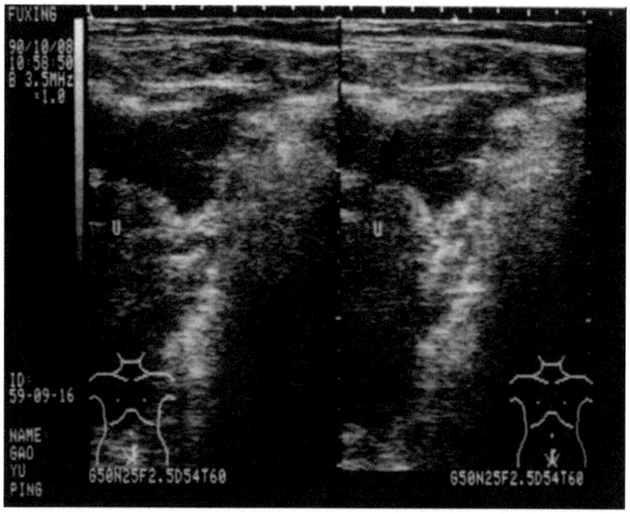

Fig. 11.20 Ultrasonography reveals interrupted echoes of uterine serosa at the site of perforation

difficulties vary because of different etiologies, illness-histories, and the operator's clinical experiences. As for ultrasonography surveillance, uterine perforation is hard to be controlled in cases of difficult intrauterine procedures, sudden changes in structure of uterine wall, high-frequency electricity interference during hysteroscopic resection, and false image created during intrauterine operation with metal devices, even for a very experienced doctor performing hysteroscopic surgery under ultrasonography guidance. As for laparoscopic surveillance, uterine perforation is also hard to be prevented because it can only observe the changes on uterine serosa and may be influenced by its viewpoint. Therefore, regardless of the application of ultrasonography or laparoscopy, the instant occurrence of uterine perforation cannot be completely avoided and sometimes uterine perforation has occurred at the instant the operator sees the crisis of perforation. Once the uterine perforation occurs, what ultrasonography reveals is indirect sign of uterine perforation, such as the interrupted echoes in the serosal layer and liquid echo-lucent areas emerging rapidly surrounding the uterus. Under the guidance of ultrasonography, the effects of medicines like oxytocin and hemostatic on the trauma of uterus may be observed and the operator may be guided to draw fluid from the abdominal cavity. Ultrasonography scan is noninvasive, and its effect is indirect. Laparoscopy can directly confirm uterine perforation and can repair the damaged uterine wall, so it is minimally invasive, and its role is direct.

11.4 The Value of Ultrasonography Guidance in Hystersocopic Surgery

The clinical applications of hysteroscopic surgeries including TCRE, EA, TCRM, TCRS, TCRA, and TCRF provide chances of cure for patients with dysfunctional uterine bleeding or intrauterine benign lesions, especially those who cannot tolerate open surgery. However, since the surgery is performed in the uterine cavity, the surgical field of vision is narrow and the electric energy used in operation has a certain penetration, the possibility of uterine perforation is the main reason for this procedure taking time to become popularized. In the early stages of carrying out this operation, the scholars have advocated laparoscopic monitoring of the operation. However, because laparoscopy cannot indicate the occurrence of posterior uterine wall perforation, uterine perforation still occurs sometimes. In 1987, Lin BL from Japan first used ultrasonography in the guidance of hysteroscopy, which was mainly used in TCRM and TCRS. In 1990, Xia EL from the Hysteroscopy Center of Fuxing Hospital, Capital Medical University, began to use ultrasonography in monitoring TCRE, and then its use is extended to TCRM, TCRS, TCRA, TCRF, and EA, which created the conditions for the development and popularization of hysteroscopic surgery in China.

Transabdominal ultrasonography monitoring can be used in simple hysteroscopic surgeries like endometrial resection and endometrial ablation to achieve the purpose of prevention of uterine perforation. Experienced surgeons did not even need any monitoring methods. However for complex hysteroscopic surgeries, such as removal of intrauterine foreign body embedded in the muscle wall, severe intrauterine adhesions, and large inward-protruding uterine intramural fibroids, it is usually necessary to use ultrasonography or laparoscopic monitoring of surgery. If the patient has a preoperative history of repeat intrauterine operations, damage to the uterine wall and intrauterine adhesions will have developed; if the patient has a history of abdominal surgery, pelvic adhesions will have been formed. Both conditions not only make the surgery more difficult, but also increase the difficulty in transabdominal ultrasonography diagnosis and intraoperative ultrasonography guidance. The trauma to uterine wall includes the uterine perforation and partial uterine perforation, and the perforation site is more common in the uterine fundus. Old uterine perforation can be detected by laparoscopic examination; partial uterine perforation is difficult to be identified by laparoscopy, hysteroscopy, or transvaginal ultrasonography, but ultrasonography in combination with hysteroscopy can improve the diagnosis rate. In addition, the recent development of laparoscopic ultrasonography makes a clearer observation of partial uterine perforation. Laparoscopic ultrasonography can distinguish the strong echo foci in the myometrium from the residual fetal bones and differentiate the strong echo formed after electric cutting of uterine wall from the residual IUD or fetal bone embedded in the muscle wall. For complex hysteroscopic surgery, laparoscopic ultrasonography can improve the diagnosis and indicate the surgical process so as to prevent uterine perforation effectively.

In short, transabdominal ultrasonography is the preferred method in the guidance of hysteroscopic surgery due to its simplicity and non-invasiveness. There is no doubt that the intervention of laparoscopy can detect timely any damage to the uterine wall and even suture the perforated uterus, which can avoid serious consequences and compensate for the absence of transabdominal ultrasonography guidance. The advent of laparoscopic ultrasonography offers chances of the successful complex hysteroscopic surgery. Being an invasive examination, laparoscopy and laparoscopic ultrasonography are not appropriate for regular methods of guidance of hysteroscopic surgery.

Suggested Reading

1. Chen C, Lu Z. Color Doppler diagnostics in obstetrics and gynecology. Beijing: People's Health Publishing House; 1998. p. 25–9. Chinese.
2. Coccia ME, Becattini C, Bracco GL, Bargelli G, Scarselli G. Intraoperative ultrasound guidance for operative hysteroscopy. A prospective study. J Reprod Med. 2000;45(5):413–8.

3. Duan H, Xia E, Duan H. TV hysteroscopic correction of uterine septum: a report of 27 cases. China J Endosc. 1998;4:48–9. Chinese.
4. Gabriele A, Zanetta G, Pasta F, Colombo M. Uterine rupture after hysteroscopic metroplasty and labor induction. A case report. J Reprod Med. 1999;44(7):642–4.
5. Graham O, Cheng LC, Parsons JH. The ultrasound diagnosis of retained fetal bones in West African patients complaining of infertility. BJOG. 2000;107(1):122–4.
6. Homer HA, Li TC, Cooke ID. The septate uterus: a review of management and reproductive outcome. Fertil Steril. 2000;73(1):1–14.
7. Kresowik JD, Syrop CH, Van Voorhis BJ, Ryan GL. Ultrasound is the optimal choice for guidance in difficult hysteroscopy. Ultrasound Obstet Gynecol. 2012;39(6):715–8.
8. Kupesic S, Kurjak A. Diagnosis and treatment outcome of the septate uterus. Croat Med J. 1998;39(2):185–90.
9. Kuzel D, Tóth D, Fucíková Z, Cibula D, Hrusková H, Zivný J. Hysteroskopická resekce submukózních myomů pri abnormálním děložním krvácení: výsledky ctyrleté prospektivní studie [Hysteroscopic resection of submucosal myomas in abnormal uterine bleeding: results of a 4-year prospective study]. Ceska Gynekol. 1999;64(6):363–7. Czech.
10. Letterie GS. Ultrasound guidance during endoscopic procedures. Obstet Gynecol Clin North Am. 1999;26(1):63–82.
11. Lin BA, Xia EL. Gynecological endoscopy. Beijing: People's Health Publishing House; 2001. p. 62–80. Chinese.
12. Salle B, Gaucherand P, de Saint HP, Rudigoz RC. Transvaginal sonohysterographic evaluation of intrauterine adhesions. J Clin Ultrasound. 1999;27(3):131–4.
13. Xia EL, Duan H, Feng L. Application of B ultrasound and laparoscopic monitoring in hysteroscopic operation. China J Endosc. 1998;4:55–6. Chinese.
14. Xia EL, Zhang M, Duan HL. Endometrial resection for menorrhagia: analysis of 400 cases. Chin J Obstet Gynecol. 1997;32:148–51. Chinese.
15. Enlan X. Progress and prospects of hysteroscopic surgery. Chin J Obstet Gynecol. 1997;5:259–62. Chinese.
16. Zhang D, Li Y, Meng Y, Liu J. Application of interventional ultrasound in transcervial resection of myomas. Chin J Med Imaging. 2001;9:268–9. Chinese.
17. Zhang D, Liu J, Meng Y. Ultrasound guidance for hysteroscopic resection of intrauterine foreign body. Chin J Med Imaging. 2000;8:438–9. Chinese.
18. Zhang D, Luo Q, Duan H. Diagnostic value of abdominal ultrasound and hysteroscopy to postmenopausal uterine bleeding. Chin J Med Imaging. 2000;8:30–1. Chinese.
19. Zhang D, Meng Y, Liu J. Application of laparoscopic ultrasonography in gynecologic surgery. Chin J Ultrasonogr. 1999;8:344–6. Chinese.
20. Zhang D, Meng Y, Liu J. Ultrasound guidance for hysteroscopic metroplasty. Chin J Med Imaging. 1998;6:197–8. Chinese.
21. Zhang D, Xia E, Li Y. Interventional ultrasound diagnosis of uterine adenomyosis. Chin J Med Imaging. 1998;6:34–6. Chinese.

Complications of Hysteroscopic Surgery

12

Enlan Xia, Rafael F. Valle, Xiaowu Huang, Dan Yu, Yuhuan Liu, and Baoliang Lin

Complications are defined as clinical incidents that occur and cause the surgery to be suspended of further treatment during operation and which requires a long time of monitoring and further laparoscopic investigation or surgery. In 2000, Propst et al. reported that in 925 cases of hysteroscopic surgery, the occurrence rate of operative complications was 2.7%. These complications involved uterine perforation, fluid overload (≥1 L), hyponatremia, hemorrhage (≥500 mL), bowel or bladder injury, difficulty in dilating the cervix, prolonged hospitalizations, etc. TCRM and TCRS had the greatest probability of complications with fluid overload the most frequent complication. TCRP and TCRE had the lowest probability of complications. Hysteroscopic operative complications, although rare, are serious. There are four kinds of major complications: (1) Hyponatremic encephalopathy, or TURP syndrome, is one of the most serious complications. It has been reported that premenopausal women are 26 times more likely to suffer neurologic sequelae from hyponatremia than postmenopausal women or men. These women will experience permanent brain damage, paralysis, and even death. To prevent this complication, premenopausal women could be transited to postmenopausal state prior to operation by using GnRH agonists in sufficient dosage and for a sufficient length of time to induce menopause. Carter reported on one healthy young woman who suffered irreversible neurological consequences from hyponatremia during a hysteroscopic resection of a small submucous myoma. (2) Uterine perforation (either with or without bowel injury). (3) Hemorrhage. (4) Infection. In addition, there may be air embolism which may cause sudden death. Therefore, to perform hysteroscopic operation safely, the surgeon must be fully aware of various complications and the ways for early detection and preventive treatment.

E. Xia (✉) · X. Huang · D. Yu · Y. Liu
Hysteroscopy Center, Fuxing Hospital, Capital Medical University, Beijing, China

R. F. Valle
Department of Obstetrics and Gynecology, Northwestern University Medical School, Chicago, IL, USA

B. Lin
Department of Obstetrics and Gynecology, Kawasaki Municipal Hospital, Kawasaki, Japan

12.1 Organ Injury

Enlan Xia

12.1.1 Uterine Perforation

Perforation of uterus is the most common complication of hysteroscopic surgery related to operators. If not found in time, large amount of irrigation fluid may flow into the abdominal cavity, and conventional instruments, or instruments with laser or electric energy may pass through the perforated uterus into pelvis and damage adjacent organs. Then uterine perforation will be concomitant with fluid overload, injuries to digestive tract and urinary tract, and rupture of major vessels, causing fatal complications such as peritonitis, fistula, heavy bleeding, and air embolism. Therefore, it is also the most serious complication (Fig. 12.1a, b).

12.1.1.1 Incidence

Perforation of the uterus is the most common complication of hysteroscopic surgery. In 2005, MacNeil reported that its occurrence rate was 1–10%. In literature reviewed over nearly 15 years, the incidence rate was 0.25–25% (Table 12.1), and the average rate was 1.22% (785/64,198).

12.1.1.2 Factors for Occurrence of Uterine Perforation

1. The operator's experience: The occurrence of uterine perforation is obviously related to operator's experience. Most perforations occur in the first stage of operation. For an inexperienced operator, the occurrence of complication is always hard to avoid and difficult to manage.

E. Xia (ed.), *Practical Manual of Hysteroscopy*, https://doi.org/10.1007/978-981-19-1332-7_12

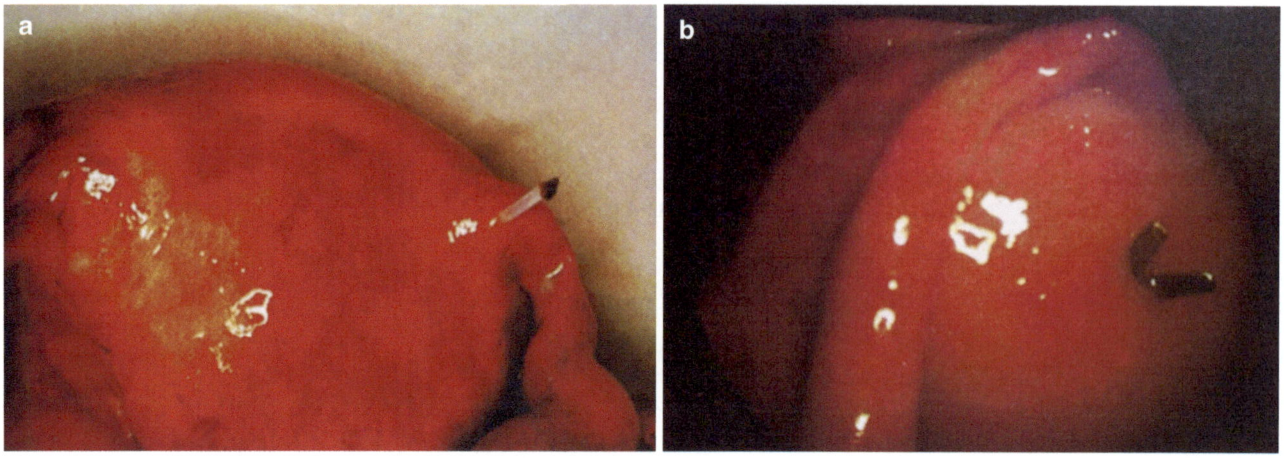

Fig. 12.1 Uterine perforation. (**a**) Caused by laser optical fiber. (**b**) Caused by scissors

Along with the progress in training, experience, and skills, less and less perforations of the uterus occur. Therefore, the operator's training is very important. The future goal is to teach the staff at the operating room how to identify and treat complications so as to ensure that patients may achieve better prognosis.

2. Anatomical location of perforation: Perforation occurs mostly at the site of uterine wall where it is prone to perforate, such as the cornua of uterus and uterine isthmus, and they are the sites most difficult to resect.
3. Active electrodes: The most commonly used electric energy and laser all may elicit accidental injury. Since the long rod device with electricity or laser is used in the narrow uterine cavity, the cooperation of eyes, brain, hands, and feet is very important. Accurate positioning is required, and only when the electrode is accurately in place, the electrode or laser can be powered up. In the currently used electrocoagulation and electroresection, the amount of thermal damage produced by its high-frequency current is beyond computation, and the distance of thermal conduction is unpredictable. The calorific value of denatured enzyme is 57 °C. Undetectable thermal necrosis will occur to the tissues at this temperature, and if it occurs to the bowel or bladder, the consequences are unimaginable. A case who suffered from generalized peritonitis after TCRE was reported. By laparotomy, the uterine wall was seen to be locally pale and degenerated, and there were two perforations in the small intestine. Application of mechanical energy is safer than using laser or electric energy, and cutting with wire loop electrode during TCRE is more likely to cause perforation than with rollerball electrode for electrocoagulation. The operator with less experience may use rollerball electrode to coagulate on the site of easy perforation, but it is not absolutely safe. In the early stage of EA, there were reports about intestine-uterine fistula.
4. Types of surgeries: TCRA and TCRS are more likely to cause perforation than TCRM, TCRE, and TCRP. In the Hysteroscopy Center of Fuxing Hospital, Capital Medical University, 2006 hysteroscopic procedures were performed, of which uterine perforation occurred in eight cases (0.4%), including three cases of intrauterine adhesions. Horak reported that the incidence of uterine perforation was 2.13%. Bukulmez et al. performed hysteroscopic lysis of total corporal synechiae caused by endometrial tuberculosis, and the incidence of uterine perforation was 25%. Roge et al. reported that the uterine perforation rate during TCRS was 5.88%. Data from Choe et al. showed that the uterine perforation rate after TCRS was 5.26%. It can be concluded that septate uterus and intrauterine adhesions are high-risk factors for intraoperative uterine perforation and should be closely monitored and precautions should be taken.
5. Past history of uterine trauma: Itzkowic and Beale reported that in three cases of uterine perforation, two cases had history of cesarean section, and one had curettage. Daniell et al. reported that 1 woman who experienced perforation during hysteroscopic surgery had a history of HEAL. Alford et al. reported that one case of perforation occurred during the second EA. Jansen et al. reported about the data on complications of diagnostic and operative hysteroscopy recorded by 82 hospitals in 1997, which were categorized into two groups: (1) approach related complications being caused by introduction of the instruments; (2) instrument related complications being caused by surgical technique with hysteroscopic instruments. Among 13,600 hysteroscopic procedures analyzed, complications occurred in 38 cases (0.28%).

Table 12.1 Uterine perforation during hysteroscopic surgery

Author	Year	No. of cases	Method	Uterine perforation		Notes
				No. of cases	%	
Peterson et al.	1990	7293	Electroresection	95	1.3	Collected by AAGL
Magos et al.	1991	250	TCRE	4	1.6	–
Pecrutto et al.	1991	54	HEAL	2	3.7	One case of bowel injury
Horak et al.	1992	141	TCRA	3	2.13	All under laparoscopic monitoring
Itzkowic and Beale	1992	–	EA	3	–	Two cases with previous cesarean section and one case with previous D&C
Daniell et al.	1992	64	EA	1	1.56	Previous history of HEAL
Hucke et al.	1992	39	TCRM	1	2.6	Small bowel injury
Choe et al.	1992	19	TCRS	1	5.26	–
Sullivan et al.	1992	–	TCRM	1	–	Suspected during operation and identified laparoscopically. By laparotomy, sigmoid perforation was discovered and was repaired
Hulka et al.	1993	17,298	Electroresection	190	1.1	Collected by AAGL, eight cases of bowel injury
Chen et al.	1994	28	Electroresection	1	3.57	–
Huvar et al.	1994	34	Electroresection	1	2.9	Perforation during TCRM
Hulka et al.	1995	14,707	Electroresection	208	1.42	Collected by AAGL
Osei et al.	1995	90	HEAL	1	1.1	Perforation suspected but was not confirmed at subsequent hysterectomy
Tapper et al.	1995	86	TCRE	1	1.16	–
Hallez et al.	1995	284	TCRM	1	0.35	–
Scottish Hysteroscopy Audit Group et al.	1995	987	Electroresection	10	1	Concomitant with obvious fluid overload
Valos et al.	1996	800	EA	7	0.88	Data from 54 hospitals
Cravello et al.	1996	395	Electroresection	1	0.25	Complicated by intraabdominal bleeding
Cravello et al.	1996	102	TCRE	1	0.98	All were menopausal women
Alford et al.	1996	–	EA	1	–	A second EA
Brian et al.	1996	126	TCRE	2	1.59	No serious consequences
Roge et al.	1996	102	TCRS	6	5.88	–
Leuschner et al.	1997	3144	Electroresection	62	2	Data from 99 hospitals
Mints	1998	70	TCRE	1	1.42	–
Castaing et al.	1999	352	Electroresection	14	4	Three cases complicated by bowel perforation
Toth et al.	1999	1410	Electroresection	1	0.7	–
Bukulmez et al.	1999	12	TCRA	3	25	Laparoscopic suturing
Jansen et al.	2000	2500	Electroresection	19	0.76	–
Schiotz	2001	348	TCRE	3	0.9	One case of investigative laparotomy
Ravi et al.	2001	70	TCRE	6	8.6	One case complicated by bladder and ureteral injury
Cravello L et al.	2002	2116	Electroresection	34	1.61	33 cases received intraoperative treatment with no sequelae
Xia Enlan	2003	3541	Electroresection	16	0.45	Data from five hospitals
Agostini	2003	2116	Electroresection	34	1.61	74 (3.5%)had complications
Parkar RB	2004	463	Electroresection	2	0.43	Both occurred during TCRM
Duan Hua	2005	4171	Electroresection	11	0.26	Seven cases of partial perforation
Boe et al.	2006	386	Electroresection	31	8	Two cases underwent laparoscopy
Shveiky D et al.	2007	600	Electroresection	6	1	The incidence of complication is 3% for an experienced operator

12.1.1.3 Identification of Uterine Perforation

Generally, intraoperative uterine perforations may be detected in the following steps.

1. Once uterine perforation occurs, the irrigation fluid may extravasate into the abdominal cavity. Ultrasonography may reveal that there is free liquid around the uterus preceding the clinical symptoms, or under ultrasonography monitoring a large amount of irrigation fluid is seen suddenly rolling into the abdominal cavity.
2. The site of perforation communicates with abdominal cavity. The peritoneum, the bowel, or omentum are visible under hysteroscope, which can be easily identified by an experienced laparoscopic operator. However, it is difficult for an operator without laparoscopic experience to make a diagnosis accordingly.
3. Under laparoscope, the serosa is seen to be translucent and blistery, and there is bleeding, hematoma, or perforation.
4. The patient is seen suddenly deteriorating, the blood pressure drops and heart rate quickens. Ultrasonography scan reveals a large amount of free fluid in the abdominal cavity.
5. The bowel is clamped out from uterine cavity: The oval forceps are introduced through the site of perforation into the abdominal cavity and clamp the bowel out, or the bowel is herniated into the uterine cavity through the site of uterine perforation and clamped out with the oval forceps.
6. Under laparoscopic monitoring, the fluid is seen to increase sharply in the abdominal cavity.
7. The operator should be alert against the progressive peritoneal expansion.

In the Hysteroscopy Center of Fuxing Hospital, Capital Medical University, 11 cases of uterine perforation were collected. Among 11 cases of uterine perforation, three perforations occurred during diagnostic hysteroscopy with the incidence rate being 0.03% and intrauterine adhesions being the indication; eight perforations occurred during operative hysteroscopy with the incidence rate being 0.4%. Their pathogeneses and treatments are seen in Tables 12.2 and 12.3.

Despite the above tips, some uterine perforations fail to be timely detected but is found only when acute abdominal pain occurs 1–2 days later. Osei et al. suspected the occurrence of perforation in one case during HEAL using laser fiber, which was not confirmed at subsequent hysterectomy. It indicates that assessment of uterine perforation by hysteroscopy is not always accurate.

12.1.1.4 Seriousness of Uterine Perforation

The seriousness of uterine perforation depends on the instrument causing perforation and the time of detection. As long as it is timely detected and treated, there will be no serious consequences.

1. The uterine perforation may be caused by surgical instrument, such as cervical dilator, resectoscope, oval forceps, curette, etc. Valos et al. reported uterine perforation occurred in one case from laminaria, four cases from dilator, and two cases from resectoscope. Magos et al. reported on one case of uterine perforation during the insertion of resectoscope. Serden and Brooks reported one perforation at the time of taking out myoma fragments. These perforations did not cause damage to the abdominal viscera and vessels. If perforation occurs in the beginning, the operation will be compelled to stop; if it occurs during operation, the laparoscopy may do with it; and if there is bleeding at the site of perforation, suturing or coagulating bleeding points can be done under laparoscope, and there is no need of laparotomy for investigation.
2. If perforation is from wire loop electrodes or laser optical fiber, it can injure the organs adjacent to uterus, such as the bowel, bladder, large blood vessels, ureter, etc., and laparotomy is needed immediately for investigation. If perforation occurs when rollerball electrode is used for electrocoagulation, electrical thermal damage can affect other adjacent organs, such as bladder and bowel. Several days later, the postoperative symptoms like diarrhea, fever, hematuria, and pain may appear.

12.1.1.5 Treatment of Uterine Perforation

First, look carefully for the site of perforation and decide on the treatment scheme. If there is uterine fundal perforation, the peritoneum, omentum, or small intestines will be visible. Since the myometrium in the uterine fundus are thick and there are relatively fewer blood vessels, there will be less bleeding, and oxytocin and antibiotics can be used under observation. The irrigation fluid into abdominal cavity may be extracted by puncture of posterior fornix and generally

Table 12.2 Occurrence and treatment of uterine perforation in three cases of diagnostic hysteroscopy

No.	Indications	Perforation instrument	Clinical manifestations	Treatment
1	IUA	Probe	No	Cured by oxytocin and antibiotics
2	IUA	Probe	Lower abdominal pain	Cured by oxytocin and antibiotics
3	IUA	Curette	Severe lower abdominal pain and generalized peritonitis 48 h later	Cured by laparotomy and hysterectomy

Table 12.3 Occurrence and treatment of uterine perforation in eight cases of operative hysteroscopy

No.	Process of the operation	Perforation instrument	Clinical manifestations	Treatment
1	TCRE with deep cutting on left cornu	Wire loop electrode	Shock. Ultrasonography reveals a large amount of fluid in abdominal cavity	Cured by oxytocin and antibiotics
2	TCRE with deep cutting on the fundus	Wire loop electrode	Peritoneum is visible under hysteroscope	Cured by oxytocin and antibiotics
3	TCRM for a submucous myoma of 7.2 cm. Too deep cutting caused sigmoid perforation of 1.8 cm	Wire loop electrode	Severe lower abdominal pain	Cured by laparotomy, subtotal hysterectomy, and repairment of bowel
4	TCRM for an inward-protruding intramural myoma of 5.4 cm, and with a narrow cavity	Wire loop electrode	Uterine injury and bleeding are discovered under laparoscope	Cured by laparotomy and hysterectomy
5	TCRA for intrauterine adhesions with a narrow cavity	Needle electrode	Ultrasonography reveals irrigation fluid into the abdominal cavity	Cured by oxytocin and antibiotics
6	TCRA and TCRF for intrauterine adhesions and fetal bone retention	Wire loop electrode	Enhanced light transmittance of uterine wall and partial uterine perforation are visible under laparoscope	Cured by oxytocin and antibiotics
7	TCRE for DUB and adenomyosis. Too deep cutting caused 1 cm injury at the bottom of bladder revealed by laparotomy	Wire loop electrode	Hysteroscopy reveals omentum majus tissues and ultrasonography reveals irrigation fluid into the abdominal cavity	Cured by laparotomy, total hysterectomy, and repairment of bladder
8	TCRA and TCRF for intrauterine adhesions and fetal bone retention	Wire loop electrode	Uterine fundal perforation is visible under laparoscope	Cured by bipolar electrocoagulation for hemostasis

there are no serious consequences. The perforations in uterine side wall and in the isthmus of the uterus are risky, which might cause damage to the uterine vasculature, so laparotomy is needed immediately for exploration. If perforation is not clear, laparoscopy shall be performed even though the general physical condition is normal, in order to observe whether there is bleeding and its sources. Bleeding at the site of perforation can be arrested by laparoscopic bipolar electrocoagulation, and for larger perforation, suturing is needed. Choe and Baggish reported that a small perforation of the uterus was caused by hysteroscopic resection of uterine septum with the Nd-YAG laser, and no treatment was required.

If the patient has 24-h pain after operation, a comprehensive examination shall be conducted, and if uterine perforation is suspected, laparoscopic exploration shall be promptly performed.

12.1.1.6 Prevention of Uterine Perforation

1. Ultrasonography and (or) laparoscopic monitoring: During ultrasonography monitoring, the heat from laser vaporization and electric cutting may cause the basal muscle tissue to dehydrate, forming a strong echo. When the strong echo reaches the serosal layer, it indicates that continued cutting at this site will induce uterine perforation. Laparoscopy is used for observation of changes in the uterine serosal surface, such as the enhanced light transmittance in local uterus and the blisters in the serosa, which is indicative of impending perforation of uterus. There were eight cases of uterine perforation analyzed in the Hysteroscopy Center of Fuxing Hospital, Capital Medical University, all of whom had been monitored by ultrasonography and (or) laparoscopy during operation, but perforation could not be completely prevented. Loffer believed that the role of laparoscopic and ultrasonography monitoring during operation was limited. Shalev et al. reported 128 women who underwent hysteroscopic surgery under ultrasonography guidance. No occurrence of intra- or postoperative complications including perforation was discovered. So it was believed that hysteroscopic surgery for intrauterine pathologies under ultrasonography guidance could avoid the application of unnecessary laparoscopy.
2. Operational problems: When there is unclear field of vision, hysteroscopic electrode must not be powered up. When cutting during TCRE, the depth of cutting must be well controlled. When activated during EA, the rollerball or vaporizing electrode must keep rolling. During TCRM, if the myoma is large, it may fully fill uterine cavity, which leads to a narrow visual space. When it is difficult to pull back the wire loop, the electrified wire loop is easy to injure the muscle wall opposite to myoma, causing perforation. The expansive growth of myoma stretches and thins the muscle wall adjacent to the edge of the myoma, and if the wire loop electrode used for resection of myoma slides here, it is also easy to cause perforation. The uterine fundus in some septate uteri are saddle-shaped, hence TCRS is likely to cause perforation in the fundus, and laparoscopic monitoring can be somewhat helpful. TCRA is most likely to cause perforation of the uterus, which is generally due to the narrow and small uterine cavity, and its occurrence may be reduced if carefully operated using a resectoscope with small outer sheath diameter (7 mm), under monitoring of ultrasonography, and by experienced doctors.

12.1.1.7 Long-Term Prognosis of Uterine Perforation

With the widespread application of operative hysteroscopy, the long-term complications have appeared gradually. In combination with the literature reported, ten cases of pregnancy after hysteroscopic surgery had uterine rupture (Table 12.4) in recent years, which included five cases after TCRS, two cases after TCRA, and one case after TCRM. Among them, 6 women had a history of uterine perforation during hysteroscopic surgery and uterine rupture occurred at the site of previous perforation scar in late pregnancy. It is worth noting that two cases having no previous uterine perforation also had uterine rupture in late pregnancy. Both cases had relatively weak uterus, including one having a history of uterine perforation caused by IUD placement and another having a history of repeated curettage. It indicates that the uterus after operative hysteroscopy has obstetric risk of uterine rupture.

12.1.2 Injury to Adjacent Organs Induced by Uterine Perforation

The most common injury to adjacent organs induced by uterine perforation is intestine injury, accounting for 2.25% of uterine perforation (14/622). More perforations occur in the colon and rectum and extremely rare in the small intestine. When perforation is discovered during operation, laparoscopic suturing can be performed. When perforation of the colon occurs, due to the extremely complex bacterial groups in colonic contents, in order to avoid the contamination of the abdominal cavity, the abdominal cavity should be thoroughly rinsed after intestinal suturing, and the drainage tube is placed in the abdominal cavity or the intestine is placed by exteriorization. Those perforations not discovered during operation may develop peritonitis within days after operation. Therefore, those who have uterine perforation should require close observation in the hospital for a few days. Bladder injury occurs occasionally with urinary leakage. Due to the urine being bacteria-free, if suturing is done in time, the patient may have a good prognosis. Laparoscopy can detect and determine the injuries to pelvic organs, but is not abso-

Table 12.4 Uterine rupture in pregnant patients after hysteroscopic surgery

Author	Year	No. of cases	Past history of surgery		Pregnancy outcomes
			Types	Perforation	
Creinin et al.	1992	1	TCRS	Yes	Term birth of twins by cesarean section, with a 7 cm defect in the uterine fundus identified
Halvorson et al.	1993	1	TCRS	No	Uterine rupture during pregnancy after surgery
Howe	1993	1	TCRS	Yes	Uterine rupture at 33 weeks of gestation, leading to neonatal death
Yaron et al.	1994	1	TCRM	Yes	Acute abdominal pain at 33 weeks of gestation and uterine rupture was detected
Lobaugh et al.	1994	1	TCRM	No	Preterm cesarean section, with a 3.5 cm × 3.5 cm perforation revealed in the uterine fundus
Gurgan et al.	1996	1	TCRA	Yes	Severe abdominal pain at 36 weeks of gestation, followed by cesarean section. A 2 cm break at the original site of perforation in the uterine fundus was detected
Tamnous et al.	1996	2	TCRS	Yes	Uterine rupture during pregnancy
			TCRA	No	Uterine rupture during pregnancy
Gabrele et al.	1999	1	TCRS	Yes	Uterine rupture during induction of labor with PGE_2
Chokri et al.	2000	1	TCRS	No	Uterine rupture during pregnancy

lutely reliable. Sullivan et al. reported that a 31-year-old woman was suspected of uterine perforation during TCRM for a pedunculated myoma. An uterine perforation was revealed under laparoscopy, but sigmoid perforation was identified by laparotomy, both of which were repaired in consequence. So they believed that laparoscopy was not sufficient in evaluating all injuries caused by perforation.

12.1.3 Large Vessel Injury Following Uterine Perforation

There has been a case report that the injury to the aorta, the external iliac, and internal iliac vessels can cause hemoperitoneum, leading to sudden death, and also case report about the injury to the mesentery and sacral vessels. If the injury to uterine blood vessels happens, there will be rapid bleeding and formation of hematoma, which can move the uterus to the opposite side.

12.1.4 Other Injuries

Valos et al. reported the formation of false passage during cervical dilatation in six cases (Fig. 12.2). There was also a case report on tearing of posterior fornix due to the unsmooth cervical dilation.

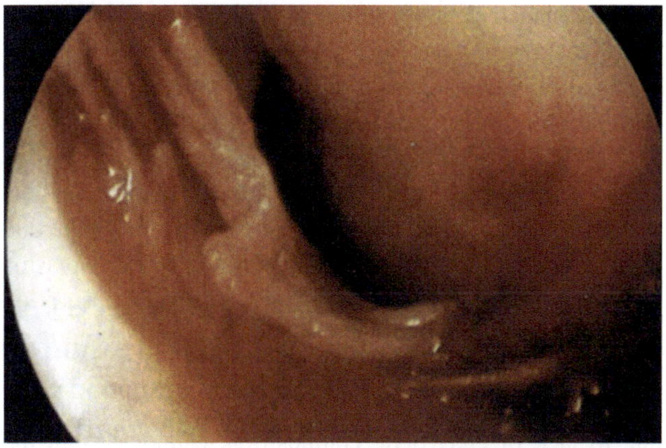

Fig. 12.2 Formation of false passage induced by hysteroscopy (The hysteroscope penetrates into the muscle wall and the false passage is produced. The normal uterine cavity is at lower left of the false passage)

12.2 Fluid Overload

Rafael F. Valle, Enlan Xia, and Xiaowu Huang

With the development of endoscopic equipment and improvement of operative instruments, operative hysteroscopy has developed rapidly in the past 20 years. Even if the bleeding disorders cannot be fully treated by blind intrauterine operation and require hysterectomy, it now may be treated effectively in a minimally invasive environment. In the early 1980s, new techniques such as resectoscope utilized the high-frequency electric energy source in hysteroscopic operation, which provides an economical, practical, and simple way in the clinical treatment of intrauterine diseases. For intrauterine operation, different hysteroscopic instruments require different low-viscosity liquid media in irrigating uterine cavity, and the media can be electrolyte or electrolyte-free fluid. However, the fluid distention media may provide a good field of vision in irrigating the uterine cavity, and meanwhile, it brings potential dangers to patients. In some of the more complex operations like endometrial resection and resection of broad-based or inward-protruding myoma, the long-time exposure of open vessels in endometrium and myometrium to the distention media during operation can cause large amounts of low-viscosity fluid absorption, resulting in fluid overload. The use of fluid without sodium ion may also cause pulmonary edema and hyponatremia. This issue has caught the attention of endoscopic doctors and preventive measures against this complication have been taken, and positive and correct treatment has been administered to the symptomatic patients.

12.2.1 Physiology of Low-Viscosity and Electrolyte Fluid

Clinically, when non-gastrointestinal tract is used for fluid replacement (such as intravenous infusion), the plasma osmotic pressure must be maintained between 280 and 300 mOsm/L. Most intravenous fluids contain substances maintaining plasma osmotic pressure. Electrolytes are the main substances to maintain the osmotic pressure in electrolyte fluids, but in electrolyte-free fluids, such as glycine, sorbitol, and mannitol, these substances will soon be metabolized in the vessels, causing a decrease in overall level of plasma osmotic pressure, thus leading to fluid overload.

In electrolyte solutions such as Ringer's lactate, saline, and 5% glucose with normal saline, sodium, chloride, and bicarbonate ions can maintain the overall level of plasma osmotic pressure. Even if there is excessive fluid absorption in some extent, patients may not present with pulmonary edema and hyponatremia. However, electrolyte-free solutions, such as 1.5% glycine, 3% sorbitol, and 5% mannitol, due to lack of electrolyte composition, cannot sustain the overall level of plasma osmotic pressure. Therefore, the early accumulation of fluid in the microcirculation can induce pulmonary edema and hyponatremia.

1.5% glycine, a non-electrolyte distention medium, being a sterile, nonpyrogenic, and low-permeability solution, is widely used in transurethral resection of the prostate. The osmolarity of this fluid is 200 mOsm/L. Ammonia and oxalate in its degradation products may cause mental disorder, and oxalate can also form deposits in the kidney in the form of crystalline.

Three percent sorbitol is also a kind of non-electrolyte distention medium, electrically nonconductive, and with osmolarity 165 mOsm/L. Being reduction of glucose, sorbitol may form carbon dioxide and water in the body and is excreted by kidneys.

Five percent mannitol is inert fluid with an osmolarity of 270 mOsm/L. It has a diuretic effect, which helps to rid the body of excess fluid absorption. Six to 10% of mannitol absorbed into the body is involved in metabolism, and the part without being metabolized is excreted by the kidneys. Although mannitol has half-life of only 15 min in the plasma, as a permeable material, there is possibly an increase in plasma volume when in use.

In the late 1970s and early 1980s, the high-viscosity liquids were commonly used as distention media in hysteroscopic surgeries, such as 32% dextran or Hyskon solution. Compared with low-viscosity liquids, this kind of fluid is viscous and has a poor flowability in the uterine cavity and cannot produce a clear vision during surgery in the absence of equipment with continuous irrigation, so currently it has been less used clinically. However, due to its high viscosity and less amount of return flow used in uterine irrigation, only a small amount of uterine distention media is needed to complete the operation, so it can also be chosen as special distention media. However, we must pay attention to the stronger permeability of high-viscosity liquids. When the intrauterine operation is implemented for a longer time, the decrease in the amount of outflow of the uterine irrigation fluid means an increase in the amount of absorption by the body. When this high-viscosity liquid enters the blood circulation, the plasma osmotic pressure may be increased and pulmonary edema may be induced. When in vivo absorption volume is more than 500 mL, it may also cause dysfunction of coagulation factors, thus leading to heavy bleeding and abnormalities of fibrinogen, coagulation factor V, coagulation factor VIII, coagulation factor IX, and VIII-Von Willebrand factor. At this time, about ten times of the amount of dextran absorbed retains in the capillary through osmotic absorption. What needs to point out is that the relative molecular weight of dextran is greater (>70,000) and cannot be filtrated by the kidneys. Moreover, it has a half-life of 6–7 days in blood circulation. Once fluid overload occurs and application of diuretics is invalid in its correction, only blood dialysis therapy can be taken.

12.2.2 Fluid Overload and Dilutional Hyponatremia

Not all hysteroscopic surgery must be performed with high-frequency electricity. The mechanical operation under hysteroscope or the surgical operation with laser as energy source is also widely used clinically. In this kind of surgery, there is no intervention of electricity, so we need not exclude the presence of conductor in the distention media. Therefore, it is better to choose the electrolyte media in irrigation of uterine cavity, such as Ringer's lactate, normal saline, and 5% glucose saline. Although the presence of electrolyte in this type of fluid is relatively less risky in causing water intoxication, excess absorption may still lead to fluid overload. Thus a close intraoperative monitoring must be conducted in the amount of inflow and outflow of irrigation fluid. When the in vivo absorption volume is more than

1.5–2 L, diuretics should be used immediately to prevent pulmonary edema (Tables 12.5 and 12.6).

When the distention fluid is used in irrigating the uterine cavity, attention must be paid to the following factors: (1) intrauterine pressure should be controlled below 100 mmHg and not exceed the level of mean arterial pressure (MAP); (2) the operating time should be controlled in no more than 1 h; (3) the excessive resection of uterine myometrial tissues should be avoided.

Although hysteroscopic fluid pump can control the intrauterine pressure, still special attention should be paid to the changes in the intrauterine pressure in the surgical treatment of lesions in the muscle wall. If the depth of myometrial resection is 3–4 mm, the amount of irrigating fluid into the blood vessels will increase along with an increase in intrauterine pressure. At this moment, the intrauterine pressure must be controlled below 100 mmHg, the amount of inflow and outflow of irrigation fluid should be accurately recorded, and the surgical treatment should be terminated as quickly as possible (Table 12.7).

In hysteroscopic surgery, the balance of fluid can be maintained by measuring the inflow and outflow of the distention fluid in a variety of ways. For example, 1% of ethanol is put into the distention fluid, and the ethanol content in the collected outflow fluid is measured through a special breath analyzer, thus in vivo absorption volume can be indirectly reasoned out. However, the accurate amount of fluid absorption cannot be calculated using this method, especially the fluid into the tissue space, which can only act as a method for auxiliary monitoring.

Table 12.5 The content and energies of sodium chloride in electrolyte media (approximate values)

Solutions	Energies (cal)	Na^+ (mmol/L)	Cl^- (mmol/L)
0.45% sodium chloride	–	77	77
5% glucose with 0.45% NaCl	170	77	77
10% glucose with 0.45% NaCl	340	77	77
Normal saline(0.9% NaCl)	–	154	154
5% glucose with 0.9% NaCl	170	154	154
10% glucose with 0.9% NaCl	340	154	154
3% sodium chloride solution[a]		513	513
5% sodium chloride solution[a]		855	855

[a]Hypertonic solution, which is not generally used in intravenous injection

Clinically, fluid overload usually occurs in the use of electrolyte-free liquid for irrigation and distention of uterine cavity. Therefore, during operation using this type of distention media, it is very important to detect continuously the concentration of electrolyte in blood, especially the concentration of blood sodium. Currently, the microcomputer-controlled testing equipment can be used to monitor various blood biochemical indexes while the operation is being performed. Using this method, only a small amount of blood can help to understand the levels of electrolyte, especially the content of sodium ion, and the results can be displayed in 2 min. This type of equipment is applicable to the monitoring of operative hysteroscopy, which not only can provide the levels of plasma electrolyte during operation, but also can guide the treatment of dilutional hyponatremia.

Compared with electrolyte distention media, the threshold value for water intoxication of electrolyte-free media is relatively low. It is very important to record accurately the amount of inflow and outflow of the fluid during operation. When the fluid deficit of inflow and outflow is ≥1 L, the concentration of electrolyte (Na^+) in blood should be immediately detected, and diuretics should be given and intravenous rehydration of solution containing electrolyte, the anesthesiologist should cooperate actively with the full range of intensive care, especially for patients under general anesthesia, such as the measurement of oxygen saturation and esophageal temperature, and the monitoring of various vital signs and urinary output (Tables 12.8, 12.9, and 12.10).

12.2.3 TURP Syndrome

TURP syndrome is a series of symptoms and signs caused by large amount absorption of electrolyte-free irrigation fluid when monopolar hysteroscopic resection is performed. Patients first present with slow heart rate and increased blood pressure, then followed by decreased blood pressure, nausea, vomiting, headache, blurred vision, anxiety, mental disorders, and lethargy. These symptoms are induced by increased blood volume, dilutional hyponatremia, and decreased plasma osmotic pressure. If diagnosis and treatment are not

Table 12.6 The energies and the contents of ion in balanced solution

Solutions	Energies (cal)	Na^+ (mmol/L)	Cl^- (mmol/L)	K^+ (mmol/L)	Ca^{2+} (mmol/L)	Lactate
Lactated Ringer's solution (HARTMANN'S)	9	130	110	4	1.5	28
5% glucose-containing Ringer's solution	179	130	110	4	1.5	28
5% glucose + 20 KCI Ringer's solution	179	130	129	24	1.5	28
5% glucose + 40 KCI Ringer's solution	179	130	149	44	1.5	28

Table 12.7 Factors influencing uterine distention media into blood circulation

Type of media: CO_2, Hyskon solution, low-viscosity distention media
Intrauterine pressure > mean arterial pressure; depth of myometrial resection >4 mm
Operating time >1 h
Amount of irrigation fluid consumption
Hysteroscopic operation without fluid outflow channel or without continuous fluid pump
Blockage of fluid outflow channel
The irrigation fluid cannot flow out due to the tight cervical orifice
Type of surgery: incision exceeds the middle layer of myometrium, reaches serosa, or forms partial uterine perforation
Excessive uterine fluid irrigation

Table 12.8 Prevention of fluid overload during TCRM

Discussion with the anesthesiologist: the complexity of operation, intraoperative venous infusion, and complications that may occur
Epidural anesthesia should be considered for patients at high risk
Indwelling catheter for monitoring of the urinary output
The fluid deficit between inflow and outflow should be accurately estimated
Observation of decompensation signs, including the change in vital signs, decrease in oxygen saturation, drop in temperature (taken by esophageal probe), and abnormal ECG
The fluid deficit of inflow and outflow is >800 mL: detecting serum electrolyte (Na^+) level, and comprehensively considering the operative process and the patient's condition
The fluid deficit between inflow and outflow is >1000 mL: if the serum electrolyte (Na^+) level decreases, the signs of functional metabolic disorder appear, and the operation cannot be completed in a short period of time, the operation should be terminated

Table 12.9 Relationship between the absorption of 1.5% glycine and the decrease of serum sodium levels

Fluid deficit (mL)	Decreased value of serum sodium (mmol/L)
<500	0–2.5
=500	4–5
=1000	8–10
=2000	16–20
>2000	>20

Table 12.10 Treatment of fluid overload during operative hysteroscopy

Decreased value of serum sodium (mmol)	Fluid deficit (mL)	Principles of treatment
0–5	≤500	No need for treatment
8–10	=1000	Close monitoring (testing serum sodium and using diuretics)
16–20	=2000	Stop the operation (dynamic observation of serum sodium, sodium replacement, and diuresis)
>20	>2000 (warning value, may cause death)	ICU (consultation, sodium replacement, and diuresis)

timely, convulsions, cardiovascular failure, or even death may also occur. This syndrome has been familiar to doctors of urology and anesthesiology. In hysteroscopic operation, for female patients, especially in the period, the functional disorders of ATP enzyme in the brain may cause a drop in their own capacity to regulate drainage, so if the timely diagnosis and treatment are not given at the onset of TURP syndrome, its risks and the likelihood of death will increase apparently. However, because the human brain itself is able to regulate body fluid balance and prevent the excess fluid absorption and hyponatremia, which manifests clinically as slow development, usually the symptoms may appear after 48 h. Therefore, clinically, doctors should be wary of hyponatremia, and once symptoms appear, positive treatment should be implemented. Notably, one must be careful of intravenous infusion of sodium, and remember the intravenous infusion of sodium should not be given fast and in a high concentration so as not to cause a temporarily low osmotic pressure inside the brain, which may transfer the brain interstitial fluid to the blood vessels, causing brain tissue dehydration, thus leading to brain damage.

In acute period of hyponatremia, the replacement of sodium at a rate of hourly increase in osmotic pressure by 1–2 mOsm/L can alleviate the symptoms, but the total increased plasma osmotic pressure must not exceed 12 mOsm/L within 24 h. In addition, the patients still need special care like continuous monitoring of plasma electrolyte concentrations and urinary output. Usually, the hypertonic saline solution should not be used in the correction of hyponatremia, but replacement of normal saline will be extremely effective, and clinical symptoms can generally recover within 12–24 h.

Based on the above reasons, if it is estimated that more tissues will be excised during operation, the regional block anesthesia should be chosen to keep the patient awake so that the doctor may discover timely the early symptoms of water intoxication such as obnubilation, tremor, nausea, and headache.

In the corrective treatment of patients with hyponatremia, the blood sodium concentration should not be made to return rapidly to normal in a rush. The serum sodium levels should be just maintained in such an extent that no serious secondary complications may occur.

Five cases with TURP syndrome had been treated in the Hysteroscopy Center of Fuxing Hospital, Capital Medical University, with the occurrence and treatment seen in Table 12.11.

12.2.4 Prevention of TURP Syndrome

1. The preoperative treatment of uterine cervix, endometrium, and uterine myomas contributes to the reduction of irrigating fluid absorption.

Table 12.11 Occurrence and treatment of TURP syndrome in five cases

No	Operations	Duration (min)	Fluid volume/deficit (mL)	Clinical manifestation	Serum sodium at the end of surgery (mmol/L)	Treatment
1	TCRE for DUB	40	21,000/1500	Lethargy, apathy, dullness	130	Intramuscular injection of furosemide 20 mg and quick intravenous injection of saline 1000 mL. The serum sodium returns to normal 16 h later
2	TCRM for 6.4 cm pedunculated submucous myoma	100	32,000/2000	Lethargy, apathy, dullness, facial swelling, headache	122	Intramuscular injection of furosemide 20 mg twice and quick intravenous injection of saline 1500 mL. The serum sodium returns to normal 24 h later
3	TCRM for 4 cm inward-protruding intramural myoma with total resection (100%)	80	6000/no result	Lethargy, facial swelling, dizziness, headache, nausea	125	Intramuscular injection of furosemide 20 mg, quick intravenous injection of 3% sodium chloride 100 mL, and normal saline 1000 mL. The serum sodium returns to normal 15 h later
4	TCRM for 4.4 cm inward-protruding intramural myoma with 80% resected	55	4000/2000	–	128	Quick intravenous injection of furosemide 20 mg and normal saline 1000 mL. The serum sodium returns to normal 4 h later
5	TCRM for two 3 cm submucous myomas resected completely, and one 4.4 cm inward-protruding intramural myoma with 20% resected	45	6000/2500	Dysphoria, pink frothy sputum, chest rales, heart rate 138 times/min, nasal flaring, indifference, oxyhemoglobin saturation 84%	105	Quick intravenous injection of furosemide 20 mg, 10% sodium chloride 40 mL, and deslanoside 0.4 mg. Facemask supply of oxygen and inhalation of 50% ethanol. The serum sodium is 125 mmol/L 4 h later and reaches 130 mmol/L after another 4 h following intravenous injection of furosemide 20 mg

2. The low-pressure irrigation should be taken on the premise of a clear vision.
3. To the patients without contraindications, intracervical injections of a dilute pituitrin solution (pituitrin 10 u + 80 mL normal saline) at 3 and 9 o'clock positions around the cervix can cause strong uterine contraction which maintains at least 20 min. Corson et al. reported that intracervical injection of vasopressin resulted in a threefold decrease in fluid absorption when compared with placebo group.
4. Excessive resection of uterine myometrial tissues should be avoided. The intrauterine pressure should be controlled below 100 mmHg and should not exceed the mean arterial pressure (MAP) levels; the operating time should not exceed 1 h. If the operation lasts more than 30 min, an intravenous injection of furosemide 20 mg can be given.
5. The fluid deficit in irrigation fluid should be closely monitored. If it amounts to 1000–2000 mL, the operation should be ended as soon as possible; if >2000 mL, the operation must be immediately stopped, and electrolyte concentration in blood should be detected.

12.2.5 Treatment of TURP Syndrome

1. If the postoperative serum sodium concentration is between 130 and 140 mmol/L, no treatment is needed.
2. If the postoperative serum sodium concentration drops to 120–130 mmol/L, intravenous injection of furosemide 10–20 mg can be administered and the intake of liquid should be limited. The amount of fluid into and out of the body should be carefully recorded, and the serum sodium concentration is detected once every 4 h until it exceeds 130 mmol/L.
3. If the serum sodium concentration is below 120 mmol/L, the treatment with hypertonic saline is required and careful care is taken.
4. For the patients with overt encephalopathy, no matter how much the serum sodium concentration is, the treatment with hypertonic saline shall be prescribed.
5. Hypertonic saline therapy: It can be seen in detail in Sect. 9.2 of Chap. 9 about the treatment of hyponatremia.

Kumar and Kumar reported that, during hysteroscopic surgery, procedures were stopped for 10 min with no intervention of glycine irrigation, which reduced the fluid absorption by 67% (38.75–85.81%). It might be due to blood clots sealing the open blood vessels which prevented further absorption of distending medium.

12.2.6 Monitoring Device for the Prevention of Fluid Overload (Portable)

During hysteroscopic operation, fluid overload often occurs in the resecting or destroying large areas of myometrial tissues, for example, resection of submucous myoma with broad pedicle, resection of the endometrium, incision or excision of large uterine septum, large areas of intrauterine adhesions, etc.

Table 12.12 Scoring criteria for high-risk fluid overload prior to EA

Score	0	1	2	3
Parous women	Yes	–	–	no
Endometrial pretreatment	Yes	No	–	–
Length of uterine cavity (cm)	<8	8	9–10	>10
Coexistence with submucous myoma	No	–	–	Yes

Table 12.13 Scores for high-risk fluid overload during TCRE (fluid absorption > 1 L)

Minor risk	0–2
Moderate risk	3–7
Severe risk	≥8

In this type of operation, if the amount of fluid absorption is more than 1 L, specialized scoring criteria can be used for the assessment of fluid overload. Molnar et al. developed a set of scoring criteria for patients with intraoperative fluid absorption of more than 1 L during TCRE (Tables 12.12 and 12.13), in which the final overall score is a very important index. Through assessment of this score, it is very helpful for the physicians to understand the overall situation of patients. It is worth stating that the operation in a larger uterine cavity makes it possible to prolong the operating time and if it is resection of larger submucosal myoma, not only the operating time is longer but also the deep layer of uterine muscle wall may be resected, and operation difficulty can be increased even without endometrial pretreatment, A long-term use of GnRH-a can constrict the endometrium and myometrial vessels and reduce the amount of intraoperative irrigation fluid absorption.

12.2.7 New Operative Device: Imitated Bipolar System

The advent of operative electrode in the electrolyte solution has attracted the great attention of endoscopic doctors. This electrode is not true bipolar coagulation electrode, but its principle is similar to that of bipolar coagulation system. The electric current flows from one side to the other and the tissues between the electrodes are destroyed by a form of vaporization through increased electric current density when operated, like the Versapoint system, which is currently used in clinical practice. It is worth mentioning that in hysteroscopic operation with the electrolyte liquid as distending medium, if there is no monitoring of the liquid, there will be excessive electrolyte fluid absorption, and it is still possible to induce pulmonary edema. And when a lot of electrolyte solution is in use and no attention is paid to monitoring the urinary output, the patients may excrete large volumes of hypertonic urine with sodium and potassium, resulting in the so-called desalination. Meanwhile, the water accumulated in the microcirculation not only can induce pulmonary edema, but also may cause delayed hyponatremia. In patients with the isotonic saline solution in use, this will eventually lead to delayed hyponatremia and even death. Therefore, when electrolyte liquid is used in distending uterine cavity with continuous monitoring system, the amount of inflow and outflow of irrigation fluid must be closely monitored, and the amount of fluid absorption may be calculated according to the fluid deficit. If the amount of distention media absorption has reached the limiting value, operation should be immediately stopped. To the patients who have electrolyte fluid absorption over 1.5–2 L, diuretic therapy should also be timely administered.

12.2.8 Conclusion

There is no doubt that great progress has been made in hysteroscopic techniques during the past 20 years, and a large number of gynecological doctors have been constantly improving their operating skills, and constantly developing and broadening new areas of treatment with operative hysteroscopy. The fantastic development of technology has greatly driven the endoscopic manufacturing enterprise to develop and produce hysteroscopy instrument with superior performance and its corollary equipment, particularly the advent of the hysteroscope with continuous irrigation and the hysteroscopic resectoscope makes intrauterine electrosurgery possible. Clinical practice has proved that low-viscosity liquid has become the main distention media in operative hysteroscopy due to its advantages of good circulation and clear vision. The electrolyte media can be used with any intrauterine operation except with intrauterine electrosurgery. However, regardless of the use of electrolyte or electrolyte-free media, prolonged intrauterine operation may cause excessive fluid absorption, and excess absorption of low-viscosity electrolyte-free solution at early stage can induce pulmonary edema and hyponatremia. Therefore, during the operation, it is very important to monitor closely the volume of inflow and outflow of uterine distention media, and the volume of liquid inflow and outflow must be recorded accurately so as to avoid the fluid deficit to be increased. At the same time, anesthesiologists, nurses in the operating room, and the operators should cooperate closely and always be alert to avoid excessive fluid absorption. Once the sign of the fluid overload appears, early diagnosis and timely treatment should be given so as to avoid serious consequences. The specialized standard procedures for hysteroscopic surgery should be established, which is of great significance for early diagnosis and proper treatment of intraoperative fluid overload so as to avoid severe complications.

12.3 Intra- and Postoperative Bleeding

Dan Yu

Bleeding complication of hysteroscopic surgeries is defined as hemorrhage with the amount being much more than that of normal blood loss during operation and in early or late postoperative period. Some measures are necessary to be taken to control the bleeding.

In the early stage of hysteroscopic applications, intra- and early postoperative bleeding was reported as the second most common complication of hysteroscopic surgeries, just following uterine perforations. Jansen et al. made a summary of 13,600 procedures of both hysteroscopy and hysteroscopic surgeries. The results showed that bleeding complication occurred in 22 procedures (0.16%), with all being associated with perforations. Agostini et al. studied 2116 hysteroscopic surgeries and found hemorrhage in 13 (0.61%). According to the data collected by the Hysteroscopy Center of Fuxing Hospital, Capital Medical University, between January 1995 and January 2001, there were 1747 cases of hysteroscopic procedures, in which, bleeding complications occurred in five (0.29%). It was believed that, in all types of hysteroscopic surgery, the highest risk of bleeding occurred in the resection of uterine myomas, especially inward-protruding intramural myomas, with the occurrence rate reaching 2–4%. It was followed by endometrial ablation with electroresection, Nd-YAG laser, or rollerball coagulation. In addition, bleeding might also occur during the resection of septum, or in cases with injuries to cervix and lower part of the uterine cavity.

Along with the development of hysteroscopic technology, the occurrence rate of bleeding complications in routine hysteroscopic surgeries decreased significantly. But in some difficult hysteroscopic surgeries, such as operations on cornual pregnancy, cervical pregnancy, scar pregnancy following cesarean section, cervical myoma, and inward-protruding intramural myoma, etc., the occurrence rate of intra- and postoperative bleeding was higher.

12.3.1 Factors and Mechanisms of Intra- and Postoperative Bleeding

12.3.1.1 The Cutting Depths of TCRE, TCRA, and TCRP Reaching the Uterine Vascular Layer

The uterus is a highly vascular organ with rich blood vessels in its muscle wall. Its vascular layer is located 5–6 mm underneath the endometrial layer, which is approximately 1/3 of the uterine muscle wall with more blood vessels running through. The cutting depths of TCRE, TCRA, and TCRP are usually above the vascular layer; therefore, massive bleeding may occur when cutting reaches this layer.

12.3.1.2 Bleeding from the Myometrium of the Fundus Because of the Injury of the Vessels When TCRS Reaches the Fundus

When the resection of TCRS gets to the fundus, heavy bleeding will be caused if the cutting is so deep that it reaches the vascular layer of the fundus, or perforation of the fundus occurs and damages the vessels of the uterine walls.

12.3.1.3 Bleeding from the Base of Myomas with Large Size and Special Location

In hysteroscopic resection of large myomas, type II submucous myomas, inward-protruding intramural myomas, or intramural myomas adjacent to the uterine cavity, because of their deep location, large vessels are easily damaged when the resection approaches or reaches the base of the myomas. In such occasions, hemostasis will be very difficult. If the myometrial wall at the base of myomas is very thin, it will be difficult to contract after resection, so the bleeding will be hard to stop. If the resection penetrates the walls at the base, which leads to perforation, massive bleeding will be caused.

Another type of myoma with special locations is cervical myoma. If the resection on cervical lateral walls is too deep during the procedure, the descending branch of uterine artery will be damaged and massive bleeding will be caused.

12.3.1.4 Bleeding from the Damaged Vessels During Hysteroscopic Operations on Intrauterine Conception in Special Locations

Intrauterine conceptions in special locations include cornual pregnancy, cervical pregnancy, cesarean scar pregnancy, etc.

In women with cornual pregnancy, the uterine cornu is enlarged due to conception. The myometrial walls in this area are filmy and plenty of blood supply, with large vessels visible. So when performing the hysteroscopic operation, it is easy to damage the vessels or get perforations, which will lead to massive bleeding.

The cervix mainly contains connective tissues, with little musculature and filmy cervical walls, therefore the cervical contractility is poor, and the opened vessels are not easy to be occluded. Therefore heavy and continuous bleeding is very prone to occur during hysteroscopic operation on cervical pregnancy.

In cases with scar conceptions following cesarean section, the probability of injury, which occurs during hysteroscopic procedures, is very high because of the filmy walls at the location of conception. Moreover, it is difficult to stop the bleeding because of the poor elasticity and low contractility of the myometrium here.

In addition, in cases with the implantation of pregnant tissues into uterine myometrium, uterine perforation or poor contraction of the uterus may occur when the hysteroscopic resection is too deep, which leads to massive bleeding.

12.3.1.5 Disturbed Contractility of the Uterus with Adenomyosis or Myoma

Uterine adenomyosis or myomas can disturb uterine contractility. Poor contractility will lead to more bleeding during intraoperative and early postoperative period when hysteroscopic surgery is performed for intrauterine lesions.

12.3.1.6 Uterine Arteriovenous Fistula

Uterine arteriovenous fistula is the connection of vascular walls between uterine artery and veins resulting from abnormal development and proliferation of uterine vessels due to congenital or acquired factors, which causes the formation of fistula. Massive bleeding might happen when arteriovenous fistula in uterine walls is damaged by hysteroscopic operations.

12.3.1.7 Coexisting with Relevant Medical Diseases

If the patients are concurrent with dysfunctional diseases of blood coagulation, such as blood disease, severe damage of liver function, hepatocirrhosis, renal failure, and long-term usage of anticoagulant after cardiac valve replacement, etc., the bleeding during hysteroscopic procedures is difficult to control.

12.3.2 Intraoperative Bleeding of Hysteroscopic Surgeries

12.3.2.1 Identification of Intraoperative Bleeding

For experienced gynecologists, massive intraoperative bleeding during hysteroscopic operation is very rare. The conventional cutting depth of TCRE is 2–3 mm underlying endometrium, which is deep enough to resect the full endometrial layer except for adenomyosis and not cut larger vessels. The vessels underneath the endometrium are so small that the resection cannot cause bleeding. Secondly, when cutting, the blended cutting current involving coagulation current may close small vessels. Furthermore, the irrigation fluid may cause an increase of intrauterine pressure, which forms the forces against vascular bleeding, thus reduces the bleeding from veins. So operations of TCRE can be regarded as “non-bleeding” procedures.

When compared with TCRE, the amount of blood loss during TCRM increases greatly. Yu et al. carried out a study and found that the volume of intraoperative bleeding was at an average of 17 mL in hysteroscopic resection of small myomas (no more than 3.5 cm in diameter), and at an average of 64 mL in large myomas (more than 3.5 cm in diameter).

A great volume of bleeding may take place when the vascular layer is damaged due to too deep resection into myometrium during hysteroscopic operations; when bigger vessels are damaged by electroresection in cases with big and deep myomas in uterine cavity; when the vessels in uterine walls are damaged due to the perforation of the uterus occurring during hysteroscopic operations; when large vessels are damaged by resection in the uterus with plenty of blood supply due to conception; when uterine arteries at the level of lateral cervical walls are damaged and perforation occurs during operations in cases with cervical lesions; and when the fistula is damaged by hysteroscopic operations in cases with uterine arteriovenous fistula.

Too much bleeding from the cutting surface during operations can seriously interfere with the vision of operating field, which results in difficult operation of hysteroscopy and prolongation of operating time. The occurrence rates of other complications such as fluid overload are increased correspondingly.

12.3.2.2 Prevention and Treatment of Intraoperative Bleeding

1. Pretreatment of medication before surgery: Many studies indicated that pretreatment of medication before hysteroscopic surgeries may lead to a thinning of endometrium and decrease of vascularizations, which reduces intraoperative bleeding. Cooper et al. held that preoperative administration of oral contraceptives or GnRH analog for a period can reduce intraoperative bleeding and help to correct anemia.
2. Intraoperative coagulation for hemostasis: For intraoperative bleeding of hysteroscopic surgery, if there is evident bleeding point, the bleeding vessels can be coagulated by electric loop electrode, and rollerball or roller cylinder electrode with the coagulation current at 40–60 W, therefore the bleeding can be arrested effectively (Figs. 12.3 and 12.4). If there is bleeding from fibroid, electrocoagulation of blood vessels may be performed around the pseudocapsule (Fig. 12.5).
3. Hemostasis by increasing the pressure distending the cavity: By increasing the distending pressure appropriately, the irrigating fluid in uterine cavity can press on the denuded broken vessels in uterine cavity to achieve hemostasis. However, it should be noted that increase of the distending pressure of the cavity and the rapid absorption of irrigating fluid can result in dilutional hyponatremia.

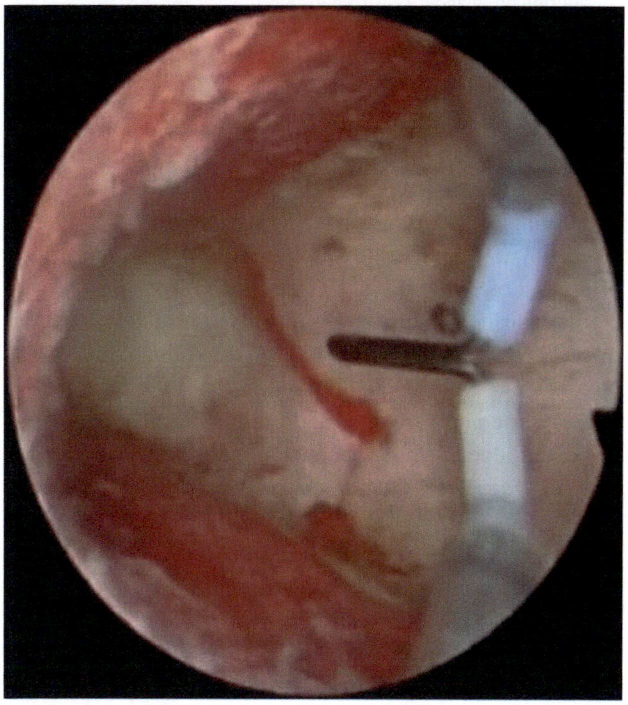

Fig. 12.3 When the resection reaches the uterine fundus during TCRS, active bleeding is visualized and coagulated by hysteroscopic needle electrode

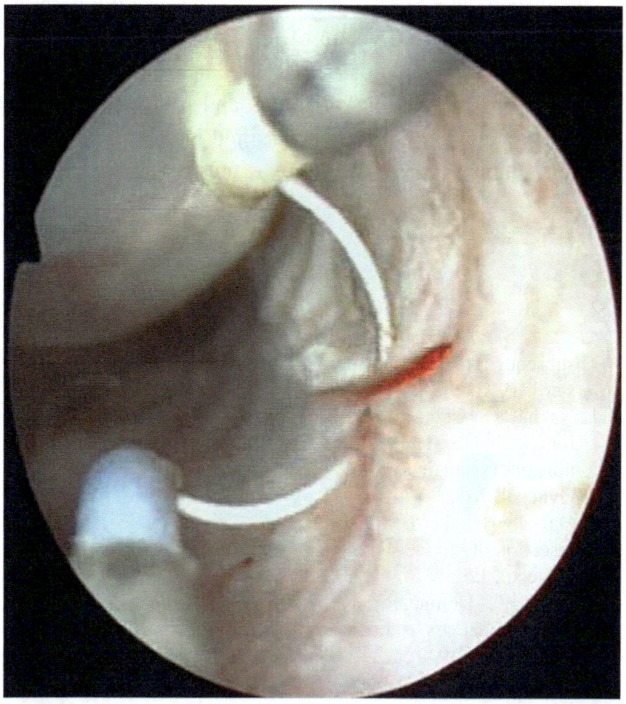

Fig. 12.4 An active bleeding is seen on lateral wall of uterine cavity during TCRE, which is stopped by coagulation with loop electrode

4. Decrease of intrauterine pressure, inspection of bleeding point, and coagulation to stop bleeding at the end of surgery: Before the operation comes to an end, the distending pressure may be reduced, which permits the visualization of bleeding from broken vessels on the surface of the cavity. Thus it is necessary to search for the bleeding points carefully under hysteroscopy and then to coagulate for precise hemostasis in conditions of pulse arterial bleeding (Figs. 12.6 and 12.7).
5. Intrauterine balloon tamponade for hemostasis: If there is blood oozing at the end of the operation, especially in operations with myoma resections, a Foley catheter can be inserted into uterine cavity and 10–30 mL of fluid may be introduced into the balloon. The balloon is kept in place for 6–8 h, which can generally achieve a good hemostasis (Fig. 12.8). In the Hysteroscopy Center of Fuxing Hospital, Capital Medical University, there have been three cases of intraoperative bleeding irresponsive to general management, and their treatment is seen in Table 12.14.
6. Prophylactic uterine artery occlusion: Laparoscopic uterine artery occlusion (LUAO) is a procedure that bilateral uterine arteries are blocked via laparoscopic approach. For hysteroscopic surgeries with high risk of bleeding, LUAO may be performed prior to the hysteroscopic operation, which can reduce the flow of blood, decrease intraoperative bleeding, make the vision of operations clear, lower the difficulty of procedures and improve its safety.

   According to different routes and regions of uterine artery occlusion, LUAO is classified into high and para-uterine approaches to occlude the uterine arteries. LUAO with high approach starts from lateral pelvic wall (the anterior leaf of the broad ligament), dissects the internal iliac, and then identifies the origin of the uterine artery,

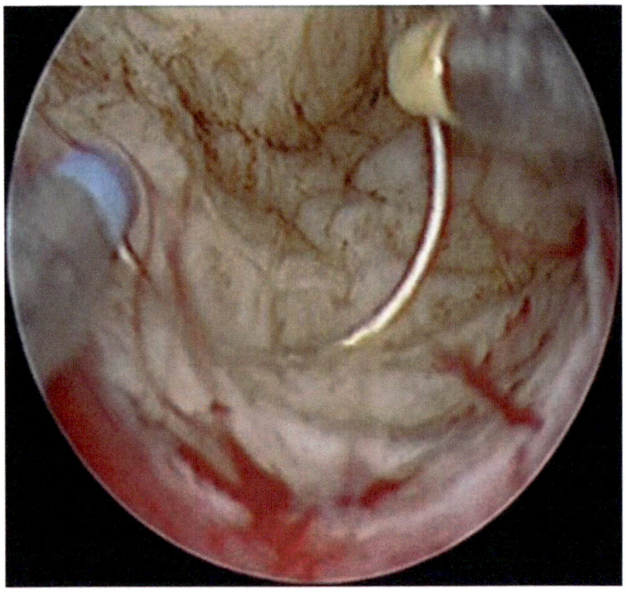

Fig. 12.5 During hysteroscopic resection of myomas, active bleedings are seen on cutting surface of pseudocapsule

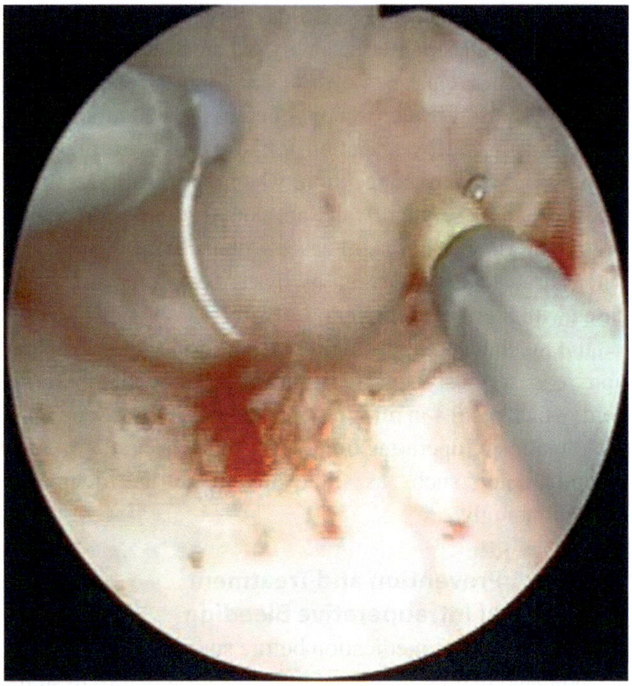

Fig. 12.6 Before the end of TCRE, the pressure in uterine cavity is reduced to inspect the cutting surface. Active bleedings are seen on posterior wall and coagulated by loop electrode

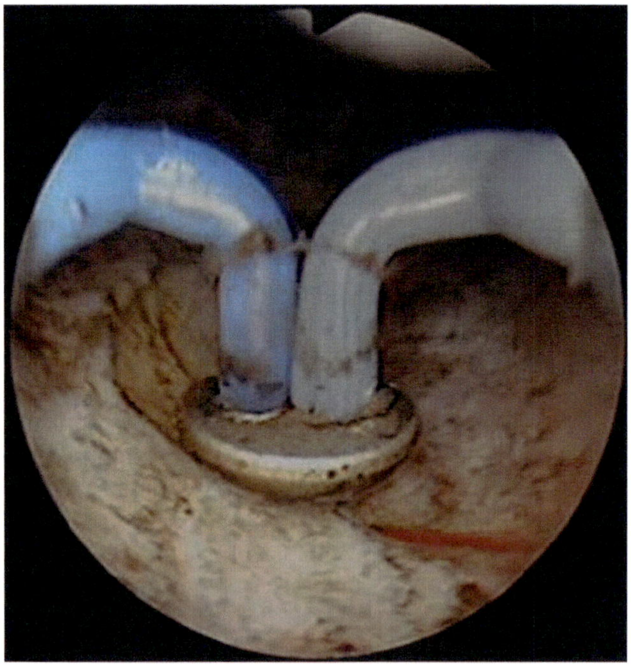

Fig. 12.7 Before the end of TCRE, the surface in uterine cavity is inspected. The active bleedings on posterior wall of uterus are coagulated with PlasmaButton vaporization

which is the first branch of internal iliac. The origin of uterine artery is isolated and coagulated to achieve occlusion. This approach is also named lateral approach and is a more commonly used occlusion method in clinic so far. LUAO with parauterine approach opened the anterior or posterior leaves of broad ligament at the level of cervical internal os, the uterine artery is identified, isolated, and then coagulated for occlusion.

7. Management of original medical diseases: In patients with concurrence of dysfunctional diseases of blood coagulation, some measures should be taken pre- or post-operatively to decrease the occurrence of bleeding complications. These measures include the management of the original medical diseases, evaluation and adjustment of the coagulation functions, preparation of intraoperative medications, and close monitoring during operations.

12.3.3 Bleeding in the Early Postoperative Period

12.3.3.1 Identification of Bleeding in the Early Postoperative Period

It is generally believed that bleeding in the early postoperative period refers to the hemorrhage within 1 week after hysteroscopic surgeries. Isaacson reported that postoperative bleeding was more common than intraoperative bleeding because of the drops of intrauterine pressure at the end of hysteroscopic procedures. In fact, there is a small volume of bleeding after almost all of the hysteroscopic surgeries. It was reported that the amount of postoperative blood loss was about 30 mL within 24 h after TCRE and was 20–80 mL within 24 h after TCRM. In conditions that the amount of bleeding is still significant at the end of procedures, some measures of hemostasis should be taken before the patients leaving the operating room.

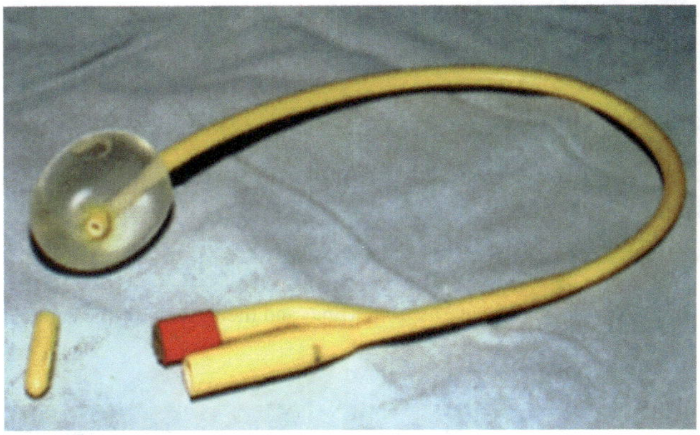

Fig. 12.8 The balloon of a Foley catheter is inflated to achieve tamponade of the cavity

12.3.3.2 Prevention and Treatment of Bleeding in the Early Postoperative Period

1. Mechanical tamponade with Foley balloon for hemostasis

   Pressing hemostasis by local tamping has been used for a long time in first aid for trauma and surgical operations. Balloon tamponade for hemostasis has been applied in transurethral resection of the prostate and treatment of esophageal varicose. In 1981, Goldrath first introduced the Foley balloon tamponade into the fields of hemorrhage in gynecology and gynecological endoscopic surgery. In a case of laser endometrial ablation with 5% glucose saline as a uterine distending medium, heavy hemorrhage of the uterus was observed when the procedure was coming to an end. After intrauterine insertion of a Foley catheter and balloon inflation with saline injection, the hemorrhage was arrested immediately.

   (a) Mechanisms of Foley balloon tamponade for hemostasis

      Application of Foley balloon tamponade can mechanically compress the uterine walls and press on the opened vessels from cutting surfaces to achieve hemostasis. Through X-ray observation with an intra-balloon injection of a contrast agent, Goldrath also discovered that the shape of the uterine cavity and the shape of the balloon were adapted to each other, and their adaptability depends on the size of the uterine cavity and the size of the balloon, respectively. Goldrath also conducted a research on

Table 12.14 Characteristics and managements of intraoperative bleeding in three cases with hysteroscopic surgeries

No.	Details in operations	Blood loss (mL)	Clinical manifestations	Managements
1	TCRM for a 5-cm broad pedicle submucous myoma with massive intraoperative bleeding. Extremely poor contraction of the uterus at the end of the operation led to ongoing bleeding	700	Dropping in blood pressure	Immediate laparotomy and removal of the uterus
2	At the end of TCRP, the uterus bled without stopping, with poor response to oxytocin	200	(–)	Bleeding stopped after balloon tamponade for 4 h
3	TCRM for a 6.5-cm intramural myoma (inward-protruding extension 30%). Sevent percent of the myoma was resected, with poor hemostasis in the base of the myoma	200	(–)	Bleeding stopped after balloon tamponade for 9 h with 120 mL of blood loss

the possibility of bleeding flowing in reverse through the fallopian tube. He concluded that the intrauterine balloon produced enough pressure to compress on the uterine cornua, and the blood clots might obturate the fallopian tubal ostia. So whatever the conditions are, there was little volume of blood in the interstice of uterine cornua flowing in reverse through the narrowed fallopian tubal canal. From other clinical observations, it was also confirmed that no case of intraabdominal hemorrhage occurred when using balloon tamponade for hemostasis. Foley balloon tamponade for hemostasis is a simple, effective, and low-cost treatment and does not need to conduct special technologies. It has gradually became one of the most commonly used methods for prevention of postoperative hemorrhage.

(b) Procedures of Foley balloon tamponade for hemostasis

- A double channel Foley catheter is applied. One to 3 mL of gas is firstly injected into the balloon to indicate the border between the balloon and the catheter, and then the tip of the catheter above the balloon is cut off with scissors (Fig. 12.9). It should be careful not to cut and break the balloon. Cutting off the top of the catheter above the balloon can make the intrauterine balloon globular, and therefore in close contact with the uterine walls, so the balloon can produce a uniform compression on uterine walls.
- At the end of operation, a Foley catheter is inserted into the uterine cavity. The Balloon is inflated with appropriate amount of sterile saline solution so that it cannot prolapse when it is pulled gently downwards. Vaginal bleeding is observed simultaneously (Fig. 12.10a, b).
- The end of the catheter is connected with a collecting bag to gather and evaluate the intrauterine bleeding.
- The Foley catheter is kept in situ for 6–8 h and removed later.
- Antibiotics are routinely given to prevent infections.

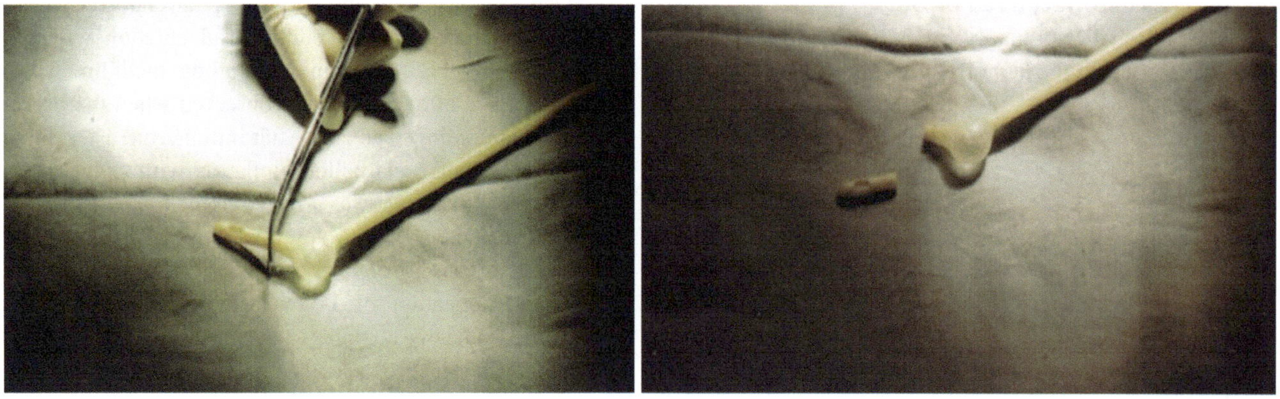

Fig. 12.9 The balloon of a double channel Foley catheter is inflated with 3 mL of a gas to indicate its borderline, and then the tip of the catheter above the balloon is cut off

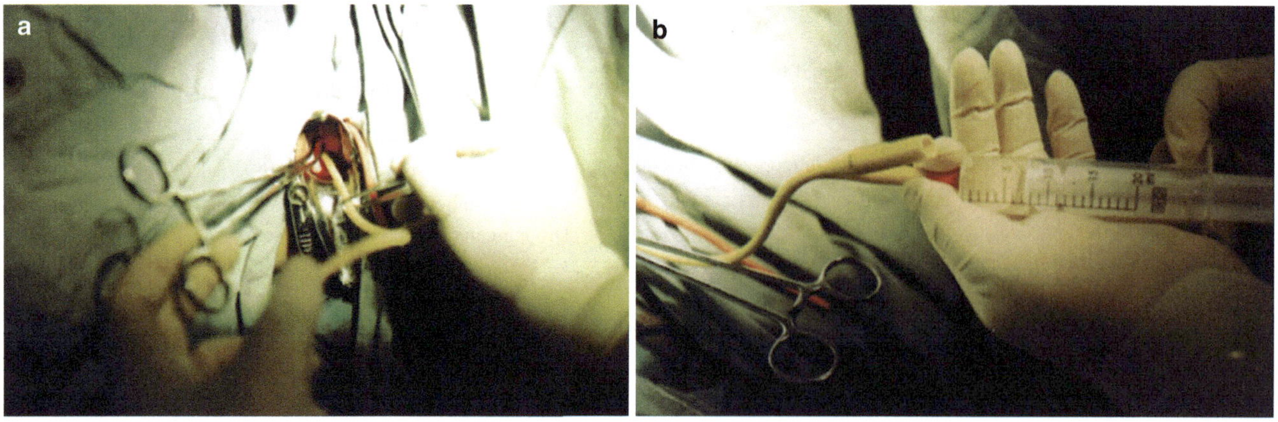

Fig. 12.10 Foley balloon tamponade. (**a**) At the end of operation, a Foley catheter is inserted into uterine cavity. (**b**) The balloon is inflated with sterile saline to achieve hemostasis

(c) Precautions

- The volume of fluid injection into the balloon: The normal capacity of uterine cavity is 5–10 mL. The volume of fluid injection is between 10 and 20 mL based on the volume of the cavity and the size of the myoma. In cases with heavy bleeding due to a larger uterus and bigger myomas, the balloon can be inflated with 15–30 mL of fluid injection. Professor Lin from Japan believed that in cases of hysteroscopic resection of myomas, the volume of fluid introduced into the balloon should be less than the weight of the excised myomas. By ultrasonography scan, the size of the balloon should be smaller than that of myomas prior to surgery (Fig. 12.11a, b). If the balloon tamponade still cannot stop bleeding, it is mostly because of insufficient injection of fluid into the balloon. In this situation, more additional injection or silk suturing of the uterine cervical os may be adopted to increase the intrauterine pressure for hemostasis. In addition, hemorrhage from cervical canal can be compressed by pulling the balloon catheter outward. At the time of withdrawing the balloon catheter, the sutures of cervical os should be removed at the same time.
- Duration of balloon tamponade: In general, the duration of intrauterine balloon tamponade is from 6 to 8 h. Prolonged and high-pressure balloon tamponade may cause avascular necrosis of endometrium or even of uterine walls. The Foley balloon can be completely removed 6–8 h later or removed after graded withdrawing of the fluid in balloon and decreasing of its pressure. In cases of using balloon tamponade, if bleeding still exists in uterine cavity, it can usually be drained away along the vagina or a Foley catheter. When the balloon is kept in situ, if the bleeding gets increased, additional measures may be conducted, such as supplementary injection of fluid into the balloon to increase the intrauterine pressure for hemostasis, suturing of the uterine cervical os with silk sutures applied for hemostasis, or pulling outward of the balloon catheter to increase the pressure on bleeding from cervical canal. There were also reports on myometrial necrosis resulting from prolonged insertion of the balloon, which supported the idea that the duration of balloon tamponade cannot be too long.
- In cases with small amount of bleeding, sufficient hemostasis can be achieved by vaginal insertion of sterile gauze. In cases with larger amount of bleeding, a Foley balloon intrauterine tamponade for hemostasis can be conducted. In cases with a big uterine cavity and heavy bleeding, two balloon catheters can be introduced into the cavity to increase the intrauterine pressures or to compress the upper and lower parts of the cavity separately.

2. Medications for hemostasis

During hysteroscopic surgeries, medications such as vasopressin and prostaglandins are also commonly used for local hemostasis.

(a) Vasopressin (VP)

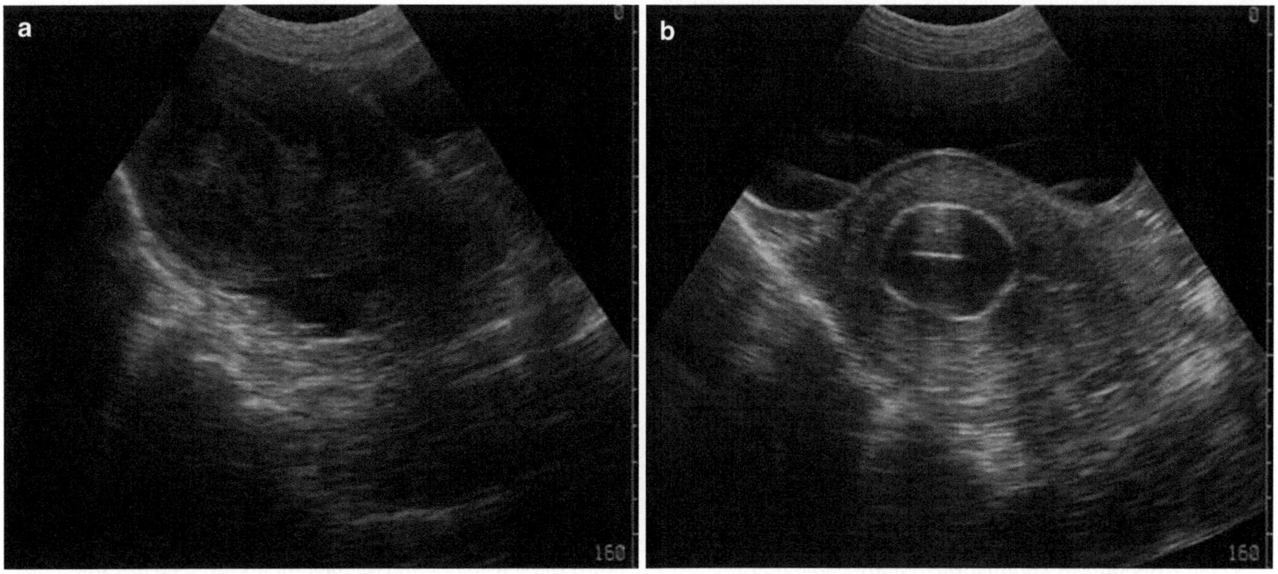

Fig. 12.11 Transabdominal longitudinal ultrasonography scan. (**a**) Before TCRM. The uterus is in anteversion, and a type II submucous myoma is located in posterior wall of the uterine cavity with 4 cm in diameter. (**b**) After TCRM. A Foley catheter is inserted into the uterine cavity, and the balloon is inflated with 30 mL of normal saline

In order to prevent and control acute or massive bleeding, natural or synthetic vasopressin has been used as a vasoconstrictor in gynecologic surgeries for a history of nearly 100 years. Pharmacological doses of vasopressin can cause the contractions of smooth muscles in gastrointestinal tract, uterus, and all vascular beds, especially the muscles in capillaries, arterioles, and venules. However it has weak effect on smooth muscular tissues in large vessels. Vasopressin injection is a water-soluble synthetic vasopressin (8-L-arginine vasopressin) with half-life of 10–20 min. Cervical injection with diluted vasopressin can cause contraction of the uterus for hemostasis. Yet many scholars believed that the administration of exogenous vasopressin could increase the abnormal secretion of antidiuretic hormone induced by the operative stress, which might increase the morbidity of dilutional hyponatremia and exacerbate the symptoms.

Philips et al. carried out a study on the effects of preoperative cervical injection with 20 mL dilute vasopressin solution (0.05 U/mL) or placebo in 106 patients who received hysteroscopic surgeries. The results showed that, in a group of patients receiving cervical injection with vasopressin solution, when compared with that in placebo group, the amount of intraoperative blood loss was significantly decreased, the volume of distending fluid absorption was greatly reduced, and the operating time was largely shortened. Furthermore, there were no significant differences between the two groups of patients in cardiac contractility, blood pressure, heart rate, or rhythm of the heart. However the vasopressin has life-threatening cardiovascular effects and may induce some serious complications, so the indications of its application must be strictly controlled in patients who have endometrial ablation and resection of myoma with the size smaller than 3 cm. Robert et al. studied the effects of preoperative paracervical injection of adrenaline in patients with TCRE. They concluded that it could decrease the amount of intra- and postoperative bleeding and reduced the application of balloon tamponade in the uterine cavity, but the routine use of it was restricted because a few patients developed paroxysmal tachycardia (>110/min).

(b) Prostaglandin derivatives

Some scholars suggested that the administration of misoprostol (prostaglandin E1 analog) orally or rectally could strengthen the uterine contractility and reduce postoperative bleeding.

3. Hysteroscopic examination and coagulation for hemostasis

During the period from 48 to 72 h to 1 week after hysteroscopic surgery, the patient occasionally encounters a sudden heavy bleeding. In this situation, hysteroscopy can be performed to identify the active bleeding on the surfaces in both cervical canal and uterine cavity. Coagulation of these bleeding points under hysteroscopy may achieve an effective hemostasis.

4. Uterine vascular occlusion and hysterectomy

If various methods of hemostasis are ineffective after hysteroscopic surgery, emergency treatments such as uterine vascular occlusion or hysterectomy should be considered. Uterine vascular occlusion mostly includes uterine artery embolization and transvaginal or laparoscopic uterine vascular occlusion. Uterine artery embolization is a procedure of selective blockage of the arteries with different substances to block the blood flow, which is mainly used in acute uterine hemorrhage. Transvaginal uterine vascular blockage is transvaginal ligation of both uterine arteries and ovarian arteries so that the blood flow of the uterus can be reduced to achieve hemostasis. Laparoscopic ligation of uterine vessels coagulates and blocks the uterine arteries under laparoscopy, which decreases the blood flow of the uterus promptly, so that the uterine bleeding can be controlled effectively.

If all of the above treatments of bleeding have failed to achieve hemostasis, transabdominal or laparoscopic hysterectomy can be conducted. With the development of medical technology, a range of conservative therapies can be taken to control the uterine bleeding effectively, which reduces the use of traumatic operations. There were four cases of postoperative bleeding that occurred in the Hysteroscopy Center of Fuxing Hospital, Capital Medical University. Their treatment process is shown in Table 12.15.

12.3.4 Bleeding in the Late Postoperative Period

Sometimes, there are patients who have massive bleeding at 1 week after operation and are referred to hospital again. In addition to intrauterine insertion of balloon catheter, suturing of the cervical os may be applied for hemostasis. Estrogen and antibiotics should be given simultaneously to promote the repair of endometrium and prevent the infections. In clinic, this situation is uncommon. Some patients may have more bleeding at their first menses after operation, and gauze packing is needed to fill the vagina for hemostasis, which is a more common situation. There were two cases with severe late postoperative bleeding that occurred in the Hysteroscopy Center of Fuxing Hospital, Capital Medical University, and both characteristics and managements are seen in Table 12.16. The hemorrhage was related to the application of sodium hyaluronate in the first case and was related to adenomyosis in the second case.

Table 12.15 Characteristics and managements of postoperative bleeding in four cases with hysteroscopic surgeries

No.	Details in operations and postoperations	Blood loss (mL)	Clinical manifestations	Managements
1	TCRS with heavy bleeding observed within 8 h after operation	800	Hemorrhagic shock	Bleeding stopped after balloon tamponade for 8 h and blood transfusion of 600 mL
2	TCRM for inward-protruding intramural myoma, with heavy bleeding observed within 6 h after operation	300	(–)	Bleeding stopped after balloon tamponade for 8 h and blood transfusion of 200 mL
3	TCRE for menorrhagia after heart valve replacement and discontinuation of warfarin. Continuous bleeding could not be stopped within 24 h after operation	1000	Hemorrhagic shock and anemia	Bleeding stopped after hysteroscopic coagulation
4	TCRM for a 5 cm myoma in posterior wall of the cervical canal. An outburst excessive bleeding occurred from the base of the myoma on the fourth day after operation	600	Hemorrhagic shock	Bleeding stopped after blood transfusion and compression with tamponade

Table 12.16 Characteristics and managements of bleeding in the late postoperative period in two cases with hysteroscopic surgeries

No.	Details in operations and postoperations	Blood loss (mL)	Clinical manifestations	Managements
1	Intrauterine injection of 3 mL sodium hyaluronate following TCRM for preventing intrauterine adhesions. An outburst of excessive bleeding occurred on the 11th day with conservative treatment being ineffective	1000	Hemorrhagic shock and anemia	Blood transfusion, laparotomy, and subtotal hysterectomy, with foreign body giant cells in the base of myoma revealed by histological examination
2	TCRE for DUB with adenomyosis diagnosed intraoperatively. Five months later, repeated heavy hemorrhage occurred after carrying a heavy load, with conservative treatment being ineffective	700	Hemorrhagic shock and anemia	Blood transfusion and subtotal hysterectomy. Severe adenomyosis was identified, which reached the serosa in right cornua

12.3.5 Prolonged Bleeding in the Postoperative Period

Very few patients may have prolonged postoperative bleeding, which may be related to inflammatory reactions, poor healings, and granulomatous foreign body reactions in the cutting surface of the uterine cavity postoperation. A thorough curettage may achieve a complete healing. Colgan et al. carried out a study on the healing process of endometrium after hysteroscopic endometrial ablation with rollerball. Findings from uterine specimen within 3 months after operations included acute inflammation, myometrial necrosis, florid foreign bodies, and granulomatous reactions. After 3 months postoperation, persistent granulomatous foreign body reaction and obvious endometrial scarring might be detected from the specimen of the uterus. They concluded that postoperative pathological reaction of hysteroscopic endometrial ablation should be recognized as granulomatous endometritis. There has been a patient with postoperative granulomatous endometritis cured by uterine curettage in the Hysteroscopy Center of Fuxing Hospital, Capital Medical University.

12.4 Infection

Yuhuan Liu

The morbidity of infection after hysteroscopic examination or surgery is very low, just between 0.01 and 2% as reported in the literature. Postoperative infection is associated with many factors, such as disinfection of operating instruments, and whether or not the patients have reproductive infectious disease, body resistance, or application of antibiotic prophylaxis, etc.

12.4.1 Characteristics of Female Genital Organs

The female genital organs are divided into internal genital organs and external genital organs. The internal genital organs communicate with the outside by way of the vagina. The normal vaginal discharge is weakly acidic, which can prevent bacteria from reproduction in the vagina; the glands in the mucosal layer of cervical canal can secrete a small amount of alkaline mucus, forming cervical mucus plug, which has a defensive function. Under normal circumstances, there are a variety of microorganisms in the female vagina, belonging to the endogenous microorganisms; the bacteria community is made up of Gram-positive or Gram-negative aerobes and anaerobes. The common aerobic bacteria include lactic acid bacillus, corynebacterium, non-hemolytic streptococcus, staphylococcus epidermidis, enterococci and Escherichia coli, vaginal Gardiner's bacteria, etc. Anaerobic bacteria include peptococcus, peptostreptococcus, bacteroides fragilis, fusobacterium, and candida as well. The vagina is established in a state of equilibrium with the microflora. When the ecological balance is destroyed by low levels of body immunity, changes in endocrine level, and some external factors (such as tissue damage), the resident flora may become pathogenic bacteria, causing infection. Therefore, endogenous microorganisms in the female lower genital tract are often pathogenic bacteria of the reproductive tract infection.

12.4.2 Factors Causing Postoperative Infection

12.4.2.1 Factors Related to Procedures

During hysteroscopic surgery, the cervical canal is dilated to 10 mm in diameter, which may cause some fibers in cervix to fracture, resulting in an open cervical orifice to communicate the uterine cavity with the outside world. At the same time of the operative procedure, repeat movements and insertion of hysteroscope can bring bacteria flora in the vagina and uterine cervix into the uterine cavity. Application of uterine distention medium may carry pathogens into the pelvic cavity through the fallopian tubes, or into local or blood system through the denuded injured endometrial or muscle tissues, which causes pelvic infection. Boubli et al. reported that in women with normal vaginal sample tests, 25% were found to have infections with pathogenic bacteria in uterine cavity at the end of hysteroscopic surgery. While in women with vaginal sample contaminated, 50% were found to have bacterial infections in uterine cavity. The relative risk of intrauterine bacterial contamination during hysteroscopic operation in women who have vaginal contamination was 8.75.

12.4.2.2 Changes in the Internal Environment of Reproductive Tract

The interference of diagnostic or operative hysteroscopy may cause obvious change and transformation of vaginal microflora. There are not only more bacteria flora species isolated from the vagina than that prior to surgery, but a decrease in positive rate of lactic acid bacillus and a significant increase in positive rate of virulent Escherichia coli and Bacteroides fragilis. Lactic acid is produced by metabolism of lactobacillus and sustains the vaginal pH of 3.8–4.2, which is advantageous to the growth of vaginal endosymbionts but disadvantageous to the growth of bacteria causing bacterial vaginosis, thus maintaining the vaginal health. Surgical wound not only provides an access for bacteria to invade into the body, but also promotes the priority growth and reproduction of virulent potential pathogens in the vagina so as to create favorable conditions for postoperative infection. If postoperative vaginal bleeding or fluid flow sustains in the vagina, the normal vaginal internal environment is disrupted; at the same time the blood is a good bacterial culture medium and is conducive to bacterial growth, resulting in pelvic infection.

12.4.2.3 Factors Related to Instrument

Since hysteroscopic instruments have fine structure, more valves, and narrow channels, which bring difficulties in cleaning, particles and protein materials remaining in the apparatus provide shelter for potentially pathogenic bacteria, and are not easy for disinfectants to infiltrate. Meanwhile, the external cables for hysteroscopy cannot be disinfected with high-pressure steam. The surgical instruments of hysteroscope are directly in contact with genital organs, if sterilization is not achieved, it is extremely easy to cause infection when examination, resection, lysis, and other procedures are performed.

12.4.3 Microbiological Characteristics of Infections After Hysteroscopy

The infections after hysteroscopy are mostly endogenous infection caused by the parasitic potentially pathogenic bacteria in the vagina. Generally, it is a mixed multiple bacterial infection, and different bacteria have synergistic effects. For example, after aerobic bacteria invade the cutting surface and oxygen is consumed, a hypoxia environment is produced, which is helpful for the anaerobic bacteria to multiply rapidly and continue to destroy the deep tissues. The main pathogenic bacteria include aerobes such as Escherichia coli and streptococcus and anaerobes such as peptostreptococcus, peptococcus, and bacteroides fragilis. Anaerobic bacteria are often pathogenic bacteria of deep pelvic infection.

12.4.4 Diagnosis and Treatment of Postoperative Infection

Infection following hysteroscopic operation is commonly mild pelvic inflammation, which is always endometritis or myometritis.

12.4.4.1 Clinical Symptoms

Postoperative temperature may exceed 37.5 °C and continue without any decline. The patients can experience persistent or paroxysmal abdominal dull pain or sharp pain, and peritoneal irritation sign may be detected in severe cases. Vaginal discharge may be increased, being bloody or purulent, and mostly with odorous smells like stinking fish.

12.4.4.2 Physical Signs

Since postoperative infection is often endometritis or myometritis, cervical motion tenderness and uterine tenderness may be detected by vaginal bimanual examination. If there are pelvic peritonitis and/or pelvic empyema, tenderness, rebound tenderness and muscular tension at lower abdomen can be obviously detected.

12.4.4.3 Auxiliary Examination

Blood routine examination can reveal an increase of white cells, with a significant rise of neutrophil granulocyte. Pelvic ultrasonography can help to discover pelvic empyema, and CT or MRI can be applied if necessary. Blood culture and drug sensitivity test should be conducted if bacteremia or septicemia is suspected.

12.4.4.4 Treatment

Since the main pathogenic bacteria of infection following hysteroscopic operation includes aerobe and anaerobe, with anaerobe often being the main pathogenic bacteria of pelvic deep infection, broad-spectrum antibiotics, especially those being very effective in killing the anaerobe, should be applied. Pelvic infection caused by chlamydia, mycoplasma, and fungus also deserves attention. Mild pelvic infection can be cured by oral antibiotics, whereas severe pelvic infection should be treated by intravenous antibiotics. For cases of pelvic abscess, surgical treatment should be considered when medication is ineffective.

12.4.5 Reports of Infections After Operative Hysteroscopy

The literature report on the incidence of infections after operative hysteroscopy varied. Aydeniz et al. reported among 21,676 hysteroscopic procedures in 92 German Hysteroscopy Centers, three cases developed endometritis, and its incidence rate of infection was 0.01%. Perez-Medina et al. reported in 6123 office diagnostic hysteroscopies, three cases (0.05) developed pelvic inflammatory disease. The blood culture was negative and the vaginal discharge culture revealed non-specific bacterial flora. Bracco et al. reported among 253 women undergoing diagnostic hysteroscopy, germs were identified preoperatively in the cervical canal in 35 cases, of which pelvic inflammatory disease developed in two cases (0.79%) and the etiological agent was Chlamydia trachomatis. Maher and Hill reported in 100 cases undergoing TCRE for AUB, two cases (2%) developed secondary infection without any detection of pathogenic bacteria. Vilos et al. reported on 800 women who underwent endometrial ablation, four cases developed endomyometritis (0.5%). Cravello et al. reported on 195 TCRP for hemorrhagic endometrial polyps, with only one case of infection occurred. Propst et al. reported on 925 women who had hysteroscopies, with two cases developing myometritis during TCRM and the incident rate of infection 0.22. Hysteroscopy postoperative infection is generally mild pelvic inflammatory disease, but serious infections also occur occasionally. Mears and Fox reported two cases of infection occurring after diagnostic hysteroscopy for irregular uterine bleeding. One case developed pelvic abscess with septicemia 6 days after diagnostic hysteroscopy, who recovered after 6 weeks of anti-infection treatment. Another case developed right tubo-ovarian abscess 2 weeks after hysteroscopic examination, who underwent abdominal excision via laparotomy. Two cases were confirmed to have a history of chronic salpingitis and were not administered prophylactic antibiotic therapy after diagnostic hysteroscopy. Amin-Hanjani and Good reported that a 47-year-old woman developed pyometra and bacteremia following endometrial resection and ablation for menorrhagia without administration of prophylactic antibiotics. Uterine cervical discharge and blood culture revealed colon bacillus. The patient was cured by placement of an intrauterine drain and intravenous antibiotic therapy. Parkin reported on a 40-year-old woman who had menorrhagia and anemia due to a small myoma in posterior uterine wall, On the second day after TCRE, she experienced diarrhea and shock. Transabdominal exploration found no bowel injury, while blood cultures and peritoneal fluid cultures discovered Staphylococcus aureus. This patient resulted in death on the eighth postoperative day due to multiple system failure and invalid rescue. Li et al. reported that a 42-year-old woman who had renal failure and required renal dialysis had a hysteroscopy for DUB. She experienced abdominal pain after operation. Candida albicans were discovered from the cultures of both a higher vaginal swab and the peritoneal dialysate effluent, which confirmed the diagnosis of fungus peritonitis. They thought it was due to the distension medium carrying the fungus into the peritoneum. McCausland et al. reported three cases of developed ovarian abscess after operative hysteroscopy, all of whom had a past history of pelvic inflammatory disease and were not given prophylactic antibiotics. Two of three underwent TCRP and one case had TCRM. Rullo et al. reported that one uterine perforation occurred in one case during operative hysteroscopy and an abscess of the left parametrium and round ligament occurred after operation. Jeanette et al. reported a case of a woman who underwent a rollerball endometrial ablation. After the procedure, she developed pelvic abscess and a Bartholin's abscess on the fourth day and hepatic abscess on the eighth day. Philips reported on one case who underwent diagnostic hysteroscopy due to menorrhagia and experienced peritonitis following the procedure. Laparoscopy revealed a normal uterus, and peritoneal exudates examination discovered white blood cells without microorganisms. The patient was cured by administration of peritoneal lavage and antibiotics. Yap et al. reported that a 41-year-old woman who suffered from late lupus nephritis and received renal dialysis underwent TCRE due to menorrhagia. Peritonitis was diagnosed one day after operation because of the turbid peritoneal fluid, and intravenous and intraperitoneal injection of antibiotics were applied. The patient then developed septicemic shock and was cured after intensive care and selecting proper antibiotics. Lin et al. reported one case of tubo-ovarian abscess and septic shock which developed following hysteroscopic diagnosis for endometrioma. Golan et al. reported that one case developed sepsis followed by DIC after hysteroscopic removal of conceptive remnants and was cured by resuscitation.

12.4.6 Preventive Measures Against Infection

Most infections are preventable. Even if the infection is inevitable, we can take preventive measures to reduce the degree of infection and should try best to eliminate the various factors inducing infection and enhance the patient's own resistance.

12.4.6.1 Strict Sterilization of Instruments

The surgical instruments of hysteroscope come into direct contact with genital tract. During examination and surgery, if sterilization is not qualified, it is extremely easy to cause infection, so the sterilization of hysteroscopic diagnostic and operative instruments is required to achieve killing germs. The methods for disinfection of instruments include: (1) High-pressure steam sterilization: It keeps a temperature at 121 °C for 20–30 min and is the most thorough disinfection method, which is applicable to metal appliances. After repeated high-pressure sterilization, the joints of some devices can be inflexible. (2) Low temperature sterilizers: The liquid used in sterilizers is sterile water and bactericidal agent which has been processed by sterilizers. It works at a low temperature between 45 and 55 °C for 30–40 min, after which the instruments should be rinsed by sterile water repeatedly so as to ensure their asepsis and cleanliness without any residual of chemical materials. Then the water is blown dry automatically. Since it has little damage to instruments, it has become a commonly used method for sterilization of hysteroscopic instruments. (3) Ethylene oxide sterilization: 800 mg/L ethylene oxide at a temperature of 55–60 °C and a relative humidity between 60 and 80% is kept for 6 h in ethylene oxide sterilizer. The advantage includes relatively less damage, and disadvantage is a longer disinfection time. (4) Immersion in chemical disinfectants: When 2% alkaline glutaraldehyde is used for sterilization, the instruments must be immersed for 10 h. Since it has corrosivity to instruments and irritation to skin, mucosa, and respiratory tract, the instruments should be rinsed in sterile water after being taken out from the disinfectants.

12.4.6.2 Strict Sterile Operation

Dhaliwal et al. counted 4032 cases who underwent obstetric and gynecological operations and found that the postoperative infection rate was 2.2% and was 0.9% in gynecological surgery, with the common pathogens involving Enterococcus, Staphylococcus, and Klebsiella species. So they held that the main source of postoperative infection was vaginal flora, which could be minimized by local sterilization. The vagina is the only way for hysteroscopic operation, so strict disinfection is more important especially in the consecutive hysteroscopic examination or surgeries, and the operators must operate under sterile conditions. Five percent iodophor disinfectant is a broad-spectrum bactericide and can kill the streptococcus, intestinal bacteria, and pathogenic yeast. It has no irritation to skin and mucosa and is applicable to disinfection of vulva and vagina, so it has been a routine disinfectant used before hysteroscopic diagnosis and surgeries.

12.4.6.3 Improvement in Patient Status

Patients with the conditions like genital inflammation, malnutrition, anemia and diabetes, or aged women with weak resistance are all underlying factors leading to infections, who should be promptly identified and treated prior to operation.

12.4.6.4 Application of Prophylactic Antibiotics

In recent years, with the development of antibiotics, great changes have taken place in the concept of preventive use of antibiotics during the operative period compared with the traditional concept. Research findings showed that the perioperative prophylaxis can reduce the occurrence of infectious complications after operation. Bhattacharya et al. studied the incidence of bacteremia following hysteroscopic surgery and found that it was 16% in the non-antibiotic group, while 2% in the group who received intravenous antibiotics at induction of anesthesia, with significant differences between them. Marchino et al. also held that even short limited operations could interfere the patient's immune system which led to lowering of her resistance. As a result, the changes in microbial flora encouraged the growth of bacteria, so the application of antibiotic prophylaxis was very important. Selection of antibiotics should meet the following criteria: broad antibacterial spectrum; high bactericidal power; high permeability of the tissues; capacity to maintain effective concentration in tissues for longer time, single drug use which can achieve the purpose of prevention; less resistant strains; few side effects; proper cost–benefit ratio. The timing of antibiotic administration is very important. If the effective concentration of the drug can be reached before contamination, it may produce the maximum effect. Although most operation is done in sterile conditions in theory, the highest risk period of the bacterial contamination is still in operation process. The reasonable time for antibiotic prophylaxis should be before possible contamination occurs, so that adequate drug concentrations in the relevant tissues can be reached in patients in order to prevent subsequent bacterial growth and reproduction. Generally, the use of prophylactic antibiotics should be prescribed once before and after operation, respectively. If the operative time is too long, an additional medication can be given during operation to maintain adequate concentrations in tissues. However, the research findings made by Hayashi et al. showed that the administration of intravenous cefotiam dihydrochloride (CTM) on the induction of anesthesia was similar in preventive effect to oral cefpodoxime proxetil (CPDX- PR) given for 3 days after operation, and there was no significant difference. It was believed that the administration of oral antibiotics appeared to be a safe, convenient, and relatively cheap postoperative prophylaxis.

Generally, the pathogens causing pelvic inflammatory disease are streptococcus, staphylococcus, Escherichia coli, and other anaerobes. However, due to specificity of the hysteroscopic pathway, pelvic inflammatory disease caused by chlamydia, mycoplasma, and fungus is also worthy of attention. For patients with pelvic inflammatory disease, the application of prophylactic antibiotics is especially important. McCausland et al. reported that in group one, four (2%) of 200 cases without using prophylactic antibiotics had a past history of pelvic inflammatory disease, three of four cases developed ovarian abscess after operative hysteroscopy; in group two, 10 (2%) of 500 cases who were given prophylactic antibiotics had a past history of pelvic inflammatory disease, no infection occurred after operative hysteroscopy.

In recent years, whether hysteroscopic diagnosis and operation must apply prophylactic antibiotics is still a controversy. Isaacson held that the application of prophylactic antibiotics was not necessary after hysteroscopic examinations. Thinkhamrop et al. reviewed six literatures to evaluate the effectiveness of antibiotics in preventing infections after hysteroscopic examination and did not make the conclusion that prophylactic antibiotics could prevent intrauterine infections posthysteroscopic procedures. In the Hysteroscopy Center of Fuxing Hospital, Capital Medical University, we strictly confine the administration of prophylactic antibiotics. For women who have neither a history of pelvic infection nor underlying susceptible factors, prophylactic antibiotics will not be used for hysteroscopic diagnosis, and for women who undergo a shorter and simple hysteroscopic surgery (e.g. TCRP), prophylactic antibiotics will not be used, and postoperative infections seldom develop.

In conclusion, hysteroscopic examination or surgery has a certain degree of risk of infection. As long as we have sufficient understanding and effective prevention, infection, especially severe infection will rarely occur or not occur, which will be more conducive to the implementation of operative hysteroscopy and beneficial to thousands of women suffering from uterine diseases.

12.5 Venous Air Embolism

Enlan Xia

Venous air embolism (VAE) or venous gas embolism (VGE) is caused by the entry of air into the venous system, which can be a consequence of trauma, iatrogenic complication (especially central venous intubation or pressurized intravenous infusion), or can also occur in some surgical procedures, being a serious, rare but fatal complication. There are three main types of gas: oxygen, CO_2, and nitrogen. Air emboli are bubbles of nitrogen gas. VAE can lead to right ventricular dysfunction and pulmonary injury, which has been reported in the research field of neurosurgery, urology, and cesarean section. The earliest VAE was documented in 1830, which was extremely rare a 100 years ago. With the rapid development of medical technology and diving under high pressure, especially as the Navy submarine escape training becomes more frequent and cardiovascular surgical operation increases in quantity and difficulty, VAE is no longer a rare disease. By estimate, there are more than twenty thousand people around the world each year suffering permanent sequelae of VAE without timely and correct treatment. Some patients suffering from VAE even die in a short time. Gottlieb et al. reported that if untreated, the patients with VAE had a mortality of as high as 93%. Therefore, it is essential to administer the timely and correct treatment to patients. In recent years, along with the universal application of operative hysteroscopy, there are reports on air embolism induced by hysteroscopic procedures, including diagnostic CO_2 hysteroscopy and transcervical resection (TCR) of uterine lesions. In a review of literature in recent 10 years, its morbidity is shown in Table 12.17.

12.5.1 Incidence

The exact incidence is uncertain, but subclinical gas emboli in hospitals may be very common. VAE clinically diagnosed

Table 12.17 VAE induced by operative hysteroscopy

Author	Year	Procedures	Cases of VAE	Notes
Pierre et al.	1995	CO_2DHS	3	Treatment with HBO and death in one case
Brooks	1997	Operative hysteroscopy	13	Death in nine cases (worldwide)
Brandner et al.	1999	CO_2 DHS	1	0.51% undiscovered
Fukuda et al.	2000	TCRM	1	The surgery suspended and the patient resuscitated
Xia Enlan	2001	5% glucose DHS	1	The patient resuscitated
Adducci and De Cosma	2001	Operative hysteroscopy	1	The patient resuscitated
Imasogie et al.	2002	Operative hysteroscopy	1	Gas caused by electroresection and the patient resuscitated
Corson	2002	Operative hysteroscopy	1	The patient resuscitated
Grove et al.	2005	Operative hysteroscopy	1	The patient resuscitated
Brugmann et al.	2007	Operative hysteroscopy	2	Discovered by anesthetist and the patient resuscitated

Note: *HBO* hyperbaric oxygen, *DHS* diagnostic hysteroscopy

following placement of central venous (CV) catheter is <2%. Research findings made by Brandner et al. showed that undetected emboli were present in 0.51% of patients. In recent years, along with the universal application of operative hysteroscopy, there are reports on venous air embolism induced by hysteroscopic surgeries, including diagnostic CO_2 hysteroscopy and transcervical resection (TCR) of uterine lesions. In 1995, Pierre et al. reported among 5140 CO_2 hysteroscopies, air embolism occurred in three cases, with its incidence rate 0.058%. In 1999, Brandner et al. reported 3932 CO_2 hysteroscopies. Air embolism occurred in one case, with its incidence rate 0.03%. In 1997, Brooks reviewed the related literature around the world and found that 13 cases had VAE in the course of hysteroscopic procedure. Some air embolisms were asymptomatic, not diagnosed, or not reported, so its exact incidence is difficult to estimate. Imasogic et al. reported that the incidence of VAE during operative hysteroscopy was 10–50%, and catastrophic outcomes occurred scarcely at a rate of three in 17,000 procedures.

Bloomstone et al. carried out a study to evaluate the frequency of gas formation with 11 cases undergoing hysteroscopic monopolar resection and three cases in control group. The formation of gases in the inferior vena cava, hepatic veins, and right heart was detected by echocardiography and serum tests. As a result, gas bubbles formed in hepatic veins and right heart were identified in ten cases of surgery group, while no gas was discovered in control group. There were no changes in coagulation function among cases in both groups. They insisted that gas bubbles could be discovered in most cases by echocardiography during hysteroscopic resection. Whether the patients had clinical presentations or not is correlative with anatomic characteristics and the volume of bubbles.

12.5.2 Etiology

The gas causing VAE may come from CO_2 in distending uterus, air in the inflow pipe, and bubbles generated in tissue vaporization, which may happen at the beginning or during the procedure. The gas enters the blood circulation through the opened veins in the cutting surface, and the increased intrauterine pressure is the promoting factor. The gas enters the right ventricle along with blood flow, and the cardiac impulse prompts the gas and intracardiac blood to mix, forming large volumes of bubbles. The cellulose, separated from "mixing," infiltrates into the pulmonary artery end, which makes the conditions more complex. The blood in pulmonary arteriole is replaced by bubbles, thus gas exchange is reduced. Intrapulmonary arteriovenous anastomoses are open in great number, arteriovenous short circuits aggravate hypoxia. Bubbles block the pathway of pulmonary artery blood flow, which leads to a rise in the pulmonary arterial pressure and a drop in end-tidal CO_2 pressure. Because the right ventricular pressure is higher than the left ventricular pressure, eventually circulatory failure results and sudden cardiac arrest occurs. The foramen ovale previously closed reopens in some adult patients, thus causing emboli to the brain and other organs.

The immediate causes of death are brain hypoxia, failure caused by right ventricular dilatation; or left ventricular failure secondary to myocardial ischemia caused by hypoxia and decreased cardiac output. After gas embolism occurs, pulmonary hypertension, arteriovenous shunt, and increased vascular permeability caused by hypoxia result in pulmonary edema and respiratory distress syndrome. If volume is greater than 300 mL, death follows.

12.5.3 Pathogenesis

In neurosurgical operations, the occurrence rate of air embolism is 25–50%. The reasons are: when neurosurgery is performed, in order to expose the head injury, the patient is placed in a sitting position. Since the heart level is below the brain, when the heart dilates each time, negative pressure is generated in the vein, which can lead to air inhalation through the opened skull and dural venous sinus. Once the air enters the venous circulation, the bubbles in the right ventricle block the blood flow, causing a rise in the pulmonary arterial pressure. In the early development of gas embolism, the end-tidal CO_2 pressure drops, and finally, circulation failure and sudden cardiac arrest occur. Because there is a higher degree of the increased right ventricular pressure than that of the left ventricular pressure, 15% of the foramen ovale previously closed in adult patients reopen, thus causing emboli to the brain and other organs. There is the same mechanism in gynecologic surgeries, but the sitting position is shifted to head-down tilt, with the level of heart lower than the level of uterus, resulting in a decrease in venous pressure, and there is significant pressure difference between the central circulation and the uterine cavity. Pressure difference comes from the intravascular negative pressure, and also the extravascular positive pressure, or both, which may be seen in trauma or when positive and negative pressure interchanged. If the head of the bed is tilted down too much and the height difference between the uterus and the heart is ≥26 cm, the pressure difference between the uterine cavity and systemic circulation may prompt the air to be inhaled into the blood circulation and accelerate the quantity and speed of air inhalation. If the large venous sinus in the deep uterine muscle wall is open and communicates with the outside, the outside air can be absorbed into the venous circulation. When the uterine distension media is infused into the uterus under pressure, this process can be aggravated. When the intrauterine pressure exceeds venous pressure, asymptomatic, symptomatic and fatal VAE may occur.

Pulmonary gas embolism can cause lung tissues to release some substances (such as smooth muscle active substance, 5-serotonin, histamine, bradykinin, prostaglandins, etc.), which may cause the bronchial smooth muscles and pulmonary vessels to constrict and lead to an increase in pulmonary capillary permeability, thus resulting in an increase in pulmonary resistance, pulmonary artery pressure, and plasma exudation, leading to pulmonary edema and difficulty in breathing. The pathogenesis of pulmonary endothelial injury may be the release of platelet-fibrin cytolymph from right heart and the activation of neutrophil, platelet, and microvascular gas–blood interface, and lipid peroxide and oxygen ion-mediated injury. When pulmonary air embolism occurs, alveolar dead space expands and the end-tidal CO_2 drops. At present, the determination of CO_2 content has been clinically regarded as an index of diagnosis of pulmonary gas embolism. The experimental findings made by Drummond showed that there was a close relationship between the change in CO_2 concentration and the amount of bubbles into the vein.

12.5.4 Pathophysiology

When the air into the venous system affects the right ventricle, pulmonary circulation, and systemic circulation (if there is a right-left shunt), symptoms and signs may develop. When embolism occurs in the vein, the blood vessels become wider and wider, and the small bubbles or a small amount of gas produces no effect on the circulation prior to its entry into the heart and arteries without development of symptoms. A large amount of gas (3–5 mL/kg body weight) can trap right ventricular ejection, leading to cardiogenic shock and cease of circulation. A moderate amount of gas accumulates in the pulmonary circulation and causes injury to the lungs, the pulmonary capillary constriction, pulmonary hypertension, vascular endothelial damage, and permeability pulmonary edema may develop. When an emboli enters the artery, because the vessels become thinner and thinner, it finally blocks the small arteries with regional blood flow occluded, leading to serious consequences. But its outcome depends on the location of the arterial embolism, if it occurs in the brain, permanent brain damage can be caused.

The brain is one of the organs in the body which requires the greatest amount of oxygen. The brain weight accounts for only 2–3% of human body, but brain oxygen consumption accounts for 20–30% of the total oxygen consumption, and 15% of cardiac output goes to the brain, and there is almost none of energy reserve in the brain tissue. If cerebral blood supply and oxygen supply completely discontinue, the patient will lose consciousness in 8–15 s, and irreversible damage will occur in 6–10 min.

In 2008, some new ideas about original reason and sudden death of gas embolism were put forward in two literatures. Chang et al. reported on death in one patient who developed VAE which resulted from ureteroscopic lithotripsy by Ho:YAG. When the procedure was coming to an end, the patient complained tightness over her chest and promptly developed into unconsciousness, followed by circulatory failure and cardiac arrest. The procedure was stopped immediately, and mask 100% oxygen inhalation, endotracheal intubation, establishing the vein passage, and cardiopulmonary resuscitation were conducted. Internal jugular vein was catheterized. The crepitus was detected when performing external chest compression, and 20–30 mL frothy blood was sucked out from the catheter, which indicated VAE. Transesophageal echocardiography revealed a large volume of gas emboli in right heart atrium and right heart ventricle. The heart contraction could not be restored after conduction of adrenalin and cardiac massage. The patient died 40 min later for failure in resuscitation. All reasons including entry of the air into the bladder by insertion and withdraw of the scope, and entry of the air via gap because of empty of the irrigating fluid, broken inflow pipe, loose connection to the sheath or replacement of inflow pipe were all excluded. The only possible reason might be the gas caused by tissue vaporization entering right heart ventricle. The entering of gas when VAE occurs is insidiously and the patient may have no characteristic symptoms; therefore, the real source of gas is uncertain.

Rademaker et al. first reported on one case of paradoxical gas embolism which occurred during hysteroscopic surgery and was detected by transesophageal echocardiography. During TCRE with bipolar electrode, at 20 min after beginning of the procedure, end-tidal carbon dioxide (ET_{CO_2}) was decreased to 2.4 kPa (1 kPa=7.5 mmHg); arterial oxygen saturation (Sa_{O_2}) was decreased below 90%, with the lowest to 40%; and a loud mill-wheel murmur was detected by precordial auscultation. VAE was diagnosed and the procedure was stopped immediately. The patient was put in Trendelenburg position and was ventilated with continuous pure oxygen. No gas was retrieved through a central venous catheter which was inserted in the internal jugular vein. At 15 min after partial pressure of CO_2 (Pa_{CO_2}) beginning to fall, a 7.4 MHz transesophageal echocardiography (TOE) probe was inserted and no gas in right atrium and right ventricle was discovered. However, echo-dense materials were identified in left atrium and left ventricle, which indicated paradoxical emboli. The paradoxical emboli described in this report might be caused by gas emboli entering left heart from right heart through atrial septal defect, open foramen ovale, pulmonary arteriovenous malformations or arteriovenous fistula. So cardiovascular and neurological complications can be promptly developed when VAE occurs, which even threatens the patients' life.

12.5.5 Clinical Manifestations

Clinical manifestations of VAE are related to the volume of embolized gas. All the early emergent symptoms are usually found by anesthesiologists, such as a sudden drop in the end-tidal CO_2 pressure, slow heartbeat and a decrease in blood oxygen saturation, and auscultation of the precordium revealing water-wheel murmur, clicking and gurgling sound, which is a typical sign of air into the heart. When more air enters, there is an increased resistance to blood flow, leading to hypoxia, cyanosis, decreased cardiac output, hypotension, and tachypnea. Cardiopulmonary failure develops rapidly and death follows due to sudden cardiac arrest. The morbidity of gas embolism induced by diagnostic CO_2 hysteroscopy reported in literatures is described in Table 12.18. Among 11 cases of VAE, three patients lost their life with the fatality rate 27.3%, and one patient was left with permanent brain damage. The morbidity of gas embolism induced by operative hysteroscopy reported in literatures is seen in Table 12.19. Among 15 cases of VAE collected, 9 patients died with the mortality rate of 60%, and one case was left with permanent neurological damage. It can be seen from two tables that the fatality rate of VAE caused by operative hysteroscopy is higher than that of diagnostic CO_2 hysteroscopy, and there is no difference between various types of surgery.

One case of VAE had occurred during diagnostic hysteroscopy in combination with ultrasonography in the Hysteroscopy Center of Fuxing Hospital, Capital Medical University. This 42-year-old woman who initially being healthy and having normal menses suffered from persistent vaginal bleeding for 2 months. No tissues were discharged with the blood. She had four pregnancies and two live births, with her last delivery 11 years ago. During operation, the patient was placed in lithotomy position, ultrasonography scan was firstly conducted and revealed that the uterus was in a horizontal position, enlarged by 70 mm × 66 mm × 56 mm, and there was an echo-free zone of 20 mm × 10 mm, which was suspected to be fetal sac. No abnormalities were found in bilateral adnexa. An HYF-XP fiber hysteroscopy (outer diameter of the tip 3.1 mm) was inserted with the application of automatic distention pump, 5% glucose as distending medium, the distension pressure set at 120 mmHg, and uterine fluid velocity at 240 mL/min. The length of uterine cavity was 10 cm. Under hysteroscope, the cavity first appeared bloody and obscure, and then bubbles were seen tumbling in the uterine cavity. When checking the distending system, no fluid was left in the container. The distention fluid was added immediately, and the procedure continued. Four minutes later, the patient suddenly felt suffocated and coughed without end, accompanied with a cyanosed face. Her blood pressure was 60/40 mmHg and heart rate 40 beats/min. She was immediately given mask with positive pressure oxygen inhalation. The veins were kept open and dexamethasone 20 mg was injected intravenously, the patient was sweating profusely and felt peripheral coldness, but kept consciousness. Lung auscultation revealed low breath sounds with no rales. Seven to 8 min later, her symptoms were relieved, and general conditions were improved with the blood pressure at 90/50 mmHg. Sixteen minutes later, her heart rate was 78 beats /min, and ECG showed no abnormalities. Then urine HCG test was taken and the result was positive. The next day, artificial abortion vacuum aspiration was performed smoothly with her blood pressure at 100/70 mmHg. This patient was found to have uterine bleeding for more than 2 months due to the early threatened abortion, so the uterus had rich blood supply and broken intrauterine mucosa. In addition, the empty container permitted the air to enter the cavity via the irrigating pipe, and intraoperative distension

Table 12.18 Characteristics and outcomes of air embolism during diagnostic hysteroscopy

Authors	Year	Distention media	Clinical manifestations	Outcomes
Nishiyama and Hanaoka	1999	CO_2	Convulsion and confusion occurred at the removal of the hysteroscope; the pulse impalpable. Treated by cardiac massage, trachea intubation, and medication	Died 16 h later
Sherlock et al.	1998	CO_2	Sudden and rapid falls in ET_{CO_2} and Sa_{O_2} on monitor; pulseless and cyanosed. Treated by oxygen inhalation and hyperbaric oxygenation	Recovered
Behnia et al.	1997	CO_2	A noncardiogenic pulmonary edema developed in the recovery room	Recovered
Ghimouz et al.	1996	CO_2	Ventricular tachycardia occurred after 2 min of CO_2 insufflation under general anesthesia, followed by a circulatory arrest. Improvement achieved by 2 min of cardiopulmonary resuscitation	Transient blindness for 3 min
Corson et al.	1996	CO_2	Bradycardia occurred suddenly after diagnostic hysteroscopy for 9 min. Transesophageal ultrasonography revealed air in four heart chambers with open oval foramen	Left with permanent brain injury
Vo Van et al.	1992	saline	A respiratory distress occurred at the end of the procedure, followed by cardiac arrest. Treated by cardio-respiratory resuscitation	Died
Crozier et al.	1991	CO_2	Three cases developed circulatory collapse and cardiac arrest 5–8 min after the start of examination. A mill-wheel murmur detected by auscultation following resuscitation and disappeared 5 min later	Recovery
Obenhaus and Maurer	1990	CO_2	Bradyarrhythmia, drop of blood pressure, metallic heart sound, and hypercapnia	Recovery
Gomar et al.	1985	CO_2	Cardiovascular collapse, cardiac arrest, and a mill-wheel murmur	Irreversible brain damage and died a week later

pressure was at 120 mmHg. Under such high pressure, the air in the irrigating pipe passed through the uterine venous sinus into the right ventricle. Due to a greater volume of air absorption, symptoms of venous air embolism appeared.

12.5.6 Diagnosis of VAE

12.5.6.1 Symptoms and Signs

VAE is characterized by sudden occurrence and rapid development. Among the typical clinical manifestations of VAE, the most sensitive monitoring method to detect VAE is the precordial Doppler ultrasonography. When more air enters the bloodstream, the end-tidal CO_2 pressure drops. The determination of ET_{CO_2} is highly sensitive and distinctive in diagnosis of VAE. At present, CO_2 level is monitored in patients under general anesthesia, and a drop in ET_{CO_2} has become the most important early sign of VAE. If the patients are at high risk prior to operation, or when difficulty arises during operation, central venous catheter may be placed to check and monitor the rise in intracardiac and pulmonary artery pressure. Suction of the bubbles contributes to the treatment of this complication.

12.5.6.2 Laboratory Tests

Arterial blood gas analysis indicates hypoxemia, hypercapnia, and metabolic acidosis. Mild symptoms may manifest as hypoxemia and hypocapnia. There are no other abnormal laboratory results.

12.5.6.3 Imaging Examination

Chest X-ray shows normal or bubbles in non-arterial system. Other X-ray reveals dilatation of the pulmonary artery, a decrease in focal blood flow (Westermark sign), and pulmonary edema. Ultrasonic cardiogram helps to determine the presence of gas in the right ventricular blood flow and can detect the tiny bubbles which cannot be located. Precordial Doppler can quickly discover bubbles. This method is simple and can quickly find out bubbles as small as 0.12–0.25 mL. Its sound quality takes on a special high-pitched tone like "rustle" or "rumble."

12.5.6.4 Electrocardiogram Examination

Tachycardia, right axis deviation, right ventricular strain, and ST segment depression might be discovered by ECG.

12.5.7 Monitoring of VAE

The onset of venous air embolism is so sudden and severe that it is extremely difficult to deal with, often leading to death and severe disability. Therefore, intraoperative monitoring should be strengthened, including continuous precordial Doppler monitoring, the end-tidal CO_2 pressure

Table 12.19 Characteristics and treatments of air embolism during operative hysteroscopy

Authors	Year	Surgery/distention media	Morbidity and treatment	Outcomes
Imasogie et al.	2002	TCRE+P	Be in lithotomy position. At 15 min after the beginning of the procedure, Sa_{O_2} declined to 87% and ET_{CO_2} dropped to 27 mmHg	Improved by 100% O_2 inhalation
Fukuda et al.	2000	TCRM	Forty-five minutes after the start of the surgery, the patient complained of severe back pain, with blood pressure 40 mmHg and Sa_{O_2} 80%. ECG showed atrial fibrillation	Improved 20 min after im. ephedrine 5 mg
Corson et al.	1996	TCRA/saline	Be in moderate lithotomy position. At the time of replacement of endoscopic sheath, the anesthetist discovered drops of the patient in heart rate, Sa_{O_2} and blood pressure, and cyanosis	Died
Corson et al.	1996	TCRS (with scissors)/CO_2	Patient was in lithotomy position. After removal of endoscope for 2 min, Sa_{O_2} and ET_{CO_2} dropped. Gas extracted by heart puncture, followed by DIC and renal failure	Gave up treatment 10 days later and died
Corson et al.	1996	Diagnostic laparoscopy after D&C	Patient was in extreme lithotomy position. The uterine manipulator with an open end was used to lift the uterus. At the end of the procedure, the blood pressure dropped. Convulsion with mill-wheel murmur revealed precordium. The patient was put in left lateral decubitus position. Foamy blood was extracted by heart puncture. The emboli were confirmed to be room air from manipulator	Died in several minutes and autopsy revealed air filling in four heart chambers
Corson et al.	1996	TCRE	Uterine aspiration performed first. Before insertion of endoscope and opening the water inflow valve, ET_{CO_2} dropped, and cardiac arrest occurred. Central venous catheter inserted and 15 mL of air extracted	Died
Nachum et al.	1992	TCRE/Hyskon solution	When changing the irrigation fluid bag, the pump still worked. The patient felt uneasy and coughed, with heart rate 50 beats/min, followed by cyanosis and apnea. Foaming blood was extracted by arterial catheter insertion, with Sa_{O_2} 16 mmHg. HBO therapy with transient improvement	Died
Perry et al.	1992	HEAL/Ringer lactate solution	After 30 min of surgery, some gas noted in the tube as irrigation bag was changed. ET_{CO_2} dropped from 34 to 22 mmHg. The operation discontinued and 100% oxygen inhalated. The ET_{CO_2} returned to normal within 3–4 min and surgery resumed. Again, the ET_{CO_2} decreased from 35 to 21 mmHg with a change in the Doppler tones characteristic of air embolism. The operation discontinued again and 100% oxygen inhalated, with subsequent recovery	Recovered
Perry et al.	1992	TCRM/1.5% glycine	After 50 min of surgery, while the uterus was irrigated using a urologic bulb syringe, the Doppler sounds suddenly increased, Sa_{O_2} decreased from 99 to 90%, ET_{CO_2} decreased from 31 to 17 mmHg, and the blood pressure decreased from 120/80 to 90/60 mmHg. The operation discontinued and 100% oxygen inhalated with subsequent recovery. The operation lasted for 150 min and hyponatremia developed	Transabdominal myomectomy
Wood and Roberts	1990	TCRE/10% glucose	Laparoscopy revealed air bubbles entering small caliber veins in the lateral pelvic wall. Sa_{O_2} dropped from 97 to 84%, her pulse rate rose from 72 to 110 beats/min. The head-down position was reversed and positive pressure ventilation started with 100% oxygen. Recovery achieved 5 min later	Complete recovered
Baggish and Daniell	1989	HEAL, cooling with air or nitrogen	Five cases. Sudden gas embolism and cardiovascular collapse developed during operation. Cardiac arrest occurred in four of the five women	Four died, and one survived with neurological deficits

monitoring, and measurement of oxygen saturation. Ultrasonic cardiogram may be the most sensitive technique in checking bubbles less than 0.5 mL within the heart, but it has not been widely used due to its high false positive rate. Now most of patients' surgery are performed under general anesthesia with carbon dioxide graphic monitoring. Insertion of central venous pressure catheter can check and monitor whether there is a rise in intracardiac and pulmonary artery pressure and can suck the bubbles out, contributing to the treatment of this complication. Figure 12.12 shows the various methods of monitoring the gas into the heart and main vessels and its secondary physiological changes. Along with the entry of more gas, abnormalities of heart and lung function may appear. Corson et al. thought that this risk might be reduced with more attention paid to operating skills and monitoring of end-tidal CO_2 levels.

12.5.8 Emergency Managements

If air embolism is suspected, the operator should immediately stop any method causing gas injection so as to prevent gas from entering. Then, invert head-down position and turn to left-side lying position, and 100% oxygen inhalation is given. For the patients with obvious dyspnea or uncontrollable hypoxemia, endotracheal intubation should be conducted. Placement of central venous pressure catheter can monitor intracardiac and pulmonary artery pressure. The catheter can be placed in the air tank to suck the bubbles out as much as possible. If cardiopulmonary failure occurs, immediate cardiopulmonary resuscitation should be performed. Closed chest massage can break the bubbles and make them smaller, thus forcing them into the pulmonary circulation and dispersing into the peripheral pulmonary venous system so as to restore ventricular functions. A large amount of normal saline is injected to promote blood circulation. If all measures (including closed chest massage) fail, thoracotomy can be performed for direct heart massage and removal of air emboli. If it is maintainable, timely hyperbaric oxygen therapy should be followed. Even after the successful management of VAE, the patient may suffer pulmonary insufficiency. VAE can appear again 30 min after air inlet pathway is blocked, so the patient must be sent to ICU for further treatment.

Head-down and left lateral decubitus position helps to limit the gas to gather in the ventricular apex and prevents the gas into the pulmonary system while maintaining the right ventricular output, thus allowing bubbles in the right ventricle to drift away from outflow tract and restore normal cardiac dynamics. But if the bubble is too large and fills up most of chambers, this may not work easily.

12.5.9 Prevention and Treatment of VAE

Air embolism is a complication from distending media during hysteroscopy. When diagnostic hysteroscopy is performed, CO_2 enters the systemic circulation, leading to gas embolism. CO_2 has a high solubility in plasma with absorption rate of 68%, so it is easy to clean. Therefore, its tolerance capacity may be up to 7.5 mL/kg, and the lethal dose is commonly between 3 and 5 mL/kg, or about 300 mL for a 70-kg patient. There is a wide safety limit for CO_2, so embolism occurs only when there is a long-time use of CO_2 or a high flow rate. Siegler and Valle proposed that when pressure was set <200 mmHg, the flow volume <100 mL/min was safe at standard temperature and pressure. Brandner et al.

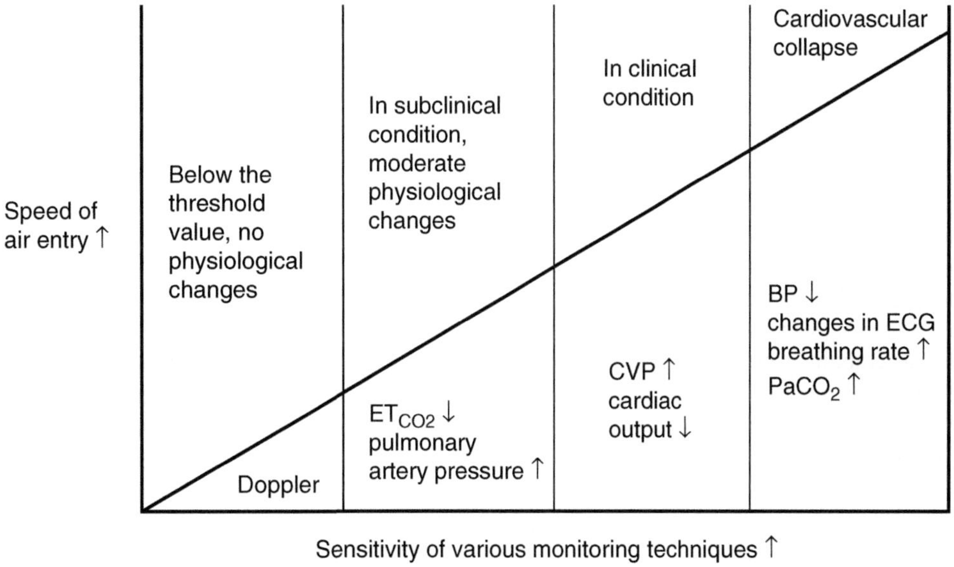

Fig. 12.12 Monitoring of VAE

studied 1261 procedures of diagnostic CO_2 hysteroscopies. The room air from the gas supply tube (about 40 mL) was deaerated before procedures and no gas embolism occurred during procedures. This indicated that emboli that occurred during CO_2 hysteroscopy were caused by room air, rather than CO_2, so it is preventable. Brundin and Thomasson reported that metallic heart sound in the systole was detected during CO_2 hysteroscopy due to the intracardiac presence of free carbon dioxide in 7 women (10%) with no history of cardiac valvular disease. The procedure was suspended immediately and the hysteroscope was withdrawn. The metallic heart sounds disappeared soon after, and the hysteroscopy continued. They suggested that monitoring with simple auscultation might avoid serious cardiovascular complications.

Nowadays it is believed that the gas of VAE may come from the inflow pipe or from the bubbles generated by vaporization of tissues. The gas in the inflow pipe enters the systemic circulation through the fractured veins in the uterine cutting surface under the intrauterine pressure. If a certain volume of air is not emptied before uterine distension, the air may enter the circulatory system at the early stage of operation. Such a small amount as 20 mL of air may produce response, so attention should be paid to emptying the gas in the inflow pipe at the time of operation. When intrauterine pressure exceeds venous pressure, asymptomatic, symptomatic, and fatal air embolism may appear, and the risk of air embolism will increase as the intrauterine pressure rises.

Nowadays, scholars have tended to reach an agreement in prevention of air embolism. Effective prevention is to aim at the cause of disease, mainly around how to block the source of intrauterine air, reduce the exposure of vascular surface, minimize the intrauterine pressure, and strengthen monitoring. The specific measures include: When at a head-down tilt position, the heart and vena cava should be avoided being lower than the level of uterus; attention should be paid to emptying the air in the irrigation pipe before operation; the cervical canal should be carefully dilated so as to avoid injury or partial penetration into the muscular wall, whose vascular network can allow air in; for nonporous women or women with previous history of cervical surgery, the osmotic dilator is used so as to reduce trauma; after cervical dilatation the vagina should be closed or wet gauze is used to tampon the cervix so as not to expose the cervix in the air; before the operator is ready to insert the hysteroscope, the last dilator must be placed in the cervical canal all the time. The risk of air embolism increases as the intrauterine pressure rises, so the effective minimal uterine pressure should be chosen at the time of operation. The flow rate of CO_2 should be controlled below 100 mL/min, and the intrauterine pressure cannot be higher than 200 mmHg. Corson reported that air embolism occurred in a case at a supine position. Therefore, at least positioning is not the only causative factor. If difficult dilatation and positioning are causative factors, the incidence rate will be higher than it is. If a change in the cardiopulmonary function takes place just when the operation begins, this indicates that air embolism may be caused by the outside air.

If air embolism is suspected, the operator should immediately stop any method using gas injection so as to prevent gas from entry. Then, invert head-down position and insert central venous pressure catheter. If cardiopulmonary failure occurs, immediate cardiopulmonary resuscitation should be performed. Left lateral decubitus position and closed chest massage can break the bubbles and force air into the pulmonary circulation so as to recover ventricular functions. Sometimes the central venous catheter can be placed in the air tank to exhaust the air as much as possible. A large amount of saline is injected to promote blood circulation and hyperbaric oxygen therapy should be administered.

In order to detect VAE timely and rescue early, in addition to the routine monitoring of blood pressure, heart rate, and oxygen saturation, it is also necessary to monitor the end-tidal CO_2 pressure. There still exist disputes over the routine application of central venous catheter and the diagnostic ultrasonography.

12.6 Intrauterine Adhesions

Dan Yu

Intrauterine adhesion is a major late postoperative complication of hysteroscopic surgery and may occur following all procedures. The severity of reformed adhesions and the likelihood of that happening are closely related to the degree and the property of previous intrauterine lesions, as well as the extent of surgical cutting. A second-look hysteroscopy in early postoperative period is a cost-effective method of diagnosing and loosening new adhesions following hysteroscopic surgery.

12.6.1 Incidence of Postoperative Intrauterine Adhesions

12.6.1.1 Hysteroscopic Endometrial Surgery

Hysteroscopic resection or ablation of endometrium usually leads to different degrees of intrauterine adhesions. Hysteroscopic endometrial surgery destroys both the basal layer of endometrium and the superficial layer of myometrium, which causes the denuded surfaces in the cavity adhering to each other so that intrauterine adhesions are developed. In the early stage of the application of hysteroscopy, Montagna et al. used second-look hysteroscopy to observe the uterine cavity after endometrial ablation. They found the uterine cavity becomes smaller in all cases, with different degrees of adhesions visible. Prof. Xia from the Hysteroscopy

Center of Fuxing Hospital, Capital Medical University carried out a study on second-look hysteroscopy in 26 patients after hysteroscopic endometrial resection. Different degrees of shortened cavity and the fibrosis of uterine walls were detected in all patients.

A variety of global endometrial ablation, i.e. second generation endometrial ablation, can also destroy the whole layer of endometrium and partial superficial layer of myometrium, which results in the formation of postoperative intrauterine adhesions. Leung et al. reported that, after thermal balloon endometrial ablation, the occurrence rate of intrauterine adhesions was 36.4% (8/22). Luo et al. analyzed 53 cases of microwave endometrial ablation and reported the occurrence rate of postoperative adhesions 52.8% (28/53).

12.6.1.2 Hysteroscopic Resection of Myomas

Just like endometrial ablations, hysteroscopic resection of myomas destroys the endometrium and may produce adhesions after the procedure. Many scholars reported the occurrence of intrauterine adhesions after hysteroscopic resection of myomas, which was shown in Table 12.20.

12.6.1.3 Hysteroscopic Surgery on Uterine Malformations

Adhesions may be produced following hysteroscopic resection of uterine septum and are usually found in the fundus and the anterior or posterior walls of the cavity. In a clinical study reported by Guida et al., the adhesions occurred in three cases (37.5%) after eight cases of TCRS. Yang et al. reported that the incidence of the adhesions after TCRS was 88% (14/16).

In recent years, with the development of hysteroscopic surgical techniques, except for TCRS, more and more women who have other congenital uterine dysplasia such as bicornuate uterus, unicornuate uterus, or T-shaped uterus, etc., apply hysteroscopic surgery for treatment and may produce postoperative adhesions.

12.6.1.4 Hysteroscopic Lysis of Intrauterine Adhesions

Intrauterine adhesions are prone to recurring after hysteroscopic adhesiolysis. In cases with initial intrauterine adhesions, the endometrium becomes fibrosis with poor ability of regeneration. By hysteroscopic lysis of adhesions, the denuded myometrium in the dissected surface of the cavity is hard to be covered by epithelium, but is prone to cohering and forming adhesions. It was reported in literature that the recurrence rate of the adhesions after hysteroscopic adhesiolysis ranged from 3.1 to 76%, and it was much higher in cases with severe adhesions (from 20 to 62.5%), which is shown in Table 12.21.

12.6.1.5 Other Hysteroscopic Surgeries

Intrauterine adhesions may be induced following other hysteroscopic surgeries, such as resection of endometrial polyps, resection of retained conceptional products, removal of intrauterine foreign bodies, etc. In a clinical study reported by Guida et al., TCRP was performed in 33 cases, with IUA occurring in 6 (18.2%). Fuchs et al. reported that the incidence of moderate and severe adhesions was 14% after hysteroscopic resection of retained products of conception in uterine cavity.

Table 12.20 The incidence of intrauterine adhesions after hysteroscopic resection of myomas

Authors	Year	Time of second-look hysteroscopy	No. of cases	No. of cases with adhesions	Incidence (%)
Taskin et al.	2000	2–4 weeks	22 (single) 13 (multiple)	8 6	36.4 46.2
Guida et al.	2004	3 months	24	8	33.3
Yang et al.	2008	1–3 months	132	2	1.5
Touboul et al.	2009	2 months	53	4	7.5
Yang et al.	2013	1 month	65	26	40

Table 12.21 The incidence of intrauterine adhesions after hysteroscopic adhesiolysis

		Preoperative intrauterine adhesions			Preoperative severe adhesions		
Authors	Year	No. of cases	No. of cases with postoperative recurrence	Incidence (%)	No. of cases	No. of cases with postoperative recurrence	Incidence (%)
Valle and Sciarra	1988	187	44	23.5	47	23	48.9
Pabuccu et al.	1997	40	8	20	10	6	60
Capella-Allouc et al.	1999	–	–	–	16	10	62.5
Preutthipan and Linasmita	2000	65	2	3.1	10	2	20
Yu et al.	2008	61	17	27.9	31	13	41.9
Yang et al.	2013	45	34	76	–	–	–

12.6.2 Mechanisms of Occurrence of Postoperative Intrauterine Adhesions

Uterus is a potential hollow organ, and under normal circumstances, even though the anterior and the posterior walls are close to each other, adhesions will not happen. This is because the endometrium has a very strong ability of regeneration under the action of ovarian hormones. In cases of intrauterine operation within a small area, as long as the basal layer of endometrium is not damaged, or even if part of the basal layer is damaged but the opposite endometrial layer is intact and without rough surfaces, the damaged areas of the endometrium can be quickly repaired by regeneration of the endometrium, thus, the formation of adhesions will not occur.

The procedures of hysteroscopic endometrial ablation extensively destroy the basal layer of endometrium and the superficial layer of myometrium. The absence of the basal layer leads to the disorder of endometrial re-growth, so some surfaces of the cavity are replaced by fibrotic scar tissues. Furthermore, the denuded surfaces in uterine cavity adhere to each other before they can be covered by the proliferated epithelium and are easy to cohere and form adhesive bands which obliterate the cavity.

Other types of hysteroscopic surgeries also can destroy the basal layer of endometrium and expose the myometrium of the uterus. The denuded surfaces, especially if they are opposite to one another, adhere together and form adhesions. When the denuded surface is concurrent with infections in uterine cavity, intrauterine adhesions are more easily developed.

12.6.3 Symptoms of Postoperative Intrauterine Adhesions

The clinical symptoms are diverse in patients who develop intrauterine adhesions after hysteroscopic surgery. Patients with mild adhesions usually present with no symptoms and generally are not easy to be diagnosed. When more endometrium is destroyed, the patients may present with menstrual disorders. Patients who produce adhesions and want to have children may present with infertility. Patients who conceive might have complications such as spontaneous miscarriage, preterm delivery, placenta adhesion, postoperative bleeding, etc. When the adhesions occlude the uterine cavity, hematometra may occur, which leads to periodic abdominal pain.

12.6.3.1 Menstrual Disorders

According to different degrees of endometrial destruction after hysteroscopic surgery, the patient may present with hypomenorrhea, prolonged and light bleeding, oligomenorrhea, or amenorrhea.

12.6.3.2 Pregnancy Disorders

Hysteroscopic endometrial ablation has an effect on artificial contraception. But postoperative conceptions were still reported in literatures. TCRE may destroy the whole endometrial layer, then the dissected surfaces heal with scar tissues; therefore, the outcomes in patients who conceive following TCRE are commonly not good. Failure of operation may happen when performing termination of pregnancy. Prof. Xia from the Hysteroscopy Center of Fuxing Hospital, Capital Medical University summarized the outcomes of 39 conceptions after TCRE in 1621 cases. The pregnancy disorders and poor outcomes discovered included tubal pregnancy, cornual pregnancy, cervical pregnancy, suction evacuation failure, hemorrhage following suction, placenta implantation, hysterectomy, etc.

Because of the presence of intrauterine adhesions, after TCRM, TCRS, TCRA, or TCRP, the patients who wish to become pregnant and produce adhesions may have infertility, and patients who achieve conception may have miscarriage, preterm delivery, placental disorders, etc.

12.6.3.3 Hematometra

When intrauterine adhesions occurring after hysteroscopic surgery obliterate the cervical os or uterine cavity partially or totally, hematometra may develop. The patients may present with periodic lower abdominal spasmodic pain, coexisting with amenorrhea or hypomenorrhea. After hysteroscopic endometrial ablation, the dissected surface is repaired by scar tissue, and new adhesions can separate the cavity into a few spaces. The residual endometrial island in scar tissues proliferates and exfoliates along with the cyclic changes of hormones, which lead to the blood gathering in the cavity and being unable to be drained off. For other hysteroscopic surgeries, new adhesions also can be developed to occlude part of the cavity, with normal endometrium in uterine cavity proliferating and exfoliating cyclically, leading to the blood gathering in the cavity and the formation of hematometra.

For those women who have also underwent tubal sterilization, after TCRE, intrauterine adhesions occurred may occlude the uterine cavity. So the menstrual blood being produced by the residual endometrium in the areas of bilateral uterine cornua cannot be discharged through the fallopian tubes, but accumulates in the space of uterine cornua, which leads to periodical abdominal pain and was named "post-ablation-tubal sterilization syndrome" (PASS).

12.6.4 Diagnosis of Postoperative Intrauterine Adhesions

Patients who get intrauterine adhesions after hysteroscopic surgery can be presumptively diagnosed by their history and clinical manifestation. Patients who are suspected of hematometra may have gynecologic ultrasonography scanning to identify irregular-shaped low echoes in uterine cavity. The accurate diagnosis of intrauterine adhesions depends on a second-look hysteroscopy.

12.6.4.1 Gynecologic Ultrasonography

Gynecologic ultrasonography may scan the uterus in the longitudinal and the transverse planes, including inspection of the contour of the uterus, the echoes of uterine walls, the echo of the endometrium, and the shape of the cavity. This has been a primary screening method for diagnosis of intrauterine adhesions.

In patients with intrauterine adhesions after hysteroscopic surgery, by ultrasonography scanning, the echoes of endometrium may appear thin, uneven, discontinuous, echolucent, or without periodical changes (Fig. 12.13). In patients with the damage of endometrium being more serious, it might be difficult to display an endometrial echo and hard to distinguish it from surrounding myometrial echoes.

When the adhesions block the cavity and produce hematometra, intrauterine adhesions divide the cavity into a few spaces with different sizes, and menstrual blood accumulates in these spaces where the endometrium remains. Under ultrasonography scanning, echolucent or low echo areas may be identified (Fig. 12.14).

12.6.4.2 Second-Look Hysteroscopy

Second-look hysteroscopy after hysteroscopic surgery can inspect the uterine cavity, identify the intrauterine adhesions, and determine the diagnosis of the adhesions under direct vision. When the adhesions occlude the cavity, hysteroscopy can only show a partial cavity below the level of the adhesions.

Under second-look hysteroscopy after hysteroscopic endometrial ablation, the normal shape of the cavity has disappeared, with its length shortened, its fundus narrowed, and the walls fibrosed. The shape of the cavity is shown as "tubiform," and sometimes constricting rings can be seen. The endometrium is present as filmy and faint or as fibrous bands (Fig. 12.15).

The characteristics of intrauterine adhesions after hysteroscopic resection of myomas are always determined by the locations, sizes, and numbers of the myomas preoperation and mostly are fibrous adhesive bands which involve the anterior and posterior walls (Fig. 12.16a, b).

After hysteroscopic resection of uterine septum, intrauterine adhesions are usually formed vertically from previous dissected surfaces, locating in the middle of the fundus or on the anterior or posterior walls (Figs. 12.17a, b and 12.18). In patients with intrauterine adhesions occurring after hysteroscopic resection of other types of uterine malformations, the

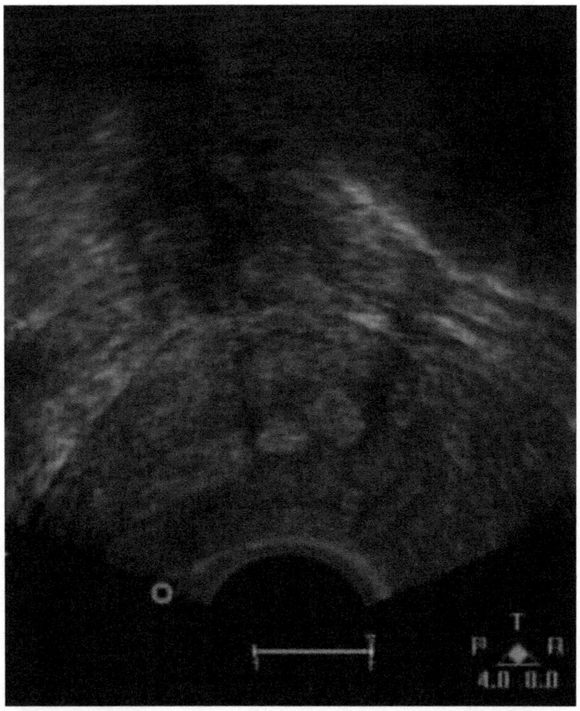

Fig. 12.13 The longitudinal scanning of the uterus by ultrasonography 1 month after hysteroscopic adhesiolysis. It shows a moderate and uneven echo of the endometrium with its thickness 7 mm. The continuity of the endometrium is interrupted, and the areas with low echoes indicate new adhesion bands

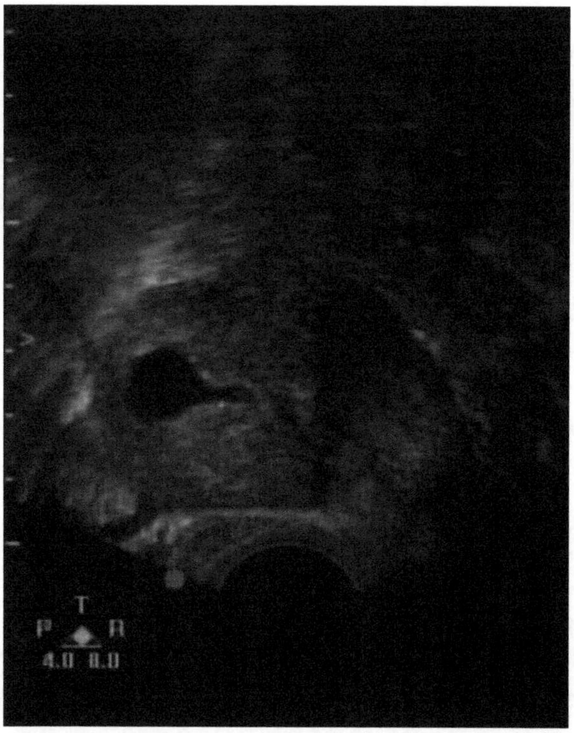

Fig. 12.14 The longitudinal scanning of the uterus by ultrasonography 3 months after hysteroscopic adhesiolysis. It shows a moderate and uneven echo of the endometrium, with its continuity interrupted. Echolucent area is shown in the fundus

uterine cavity may be narrow, with the top of the cavity occluded, and the adhesions may block both cornual areas (Fig. 12.19a, b).

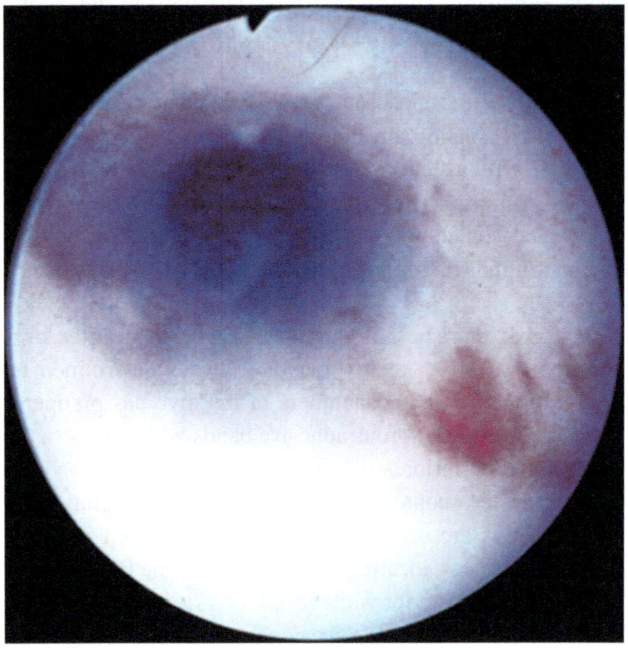

Fig. 12.15 Second-look hysteroscopy after hysteroscopic endometrial ablation. The uterine cavity presents a narrowed shape, with the endometrium being filmy and pale

After hysteroscopic adhesiolysis, the recurrence of intrauterine adhesions may show a variety of presentations, such as the reformation of the adhesions from the area of the original adhesions which has been divided or formation of new adhesions from other traumatic areas (Figs. 12.20 and 12.21).

12.6.5 Prevention of Postoperative Intrauterine Adhesions

For patients who are prone to having intrauterine adhesions after hysteroscopic surgery, some measures are taken during and following operations to prevent the formation of intrauterine adhesions.

12.6.5.1 Reduction of the Surgical Trauma During Hysteroscopic Surgery

The cutting of hysteroscopic endometrial resection should stop above the level of cervical os, to avoid the injury to cervical canal. Trauma to cervical canal may lead to cervical atresia and hematometra.

Procedures of other types of hysteroscopic surgery should try to minimize the extent and the depth of injury to endometrium so as to avoid too large areas of injured surface in uterine cavity. If more fibroids are in the cavity, complete resection of myomas through primary operation will lead to too large areas of dissected surface and is prone to develop-

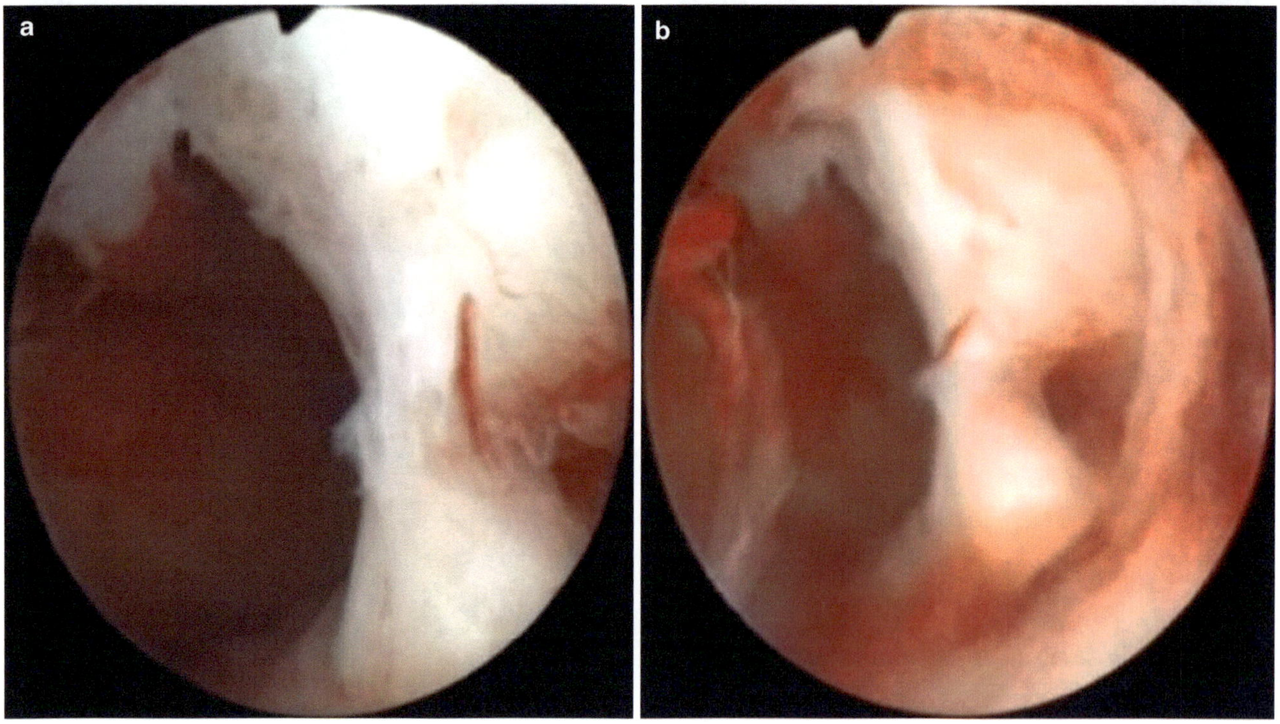

Fig. 12.16 Second-look hysteroscopy 9 months after hysteroscopic resection of multiple myomas. The normal shape of the cavity is disappearing and a vertical adhesive band is seen on the left, which is the adhesion produced from the previous dissected surfaces between anterior and posterior walls. (**a**) Image with close view. (**b**) Image with far view

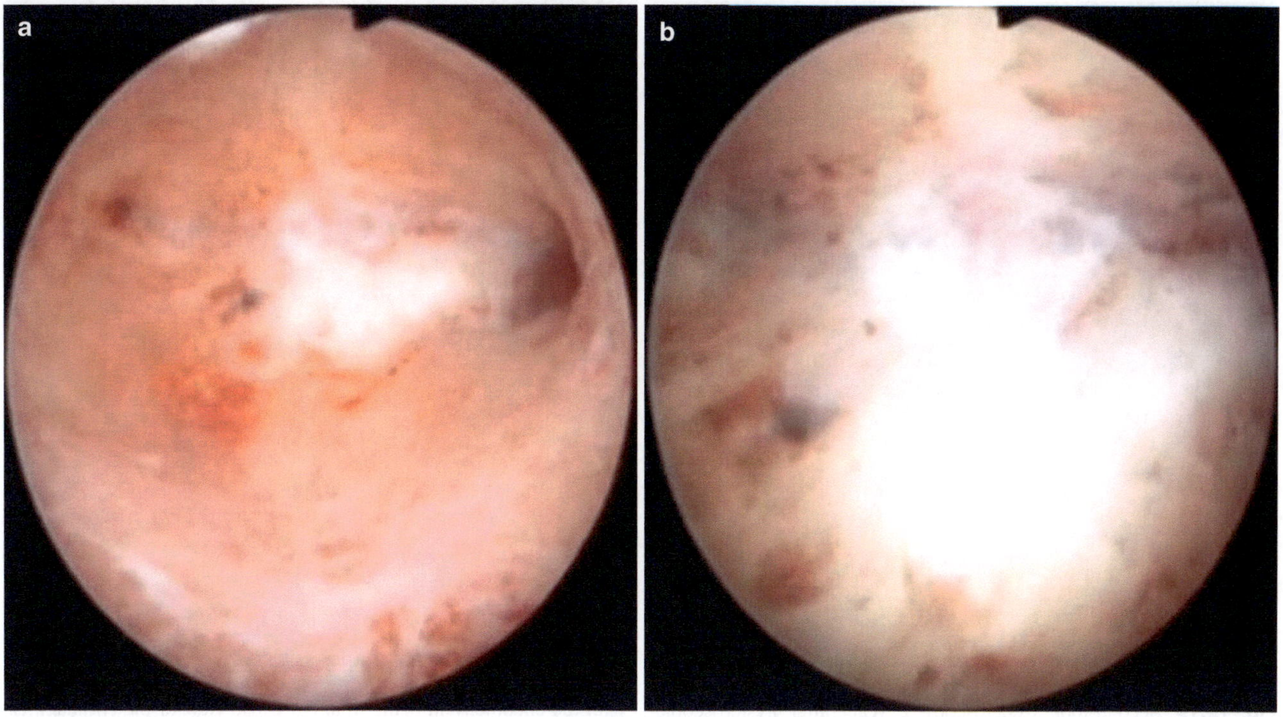

Fig. 12.17 Second-look hysteroscopy 4 years after hysteroscopic resection of uterine septum. (**a**) The uterine cavity is near normal, with both tubal ostia visible. (**b**) Close view of the fundus, with vertical scars seen

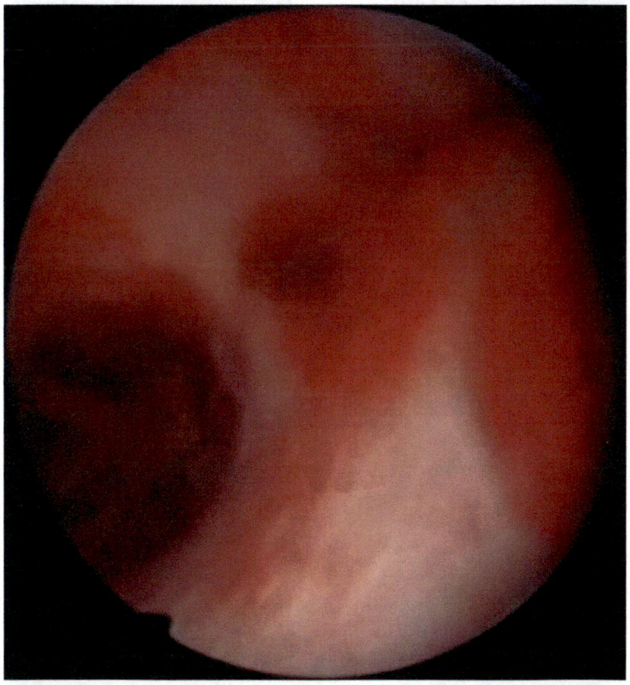

Fig. 12.18 Second-look hysteroscopy 2½ years after hysteroscopic resection of uterine septum. The left wall in the cavity constricts, with visualization of vertical adhesive bands between the anterior and posterior walls of the cavity

ing postoperative intrauterine adhesions. In this situation, multiple procedures may be conducted. Partial resection of intrauterine myomas is performed during the first operation, and the complete resection is performed by repeated operations after the recovery of the dissected surface.

Selection of a suitable hysteroscopic instrument may also reduce the surgical injury to endometrium. Operations without energy sources such as scissors and biopsy forceps may achieve precise incisions and avoid the injury to endometrium caused by energy sources. Hysteroscopic electrosurgery can resect the lesions precisely and stop the bleeding effectively, but the thermal damage caused by energy surgery can induce the formation of scar tissues and the injury to adjacent normal endometrium, which results in the formation of adhesions.

12.6.5.2 Artificial Cyclic Hormone Treatment After Hysteroscopic Surgery

A certain dose of sex hormone treatment after hysteroscopic surgery can stimulate the proliferation of endometrial glands and stroma, which accelerates the repair of endometrium. So artificial cyclic treatment with sex hormones, which enhances the re-growth of endometrium, has become a common adjuvant therapy for hysteroscopic surgeries, such as the resection of uterine septum, the lysis of adhesion, etc. A routine

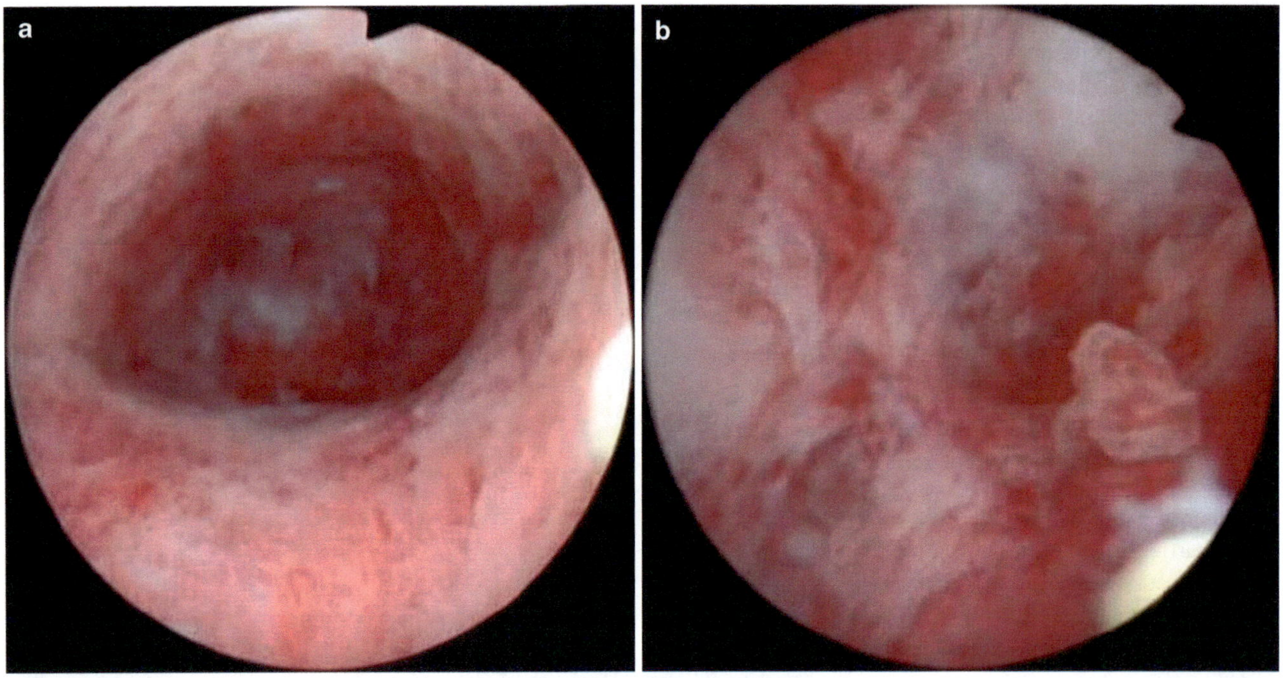

Fig. 12.19 Second-look hysteroscopy 2 years after hysteroscopic metroplasty of right unicornuate uterus. (**a**) The cavity is narrow-shaped, with the top of the cavity occluded. The cavity is to the right, with the endometrium being thin. (**b**) Close view of the cornual area. The tubal ostium is invisible, with vertical mild adhesive band visualized

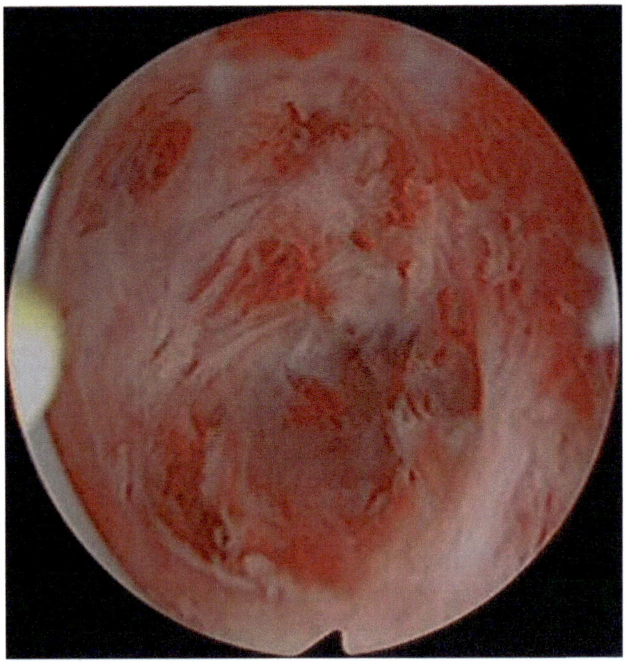

Fig. 12.20 Second-look hysteroscopy 2 years after hysteroscopic adhesiolysis. The shape of the cavity is distorted as narrow-shaped, with the top of the cavity occluded and adhesive band visualized

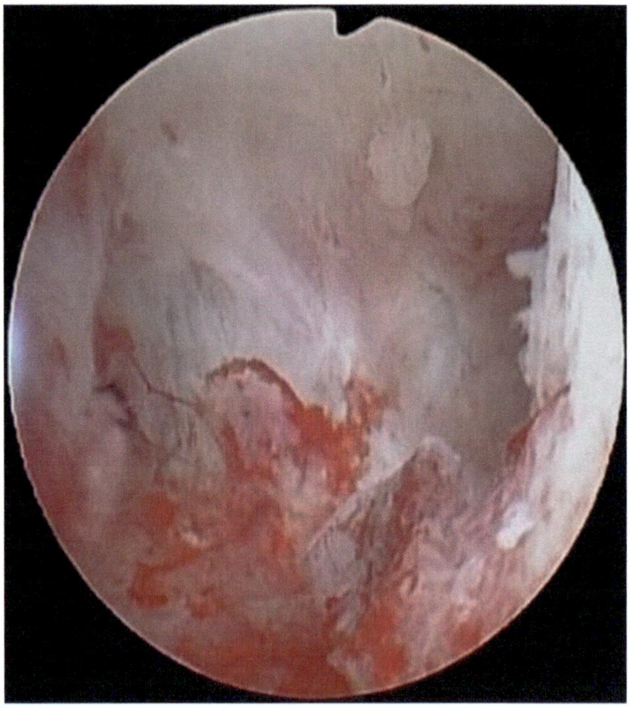

Fig. 12.21 Second-look hysteroscopy 4 months after hysteroscopic adhesiolysis. The shape of the cavity is distorted, with vertical adhesive bands in the fundus and on left lateral wall. The endometrium is thin and pale

regime is the use of a sequential therapy of estrogen and progesterone for 2 or 3 cycles, with estrogen 4 mg/day for 4 weeks, and the addition of progesterone in the last 2 weeks of the treatment cycle.

12.6.5.3 Intrauterine Insertion of Barriers After Hysteroscopic Surgery

At the end of hysteroscopic procedures such as the resection of septum, the lysis of adhesions, etc., intrauterine insertion of an IUD for 1–3 months, concurrent with the administration of cyclic hormone treatment, is a common used therapy to promote the healing of injured surfaces and prevent the formation of adhesions.

Some scholars attempted intrauterine instillation of ACP gel after hysteroscopic surgery to prevent the formation of intrauterine adhesions. Guita et al. studied the use of Hyalobarrier gel at the end of hysteroscopic surgeries including the resection of myomas, polyps, and septa. Second-look hysteroscopy was applied to detect the formation of postoperative intrauterine adhesions. The incidence of the adhesions was found to be 10.44% (7/67) in patients with ACP gel and was 26.2% (17/65) in the control group ($P < 0.05$).

12.6.5.4 Prophylactic Antibiotics

The routine use of antibiotics is not usually recommended for preventing infections following hysteroscopic surgery. In patients with the use of IUD or ACP gel, broad-spectrum antibiotics should be routinely used to prevent infections. In general, it is taken for 3–7 days.

12.6.5.5 Second-Look Hysteroscopy After Hysteroscopic Surgery

The crucial healing period of the injured surfaces after hysteroscopic surgery is 1–2 months postoperatively. When the withdrawal bleeding is stopped after 1–3 months of hormone treatment, a second-look hysteroscopy may be conducted, and new filmy adhesions can be divided simultaneously and mechanically by hysteroscope, but moderate and severe adhesions must be dissected by operative hysteroscopy afterwards.

12.6.6 Treatment of Postoperative Adhesions

For hysteroscopic endometrial ablation and other types of hysteroscopic surgeries in women without the desire to become pregnant, the postoperative adhesions should be managed only when the woman has developed clinical symptoms. The therapy regimes include dividing the adhesions of the uterine cavity, draining the hematometra and fluid accumulation in uterine cavity, and reducing the periodical abdominal pain.

For patients who want to get pregnant and have intrauterine adhesions following hysteroscopic surgery, an operative hysteroscopy is needed so as to restore the normal shape of the cavity and expose bilateral tubal ostia, as well as avoid the damage to normal endometrium.

It is easy to develop recurrent adhesions after lysis of intrauterine adhesions, so adjuvant measures, such as cyclic hormone treatment and intrauterine placement of IUD, should be conducted following adhesiolysis. A second-look hysteroscopy may be performed to divide the reformed adhesions in the early postoperative period.

12.6.6.1 Division of Adhesions During Second-Look Hysteroscopy Under Ultrasonography Guidance

The mild and loose intrauterine adhesions may be divided by diagnostic hysteroscope during second-look hysteroscopy. For those patients who have adhesions in cervical os after hysteroscopic surgery, the probe may be applied to investigate the uterine cavity under abdominal ultrasonography guidance. After the drainage of dark red or coffee-like old blood, Hegar dilators can be used to dilate the cervix to No. 6 or 7, and then diagnostic hysteroscopy is performed to inspect the uterine cavity. Antibiotics should be administered postoperatively to prevent infections.

12.6.6.2 Hysteroscopic Lysis of Adhesions

If intrauterine adhesions are too thickened to be divided by diagnostic hysteroscope, operative hysteroscopy can be conducted to excise the adhesions. Usually it uses wire loop electrode to cut or the needle electrode to divide under direct vision. Adhesions which are formed following hysteroscopic endometrial resection are mostly fibromuscular adhesions. Due to the extensive areas of adhesions and insufficient identifications of endometrium, the dividing process must be guided by ultrasonography so as to avoid undue injury to uterine walls caused by blind division. This undue injury might result in massive intraoperative bleeding or uterine perforation. It should be noted that the purpose of dividing intrauterine adhesions after TCRE is not to reconstruct the uterine cavity but to release the uterine hematometra or fluid accumulation and then to alleviate periodical abdominal pain. In the process of division, there is no need to expose the bilateral fallopian tubal openings, but is enough to have the residual hematometra released completely.

For patients who develop intrauterine adhesions after TCRM, TCRP, TCRS, and TCRA, if they wish to become pregnant, attention should be paid to restoring a normal cavity, opening both tubal ostia, and trying to avoid the destruction of normal endometrium. Details of operative procedures can be seen in Sect. 9.6 of Chap. 9.

12.6.6.3 Hysterectomy

Hysterectomy may be considered in the conditions that if all the above therapies are ineffective, if there are thickened and extensive adhesions in the cavity, or if the patients have severe dysmenorrhea due to hematometra in the areas of fallopian tubal ostium.

12.7 Postoperative Pregnancy

Enlan Xia

In the early stage of application of TCRE technique, it was thought that the implantation of fertilized eggs was difficult due to the postoperative uterine scarring after TCRE, so patients who do not require fertility are listed as operative indications. In 1990, Skar and Nesheim reported that TCRE technique might be used for contraception. However, with the wide application of this procedure, there are more and more reports about pregnancy after TCRE and EA. Greater difficulty in induced abortion for postoperative pregnancy and more obstetric complications occurring in pregnant women after hysteroscopic surgery should attract the attention of the doctors and patients.

12.7.1 Possibility of Pregnancy After TCRE

Although postoperative pregnancy after EA is rare, it is possible. Kir and Hanlon-Lundberg calculated that the pregnancy rate after endometrial ablation was 0.24–0.68%. It has been reported that due to the narrowed and scarred cavity following endometrial surgery, pathologic placental adherence and fetal demise developed in postoperative pregnant woman. In theory, the resected endometrium cannot regenerate and there should be long-term contraceptive effects. DeCherney et al. reported that two cases died of medical diseases within half a year after operation, and autopsy revealed that the endometrium was completely replaced by collagen scar tissues. Magos et al. reported that second-look hysteroscopy was performed at the third and 12th month after operation in 68 cases which revealed a small uterine cavity and fibrotic endometrium. However, since the ability of endometrium to regenerate is amazing, the anatomic morphology of uterine cornua is invaginated and histological structure of muscle wall is thin, perforation of the uterus may occur easily. Uterine fundus is located in the upper portion of uterus, the wire loop electrode is needed to do the transverse cutting, which is difficult technically. The endometrial ablation by electroresection or rollerball electrocoagulation is usually not complete, so if the residual endometrium retains or regenerates, intrauterine pregnancy is possible. Turnbull et al. studied the uterus using MRI after endometrial resection in 59 women, of whom 22 were amenorrheic. The results showed that residual endometrium was in all except three cases, but not all those with residual endometrium have menses. Therefore, there are patients occasionally with postoperative pregnancy in clinical practice, which may be intrauterine or ectopic pregnancy with the occurrence rate of 0.7–2%. Xia et al. from the Hysteroscopy Center of Fuxing Hospital, Capital Medical University, analyzed 1341 TCRE procedures from May 1990 to November 2001 with a follow-up of 3 months to 11 years and 6 months. There were 32 pregnancies in 26 patients after operation with the occurrence rate of 2.39%. Among 32 pregnancies, there was one cervical pregnancy, two tubal pregnancies, and one right cornual pregnancy. Among 28 intrauterine pregnancies in 22 women, there were three pregnancies in two women and two pregnancies in two women. Its occurrence was related to the age of the patient, the ability of endometrial regeneration, and the depth and extent of endometrial resection. The probability of intrauterine pregnancies was decreased with the extension of postoperative duration. Among pregnancies following TCRE, 62.5% occurred within the first year, 21.88% in the second year, 9.38% in the third year, and 3.11% in both the fourth and fifth years. Of them, 7% occurred in the first 100 procedures, and among the rest 1241 procedures, postoperative pregnancy rate fell to 1.69%. The higher rate of occurrence in the first 100 procedures was obviously related to shallow resection of endometrium in the initial stage of the application of the procedure. The second generation endometrial ablation is safe and easy to operate compared with TCRE procedure, but in recent years its postoperative pregnancies have also been reported. Ismail et al. reported on one case of intrauterine pregnancy after thermal balloon endometrial ablation. In 1992, Whitelaw and Sutton first reported on ectopic pregnancy after TCRE. Dicker et al. reported on five cases of cervical pregnancy and held that its etiology was related to the damage to the endometrium caused by induced abortion and traumatic curettage. Two of five cases had severe intrauterine adhesions, which produced partial or total occlusion of the uterine cavity, and this kind of adhesion might be an important cause of cervical pregnancy.

In short, endometrial resection/ablation does not mean sterilization and also cannot ensure sterilization. In addition, those with no menstruation are still likely to conceive; therefore, we should have a due and sufficient understanding of pregnancy after endometrial ablation and advocate contraception in patients after operation. The doctors should warn the patients who had amenorrhea, dripping bleeding and abdominal pain of the possibility of intrauterine and ectopic pregnancy.

12.7.2 Risk of Pregnancy After TCRE

12.7.2.1 Abnormal Placenta Implantation

After endometrial resection, due to lack of decidual membrane support, the fertilized egg is likely to result in first-trimester miscarriages. Goldberg, McLucas, Mints, and other scholars have had reports about spontaneous miscarriages of pregnancy after TCRE or EA procedure. During late pregnancy, the disorder of blood supply to placenta can cause placental development and implantation abnormalities, intrauterine fetal growth retardation and intrauterine fetal death, and abnormalities of the third stage of labor. Kucera et al. reported that severe complications of postoperative pregnancy after EA and TCRS occurred in three cases. In the first case, pregnancy occurred after TCRS and uterine rupture occurred in the second stage of labor. In the other two cases, one case each occurred after TCRS and EA, respectively, and heavy bleeding occurred during the middle of pregnancy. Maouris reported on one case of pregnancy who underwent cesarean section at 30 weeks of gestation due to abnormal fetal position and premature rupture of fetal membranes, with partial adhesions between the placenta and the fundus. In the Hysteroscopy Center of Fuxing Hospital, Capital Medical University, one woman had amenorrhea achieved within 2 years after TCRE, followed by oligomenorrhea. After about 6 months of amenorrhea, a grossly distended abdomen was present, and ultrasonography indicated intrauterine pregnancy for about 6 months. At 39 weeks of gestation, a female liveborn infant was delivered by cesarean section, weighing about 2500 g. Subtotal hysterectomy was conducted due to deep implantation of the placenta into the uterine myometrium. Placenta increta was confirmed by histopathology. More seriously, there is the obstetric risk of uterine rupture after hysteroscopic electroresection. There have been nine cases reported in recent literature. Although none of them occurred following endometrial ablation, the electroresection injury should be obstetric risk factors for uterine rupture. The scarred and narrowed cavity after TCRE is quite similar to that of Asherman syndrome. Friedman et al. reported that severe obstetric complications of intrauterine adhesions are preterm birth (12%), placenta increta, sacculated uterus, and uterine dehiscence. Intrauterine adhesion after TCRE may obstruct the implantation of fertilized eggs, leading to ectopic pregnancy. If the ruptured ectopic pregnancy cannot be detected and treated timely, intraperitoneal bleeding is likely to threaten life. So patients with postoperative pregnancy after TCRE should be considered as high-risk population.

12.7.2.2 High Incidence of Ectopic Pregnancy

Xia et al. made a retrospective analysis of 1621 cases who had DUB, were unresponsive to medication, and had no desire for future pregnancy. All women underwent TCRE from 1990 to 2005 with a follow-up of 1–14 years and 8 months. There were 39 pregnancies in 32 women, of which there were five ectopic pregnancies, including one cervical pregnancy, two tubal pregnancies, one right cornual pregnancy, and one left cornual pregnancy, and they were all cured by operation. The ectopic pregnancy rate following TCRE was 12.8% (5/39) of all pregnancies. There were severe intrauterine adhesions in two cases of cornual pregnancy and one case of suspected cornual pregnancy, producing partial uterine cavity occlusion, which might be the major cause of cornual pregnancy and ectopic pregnancy. In 2007, Giarenis et al. reported on one case of cervical pregnancy after EA, who was cured with conservative treatment by ammonia armor pterin.

12.7.2.3 High-Risk Population Related to Induced Abortion

Most induced abortions after TCRE can be uneventfully performed, but they are also likely to encounter difficulties. In a follow-up of 28 cases of induced abortion in the Hysteroscopy Center of Fuxing Hospital, Capital Medical University, one case was transferred from another hospital due to a failed induced abortion and a diagnosis of right cornual pregnancy. All 28 cases underwent electric suction curettage smoothly with difficulties occurred in 4. The first case was 32 years old, who had only periodical dripping bleeding for more than 1 year after TCRE and was transferred to our hospital due to a failed induced abortion and diagnosis of right cornual pregnancy in another hospital. Gynecological examination showed an enlarged uterus with 8 weeks of gestation, and hysteroscopy revealed intrauterine adhesions and stenosis 4 cm away from the cervical os. A 7 mm resectoscope with a closed-loop electrode was used to move forward along the longitudinal axis of uterus under ultrasonography guidance with the incision of the adhesive tissues about 2 cm deep, so as to move the fetal sac into the uterine cavity and be followed by suction curettage. The second case was 38 years old, who had TCRE 4 years ago and suffered hypomenorrhea after operation. She underwent electric suction curettage after 59 days of amenorrhea. Gynecological examination revealed the uterus was enlarged to a size consistent with 8 weeks of pregnancy. Preoperative laboratory tests results: Hb 115 g/L; bleeding time 2 min; coagulation time 4 min; platelet 143 × 10^9/L; blood HbsAg(+); anti-HBc (+). There was heavy arterial bleeding after the gestational sac was aspirated totally. Cervical injection of oxytocin and combined use of hemostat for hemostasis obtained little effectiveness. The total amount of bleeding was up to 700 mL with a drop in blood pressure. A 16Fr Foley balloon was inserted into the uterine cavity, and after injection of 13 mL of sterile saline into the balloon, the bleeding was arrested. The third case was 42 years old, who had TCRE and TCRP 1 year and 5 months ago. She suffered hypomenorrhea after operation. Ultrasonography indicated intrauterine pregnancy after 40 days of amenorrhea. But when electric suction curettage was performed, only a small amount of decidual and villous tissues were aspirated by suction with the pathological report being decidua and highly secretory endometrium and placental villus. Intraoperative ultrasonography revealed that there was a dark area of fluid about 3.5 cm × 2 cm in proximal right posterior wall, which could not be touched by a probe or a suction tube. The vaginal color Doppler performed 5 days later suggested that the uterus was 7.7 cm × 6.8 cm × 4.8 cm, and the gestational sac was visible in the right posterior wall with the size 4.3 cm × 1.6 cm, in which fetal bud and fetal heart beating rhythmically were visible, and the distance between the outer brim of gestational sac and serosa was only 1.8 mm. Two days later, subtotal hysterectomy was performed, with the right uterine cornu detected outward-protruding. A "Y-shape" incision was made in the anterior wall of the uterine corpus, with fibrous scar in the uterine cavity, adhesions near the fundus, endometrium visible in the bilateral cornua, and a gestational sac about 3.5 cm in diameter seen at the right cornua with a thickness of 5 mm between the outer brim and serosa. The fourth case was 40 years old, who had the third pregnancy complicated by multiple fibroids after TCRE. She developed acute abdominal pain and low fever after 62 days of amenorrhea. She had a uterus about 11 weeks of pregnancy, diagnosed as early pregnancy complicated by uterine fibroid red degeneration. Electric suction curettage was performed under intravenous anesthesia. Due to obliteration from intrauterine scar and myomas, the uterine cavity became bended with a depth of 13 cm. The gestation sac was aspirated by suction under the guidance of ultrasonography and abdominal pain disappeared after operation.

During induced abortion in pregnant women after TCRE, heavy hemorrhage, intrauterine adhesions, cornual pregnancy, and even cervical pregnancy may be encountered. The contracture of uterine scars may cause the distortion of uterine cavity. Even with ultrasonography intervention, it is very difficult for a probe or suction tube to uneventfully enter the uterine cavity. If cervical pregnancy is not diagnosed before operation and curettage is performed hastily, the bleeding after curettage is often difficult to control. Therefore, the surgical history of TCRE should be regarded as risk factors for induced abortion.

12.7.3 Diagnosis and Management of Pregnancy After TCRE

12.7.3.1 Diagnosis

There may be improvement in menstruation after TCRE, which may be amenorrhea, spotting, hypomenorrhea, normal menstruation, and oligomenorrhea, and could also be different forms of transition like from menstruation to amenorrhea or from amenorrhea to menstruation, and there may also be dripping bleeding during the transition period. In the Hysteroscopy Center of Fuxing Hospital, Capital Medical University, the patients' menstruations from the time after TCRE to the time before pregnancy were analyzed, with hypomenorrhea in one cervical pregnancy, two tubal pregnancies, and one right cornual pregnancy. Among 32 pregnancies in 26 women, hypomenorrhea occurred in two women with three pregnancies; in two women with two pregnancies, one case had postoperative hypomenorrhea, and the other had no menstruation for 6 months after induced abortion and became pregnancy again; in 24 women each with one pregnancy, 14 cases had postoperative hypomenorrhea, six cases had no menstruation within 3–6 months after operation and small amount of period afterwards, three cases had amenorrhea for 7 months to 2 years after operation and irregular or small amount of period thereafter, and one case had amenorrhea within 3 months after operation and developed pregnancy shortly thereafter. The change in menstruation led to difficulty in timely diagnosis during the early pregnancy, so the early diagnosis of pregnancy after TCRE depends on careful attention of doctors and patients to pregnancy and the regular follow-up.

12.7.3.2 Management

Generally, the patients who accept TCRE procedure have no desire for future pregnancy. If pregnancy occurs, mostly it will end up in induced abortion. Therefore, both the hospitals and doctors receiving patients should be well prepared to deal with a variety of difficult conditions during induced abortion. The location of gestational sac must be accurately determined by ultrasonography prior to operation, and the difficulty of the operation should be estimated through a careful observation of uterine cavity. For patients with obscure uterine lining or migrated gestational sac, it is better to perform the cervical catheterization before operation, administer anesthesia during operation, and carry out suction aspiration under ultrasonography monitoring. If the insertion of the probe or the suction tube is difficult, diagnostic hysteroscopy can be performed to inspect the cervical canal and the uterine cavity. If stenosis, adhesion, or distortion occurs, incision under ultrasonography guidance can make the uterine cavity unblocked. Hysteroscopy can be performed to check whether the embryo is aspirated by suction completely or not at the end of the procedure. There is profuse bleeding at the end of suction evacuation in the second case mentioned above. In order to avoid removal of the uterus, Foley balloon compression is an effective alternative before implementation of radical therapy. After termination of pregnancy in the fourth case, abdominal pain disappeared.

Baumann et al. first reported on a successful pregnancy with good outcomes after tubal sterilization by bipolar coagulation and TCRE. Pugh et al. reported on a viable pregnancy after EA. Pinette et al. reported on a successful pregnancy after YAG laser ablation. There is also report about treatment of infertility with TCRE. Cravello et al. reported that endometrial ablation was performed in patients with AUB who failed in progestin therapy. Patients who conceived after recovery from bleeding might have term deliveries. There was one case of full term pregnancy after TCRE at the Hysteroscopy Center of Fuxing Hospital, Capital Medical University. A small infant was delivered by cesarean section. Due to total implantation of placenta, the uterine corpus was removed at the same time. So if pregnancy is detected during the second or the third trimester of pregnancy and the patients have desire for delivery, continuation of pregnancy may be considered. In order to achieve a better obstetric prognosis, a close and strict pregnancy care should be carried out to monitor the fetal development and the placental function. For the patients who want a vaginal delivery, the third stage labor should be handled properly; for the patients who want a cesarean section delivery, the possibility of hysterectomy should be considered.

12.8 Postablation-Tubal Sterilization Syndrome

Enlan Xia

Postablation-tubal sterilization syndrome (PASS) is a late complication of TCRE procedure. In 1993, Townsend et al. first reported that 6 women who had a history of tubal sterilization followed by endometrial ablation suffered postoperative lower abdominal pain and dripping vaginal bleeding. In all patients, hysteroscopy revealed obvious scarring of endometrium, and laparoscopy showed one or two tubal swollen and hematocele in the proximal portion. As all the patients have a history of tubal sterilization, it is named as postablation-tubal sterilization syndrome. In 1996, Bae et al. reported on characteristic pathologic findings in six cases with postablation-tubal sterilization syndrome, which included hematosalpinx, and some changes under microscope such as endometriosis, acute and chronic inflammation of the fallopian tubes, and acute and chronic myometritis. In the same year, Webb et al. reported one case of such conditions. This patient had previous tubal sterilization and previous dysmenorrhea which had been relieved with leuprorelin, who developed cyclic abdominal pain 6 months after endometrial ablation, followed by vaginal spotting. Ultrasonography revealed an echo-free zone in uterine fundus. She was treated by total hysterectomy and bilateral oophorectomy, with hematosalpinx and dilation of proximal tubes identified at the time of operation, as well as endometriosis detected in the right fallopian tube, which was considered to be the cause of preoperative dysmenorrhea. However, postoperative pain was far serious than the preoperative pain, leading to hysterectomy required. In 1999, Xia reported four cases of PASS who underwent TCRE 1–8 years after tubal sterilization. Serious cyclic or persistent lower abdominal pain concomitant with hydrosalpinx developed within 3–11 months following TCRE. The features of the cases are shown in Table 12.22. The first three cases had no history of dysmenorrhea prior to TCRE and had a slight large uterus, and the fourth case had mild dysmenorrhea with a normal uterus. Ultrasonography revealed uneven echo in the myometrium in the first case. At the time of TCRE, adenomyosis, which was not suspected in all the four cases, was confirmed in the first three cases by pathology and might be one of the causes of severe abdominal pain.

12.8.1 Etiology of PASS

After TCRE, cyclic bleeding still occurs in the residual functional endometrium or future regenerative endometrium in the uterine cavity. The uterine scarring or distortion may block the discharge of menstrual blood, and if the blockage occurs at the distal end of fallopian tubes, the upstream of menstrual blood leads to hematosalpinx, thus causing PASS.

Table 12.22 Characteristics of PASS in four cases

No.	Postoperative menstruation	Onset of PASS	Treatment	Histological results
1	Amenorrhea for 3 months, followed by spotting	Five months after operation	Total hysterectomy, both oophorectomy, and appendix	Adenomyosis, mild hyperplasia endometrium, bilateral chronic salpingitis, chronic appendicitis
2	Amenorrhea	Five months after operation	Total hysterectomy, left salpingectomy, right oophorectomy, and appendectomy	Adenomyosis, endometrium at proliferative stage; left chronic salpingitis; chronic appendicitis
3	Amenorrhea for 3 months, followed by spotting	Three months after operation	Resection of intrauterine adhesion and residual endometrium	Adenomyosis
4	Amenorrhea for 9 months, followed by spotting	11 months after operation	Exploration of the cavity and discharge of hematocele	No

12.8.2 Diagnosis of PASS

PASS may be one of the various causes of abdominal pain in the late postoperative period, which usually occurs a few months after operation, and manifests as cyclic unilateral or bilateral abdominal pain. The pain may exacerbate due to the tubal distention and may be combined or not combined with vaginal spotting. The severity of pain is related to the length of proximal fallopian tube, the area of residual endometrium, and the volume of hemorrhage. The late onset of symptoms may be explained by the slow endometrial regeneration. Ultrasonography may reveal an echolucent area in the uterine fundus. Diagnosis can be determined by tubal dilation detected via ultrasonography, laparotomy, or laparoscopy (Fig. 12.22).

12.8.3 Treatment of PASS

PASS is a late complication of fallopian tubal ligation and endometrial ablation. So the earlier detection and management are undertaken, the better the outcomes are. Gannon thought that the patients who underwent endometrial ablation after tubal sterilization should conduct ultrasonography examination 4 months after operation for timely detection and elimination of uterine hematocele or resection of residual endometrium, and if ineffective, the patients should undergo hysterectomy. Townsend et al. suggested that laparoscopy should be the first choice for treatment. Since the pathological changes of hematosalpinx might be bilateral, even if there was only unilateral pain, the bilateral salpingectomy should be undergone. Among six cases of PASS, five responded well to laparoscopic salpingectomy or electrocauterization of the compromised fallopian tubes, and the last case underwent transvaginal removal of uterus due to the recurrence of the symptom. After treatment of six cases of postoperative cyclic pain, Bae et al. held that laparoscopic tubal resection assisted with selective hysterectomy could successfully relieve the symptoms. Webb et al. believed that when there was an extensive understanding of this syndrome, a more conservative method than transvaginal resection of total uterus and bi-adnexa might be taken, including laparoscopic salpingectomy or hysteroscopic repeat resection of the residual endometrium. Among four cases treated by Xia, the first case achieved no improvements after undergoing the exploration of the uterine cavity twice and consistently applying nemestran and danazol after eliminating the hematometra. Laparotomy was performed 15 months after operation and the resected specimen revealed hematometra in two small cavities in the left uterine cornu and uterine fundus with bits of endometrium and hematometra in the left fallopian tube. The second case developed cyclic spasmodic pain in the lower abdomen as of 5 months after surgery, which comes and goes, mild or serious, with intramuscular injection of pethidine hydrochloride (dolantin) ineffective in severe cases. Laparotomy was performed 23 months after surgery and the resected specimen revealed that the majority of the uterine cavity was occluded due to adhesions and there was hematometra in three small cavities in the left uterine cornu and swelling and hematometra in the left fallopian tube. The third case developed sharp pain in the left lower quadrant of abdomen during menstrual period since the return of menses. The diagnostic hysteroscope was inserted and gained access only 4 cm into the uterine cavity due to occlusion of the upper segment of uterine cavity. The operative hysteroscopy was applied to incise the adhesive band and the uterine cavity was unblocked with a whole length of uterine cavity 7.8 cm. The right tubal opening and some hematometra were visible, while the left tubal opening was not clear, and left lower abdominal pain disappeared. The fourth case developed cyclic sharp pain in the lower abdomen 3 months after the return of menses and then was concomitant with amenorrhea for 40 days with enlarged uterus. Ultrasonography revealed bilateral hydrosalpinx and hydrohystera. The uterine cavity was investigated under ultrasonography guidance, with resistance encountered at 4 cm of insertion. A slight force forward brought a sense of breakthrough and lead to the outflow of old and fresh blood about 200 mL. Then the acoustic image of dilated bilateral fallopian tubes disappeared, and abdominal pain was relieved immediately.

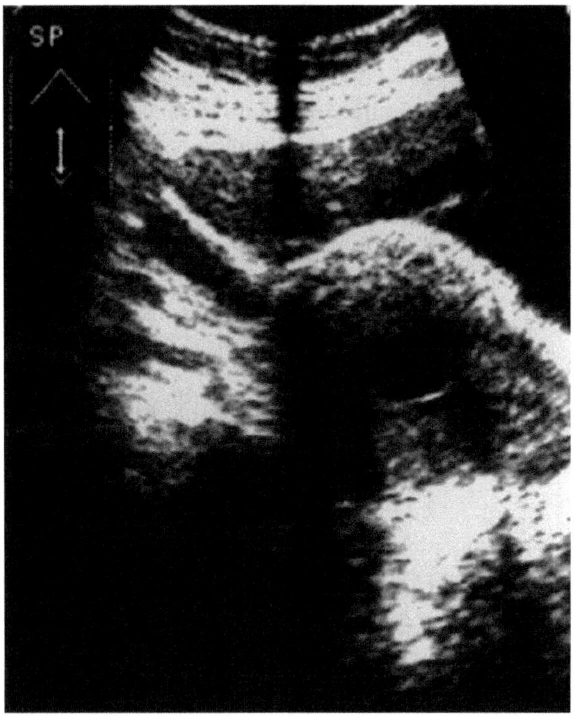

Fig. 12.22 Uterine cavity and hematosalpinx with PASS under ultrasonography

12.8.4 Prevention of PASS

In order to avoid perforation of uterus, there may be insufficient resection of the endometrium at the easily perforated sites like the uterine fundus and uterine cornua at the time of TCRE, leading to the presence of active endometrium in this area continuously. Its cyclic bleeding is obstructed in the remaining parts of uterine cavity by the surgical scar and synechia and enters the obliterated fallopian tubes via the tubal orifices, leading to the dilation of proximal fallopian tubes, resulting in pain. The severity of the symptom may depend on the length of proximal tubes, the extent of functional endometrium, and the volume of hemorrhage. Therefore, the operator should remove the endometrium at the uterine cornua and uterine fundus as completely as possible, and if not sure, electrocautery may be used, which is relatively safer than electroresection. The data presented by Gannon et al. suggested that the incidence of PASS after rollerball endometrial ablation was far less than that of TCRE ($P < 0.007$). Bae et al. proposed that when electroresection and laparoscopic sterilization were performed at the same time, laparoscopic electrocoagulation of the proximal fallopian tube and destruction of uterine cornua should be performed so as to prevent this syndrome.

Other authors have reported on the similar clinical manifestations. Magos et al. made a retrospective study that, in 234 patients after TCRE, 16 cases had hysterectomy for a variety of reasons, including two cases undergoing hysterectomy at the ninth and 12th months after surgery due to severe abdominal pain. Of them, one case had hematometra at the left cornu which was similar to that of PASS and had recurrence following hysteroscopic drainage. Sorensen et al. reported on one case who had hematosalpinx and dilated fallopian tube after EA which was similar to that of PASS, and worsening cyclic abdominal pain within 8 months after surgery. However, these two authors did not indicate whether those patients had histories of tubal sterilization or not. Nowadays, with the wide application of TCRE, an increase in the number of procedures and the prolonged duration of follow-up sheds light on the late complications of postoperative abdominal pain. Steffensen and Schuster presented explanations of its causes as following: (1) intrauterine adhesions; (2) the regeneration of the residual endometrium at the uterine fundus leads to hematometra; (3) the covering of the basal layer of endometrium by scar leads to iatrogenic adenomyosis and progressive dysmenorrhea; (4) the functional endometrium is squeezed into the myometrium under the intrauterine pressure at the time of operation, leading to adenomyosis; (5) the endometrium at the uterine cornua is not completely destroyed. Therefore, whether PASS is one independent syndrome requires further discussions. Wortman held that the prevention of this syndrome was similar to the prevention of uterine hematometra after TCRE/EA, that is, careful resection of all sites of endometrium at the time of operation, including the uterine cornua. The uterine cornua may be deeply concaved in some cases, so its removal may be neglected, and if the patient had a history of previous tubal sterilization, PASS will occur.

12.9 Accidental Electrical Injuries

Baoliang Lin

In recent years, great improvements on high-frequency electric devices have been made not only in quality but also in safety, and there is a significant decrease in accidental electrical injuries. However there is still risk of the occurrence of accidental electrical injuries in the hospitals using the old type of high-frequency devices. Therefore, the doctors and nurses who manipulate high-frequency electric devices must understand the accidents that may be caused by high-frequency waves.

12.9.1 Electrical Burn Accidents

Electrical burn accidents are mainly caused by high intensity of high-frequency wave current, which can be divided into two types as follows.

12.9.1.1 Burns Around the Negative Plate

Generally, in order to avoid a very high local current density, a large negative plate is required for use. This negative plate needs to be connected to the human body comprehensively and intensively and a close connection with the muscles rich in bloodstream can ensure a return current of high-frequency wave; otherwise, electrical burns will occur. In addition, the closer the connection of the negative plate to the surgical site, the shorter is the running distance for the high-frequency wave in the human body.

1. Negative plate: Being easily bent, a negative plate can be fixed at the bending positions like the thigh. However, if the negative plate of lead is bent several times, its surface will become uneven, which will lead to a decrease in the contact area with the human body. In addition, due to metal fatigue, the negative plate may crack or break, leading to a decrease in the effective area of the negative plate, and high intensity of return current of the high-frequency wave current may result in electrical burn.
2. Negative plate for younger children: due to the small area, it is easy to cause burns.
3. Stainless steel negative plate: It is more commonly used because it has advantages of no corrosion and easy cleaning after use. In order to increase the electrical conductivity, it is often wrapped with saline-soaked gauze when in

use. If it is wrapped with dry gauze, or soaked with common water instead of saline, there will be a decrease in the electric conductivity. Once the return current is intensified at one site, it is easy to cause local burns. The stainless steel negative plate is hard in texture, if connected to the protruding positions like the sacrum, scapula, and so on, the contact area will be reduced. If the patient's position changes, the negative plate migrates, there will also be a decrease in the contact area, thus causing burns.

4. The electrolyte-free disinfectant liquid may flow in between the well-connected negative plate, and there will be a decrease in the contact area between the negative plate and the human body, resulting in burns.
5. The disinfectant liquid may flow in between the well-connected negative plate, which corrodes the negative plate, resulting in a decrease in the contact area, thus causing burns.

12.9.1.2 Burns Outside the Site of Negative Plate

High-frequency wave is very likely to stray, and burns occur when the stray current passes through the site outside the negative plate. More common causes are: the negative plate being abnormal, the patient touching the metal parts of the operating table, the stray current being caused by blood and saline on the operating table, and stray currents being induced by resectoscope via speculum. In addition, stray currents are also generated by electrode via the ECG and electroencephalography (EEG). Vilos et al. reported 13 cases of genital tract electrical burns due to the stray currents generated by speculum of resectoscope.

12.9.2 Electric Shock Accidents

Electric shock accidents are caused by electricity leakage. There are two types of electric shock: macro- and micro-shock. Macro-shock occurs when electric current runs from outside through the skin or human body and runs out of the body, micro-shock involves the running of an electric current through the body tissues into the heart. Both types of shock may endanger life.

12.9.3 Accidents Caused by Electromagnetic Interference

High-frequency electric device is one that can generate high-power high-frequency wave. When high-frequency electric device is in use, its powerful electromagnetic wave can affect a variety of electronic instruments, such as ECG, EEG, computer, and artificial pacemakers, and cause disorders induced by random wave to interfere with normal function of electronic instrument. A more serious consequence is the interference with the artificial pacemaker which can endanger life.

12.9.4 Accidents Caused by Sparks

As flammable anesthetic gas is no longer used, explosive accidents would not now occur, but under the conditions of high concentration oxygen, the use of electric knife could also be dangerous.

12.10 Other Complications

Enlan Xia

12.10.1 Hematometra

Hematometra is a rare complication following TCRE and EA. Uterine fundus and bilateral uterine walls are with folds, which are easy to develop synechiae after operation, resulting in a small or narrow uterus. The anterior and posterior uterine walls adhere to each other when uterine contraction occurs, if such condition lasts long, synechia may occur. Most of such uterine synechia are asymptomatic, and abdominal pain is the major symptom which prompts the patient to go to see a doctor. The uterine synechia in some patients is detected when hysteroscopy is performed for other indications, so its incidence is unknown. The lower segment of uterine cavity is occluded due to synechiae, and when there is active endometrium in the upper segment still responsive to ovarian hormone, the menstrual blood accumulates, leading to hematometra. Regular postoperative exploration of uterine cavity and (or) diagnostic hysteroscopy may prevent or detect the occurrence of this disease. Theoretically, the cervical stenosis at isthmus can cause hematometra, so Hamou proposed that partial endometrial ablation should be performed and the endometrium of 1 cm at lower end of uterine cavity should be retained. In fact, even after resection of the mucous membrane at the upper segment of cervix, cervical stenosis and secondary hematometra are also extremely rare. On the contrary, all hematometra occurs in the uterine fundus, as long as there is still active endometrium in the fibrotic uterine cavity after endometrial ablation, there is equal chance of occurrence of hematometra after total or partial resection of the endometrium. This condition occurs 2–16 months after operation and the reported incidence is 1.8% according to some scholars. Tapper and Heinonen reported that in 84 cases of TCRE, there were four cases of postoperative hematometra occurring in first few days after TCRE. Postoperative treatment with HRT following TCRE might also cause hematometra, whose symptoms are cyclic or persistent abdominal pain and intermittent vaginal bleeding. A uterine probe could not get to the uterus, but under ultrasonography hematocele in the uterus is visible, which is easy to diagnose. If exploration of uterine cavity, elimination of hematocele, and maintaining a smooth drainage of uterine cavity produce good treatment effects, hysteroscopic resection of intrauterine adhesions and residual endometrium under ultrasonography intervention can prevent its recurrence. Romer et al. reported that one case experienced cyclical abdominal pain 13 months after TCRE and hematometra occurred due to obliteration of the cervical internal ostium. They pointed out that all patients should have a regular clinical and sonographical follow-up after operation. But it still remains to be confirmed whether it is necessary to perform regular exploration of uterine cavity within weeks after operation so as to reduce its occurrence, while it may cause infection and perforation of the uterus. The incomplete drainage of uterine cavity after operation may also cause hematometra and spasmodic pain in the lower quadrant of abdomen. Among 149 cases of TCRE performed by Lin, regular outpatient treatment by dilation of the cervix was administered all within 1 month after operation and there was no occurrence of hematometra. Among 1100 TCRM procedures, one case developed cervical adhesion and hematometra due to the resection of myoma near the cervix and cured after cervical dilation and elimination of hematocele. Hill et al. reported on 24 cases of hematometra who received treatment by puncture, drainage, flushing with irrigation fluid via hysteroscopy, of which one case was treated by vaginal hysterectomy. He pointed out that any patient who underwent TCRE and EA should be informed of the potential complications. McCausland et al. reported partial endometrial ablation could successfully treat menorrhagia in patients without deep adenomyosis, and it did not cause intrauterine adhesions and hematometra. In 2002, McCausland et al. undertook a study of the frequency, diagnosis, treatment, and prevention of symptomatic cornual hematometra and PASS in 50 patients who received total rollerball endometrial ablation. After a follow-up of 4–90 months, 5 (10%) were diagnosed by ultrasonography or MRI, with two patients with cornual hematometra and 3 patients with PASS. Subsequent GnRH-a or hysteroscopic drainage achieved limited effect, and hysterectomy with salpingectomy was performed in recurrent cases. They suggested that the incidence of hematometra was not uncommon (10%) and could be decreased by partial EA.

12.10.2 Abdominal Pain

Severe lower abdominal pain is the condition related to the occurrence of hematometra, which is often cyclical, but there is pain without hematocele in the uterine cavity and even without menstruation, which may occur in a small number of women. There is a postoperative decrease in menstrual blood and an increase in abdominal pain in some patients but the reasons remain unknown. Laparoscopic examination may reveal endometriosis and other causes of pelvic pains. However, there is still a lack of evidence for extrinsic endometriosis caused by hysteroscopic operations, and it is most likely to cause internal endometriotic foci and the small ectopic foci buried in the myometrium. This condition is similar to intrauterine adhesions with abdominal pain described by Asherman, and 25% of the patients with Asherman's intrauterine adhesions have pelvic pain. In respect to treatment, only analgesics are ineffective to relieve the severe abdominal pain, and there is no report about the effect of laparoscopic presacral neurectomy, so its efficacy is unclear, some patients require hysterectomy. Mints et al. reported that in 97 cases who were followed with a mean period of 29 months, 11 women (11%) suffered from postoperative dysmenorrhea. The following theories can explain the abdominal pain after TCRE: (1) Intrauterine adhesions; (2) The regeneration of residual endometrium at the uterine fundus leads to hematometra; (3) The covering of the basal layer of endometrium by scar leads to iatrogenic adenomyosis and progressive dysmenorrhea; (4) The active endometrium is squeezed into the myometrium under the increased intrauterine pressure at the time of operation, leading to adenomyosis; (5) The endometrium at the uterine cornua is not completely destroyed. Steffensen and Hahn held that resection of a submucous adenomyoma during TCRE increased the risk of distention fluid absorption. Later cyclic pelvic pain after operation was associated with large amount of intraoperative fluid absorption and postoperatively persistent menstrual bleeding.

12.10.3 Iatrogenic Uterine Adenomyosis

As there are more and more surgical cases, scholars have come to realize the presence of adenomyosis confirmed by subsequent hysterectomy that might cause the postoperative abdominal pain which is hard to explain. In UK, a large scale of cross-sectional study was undertaken in thirteen hospitals of Scottish Health Board to assess the satisfaction in 978 cases at 12 months postoperatively by questionnaire between December 1991 and December 1993 who had hysteroscopic surgery for menstrual disorder. The criterion for satisfaction was that there was postoperative menstrual improvement and no need for any form of treatment. Eighty-four percent of those returning their questionnaires were satisfied or very satisfied. The main reason for dissatisfaction was exacerbation of pain. There was no constant relationship between the satisfaction rate and postoperative amenorrhea rate. Adenomyosis was hard to determine except for triple symptom complex prior to operation. Bae et al. held that it still remained to be explored whether the postoperative exacerbation of abdominal pain was caused by worsening of previous adenomyosis or by surgery. Some scholars thought that postoperative adenomyosis should have developed before TCRE or EA and had no relation with the surgery. Mints et al. reported that 29% of cases suffered from adenomyosis after operation. Data reported proved that adenomyosis was easier to occur when electric cutting loop was applied in TCRE than that when rollerball or laser in EA was applied. The reason might be that endometrium is more easily retained in TCRE than in EA and is covered by scarring tissues subsequently, leading to iatrogenic endometriosis. Another reason might be that at the time of endometrial resection, the endometrium enters through the traumatized vessels or muscle layers into the uterine myometrium, causing this disorder. Keckstein reported that adenomyosis was a disease of the myometrium, which could be diagnosed by hysteroscopy. The depth of the adenomyosis might be investigated by transcervical punch biopsies or loop resection. Superficial adenomyosis could be managed by transcervical coagulation or resection of endometrium, which could lead to iatrogenic adenomyosis. However, it could be treated by second-look hysteroscopy. Adenomyosis might also be caused by partial EA or TCRE. In selected cases, it was possible for hysteroscopic treatment of symptomatic focal adenomyosis. Some scholars have noticed that the purple blue dots were visible in the superficial myometrium in patients who had hysterectomy following TCRE, which was ectopic endometrium. There are two kinds of explanation for it. At the beginning of advocating hysteroscopic resection, it was discovered when patients asked treatment for abdominal pain. So, it was thought that when the endometrium was compressed into the myometrial wall during operation, if survived, adenomyosis occurred, which was a complication of TCRE. However, due to an increase in the number of cases, pathological findings showed that adenomyosis foci were found in 8% of the resected muscle strips in which adenomyosis was not preoperatively diagnosed. Recently, doctors had been trying deep cutting in transcervical resection of the endometrium, which reached 4–5 mm underlying the endometrium, and the detection rate of adenomyosis had been increased up to 46%. So, it was thought that there were more patients with adenomyosis prior to operation, but we could not explain why they were preoperatively asymptomatic while abdominal pain occurred postoperatively.

12.10.4 Treatment Failure and Recurrence of Symptoms

In the short-term after operation, clinically, there should be clear distinctions in treatment failure, lack of improvement of symptom, and recurrence of symptom. In cases performed by most operators, the improvement of menstruation is achieved in 80–90% of patients after one surgery, and the recurrence of symptoms after a successful electroresection or laser surgery is extremely rare. Although it is a novel procedure and the follow-up data are limited, the majority of women benefit from this surgery, and there are still exceptional patients who have amenorrhea after total resection of endometrium but heavy bleeding occurs suddenly 2 years later. If initial treatment fails and the symptom recurs, a second operation may be performed. Hysterectomy should be reserved as a last resort, and this novel procedure should not be performed by force against the patient's wishes. The incidence of postoperative abnormal uterine bleeding is 5–10%, which occurs more often when there is endometrial regeneration. However, there is such case on earth who has bleeding but without endometrium confirmed by hysteroscopy or hysterectomy, which was thought to be induced by uterine vascular dysplasia according to the father of hysteroscopy—Hamou from France. Such kind of hemorrhage is always sudden and transient, and sometimes may heal spontaneously. There has been no good way in its prevention and treatment up to now.

12.10.5 Malignant Lesions of the Uterus

There are two types of malignant lesions to be discussed, namely the latent endometrial carcinoma and the long-term risk of canceration. Electroresection can provide tissues for histological examination, which is superior to other procedures in this respect. It still is a purely theoretical issue whether subsequent canceration occurs in buried endometrial island, or whether endometrial cancer is concealed by intrauterine adhesion or cervical stenosis. However, it is most important that the ablation of the endometrium reduces the risk of endometrial canceration. If there are still bits of tissues of endometrium in situ at the end of the operation, the chances of development of endometrial cancer are slim. There is no change in the probability of occurrence of uterine sarcoma, cervical cancer, and ovarian tumor. In the Hysteroscopy Center of Fuxing Hospital, Capital Medical University, there has been a case of endometrial cancer developed 8 years after hysteroscopic electroresection. This 60-year-old woman underwent TCRP and TCRE for menopausal bleeding and endometrial polyps, with the pathological examination of excised tissues showing endometrium and endometrial polyps. At the postoperative follow-up, there was no bleeding and fluid discharge all the time until vaginal spotting occurred 8 years later. Hysteroscopic examination and biopsy were performed 3 days later and revealed thickened endometrium with the length of uterine cavity 7 cm. Histological findings showed atypical endometrial hyperplasia and suspicion of cancer. Extensive removal of total uterus and both adnexa was performed and no enlarged lymph nodes in pelvic cavity were detected. Postoperative histological examination revealed diffuse well-differentiated endometrial adenocarcinoma, which invaded 1/2 of myometrial layer and involved bilateral cornua, and no abnormalities were found in bilateral ovaries and fallopian tubes. At present, there are eight cases of occurrence of endometrial cancer after TCRE reported worldwide, and all cases had preoperative conditions of endometrial simple or complex hyperplasia. So, to these patients, postoperative treatment with high progesterone should be administered.

12.10.6 Uterine Necrosis

Rousseau et al. reported on one case with uterine myometrial coagulative necrosis occurring after Nd-YAG laser endometrial ablation. This patient had initial adenomyosis and was treated preoperatively with Luteinizing Hormone-Releasing Hormone (LH-RH).

12.10.7 Pulmonary Hemorrhage

In 2007, Su et al. reported for the first time a rare fatal complication of lung collapse resulted from pulmonary hemorrhage after hysteroscopic operation.

12.10.8 Transient Blindness

It is known to urologists that transient blindness may be induced after transurethral resection of the prostate with 1.5% glycine as the irrigating fluid, which was first reported by Israeli Dr. Levin and Ben-David in 1996. In 1999, Indian Dr. Motashaw and Dave reported a case of postoperative transient blindness in a 38-year-old woman who underwent TCRM and TCRE with 1.5% glycine as distention medium. In 2003, Turkish Karci and Erkin also reported one case of transient blindness occurring after TCRM.

12.10.9 Nerve Injury

Nerve injury is often caused by fibular nerve compression or overstretching of the sciatic nerve with its occurrence rate of 0.01–0.04%. Most of the nerve injuries are caused by incorrect lithotomy position during hysteroscopic surgery or long-time compression from the leg holders and equipment. Its symptoms include pain or paralysis, which can recover completely, but sometimes takes longer time. To avoid this trouble, the operator should check in person the patient's positioning and body posture before operation.

12.10.10 Death

The greatest risk of TCRE does not lie in the operation, but in the operator. There are two reports about 27 cases who died of severe hyponatremia induced by body fluid overload and died due to the fatal intraabdominal bleeding caused by uterine perforation. Among them, the common feature is that the operators are inexperienced and lack either the basic knowledge or the basic skills, so hysteroscopic surgery is not suitable for the beginners. In Scotland, it was reported that among 978 cases having hysteroscopic surgery, there was one death from toxic shock syndrome. Hulka et al. concluded that among 17,298 hysteroscopies, there were three deaths. Bae et al. pointed out that when the uterine cavity was dilated to 10–11 mm using laminaria and the intrauterine pressure was maintained constantly below 70–75 mmHg, there would be a better uterine distention and vision field and might reduce the occurrence rate of the major potential complications like perforation of the uterus. The prerequisite to avoid death is the confident diagnostic techniques in using hysteroscopy. On the contrary, an operator who is expert in laparoscopy cannot replace the one expert in hysteroscopy in that these two kinds of procedures are so different from each other. TCRE and other endometrial ablation procedures are considered as "minimally invasive," but in the hands of a wrong operator, it will become "the greatest trauma."

12.10.11 Complications of the Second Generation Endometrial Ablation

The second generation endometrial ablation is performed with a disposable device which is inserted into the uterine cavity to ablate, lyse, or destroy the endometrium, so it is also called global endometrial ablation. In contrast to first generation endometrial ablation, the global endometrial ablation does not require uterine distention and uses heat instead of electricity. Its device is computer-controlled, which can display pressure, temperature, and time. So it is relatively safe in general, but there are also complications. In 2003, Gurtcheff and Sharp reported about the complications of global endometrial ablation present in Medline and references, which included hemorrhage (two cases), pelvic infection (one case), endometriosis (20 cases), skin burns (two cases of grade 1), hematometra (nine cases), vaginitis and(or) cystitis (16 cases). Data from the Food and Drug Administration and User Facility Device Experience (MAUDE) showed that there were 85 complications in 62 patients, which included bowel thermal injuries in eight cases, uterine perforation in 30 cases, of which 12 cases required immediate laparotomy, three cases were transferred into ICU, one case developed necrotizing fasciitis leading to genital mutilation, ureteral stoma, and bilateral below-knee amputations, and one case died of bowel thermal injury. None of these complications has been reported in published literature. There were more reports about the complications following thermal balloon endometrial ablation, with hematometra followed this procedure in <3% of patients, but risk factors for this complication were still unclear. In 2001, Hubert et al. reported that a woman who had a history of cervical incompetence at the time of pregnancy experienced cervical atresia and hematometra following UBT, which was treated by cervical dilatation and temporary insertion of a stent. It was thought that the normal resistance of the internal os might be important in preventing injuries to cervical canal caused by heat of UBT. It was suggested from this case that a history of cervical incompetence might be a clinical indicator of decreased cervical resistance. In 2007, Robson and Devine reported two cases of necrosis of uterine myoma after thermal balloon EA. In the same year, Schlumbrecht et al. reported on a case who subsequently developed pyometra after thermal endometrial ablation that induced sepsis and cervical necrosis. In 2004, Roth and Rivlin reported a case of thermal ablation with bilateral tubo-ovarian abscesses being developed 50 days later, and the patient was treated by total abdominal hysterectomy and bilateral salpingo-oophorectomy. In 2006, Leung and Yuen reported one case of PASS following thermal balloon endometrial ablation. In 2004, Kir and Hanlon-Lundberg reported that a 38-year-old woman had a three-chambered uterus due to adhesions after thermal balloon uterine endometrial ablation. She got pregnant at the 11th months after the operation. She spontaneously delivered a liveborn infant without complication at 35 weeks of gestation. In 2007, Foote et al. reported a pregnancy in a 43-year-old woman after thermal balloon endometrial ablation and uterine artery embolization. A livebirth infant weighing 2466 g was delivered by cesarean section. In 2003, El-Toukhy and Hefni first reported that a woman who had laparoscopic tubal sterilization 4 years ago experienced conception and miscarriage following HTA. In 2006, Moukarram et al. reported a case of pregnancy after MEA. In 2005, Gandhi et al. reported a case of cervical pregnancy after Cavaterm. It can be concluded that complications occurred following the first generation EA could occur following the second generation EA. There is still no report about the occurrence of gas embolism after second generation EA.

Suggested Reading

Organ Injury

1. A Scottish audit of hysteroscopic surgery for menorrhagia: complications and follow up. Scottish Hysteroscopy Audit Group. Br J Obstet Gynaecol. 1995;102(3):249–54.
2. Alford WS, Hopkins MP. Endometrial rollerball ablation. J Reprod Med. 1996;41:251–4.
3. Boe Engelsen I, Woie K, Hordnes K. Transcervical endometrial resection: long-term results of 390 procedures. Acta Obstet Gynecol Scand. 2006;85(1):82–7.
4. Bukulmez O, Yarali H, Gurgan T. Total corporal synechiae due to tuberculosis carry a very poor prognosis following hysteroscopic synechia lysis. Hum Reprod. 1999;14:1960–1.
5. Carter JE. Hysteroscopic surgery – avoid the complication of hyponatraemic encephalopathy. Minim Invasive Ther Allied Technol. 1997;6(3):241–8.
6. Castaing N, Darai E, Chuong T, Benifla JL, Bernard G, Meneux E, Tardif D, Batallan A, Madelenat P. Complications mécaniques et métaboliques de l'hystéroscopie opératoire: à propos d'une étude rétrospective de 352 interventions [Mechanical and metabolic complications of hysteroscopic surgery: report of a retrospective study of 352 procedures]. Contracept Fertil Sex. 1999;27(3):210–5. French.
7. Chen MY, Edwards VH, Ott DJ, Fayez JA. Hysterosalpingography after hysteroscopic surgery. Abdom Imaging. 1994;19(5):477–80.
8. Choe JK, Baggish MS. Hysteroscopic treatment of septate uterus with Neodymium-YAG laser. Fertil Steril. 1992;57:81–4.
9. Chokri A, Chekib M, Fethi Z, Anis F, Sadok M. Rupture utérine au troisième trimestre aprés metroplastie hysteroscopique [Uterine rupture in the third trimester after a hysteroscopic metroplasty]. Tunis Med. 2000;78(8–9):527–9. French.
10. Cravello L, de Montgolfier R, D'Ercole C, Boubli L, Blanc B. Hysteroscopic surgery in postmenopausal women. Acta Obstet Gynecol Scand. 1996;75(6):563–6.
11. Cravello L, D'Ercole C, Roge P, Boubli L, Blanc B. Hysteroscopic management of menstrual disorders: a review of 395 patients. Eur J Obstet Gynecol Reprod Biol. 1996;67(2):163–7.
12. Creinin M, Chen M. Uterine defect in a twin pregnancy with a history of hysteroscopic fundal perforation. Obstet Gynecol. 1992;79:879–80.
13. Daniell JF, Kurtz BR, Ke RW. Hysteroscopic endometrial ablation using the rollerball electrode. Obstet Gynecol. 1992;80(3Pt1):329–32.
14. Duan H, Xia EL, Zhang M, Yu D, Peng XB, Cheng J, Zheng J. Clinical analysis of 36 cases with complications of operative hysteroscopy. Chin J Obstet Gynecol. 2005;40(7):435–7. Chinese.
15. Erian MM, Goh JT. Transcervical endometrial resection. J Am Assoc Gynecol Laparosc. 1996;3:263–6.
16. Gabriele A, Zanetta G, Pasta F, Colombo M. Uterine rupture after hysteroscopic metroplasty and labor induction. A case report. J Reprod Med. 1999;44(7):642–4.
17. Gürgan T, Yarali H, Urman B, Dagli V, Dogan L. Uterine rupture following hysteroscopic lysis of synechiae due to tuberculosis and uterine perforation. Hum Reprod. 1996;11(2):291–3.
18. Hallez JP. Single-stage total hysteroscopic myomectomies: indications, techniques, and results. Fertil Steril. 1995;63:703–8.
19. Halvorson LM, Aserkoff RD, Oskowitz SP. Spontaneous uterine rupture after hysteroscopic metroplasty with uterine perforation: a case report. J Reprod Med. 1993;38:236–8.
20. Horak S, Blecharz A, Rzempołuch J, Grochal S. Powikłania zabiegów endoskopowych w ginekologii [Complications of endoscopy in gynecology]. Ginekol Pol. 1992;63(12):619–22. Polish.
21. Howe RS. Third-trimester uterine rupture following hysteroscopic uterine perforation. Obstet Gynecol. 1993;81:827–9.
22. Hucke J, Campo RL, De Bruyne F, Freikha AA. Die hysteroskopische Resektion submuköser Myome [Hysteroscopic resection of submucous myoma]. Geburtshilfe Frauenheilkd. 1992;52(4):214–8. German.
23. Hulka JF, Peterson HA, Phillips JM, Surrey MW. Operative hysteroscopy: American Association of Gynecologic Laparoscopists'

1993 membership survey. J Am Assoc Gynecol Laparosc. 1995;2(2):131–2.
24. Hulka JF, Peterson HB, Phillips JM, Surrey MW. Operative hysteroscopy. American Association of Gynecologic Laparoscopists 1991 membership survey. J Reprod Med. 1993;38(8):572–3.
25. Huvar I, Tinga D, Pilka L. Hysteroscopic resection of myomas. Ceska Gynekol. 1994;59:114–6.
26. Itzkowic D, Beale M. Uterine perforation associated with endometrial ablation. Aust N Z J Obstet Gynaecol. 1992;32:359–61.
27. Jansen FW, Vredevoogd CB, van Ulzen K, Hermans J, Trimbos JB, Trimbos-Kemper TC. Complications of hysteroscopy: a prospective, multicenter study. Obstet Gynecol. 2000;96(2):266–70.
28. Leuschner H, Riedel HH, Anders M. Hysteroscopic survey from 1994 to 1996 in the eastern part of Germany. J Am Assoc Gynecol Laparosc. 1997;4(Suppl 4):S28.
29. Lobaugh ML, Bammel BM, Duke D, Webster BW. Uterine rupture during pregnancy in a patient with a history of hysteroscopic metroplasty. Obstet Gynecol. 1994;83(5 Pt 2):838–40.
30. Loffer FD. Complications of hysteroscopy—their cause, prevention, and correction. J Am Assoc Gynecol Laparosc. 1995;3:11–26.
31. MacNeil JS. Uterine perforation is the most common complication of operative hysteroscopic, occurring in 1%-10%. OB/GYN News; 2005. p. 15.
32. Magos AL, Baumann R, Lockwood GM, Turnbull AC. Experience with the first 250 endometrial resections for menorrhagia. Lancet. 1991;337(8749):1074–8.
33. Magos AL, Baumann R, Turnbull AC. Transcervical resection of endometrium in women with menorrhagia. Br Med J. 1989;298:1209–12.
34. Osei E, Tharmaratnam S, Opemuyi I, Cochrane G. Laser endometrial ablation with the neodymium: yttrium-aluminium garnet (Nd-YAG) laser: a review of ninety consecutive patients. Acta Obstet Gynecol Scand. 1995;74(8):619–23.
35. Parkar RB, Thagana NG. Hysteroscopic surgery at the Aga Khan Hospital, Nairobi. East Afr Med J. 2004;81(7):336–40.
36. Peterson HB, Hulka JF, Phillips JM. American Association of Gynecologic Laparoscopists' 1988 membership survey on operative hysteroscopy. J Reprod Med. 1990;35(6):590–1.
37. Petrucco OM, Gillespie A. The neodymium:YAG laser and the resectoscope for the treatment of menorrhagia. Med J Aust. 1991;154(8):518–20.
38. Propst AM, Liberman RF, Harlow BL, Ginsburg ES. Complications of hysteroscopic surgery: predicting patients at risk. Obstet Gynecol. 2000;96(4):517–20.
39. Ravi B, Schiavello H, Chandra P, Takeshige T. Safety and efficacy of hysteroscopic endomyometrial resection-ablation for menorrhagia. J Reprod Med. 2001;46(8):717–23.
40. Roge P, D'Ercole C, Cravello L, Boubli L, Blanc B. Hysteroscopic management of uterine synechiae: a series of 102 observations. Eur J Obstet Gynecol Reprod Biol. 1996;65(2):189–93.
41. Schiøtz HA. Transcervikal endometrieresekjson [Transcervical resection of the endometrium]. Tidsskr Nor Laegeforen. 2001;121(23):2706–9. Norwegian.
42. Serden SP, Brooks PG. Treatment of abnormal uterine bleeding with the gynecologic resectoscope. J Reprod Med. 1991;36(10):697–9.
43. Shalev E, Shimoni Y, Peleg D. Ultrasound controlled operative hysteroscopy. J Am Coll Surg. 1994;179(1):70–1.
44. Shveiky D, Rojansky N, Revel A, Benshushan A, Laufer N, Shushan A. Complications of hysteroscopic surgery: "beyond the learning curve". J Minim Invasive Gynecol. 2007;14(2):218–22.
45. Sullivan B, Kenney P, Seibel M. Hysteroscopic resection of fibroid with thermal injury to sigmoid. Obstet Gynecol. 1992;80(3 Pt 2):546–7.
46. Tannous W, Hamou J, Henry-Suchet J, Achard B, Lelaidier C, Belaisch-Allart J. Ruptures utérines lors d'accouchements après hystéroscopie opératoire [Uterine rupture during labor following surgical hysteroscopy]. Presse Med. 1996;25(4):159–61. French.
47. Tapper AM, Heinonen PK. Hysteroscopic endomyometrial resection for the treatment of menorrhagia follow-up of 86 cases. Eur J Obstet Gynecol Reprod Biol. 1995;62:75–9.
48. Tóth D, Kuzel D, Fucíková Z, Cibula D, Zivný J. Význam operacní hysteroskopie v resení intrauterinních patologií: metoda první volby [Importance of operative hysteroscopy in the treatment of intrauterine pathology: method of first choice]. Ceska Gynekol. 1999;64(4):234–8. Czech.
49. Valos GA, Valos EC, King JH. Experience with 800 hysteroscopic endometrial ablations. J Am Assoc Gynecol Laparosc. 1996;4:33–8.
50. Ven Herendael BJ. Hazard and dangers of operative hysteroscopy. In: Sutton C, Diamond MP, editors. Endoscopic surgery for gynecologists. 2nd ed. London: WB Saunders; 1998. p. 641–8.
51. Xia EL, Duan H, Zhang J, Chen F, Wang S, Zhang P, Yu D, Zheng J, Huang XW. An analysis of 16 cases of uterine perforation after hysteroscopic electric resection. Chin J Obstet Gynecol. 2003;38(5):280–3. Chinese.
52. Yaron Y, Shenhav M, Jaffa AJ, Lessing JB, Peyser MR. Uterine rupture at 33 weeks' gestation subsequent to hysteroscopic uterine perforation. Am J Obstet Gynecol. 1994;170(3):786–7.

Fluid Overload

53. Arieff AI, Ayres JC. Endometrial ablation complicated by fatal hyponatremic encephalopathy. JAMA. 1993;270:1230–2.
54. Baggish M, Davauluri C, Rodriquez F, Camporesi E. Vascular uptake of Hyskon (Dextran 70) during operative and diagnostic hysteroscopy. J Gynecol Surg. 1992;8:211–7.
55. Baggish MS, Brill AI, Rosenweig B, Barbot JE, Indman PD. Fatal acute glycine and sorbitol toxicity during operative hysteroscopy. J Gynecol Surg. 1993;9:137–43.
56. Corson SL, Brooks PG, Serden SP, Batzer FR, Gocial B. Effects of vasopressin administration during hysteroscopic surgery. J Reprod Med. 1994;39(6):419–23.
57. Garry R, Hasham F, Kokri MS. The effect of the pressure on fluid absorption during endometrial ablation. J Gynecol Surg. 1992;8:1–10.
58. Hahn RG. Ethanol monitoring of irrigation fluid absorption. Eur J Anesthesiol. 1996;13:102–15.
59. Hasham F, Garry R, Kokri MS, Mooney P. Fluid absorption during laser ablation of the endometrium in the treatment of menorrhagia. Br J Anaesth. 1992;68(2):151–4.
60. Hulka JF, Peterson HB, Philips JM. American Association of Gynecologic Laparoscopists 1991 Membership Survey. J Reprod Med. 1993;38:572–3.
61. Indam PD, Brooks PG, Cooper JM. Complications of fluid overload from resectoscopic surgery. J Am Assoc Gynecol Laparosc. 1998;5:63–7.
62. Istre O, Bjoennes J, Naess R. Postoperative central oedema after transcervical endometrial resection and uterine irrigation with 1.5% glycine. Lancet. 1994;344:187–9.
63. Istre O, Skajaa K, Schjoensby AP. Changes in serum electrolytes after transcervical resection of endometrium and submucous fibroids with use of glycine 1.5% for uterine irrigation. Obstet Gynecol. 1992;80:218–22.
64. Kumar A, Kumar A. A simple technique to reduce fluid intravasation during endometrial resection. J Am Assoc Gynecol Laparosc. 2004;11(1):83–5.
65. Loffer FD. Complications from uterine distention during hysteroscopy. In: Corfman RS, Diamond MP, DeCherney A, edi-

tors. Complications of laparoscopy and hysteroscopy. London: Blackwell Scientific; 1993. p. 177–86.
66. Mclucas B. Hyskon complications in hysteroscopic surgery. Obstet Gynecol Surv. 1991;46:196–200.
67. Molnar BG, Broadbent JAM, Magos AL. Fluid overload risk score for endometrial resection. Gynaecol Endosc. 1992;1:133–8.
68. Molnar BG, Magos AL, Kay J. Monitoring fluid absorption using 1% ethanol tagged glycine operative hysteroscopy. J Am Assoc Gynecol Laparosc. 1997;4:357–62.
69. Wortman M. Complications of hysteroscopic surgery. In: Isaacson K, editor. Complications of gynecologic endoscopic surgery. Philadelphia: Saunders Elsevier; 2006. p. 192.
70. Peterson HB, Hulka JF, Phillips JM. American Association of Gynecologic Laparoscopists' 1988 membership survey on operative hysteroscopy. J Reprod Med. 1990;35(6):590–1.
71. Steele A, Gowrishankar M, Abrahamson S, Mazer CD, Feldman RD, Halperin ML. Postoperative hyponatremia despite near-isotonic saline infusion: a phenomenon of desalination. Ann Intern Med. 1997;126(1):20–5.
72. Taskin O, Buhur A, Birincioglu M. Endometrial Na+, K+-ATPase pump function and vasopressin levels during hysteroscopic surgery in patients pretreated with GnRH agonist. J Am Assoc Gynecol Laparosc. 1998;5:119–24.
73. Valle RF. A manual of clinical hysteroscopy. New York: Parthenon Publishing; 1998. p. 41–6.
74. Vugaropulos SP, Haley AC, Hulka JF. Intrauterine pressure and fluid absorption during continuous flow hysteroscopy. Am J Obstet Gynecol. 1992;167:386–91.
75. Witz CA, Sliverberg KM, Burns WN. Complications associated with the absorption of hysteroscopic fluid media. Fertil Steril. 1993;60:745–56.

Intra- and Postoperative Bleeding

76. Agostini A, Bretelle F, Cravello L, Ronda I, Roger V, Blanc B. Complications de l'hystéroscopie opératoire [Complications of operative hysteroscopy]. Presse Med. 2003;32(18):826–9. French.
77. Azar D, Thomford NR, Pace WG, Sirinek KR. Intra-arterial vasopressin administration complicated by adverse cardiodynamic effects. Rev Surg. 1977;34(2):140–4.
78. Baggish MS, Sze EHM. Endometrial ablation: a series of 568 patients treated over an 11-year period. Am J Obstet Gynecol. 1996;174:908–13.
79. Birinyi L, Kalamász N, Juhász AG, Major T, Borsos A, Bacskó G. Follow-up study on the effectiveness of transcervical myoma resection (TCRM). Eur J Obstet Gynecol Reprod Biol. 2004;113(1):78–82.
80. Colgan TJ, Shah R, Leyland N. Post-hysteroscopic ablation reaction: a histopathologic study of the effects of electrosurgical ablation. Int J Gynecol Pathol. 1999;18:325–31.
81. Cooper JM, Brady RM. Intraoperative and early postoperative complications of operative hysteroscopy. Obstet Gynecol Clin North Am. 2000;27:347–66.
82. Corson SL, Brooks PG, Serden SP, Batzer FR, Gocial B. Effects of vasopressin administration during hysteroscopic surgery. J Reprod Med. 1994;39(6):419–23.
83. Galka E, Goldfarb HA. Disseminated intravascular coagulation as a complication of intrauterine balloon tamponade for posthysteroscopic acute uterine bleeding. J Am Assoc Gynecol Laparosc. 2000;7:573–6.
84. Goldrath MH, Fuller TA, Segal S. Laser photovaporization of endometrium for the treatment of menorrhagia. Am J Obstet Gynecol. 1981;104:14.
85. Goldrath MH. Uterine tamponade for the control of acute uterine bleeding. Am J Obstet Gynecol. 1983;147:869–72.
86. Hulka JF, Peterson HA, Phillips JM, Surrey MW. Operative hysteroscopy: American Association of Gynecologic Laparoscopists' 1993 membership survey. J Am Assoc Gynecol Laparosc. 1995;2(2):131–2.
87. Isaacson KB. Complications of hysteroscopy. Gynecol Oper Endosc. 1999;26:39–51.
88. Jansen FW, Vredevoogd CB, van Ulzen K, Hermans J, Trimbos JB, Trimbos-Kemper TC. Complications of hysteroscopy: a prospective, multicenter study. Obstet Gynecol. 2000;96(2):266–70.
89. Loffer FD. Removing intrauterine lesions: myomectomy and polypectomy. In: Bieber EJ, Loffer FE, editors. The gynecologic resectoscope. Cambridge: Blackwell Scientific; 1994. p. 168–94.
90. Martin JD, Shenk LG. Intraoperative myocardial infarction after paracervical vasopressin infiltration. Anesth Analg. 1994;79:1201–2.
91. Phillips DR, Nathanson HG, Milim SJ, Haselkorn JS, Khapra A, Ross PL. The effect of dilute vasopressin solution on blood loss during operative hysteroscopy: a randomized controlled trial. Obstet Gynecol. 1996;88(5):761–6.
92. Propst AM, Liberman RF, Harlow BL, Ginsburg ES. Complications of hysteroscopic surgery: predicting patients at risk. Obstet Gynecol. 2000;96(4):517–20.
93. Roberts M, Walton SM. The effect of paracervical adrenaline on blood loss in patients undergoing transcervical resection of the endometrium. Gynaecol Endosc. 2000;9:153–6.
94. Sowter MC, Singla AA, Lethaby A. Pre-operative endometrial thinning agents before hysteroscopic surgery for heavy menstrual bleeding. Cochrane Database Syst Rev. 2000;(2):CD001124.
95. Townsend DE. Vasopressin pack for treatment of bleeding after myoma resection. Am J Obstet Gynecol. 1991;165:1405–7.
96. Yu D, Li TC, Xia EL, Huang XW, Zheng J. A prospective randomized controlled trial on the effectiveness of routine Foley balloon tamponade on the reduction of bleeding after hysteroscopic resection of myoma. Gynecol Surg. 2006;3:93–6.

Infection

97. Amin-Hanjani S, Good JM. Pyometra after endometrial resection and ablation. Obstet Gynecol. 1995;85(5 Pt 2):893–4.
98. Aydeniz B, Gruber IV, Schauf B, Kurek R, Meyer A, Wallwiener D. A multicenter survey of complications associated with 21,676 operative hysteroscopies. Eur J Obstet Gynecol Reprod Biol. 2002;104(2):160–4.
99. Bartlett JG, Moon NE, Goldstein PR, Goren B, Onderdonk AB, Polk BF. Cervical and vaginal bacterial flora: ecologic niches in the female lower genital tract. Am J Obstet Gynecol. 1978;130(6):658–61.
100. Bhattacharya S, Parkin DE, Reid TM, Abramovich DR, Mollison J, Kitchener HC. A prospective randomised study of the effects of prophylactic antibiotics on the incidence of bacteraemia following hysteroscopic surgery. Eur J Obstet Gynecol Reprod Biol. 1995;63(1):37–40.
101. Boubli L, Porcu G, Gandois JM, d'Ercole C, Blanc B. Risque infectieux de l'hystéroscopie [Hysteroscopy infection risk]. J Gynecol Obstet Biol Reprod (Paris). 1997;26(3):250–5. French.
102. Bracco PL, Vassallo AM, Armentano G. Infectious complication of diagnostic hysteroscopy. Minerva Ginecol. 1996;48(7–8):293–8.
103. Cravello L, Stolla V, Bretelle F, Roger V, Blanc B. Hysteroscopic resection of endometrial polyps: a study of 195 cases. Eur J Obstet Gynecol Reprod Biol. 2000;93(2):131–4.
104. Dhaliwal JK, El-Shafei AM, Al-Sharqi MR, Jothy KR, Vijayan U, Qadri A. Hospital morbidity due to post-operative infections in obstetrics & gynecology. Saudi Med J. 2000;21(3):270–3.

105. Hayashi H, Yaginuma Y, Yamashita T, Morizaki A, Ishiya T, Katou Y, Ishikawa M. Prospective randomized study of antibiotic prophylaxis for nonlaparotomy surgery in benign conditions. Chemotherapy. 2000;46(3):213–8.
106. Jeanette SC, Chen and Charles WFM. A case of pelvic and hepatic abscesses following rollerball endometrial ablation. Gynaecol Endosc. 1999;8:183–5.
107. Li PK, Leung CB, Leung AK, Luk WK, Lai KN. Posthysteroscopy fungal peritonitis in a patient on continuous ambulatory peritoneal dialysis. Am J Kidney Dis. 1993;21(4):446–8.
108. Maher PJ, Hill DJ. Transcervical endometrial resection for abnormal uterine bleeding-report of 100 cases and review of the literature. Aust N Z J Obstet Gynaecol. 1990;30(4):357–60.
109. Marchino GL, Mazza O, Baccarini G, Zaccheo F, Grio R. Profilassi antibiotica con cefotaxime nell'endoscopia ginecologica [Antibiotic prophylaxis with cefotaxime in gynecological endoscopy]. Minerva Ginecol. 1994;46(6):337–41. Italian.
110. McCausland VM, Fields GA, McCausland AM, Townsend DE. Tuboovarian abscesses after operative hysteroscopy. J Reprod Med. 1993;38(3):198–200.
111. Mears J, Fox R. Severe pelvic infection following diagnostic hysteroscopy in women with pre-existing tubal disease. J Obstet Gynaecol. 2005;25(3):317.
112. Parkin DE. Fatal toxic shock syndrome following endometrial resection. Br J Obstet Gynaecol. 1995;102(2):163–4.
113. Perez-Medina T, Bajo JM, Martinez-Cortes L, Castellanos P, Perez de Avila I. Six thousand office diagnostic-operative hysteroscopies. Int J Gynaecol Obstet. 2000;71(1):33–8.
114. Propst AM, Liberman RF, Harlow BL, Ginsburg ES. Complications of hysteroscopic surgery: predicting patients at risk. Obstet Gynecol. 2000;96(4):517–20.
115. Redondo-Lopez V, Cook RL, Sobel JD. Emerging role of lactobacilli in the control and maintenance of the vaginal bacterial flora. Rev Infect Dis. 1990;12:856–72.
116. Rullo S, Boni T. Broad ligament abscess after operative hysteroscopy. Clin Exp Obstet Gynecol. 1995;22(3):240–2.
117. Thomason JL, Gelbart SM, Scaglione WJ. Bacterial vaginosis: current review indications for asymptomatic therapy. Am J Obstet Gynecol. 1991;165:1210–7.
118. Vilos GA, Vilos EC, King JH. Experience with 800 hysteroscopic endometrial ablations. J Am Assoc Gynecol Laparosc. 1996;4(1):33–8.

Venous Air Embolism

119. Adcock J, Maartin DC. Air embolus associated with tubal insufflation. J Am Assoc Gynecol Laparosc. 1999;6:505–7.
120. Adducci E, De Cosmo G. Gas embolism during hysteroscopy. A case report. Minerva Anestesiol. 2001;8(2):181–92.
121. Albin MS, Ritter RR, Reinhart R, Erickson D, Rockwood A. Venous air embolism during radical retropubic prostatectomy. Anesth Analg. 1992;74(1):151–3.
122. Baggish MS, Daniell JF. Catastrophic injury secondary to the use of coaxial gas cooled fibers and artificial sapphire tips for intrauterine surgery: a report of five cases. Lasers Surg Med. 1989;9:581–4.
123. Behnia R, Holley HS, Milad M. Successful early intervention in air embolism during hysteroscopy. J Clin Anesth. 1997;9:248–50.
124. Bloomstone J, Chow CM, Isselbacher E, VanCott E, Isaacson KB. A pilot study examining the frequency and quantity of gas embolization during operative hysteroscopy using a monopolar resectoscope. J Am Assoc Gynecol Laparosc. 2002;9(1):9–14.
125. Brandner P, Neis KJ, Ehmer C. The etiology, frequency, and prevention of gas embolism during CO_2 hysteroscopy. J Am Assoc Gynecol Laparosc. 1999;6:421–8.
126. Brooks PG. Venous air embolism during operative hysteroscopy. J Am Assoc Gynecol Laparosc. 1997;4:399–402.
127. Brügmann AH, Kristoffersen SE, Hansen AK, Nielsen JB. Gasemboli som komplikation i forbindelse med hysteroskopisk kirurgi [Gas embolization as a complication of hysteroscopic surgery]. Ugeskr Laeger. 2007;169(23):2226–7. Danish.
128. Brundin J, Thomasson K. Cardiac gas embolism during carbon dioxide hysteroscopy: risk and management. Eur J Obstet Gynecol Reprod Biol. 1989;33:241–5.
129. Chang CP, Liou CC, Yang YL, Sun MS. Fatal gas embolism during ureteroscopic holmium: yttrium-aluminium-garnet laser lithotripsy under spinal anesthesia - a case report. Minim Invasive Ther Allied Technol. 2008;17(4):259–61.
130. Corson SL, Brooks PG, Soderstrom RM. Gynecologic endoscopic gas embolism. Fertil Steril. 1996;65:529–33.
131. Corson SL. Venous air and gas emboli in operative hysteroscopy. J Am Assoc Gynecol Laparosc. 2001;8(2):181–92.
132. Crozier TA, Luger A, Dravecz M, Sydow M, Radke J, Rath W, Kuhn W, Kettler D. Gasembolie mit Kreislaufstillstand bei Hysteroskopien: Fallberichte von drei Patientinnen [Gas embolism with cardiac arrest during hysteroscopy. A case report on 3 patients]. Anasthesiol Intensivmed Notfallmed Schmerzther. 1991;26(7):412–5. German.
133. Edmonds C, Lowry C, Pennefather J. Diving and subaquatic medicine. 3rd ed. Oxford: Butterworth-Helneman; 1992. p. 95–114.
134. Fisher B. Handbook of hyperbaric oxygen therapy, vol. 6. Berlin: Springer; 1988. p. 976.
135. Fukuda T, Fujii T, Saito S, Nishida M, Toyooka H. [Complications of hysteroscopical myomectomy: a report of two cases]. Masui. 2000;49(9):1033–5. Japanese.
136. Ghimouz A, Loisel B, Kheyar M, Fried D, Bouret JM. Embolie de CO2 lors d'une hystéroscopie suivie de cécité transitoire [Carbon dioxide embolism during hysteroscopy followed by transient blindness]. Ann Fr Anesth Reanim. 1996;15(2):192–5. French.
137. Gomar C, Fernandez C, Villalonga A, Nalda MA. Carbon dioxide embolism during laparoscopy and hysteroscopy. Ann Fr Anesth Reanim. 1985;4(4):380–2.
138. Gottlieb JD, Ericsson JA, Sweet RB. Venous air embolism: a review. Anesth Analg. 1965;44(6):773–9.
139. Grove JJ, Shinamam RC, Drover DR. Noncardiogenic pulmonary edema and venous air embolus as complications of operative hysteroscopy. J Clin Anesth. 2004;16(1):48–50.
140. Hart GB. Treatment of decompress on illness and air embolism with hyperbaric oxygen. Aerosp Med. 1974;45:1190.
141. Imasogie N, Crago R, Leyland NA, Chung F. Probable gas embolism during operative hysteroscopy caused by products of combustion. Can J Anaesth. 2002;49(10):1044–7.
142. Levy B. Air embolism during gynecologic endoscopic surgery. J Am Assoc Gynecol Laparosc. 1997;4:291–2.
143. Li YT, Tsui MS, Lin HM, Sun LS, Tu FC, Chen PC, Chan PF, Yang CH. [Transcervical resection of endometrium and submucous myomas]. Zhonghua Yi Xue Za Zhi (Taipei). 1992;50(5):434–8. Chinese.
144. Loffer FD. Complications of hysteroscopy-their cause, prevention, and correction. J Am Assoc Gynecol Laparosc. 1995;3:11–26.
145. Lowenwirt IP, Chi DS, Handwerker SM. Nonfatal venous air embolism during cesarean section: a case report and review of the literature. Obstet Gynecol Surv. 1994;49:72–6.
146. Mader JT, Hulet WH. Delayed hyperbaric treatment of cerebral air embolism report of a case. Arch Veurol. 1979;36:504.
147. Nachum Z, Kol S, Adir Y, Melamed Y. Massive air embolism--a possible cause of death after operative hysteroscopy using a 32% dextran-70 pump. Fertil Steril. 1992;58(4):836–8.
148. Nishiyama T, Hanaoka K. Gas embolism during hysteroscopy. Can J Anaesth. 1999;46(4):379–81.

149. Obenhaus T, Maurer W. CO2 embolism during hysteroscopy. Anaesthesist. 1990;39:243–6.
150. Paddison K. Menorrhagia: endometrial ablation or hysterectomy? Nurs Stand. 2003;18(1):33–7.
151. Perry PM, Baughman VL. A complication of hysteroscopy: air embolism. Anesthesiology. 1990;75:546–7.
152. Pierre F, Lansac J, Soutoul JH. Embolie gazeuse et hystéroscopie exploratoire: mythes ou réalités? Note préliminaire [Air embolism and exploratory hysteroscopy: myths or realities? Preliminary results]. J Gynecol Obstet Biol Reprod (Paris). 1995;24(1):19–23. French.
153. Rademaker BM, Groenman FA, van der Wouw PA, Bakkum EA. Paradoxical gas embolism by transpulmonary passage of venous emboli during hysteroscopic surgery: a case report and discussion. Br J Anaesth. 2008;101(2):230–3.
154. Serden SP, Brooks PG. Treatment of abnormal uterine bleeding with the gynecologic resectoscope. J Reprod Med. 1999;36(10):697–9.
155. Sherlock S, Shearer WA, Buist M, Rasiah R, Edwards A. Carbon dioxide embolism following diagnostic hysteroscopy. Anaesth Intensive Care. 1998;26(6):674–6.
156. Siegler AM, Valle RF. Therapeutic hysteroscopic procedures. Fertil Stetil. 1988;50:685–701.
157. Simo Moyo J, Adnet P, Wambo M. Detection of gas embolism in neurosurgery by capnography. Apropos of 32 patients surgically treated in seated position. Cah Anesthesiol. 1995;43:77–9.
158. Vo Van JM, Nguyen NQ, Le Bervet JY. A fatal gas embolism during a hysteroscopy curettage. Cah Anesthesiol. 1992;40:617–8.
159. Wood SM, Roberts FL. Air embolism during transcervical resection of endometrium. BMJ. 1990;300:945.
160. Xia EL, Duan H, Feng LM. Air embolism during diagnostic hysteroscopy: a case report and literature review. Chin J Obstet Gynecol Clin. 2000;1:45–57. Chinese.
161. Zlatkov V, Bŭrzakov G, Cholakova A, Miloshov V, Radeva V, Velinov E, Mikhova A. [Diagnostic possibilities of the flexible hysteroscopy in irregular uterine bleeding]. Akush Ginekol (Sofiia). 2006;45(1):36–40. Bulgarian.

Intrauterine Adhesions

162. Fuchs N, Smorgick N, Ben Ami I, Vaknin Z, Tovbin Y, Halperin R, Pansky M. Intercoat (Oxiplex/AP gel) for preventing intrauterine adhesions after operative hysteroscopy for suspected retained products of conception: double-blind, prospective, randomized pilot study. J Minim Invasive Gynecol. 2014;21(1):126–30.
163. Guida M, Acunzo G, Di Spiezio SA, Bifulco G, Piccoli R, Pellicano M, Cerrota G, Cirillo D, Nappi C. Effectiveness of autocrosslinked hyaluronic acid gel in the prevention of intrauterine adhesions after hysteroscopic surgery: a prospective, randomized, controlled study. Hum Reprod. 2004;19(6):1461–4.
164. Leung PL, Tam WH, Yuen PM. Hysteroscopic appearance of the endometrial cavity following thermal balloon endometrial ablation. Fertil Steril. 2003;79:1226–8.
165. Luo X, Lim CE, Li L, Wong WS. Hysteroscopic appearance of endometrial cavity after microwave endometrial ablation. J Minim Invasive Gynecol. 2010;17(1):30–6.
166. McCausland AM, McCausland VM. Partial rollerball endometrial ablation: a modification of total ablation to treat menorrhagia without causing complications from intrauterine adhesions. Am J Obstet Gynecol. 1999;180:1512–21.
167. Montagna S, Zacchè G. L'ablazione endometriale con resettoscopio. Esperienza personale [Endometrial ablation with the resectoscope. The authors' experience]. Minerva Ginecol. 1995;47(1–2):17–21. Italian.
168. Mukul LV, Linn JG. Pregnancy complicated by uterine synechiae after endometrial ablation. Obstet Gynecol. 2005;105:1179–82.
169. Robbins ML. Lysis of uterine adhesions with the four-channel hysteroscope. J Gynecol Surg. 1995;11:7–9.
170. Stefanescu A, Marinescu B. Diagnostic hysteroscopy - a retrospective study of 1545 cases. Maedica (Buchar). 2012;7:309–14.
171. Taskin O, Onoglu A, Inal M, Turan E, Sadik S, Vardar E, Postaci H, Wheeler JM. Long-term histopathologic and morphologic changes after thermal endometrial ablation. J Am Assoc Gynecol Laparosc. 2002;9(2):186–90.
172. Taskin O, Sadik S, Onoglu A, Gokdeniz R, Erturan E, Burak F, Wheeler JM. Role of endometrial suppression on the frequency of intrauterine adhesions after resectoscopic surgery. J Am Assoc Gynecol Laparosc. 2000;7(3):351–4.
173. Touboul C, Fernandez H, Deffieux X, Berry R, Frydman R, Gervaise A. Uterine synechiae after bipolar hysteroscopic resection of submucosal myomas in patients with infertility. Fertil Steril. 2009;92(5):1690–3.
174. Xia E, Li TC, Yu D, Huang X, Zheng J, Liu Y, Zhang M. The occurrence and outcome of 39 pregnancies after 1621 cases of transcervical resection of endometrium. Hum Reprod. 2006;21(12):3282–6.
175. Xia EL, Zhang M, Duan H. Endometrial resection for menorrhagia: analysis of 400 cases. Chin J Obstet Gynecol. 1997;32:148–51. Chinese.
176. Yang JH, Chen MJ, Chen CD, Chen SU, Ho HN, Yang YS. Optimal waiting period for subsequent fertility treatment after various hysteroscopic surgeries. Fertil Steril. 2013;99(7):2092–6.e3.
177. Yang JH, Chen MJ, Wu MY, Chao KH, Ho HN, Yang YS. Office hysteroscopic early lysis of intrauterine adhesion after transcervical resection of multiple apposing submucous myomas. Fertil Steril. 2008;89(5):1254–9.
178. Yu D, Wong YM, Cheong Y, Xia E, Li TC. Asherman syndrome--one century later. Fertil Steril. 2008;89(4):759–79.
179. Zhang D, Meng Y, Liu J, Zhai L. Ultrasound guidance: hysteroscopic metroplasty. Chin J Med Imaging. 1998;6:197–8. Chinese.

Postoperative Pregnancy

180. Baumann R, Owerdieck W, Reck G. Pregnancy following sterilization and endometrium resection. Geburtshilfe Frauenheilkd. 1994;54(4):246–9.
181. Cravello L, Porcu G, Roger V, D'Ercole C, Blanc B. Hystéroscopie opératoire et fertilité [Hysteroscopic surgery and fertility]. Contracept Fertil Sex. 1998;26(7–8):589–92. French.
182. DeCherney AH, Diamond MP, Lavy G, Polan ML. Endometrial ablation for intractable uterine bleeding: hysteroscopic resection. Obstet Gynecol. 1987;70(4):668–70.
183. Dicker D, Feldberg D, Samuel N, Goldman JA. Etiology of cervical pregnancy. Association with abortion, pelvic pathology, IUDs and Asherman's syndrome. J Reprod Med. 1985;30(1):25–7.
184. Friedman A, DeFazio J, DeCherney A. Severe obstetric complications after aggressive treatment of Asherman syndrome. Obstet Gynecol. 1986;67(6):864–7.
185. Giarenis I, Shenoy J, Morris E. Cervical ectopic pregnancy after endometrial ablation: a case report. Arch Gynecol Obstet. 2008;277(6):567–9.
186. Goldberg JM. Intrauterine pregnancy following endometrial ablation. Obstet Gynecol. 1994;83:836–7.
187. Ismail MS, Torsten U, Serour GI, Weitzel H, Berlien HP. Is endometrial ablation a safe contraceptive method? Pregnancy following endometrial ablation. Eur J Contracept Reprod Health Care. 1998;3(2):99–102.

188. Kir M, Hanlon-Lundberg KM. Successful pregnancy after thermal balloon endometrial ablation. Obstet Gynecol. 2004;103(5 Pt 2):1070–3.
189. Kucera E, Krepelka P, Krofta L, Feyereisl J, Hejda V. Tehotenské komplikace po intrauterinní hysteroskopické chirurgii [Pregnancy complications after intrauterine hysteroscopic surgery]. Ceska Gynekol. 2005;70(4):312–6. Czech.
190. Magos AL, Baumann R, Lockwood GM, Turnbull AC. Experience with the first 250 endometrial resections for menorrhagia. Lancet. 1991;337(8749):1074–8.
191. Magos AL, Baumann R, Turnbull AC. Transcervical resection of endometrium in women with menorrhagia. Br Med J. 1989;298:1209–12.
192. Maouris P. Pregnancy after planned partial endometrial resection. Aust N Z J Obstet Gynaecol. 1994;34:122–3.
193. McLucas B. Pregnancy after endometrial ablation: a case report. J Reprod Med. 1995;40(3):237–9.
194. Mints M, Radestad A, Rylander E. Follow up of hysteroscopic surgery for menorrhagia. Acta Obstet Gynecol Scand. 1998;77(4):435–8.
195. Pinette M, Katz W, Drouin M, Blackstone J, Cartin A. Successful planned pregnancy following endometrial ablation with the YAG laser. Am J Obstet Gynecol. 2001;185(1):242–3.
196. Pugh CP, Crane JM, Hogan TG. Successful intrauterine pregnancy after endometrial ablation. J Am Assoc Gynecol Laparosc. 2000;7(3):391–4.
197. Skar O, Nesheim BI. Operative hysteroscopy in the treatment of intrauterine disorders. Acta Obstet Gynecol Scand. 1990;69(7–8):565–6.
198. Turnbull LW, Jumaa A, Bowsley SJ, Dhawan S, Horsman A, Killick SR. Magnetic resonance imaging of the uterus after endometrial resection. Br J Obstet Gynaecol. 1997;104(8):934–8.
199. Whitelaw NL, Sutton CJ. Ruptured ectopic pregnancy in an amenorrhoeic women after transcervical resection of the endometrium. Aust N Z J Obstet Gynaecol. 1992;32(4):387.
200. Xia E, Li TC, Yu D, Huang X, Zheng J, Liu Y, Zhang M. The occurrence and outcome of 39 pregnancies after 1621 cases of transcervical resection of endometrium. Hum Reprod. 2006;21(12):3282–6.
201. Xia EL. Gynecological endoscopy. Beijing: People's Medical Publishing House; 2001. p. 214–5. Chinese.
202. Xia EL. Uterine balloon compression for hemostasis in 1 case of induced abortion. Chin J Clin. 2000;28:42. Chinese.

Postablation-Tubal Sterilization Syndrome

203. Bae IH, Pagedas AC, Perkins HE, Bae DS. Postablation-tubal sterilization syndrome. J Am Assoc Gynecol Laparosc. 1996;3(3):435–8.
204. Gannon MJ, Johnson N, Watters LK. Haematometra-endometrial resection sterilization syndrome. Gynaecol Endosc. 1997;6:45–6.
205. Leung PL, Yuen PM. Postablation-tubal sterilization syndrome following thermal balloon endometrial ablation. Acta Obstet Gynecol Scand. 2006;85(4):504–5.
206. Magos AL, Baumann R, Lockwood GM, Turnbull AC. Experience with the first 250 endometrial resections for menorrhagia. Lancet. 1991;337(8749):1074–8.
207. Sorensen SS, Andersen LF, Lose G. Endometriosis by implantation: a complication of ablation. Lancet. 1994;343:1226.
208. Steffensen AJ, Schuster M. Endometrial resection and later reoperation in the treatment of menorrhagia. J Am Assoc Gynecol Laparosc. 1997;4:325–9.
209. Townsend DE, McCausland V, McCausland A, Fields G, Kauffman K. Post-ablation-tubal sterilization syndrome. Obstet Gynecol. 1993;82(3):422–4.
210. Webb JC, Bush MR, Wood MD, Park GS. Hematosalpinx with pelvic pain after endometrial ablation confirms the postablation-tubal sterilization syndrome. J Am Assoc Gynecol Laparosc. 1996;3(3):419–21.
211. Wortman M. Complications of hysteroscopic surgery. In: Isaacson K, editor. Complications of gynecologic endoscopic surgery. Philadelphia: Saunders Elsevier; 2006. p. 198.
212. Xia EL. Postabortion-tubal sterilization syndrome. Chin J Pract Gynecol Obstet. 1999;15:759–60. Chinese

Accidental Electrical Injuries

213. Vilos GA, Brown S, Graham G, McCulloch S, Borg P. Genital tract electrical burns during hysteroscopic endometrial ablation: report of 13 cases in the United States and Canada. J Am Assoc Gynecol Laparosc. 2000;7(1):141–7.

Other Complications

214. Bae IH, Pagedas AC, Barr CA, Alexander C, Bae DS. Retrospective analysis of 305 consecutive cases of endometrial ablation and partial endomyometrial resection. J Am Assoc Gynecol Laparosc. 1996;3(4):549–54.
215. Colgan TJ, Shah R, Leyland N. Post-hysteroscopic ablation reaction: a histopathologic study of the effects of electrosurgical ablation. Int J Gynecol Pathol. 1999;18:325–31.
216. Cooper JM, Brady RM. Late complications of operative hysteroscopy. Obstet Gynecol Clin North Am. 2000;27:367–74.
217. Dwyer N, Fox R, Mills M, Hutton J. Haematometra caused by hormone replacement therapy after endometrial resection. Lancet. 1991;338(8776):1205.
218. Edwards A, Tippett C, Lawrence M, Tsaltas J. Pregnancy outcome following endometrial ablation. Gynaecol Endosc. 1996;5:349–51.
219. El-Toukhy T, Hefni M. Pregnancy after hydrothermal endometrial ablation and laparoscopic sterilisation. Eur J Obstet Gynecol Reprod Biol. 2003;106(2):222–4.
220. Feng LM, Xia EL. Pregnancy after transcervical resection of endometrium: a report of 16 cases. Chin J Obstet Gynecol. 1998;33:368. Chinese.
221. Foote M, Rouse A, Gil KM, Crane S, Lavin JP Jr. Successful pregnancy following both endometrial ablation and uterine artery embolization. Fertil Steril. 2007;88(6):1676.e15–7.
222. Gandhi SV, Habiba MA. Ectopic pregnancy presenting as haematometra following Cavaterm balloon endometrial ablation. J Obstet Gynaecol. 2005;25(6):614–5.
223. Goldberg JM. Intrauterine pregnancy following endometrial ablation. Obstet Gynecol. 1994;83:836–7.
224. Gurtcheff SE, Sharp HT. Complications associated with global endometrial ablation: the utility of the MAUDE database. Obstet Gynecol. 2003;102(6):1278–82.
225. Hill DJ, Maher PJ, Davison GB, Wood C. Haematometra--a complication of endometrial ablation. Aust N Z J Obstet Gynaecol. 1992;32(3):285–6.
226. Hill DJ, Maher PJ. Pregnancy following endometrial ablation. Gynaecol Endosc. 1992;1:47.
227. Hopkisson JF, Kennedy SH, Ellis JD. Caesarean hysterectomy for intrauterine death after failed endometrial resection. Br J Obstet Gynaecol. 1994;101:810–1.

228. Hubert SR, Marcus PS, Rothenberg JM, Schilder JM, Hurd WW. Hematometra after thermal balloon endometrial ablation in a patient with cervical incompetence. J Laparoendosc Adv Surg Tech A. 2001;11(5):311–3.
229. Hulka JF, Peterson HB, Phillips JM, Surrey MW. Operative hysteroscopy. American Association of Gynecologic Laparoscopists 1991 membership survey. J Reprod Med. 1993;38(8):572–3.
230. Indman PD, Brooks PG, Cooper JM, Loffer FD, Valle RF, Vancaillie TG. Complications of fluid overload from resectoscopic surgery. J Am Assoc Gynecol Laparosc. 1998;5(1):63–7.
231. Istre O. Transcervical resection of endometrium and fibroids: the outcome of 412 operations performed over 5 years. Acta Obstet Gynecol Scand. 1996;75:567–74.
232. Karci A, Erkin Y. Transient blindness following hysteroscopy. J Int Med Res. 2003;31(2):152–5.
233. Keckstein J. Hysteroscopy and adenomyosis. Contrib Gynecol Obstet. 2000;20:41–50.
234. Kir M, Hanlon-Lundberg KM. Successful pregnancy after thermal balloon endometrial ablation. Obstet Gynecol. 2004;103(5 Pt 2):1070–3.
235. Lam AM, Al-Jumally RY, Holt EM. Ruptured ectopic pregnancy in an amenorrhoeic woman after transcervical resection of the endometrium. Aust N Z J Obstet Gynaecol. 1992;32:81–2.
236. Leung PL, Yuen PM. Postablation-tubal sterilization syndrome following thermal balloon endometrial ablation. Acta Obstet Gynecol Scand. 2006;85(4):504–5.
237. Levin H, Ben-David B. Transient blindness during hysteroscopy: a rare complication. Anesth Analg. 1995;81(4):880–1.
238. Magos AL, Baumann R, Lockwood GM, Turnbull AC. Experience with the first 250 endometrial resections for menorrhagia. Lancet. 1991;337(8749):1074–8.
239. Maouris P. Pregnancy after planned partial endometrial resection. Aust N Z J Obstet Gynaecol. 1994;34:122–3.
240. McCausland AM, McCausland VM. Frequency of symptomatic cornual hematometra and postablation tubal sterilization syndrome after total rollerball endometrial ablation: a 10-year follow-up. Am J Obstet Gynecol. 2002;186(6):1274–80.
241. McCausland AM, McCausland VM. Partial rollerball endometrial ablation: a modification of total ablation to treat menorrhagia without causing complications from intrauterine adhesions. Am J Obstet Gynecol. 1999;180(6 Pt 1):1512–21.
242. McLucas B, Perrella R. Does endometrial resection cause adenomyosis? Gynaecol Endosc. 1995;4:123–7.
243. Mints M, Radestad A, Rylander E. Follow up of hysteroscopic surgery for menorrhagia. Acta Obstet Gynecol Scand. 1998;77:435–8.
244. Mongelli JM, Evans AJ. Pregnancy after transcervical endometrial resection. Lancet. 1991;338:578–9.
245. Motashaw ND, Dave S. Vision disturbances after operative hysteroscopy. J Am Assoc Gynecol Laparosc. 1999;6:213–5.
246. Moukarram H, Chia KV, Jilumudi J. Intrauterine pregnancy after microwave endometrial ablation. J Obstet Gynaecol. 2006;26(8):818.
247. Parkin DE. Fatal toxic shock syndrome following endometrial resection. Br J Obstet Gynaecol. 1995;102:163–4.
248. Robson S, Devine B. Two cases of leiomyoma necrosis after thermal balloon endometrial ablation. J Minim Invasive Gynecol. 2007;14(2):250–2.
249. Romer T, Campo R, Hucke J. Hematometra after hysteroscopic endometrium ablation: a case report. Zentralbl Gynakol. 1995;117:278–80.
250. Roth TM, Rivlin ME. Tuboovarian abscess: a postoperative complication of endometrial ablation. Obstet Gynecol. 2004;104(5 Pt 2):1198–9.
251. Rousseau E, Jourdain O, Rabreau M, Cambon D, Dallay D. Nécrose utérine après réduction d'endomètre au laser nd:YAG. A propos d'un cas [Uterine necrosis after Nd-YAG laser ablation of the endometrium. A case report]. J Gynecol Obstet Biol Reprod (Paris). 1996;25(3):264–6. French.
252. Schenker JG, Margalioth EJ. Intrauterine adhesions: an updated appraisal. Fertil Steril. 1982;37:593–610.
253. Schlumbrecht M, Balgobin S, Word L. Pyometra after thermal endometrial ablation. Obstet Gynecol. 2007;110(2 Pt 2):538–40.
254. Scottish Hysteroscopy Audit Group. A Scottish audit of hysteroscopic surgery for menorrhagia: complications and follow up. Br J Obstet Gynecol. 1995;102:249–54.
255. Sorensen SS, Andersen LF, Lose G. Endometriosis by implantation: a complication of endometrial ablation. Lancet. 1994;343:1226.
256. Steffensen AJ, Hahn RG. Fluid absorption and the long-term outcome after transcervical resection of the endometrium. Acta Obstet Gynecol Scand. 1998;77(8):863–8.
257. Steffensen AJ, Schuster M. Endometrial resection and late reoperation in the treatment of menorrhagia. J Am Assoc Gynecol Laparosc. 1997;4:325–9.
258. Su HW, Wu CF, Chou SY, Chen TG, Hsu CS. Lung collapse induced by pulmonary hemorrhage: a rare complication of hysteroscopy. Gynecol Obstet Invest. 2007;63(1):11–4.
259. Tapper AM, Heinonen PK. Hysteroscopic endomyometrial resection for the treatment of menorrhagia follow-up of 86 cases. Eur J Obstet Gynecol Reprod Biol. 1995;62:75–9.
260. Valle RF, Baggish MS. Endometrial carcinoma after endometrial ablation: high-risk factors predicting its occurrence. Am J Obstet Gynecol. 1998;179:569–72.
261. ven Herendael BJ. Hazard and dangers of operative hysteroscopy. In: Sutton C, Diamond MP, editors. Endoscopic surgery for gynecologists. 2nd ed. London: WB Saunders; 1998. p. 641–8.
262. Whitelaw N, Garry R, Sutton CJG. Pregnancy following endometrial ablation: two case reports. Gynaecol Endosc. 1992;1:129–32.
263. Wood C, Rogers P. A pregnancy after planned partial endometrial resection. Aust N Z J Obstet Gynaecol. 1993;33:316–8.
264. Xia EL, Zhang M, Duan H. Endometrial resection for dysfunctional uterine bleeding. Chin J Obstet Gynecol. 1992;27:200–3. Chinese.
265. Yin CS, Wei RY, Chiao TC. Hysteroscopic endometrial ablation without endometrial preparation. Int J Gynaecol Obstet. 1998;62:167–72.
266. Yuen PM. Adenomyosis following endometrial rollerball ablation. Aust N Z J Obstet Gynaecol. 1995;3:335–6.

Hysteroscopy for Other Purposes

13

Jie Zheng and Enlan Xia

13.1 Vaginoscopy

Vaginoscopy is also named non-touch hysteroscopy, which applies hysteroscopic instruments and non-invasive techniques (such as no placement of speculum, no holding of cervix, no dilation of cervical canal, no probe of the length of uterus, distension of the cavity with low pressure, and use of mini instruments) to accomplish the hysteroscopic examination so as to reduce the pain and discomfort which are caused by traditional hysteroscopy such as placing the speculum and cervical forceps, using the scope with large diameter, and requiring local or general anesthesia. With the extensive use of office hysteroscopy, vaginoscopy has been gradually favored by both doctors and patients. The application of it cannot only replace the traditional hysteroscopy, but also favor the female infants, young girls, and unmarried women of child-bearing age because of no damage to the hymen.

Vaginoscopic examination and operation are conducted by inserting a diagnostic, therapeutic, or operative hysteroscope into vagina under the condition without placement of speculum, irrigating and dilating the vagina with normal saline, clearly visualizing the vaginal wall and cervix, and then entering the uterine cavity via cervical canal, and inspecting and treating vaginal, cervical, and uterine abnormalities. During the procedure of vaginoscopy, it does not place the speculum, not dilate the cervix, and not probe the length of uterine cavity, and it can preserve the integrity of the hymen for young girls or unmarried women, so it can greatly reduce the injuries and pain caused by speculum to young girls, unmarried women, and postmenopausal women. Therefore, it has been a commonly used diagnostic and operative method for those patients in recent years.

13.1.1 Indications of Vaginoscopic Diagnosis and Operation

Vaginal diagnosis and operation may be conducted in young girls, unmarried women, or postmenopausal old women who experience vaginal bleeding or abnormal discharge. Diseases which can be discovered and managed by vaginoscopy include:

1. Discovering and removing vaginal foreign bodies. In the Hysteroscopy Center of Fuxing Hospital, Capital Medical University, vaginal foreign bodies such as small glass balls, condoms, nut shells, pen caps, buttons, sands, cotton, small bottle caps, spring rings, plastic toy fragments, sausage wrapping buttons, small metal rings, etc. have been detected and removed.
2. Discovering vaginal infection and treating by vaginal irrigation.
3. Discovering benign lesions including vaginal mucosal adhesions, vaginal granulation, vaginal polyps or cervical polyps, etc., and treating by vaginal operations.
4. Discovering, sampling, and diagnosing vaginal or cervical neoplasms, and following up postoperative outcomes. In our Hysteroscopy Center, endodermal sinus tumor, rhabdomyosarcoma, hemangioma, botryoid sarcoma, Mullerian papilloma, etc. in young girls have been diagnosed.
5. Vaginoscopy can be placed into uterine cavity, and discover, diagnose and treat intrauterine lesions.

13.1.2 Contraindications of Vaginoscopic Diagnosis and Operation

1. Acute or subacute genital tract infection.
2. Severe adhesions in vagina.

J. Zheng (✉) · E. Xia
Hysteroscopy Center, Fuxing Hospital, Capital Medical University, Beijing, China

E. Xia (ed.), *Practical Manual of Hysteroscopy*, https://doi.org/10.1007/978-981-19-1332-7_13

13.1.3 Procedures of Vaginoscopic Diagnosis and Operation

13.1.3.1 Vaginoscopic Examination

Vaginoscopic examination applies diagnostic hysteroscope with the diameter of the outer sheath being 3.1 mm, 4.5 mm, or 5.5 mm. 0.9% normal saline is used as media for dilating the vagina, with the distention pressure set at 60–80 mmHg. Vaginoscopic operations can use 6.5 mm therapeutic hysteroscope, 8 mm or 9 mm monopolar hysteroscopic resectoscope, or 8.5 mm bipolar hysteroscopic resectoscope.

13.1.3.2 Vaginoscopic Diagnosis and Operation

A diagnostic hysteroscope is introduced into the vagina via the hymen, and proceed slowly from the vaginal external os to cervix under direct vision. Then vaginal walls, vaginal fornix, and ectocervix were inspected in sequence (Fig. 13.1a, b). After examining the vagina and cervix, the hysteroscope goes upwards from vaginal posterior fornix over the posterior lip of the cervix into cervical os, and observing the cervical canal. Then it goes through the cervical canal to the internal os and progressively inspects the whole cavity. The hysteroscope is then retrieved slowly and detects the whole vagina again under its expansion. Based on the results of vaginoscopy, vaginal irrigation and target biopsy may be conducted. Abnormal conditions which may be discovered by vaginoscopy include:

1. Vaginal foreign bodies: Vaginoscopy may detect vaginal foreign bodies such as hair, button, cotton, pen caps, sand, bottle caps, string rings, etc. which lie in the fornix, middle segment, or external os of vagina (Fig. 13.2a–d). Because of long-term detention of vaginal foreign bodies, the vaginal wall where the foreign body locates commonly present inflammatory changes. The vaginal foreign bodies can be removed with hysteroscopic foreign forceps under the direct vision of the hysteroscope.
2. Vaginitis in children: Vaginoscopy in female children sometimes can visualize purulent secretion in vagina, yellow membranous tissues which cover the vaginal wall, congestive, punctate hemorrhage, erosion, and granulation proliferation on vaginal mucosa, and even inflammatory polyps (Fig. 13.3). Repeated onset of vaginitis may also lead to adhesions of vaginal mucosa (Fig. 13.4). Vaginitis can be treated by regular vaginal irrigation with normal saline, 0.05% iodophor or antibiotics. Histological examination of sampling biopsy may indicate inflammatory tissues, and even inflammatory polyps.
3. Vaginal and cervical neoplasm: Vaginoscopy for neoplasm may discover vaginal or cervical space-occupying lesions, which can be polyps, granulation proliferation, focal proliferation, cervical or vaginal tumors (Figs. 13.5, 13.6 and 13.7). Sampling of the neoplasm can be obtained by hysteroscopic biopsy forceps and be sent for histological examination, or the neoplasm can be completely excised for histological examination. Alternatively a loop electrode of hysteroscopic resectoscope is used for resection and the resected tissues are sent for histological examination.

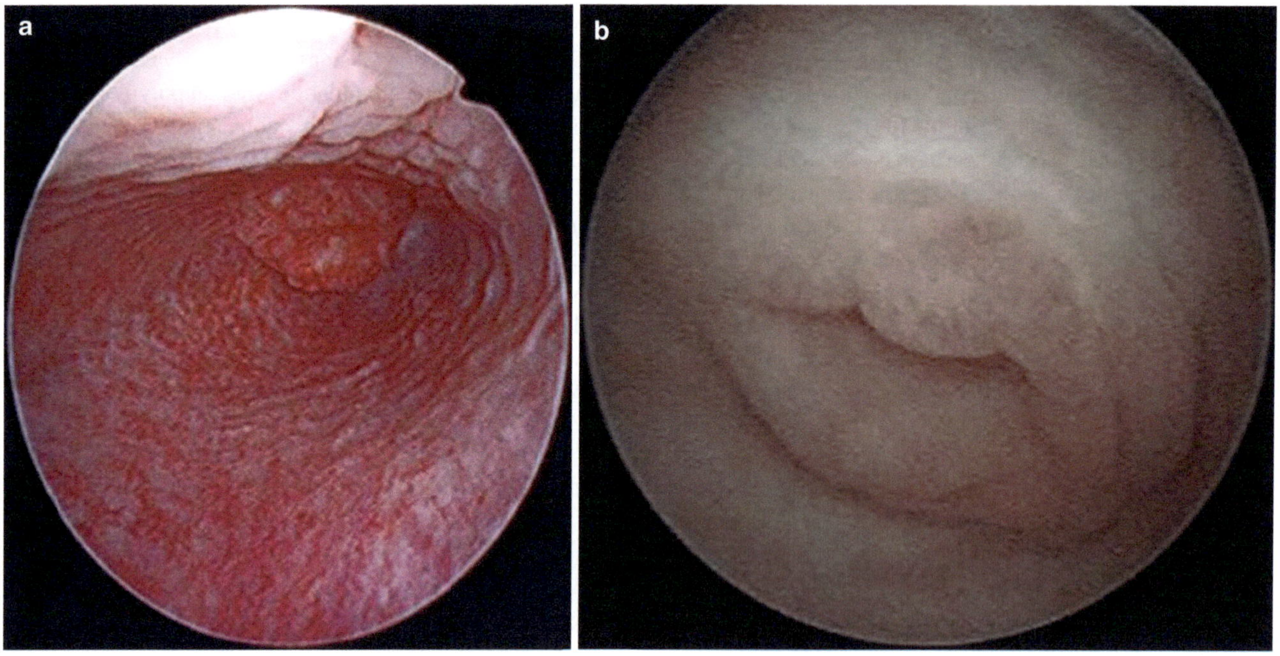

Fig. 13.1 (a) Whole picture of vagina with vaginoscopy. (b) Normal cervix with vaginoscopy

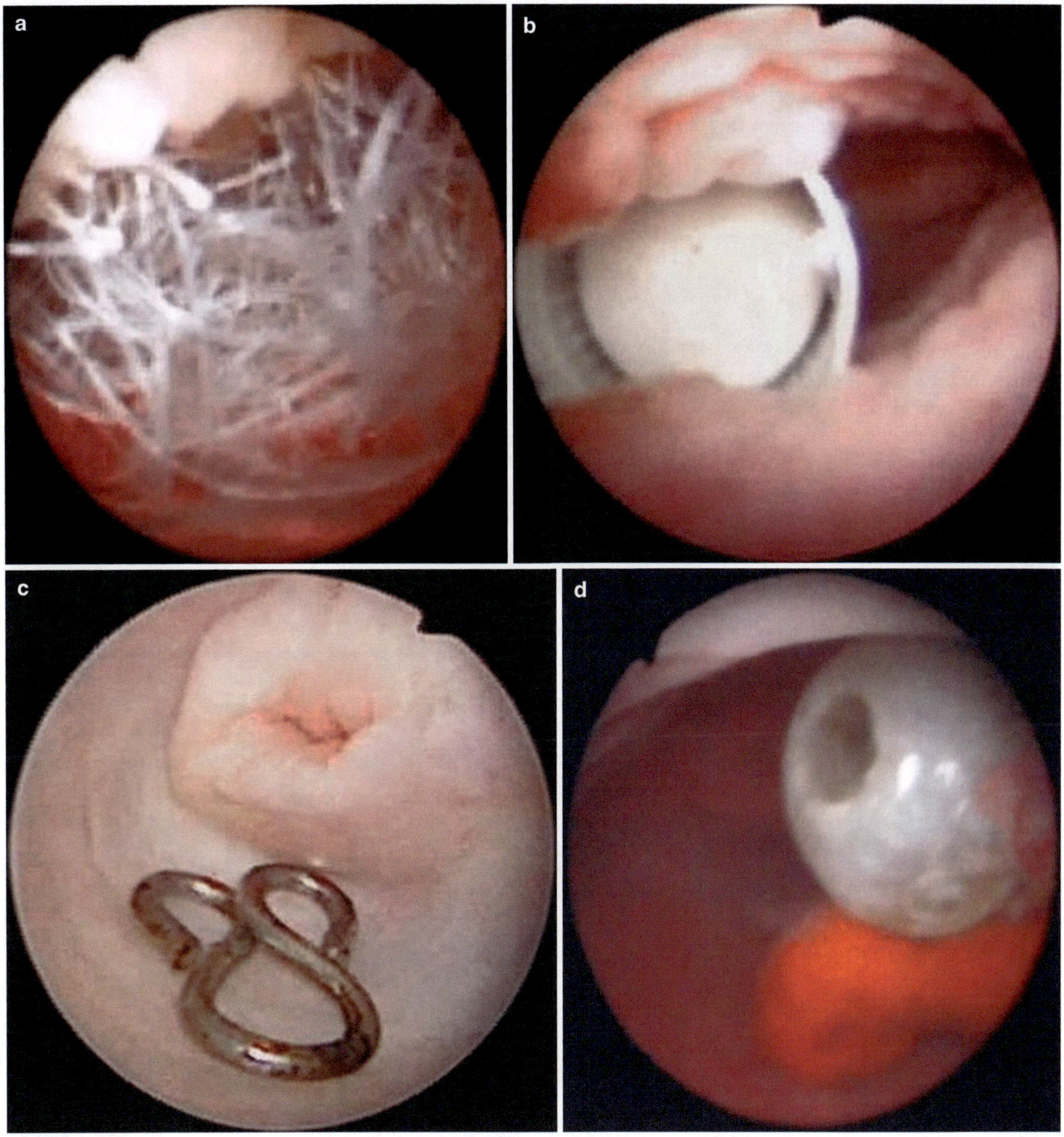

Fig. 13.2 Vaginal foreign bodies in young girls. (**a**) Cotton. (**b**) Pen cap with rubber and metal sheath. (**c**) Curvy metal ring. (**d**) Plastic ball

13.1.3.3 Vaginoscopic Removal of Vaginal Foreign Bodies

Vaginal foreign bodies can be removed by grasping with foreign forceps which is introduced through hysteroscopic working channel or is inserted beside the hysteroscope. Or a surgical forceps is introduced into vagina, and grasps and removes the foreign bodies under the direct vision of vaginoscope (Fig. 13.8a, b). After the removal of the foreign bodies, vaginal walls should be inspected to determine condition of traumatic surface, and whether there are bleeding and fistula formation or not. If there is bleeding, rollerball electrode can be used to coagulate for hemostasis. And vaginal irrigation should be determined according to the condition of vaginal inflammation.

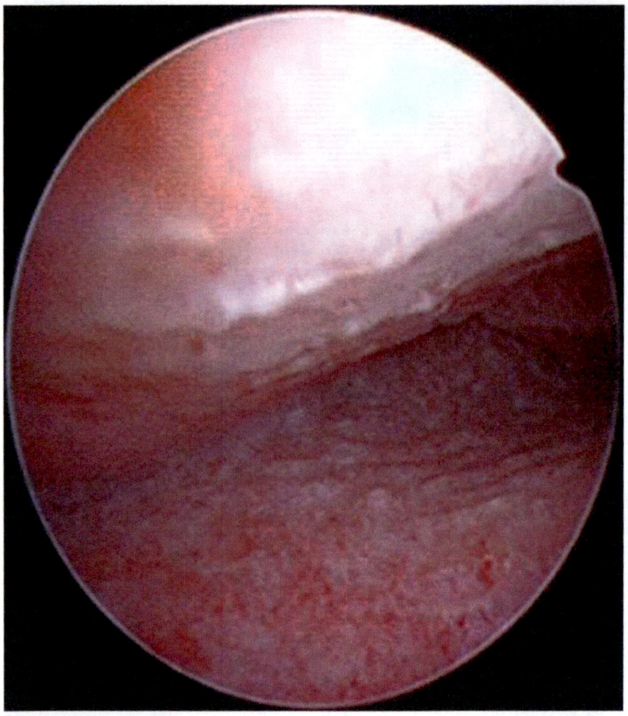

Fig. 13.3 Vaginal mucosal congestion with punctate hemorrhage visualized with vaginoscopy

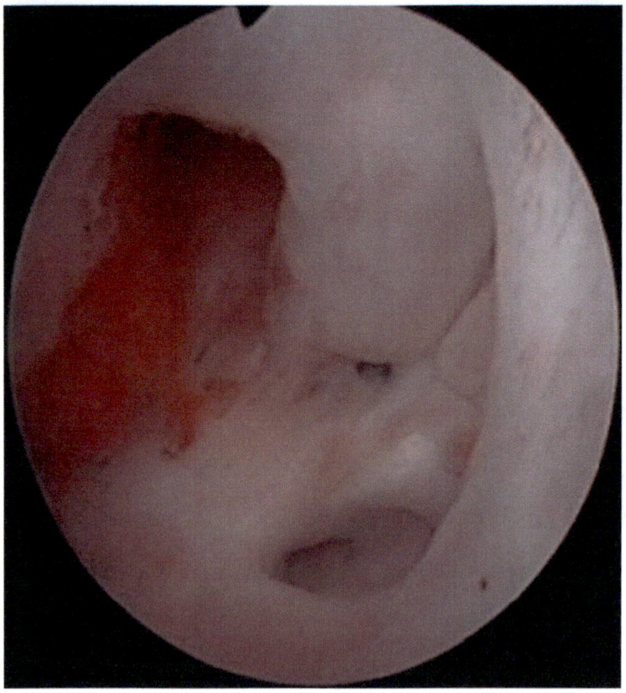

Fig. 13.4 The inflammation occurs repeatedly after the removal of vaginal foreign bodies. Vaginoscopy reveals adhesions between cervical posterior lip and vaginal posterior fornix

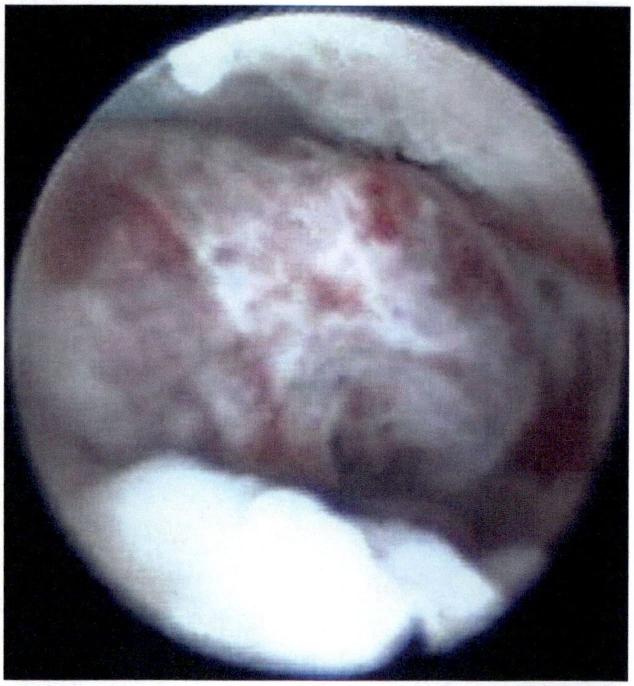

Fig. 13.5 Vaginoscopy reveals vaginal polyps with 2 cm in diameter

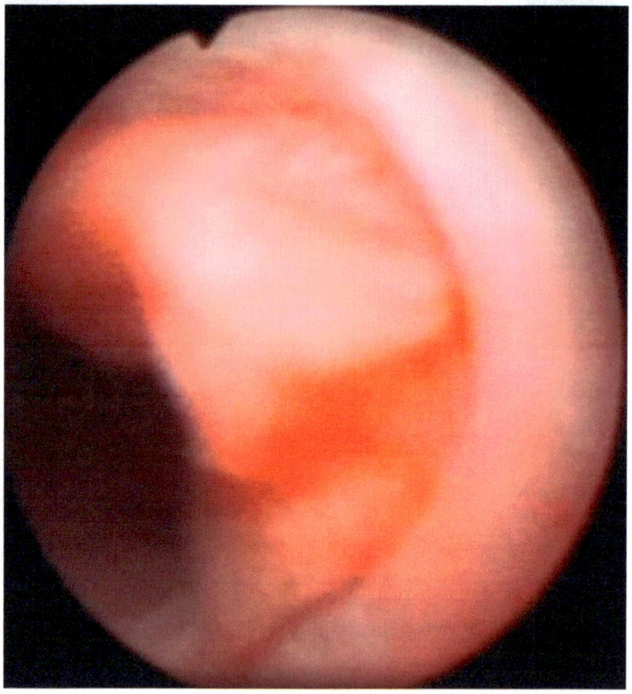

Fig. 13.6 Vaginoscopy for vaginal foreign body. An inflammatory polyp with 1 cm in diameter is detected at left wall of vaginal lower segment

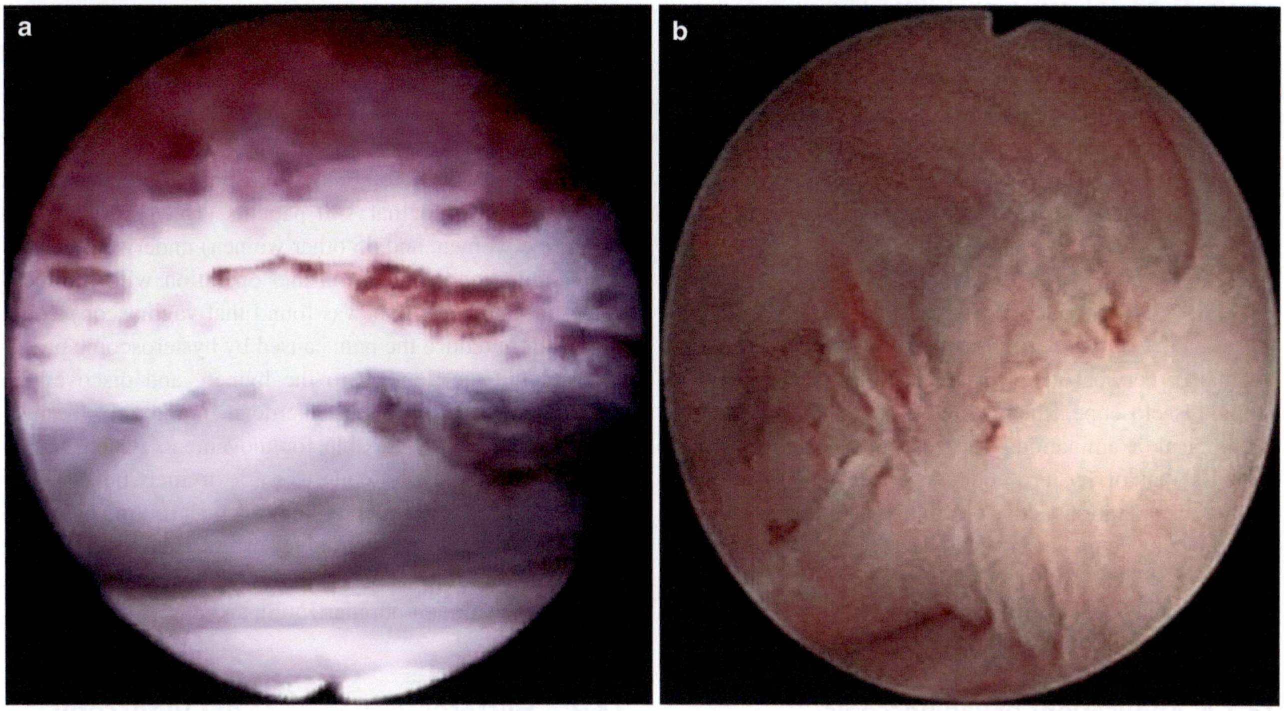

Fig. 13.7 (**a**) Vaginoscopy for hemangioma. A space-occupying lesion is detected with plenty of spotty vessels on its surface which appears as a strawberry-like change. (**b**) Vaginoscopy for Mullerian papilloma. An irregular clustery hyperplastic tissue with a fragile surface and thickened vessels is detected at left-posterior vaginal wall

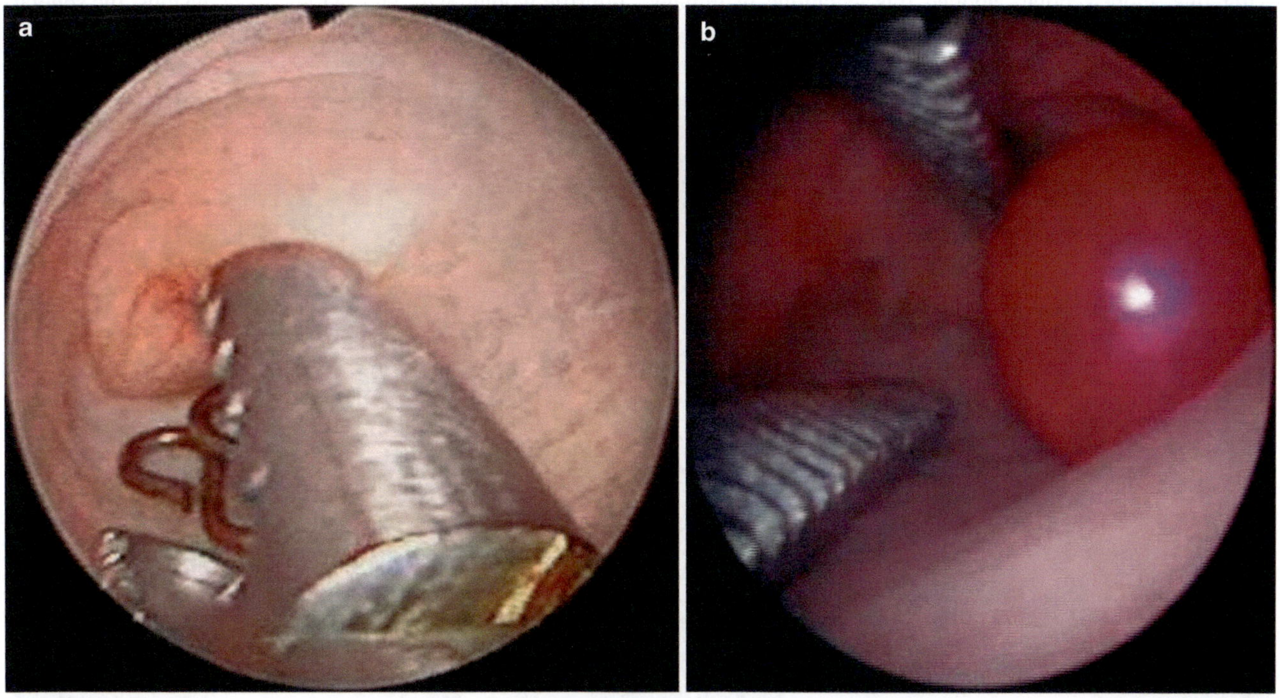

Fig. 13.8 (**a**) Hysteroscopic foreign forceps is grasping the vaginal foreign body. (**b**) A surgical forceps is introduced into the vagina to grasp the foreign body—a pink plastic ball

13.1.3.4 Vaginal Wall Biopsy Under Vaginoscopy

A hysteroscopic biopsy forceps can be inserted through working channel of the hysteroscope, or be parallelly inserted beside the hysteroscope, and grasps the vaginal wall or vaginal/cervical neoplasm, with a small amount of tissues removed and sent for histological examination (Fig. 13.9a, b).

13.1.3.5 Hysteroscopic Resection or Coagulation Vaginoscopically

Vaginal or cervical neoplasms can be excised by hysteroscopic resectoscope. The resected tissues should be sent for histological examination. The resecting technique is the same as that of hysteroscopic resection (Fig. 13.10a, b). During the operation, active bleeding on cutting surface may be stopped by coagulation with hysteroscopic rollerball electrode (Fig. 13.11). Adhesions in vagina can be divided with hysteroscopic needle electrode (Fig. 13.12).

13.1.4 Applications of Vaginoscopic Examination and Operation

Early in 1997, Paschopoulos et al. reported that in 324 cases of vaginoscopy, 211 procedures (65%) achieved success. After this, more scholars applied this technique in female infants, young girls, and unmarried women and achieved good effects. In 2010, Cooper et al. reviewed many good, relevant articles and discovered that when compared with traditional hysteroscopy, vaginoscopy could significantly reduce the pain and should be considered as a standard method of office hysteroscopy. In 2012, Zheng et al. from the Hysteroscopy Center of Fuxing Hospital, Capital Medical University reported that 140 patients (15 young girls, 20 unmarried women, and 55 other women) underwent vaginal and intrauterine examination and operation with the technique of vaginoscopy. It was found that vaginoscopy could significantly reduce the pain caused by hysteroscopic procedures, avoid the damage to the hymen, and discover the bleeding caused by vaginal disorders. In addition, the hysteroscope was more flexible for movement, which was in favor of the patient whose uterus was extremely flexed. They held that vaginoscopy had less trauma than routine hysteroscopy and was especially suitable for investigation in young girls and unmarried women with low genital tract disorders, so it had the value of popularization and application.

13.2 Hysteroscopy in Place of Culdoscopy in Fertiloscopy

Laparoscopy is an effective means in the diagnosis of pelvic factor infertility. Due to its seemingly great trauma to the infertile women without obvious pelvic lesions, the scholars have begun to try transvaginal hydrolaparoscopy (THL) on

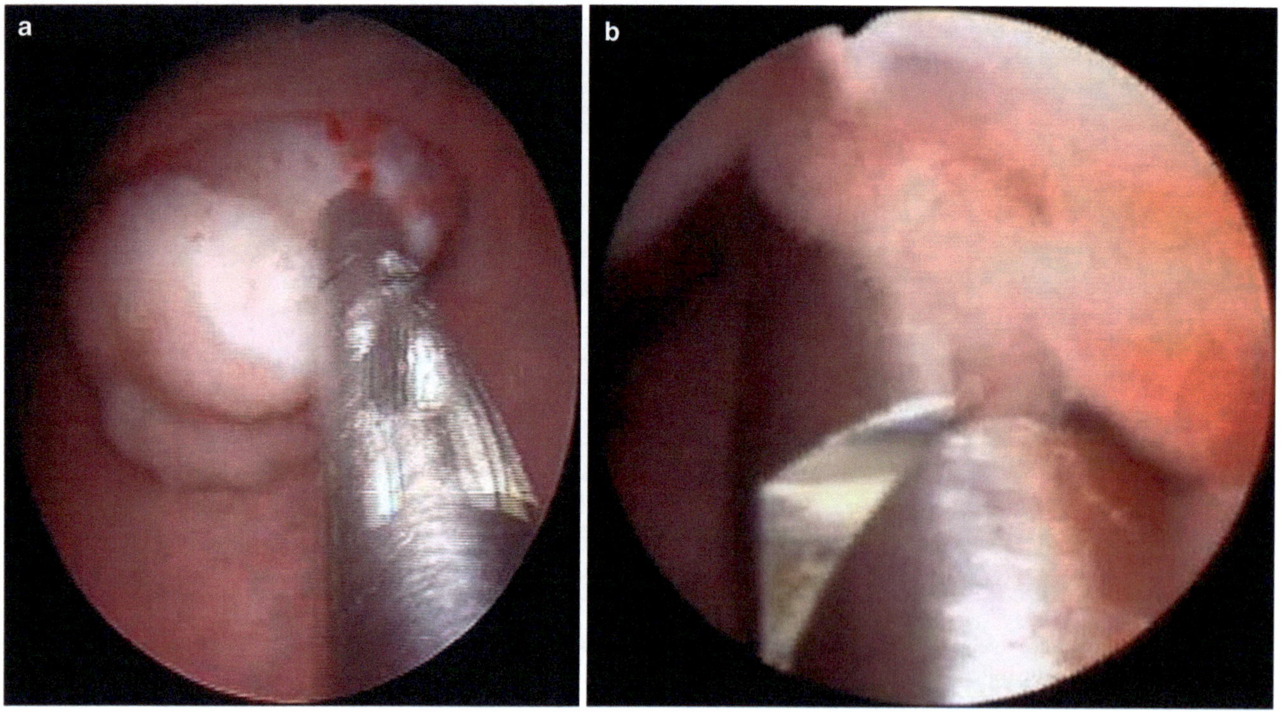

Fig. 13.9 (a) Hysteroscopic biopsy forceps is grasping the vaginal anterior wall to get some tissues for histological examination. (b) Hysteroscopic biopsy forceps is grasping the membranoid neoplasm to get some tissues for histological examination

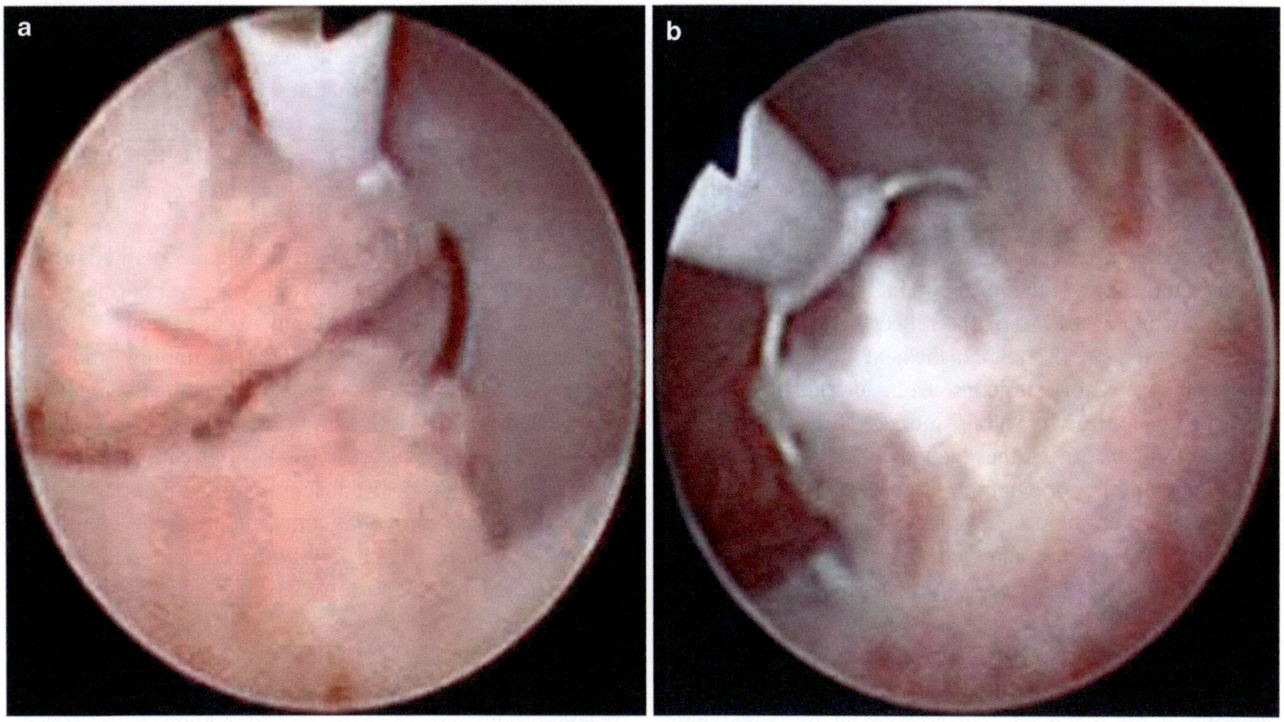

Fig. 13.10 (**a**, **b**) Vaginoscopically resection of vaginal lesions with a 7 mm hysteroscope and a closed-loop electrode

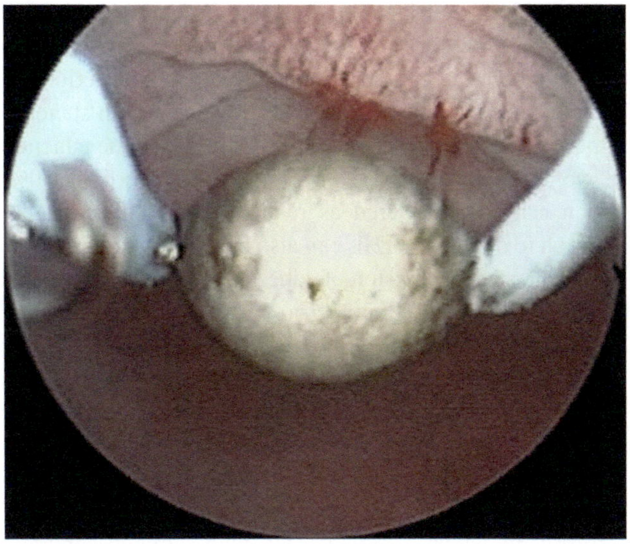

Fig. 13.11 Hysteroscopic rollerball electrode is coagulating the active bleeding points on vaginal anterior wall

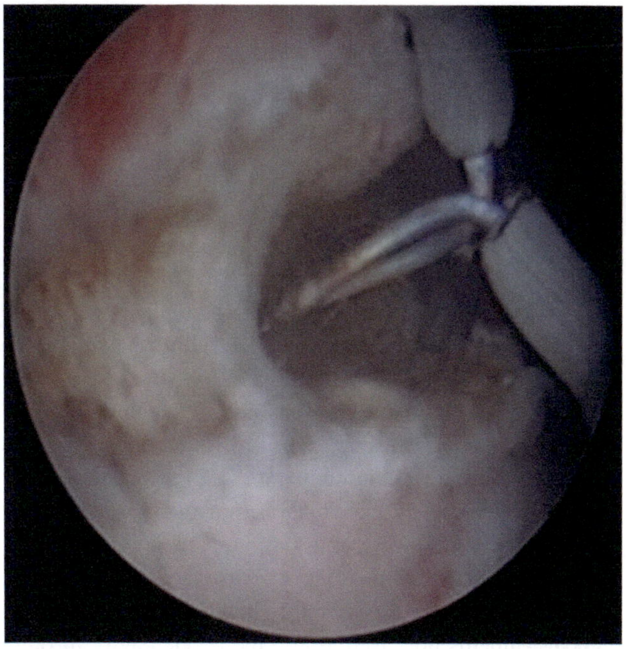

Fig. 13.12 Hysteroscopic needle electrode is dividing the adhesions on right vaginal wall

patients who had unexplained infertility with normal gynecological examination and TVS and without a history of pelvic disease or pelvic surgery. The results suggest that the advantages of THL include repeatability of pelvic examination and safety, and 40% of the patients who have undergone THL can avoid laparoscopy. Fertiloscopy, born in twenty-first century, combines transvaginal hydrolaparoscopy (culdoscopy, lap and dye, and hysteroscopy), salpingoscopy, and microsalpingoscopy, which forms a new minimally invasive diagnostic technique. Fertiloscopy is not fundamentally different from laparoscopy in diagnostic function. Due to its simplicity, safety, and minimal invasiveness, it is considered to be a good alternative to diagnostic laparoscopy, and its application is becoming more and more popular.

The basic procedure of fertiloscopy is to introduce the endoscope through the posterior vaginal fornix into the pelvic cavity as that of transvaginal hydrolaparoscopy, and to observe pelvic anatomy and tubal lesions in infertile women with saline as distention medium. The development of this minimally invasive diagnostic method can be traced back to culdoscope in the early twentieth century. In 1901, von Ott was the first to inspect the pelvic cavity of a pregnant woman through an incision in the posterior vaginal fornix via cystoscope by using a head mirror to reflect light. Thereafter, he became the first culdoscopist. In the next 40 years, there have been physicians or surgeons from Germany, Sweden, Switzerland, Denmark, South America, Britain, the United States, Hungary, and other countries committed to the exploration and development of laparoscopy. Just as laparoscopic techniques were developing rapidly, the outbreak of the Second World War restricted the international technical exchanges and cooperation. As of the early 1940s to the late 1960s, many medical centers used culdoscopy to replace laparoscopy. Culdoscopy, which was introduced as a minimally invasive procedure in 1944, became an alternative to laparotomy for diagnosis and assessment of pelvic pain, infertility and pelvic mass. After the Second World War, under the influence of Raoul Palmer and Hans Frangenheim, the "father of modern operative laparoscopy," laparoscopic technology began to boom again in Europe. As there were some further development and improvements on the laparoscopic system and surgical instruments, diagnostic laparoscopy has begun to mature since the 1970s. Due to wide field of vision, laparoscopy has become an effective means of endoscopic diagnosis while culdoscopy has fallen into oblivion in history. A large number of diagnostic laparoscopies revealed no pelvic abnormalities in 49%–70% of patients. This phenomenon urged doctors to contemplate and seek a less traumatic pelvic examination procedure to replace the standard laparoscopy. Not until late 1990s, the company Circon developed a special Veress needle-cannula system, which makes THL possible. THL is a new culdoscopy. The difference between culdoscopy and THL is that when culdoscopy is performed, the patient is in a knee-chest position with air as distention medium, but the patient is placed in a lithotomy position when THL is performed with peritoneal distention by saline. The similarity between them lies in that both instruments are inserted into the pelvic cavity through the rectouterine pouch. In 1998, Belgian Gordts et al. reported on THL for the first time. But its application was far less common than that of laparoscopy and hysteroscopy, which might be related to its limited indications. At present, the application of HSG and laparoscopy to investigating the causes of infertility is greatly controversial. THL may avoid the real surgical operation like laparoscopy and HSG may induce improper X-ray exposure. The combined application of hysteroscopy and dye tubal patency can complete one-stop endoscopic pelvic exploration in infertile women. Its standard procedure is not only harmless but also can detect the posterior pelvic abnormalities in asymptomatic patients, including lesions on uterine posterior wall, ovary, small intestine, and rectum. Under general or local anesthesia, the patients may have good tolerability, and it can be performed in an office setting.

Indications for THL: (1) Early stage unexplained primary or secondary infertility, no obvious pelvic abnormalities by gynecological and ultrasonography examination; (2) Infertile women with HSG or ultrasonography findings indicating intrauterine abnormalities, which requires diagnostic hysteroscopy and (or) operative hysteroscopy; (3) Women who cannot conceive after at least 3 cycles of treatment but with a normal HSG result; (4) Endoscopic follow-up after abdominal or laparoscopic myomectomy, tubal surgery, and grade III or IV endometriosis surgery, with THL taking the place of HSG or standard second-look laparoscopy; (5) An alternative to standard laparoscopy so that a simple laparoscopic diagnosis can be done for hysteroscopic surgery. THL can be considered as a first-line investigation method, and diagnostic laparoscopy will be as the second method.

Contraindications for THL: (1) Significant pelvic lesions and lower genital tract infection; (2) Uterine retroversion and fixation, closure of Douglas' pouch; (3) Patients who have indications for laparoscopy should not try to undergo THL. Verhoeven and Brosens pointed out that posterior fornix puncture may be unsuccessful in women with stenosed upper vagina and obesity, and the failure rate of the puncture in women with a retroverted but not fixed uterus is 50%, which can be considered as relative contraindications. In addition to diagnosis, THL can also be used for some simple treatment, such as division of adhesions, ovarian drilling and electrocoagulation of endometriotic foci, etc.

The maturity and wide application of IVF technology provides options of surgery or IVF in the treatment of the fallopian tubal diseases. The evaluation of the fallopian tubal lesions includes the condition of tubal mucosa and tuboperitoneal environment, so only HSG and laparoscopic diagnosis are obviously inadequate. Therefore, this leads to the birth of fertiloscopy, which combines THL with salpingoscopy and microsalpingoscopy.

In 1997, Watrelot et al. proposed the concept of fertiloscope, and defined it as the combination in one investigation of transvaginal hydropelviscope, dye-test, optional salpingoscope, and eventually hysteroscope, which can be performed on an outpatient basis under local or block anesthesia. In 1999, Watrelot published his experience with fertiloscope in English, which was performed on 160 infertile patients with unknown reason. Fertiloscope was successfully performed in 154 patients (96.2%) and failed in five because of technical problem or adhesions in the pouch of Douglas. It was normal in 60 patients (37.5%) under fertiloscope. One patient encountered rectal injury (0.6%) and was treated with antibiotics for 2 days conservatively. Findings of fertiloscopy included endometriosis in 21 patients (13.1%), inflammation in deep pelvic cavity in 58 cases (36.2%), tubo-ovarian adhesions in 27 cases (16.8%), and mini abnormalities in 15 cases (9.3%). For women with pelvic inflammatory lesions detected, salpingoscopy was performed, with 39% of cases undergoing partial examination due to external tubal adhesions but clearly visualizing the fimbriae. IVF procedures were undertaken directly in 74 patients (46.2%) so as to avoid a further laparoscopy. The case of rectal perforation was the 26th among 160 cases, who suffered from severe deep infiltrating endometriosis of the rectovaginal septum. Thereafter, a Veress needle puncture injection was used, and then the trocar was inserted, no rectal perforation occurred again. The insertion of salpingoscope in the procedure of fertiloscopy is much easier than that of laparoscope, and can obtain more information about mucosal adhesions in tubal fimbriae and ampullary. The main advantages of fertiloscopy are safety and minimal invasiveness. Compared with laparoscopy, it will not damage the large blood vessels, not require Trendelenburg position and not need CO_2 pneumoperitoneum, so there will be no acidosis induced by CO_2, thus attracting attention of the academic field. In the next year, Messin from Italy reported his experience with fertiloscopy and held that fertiloscopy was a useful first-line alternative procedure in diagnosing infertility. Fertiloscopy has the advantage of strictly limiting the indications of culdoscopy and maintaining a high diagnostic quality. Furthermore, it is cost-effective, economizes on manpower and decreases the surgical risks, and the patient has a better compliance. In 2002, Watrelot et al. reported the results of fertiloscopy in 500 infertile women with unknown reason, of whom 85% had salpingoscopy. Of those with no pathology detected by fertiloscopy, abnormalities were found in 8.2% with salpingoscopy, and 37% with microsalpingoscopy. They held that intratubal exploration should be conducted when evaluating the infertility. In 2004, Fernandez et al. from French developed ovarian drilling by transvaginal fertiloscopy for the first time. They conducted a prospective study to evaluate the outcomes of ovarian drilling with bipolar energy under fertiloscopy in women who had PCOS and resisted to clomiphene citrate. During a mean follow-up of about 18 months, 73 women (91%) got recovery of ovulatory menstruation, and 44 women got pregnancy with the mean time to conceive 4 months. Delayed miscarriages occurred in 8 women, and there were no ectopic pregnancies or multiple pregnancies, and no complications. They thought that this procedure appeared to be an effective in patients with clomiphene citrate resistant PCOS.

There were few reports about the complications following fertiloscopy, let alone the reports about the severe complications. In 2001, Gordts et al. from Belgium made a retrospective survey of four centers on complications of full-layer bowel injury following THL and fertiloscopy. A total of 3667 procedures were included, among them 24 bowel injuries (0.65%) occurred. The occurrence rate of bowel injury decreased to 0.25% when the initial period of application is excluded. All the injuries were recognized during surgery and 22 cases were successfully treated without poor outcomes. In 2004, Chiesa-Montadou et al. reported on two complications of ovarian drilling by fertiloscopy. Among 43 women who underwent fertiloscopy, 15 women were treated by ovarian drilling during fertiloscopy because of PCOS with two complications occurring. The first case had a delicate operation with an ovarian incision only about 0.5 cm, but was converted to laparoscopy due to heavy hemorrhage. The second case underwent drilling procedure with small-bowel loops and ovaries intertwined, and suffered nausea, vomiting, and radiating pain in left shoulder on the first day after operation. Laparoscopic examination revealed intestinal perforation and laparotomy was performed immediately to resect the intestinal segment. They indicated that ovarian drilling for fertiloscopy is just a beginning, but these two cases suggested no procedure is without adverse effects and risks. So it was necessary to carry out further study with longer follow-up to properly access the effectiveness and risks of fertiloscopy.

The recent studies have ascertained the role of fertiloscopy. In 2007, Nohuz et al. made a retrospective study of 229 women with primary or secondary infertility without pathology, with successful fertiloscopic examination procedures in 203 women (88.6%). Fifty eight patients required a laparoscopic intervention because of pelvic lesions revealed by fertiloscopy, which included pelvic adhesions, endometriosis, tubal disease, failure in visualizing the adnexa and ovarian cysts. Complications occurred in 5 patients including two rectal injuries, two hemorrhages and a postoperative salpingitis. The authors held that fertiloscopy was safe and reliable, and can be considered as a substitute for laparoscopy when evaluating infertile women with unknown reason. In the same year, Watrelot from France pointed out that in the treatment of fallopian tubal diseases, the option of tubal surgery or IVF was based on tubal lesions, which included the conditions of both tubal mucosa and tuboperitoneal environment. Endoscopic examination could accomplish their assessment, but fertiloscopy could take its place due to its minimal invasiveness, repeatability, and accuracy which was similar to laparoscopy and dye. Furthermore, salpingoscopy and microsalpingoscopy can be performed routinely during the procedure. So he insisted to adopt fertiloscopy as the standard procedure for tubal evaluation. This new diagnostic technique requires the use of special disposable instruments.

13.3 Hysteroscopy in Place of Laparoscopy

Hysteroscope has three kinds of telescopes according to different diameter, namely, 1.9 mm, 3 mm, 4 mm, and two types of telescopes according to its materials, namely, columnar crystal and glass fiber. The columnar crystal optical tube is thin, not resistant to bending and not easy to break under the protection of outer sheath when used as hysteroscope, but the operator should take care when used as laparoscope. The glass fiber optic tube has a certain anti-bending performance, and is more suitable to be used as laparoscope. At present, the trocar has four types, 2 mm, 3 mm, 5 mm, and 10 mm. So when a 4 mm optical tube is inserted with 5 mm trocar, there will be leakage of air. 1.9 mm and 3 mm optical tubes have exclusive trocar, which is more often used in laparoscope. Most of the occasions where the hysteroscope is used as laparoscope are there is laparoscopic monitoring or simple pelvic operation, so that a telescope can be used as either a hysteroscope or a laparoscope. It can solve the problem of shortage of laparoscopes and avoid being left unused and waste of money due to a purchase of a large number of laparoscopes.

13.4 Hysteroscopy in Place of Cystoscopy

Modern hysteroscope and cystoscope share a common origin and there have been many similarities in their structure and basic manipulation of the instruments so far. For example, the inspectoscope with hysteroscopy and cystoscopy is made up of sheath and optical tube; there are diverters similar in structures at the front end of catheterizing ureteroscope and tubal cannulation falloposcope, which can control the up and down direction through the controller on the handle, thereby changing the direction of ureteral catheter or fallopian tube catheterization; the electrode on the surgical endoscope is mostly wire loop electrode and rollerball electrode. However, these two instruments are slightly different, for example, there is a special structure at the front end of some cystoscopic sheath, which is round and blunt in appearance, and looks like beak, forming an obtuse angle with the rod. It has two types, concaved and convex, which is easy to be introduced into the scope without damage to the urethra, but hysteroscope has no such structure. There are two cannula bores on the handle of catheterizing ureteroscope but there is only one cannulation hole with hysteroscope. In the process of introduction of endoscopic body, the obturator with cystoscope will be used more often. These subtle differences do not affect the similarity in their manipulation, which provides convenient conditions for the application of hysteroscope in cystoscopic operation.

Although bladder and uterus are hollow elastic muscular organs, these two organs are different in many respects. Bladder mucosa has poor ability to regenerate, cannot shed and repair periodically as the endometrium; bladder wall is thin and more flexible compared with the uterine wall, which enables the bladder capacity above 400 mL, and even 1000 mL, but even with a wider uterus, the volume of uterine cavity seldom exceeds 20 mL; urethral mucosa is more vulnerable and more prone to injury than cervical mucosa. The difference in anatomical structure between bladder and uterus requires the operator to be gentle and slow in the application of hysteroscopy for cystoscopy so as to avoid injury to the urethra and bladder mucosa, and the requirements on equipment and operating area should also be more rigid in order to avoid causing urinary tract infection.

Because the cystoscopy and intrauterine operation are performed mostly in special situations or emergencies, we need to understand the indications and contraindications for cystoscopy.

13.4.1 Indications for Hysteroscopy in Place of Cystoscopy

1. Excluding bladder and ureteral injuries in hysteroscopic and laparoscopic surgery: During cystoscopy, on the one hand, an observation of the integrity of bladder wall and whether there is active bleeding in the bladder wall can be conducted to verify whether there is injury to bladder wall or not. On the other hand, an observation of color and quantity of ureteral jet can help to understand whether the ureter is damaged or not.
2. Etiology of chronic pelvic pain: Since interstitial cystitis and endometriosis are the two major causes of chronic pelvic pain, there is a strong correlation (the reported correlation as high as 96.6%) between interstitial cystitis and chronic pelvic pain. Therefore, for patients with chronic pelvic pain, it is absolutely necessary to undergo two kinds of endoscopic examination simultaneously—cystoscopy and hysteroscopy under one anesthesia in order to avoid unnecessary delays in the diagnosis and treatment so that the patients can have timely and exact diagnosis at first diagnosis.
3. Ureteral intubation: In the past, ureteral intubation was peculiar to urological surgeons. In gynecological laparoscopic surgery, gynecologists may save a lot of valuable time by ureteral intubation via hysteroscope and provide important guide in the lysis of pelvic adhesions so as to avoid injury to the ureter. On the other hand, when there is suspected ureteral injury, ureteral intubation can be performed for verification. In addition, when inadvertent clamping and pulling of ureter induce hematuria in patients, the placement of double pigtail stent in the ureter can support and dredge the ureteral wall in order to prevent occurrence of ureteral stricture in future.

4. Monitoring of the treatment of stress urinary incontinence: At present, more and more patients with stress urinary incontinence choose tension-free vaginal tape (TVT) surgery or laparoscopic Burch procedure for treatment of stress urinary incontinence. These two procedures both require cystoscopic examination and monitoring so as to prevent the suture from penetrating the bladder wall and understand the postoperative urethral tension and straining angles.
5. Cystoscopic examination and auxiliary removal of the lost IUD: Part of IUD can slip out of the uterine wall, and may also penetrate the bladder wall partly or completely into the bladder cavity. Hysteroscopy combined with cystoscopy can be performed under anesthesia to locate such lost IUD precisely and assist each other in removing the foreign bodies.
6. Other conditions: Serious deformities of the bladder cavity can be found when cystoscopy is performed for urological examination in some female patients with frequent urination, especially with frequent nocturnal urination, and furthermore, uterine fibroids may be detected in these patients. So, such kind of inspection should also be the gynecological endoscopic doctors' duty.

13.4.2 Contraindications for Hysteroscopy in Place of Cystoscopy

1. Urethral Stricture: Urethral stricture is the main reason for the failure of cystoscopy. If there is severe urethral stenosis and insufficient consideration about the urethral stricture before examination, and if the telescope is still inserted with force despite resistance, urethral perforation can be caused.
2. Too Small Bladder Capacity: If a bladder capacity is less than 50 mL, it will not be suitable for cystoscopy. On the one hand, if the bladder is introduced with some fluid, the patient may have a sense of discomfort, which makes observations unsatisfactory. On the other hand, if the operator has no knowledge of the patient's bladder capacity, the insertion of the telescope may cause bladder perforation.
3. Acute inflammatory stage: Hysteroscopy is not advisable when there is acute inflammatory, nor is cystoscopy.
4. If cystoscopy has been done in 1 week, a repeat examination should be avoided, because the impact of the previous examination on bladder has not been eliminated, which may affect the effect of observation.
5. The patients with severe systemic disease or renal impairment.
6. Other conditions: Cystoscopy cannot be performed due to such conditions as the bone and joint disease, deformity, and problem of patient's position.

13.4.3 Matters Need Attention for Using a Hysteroscope as a Cystoscope

There have had incisive descriptions on some of the basic skills about cystoscopic examination in the relevant professional books, so here are a few specifications for some problems to which gynecological endoscopic doctors should pay special attention.

1. When cystoscopy is performed, anesthetic should be applied to the mucosal surfaces.
2. The obturator should be used when a larger diameter hysteroscope is in use for examination.
3. Whatever diameter hysteroscope is used for cystoscopy, sterile glycerol or liquid paraffin should be coated in the front part of the telescope to lubricate the urethra.
4. In the process of inserting hysteroscope, the telescope should be prevented from slipping into the vagina, particularly for older women or the patients whose urethral orifice is narrow and close to the vaginal orifice. If the telescope slips into the vagina, it should be disinfected carefully after its retrieval. This also suggests that when endoscopy is performed, it is very important to disinfect carefully the vulva, around the urethra and in the vagina.
5. The bladder base is mostly jacked up by uterus, especially when there is leiomyoma growing in the anterior uterine wall. After the entry of telescope into the urethra, if the telescope continues to be inserted horizontally, damage to the bladder base may be caused, so operation inside the bladder should be gentle and slow, and the end of telescope should be tilted slightly upward after entry so as to avoid unnecessary injury.
6. Since the bladder has good elasticity, there is no need to use distention pump during examination. As long as the transfusion bottle is hung about 1 m above the operating table. The irrigating fluid can be saline, 5% glucose solution, 5% mannitol, 3% sorbitol, and 1.2%–1.5% glycine. But if there is any electrosurgical operation in the bladder, electrolyte-containing fluids like saline should not be used. As the bladder has larger capacity, if the operator forgets drainage while irrigating, this can cause overfilling of bladder, resulting in patients' discomfort. Thus, the fluid inflow and the drainage must be conducted together and fluid irrigation should be stopped when the folds of bladder mucosa are seen to become flat.
7. When the ureteral intubation is to be performed and the telescope is being inserted into the urethra, it is important to keep the controller (diverter) in a turned-off or reset state so as to avoid scratching the urethra. Intubation should not start until the tip of the ureteral catheter is close to ureteral orifice through moving the telescope. Do not use the diverter frequently in order to avoid injury to bladder mucosa. We must see clearly the ureteral orifice

before intubation lest mucosal edema may occur due to a forceful intubation.

8. Since the ordinary hysteroscope is a rigid telescope with a smaller and fixed angle, a fiber hysteroscope should be chosen if an all-round inspection of the bladder is required. Take Olympus hysteroscope for example, HYF-XP fiber hysteroscope has a telescope of 3.1 mm in diameter and 100° of view angle, while HYF-IT fiber hysteroscope has a view angle up to 120°, with biopsy capability and the telescope 4.9 mm in diameter. Both are very suitable for all-round inspection of the bladder.
9. Through an observation of the color and quantity of ureteral jet, we can understand whether the ureter is impaired or not. If the patient is given intravenous infusion of 1 or 2 ampoules of methylene blue solution, which can make the urine turn blue, it will be easier to observe the patency of the ureter. In such a case, it is more appropriate to choose 5% glucose as the irrigating fluid, because saline is easy to be mixed instantaneously with urine containing blue color, it will be not easy for observation in a blue vision field. However, 5% glucose solution is not easy to be mixed with urine within a short time and more convenient for observation.

With the development of modern medical science, there are more and closer relationships between each individual division of medicine. With the emergence and boom of a new discipline—Female Urology, we believe that more and more gynecologic endoscopists will also be competent in cystoscopic examination and surgery, and will harvest more experiences and skills.

Suggested Reading

1. Almeida ZM, Pontes R, Costa HL. Evaluation of pain in diagnostic hysteroscopy by vaginoscopy using normal saline at body temperature as distension medium: a randomized controlled trial. Rev Bras Ginecol Obstet. 2008;30:25–30.
2. Chiesa-Montadou S, Rongières C, Garbin O, Nisand I. A propos de deux complications au cours du drilling ovarien par fertiloscopie [About two complications of ovarian drilling by fertiloscopy]. Gynecol Obstet Fertil. 2003;31(10):844–6. French.
3. Cooper NA, Smith P, Khan KS, Clark TJ. Vaginoscopic approach to outpatient hysteroscopy: a systematic review of the effect on pain. BJOG. 2010;117(5):532–9.
4. Dechaud H, Ali Ahmed SA, Aligier N, Vergnes C, Hedon B. Does transvaginal hydrolaparoscopy render standard diagnostic laparoscopy obsolete for unexplained infertility investigation? Eur J Obstet Gynecol Reprod Biol. 2001;94(1):97–102.
5. Di Spiezio SA, Di Carlo C, Spinelli M, Zizolfi B, Sosa Fernandez LM, Nappi C. An earring incidentally diagnosed and removed through two-step vaginoscopy in a pubertal virgin girl with miliary tuberculosis. J Minim Invasive Gynecol. 2014;21(2):176–7.
6. Feng Z, Shao J. Practical hysteroscopy. Shanghai: Shanghai Medical University Publishing House; 1999. p. 120. Chinese.
7. Fernandez H, Watrelot A, Alby JD, Kadoch J, Gervaise A, deTayrac R, Frydman R. Fertility after ovarian drilling by transvaginal fertiloscopy for treatment of polycystic ovary syndrome. J Am Assoc Gynecol Laparosc. 2004;11(3):374–8.
8. Garbin O, Kutnahorsky R, Göllner JL, Vayssiere C. Vaginoscopic versus conventional approaches to outpatient diagnostic hysteroscopy: a two-centre randomized prospective study. Hum Reprod. 2006;21(11):2996–3000.
9. Gordts S, Campo R, Rombauts L, Brosens I. Transvaginal salpingoscopy: an office procedure for infertility investigation. Fertil Steril. 1998;70(3):523–6.
10. Gordts S, Watrelot A, Campo R, Brosens I. Risk and outcome of bowel injury during transvaginal pelvic endoscopy. Fertil Steril. 2001;76(6):1238–41.
11. Gorts S, Campo R, Brosens I. Office transvaginal Hydrolaparoscopy for early diagnosis of pelvic endometriosis and adhesions. J Am Assoc Gynecol Laparosc. 2000;7(1):45–9.
12. Guida M, Di Spiezio SA, Acunzo G, et al. Vaginoscopic versus traditional office hysteroscopy: a randomized controlled study. Hum Reprod. 2006;21:3253–7.
13. Guo H, Lan J, Zhao S, Gao J, Bie Y, Hu X. Comparison of no-touch hysteroscopy with traditional hysteroscopy. Chin J Obstet Gynecol. 2011;46(4):281–2. Chinese.
14. Guo Y. Intrauterine urology. Beijing: People's Medical Publishing House; 1992. p. 105–26. Chinese.
15. Ma J, Xia E. The clinical application of vaginoscopy in diagnosis and treatment of vaginal abnormal discharge in young girls. China J Endoscopy. 2009;15:730–2. Chinese.
16. Messini S. Fertiloscopy. Minerva Ginecol. 2000;52(9):363–6.
17. Paschopoulos M, Paraskevaidis E, Stefanidis K, Kofinas G, Lolis D. Vaginoscopic approach to outpatient hysteroscopy. J Am Assoc Gynecol Laparosc. 1997;4(4):465–7.
18. Verhoeven HC, Brosens I. Transvaginal hydrolaparoscopy, its history and present indication. Minim Invasive Ther Allied Technol. 2005;4(3):175–80.
19. Watrelot A, Dreyfus JM, Andine JP. Evaluation of the performance of fertiloscopy in 160 consecutive infertile patients with no obvious pathology. Hum Reprod. 1999;14(3):707–11.
20. Watrelot A, Dreyfus JM, Cohen M. Systematic salpingoscopy and microsalpingoscopy during fertiloscopy. J Am Assoc Gynecol Laparosc. 2002;9(4):453–9.
21. Watrelot A. Fertiloscopie: l'expérience clermontoise [Fertiloscopy: Clermont-Ferrand's experiment]. Gynecol Obstet Fertil. 2007;35(3):281–2.
22. Watrelot A, Gordts S, Andine JP, Brosens I. Une nouvelle approche diagnostique: la fertiloscopie. Endomag. 1997;21:7–8. French.
23. Watrelot A. Place of transvaginal fertiloscopy in the management of tubal factor disease. RBM Online. 2007;15:389–95.
24. Xia EL, Felix W, Li Z. Gynecologic endoscopy. Beijing: People's Medical Publishing House; 2001. p. 10–5. Chinese.
25. Xia EL. Hysteroscopy: office evaluation and management of the uterine cavity. 1st ed. Beijing: Peking University Press; 2013. p. 1. Chinese.
26. Xia EL. The clinical application of endoscopy in female infants of gynecological disorders. Chin J Pract Gynecol Obstetr. 2004;20:529–31. Chinese.
27. Zheng J, Xia EL. Evaluation of vaginoscopy in clinical application. China J Endoscopy. 2012;18:350–3. Chinese.

Hysteroscopy Training

14

Enlan Xia and Xiaowu Huang

Before widespread clinical application, any kind of diagnostic and treatment technique must involve a set of systematic learning methods to guide operators to understand and grasp its operating principles step by step. Through clinical practice, its application methods, operating skills, and safety are constantly improved and perfected. Therefore, systematic training is important for the completion and implementation of endoscopic training program, and all the gynecologists to be engaged in this program must be qualified in this planned standard training so as to achieve the expected level of expertise.

14.1 Training Procedures

The training of hysteroscopic operating system should start with a comprehensive understanding of its varied instruments and their components, followed by the practice on the models, animal specimens, isolated uterus, or other simulated environment in order to achieve hand-eye coordination and learn to complete the surgical procedure through endoscopic images. On this basis, the gynecologists must learn its indications, contraindications, and potential complications. Through attending workshops, seminars, tutorials and reading relevant books and their matching atlas in combination with simulated training, the unity of theory and practice can be achieved. Its training procedures are as follows.

1. To acquire relevant knowledge in this field through reading and reviewing the relevant teaching materials about hysteroscopic operation such as atlas, teaching video, slide and CD, etc. Only when gynecologists have a good understanding of the uterine anatomy and pathology, can they distinguish normal tissues from diseased ones, and then make a definite diagnosis.
2. To familiarize with the instruments and equipment, and master the indications, contraindications, and complications.
3. To learn the basic knowledge through the relevant data, photos, and videos and master operating skills by attending workshops, seminars, and tutorials.
4. To practice hysteroscopic examination in simulation on the uterine model and removed uterine specimens, and then practice diagnostic hysteroscopy in living bodies prior to diagnostic curettage or vaginal hysterectomy. Only when the operators are completely proficient in hysteroscopic examination, can they start the practice of hysteroscopic tubal cannulation and hydrotubation.
5. To learn hysteroscopic surgeries after being proficient in hysteroscopic diagnosis and treatment.

14.2 Requirements for an Operator

Hysteroscopy is a specific procedure in gynecological field. Its safety and efficacy are closely related to the operating level of operators. Hysteroscopic surgery needs special instruments. During surgery, doctors operate by using monocular view or 2D images on a television screen instead of three-dimensional observation, which adds difficulty to operation. So, operators must pass strict technical training to achieve a safe procedure. The requirements for operators in hysteroscopy are as follows.

1. Operators must have good basic surgical trainings, in-depth knowledge about anatomical uterine markers, and rich experience in open surgery, and can handle the surgical complications and intraoperative accidental events.
2. Operators must have sufficient experience and strong ability in diagnostic hysteroscopy.
3. Operators must have skillful hands, can coordinate hands, feet, eyes, and brain to work in harmony, can manipulate the resectoscope proficiently and have a good control of cutting depth.

E. Xia (✉) · X. Huang
Hysteroscopy Center, Fuxing Hospital, Capital Medical University, Beijing, China

E. Xia (ed.), *Practical Manual of Hysteroscopy*, https://doi.org/10.1007/978-981-19-1332-7_14

4. Operators must have a clear and quick mind to deal with various accidental situations rapidly during the operation.
5. Operators must have knowledge of energy source so as to clear troubles timely.

14.3 How to Teach Beginners

Because hysteroscopic surgery may be rather difficult and performed in a very narrow vision field, it is not easy for beginners to learn. So attention should be paid to the following points.

1. To begin with, do some resection exercises for a certain period of time on the real objects, such as meat, apple, soap, or corpse so as to manipulate the resectoscope and resectional techniques of tissue proficiently.
2. To observe how teachers handle electric cutting with the aid of teaching endoscope or TV video.
3. Under the guidance of teachers and surveillance of teaching endoscope or TV, the beginners can perform short-time electric coagulation and (or) resection of a small amount of cervical tissues.
4. After a good command of basic operations, the beginner may choose to perform electroresection in a slightly larger uterus monitored by the teacher through a teaching endoscope or television. If only a small portion is excised in half an hour, the teacher should change position with the beginner in order to try to complete the operation within the second half hour.
5. When the beginner starts to perform electroresection, after the completion of the operation, the teacher should conduct inspection and supplements.

14.4 How to Cut Tissues

In hysteroscopic surgery, electric cutting is a crucial step, and also a key indicator to evaluate the success or failure of operation and operator's level. So, how to cut tissue is the focus of training.

1. Place the electric cutting loop at the distal side and on the surface of the tissues to be excised. Before moving the loop electrode to start cutting, the first step is to step on the foot pedal. Then moving the cutting handle or spring when the hands have a sense of cutting, and cutting into tissues according to the requirements and resecting the tissues based on the required cutting depth. The moving speed is usually 1 cm/s.
2. After each cut, there should be tissues visible from a cutting surface. Only when the loop electrode moves into the sheath and the foot is released, will it be possible to resect the tissues fully.
3. Generally, the resected tissue appears to be stripped. It is slightly thinner at either end and thicker in the center, like a small boat. The thickness of tissue slice is directly proportional to the placement depth of loop electrode, and its length depends on the moving distance of the loop electrode and the endoscopic sheath.
4. Taking the internal cervical os as a pivot, the depth of cutting is adjustable.
5. If the tissue to be resected is thick, the operator should lean the tip of resectoscope sheath slightly forward so that the loop electrode may cut into the tissue and then cut slightly and deeply in arcing movement until the end of cutting. Then raise the sheath slightly, and excise the tissue successfully.

Hysteroscopic training must start from a simple procedure to complex ones. Simple procedures include removal of IUD, polyps, foreign bodies, etc.; complex procedures include division of intrauterine adhesions, resection of septum or myoma, and resection of endometrial polyps or endometrium.

Suggested Reading

1. Xia EL. Specifications of gynecological endoscopic operation. Chin J Obstet Gynecol. 1997;32:267–75.

The Future of Hysteroscopy

15

Enlan Xia

In the past 30 years, rapid development of hysteroscopic technique and great progress in its equipment have turned hysteroscopic examination and surgery into an effective means of diagnosis and treatment of intrauterine lesions for gynecologists. It can be foreseen that there is a great deal of hope for hysteroscopy. Not only the indications for hysteroscopic diagnosis and treatment are well established nowadays, but they have also been extended and have replaced some other operations performed by gynecologists, such as curettage, removal of uterine submucous myoma by hysterotomy and blind division of intrauterine adhesions, and so on. The main aspect for future research will be the new second generation endometrial ablation technique. The ideal second generation technique should be accomplished more easily, require less skills and less training, and can be done under local anesthesia, but its effect can be comparable to classic hysteroscopic surgery, which can be adapted to all intrauterine operations including fibroids, and there are fewer complications compared with TCRE and EA. There is still more need for analysis of randomized controlled trials on various endometrial ablation techniques as much as possible so as to evaluate its effectiveness and safety. If there is no solid credible evaluation, new technique and new equipment cannot be applied routinely in clinic and be introduced in the market. In the treatment of obstetric and gynecological diseases, the costly endometrial pretreatment with drugs has gradually given way to mechanical pretreatment for economic reasons.

The future begins today. Everything will move forward as time goes by. Future instruments will be more simplified and future energy will be more secure. Intraoperative use of micro-morcellator not only disturbs uterine distention, but also makes a clearer vision field, which extends its therapeutic indications. And more and more various kinds of auxiliary devices and electrodes will emerge, and hysteroscopic examination and surgery will be more suitable in an outpatient setting. With the simplification of procedure, this surgery will be more practical, more secure and the operative time will also be shortened, and its accuracy will also be improved. These tendencies will lead to simplification of many surgical procedures. With the advent and application of ultrasonography control technology and with the perfection and practicality of the modern operating room facilities, labor intensity of doctors will be greatly reduced so that the range of diagnostic and operative hysteroscopy will be further extended.

In 2001, scholars at the tenth annual meeting of the International Society for Gynecologic Endoscopy held in San Francisco of America pointed out that, by 2025, most of gynecological operations will be replaced by endoscopic operation.

We must learn from history, continue to innovate and create so as to make medical techniques simpler, safer, and more beneficial to patients. Since the initial objective has not yet been achieved completely, the innovation and creation in hysteroscopy should never stop.

Suggested Reading

1. Baggish MS, Valle RF. Future of hysteroscopy. In: Baggish MS, Barbot J, Valle RF, editors. Diagnostic and operative hysteroscopy. 2nd ed. St. Louis: Mosby; 1999. p. 391–401.
2. Parkin DE. Endometrial resection and ablation: past, present and future. Gynaecol Endosc. 2000;9:1–7.

E. Xia (✉)
Hysteroscopy Center, Fuxing Hospital, Capital Medical University, Beijing, China

E. Xia (ed.), *Practical Manual of Hysteroscopy*, https://doi.org/10.1007/978-981-19-1332-7_15

16 Digital Storage and Application of Endoscopic Image

Baijiang He

The storage and application of endoscopic image data had been problems difficult to resolve properly before the introduction of computer technology. In order to save a valuable picture on the monitor as a static image, it is unimaginable to directly face the monitor and shoot. Some endoscopic manufacturers developed special equipment for shooting the endoscopic images with optical camera. After being filmed and processed, photographs are created for preservation. The dynamic images can only be stored in video tape, CD, or DV (digital video cassette). The shortcomings of doing so are that there will be loss in video quality after being preserved for long term or being replicated for many times, and that it is not possible or difficult to effectively edit and modify freely without professional equipment. For example, if we would like to produce a short teaching video about endoscopic surgery, there was a need to edit the original video data, such as editing videos, adding captions, and putting both narration and music. Its completion not only requires professional equipment worth of hundreds of thousands of dollars in the television station or publishing house but also assistance of the professional and technical personnel.

Since the rapid development of computer multimedia technology, there have been radical changes in the situation. Especially, today's desktop computer performance is similar to small video workstation performance. So, we are fully conditioned to conduct endoscopic static and dynamic image collection in the hospital with simpler devices, and edit and modify in the late stage so as to produce the surgical atlas and short teaching videos of our own style. Mastery of this technique has become one of the necessary skills for endoscopic doctors.

B. He (✉)
Endoscope Marketing Department, Olympus (Beijing) Sales and Service Co., Ltd, Beijing, China

16.1 Basic Concept

A static image is composed of a large number of pixels arranged in a matrix form. The smaller the pixels per unit area is and the more number of pixels is, the higher the image resolution will be, and it looks more realistic as we see. A dynamic image is composed of a series of rapid continuous play of static images based on the theory of visual persistence. Usually, a film consists of 24 static frames per second and TV consists of 25 frames per second. Human eyes cannot detect such rapid image shift but can produce a smooth sense of reality. Every pixel of color image is formed by the color and luminance information. The analog signal is to use the voltage values to simulate the color and brightness of each pixel while the digital signal is to use binary digits to represent the color and brightness of each pixel. Either analog or digital signals, as long as they follow their putative coding rules, can encode any static and dynamic image and transfer the codes through the transmission media to the destination and represent them as video image. Analog signals may be subject to outside interference in the process of encoding, transmission, transcription, and representation, resulting in mild offset voltage value, thereby leading to distortion in the represented image. Since digital signals have only two values of 0 and 1, and there is check mechanism in the every process above, it will not be distorted no matter how many times it is transcribed or how far it is transmitted. Theoretically speaking, as long as the original capturing rate is high enough and data has not lost (lossy compression) in the late procession, the digital signal can be taken to be exactly the same image as the original at any time, on any occasion and in any form. This is the reason why the digital image technique is superior and will eventually replace simulation technique.

At present, the host computer with endoscopic imaging system can provide three kinds of analog video signal output, namely, composite video, Y/C, and RGB, in which the signal quality is in succession upgraded. In some high-end models, YPbPr output can also be provided. The digital

E. Xia (ed.), *Practical Manual of Hysteroscopy*, https://doi.org/10.1007/978-981-19-1332-7_16

storage and application of these analog video signals must go through analog-to-digital conversion, and this process is completed in the video capture card (connected to the card in the computer PCI expansion slot). The digital image quality formed depends on the type and quality of original analog video signals and the quality of analog/digital conversion equipment (i.e., video capture card). With advances in technology, we can obtain very easily the universal digital video signals from the endoscopic instruments so that the formation of endoscopic image from production to final application is a purely digital process. Now we have been able to record digital images in multiple formats through extensive recording media. For example, the pioneer of digital video signal host computer—Olympus Corporation, after launching VISERA camera system which meets the requirement for a variety of endoscopic surgeries, developed the latest Exera II system in accordance with 1080i HDTV standard. They can all provide a universal digital video signal output, IEEE1394.

16.2 Storage and Application of Static Images

The static image formed instantly in an endoscopic imaging host computer may be saved as a file in a universal computer format and used for exchange. Such image file can be added directly to the PowerPoint slide for academic exchanges, and can be directly used for publication in a book, can be printed as photos, but also can be edited and modified with software like PhotoShop, for example, adding annotations.

OTV-S7 digital camera system (Fig. 16.1) produced by Olympus Corporation can directly save the images in a size of 3.7 mm × 4.5 mm × 0.1 mm SmartMedia card (Fig. 16.2) in a JPEG or TIFF format. A 256 MB SmartMedia card can hold about 2400 low-quality images, or about high-quality 960 images. These image files can be stored into the hard disk or CD-ROM for various uses.

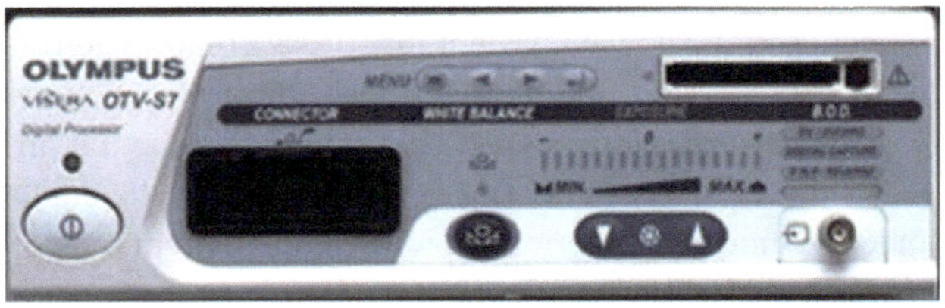

Fig. 16.1 OTV—S7

16.3 Storage and Application of Dynamic Images

The digital processing of dynamic images is complex. When we receive Video or Y/C analog video signals from endoscopic imaging host computer, they are input into the video signal capture card, and then the video signals are captured and encoded, thus forming the video files in the computer hard disk. Later, we can use the corresponding player software to play on the computer screen or projector, and also use the software and (or) hardware for editing.

Before the digital video files cannot be effectively compressed with high quality, huge amounts of data may overload the computer system. The data volume of digital video signals up to 216 MB/s (component video) or 142 MB/s (composite video) can only be processed in high-end digital video workstation. Nowadays, the digital video compression algorithm is becoming more mature day by day and the PC performance is improved constantly. All these have made the processing of the digital video files in a desktop computer or a notebook computer possible. The common compression formats are Motion-JPEG, MPEG1, MPEG2, MPEG4, as well as VCD/ MPEG1 format and DVD/MPEG2 format.

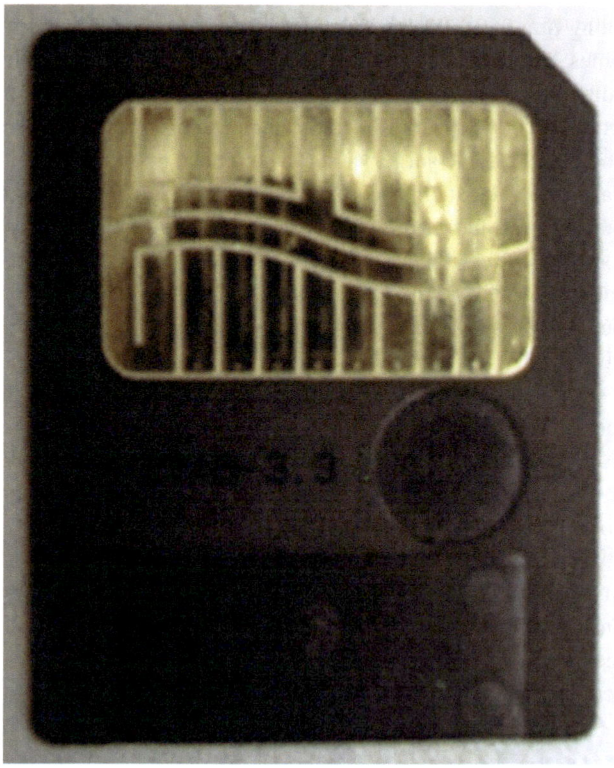

Fig. 16.2 SmartMedia card

Different video cards offer different combinations of three different functions: capture, compression, and editing (thus named differently), offer different number and types of interfaces (composite, Y/C, component, IEEE 1394) and offer different compression algorithms, so different types of video files may be generated for selection according to actual needs. Generally, to provide one or two composite or Y/C signal input is suitable for hospital use in any one format or more formats among MPEG1, VCD, MPEG2, Motion-JPEG and AVI, and the hardware video editing card for special effects is essentially not needed. MPEG1 and VCD files can be directly burned into VCD disk, and simple operation can be completed with VideoPack burning software. Its weakness is ordinary effect with playback on computer. MPEG2 is DVD quality digital video format. PC has optical disk drive supporting DVD burning function, which can make DVD disk with the appropriate software. Motion-JPEG and AVI is a commonly used video editing format with very high image quality, its frame accurate editing can be realized, but the file is bigger, the requirement for computer system is relatively high, and its operation is slightly more complex. Therefore, if we want to use the most convenient way to get VCD disk, the first scheme can be adopted; if we wish to obtain higher playback quality on a computer screen or projector, the second type of scheme can be adopted; the third scheme is applicable to relatively professional users, which can be used to edit admirable personalized teaching short videos. In addition, when choosing video card, we should not choose one with recording time limits, otherwise it will bring us trouble in the recording and processing in the late stage. No matter which kind of format is adopted in file compression, the most frequent needs are to edit the surgical process and remove unnecessary parts, and add text captions and sync sounds as well. These operations can be completed by using Adobe Premiere or Ulead Media Studio, VideoStudio (true to like), and others. And we can also choose from varied domestic software, which is very easy to use.

If the endoscopic imaging host computer provides IEEE1394 digital video output (such as Olympus Visera or Exera II system), it can be connected directly with IEEE 1394 (Firewire) interface on the notebook computer, and digital video capturing and simple editing can be conducted by using Windows MovieMaker software. This is the most convenient solution.

16.4 Concept and Composition of Nonlinear Editing System

Colloquially, nonlinear editing system is the incorporation of hardware and software system for digital processing of the above video signals. The traditional image editing is to record the analog video signals to videotape, and then edit, synthesize, add captions or sync sounds by using the equipment like editing machine, subtitling machine and mixer which are worth hundreds of thousands of yuan, and all operations must be implemented in strict accordance with the timing sequence instead of at will. Nonlinear editing system is to code the digital video source by using high-performance computer and then to store them in the high-speed digital hard disk. When editing, creating stunts, adding captions and sync sounds are being conducted, it is actually calculating and rewriting the digital codes. Then, the dynamic images generated from these codes are played on computer, television, projectors, and other devices. The digital images will not be distorted even with frequent transcription and passage of time. During the processing, there is no need to be confined to the video data sequence, so the nonlinear editing system has incomparable superiority compared with the traditional linear editing system. More important is that very little investment in equipment can allow the work to be completed in high quality, which would require 10 times the price if the original equipment is used. Now in the professional institutions, nonlinear editing system has been widely used and has also become readily available in individual applications.

The basic nonlinear video editing system is made up of the high-performance computer (including high-speed video storage system), analog (digital) video (audio) capture, editing, playback device, optical disk recorder, scanner and the corresponding software package, and other equipment can be added depending on the specific uses. The video processing computer has higher requirements on the system performance, in addition to good overall performance, still a large memory space, high speed and large capacity hard disk and stronger multimedia processing capability are needed, to which attention should be paid in the configuration of a computer system.

16.5 Clinical Applications of Digital Video Image Data

1. The unedited original surgery data can be burnt to a CD for long-term preservation or play in VCD and DVD player at any time.
2. The edited endoscopic video images, X-ray imaging, ultrasonography imaging, live surgery or surgery-explained video can be used for academic exchanges, teaching, demonstration and being made into a CD-ROM for permanent preservation.
3. Thc live video image or video image data may be transmitted through the broadband network so as to accomplish video conferencing, telemedicine, and online teaching.

Appendix 1: Routine Orders in a Hysteroscopic Ward

Doctor's Orders on Admission

Standing Orders

1. Gynecological Usual Care.
2. Nursing care second grade.
3. General diet.
4. Prescription orders according to the patient's conditions and requirements.

Stat Orders

1. Routine blood tests, ABO and RH blood grouping.
2. Routine urine tests.
3. Liver and kidney function tests, biochemistry tests, and lipid blood tests.
4. Tests for surface antigen of the hepatitis B virus (HBV).
5. Coagulation tests (four items).
6. Cervical smear (which can be ignored if having TCT results).
7. Tests for vaginal cleanliness, Monillia, and bacterial vaginosis.
8. Chest X-ray PA (posteroanterior) & LAT (lateral).
9. Electrocardiogram (ECG).
10. Abdominal pelvic ultrasonography (within 1 month).
11. Gynecological examination.
12. Tumor-associated antigens (in patients with adnexal mass): AFP, CEA, CA125, CA199
    And: serum HCG, AKP, LDH.
13. Tests for hepatitis C virus (HCV) antibody and treponema pallidum hemagglutination assay (TPHA) and HIV antibody.

Hysteroscopic Operations

Orders on the Day Before Operation

1. Time and type of operation.
2. No eating and drinking on the morning of operation.
3. Insertion of cervical osmotic tent.
4. Anal tampon with indomethacin 100 mg 30 min before insertion of osmotic tent.
5. Prescription orders according to the patient's conditions, antibiotics when needed.
   Notes: Cervical ripening of (3) and (4) can be replaced by the following methods:

1. Misoprostol 400 μg is inserted into posterior fornix of the vagina 2 h prior to the operation.
2. Phloroglucinol (smooth muscle antispasmodic agent), 40–80 mg, is applied by intravenous drip 15 min prior to operation, which should be finished in 5 min.

Postoperative Orders

1. Postoperative care following TCR__ under anesthesia.
2. First grade nursing care for 1 day, then second grade nursing care.
3. Fasting for 6 h, then regular diet.
4. Prescription orders according to the patient's conditions, including antibiotics.
5. Orders for special conditions and treatment.
6. 1–3 days after operation: routine blood tests and leukocyte differential count (DC).
   Note: please write down the abbreviated English name of the surgery in the first item.

Special Management After TCRS and TCRA

1. Vulva washing one or two times (if a balloon catheter is retained).
2. Hormone replacement therapy (For reference).
   (a) Estradiol Valerate (Progynova) 2 mg, take orally (p.o.), twice a day (b.i.d), from the fifth day of menstruation and continued for 21 days.
   (b) Provera (medroxyprogesterone acetate) 4 mg, p.o., b.i.d, or Dydrogesterone 10 mg, b.i.d, taken from the 19th day of the menstrual cycle for 7 days.
   (c) A menstrual period may resume 3–7 days after simultaneous discontinuation of these two drugs. In the next menstrual cycle, the medication is administered the same as the last, and there are two artificial cycles in total.
3. Second-look hysteroscopy is performed 4 weeks after operation.

E. Xia (ed.), *Practical Manual of Hysteroscopy*, https://doi.org/10.1007/978-981-19-1332-7

Conditions on Discharge

1. Histological results.
   (a) There must be histological report in principle.
   (b) The patient should be informed and given explanation by her doctor.
2. Routine blood test is normal.
3. The temperature is normal. The patient's condition is stable and there is no much bleeding.
4. A discussion must be held before an early discharge from hospital.

Precautions After Hysteroscopic Operation

1. It is normal that there is a small amount of bleeding and discharge within 2 months after operation, during which sexual intercourse should be banned. If there is too much bleeding and discharge, timely follow-up is needed.
2. If there is bleeding in patients within the third month after resection of endometrium, it is menstrual blood.
3. Outpatient check-up should be conducted in the first and third month after operation, and re-check should be followed once every half a year thereafter.
4. TCRE may produce certain contraceptive effects with a low failure rate like all other contraceptive measures, so if there is abnormal condition, please come quickly to the hospital for a diagnosis. However, this does not belong to the scope of family planning.
5. The patients may get pregnant after removal of IUD 2 months following resection of septum.
6. The patients may get pregnant 3 to 6 months after resection of submucous myoma.
7. Menstruation can return to normal in patients 1 month or so after TCRP, TCRA, and TCRF.
8. Comply with doctor's orders given other conditions.

Laparotomy Surgery

Orders on the Day Before Operation

1. Time and type of operation, and method of anesthesia.
2. Skin preparation.
3. 200–400 mL of blood preparation (according to the patient's conditions).
4. Semi-liquid diet on the night before operation, and no eating and drinking on the next morning.
5. Enema with drugs (glycerin bowel enema) twice at the night before surgery and the morning of surgery.
6. Cleaning the vagina with 0.5% povidone-iodine once at 3 p.m. before surgery and once on the morning of surgery.
7. Antibiotics are administered via intravenous infusion 30 min prior to operation (see clinical medications).
8. Urethral catheterization on the morning of surgery.
9. Antibiotics and fluid according to the patient's conditions (postoperative medications).

Postoperative Orders

1. Postoperative care for the surgery and anesthesia.
2. First grade nursing care for 3 days, then second grade nursing care.
3. Fast for 6 h, then semi-liquid diet, regular diet 2 days later.
4. A companion for 3 days.
5. The catheter is retained for 24–48 h (according to the patient's conditions), then removed.
6. Scrubbing vulva once a day (after hysterectomy, usually for 3 days).
7. Antibiotics and liquid according to the patient's conditions (see clinical medications).
8. Timely discontinuation or modification of medication according to patients' conditions.
9. Removal of sandbag after 6 h of abdomen compression.
10. In the patient with an abdominal drainage, its removal is determined by her condition and materials drained.
11. 1–3 days after operation:
    (a) Routine blood test and leukocyte DC.
    (b) Routine urine test (10 items).
    (c) Changing the abdominal wound dressing.

Precautions After Operation

1. An outpatient check-up should be conducted 1 month after surgery.
2. Sexual intercourse should be banned within 1–2 months after total hysterectomy and 1 month after other surgery, or follow the doctor's advice.
3. There might be a small amount of vaginal bleeding 2–4 weeks after hysterectomy. If the bleeding volume is equal to that of a menstrual period or there is vaginal discharge, please return quickly to see the doctor.
4. The patient has a poor physical strength within 3 months after hysterectomy, and returns to preoperative health status after 6 months, and is significantly improved in health status 1 year later.
5. Menstruation may return to normal about 1 month after myomectomy. Pregnancy is feasible after 1–2 years of contraception.
6. The regular menstruation may be resumed about 1 month after adnexa surgery.
7. Comply with doctor's orders given other conditions.

Conditions on Discharge

1. The incision heals well.
2. The temperature is normal for more than 2 days.
3. The routine blood and urine tests are normal.
4. Record of gynecological examination before discharge.

5. There must be histological report. In special cases, the patient should obtain permission before discharge from hospital after discussion. The patient should be informed and given explanation by her doctor.

Routine Orders of Diagnostic or Operative Laparoscopy

Orders on the Day Before Operation

1. Full liquid diet on the morning and afternoon, and fasting on the night before surgery. Nil by mouth on the morning of surgery.
2. Time and type of operation under general anesthesia.
3. Liquid paraffin 30 mL, or polyethylene glycol electrolytes powder 2–3 boxes, 4:30 p.m. p.o., or soapsuds or glycerin enema once the night before surgery and once the morning of surgery.
4. Cleaning the umbilical stump. Intravenous antibiotics injection (i.v.), 30 min prior to operation (see clinical medications).
5. Postoperative medications (supplement fluid 1000–1500 mL i.v.).
6. Medications according to the patient's conditions.

Bowel Preparation

1. Bowel preparation is needed when the surgery might be associated with intestines.
2. The surgeries requiring bowel preparation include:
   (a) LAVH, large ovarian cyst.
   (b) A history of abdominal surgery.
   (c) Chocolate cyst with suspected adhesions.
   (d) There may be intraoperative bowel injury.

Methods of Bowel Preparation (See Table- Appendix 1)

Three Days Before Operation

1. Semi-liquid diet.
2. Oral medicines: (1) metronidazole 0.4 g, 3 times a day (t.i.d). (2) gentamicin 80 mg, b.i.d.

Two Days Before Operation

1. Total liquid diet.
2. Senna 10 g, taken as tea, once a day for 2 days.

On the Day Before Operation

1. Nil by mouth.
2. 2500–3000 mL rehydration.
3. Liquid paraffin 30 mL, or polyethylene glycol electrolytes powder 2–3 boxes, 4:30 p.m. p.o.; or soapsuds or glycerin enema 1–3 times at 3:30 p.m. before surgery and 6:30 a.m. on the day of surgery.

Postoperative Orders

1. Postoperative care for the surgery and general anesthesia.
2. First grade nursing care for 1 day, then second grade nursing care.
3. Fast for 6 h, then semi-liquid diet, regular diet 2 days later. (Fast for 6 h, then regular diet after diagnostic laparoscopy.)
4. A companion for 1 day.
5. The catheter is retained, and is removed after intravenous infusion.
6. Antibiotics according to the patient's conditions (see clinical medications). If necessary, an indwelling catheter is used. If there is external suture, stitches are removed in 5–7 days.
7. If laparoscopic cervical cerclage is performed in mid trimester of pregnancy, medications should be prescribed as follows: 5% glucose (GS) 250 mL with 25% Magnesium Sulfate 5 g, i.v. given within 1 h. Then 5% GS 500 mL with 25% Magnesium Sulfate 7.5 g, i.v. given within 4–6 h. Respiration and patellar reflex should be monitored. Medications on the next day prescribed according to patient's condition.
8. In the patient with an abdominal drainage, its reservation and removal is determined by her condition and materials drained.
9. 1–3 days after operation:
   (a) Routine blood test and leukocyte DC.
   (b) Routine urine test (10 items).
   (c) Changing the abdominal wound dressing.

Conditions on Discharge

1. The incision heals well.
2. The temperature is normal for more than 2 days.
3. The routine blood and urine tests are normal.
4. Record of gynecological examination before discharge.
5. There must be histological report. In special cases, the patient should obtain permission before discharge from hospital after discussion. The patient should be informed and given explanation by her doctor.

Routine Orders of Transvaginal Surgery

Preoperative Preparation for Transvaginal Surgery

1. 1/5000 potassium permanganate solution, hip bath, b.i.d. (4 g potassium permanganate on the doctor's order).
2. The pubic hair should be shaved clean before a hip bath.
3. Vagina scrubbing, b.i.d. for 3 days before surgery (standing orders).

Notes: if colporrhaphy is done in old women, estrogen should be applied for period of time to pretreat the vaginal mucosa.

Orders on the Day Before Operation

1. Time and types of operation and anesthesia.
2. Skin preparation.
3. 200–400 mL blood is prepared (according to the patient's conditions).
4. Semi-liquid diet on the night before operation, nil by mouth on the morning of operation.
5. Soapsuds enema once the night before surgery and once the morning of surgery.
6. Antibiotics (see clinical medications) and fluids are prescribed according to the patient's conditions, i.v. 30 min before operation.

Standing Orders After Transvaginal Surgery

1. Postoperative care for the surgery and anesthesia.
2. First grade nursing care for 3 days, then second grade nursing care.
3. A companion for 3 days.
4. The catheter is retained for 24–48 h (according to the patient's conditions).
5. Vulva scrubbing 1–2 times a day (according to the patient's conditions).
6. Fast for 6 h, then semi-liquid diet, regular diet 2 days later.
7. Antibiotics (see clinical medications) and other drugs are prescribed according to the patient's conditions.

Documents Provided to the Patients on Discharge

1. A certificate of in-patient diagnosis, on which the admission date, the discharge date, the surgery performed, the diagnosis and the duration of restoration should be stated clearly.
2. Writing postoperative precautions, medications, and time of check-up on patient's medical recording book.
3. Medical files including discharge abstract.

Clinical Medication

Antibiotics in Common Usage

1. Cefoxitin 2.0 g diluted in 0.9% N.S. 100 mL, iv drip (intravenous drip), Bid.
2. If the patient is allergic to penicillin or cephazoline, alternatives may be:

Clindamycin 0.6 g iv drip Bid.

Fluid replacement

1. MG3 (Compound Electrolytes and Glucose Injection) 500 mL.
2. 5% G.S. 500 mL.
3. 10% G.S. 500 mL q.i.d (once a day) iv drip.
4. Vit C 1 g.

Addendum

1. Pretreatment of hysteroscopic surgery (Or apply intraoperative suction-mechanical thinning of endometrium).
   (a) Gestrinone 2.5 mg p.o., twice per week. (stat order)
   (b) GnRH-a once per 28 days.
2. Progesterone hormone therapy for endometrial carcinoma (for reference).

Medroxyprogesterone	100 mg	p.o.	b.i.d	× 3 months
Progesterone caproate	250 mg	im	q.i.d	× 3 months
Medroxyprogesterone	250 mg	p.o.	q.i.d	× 3 months
Medroxyprogesterone	500 mg	p.o.	q.i.d	× 3 months
Medroxyprogesterone	100 mg	im	q.i.d	× 3 months

BMI body weight/height^2, the range of normal value is from 22 to 24
im intramuscular

3. Medication routines for atypical endometrial hyperplasia following resection of endometrium (For reference).
   (a) Mild: medroxyprogesterone 30 mg, q.i.d × half a year.
   (b) Moderate: medroxyprogesterone 100 mg, q.i.d × 3 months, and half dose for another 3 months.
   (c) Severe: Medroxyprogesterone 250 mg, q.i.d × 3 months, and half dose for another 3 months.
   (d) Reexamination is done every 3 months including second look hysteroscopy and target biopsy.

   Notes: The conservative treatment of endometrial cancer should be well explained and the patient's consent must be obtained. It can apply a combined treatment of GnRH-a and LNG-IUS, and diagnostic hysteroscopy and curettage for histological examination should be performed every 2 to 3 months
4. Hemostasis.
   (a) Hemostatic triple injections (5% GS 500 mL + Etamsylate 3.0 g + Vit C 3 g + *p*-aminomethyl benzoic acid 0.3 g), iv drip, q.i.d.
   (b) Hemocoagulase 1 U, im or iv.
   (c) Tranexamic acid and sodium chloride injection, 100 mL, iv drip.
5. Use of anticoagulants in patients with artificial valve replacement.
   (a) Patients with mechanical heart valves need lifelong anticoagulation (warfarin).
   (b) The use of anticoagulants should be regulated according to the patient's conditions.

(c) The international normalized ratio (INR) of prothrombin time may be 1.5–2 times of normal value after taking anticoagulants. If it is lower than 1.5 times, it should be appropriate to increase the dosage, and if it is 2.5 times or higher, the dosage should be appropriately reduced.
(d) During medication, attention should be paid to bleeding tendency; if there is skin petechiae, epistaxis, gingival bleeding, hematuria, and other symptoms, it should be appropriate to reduce the dosage, and stop if necessary (INR > 5 or 2.5 times more than that of average person). Vitamin K_1 antagonists cannot be injected casually unless in a special emergency.
(e) If there is traumatic bleeding, hemostasis can be achieved by local compression, and there is no need to discontinue the anticoagulant. If an urgent surgery is required, it may be done with intravenous injection of vitamin K_1.
(f) In case of an elective surgery, first discontinue the medication for 2–3 days and if the prothrombin time returns to normal, the operation may be undertaken. 36–72 h later, the medication is resumed at an initial dose of 2.5 mg, and then discontinue the medication for 1 day. On the third day, a dose of 2.5–5 mg is administered and its dosage should be adjusted according to the prothrombin time.
(g) If there is more vaginal bleeding, the patient can be given intramuscular injection of oxytocin or symptomatic treatment like D&C, and there is no need to discontinue anticoagulants. If an emergency surgery is needed and INR value is higher, injection of vitamin K_1 antagonism may be given when necessary.
(h) In case of an elective surgery, warfarin should be discontinued 5 days before surgery and an injection of low molecular heparin is administered instead, such as subcutaneous injection of fraxiparine 1 mg/kg, per 12 h, given and stopped on the day of surgery (usage: For a patient with weight of less than 70 kg, each injection 0.4 mL is given; for a patient with weight greater than 70 kg, each injection 0.6 mL is given). The ratio of INR at operation is preferably less than 2.
(i) If there is not much bleeding from the wound after surgery, an injection of low molecular heparin is administered on the first day after operation (the usage is same as above). Three days later, warfarin (2.5 mg, q.i.d) is added. After combined use for 3 days, the use of low molecular heparin is discontinued. Four items of coagulation tests are checked once every 3–5 days. The dosage of anticoagulants is adjusted according to INR value, and when its value becomes stable, the reexamination is conducted once in a month. The INR value is maintained between 2 and 3.

6. One-day treatment program for ovarian cancer (CAP).
   (a) 5% G.N.S. 1000 mL, from the night before surgery till the next morning.
   (b) 5% G.N.S. 250 mL+ furosemide 20 mg, by small pot.
   (c) 20% Mannitol 125 mL (finishing in 30 min).
   (d) 5% G.N.S. 750 mL+ amycin 50 mg (into 50 mL N.S. solution), by small pot.
   (e) 5% G.N.S. 500 mL + D.D.P 50 mg (into 50 mL N.S. solution), by small pot.
   (f) 5% G.N.S. 500 mL + CTX 500 mL (into 50 mL N.S. solution), by small pot.
   (g) 15% KCl 10 mL + 5%G.S. 500 mL + Vitamin B6 100 mg + Vitamin C 2 g + Metoclopramide 10 mg, iv drip, q.i.d. Daily rehydration of fluid above 3000 mL.
7. VAC treatment program for ovarian cancer.
   (a) V (Vincristine): 5% G.S. 500 mL + vincristine 1–1.5 mg, once a week × 12 weeks.
   (b) A (Actinomycin): 5%G.S. 500 mL + dactinomycin 400 mg, iv drip × 5 days.
   (c) C (Cyclophosphamide): cyclophosphamide 5–7 mg/(kg • day) or 500 mg/day, into the pot, iv drip, × 5 days.
   (d) Once a month for two consecutive years.
   (e) If actinomycin is unavailable, amycin 500 mg may be used once a month for 2 consecutive years.
   (f) Zofran 8 mg into a small pot is given daily prior to infusion.
8. Hysterosalpingography with iodine oil
   (a) 76% meglumine diatrizoate 20 mL × 1.
   (b) 76% meglumine diatrizoate 2 mL for test sensitivity (for intravenous injection).
9. Bowel preparation with polyethylene glycol electrolytes powder.
   (a) Ordinary bowel preparation in gynecology.
      - Diet preparation.
         – On the day before surgery, taking soft food at noon and liquid diet at night (such as lotus root starch, various soups, but excluding food easy to produce flatulence like beans, milk, sugar, and others). Two packs of polyethylene glycol electrolytes powder are taken around 4 p.m. Fasting starts on the morning of surgery.
         – If reactive hypoglycemia like dizziness, palpitations, hunger, and others appear, please tell the doctor and nurse (some fluid rehydration may be applied).
      - Oral whole-gut lavage fluid.
         – The preparation of the whole-gut lavage fluid: 1 pack of polyethylene glycol electrolytes powder is poured into the large pot (provided by nursing department), and warm water is

added up to 1000 mL, then it is stirred so as to dissolve completely.

- How to take: Two packs of polyethylene glycol electrolytes powder with a total volume of 2000 mL are taken. 1000 mL fluid is taken orally every hour until all the fluid is consumed completely or a clear watery stool is discharged. During medication, the upper body should be maintained upright, and the patient can also drink while going about and can do abdominal massage gently clockwise. The fluid should be finished in approximately 2 h.

• Precautions.
  - Some patients may develop abdominal distention, abdominal pain, nausea, vomiting, and other reactions after taking polyethylene glycol electrolytes powder. The patient with mild symptoms may be relieved when slowing down the drinking speed appropriately. If necessary or with severe symptoms, tell your doctor and nurse in charge.
  - If you usually have dry stool, please take laxative ahead of time before taking polyethylene glycol electrolytes powder.
  - Generally the patient will defecate within 1 h after taking the medicine. If it does not occur at 3 h, the patient should tell the nurse in charge and the intestinal tract should be cleaned combined with other ways.
  - The patient should tell the nurse about the number of defecation and the texture of stool (such as formed stool, paste stool, loose stool, watery stool, and clear watery stool).
  - After taking polyethylene glycol electrolytes powder or anal enema, the fluids inside the intestinal tract should be emptied as far as possible.

(b) Cleaning the intestinal tract as preparation for gynecologic surgery.
  • Diet preparation.
    - On the day before surgery, liquid food without residue is eaten at noon (such as porridge, noodles, but excluding foods easy to produce flatulence like beans, dairy, sugar, and others) and fasting in the evening. Two packs of polyethylene glycol electrolytes powder are taken on an empty stomach around 11 a.m., and another two packs of polyethylene glycol electrolytes powder are taken around 4 p.m. Fasting starts on the morning of surgery.
    - If reactive hypoglycemia symptoms like dizziness, palpitations, hunger, and others appear, please tell the doctor and nurse (Fluid rehydration can be given). A companion can be with the patient to observe any sign of hypoglycemia if she has diabetes.
  • Oral whole-gut lavage fluid (as stated above).

Table-Appendix 1 Guideline of Preoperative bowel preparations for laparoscopic surgery

	1. Laparoscopic examination or monitoring		*2. Simple laparoscopic surgery:* Simple adnexal surgery, simple ovarian cyst, small subserous myoma, estimated adhesion-free surgery, and so on
The day before surgery	Semi-liquid diet at noon, fasting in the evening, fasting and water deprivation on the morning of surgery Liquid paraffin 30 mL 4 p.m. p.o.		Semi-liquid diet at noon, fasting in the evening, nil by mouth on the morning of surgery Folium sennae 10 g is taken with water Liquid paraffin 30 mL 4 p.m. p.o.
	3. More complex laparoscopic surgery: LAVH, TLM, large ovarian cyst, with a history of open surgery, chocolate cyst with suspected adhesions, suspected bowel injury during surgery		*4. With severe pelvic adhesions and suspected bowel injury*
	Ordinary surgery	Complex surgery with possible bowel injury	
3 days before surgery	Regular diet Metronidazole 0.4 g t.i.d Gentamicin 80,000 u b.i.d × 3 days		Liquid diet without residue Gentamicin 80,000 u b.i.d Metronidazole 0.4 g b.i.d Vit K_1 10 mg im q.i.d or small pot × 3 days
2 days before surgery	Semi-liquid diet Folium sennae 10 g, taken with water for 2 days	Semi-liquid diet	Liquid diet without residue 50% $MgSO_4$ 30 mL

The day before surgery	Full liquid diet on the morning and at noon, and fasting on the evening; Nil by mouth on the morning of surgery; Liquid paraffin 30 mL 4 p.m. p.o. Fluid replacement 1500 mL(MG3 1000 mL + lactated Ringer's solution 500 mL)	Full liquid diet on the morning and at noon, and fasting on the evening; Nil by mouth on the morning of surgery, Cleansing the intestinal tract at 3 p.m. the day before surgery and at 6 a.m. on the morning of surgery Fluid replacement 2000 mL (MG3 1000 mL + lactated Ringer's solution 1000 mL)	Fasting Cleansing the intestinal tract on the night before surgery and on the morning of surgery Rehydration 3000 mL Replacement of potassium: 15%KCl 10 mL Note: For the patient with poor nutrition: Ensure 1 tin p.o.

Basic hospital diet

1. Semi-liquid diet: porridge, noodles, dumplings, steamed egg, tofu, etc. 4–5 times daily
2. Liquid diet: rice soup, sugar-free lotus root starch, gravy, vegetable juice, etc. 5–6 times daily

Appendix 2: A Practical Manual of Hysteroscopic Surgery

Facilities of Operating Room and Patient's Body Position

1. Operating room: An operating room should be spacious, and the operating table should be put in the center, at the head of which can be placed the anesthesia machine and monitors manipulated by the anesthetists. On one side of the patient are placed a multi-layer cart or supplies boom with TV monitor, video camera, recorder, fluid distending pump, and other equipment on it, and also placed instrument tables and B-mode ultrasonography machine; on the other side are current generator and cold light source. There are at least 3 sockets in the wall which are powerful enough to meet the demand of electricity for operation.
2. Gynecologic operating table: It should have the following functions:
   (a) The patient's position can be changed quickly with the requirement of operation in order to meet the objective need that the resecting time is restricted.
   (b) There should be enough space in the operating area so as to facilitate the resecting surgery smoothly.
   (c) There should be a complete system of irrigation and collection of distention medium so as to adapt to the massive requirement of fluid by resection surgery.
   (d) It should have a wide variety of applications, on which any gynecological operation can be performed so that the operation can be immediately transferred to laparotomy in case of need.
3. Position: The patient is placed in a modified lithotomy position, that is, supporting the legs with the relaxed knees, the thigh at an angle of 45° to the horizontal line, abduct legs to an extreme degree in order to increase the available space. Compared with full lithotomy position, this position is advantageous in small intra-abdominal pressure, no interference with breathing and easy access to the tubal ostia. If laparoscopy is at the same time performed, make the thigh at 30° angle to the horizontal line so as not to affect the laparoscopic procedure. Generally, a slightly low head position is taken.
4. The distance between the height of distention medium and the patient's pubic symphysis is from 100 cm to 120 cm so as to maintain a certain intrauterine distention pressure. If the automatic uterine distending pump is applied, the pressure can be adjusted to the mean pulse pressure. When operation starts, if hypertrophic endometrium or large submucous myomas occupy the uterine cavity, and narrowed septate uterus or intrauterine adhesions restrict distention medium into the uterine cavity leading to obscure vision, the intrauterine pressure can be elevated instantly, but only transiently.
5. Be sure to open the inflow and outflow switch, and empty the gas out of fluid irrigation tube. When operation begins, switch on continuous perfusion system to irrigate and wash off intrauterine tissue fragments and blood. Sometimes, if there is larger blood clot blocking the sheath and hindering the circulation of distention medium, the hand piece and the scope or the inner sheath must be taken out and cleaned. After one has a clear vision of the uterine cavity, then connect the cables and start the operation.
6. At present, the commonly used intrauterine electrosurgery is a monopolar circuit loop. Before switching on the power for operation, remember to check the loop electrode in the patient to ensure a complete current cycle. If nonelectrolyte liquid can be used as distending medium only, prepare some active electrodes for spare use before each operation, in order that the active electrode is changed in time if tissue fragments adhere to the electrode. The replaced electrode can be reused after being cleaned. The usual power is set at 80 W for electroresection and 60 W for electrocoagulation, and may be regulated according to intraoperative conditions. If a hysteroscopic plasma bipolar working element is applied, the power is set at 250–310 W for electroresection and 90 W for electrocoagulation.

E. Xia (ed.), *Practical Manual of Hysteroscopy*, https://doi.org/10.1007/978-981-19-1332-7

Preoperative Preparations

1. Preparation on the day before operation.
   (a) Disinfection of hysteroscope and its instruments.
   (b) Cervical dilator or laminaria tent is introduced into cervix on the night before operation to soften and dilate the cervix. When insertion is difficult, 100 mg indomethacin can be used per rectally. Or misoprostol 400 μg is placed into posterior fornix of the vagina 2 h prior to the operation. Also phloroglucinol (smooth muscle antispasmodic agent), 40–80 mg is given by intravenous drip 15 min prior to operation, which should be finished in 5 min.
2. Preparation on operation day
   On the morning, the patient should have fasting and have a full bladder so as to facilitate ultrasonographic monitoring during operation.
3. The transparency and activity of the operating frame, whether the connectors on current generator, cables, and the electrode plate are loose or not should all be checked. If there is malfunction with the equipment, it should be repaired timely prior to operation. There should be a certain number of wire loops for spare use.

Transcervical Resection of Endometrium (TCRE)

Indications

1. Persistent abnormal uterine bleeding, and malignant diseases have been excluded.
2. The uterus is enlarged to 8–9 weeks of gestation, and uterine cavity is 10–12 cm in length.
3. submucous myoma with 4–5 cm in diameter.
4. No requirement for fertility.

Contraindications

1. Cervical scar and the cervix cannot be well dilated.
2. Acute uterine flexion and the hysteroscope cannot reach the uterine fundus.
3. Acute stage of reproductive tract infection.
4. Acute period of heart, liver, and kidney failure.
5. One has no good psychological capability to bear the fact that this operation is to relieve symptoms rather than a radical cure.

Timing of Operation

1. After menstruation, the endometrium is at its early proliferative stage, which is the optimal time for operation.
2. For those who have completed endometrial pretreatment, operation may also be performed during non-menstrual phase.
3. If there is an uncontrollable bleeding, emergency operation should be done.

Anesthesia

Commonly, general intravenous anesthesia or continuous epidural anesthesia is conducted.

Operating Procedures

1. The patient is placed in lithotomy position on the operating table, and the vulva and vagina are disinfected routinely with 0.25%–0.5% iodophor solution. If cervical dilatation rod is inserted, the assistant should wear sterile gloves and remove it from the vagina, which can avoid fracture of cervical dilator by other methods and partial retention in the uterine cavity. After placement of surgical drape sheets, the external orifice of urethra is disinfected and urinary catheter is inserted. An injection of distention medium (5% glucose or 5% mannitol) is introduced into the bladder to fill the bladder properly so as to push the bowel covering the uterine surface aside. The uterus is clearly displayed with acoustic beam through the acoustic window formed by the filling bladder. The amount of distension of the bladder varies from person to person. For those who have no history of pelvic surgery, the upper half of the uterine corpus needs to be shown. During hysteroscopy, the cervical forceps is used to pull the cervix downward and the uterine fundus is exposed, and this will not affect the surgeon's operation due to the overfilling of bladder. For those who have history of pelvic surgery, if there are pelvic adhesions, when the cervical forceps is pulled downward, the mobile extent of the uterus will be small. Therefore, there should be slightly more bladder filling than those with no pelvic surgery, and it is enough to expose the uterine fundus.
2. Then go on to disinfect the vagina and cervix, place the vaginal speculum and clamp the cervical anterior lip with cervical clamp, detect the depth of uterine cavity under ultrasonography surveillance, and then dilate the internal cervical os gradually enough to insert the operative hysteroscope, usually 10–11 mm. Then, install light sources, irrigation tubing, cables (its surface is scrubbed with 75% ethanol), and manipulator control. If the cervical internal os is tight and difficult to dilate, the obturator can be inserted with the sheath into the cervix so that its front end may further dilate cervical internal os. After entering the uterine cavity, the obturator can be taken out, and then introduce hysteroscope and manipulator control into the uterine cavity for operation.

3. If endometrium is found to be thick, suction aspiration can be first used.
4. The resection of endometrium must follow a certain procedure. First, use vertical wire loop electrode to cut the portion of uterine fundus. This area is the hardest to resect, but easy to perforate, therefore the operator must be very careful. The uterine fundus is easy to be covered by the resected fragments, thus the vision is hindered. So, some people prefer to use rollerball electrode to coagulate the fundal endometrium and then use wire loop to do with the rest parts. Some would like to use a wire loop with an angle of oblique forward 10° to resect the uterine fundus, and a wire loop with an angle of oblique backward to resect the rest of the uterine cavity. During the operation, one or two wire loop electrodes suitable for management with the uterine fundus and uterine cornua should be prepared. Since the endometrium resected at two cornua appears to be fragmented, therefore the operator must be very careful not to push the wire loop too far into the myometrium. Especially after resecting the portion of two cornua which is the thinnest, the operator must cut and shave shallow each time until all the endometrium is removed completely, which is at a less risk of perforation than a deep cut.
5. After management with the uterine fundus, the 90° wire loop is pushed out of sheath and extended to the distant position. According to the requirements on the depth and length of resection, a parallel cutting is done from the distal to the proximal. First the sheath is pulled back and anterograde resection is undertaken. Then the spring of the cutting handle is loosened slowly. Only when the wire loop electrode is moved into the sheath and the foot pedal is released will the tissues be possibly resected completely. For the beginners, the moveable distance of wire loop electrode is confined within 2.5 cm, and a systemic resection of endometrium is resected from 9 o'clock position in a counterclockwise direction. First, resect endometrium of upper 1/3 portion of uterus, then resect middle 1/3 portion of uterus. If total endometrial resection is to be done, resect the lower 1/3 portion of uterus until the cervical canal. If the operator is skilled and proficient, he can increase the cutting distance through moving the hysteroresectoscope from the uterine fundus to the uterine isthmus, and take out the resected tissue strips immediately.
6. The resection of endometrium in uterine walls is preferably to begin with the posterior wall because the resected debris is likely to gather and cover in the posterior wall. Although the tissue fragments can be clamped out piece by piece from the cavity, the distention fluid will flow out from the cervical os each time. Each dilation and collapse of uterine cavity may cause uterine bleeding, thus hindering the hysteroscopic view. So the tissue fragments are better to be retained in the uterine cavity and be pushed at uterine fundus until the end of surgery.
7. The depth of the resection depends on the endometrial thickness, and the aim is to cut into the superficial myometrium 2–3 mm underlying endometrium. This depth is sufficient to remove the full layer of endometrium except for the extremely deep endometrium without cutting the larger vessels. If endometrium has been pretreated previously, generally it rarely requires cutting more than once and can reach the desired depth. If endometrium is thicker, electrocoagulation can be repeated following the electric cutting, by which the efficacy can be improved. There is no difficulty concomitant with resection of submucous myoma <3 cm, and a larger myoma may also be resected with necessary devices. After resection, the electro-resectoscope is retrieved and the oval forceps or curette is used to remove endometrial fragments, and a small amount of endometrial fragments can be discharged spontaneously several days after operation. The endometrial fragments are sent for histological examination.
8. After the uterine cavity is made empty, the hysteroresectoscope is put back to check whether there is residual endometrium or large bleeding points. The former needs to be resected while the latter needs electrocoagulation with wire loop or rollerball electrode. The irrigation system prompts an increase in the intrauterine pressure and intraoperative bleeding is rare. When uterine distention pressure drops, the bleeding points become evident. Unless there is a large amount of bleeding, there is no need to waste time in electrocoagulation.
9. The total resection includes the resection of total uterine cavity and upper cervical canal. Partial resection is the resection of full-layer endometrium in the upper 2/3 portion of uterine cavity. The left untreated endometrial edge is 1 cm in width, located above the isthmus of uterus. The patients who undergo routine partial resection are afraid that the total resection may induce the cervical stenosis, and if there is functional endometrium in the uterine cavity, secondary intrauterine hematometra may occur. The hematocele is more often at the uterine fundus clinically rather than on the isthmus, therefore, it is unnecessary to undertake partial resection unless there is still desire for menstruation after operation.

Intraoperative Ultrasonography Monitoring and Guidance

1. The operator may observe the probe entering the uterine cavity, determine the direction of the probe reaching the fundus and guide the hysteroscope to be placed at the cervical internal os. The distention medium injected into the uterine cavity and the filling bladder form acoustic windows for double contrast.

2. From the beginning of surgery to the end, the two-dimensional double-contrast ultrasonographic imaging is performed in continuous monitoring of surgical process. The following contents should be included in observation. (a) Changes in the thickness of uterine wall and the location of resectoscope should be observed in order to prevent uterine perforation. (b) Signs in the changes of the echo under the effect of electric heat on the inner lining of the uterus and the muscle wall should be observed so as to determine the electric cutting depth, extent, and intramural lesions as well. (c) The location and size of the intrauterine lesions and the relationship between the pathological changes in the uterine muscle wall and the uterine cavity should be determined and the resection of intrauterine and intramural lesions should be monitored. (d) Whether there is previous uterine malformation and old injury in the uterine muscle wall which are difficult to diagnose should be explored before surgery. (e) Observation of uterus and monitoring whether there is distention medium flowing via the fallopian tubal ostia into abdominal cavity or not and its volume should be conducted.
3. The resected uterine lining may dehydrate and shrink due to heat produced by the high-frequency thermal effect of the wire loop during TCRE procedure, and the strong linear echo in the inner lining of the uterus turns into strong echogenic band of 3–4 mm in breadth. When cutting reaches myometrium, the strong echogenic band may fade away after 15–40 min of resection. In case of patients with DUB, when the cutting depth is confined to the mucosal layer, the strong echogenic band formed may disappear rapidly. During operation, the important indication for prevention of missed resection is whether the strong echogenic light band is intact or not. The duration of the strong echogenic light band is the ultrasonic indication suggestive of the cutting depth. The location of resectoscope is closely monitored so as to prevent the wire loop from leaning tight against or penetrating the uterine wall. When the outer edge of the strong echogenic band reaches the deep myometrium, it suggests that the operator should stop the local cutting, which may prevent uterine perforation effectively.

Postoperative Precautions

1. A small amount of bleeding and discharge are normal within 2 months after operation. If there is too much bleeding and discharge, a follow-up is needed.
2. If there is bleeding in patients at the third month after resection of endometrium, it is menstrual blood.
3. Outpatient reexamination should be conducted in the first and third month after operation, and re-check should be followed once every half a year thereafter.
4. Transcervical resection of endometrium may produce certain contraceptive effects with a low failure rate like all other contraceptive measures, so if there is abnormal condition, please come quickly to the hospital for a diagnosis. However, this does not belong to the scope of family planning.
5. Sexual intercourse should be banned for 2 months after operation.
6. The patients who have adenomyosis diagnosed postoperatively require medication therapy, such as gestrinone, danazol, and GnRH-analogs for 3 months. After administration of danazol and gestrinone for 1 month, the patients should take liver function tests. If there is abnormality, the medication is discontinued.

Transcervical Resection of Myoma (TCRM)

Indications

TCRM procedure is suitable for symptomatic submucous myoma, inward-protruding intramural myomas, and cervical myoma.

1. Menorrhagia or abnormal bleeding.
2. The size of the uterus is generally limited to 10 weeks of gestation and the length of uterine cavity is limited to 12 cm.
3. The size of submucosal or inward-protruding intramural myoma is generally limited to less than 5 cm.
4. No cancerous changes in uterus.

More than one procedure may be required to complete the removal of submucous myomas deeply embedded into myometrial layer and inward-protruding intramural myomas. As to the submucosal myomas which prolapse into the vagina, its size or thickness of the pedicle is not restricted.

Contraindications

1. Cervical scar and the cervix cannot be fully dilated.
2. Acute uterine flexion and the hysteroscope cannot reach the uterine fundus.
3. Acute stage of reproductive tract infection.
4. Acute period of heart, liver, and kidney failure.
5. Patients who have no good psychological capability to bear the fact that this procedure may relieve symptoms of hemorrhage but recurrent myomas after operation.

Preoperative Preparations

1. Preoperative medication pretreatment (if there is larger myoma and difficult operation in patients) is administered with GnRH-a, once every 28 days for a consecutive 3–6 months. The surgery is performed within 3–6 weeks after the last medication.

2. If myoma is not prolapsed out of the cervical canal, cervical ripening is conducted on the night before surgery. Indomethacin 100 mg can be used per rectally and 30 min later the uterine cervical dilator or laminaria tent is inserted into the cervix.
3. On the morning of surgery, the patient should be fasted and ace a full bladder so as to facilitate ultrasonographic intraoperative monitoring.

Timing of Operation

The ideal time for operation is at the first half of menstrual period. If there is excessive bleeding, the operation must be done even in the secretary phase. If there is uncontrollable bleeding, an emergency surgery may be performed.

Anesthesia

Continuous epidural anesthesia is generally administered.

Operating Procedures

1. The patient is placed in lithotomy position, and the assistant should remove the cervical dilator from the vagina with sterile gloves. The patient's vulva and vagina are regularly disinfected with 0.25%–5% iodophor, and surgical drape sheets are placed under the buttocks. The negative plates are attached to the patient's buttocks or thighs (with rich muscles), turn on the power switch and set at 80 W for electric cutting and 60 W for electrocoagulation.
2. After disinfecting the hands, the operator puts on sterile gloves, insert the vaginal speculum, disinfect the vagina again, clamp the anterior lip of cervix with the cervical clamp, disinfect the cervical canal, and dilate the cervix to 11–12 mm.
3. Install the irrigation tubing, cables, light source and adapter and disinfect with 75% ethanol twice, and empty the gas out of the irrigation tubing, install them in turn onto the manipulator's handle. Adjust the camera focus, color, and definition before inserting it into the uterine cavity. Check the negative plate, open the inflow and outflow switch, then insert the endoscope into the uterine cavity.
4. To begin with, diagnostic hysteroscopy is performed. By ultrasonography, the location of intrauterine myoma and the status of pedicles are examined carefully. Then, the surgery is performed according to the types of the myomas. First, the wire loop electrode and rollerball electrode are used to coagulate the large vessels in the surface of myoma and blood vessels in the tumor pedicle, which may reduce intraoperative bleeding. The wire loop electrode is placed at the distal side and step on the foot pedal. When the hands have a sense of cutting, move the cutting handle or spring and then start resection of tissues. When the wire loop electrode is moved into the sheath and the foot pedal is released, the tissues are excised. With this repeat action, the tumor is cut piece by piece, and the size of the myoma is shrunk, thus dissecting the myoma completely. Alternatively, the forceps are used to clamp the myoma and screw out by twisting. The myoma is removed completely by repeat cutting and clamping of the myoma or clamped out by cutting off the tumor pedicle. Intraoperative administration of oxytocin via intravenous injection and surgical operation may increase the protruding degree of submucous myoma into uterine cavity, and even some intramural myomas as well, which may be transformed into submucous myomas and can be removed.
5. As to pediculated submucous myomas, the tumor is made smaller by cutting or its pedicle is cut off and then is removed with forceps. If there is larger myoma or there is no way to clamp out the myoma because of its smooth surface, the tumor needs cutting and its size is to be shrunk. It is better to cut grooves in the tumor so as to facilitate the clamping.
6. As to sessile submucosal myoma, the wire loop electrode of 9 mm hystero-resectoscope is used to cut gradually along the tunica at the bottom of the myoma under intensive monitoring of the ultrasonography. The distal end of the telescope may be used to press myomas so as to blunt dissect the muscular layer. When the resection has been conducted to a certain degree, myomas may be clamped with myoma forceps, twisted and pulled while viewing the ultrasonic image to separate the myomas from the wall of uterine cavity. Clamping and cutting are repeated until the total removal of myomas. As to the myoma with protruding degree <20%, when resection starts, the myoma begins to protrude into the uterine cavity, so a complete resection is possible. If not completely resected, use a 9 mm hystero-resectoscope to resect the myoma in uterine cavity and the residual myoma in the myometrium more than 5 mm; after 2 to 3 months of operation, conduct reexamination by hysteroscopy, and then perform TCRM again to resect the myoma protruding into the uterine cavity completely.
7. As to multiple submucous and intramural myomas, it should be resected as much as possible at a time. When the operation ends, IUD should be placed in the uterine cavity, and taken out 2 months later.
8. Cervical myomas are all coated. As to the cervical myomas prolapsed from the cervical canal, wire loop electrode can be used to cut off the pedicle and remove it completely or cut open the capsule and screw it out. As to the myomas embedded in the cervical tissues, as long as its outline is made clear, the wire loop electrode is used to cut from the thinnest part of the embedded tissues, when cutting reaches the myoma, the incision can be appropriately extended, and the myoma can be stripped out from the capsule completely. After the removal of myomas, generally the tumor bed does not

bleed. If the tumor bed is larger or the outline of cervix is not integrated, absorbable catgut can be used for suture. As to sessile submucous myoma in the cervical canal, since the cervical canal wall has become very thin, it is extremely easy to cause perforation.

9. As to the large fibroid of more than 6 cm in diameter, preoperative treatment with GnRH-analogs should be administered.
10. It should be noted that the operative time should be limited within 1 h and absorption volume of irrigation fluid should be limited in 2000 mL so as to avoid TURP syndrome.
11. After operation, the uterine cavity is inspected, and hemostasis is achieved by electrocoagulation of the bleeding points. If there is more hemorrhage, a balloon catheter may be placed into the uterine cavity to achieve hemostasis by compression, and saline of 15–40 mL is introduced into the balloon, and the balloon is taken out after 4–6 h. Meanwhile, uterine contraction agents and hemostatic agents can be used.
12. The specimens are measured in weight and sent for histological examination.

Postoperative Management

1. Antibiotics is administered via intravenous dripping so as to prevent infection.
2. Observation of the vital signs.
3. Observation of hemorrhage. If there is more bleeding, oxytocin and (or) hemostasis with 5% glucose solution 500 mL, vitamin C 3 g, dicynone 3 g, and pamba 0.3 g can be administered by intravenous route. If there is acute active bleeding, electrocoagulation hemostasis should be applied again under hysteroscope.
4. After 6 h of fasting, regular diets are administered.
5. Attention should be paid to the electrolyte and acid-base balance.

Postoperative Precautions

1. It is normal that there is a small amount of bleeding and discharges in patients within 2 months after the surgery.
2. Sexual intercourse should be banned for two months.
3. Regular reexamination should be done in an outpatient setting.

Transcervical Resection of Endometrial Polyp (TCRP)

Indications

This procedure is suitable for the removal of symptomatic uterine endometrial polyps, with the exception of malignant change of polyps.

Contraindications

1. Cervical scar and the cervix cannot be dilated fully.
2. Acute uterine flexion and the hysteroscope cannot gain an access into the uterine fundus.
3. Acute stage of reproductive tract infection.
4. Acute period of heart, liver, and kidney failure.

Preoperative Preparation

1. Cervical ripening is conducted on the night before surgery. Indomethacin 100 mg can be used per rectally and 30 min later the uterine cervical dilator or laminaria is inserted into the cervix.
2. On the morning of surgery, the patient should be fasted and have a full bladder so as to facilitate B ultrasonographic intraoperative monitoring.

Timing of Operation

1. After menstruation, the endometrium is at its proliferative stage, which is the optimal time for operation.
2. For those who have had endometrial pretreatment, operation may also be performed during non-menstrual phase.
3. If there is an uncontrollable bleeding, emergency operation should be done.

Anesthesia

The time for TCRP procedure is short, so intravenous anesthesia can be administered. If the expected operative time is longer, continuous epidural anesthesia can be given.

Operating Procedures

1. The patient is placed in lithotomy position, and the assistant should remove the cervical dilator from the vagina. The patient's vulva and vagina are regularly disinfected with 0.25%–5% iodophor, and surgical drape sheets are placed under the buttocks. The negative plates are attached to the patient's buttocks or thighs (with rich muscles), turn on the power switch and adjust it at 80 W for electric cutting and 60 W for electrocoagulation.
2. After disinfecting the hands, the operator puts on sterile gloves, inserts the vaginal speculum, disinfects the vagina again, clamps the anterior lip of cervix with the cervical pliers, disinfects the cervical canal, and dilates the cervix to 9–10 mm so that the operative hysteroscope can be inserted.
3. Install the irrigation tubing, cables, light source, and adapter and disinfect with 75% ethanol twice, and empty the gas out of the irrigation tubing, install them in turn onto the manipulator's handle. Adjust the camera focus, color, and definition before inserting it into the uterine cavity. Check the negative plate, open the inflow and outflow switch, then insert the endoscope into the uterine cavity.

4. First, a diagnostic hysteroscopy is performed to determine the number, size, and pedicle location of the polyp.
5. The wire loop electrode is extended to the distal side of the basal pedicle of the polyp to be resected and step on the foot pedal. When the hands have a sense of cutting, move the cutting handle or spring and then start resection of tissues. When the wire loop electrode is moved into the sheath and the foot pedal is released, the tissues are excised. Make sure that the pedicle is removed totally lest it may recur later.
6. As to multiple polyps, resection of part of the polyp may also be done. Then the negative pressure suction aspirator can be used to suck out the endometrium and polyps. If the endometrium lining the surface of polyps is sucked out, there will be only the interstitial tissue of the polyps left with its size and diameter explicitly shrunk. With the inflow of irrigation fluid, its resection is made easy.
7. If there are larger blood vessels on the surface of the tissues to be excised, vascular electrocoagulation should be done before cutting tissues.
8. After operation, the uterine cavity is inspected, and hemostasis is achieved by electrocoagulation of the bleeding points. If there is more hemorrhage, a balloon catheter may be placed into the uterine cavity to achieve hemostasis by compression, and antibiotics may be administered, and the intrauterine residues are to be emptied in combination with the administration of uterine contraction agents and hemostatic agents. The balloon catheter should be taken out 4–6 h later.
9. The specimens are measured in weight and sent for examination.

Postoperative Management

1. Antibiotics is administered via intravenous route so as to prevent infection.
2. Observation of the vital signs.
3. Observation of hemorrhage. If there is more bleeding, oxytocin and (or) hemostasis with 5% glucose solution 500 mL, vitamin C 3 g, dicynone 3 g, and pamba 0.3 g can be administered by intravenous drip. If there is acute active bleeding, electrocoagulation hemostasis should be applied again under hysteroscope.
4. After 6 h of fasting, regular foods are administered.
5. Attention should be paid to the electrolyte and acid-base balance.

Postoperative Precautions

1. It is normal that there is a small amount of bleeding and discharges in patients after 2 months of surgery.
2. Sexual intercourse should be banned for 2 months.
3. Regular reexamination should be done in an outpatient setting.

Transcervical Resection of Uterine Septum (TCRS)

Indications

The procedure is suitable for symptomatic complete and partial septate uterus.

Preoperative Preparations

The operation should be performed within 3–7 days after menstruation. The surgery is usually performed under laparoscopic diagnosis and monitoring. Liquid paraffin 30 mL is taken orally at 4 p.m., semi-liquid food is allowed for dinner and at 7 p.m., the cervical dilator is inserted into the cervix on the day before surgery. On the morning of surgery, the patient should be fasting and antibiotics are administered for prevention on the day of surgery.

Operating Procedures

1. After a successful general anesthesia, the patient is placed in lithotomy position, and regular disinfection of the laparoscopic operating field is performed. The cervical dilator is removed from the vagina, and the patient's vulva and vagina are disinfected with 0.25%–5% iodophor.
2. The negative plates are attached to the patient's buttocks or thighs (with rich muscles), turn on the electric knife switch and adjust laparoscopy at a power of 30 W for electric cutting and electrocoagulation, and the hysteroscopy is adjusted at a power of 80 W for electric cutting and 60 W for electrocoagulation.
3. After placement of surgical drapes and sheets, diagnostic laparoscopy is performed first to obtain information about the location and size of the uterus and the concave of uterine fundus and exclude the condition of didelphic uterus, bicornuate uterus, unicornuate uterus, and rudimentary horns. If it is didelphic uterus, bicornuate uterus, unicornuate uterus, and rudimentary horns, the hysteroscopic surgery is canceled.
4. Under ultrasonography monitoring, a proper volume of fluid is introduced into the bladder so as to obtain a clear image of uterus. The surface of irrigation fluid catheter, camera, and cable is scrubbed with 75% ethanol twice by the assistant, and then they are installed with the manipulator's handle.
5. When resecting incomplete uterine septum, first, the shape and location of septum is observed. When endometrium is thicker, leading to an obscure vision, suction aspiration can be first done to make the endometrium thinner. The wire loop electrode is used to cut the septum. When cutting, the wire loop electrode is placed on one side of septum, and under ultrasonography monitoring a transverse cutting towards the opposite side is carried out,

and then a backward cutting from the opposite side is done. Attention should be paid to the penetrating depth, the direction of the electrode, and the left-right equivalent cutting. The operator should be watchful on the symmetry of the uterine cavity and try to avoid the deeper cutting of one side, leading to the deformation of the uterus. When cutting reaches the base of septum, much attention should be paid to avoidance of deep cutting and injury to the uterine fundus. If necessary, the needle electrode is used to incise the junction site between the septum and anterior-posterior uterine wall so as to restore the normal uterine cavity maximally. If there is bleeding, an optional electrocoagulation can be performed.

6. As to resection of complete septate uterus, a 4 mm Hegar dilator or a balloon is placed in one side of uterine cavity, and the septum from the upper portion of internal orifice of uterine cavity opposite to the Hegar uterine dilator or the balloon is cut, then the uterine dilator or the balloon is taken out and the surgery is continued. The subsequent procedures are the same as resection of subseptate uterus.
7. As to the resection of double cervix concomitant with septate uterus, the surgical method is basically the same as hysteroscopic resection of the complete uterine septum. The surgery does not destroy the structure of double cervix, and attention should be paid to retention of tissues 0.5–1.0 cm above the internal orifice of uterus.
8. Mechanical resection with scissors under hysteroscope is undertaken and the irrigating fluid may contain electrolyte. Hysteroscopic scissors can be classified into soft, semi-rigid, and rigid scissors. The soft scissors are not easy to manage, so the semi-rigid scissors are most commonly used, which can divide the tissues directly, an accurate cutting in the midline of septum and fibrosis site without the blood vessels should be started. Uterine myometrial vessels run from the uterine posterior-anterior wall into the septate tissues, the posterior and anterior wall of uterus should be avoided so as to prevent unnecessary bleeding. The cutting should start from one side, and cut gradually towards the opposite side, and cut off a small piece each time. Once the fallopian tube ostia are seen, the cutting should be shallow. The operator should watch carefully the small blood vessels from the myometrial layer to avoid penetrating uterine myometrium. After resection of septa, the operator should observe the uterine fundus under hysteroscope before the exit of the equipment and decrease the intrauterine pressure to observe whether there is obvious bleeding. If there is arterial bleeding, selective electrocoagulation can be carried out. The wide and large septum may affect the hysteroresectoscopic operation and make the resection of septum difficult, the mechanical resection by microscissors or division by laser optical fiber can be implemented.
9. When the operation comes to an end, the objective lens is retrieved to the internal os, and symmetry of uterus is observed. Then IUD is placed.

Postoperative Precautions

1. A slight lower abdominal pain may develop 1–3 days after operation. A two-week rest and prophylactic use of antibiotics should be prescribed.
2. The IUD placed in the uterine cavity should be removed 2 months after operation, and at the same time diagnostic hysteroscopy is performed so as to obtain information about the uterine cavity. If necessary, a supplementary cutting of the residual septum is undertaken.
3. Sexual intercourse is banned within 8 weeks after operation.
4. Hormone therapy is administered for three months after operation.

Transcervical Resection of Adhesions (TCRA)

Indications

This procedure is applicable to the symptomatic patients with intrauterine adhesion.

Preoperative Preparations

The operation should be performed within 3–7 days after menstruation. The operation on patients with severe adhesions should be performed under laparoscopic monitoring. Liquid paraffin 30 mL is taken orally at 4 p.m., semi-liquid food is allowed for dinner, and at 7 p.m., the cervical dilator is inserted into the cervix on the day before surgery. If there is difficulty in inserting cervical dilator, a fine catheter or laminaria is used to soften the cervix. On the morning of surgery, the patient should be fasted and antibiotics are administered for prevention of infection on the day of surgery.

Operating Procedures

1. After a successful general anesthesia under laparoscopic monitoring, the patient is placed in lithotomy position, and regular disinfection of the laparoscopic operating field is performed. The cervical dilator is removed from the vagina, and the patient's vulva and vagina are disinfected with 0.25%–5% iodophor.
2. The negative plates are attached to the patient's buttocks or thighs (with rich muscles), turn on the power switch and set at a power of 30 W for electric cutting and electrocoagulation, and the hysteroscopy is adjusted at a power of 80 W for electric cutting and 60 W for electrocoagulation.

3. After placement of surgical drapes and sheets, diagnostic laparoscopy is performed first to obtain information about the location and size of the uterus. If there is pelvic adhesion, laparoscopic adhesiolysis is performed simultaneously.
4. Under ultrasonography monitoring, a proper volume of fluid is introduced into the bladder by the operator so as to obtain a clear image of uterus. The surface of irrigation tubing, camera, and cable is scrubbed with 75% ethanol twice by the assistant, and then they are installed with the manipulator's handle.
5. Resection with hystero-resectoscope. First the shape and location of adhesions is observed. The filmy, loose adhesions can be divided by pushing with the tip of diagnostic hysteroscope and there is not necessarily a need to dilate the cervix, which is generally applicable to fresh adhesion or old adhesions at cervical internal os. The old and complex adhesions found in the uterine fundus and bilateral walls of the uterine cavity require removal with microscissors and wire loop electrode. As for horizontal or longitudinal adhesive zone in a basically normal uterine cavity, the wire loop electrode may be used to remove the adhesions under ultrasonography monitoring. If necessary, retrograde resection of adhesive zone can be performed so as to restore the normal morphology of uterine cavity. In case of total uterine cavity occlusion or severe deformity of uterine cavity, a dissection of the adhesions should begin from the internal cervical os until a new cavity is created. The aim of surgery is to restore the normal morphology of uterine cavity maximally. The needle electrode is first used to incise the uterine cavity, and under ultrasonography monitoring, a 7 mm or 8 mm resectoscope is properly inserted to excise the adhesive tissues antegrade or retrograde, and the resection extends gradually in the uterine cavity till the uterine fundus, and then the cornua. The bent-forward wire loop electrode may also be used to divide directly or excise adhesions. If there is bleeding, an optional electrocoagulation may be performed. If there are extensive adhesions, the operator should be alert to the perforation of uterus. When the operation comes to an end, the objective lens is retrieved to the internal orifice of uterus, and symmetry of uterus is observed. And then an IUD is placed.
6. For the patients with stenosis of uterine cavity and amenorrhea due to scarred uterine walls resulting from intrauterine adhesions, the needle electrode is used to cut 4 to 5 strips along the long axis of the uterus to expand the uterine cavity, and postoperatively the hormone therapy is administered to resume their menstrual cycle.
7. Under laparoscopic monitoring, the methylene blue solution can be injected into the uterine cavity to do a test on the fallopian tube patency.
8. The bendable semi-rigid or rigid scissors may be used to divide the adhesions from the center of the uterine cavity to expand the uterine cavity. In case of total uterine cavity occlusion, a division of the adhesions begins from the internal cervical os until a new cavity is created and then the cornua are opened. The continuous thicker adhesive tissues are not easy to divide and resect, a sharp biopsy forceps may be used to open the uterine cavity step by step and make it symmetrical. If there is extensive adhesion, the operator should be aware of the occurrence of the perforation of uterus. At the end of surgery, diluted methylene blue solution is injected through the cervix for detection of tubal patency.
9. After operation, an IUD is placed into the uterine cavity.

Postoperative Precautions

1. A slight lower abdominal pain may develop 1–3 days after operation. A 2-week rest and prophylactic use of antibiotics should be prescribed.
2. The IUD placed in the uterine cavity should be removed 2 months after operation, and at the same time diagnostic hysteroscopy is performed so as to obtain information about the uterine cavity. If necessary, a second surgery should be performed.
3. Sexual intercourse is banned for 8 weeks after operation.
4. Hormone therapy is administered for three months after operation.

Transcervical Removal of Uterine Foreign Body (TCRF)

The common intrauterine foreign bodies include IUD, trophoblastic remnants, fetal bone and retained suture strings.

Removal of IUD

Indications

Under the following conditions, the removal of IUD is needed with an aid of hysteroscope or ultrasonography intervention:

1. IUD with broken tail string, with stenosis or adhesion in uterine cervix and uterine cavity.
2. When blind removal is difficult and IUD embedment is suspected, and only parts of IUD are taken out or fragments of IUDs still remain within the uterus.
3. When reversible fallopian tube contraceptive device is deeply embedded in uterine cornua or its fragments are still retained.
4. When the women are at menopause (the longer duration of menopause, the more serious the atrophy of reproductive organ), the removal of IUD will be much more difficult and prone to infection.

Methods

1. The therapeutic hysteroscope, which is equipped with alligator forceps or grasping forceps, can be used to clamp foreign bodies under direct vision. If it is not powerful enough, or if there is embedment, a hysteroscopic resectoscope needs to be replaced. The open type of semi-wire loop can be put onto the stainless steel ring to hook it out.
2. If an IUD is imbedded in the uterine wall or migrates through the fibroids or is wrapping around the fibroids, the wire loop electrode can be used to incise the myometrium of the uterine wall around the embedded IUD or the fibroid is resected to remove IUD or to clamp out IUD under ultrasonographic positioning.
3. If the IUD is embedded deep, laparoscopic examination should be performed simultaneously to determine whether the IUD has passed through the uterine serosal layer or not.
4. The spring and tail string of the reversible fallopian tube contraceptive device are often embedded in tubal ostia and uterine horns. Once the tail string is broken, the IUD will be extremely difficult to remove. In such circumstances, the 21Fr operative hysteroscope and a closed electrode can be used to plough deep into the uterine cornua and take it out. Alternatively a hook or a long curved hemostat is placed in its side and it is hooked out or pulled out under direct vision of resectoscope.

Removal of the Residual Trophoblastic Remnants

The residual remnants of missed abortion, incomplete abortion, adherent placenta, and placenta accreta in the uterine cavity can cause intrauterine adhesions, amenorrhea, or irregular bleeding. By D&C, the residual trophoblastic remnants may not be removed completely or may not be detected due to adhesions. The trophoblastic remnants confirmed by hysteroscopy and fixed biopsy may be scraped or excised with wire loop electrode under ultrasonography monitoring. The excised tissues may be sent for pathologic examination. In the management of the residual trophoblastic remnants, this procedure is characterized by easy operation and short operating time, accurate location, and can remove the residual trophoblastic remnants completely, and obviously superior to conventional D&C.

Removal of Residual Fetal Bone

The retention of fetal bone after abortion is a rare complication. Fetal bone remnants may sometimes occur in a late-term induced abortion, and may often cause abnormal uterine bleeding and infertility. The retained fetal bones sometimes take up most of the uterine cavity. Strong intrauterine echo may be identified by ultrasonography and the retained fetal bones may be observed directly under hysteroscope. Under transabdominal ultrasonography guidance, the fetal bone is removed with the wire loop electrode of hysteroscope. The fresh residual fetal bones are easy to be taken out by hysteroscopy. The embedded fetal bones in the myometrium may not be removed completely. Patients who failed to completely remove the embedded fetal bones may conceive after operation, hence the removal of embedded fetal bones should not be roughly so as to avoid uterine perforation when clamping.

Removal of Remaining Sutures

When the non-absorbable sutures were used at cesarean section or resection of uterine corpus, the residual thread or thread node may be seen at the internal cervical os during diagnostic hysteroscopy, and this foreign body may cause endometrial bleeding or inflammation. The residual thread or thread node may be pulled out by alligator forceps or removed by wire loop electrode under hysteroscope.

Monitoring of TCRF

At the removal of foreign bodies, precise positioning is required and uterine perforation should be avoided, so the surgery should be performed under ultrasonography and (or) laparoscopic monitoring.

1. Transabdominal ultrasonography monitoring: The double or triple contrast transabdominal ultrasonography monitoring is employed, which may have a guiding effect on the uterine probe, uterine dilator and the insertion of hysteroscope and avoid the occurrence of uterine perforation. Ultrasonography intervention can suggest the location, size, and number of intrauterine foreign bodies, especially can locate the foreign bodies embedded in the uterine wall, help to learn about its embedded depth, and decide on the ways to remove by resection, incision, or clamping of the foreign bodies; and it may detect the fetal bones, small IUD fragments and broken hook buried in the endometrial layer or the myometrium, which cannot be revealed by hysteroscopy or laparoscopy. At the time of surgery, ultrasonography can guide the intrauterine hysteroscopic operation with wire loop. After resection with the wire loop electrode, its basal layer may dehydrate due to heat, forming strong echo, which can guide the direction of the resection of cervix and intrauterine adhesions, suggest and guide the cutting depth and assess whether the embedded foreign bodies have been removed completely or not. During the removal of residual fetal bone or metal IUD fragments, since the fetal bones and metal fragments all have strong echo, ultrasonography cannot distinguish easily the strong echo formed by electroresection or by residual fetal bone and metal fragments because of its resolution, and this is its weakness. Ultrasonography intervention is non-invasive, inexpensive, convenient, and is the most commonly used and effective way in monitoring hysteroscopic surgery.

2. Laparoscopic monitoring: By laparoscopy the changes in the uterine surface can be directly observed. If the uterine wall is seen to be translucent or the surface of serosa is blistery, it indicates that the uterine perforation is imminent. Once uterine perforation occurs, the detection of wound, timely electrocoagulation and repairing of the uterine wound by suturing can be performed by laparoscopy, which cannot be accomplished by ultrasonography. Compared with ultrasonography, laparoscopic monitoring cannot indicate the conditions of uterine cavity, and cannot guide the intrauterine operation, and cannot display intraoperative changes in the uterine wall thickness, so it must be applied in combination with hysteroscopy. Laparoscopy is invasive and expensive. After all, there are rare cases of uterine perforation following TCRF, therefore, the patients who have higher risk factors for uterine perforation may choose laparoscopic monitoring.
3. Laparoscopic ultrasonography monitoring: Laparoscopic ultrasonography (LUS) is higher in resolution than ultrasonography. Its operative method is to first establish a pneumoperitoneum, then introduce a laparoscope, instill saline 200 to 300 mL into the pelvic cavity, and then the laparoscopic ultrasonography probe (Sharplan probe scanning range 180°, frequency of 8 mHz, 10 mm in diameter, probing depth of up to 6 cm) is introduced under direct vision of laparoscopy via the cannula beneath the umbilicus or lateral side of lower abdomen into the abdominal cavity, allowing for a free scanning of uterus. The laparoscopic imaging and ultrasonography imaging are displayed on a monitor via a mixer, which is helpful to accurate understanding of uterine morphology, size, and identification of the lesions and the cutting range. For TCRF, laparoscopic ultrasonography can accurately locate in patients the small lesions, detect or rule out invasive intramural lesions and foreign bodies embedded in the myometrial layer, and can also avoid the influence of intestinal gas. It can view the appearance of uterus via laparoscope, but also can guide the intrauterine operation via laparoscopic ultrasonography. Laparoscopic ultrasonography has a high frequency probe, which improves the ability to penetrate tissues, can observe the adhesive tissues and dead cavity formed after adhesions, distinguish between the calcification focus and the residual fetal bone, and distinguish the strong echo formed after electroresection of muscular wall from the intrauterine residual ring or fetal bones. So, it is helpful to make a definite diagnosis and also to guide exactly the operating process. Since laparoscopic ultrasonography is invasive procedure, it can be applied only when a definite diagnosis is hard to make combined with diagnostic laparoscopy or transabdominal or transvaginal ultrasonography.

Transcervical Resection of Cervix (TCRC)

Preoperative Preparations

1. TCRC procedure should be performed within 3 to 7 days after menstruation. On the morning of surgery, the patient should be fasting.
2. If cervicitis is at the stage of acute inflammation, the drugs (such as policresulen vaginal suppositories, confort pessaries) should be generally applied locally for 2–4 weeks, and surgery can be performed after the control of acute inflammation.

Operating Procedures

1. The patient is placed in lithotomy position, and the patient's vulva and vagina are disinfected regularly with 0.25%–5% iodophor. The surgical drapes are placed. The negative plates are attached to the patient's buttocks or thighs (with rich muscles), the power switch is turned on and set at a power of 60 W for electric cutting and 40 W for electrocoagulation.
2. The surface of irrigation tubing, camera, and cable is scrubbed with 75% ethanol twice, and then they are installed with the manipulator's handle.
3. The uterine cervical canal is disinfected with iodophor cotton stick, the cervical lesion is examined, and the range of resection is decided in combination with the previous results of CCT or TCT and cervical biopsy. For the patients with cervical intraepithelial neoplasia (CIN), cervical smear with 2.5% iodine tincture is done to judge the risk of cervical lesions. The resected tissues and other tissues are separately examined pathologically. If necessary, several biopsy positions are recorded.
4. Generally, the extent of resection is 1 mm more than the normal tissues, and the ideal cutting depth is 7 mm. If coexisting with cervical canal polypoid or polyps, resection should be done under direct vision of hysteroscope. In case of CIN2 and CIN3 lesions less than 2.5 cm in diameter, a cold knife conization should be performed.[1]
5. The wire loop electrode is pushed out totally, and the posterior lobe of vaginal speculum is taken for fulcrum at the cutting of the anterior lip, and there is no exact fulcrum at the cutting of posterior lip.
6. The cutting usually starts from the 6 o'clock position in a clockwise direction (if cutting starts from anterior lip, the occurrence of lots of bleeding may affect the cutting of

[1]For reference: Bian Meilu, Liu Shufan. Diagnosis and treatment of cervical diseases. Beijing: Scientific and Technical Documentation Press. 2001,5.

posterior lip). First, step on the foot pedal, and when the hands feel a sense of cutting action, move the cutting handle or spring, and excise the tissues according to the expected cutting depth. When doing with "arc cutting" from the inside to the outside, the cutting speed should not be fast, or the electrocoagulation applied in the blended current cannot play its function well, resulting in bleeding. In principle, the wire loop electrode is used under direct vision to coagulate the bleeding points, and the wound oozing may be stopped by electrocoagulation with rollerball electrode. If there is severe erosion and congestion in the cervix, the rollerball electrode is first used to coagulate the cervix, and then the wire loop electrode is used instead so as to reduce bleeding. Sometimes, there are multiple Nabothian cyst underlying the smooth epithelium, the cutting may be properly extended to destroy the Nabothian cyst so as to ensure a thorough treatment.

7. After cutting, the cervix appears to be "shallow urn-shaped" or "mushroomhead" in shape.

Postoperative Precautions

1. A slight lower abdominal pain may develop 1–3 days after operation. A two-week rest and less exercise should be prescribed.
2. Vaginal discharge for 2–3 weeks after operation is bloody, and hemorrhagic during decrustation.
3. After operation, there is exudate from the cutting surface and more vaginal discharges, which may last about 4 weeks.
4. Generally, it takes 8 weeks for the cutting surface to heal completely, so sexual intercourse is banned during this period.
5. When the amount of bleeding is more than that of menses, vaginal examination should be undertaken. If there is active bleeding, iodoform gauze can be placed on the cutting surface for hemostasis by compression and be removed after placement for up to a maximum of 1 week. If it still cannot stop bleeding, electrocoagulation should be performed under direct vision of hysteroscope, simultaneously antibiotics should be administered to prevent infection.

Appendix 3: Patient Consent Form for Hysteroscopic Operation in the Hysteroscopy Center of Fuxing Hospital, Capital Medical University

Patient Consent Form for Hysteroscopic Operation

Name: Age: Admission number:

1.Preoperative Diagnosis: menorrhagia dysfunctional uterine bleeding uterine fibroid

cervical polypoid hyperplasia others

2.Diagnostic foundations: history of illness physical examination ultrasonography

laboratory tests diagnostic hysteroscopy

3.Proposed surgery: TCR-

4.Indications: menorrhagia anemia or leucorrhea which affects health

5.Anesthesia: venous continuous epidural anesthesia

6.Intraoperative and postoperative complications and managements

1) Bleeding: strict hemostasis, blood matching preparation for spare use.

2) Infections: Strict sterile operation, preoperative and postoperative use of antibiotics.

3) Injuries: Distinguish anatomical structure and operate carefully to avoid side injuries as far as possible. Once an injury occurs, timely repair or delayed repair will be conducted,or hysterectomyif necessary.

4) TURP syndrome.

5) If there is much bleeding during surgery, and cannotbe controlled after measures are taken, conversion to laparotomy is required if necessary.

6) Air embolism: Promptly rescue.

7) The patients who had previous tubal sterilization may develop PASS syndrome following TCRE. Successive intrauterine exploration may be conducted for 2 months.

8) Anesthetic accidents: Promptly rescue.

7. Postoperative outcomes

1) Amenorrhea.

2) Significantly reduced period.

3) The patients with no significantly improved period or recurrence require further treatment.

4) The patient's ovarian function is not affected.

5) The patient with myomas that could not be resected or failed to be removed completely needs continued observation or treatment.

8. Preoperative preparations

Skin preparation, blood matching, preoperative cervical intubation

9. Patient`s consent and signature:

Physician:

Month Day Year

E. Xia (ed.), *Practical Manual of Hysteroscopy*, https://doi.org/10.1007/978-981-19-1332-7

Appendix 4: Patient Consent Form for Hysteroscopic Diagnosis in the Hysteroscopy Center of Fuxing Hospital, Capital Medical University

Patient Consent Form forHysteroscopic Diagnosis

Name: Age: Diagnosis:

Diagnostic hysteroscopy is a minimal invasive examination for diagnosing lesions in uterine cavity and cervical caal. It can directly observe the abnormalities in cervix and uterine cavity, and take target biopsy of suspected lesions. However, the uterine cavity is narrow and small with plenty of blood supply of uterine walls. The pathology causes changes in normal anatomy of the uterus, so there may be some conditions occurring during diagnostic procedure as follows:

1. Bleeding.
2. Perforation and damage to other organs.
3. Reaction of artificial abortion syndrome.
4. Air embolism.

The following conditions may occur after procedure:

1. Bleeding.
2. Infection.

It is common responsibility of doctors and patients to understanding these information. Surgeons will strictly obey the operating rules during diagnostic procedures to maximally avoid the occurrence of above accidents. Since the patient may have her own features of health conditions, individual difference, and some unpredictable factors, it is possible to develop some accidents during hysteroscopic diagnosis. The doctors will deal with it promptly and conduct repair if necessary. The patient and her relatives are supposed to understand and accept these issues.

The patient signs to confirm that: ① I haveread the content of this protocol; ② I give consent to undergo diagnostic hysteroscopy; ③ I understand and agree with the hysteroscopic process explained in this protocol, including the risksof diagnostic hysteroscopy, ④ Therefore, I sign as follows:

Patient`s signature: Doctor`ssignature:

Date: Date:

E. Xia (ed.), *Practical Manual of Hysteroscopy*, https://doi.org/10.1007/978-981-19-1332-7

Appendix 5: Report of Diagnostic Hysteroscopy

International Hysteroscopy Training Center
Hysteroscopy Center of Fuxing Hospital, Capital Medical University
Report of diagnostic hysteroscopy combined with B-ultrasonography

Serial number:

Name: Age: Case No.: Date:13th August 2014

Indications:

Menstrual and obstetrical history: MC: LMP: G/P:

Gynecological examination: Vulva:married type; Vagina: unobstructed; Cervix: smooth; Uterus: anteverted, normal size, movable and without tenderness; Adnexa: no abnormalities in both sides.

Clinical diagnosis: uterine malformation

Preoperative preparation:Anesthesia: local infiltration anesthesia Dilation of cervix: length of uterine cavity: cm

Findings under hysteroscope:

Intraoperative intervention: Curettage: g; Endometrialthickness: mm; IUD removal:

Combined diagnosis:

Postoperative treatment:waiting for histological result; out-patient re-check one week later;

Examining physicians: Recording physician:

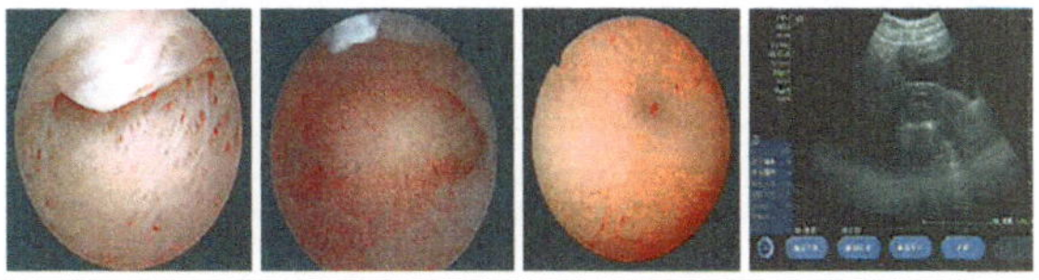

Precautions after hysteroscopy:

1. Please read these items carefully after hysteroscopy.
2. A small amount of bleeding within one weekfollowing hysteroscopy is normal. Please come and see your doctor if it reaches the amount of period.
3. Please come and see your doctor or call your doctor if your experiences abdominal pain and fever.
4. Sexual intercourse and bathare banned within one month.
5. Please come and have further consultation with your doctor one week later and get your histological report.
6. Contact number: 88062548.

E. Xia (ed.), *Practical Manual of Hysteroscopy*, https://doi.org/10.1007/978-981-19-1332-7

Batch number: 10731661

Printed by Printforce, the Netherlands